D0370503

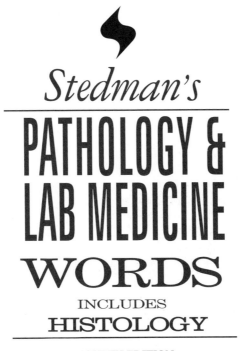

Stedman's

PATHOLOGY & LAB MEDICINE

WORDS

INCLUDES

HISTOLOGY

FOURTH EDITION

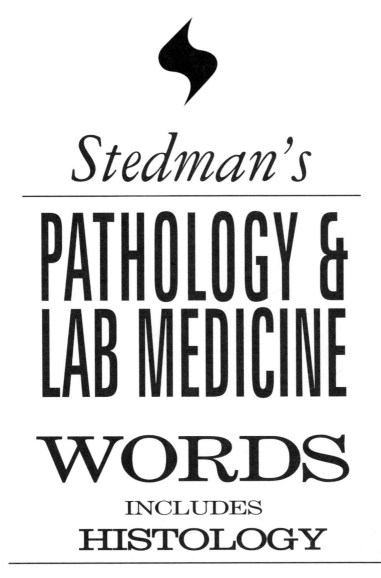

Stedman's

PATHOLOGY & LAB MEDICINE

WORDS

INCLUDES

HISTOLOGY

FOURTH EDITION

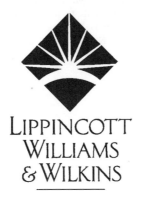

LIPPINCOTT
WILLIAMS
& WILKINS

Publisher: Julie K. Stegman
Senior Product Manager: Eric Branger
Associate Managing Editor: Amy Millholen
Production Coordinator: Jason Delaney
Typesetter: Josephine Bergin
Printer & Binder: Malloy Litho, Inc.

Copyright © 2005 Lippincott Williams & Wilkins
351 West Camden Street
Baltimore, Maryland 21201-2436

All rights reserved. This book is protected by copyright. No part of this book may be reproduced in any form or by any means, including photocopying, or utilized by any information storage and retrieval system without written permission from the copyright owner.

Printed in the United States of America

2005

Library of Congress Cataloging-in-Publication Data

Stedman's pathology & lab medicine words : includes histology.— 4th ed.
    p. ; cm.— (Stedman's word books)
Includes bibliographical references.
  ISBN 978-0-7817-6176-5
  ISBN 0-7817-6176-X
  1. Pathology—Terminology. 2. Diagnosis, Laboratory—Terminology. I. Title: Stedman's pathology and lab medicine words. II. Title: Pathology & lab medicine words. III. Stedman, Thomas Lathrop, 1853-1938. IV. Lippincott Williams & Wilkins. V. Series.
  [DNLM: 1. Pathology—Terminology—English. 2. Laboratory Techniques and Procedures—Terminology—English.]
RB115.S73 2005
616.07'01'4--dc22

2005000394
07
2 3 4 5 6 7 8 9 10

Contents

Acknowledgements

An important part of our editorial process is the involvement of medical transcriptionists—as advisors, reviewers, and editors.

We extend special thanks to Ellen Atwood and Amy Stummer for editing the manuscript and helping to resolve many difficult questions, to Jeanne Bock for helping to revise and develop the appendices, and to Jo-Ann Clarke for her assistance with the appendices. We are grateful to advisory board members Beth Pessetto, Kim Hamacher, Kristine Krafts, Lynn R. Price, and Janet West, who shared their valuable judgment, insight, and perspective.

Our appreciation goes to the following reviewers who helped to enhance the A-Z content for this edition: Ellen Atwood; Jeanne Bock, CSR, MT; Kim Buchanan, CMT, FAAMT; R. Jo-Ann Clarke; Robin Koza; Kristine P. Krafts, MD; Richard MacPherson; Beverly S. Oberline, CMT; Beth Pessetto; Lynn R. Price, CMT; Deborah Randolph; Julie Trenary, CMT; Janet West; Patricia Lee White, CMT, FAAMT; and Chiara Zaratkiewicz. We thank Barb Ferretti, who played an integral role in the process by reviewing the content files for format and updating the manuscript. We also extend thanks to Helen Littrell for performing the final prepublication review.

As with all our Stedman's word references, this resource incorporates the suggestions and expertise of our many contacts in the medical transcriptionist community. Thanks to all of our advisory board participants, reviewers, and editors; AAMT meeting attendees; and others who have written us with requests and comments—keep talking, and we'll keep listening.

Editor's Preface

Pathology and laboratory medicine language is unusually rich, challenging, even exciting. For many years, physicians needed to know the entire body of science, perform their own lab tests and postmortems, and engage, joyfully, in research and discovery. True, these were remarkable people, but it was just a hundred years ago that the entire body of medical, biological, and chemical knowledge could fit in a relatively small book!

Today, it is clinical laboratory medical professionals, particularly those engaged in postmortem evaluations, who come closest to encyclopedic understanding and use of such an extensive base knowledge. Pathology and laboratory medicine encompasses the entire spectrum of medical language: anatomy, both gross and microscopic; physiology; histology; chemistry; physics; and animal and plant life are only a few examples. These studies tell how we live and the manner and cause of death. Laboratory medicine and pathology contribute to both wellness and disease.

Scientific medicine in its formative period relied upon the languages of the educated and elite of the mid 19th century: Latin, Greek, German, and French, with a smattering of Russian and Italian and a dab of Spanish and Portuguese. Mere English would not do! Dating from the very beginnings of scientific medicine, laboratory procedures, tissue examination, and organisms were labeled with descriptive terms derived from everyday life. This tradition continues, with such examples as pizza lung or Legionnaires disease.

Individuals, professional as well as wealthy science hobbyists, were immortalized by having their "discovery"—a cell, a particular formation, a dye, a bacteria, a disease or syndrome—named in their honor. We find the same handful of names scattered widely among many disciplines that are now considered specialties and subspecialties. Now, we have a 20th century trend away from eponymous terms to common descriptive terms, acknowledging the sad fact that the true "discoverer" was not always properly represented or even known. This trend, however, is moving ahead slowly. Old habits are hard to break, so along with an explosion of new words, we still need to know those endless lists of eponyms and try to understand the common descriptive name.

Naming conventions are only a part of laboratory medicine and pathology. There is a widespread fascination with the medical detectives who can delve into the microscopic secrets of injury and death. DNA has become a staple of the courtroom. A couple of best-seller series feature a medical examiner and a forensic anthropologist. Several widely popular TV shows feature laboratory medicine and forensics solving criminal cases. Forensic medicine, autopsy, toxicology, and histopathological evaluations identify the clues left behind in unnatural or suspicious death. Traditional detective work is vastly aided by findings from the laboratory.

One area not quite so well-known, but of intense interest since the 9-11 attacks, is weapons of mass destruction, including biological, chemical, and nuclear warfare. Laboratory medicine is involved in identifying rare organisms, toxic gases, and drugs that inflict mass casualties and their characteristic lesions and patterns. The descriptive terms of biological and chemical terrorism are included in this book. Since writing this preface, the unparalleled (in modern times) disaster of the Asian tsunami has occurred. Undoubtedly, the next edition of this book will contain a multitude of new descriptive terms derived from the effects of killer waves and the sequelae on humankind.

Laboratory hematology, the study of the blood and its components, is the primary aim of this word book. Hematology, the clinical identification, diagnosis, and treatment of blood diseases, is sparsely represented. For diagnosis and treatment options of blood diseases such as anemias, cancers, and other disorders, please consult *Stedman's Oncology Words, Fourth Edition*; *Stedman's Internal Medicine & Geriatric Words*; and *Stedman's Medical Speller, Fourth Edition*. "Cardiology lab" terms and "GI lab" terms will be found in their corresponding specialty books.

Many thanks to Amy Stummer who tackled this highly technical subject matter with care and dedication. Barb Ferretti performed her usual magical (but very brain- and labor-intensive) massage of the database to provide consistent results. Jeanne Bock, who made major contributions to the appendices, also receives our grateful acknowledgment.

Ellen Atwood

Publisher's Preface

Stedman's Pathology & Lab Medicine Words, Fourth Edition, offers an authoritative assurance of quality and exactness to the wordsmiths of the healthcare professions—medical transcriptionists, medical editors and copyeditors, health information management personnel, court reporters, and the many other users and producers of medical documentation.

Users will find an extensive array of clinical pathology, anatomical pathology, hematology, medical technology, blood banking, clinical chemistry, histology, bacteria, fungi, parasites, viruses, and bioterrorism terminology. The appendix sections in this edition include labeled anatomical illustrations; culture media; stains, dyes, and fixatives; sample reports; and common terms by procedure; plus these new appendices: the Greek alphabet; elements and symbols; units of measure for pathology; sample immunodiagnostic panels; common lab tests; and drugs of abuse, toxicology, and therapeutic drug levels.

This new edition, with more than 100,000 entries, includes the *Stedman's Word Book Series* trademarks: cross-indexing by first and last word, A-Z format with main entries and subentries, and appendix material for additional comprehension and application of the terminology.

We at Lippincott Williams & Wilkins strive to provide you with the most up-to-date and accurate word references available. Your use of this *Word Book* will prompt new editions, which we will publish as often as updates and revisions justify. We welcome your suggestions for improvements, changes, corrections, and additions—whatever will make this Stedman's product more useful to you. Please complete the postage-paid card in this book for future suggestions and recommendations, or visit us online at www.stedmans.com.

Explanatory Notes

Medical transcription is an art as well as a science. Both approaches are needed to correctly interpret the dictation of a physician, whose language is a product of education, training, and experience. This variety in medical language means that there are several acceptable ways to express certain terms, including jargon. *Stedman's Pathology & Lab Medicine Words, Fourth Edition*, provides variant spellings and phrasings for many terms. These elements, in addition to complete cross-indexing, make *Stedman's Pathology & Lab Medicine Words, Fourth Edition*, a valuable resource for determining the validity of terms as they are encountered.

Alphabetical Organization

Alphabetization of main entries is letter by letter as spelled, ignoring punctuation, spaces, prefixed numbers, or other characters. For example:

methylbutane fixative/solution
3-methylcrotonylglyinuria
methylcytosine
5-methylcytosine (5-MeC)

Terms beginning or ending with Greek letters show the Greek letters spelled out and listed alphabetically. For example:

alpha
   a. antitrypsin (AAT)
   a. chain
   a. thalassemia
   a. unit

In subentry alphabetization, the abbreviated singular form or the spelled-out plural form of the noun main entry word is ignored.

Format and Style

All main entries are in **boldface** to expedite locating a sought-after term, to enhance distinction between main entries and subentries, and to relieve the textual density of the pages.

Irregular plurals and variant spellings are shown on the same line as the singular or preferred form of the word. For example:

mycobacterium, pl. **mycobacteria**
teniacide, taeniacide

Capitalization

Trade/brand names (proprietary) and proper names (eponyms) begin with a capital letter.

Barrett esophagus
Clarke fluid
Dakin solution
Malpighi capsule

However, word formations using a proper name are not capitalized.

malpighian capsule

Product names that are represented in all upper case by the manufacturer are represented with an initial upper case in this book as shown in bold below.

Takara Biomedicals SUPREC tube = **Takara Biomedicals Suprec tube**

An all upper case product name that is an acronym remains all upper case.

NIXIE tube

Irregular capitalization used by the manufacturer is maintained as shown below.

AvoSure INR test device
AxSYM analyzer
Cardiac STATus rapid assay

In the formal representation of bacteria genus and species names, the genus is capitalized and both genus and species are italicized. A general reference is not capitalized or italicized.

Staphylococcus aureus
staphylococcus culture

Hyphenation

As a rule of style, multiple eponyms (e.g., **von Hippel-Lindau gene**) are hyphenated. Terms combining an eponym and a manufacturer's name may be hyphenated (e.g., **Abbé-Zeiss counting chamber**). Some eponyms are actually first and last names and thus not hyphenated (e.g., **Pierre Robin syndrome**). Please note that in many cases, hyphenation is a question of style, not of accuracy, and thus is a matter of choice.

Possessives

Possessive forms have been dropped in this reference for the sake of consistency and conformance with the guidelines of the American Association for Medical Transcription (AAMT) and other groups. Please note, however, that in many cases, retaining the possessive, like hyphenating, is a question of style, not of accuracy, and thus is a matter of choice. To form the possessive of a word, simply add the apostrophe or apostrophe "s" to the end of the word.

Cross-indexing

The word list is in an index-like main entry-subentry format that contains two combined alphabetical listings:

(1) A noun main entry-subentry organization, which is typical of the A-Z section of medical dictionaries like Stedman's:

cell	death
carrier c.	black d.
flat c.	brain d.
resident c.	crib d.
target c.	natural d.

(2) An adjective main entry-subentry organization, which lists words and phrases as you hear them. The main entries are the adjectives or modifiers in a multiword term. The subentries are the nouns around which the terms are constructed and to which the adjectives or modifiers pertain:

active
  a. electrode
  a. immunity
  a. medium
  a. transport

nuclear
  n. antibody
  n. chain
  n. membrane
  n. pore

This format provides the user with more than one way to locate and identify a multiword term. For example:

activated
  a. charcoal

charcoal
  activated c.

antibiotic
  a. sensitivity

sensitivity
  antibiotic s.

It also allows the user to see together all terms that contain a particular descriptor, as well as all types, kinds, or variations of a noun entity. For example:

hepatitis
  acute viral h.
  h. A virus
  epidemic h.
  h. virus

marrow
  bone m.
  m. cell
  m. fibrosis
  lymphocytic m

Wherever possible, abbreviations are separately defined and cross-referenced. For example:

ORD
optical rotary dispersion

optical
o. rotary dispersion (ORD)

dispersion
optical rotary d. (ORD)

Special Note

Virus nomenclature is evolving into a standardized form, and during the transition phase some viruses are referred to with both their former and new names. These former names are included in this edition, enclosed in quotes with some using Greek characters, the same format the International Committee on Taxonomy of Viruses (ICTV) uses:

"L5-like viruses"
" 29-like viruses"
"Sulfolobus SNDV-like viruses"

References

In addition to the manufacturers' literature we gather at various medical meetings, scientific reports from hospitals, and the lists of our MT Editorial Advisory Board members (from their daily transcription work), we used the following sources for new terms in *Stedman's Pathology & Lab Medicine Words, Fourth Edition*:

Books

Anderson WR. Forensic Sciences in Clinical Medicine: A Case Study Approach. Philadelphia: Lippincott-Raven, 1998.

Bishop ML, Duben-Engelkirk JL, Fody EP (eds.). Clinical Chemistry: Principles, Procedures, Correlations, 4th ed. Philadelphia: Lippincott Williams & Wilkins, 2000.

Chernecky CC, Berger BJ (eds.). Laboratory Tests & Diagnostic Procedures, 4th ed. Philadelphia: Saunders, 2004.

Clinical Laboratory Tests: Values and Implications, 3rd Edition. Springhouse, PA: Springhouse, 2001.

Desai SP. Clinician's Guide to Laboratory Medicine: A Practical Approach. Hudson, OH: Lexi-Comp, 2004.

Desai SP. Clinician's Guide to Laboratory Medicine Pocket. Hudson, OH: Lexi-Comp, 2004.

Dorland's Laboratory/Pathology Word Book for Medical Transcriptionists. St. Louis: Saunders, 2002.

Drake E. Sloane's Medical Word Book, 4th ed. Philadelphia: Saunders, 2002.

Dudek RW. High-Yield Histology, 3rd Edition. Baltimore: Lippincott Williams & Wilkins, 2004.

Eroschenko VP. diFiore's Atlas of Histology with Functional Correlations, 10th ed. Baltimore: Lippincott Williams & Wilkins, 2005.

Fischbach F. A Manual of Laboratory and Diagnostic Tests, 7th ed. Philadelphia: Lippincott Williams & Wilkins, 2004.

Goljan EF (ed.). Rapid Review Series: Pathology. Philadelphia: Mosby, 2004.

Handbook of Diagnostic Tests, 3rd ed. Springhouse, PA: Lippincott Williams & Wilkins, 2003.

Jacobs DS, DeMott WR, Oxley DK (eds.). Laboratory Test Handbook, 5th ed. Hudson, OH: Lexi-Comp, 2001.

Jakob M. Normal Values Pocket. Hermosa Beach, CA: Börm Bruckmeier, 2002.

Jones SL (ed.). Clinical Laboratory Pearls. Philadelphia: Lippincott Williams & Wilkins, 2001.

Keyes DC, Burstein JL, Schwartz RB, Swienton RE. Medical Response to Terrorism: Preparedness and Clinical Practice. Philadelphia: Lippincott Williams Wilkins, 2005.

McClatchey KD (ed.). Clinical Laboratory Medicine, 2nd ed. Philadelphia: Lippincott Williams & Wilkins, 2002.

Michota FA (ed.). Diagnostic Procedures Handbook, 2nd ed. Hudson, OH: Lexi-Comp, 2001.

Professional Guide to Diagnostic Tests. Ambler, PA: Lippincott Williams & Wilkins, 2005.

Raab SS, Grzybicki DM, Bejarano PA, Bissell MG, Stanley MW (eds.). Year Book of Pathology and Laboratory Medicine 2004. Philadelphia: Mosby, 2004.

Rubin E, Farber JL (eds.). Pathology, 3rd ed. Philadelphia: Lippincott-Raven, 1999.

Rubin E, Gorstein F, Rubin R, Schwarting R, Strayer D (eds.). Rubin's Pathology: Clinicopathologic Foundations of Medicine. Baltimore: Lippincott Williams & Wilkins, 2005.

Schneider AS, Szanto PA. Board Review Series Pathology, 2nd ed. Baltimore: Lippincott Williams & Wilkins, 2002.

Sloane SB, Dusseau JL. A Word Book in Pathology & Laboratory Medicine, 2nd ed. Philadelphia: Saunders, 1995.

Stedman's Medical Dictionary, 27th ed. Baltimore: Lippincott Williams & Wilkins, 2000.

Sternberg SS, Antonioli DA (eds.). Diagnostic Surgical Pathology, 3rd Edition. Philadelphia: Lippincott Williams & Wilkins, 1999.

Turgeon ML. Clinical Hematology, Theory and Procedures, 3rd ed. Philadelphia: Lippincott Williams & Wilkins, 1999.

Vera Pyle's Current Medical Terminology, 8th ed. Modesto, CA: Health Professions Institute, 2000.

Journals

ADVANCE for Health Information Professionals. King of Prussia, PA: Merion, 2003-2004.

Advances in Anatomic Pathology. Philadelphia: Lippincott Williams & Wilkins, 1999-2000.

American Journal of Clinical Pathology. Philadelphia: Lippincott Williams & Wilkins, 2004.

The American Journal of Forensic Medicine and Pathology. Philadelphia: Lippincott Williams Wilkins, 2003-2004.

The American Journal of Pathology. Bethesda, MD: American Society for Investigative Pathology, 2003.

American Journal of Surgical Pathology. Philadelphia: Lippincott Williams & Wilkins, 1998-1999.

Applied Immunohistochemistry & Molecular Morphology. Philadelphia: Lippincott Williams & Wilkins, 2003-2004.

Archives of Pathology & Lab Medicine. Northfield, IL: College of American Pathologists, 2003.

Blood. Washington, DC: The American Society of Hematology, 2003.

Clinical Lab Products. Amherst, NH: Clinical Lab Products, 2000-2002.

The Endocrinologist. Baltimore: Lippincott Williams & Wilkins, 2000.

Internal Medicine. Montvale, NJ: Medical Economics, 2000.

JAAMT. Modesto, CA: American Association for Medical Transcription, 2001-2003.

Journal of Clinical Pathology. London: BMJ Publishing Group, 2003.

The Journal of Pathology. Hoboken, NJ: John Wiley & Sons, 2003.

Laboratory Medicine. Chicago: American Society of Clinical Pathologists, 1998.

The Latest Word. Philadelphia: Saunders, 1999, 2002-2004.

Modern Pathology. Baltimore: Lippincott Williams & Wilkins, 1999-2000.

Pathology Case Reviews. Philadelphia: Lippincott Williams & Wilkins, 2003-2004.

Pathology Patterns. Chicago: American Society of Clinical Pathologists, 1994, 1997.

Perspectives. Modesto, CA: Health Professions Institute, 2001-2004.

Images

Hardy NO. Westport, CT. Stedman's Medical Dictionary, 27th ed. Baltimore: Lippincott Williams & Wilkins, 2000.

LifeART Nursing 1, CD-ROM. Baltimore: Lippincott Williams & Wilkins.

LifeART Nursing 2, CD-ROM. Baltimore: Lippincott Williams & Wilkins.

LifeART Nursing 3, CD-ROM. Baltimore: Lippincott Williams & Wilkins.

LifeART Pediatricts 1, CD-ROM. Baltimore: Lippincott Williams & Wilkins.

LifeART Super Anatomy Collection 2, CD-ROM. Baltimore: Lippincott Williams & Wilkins.

References

LifeART Super Anatomy Collection 5, CD-ROM. Baltimore: Lippincott Williams & Wilkins.

MediClip Clinical Cardiopulmonary, CD-ROM. Baltimore: Lippincott Williams & Wilkins.

MediClip Clinical OB/GYN, CD-ROM. Baltimore: Lippincott Williams & Wilkins.

Smeltzer SC, Bare BG. Textbook of Medical-Surgical Nursing, 9th ed. Philadelphia: Lippincott Williams & Wilkins, 2000.

Ward L. Salt Lake City, UT. Fuller J, Schaller-Ayers J. Health Assessment: A Nursing Approach, 2nd ed. Philadelphia: J.B. Lippincott Company, 1994.

Willis MC. Medical Terminology: A Programmed Learning Approach to the Language of Health Care. Baltimore: Lippincott Williams & Wilkins, 2002.

Websites

http://arpa.allenpress.com

http://jama.ama-assn.org

http://menopause.home.test.biolifedynamics.com

http://perso.wanadoo.fr/alzheimer.lille/pdf/2000/2000DelacourteBueeCOIN.pdf

http://quickmedical.com

http://us.labsystem.roche.com

http://www.abbottdiagnostics.com

http://www.abbottdiagnostics.com

http://www.accutech-llc.com

http://www.acrometrix.com

http://www.aerocrine.com

http://www.afip.org

http://www.ascp.org

http://www.bacterio.cict.fr/allnamestwo.html

http://www.beckman.com

http://www.brinkmann.com

http://www.cap.org

http://www.ciphergen.com

http://www.compumed.net

http://www.dakocytomation.us

http://www.dpcweb.com

http://www.fda.gov

http://www.hemametrics.com

http://www.hematology.org

http://www.hpisum.com

http://www.jimro.com

http://www.medtox.com

http://www.mtdesk.com

http://www.mtmonthly.com

http://www.orasure.com

http://www.orthoclinical.com

http://www.prometheuslabs.com

http://www.quidel.com

http://www.quidel.com

http://www.responsebio.com

http://www.roche-diagnostics.com

http://www.spectraldx.com

http://www.stanford.edu/group/hopes/sttools/gloss

http://www.statspin.com

http://www.tapestrypharma.com

http://www.thermo.com

http://www.vielle.info/menopause

http://www.vysis.com

A
   adenine
   ampere
      acetylcoenzyme A (acetyl-CoA)
      amyloid protein A
      A antigen
      arylsulfatase A (ARS A)
      azure A
      A band
      A or B isozyme of G6PD
      A cell
      chromogranin A (CgA, ChrA)
      clostridiopeptidase A
      concanavalin A (Con A)
      A disc
      A fiber
      A virus hepatitis
A1
   angiotensin 1
A2
   angiotensin 2
      cytosol phospholipase A2 (cPLA2)
      lipoprotein-associated phospholipase A2
      A2 MicroArray system
A3
   angiotensin 3
      chromomycin A3
Å
   angstrom
a
      a disintegrin and metalloprotease (ADAM)
      a disintegrin and metalloproteinase with thrombospondin domain 13 (ADAMTS 13)
      a hypotonic environment
A1c
      A1c At·Home testing kit
      hemoglobin A1c
A$_2$
   hemoglobin A$_2$
A549 human lung carcinoma cell
A5B7 monoclonal antibody
A68 protein
AA
   amyloid A
   arachidonic acid
      AA amyloidosis
AAA
   abdominal aortic aneurysm
   androgenic anabolic agent
AAC
   antibiotic-associated colitis

A1AC
   alpha-1 antichymotrypsin
AAD
   antibiotic-associated diarrhea
AADC
   aromatic l-amino acid decarboxylase
AAH
   atypical adenomatous hyperplasia
AAN
   amino acid nitrogen
      AAN test
AAO
   automated assay optimization
Aarskog-Scott syndrome
Aarskog syndrome
AAS
   aminoalkylsilane
   atomic absorption spectrophotometer
   atomic absorption spectrophotometry
AAT
   alpha antitrypsin
A1AT
   alpha$_1$ antitrypsin
      A1AT deficiency
      A1AT deficiency panniculitis
AAV
   adeno-associated virus
AB
   abortion
   Alcian blue
   asbestos body
   asthmatic bronchitis
      AB decalcification
A:B
   acid-base ratio
A/B
      FLU OIA A/B rapid test
Ab
   antibody
abacterial thrombotic endocarditis
abarticular gout
abarticulation
abattoir worker
ABB
   acute bronchitis/bronchiolitis
abbau
Abbé test plate
Abbé-Zeiss
      A.-Z. apparatus
      A.-Z. counting chamber
ABBI
   advanced breast biopsy instrumentation
Abbott
      A. AxSYM Prizm HCV assay
      A. Cell-Dyn hematology analyzer

ABC
  aneurysmal bone cyst
  aspiration biopsy cytology
  ATP-binding cassette
  avidin-biotin peroxidase complex
    ABC immunodetection system
    ABC staining method
    ABC technique
abdominal
    a. anthrax
    a. aortic aneurysm (AAA)
    a. dropsy
    a. fat pad biopsy
    a. fibromatosis
    a. fistula
    a. muscle deficiency syndrome
    a. viscera
Abell-Kendall method
Abelson
    A. murine leukemia virus
    A. oncogene
abequose
Abercrombie syndrome
aberrans
    Haller vas a.
aberrant
    a. angiogenesis
    a. crypt focus
    a. duct
    a. ductule
    a. ganglion
    a. germ
    a. goiter
    a. hemoglobin
    a. pancreas
    a. renal vessel
    a. rest
    a. ribonucleic acid
    a. tissue
aberrantes
    ductuli a.
    ductus a.
aberrantia
    Ferrein vasa a.
    vasa a.
aberrata
    struma a.
aberration
    chromatic a.
    chromosomal a.
    chromosome a.
    heterosomal a.
    interchromosomal a.
    intrachromosomal a.
    karyotype a.
    penta X chromosomal a.
    tetra-X chromosomal a.
    triple-X chromosomal a.
abetalipoproteinemia (ABL)

ABG
    arterial blood gas
ABH antigen
abietic acid
ability
    shattering a.
ab initio
Abiotrophia
abiotrophy
ABI Prism 3100 Genetic Analyzer
abiuret
abiuretic
ABL
    abetalipoproteinemia
ablastin
ablatio
    a. placentae
    a. retinae
ablative chemotherapy
ablepharon
abluminal surface
ABMT
    autologous blood and marrow
      transplantation
    autologous bone marrow transplantation
ABN
    abnormal
abnormal (ABN)
    a. banding region
    a. beta cell function
    a. chorion
    a. chorionic villus
    a. clinical manifestation
    a. endochondral ossification
    a. flow
    a. mitosis
    a. shortening
abnormality
    adrenocortical a.
    bell-clapper a.
    bone marrow a.
    bronchial wall a.
    cartilaginous a.
    chromosomal a.
    cytologic a.
    endotracheal a.
    fetal a.
    gain-of-function a.
    genetic a.
    joint a.
    morphologic a.
    no histopathologic a. (NHPA)
    nonspecific hepatocellular a.
    no serious a. (NSA)
    no significant a. (NSA)
    sex chromosome a.
    transient enzyme a.
    traumatic a.
    wire-loop a.

abnormally localized immature precursor (ALIP)
ABO
    ABO antibody
    ABO antigen
    ABO blood group
    ABO compatibility
    ABO factor
    ABO hemolytic disease of the newborn
    ABO incompatibility
    ABO typing
ABO-Rh typing
aborted ectopic pregnancy
abortion (AB)
    afebrile a.
    ampullar a.
    artificial a.
    cervical a.
    complete a.
    criminal a.
    habitual a.
    imminent a.
    incomplete a.
    induced a.
    inevitable a.
    infected a.
    justifiable a.
    missed a.
    placenta previa a.
    septic a.
    spontaneous a.
    therapeutic a. (TA)
    threatened a.
    tubal a.
abortive
    a. infection
    a. neurofibromatosis
    a. transduction
    a. viral disease
abortus
    Brucella a.
    Chlamydophila a.
    a. fever
    hydropic a.
ABP
    androgen-binding protein
ABPA
    allergic bronchopulmonary aspergillosis
ABPM
    allergic bronchopulmonary mycosis
abraded wound

Abrams test
abrasion
    a. collar
    muzzle a.
    punctate a.
    a. rim
    a. ring
    tattooing a.
abrasive cytology
Abrikosov tumor
abrin
abruption
    placental a.
abruptio placentae
Abrus precatorius
ABS
    alkylbenzene sulfonate
abscess
    acute a.
    a. aerobic culture
    alveolar a.
    amebic brain a.
    apical a.
    appendiceal a.
    Bartholin a.
    Bezold a.
    bicameral a.
    bone a.
    brain a.
    Brodie a.
    bursal a.
    caseous a.
    cerebral epidural a.
    cholangitic a.
    chronic a.
    cold a.
    collar button a.
    crypt a.
    diffuse a.
    Douglas a.
    dry a.
    Dubois a.
    embolic a.
    eosinophilic a.
    epidural a.
    fecal a.
    follicular a.
    gas a.
    gravitation a.
    gummatous a.
    hematogenous a.
    hepatic a.

NOTES

abscess *(continued)*
    hot a.
    hypostatic a.
    ischiorectal a.
    Kogoj a.
    lacunar a.
    liver a.
    lung a.
    mastoid a.
    metastatic a.
    migrating a.
    miliary a.
    Munro a.
    mycotic a.
    orbital a.
    otic a.
    otitic a.
    pancreatic a.
    parafrenal a.
    parametric a.
    paranephric a.
    parotid a.
    Pautrier a.
    pelvic a.
    perforating a.
    perianal a.
    periapical a.
    periappendiceal a.
    periarticular a.
    perinephric a.
    perirectal a.
    peritonsillar a.
    periureteral a.
    periurethral a.
    phlegmonous a.
    Pott a.
    premammary a.
    psoas a.
    pyemic a.
    pylephlebitic a.
    pyogenic a.
    radioisotope liver-lung scan for subdiaphragmatic a.
    renal a.
    residual a.
    retrobulbar a.
    retrocecal a.
    retropharyngeal a.
    satellite a.
    septicemic a.
    shirt-stud a.
    stellate a.
    stercoral a.
    sterile a.
    stitch a.
    subacute a.
    subdiaphragmatic a.
    subepidermal a.
    subhepatic a.
    subphrenic a.
    subungual a.
    sudoriferous a.
    sudoriparous a.
    syphilitic a.
    testis a.
    thecal a.
    thymic a.
    Tornwaldt a.
    tropical a.
    trunk a.
    tuberculous a.
    tuboovarian a. (TOA)
    verminous a.
    wandering a.
    worm a.

abscessus
    Mycobacterium chelonae subsp. *a.*
    Nocardia a.

absence
    congenital a.
    a. of estrogen
    a. of glucose-6-phosphatase
    a. of hemolysis

absent regression

Absidia
    A. corymbifera
    A. ramosa

absolute
    a. alcohol
    atmosphere a.
    a. cell increase
    a. eosinophil count
    a. erythrocytosis
    a. granulocyte count (AGC)
    a. iodine uptake (AIU)
    a. leukocytosis
    a. polycythemia
    a. retention time (ART)
    a. system of units
    a. temperature scale
    a. terminal innervation ratio
    a. value
    a. viscosity
    a. zero

absorbed
    anthrax vaccine a.
    a. dose

absorbefacient
absorbency index
absorbent
    carbon dioxide a.
absorber
absorptiometer
absorption
    atomic a.
    a. cavity
    a. cell
    a. coefficient

a. constant
disjunctive a.
D-xylose a.
a. of erythrocyte antibody
fat a.
intestinal a.
iron a.
a. peak
percutaneous a.
protein a.
a. spectrum
absorptive
a. cell
a. cell of intestine
a. disorder
a. lipemia
a. state
absorptivity
molar a.
specific a.
abstinence
alimentary a.
abstriction
abundant cytoplasm
abuse
drugs of a. (DOA)
InstaCheck Med+ immunoassay for drugs of a.
abyssalis
Idiomarina a.
abyssi
Caldithrix a.
Deferribacter a.
Moritella a.
AC
adenocarcinoma
anticoagulant
anticomplementary
antiinflammatory corticoid
autoclave
NATO code for HCN
A:C
amylase/creatinine clearance ratio
Ac
actinium
ACA
adenocarcinoma
anticardiolipin antibody
acalculous cholecystitis
acanthamebiasis
Acanthamoeba
A. astronyxis

A. castellanii
A. culbertsoni
A. hatchetti
A. keratitis
A. medium
A. polyphaga
A. rhysodes
Acanthella
Acanthia lectularia
Acanthobdella
Acanthocephala
acanthocephaliasis
Acanthocheilonema
A. perstans
A. streptocerca
acanthocyte, acanthrocyte
acanthocytosis
hereditary a.
acanthoid cell
acantholysis
acantholytic dermatosis
acanthoma
a. adenoides cysticum
basal cell a.
clear cell a.
large-cell a.
pilar sheath a.
a. verrucosa seborrheica
acanthomatous ameloblastoma
acanthopodia
acanthor
acanthorrhexis
acanthosis
glycogen a.
glycogenic a.
a. nigricans
verrucous a.
acanthotic
acanthrocyte (*var. of* acanthocyte)
acanthrocytosis
acapnia
acapnial alkalosis
acarbia
acardiacus
acardius
acari (*pl. of* acarus)
acariasis
acaricide
acarid
Acaridae
acaridan
acaridiasis

NOTES

Acarina
acarine
acarinosis
acarodermatitis
acaroid
acarology
Acarus
   A. folliculorum
   A. gallinae
   A. hordei
   A. rhizoglypticus hyacinthi
   A. scabiei
   A. siro
acarus, pl. **acari**
acaryote (*var. of* akaryote)
ACAT
   acyl-CoA acyltransferase
acatalasemia
acatalasia
acathectic
acathexia
Acaulium
ACB
   albumin cobalt binding
   ACB test
ACC
   acinar cell carcinoma
   adenoid cystic carcinoma
Acceava
   A. hCG Basic
   A. hCG Combo
   A. *Helicobacter pylori*
   A. MONO
   A. Strep A
accelerant
accelerated
   a. reaction
   a. rejection
   a. villous maturation
acceleration
   angular a.
   growth a.
   linear a.
   serum prothrombin conversion a.
   (SPCA)
accelerator
   a. factor
   a. globulin (AcG)
   proserum prothrombin conversion a.
   (PPCA)
   prothrombin a.
   serum prothrombin conversion a.
   (SPCA)
   serum thrombotic a. (STA)
   thromboplastin generation a.
accelerin
Accelon Combi biosampler
accentuator

acceptor
   hydrogen a.
   oxygen a.
   proton a.
access
   A. AccuTnI test
   A. AFP immunoassay analyzer
   exit a.
   A. Hybritech PSA test
   A. 2 immunoassay system
   multiple a.
   A. Ostase test
   sequential a.
   A. testosterone assay
   a. time
accessible antigen
accessoria, pl. **accessoriae**
   glandulae lacrimales accessoriae
   glandulae suprarenales accessoriae
   glandula parotidea a.
   glandula parotis a.
   glandula thyroidea a.
   thyroidea a.
accessorius
   ductus pancreaticus a.
   lien a.
   splen a.
accessory
   a. adrenal
   a. atrium
   a. cell
   a. chromosome
   a. lacrimal gland
   a. molecule
   a. organ
   a. pancreas
   a. pancreatic duct
   a. parotid gland
   a. spleen
   a. suprarenal gland
   a. thyroid
   a. thyroid gland
accident
   cerebrovascular a. (CVA)
   Chernobyl nuclear plant a.
   neonatal cerebrovascular a.
   serum a.
accidental
   a. host
   a. parasite
acclimation
accolé form
accommodation
   histologic a.
   spasm of a.
account
   dose a.
accreta
   placenta a.

accretionary growth
accretion line
AccuDx test
accumbens
　　nucleus a.
AccuMeter
　　A. fructosamine
　　A. HDL
　　A. theophylline
accumulation
　　a. of carbohydrates
　　a. of complex lipids
　　a. disease
　　extensive a.
　　forskolin-stimulated intracellular
　　　cAMP a.
　　a. of glycogen
　　intracellular a.
　　a. of lactate
　　lipofuscin a.
　　a. of pigment
　　a. of protein
　　pulmonary a.
accumulator
AccuProbe method
accuracy
　　photometric a.
　　Standards for Reporting of
　　　Diagnostic A. (STARD)
　　wavelength a.
Accurun 515 drug resistant mutant
　control series
AccuTnI test
ACD
　　acid-citrate-dextrose
ACE
　　adrenocortical extract
acellular
　　a. basement membrane
　　a. mucus lake
　　a. tumor
acelom
acelomate
acentric
acephaline
acephalocyst
acephalous
acephalus
　　holoacardius a.
acerina
　　Centrospora a.
　　Mycocentrospora a.

acervulus
acestoma
acetabulum, pl. acetabula
　　protrusio a.
acetal
acetaldehydase
acetaldehyde
acetamide
acetaminophen
　　a. assay
　　a. hepatic toxicity
acetanilid poisoning
acetarsol
　　sodium a.
acetate
　　aqueous uranyl a.
　　cellulose a.
　　cresyl violet a.
　　deoxycorticosterone a. (DOCA)
　　ethyl a.
　　methyl a.
　　phorbol myristate a.
　　potassium a.
　　sodium a.
acetazolamide
　　sodium a.
Acetest
aceti
　　Acetobacter a.
　　Turbatrix a.
acetic
　　a. acid-alcohol-formalin
　　a. acid-induced writing test
　　a. acid and potassium ferrocyanide
　　　test
　　a. aldehyde
　　a. anhydride
　　a. orcein
aceticus
　　Acidilobus a.
acetigenes
　　Sporanaerobacter a.
acetiphilus
　　Denitrovibrio a.
acetoacetate
acetoacetic
　　a. acid
　　a. acid test
　　a. aciduria
acetoacetyl

NOTES

acetoacetyl-CoA
a.-CoA reductase
a.-CoA thiolase
Acetobacter
A. *aceti*
A. *cerevisiae*
A. *cibinongensis*
A. *estunensis*
A. *indonesiensis*
A. *lovaniensis*
A. *malorum*
A. *orientalis*
A. *orleanensis*
A. *syzygii*
A. *tropicalis*
A. *xylinus*
Acetobacterium tundrae
acetobutylicum
Clostridium a.
acetocarmine
acetoin test
acetolysis
acetonation
acetone
a. body
a. compound
a. fixative
a., methylbenzoate, xylene (AMeX)
a. test
acetone-insoluble antigen
acetonemia
acetonemic
acetonitrile
acetonuria
acetoorcein stain
acetosoluble albumin
acetous
acetowhite test
acetoxidans
Desulfobacca a.
aceturate
diminazene a.
acetyl
a. group
a. value
acetylated low-density lipoprotein (AcLDL)
acetylation
acetylator
acetylcholine receptor antibody (AChRAb)
acetylcholinesterase assay
acetyl-CoA
acetylcoenzyme A
acetyl-CoA acetyltransferase
acetyl-CoA acyltransferase
acetyl-CoA carboxylase

acetyl-CoA hydrolase
acetyl-CoA synthetase
acetylcoenzyme A (acetyl-CoA)
acetylene trichloride
acetylhydrolase
platelet-activating factor a. (PAF-AH)
acetylization
acetylmethylcarbinol
acetylsalicylic acid (ASA)
acetylsulfadiazine
acetylsulfaguanidine
acetylsulfathiazole
acetyltransferase
acetyl-CoA a.
choline a.
AcG
accelerator globulin
aCGH
array-based comparative genomic hybridization
ACH
adrenocortical hormone
Achaetomium
achalasia
biliary a.
esophageal a.
pelvirectal a.
sphincteral a.
Achard syndrome
Achard-Thiers syndrome
Achatina
Achenbach syndrome
Achillea
achiral
achlorhydria
watery diarrhea, hypokalemia, a. (WDHA)
achlorhydric anemia
achlorophyllous
Acholeplasma
A. *axanthum*
A. *granularum*
A. *laidlawii*
A. *vituli*
Acholeplasmataceae
Acholeplasmatales
acholic stool
acholuria
acholuric jaundice
achondrogenesis
achondroplasia
homozygous a.
achondroplastic
a. dwarf
a. dwarfism
Achorion
AChRAb
acetylcholine receptor antibody

achrestic anemia
achroacyte
achroacytosis
achrodextrin (*var. of* achroodextrin)
achromacyte (*var. of* achromocyte)
achromasia
achromate
Achromatiaceae
achromatic
    a. apparatus
    a. lens
    a. objective
    a. spindle
achromatin
achromatinic
achromatism
achromatize
achromatocyte
achromatolysis
achromatophil, achromophil
achromatophilia
achromatopsia
achromatosis
achromatous
achromaturia
achromia
    central a.
    congenital a.
    cortical a.
    a. parasitica
    a. unguium
achromians
    incontinentia pigmenti a.
achromic
Achromobacter
    A. denitrificans
    A. insolitus
    A. lwoffi
    A. spanius
Achromobacteraceae
achromocyte, achromacyte
achromophil (*var. of* achromatophil)
achromophilic, achromophilous
achrooamyloid
achroodextrin, achrodextrin
achrotrichium
Achucarro stain
achylia
Aciculoconidium
acid
    aberrant ribonucleic a.
    abietic a.

acetoacetic a.
acetylsalicylic a. (ASA)
acrylic a.
adenylic a.
agaric a.
a. agglutination
a. albumin
a. alcohol
alcohol-formaldehyde-acetic a.
  (AFA)
aldaric a.
aldonic a.
alginic a.
aliphatic a.
allantoic a.
all-*trans*-retinoic a. (ATRA)
alpha amino a.
alpha ketoglutaric a.
alpha-linolenic a. (ALA)
amino a.
aminoacetic a.
aminocaproic a.
aminoglutaric a.
aminolevulinic a. (ALA)
aminopenicillanic a. (APA)
aminosuccinic a.
a. anhydride method
anthranilic a.
apurinic a.
arachidonic a. (AA)
argininosuccinic a.
aromatic amino a.
ascorbic a.
asparaginic a.
aspartic a. (Asp)
aurin tricarboxylic a.
basic amino a.
behenic a.
benzoic a.
benzoylaminoacetic a.
bile a.
binary a.
blauseare (Berlin blue a.)
boric a.
branched-chain amino a. (BCAA)
branched-chain keto a. (BCKA)
Brönsted-Lowry a.
butanoic a.
butyric a.
cacodylic a.
carbolic a.
carbonic a.

NOTES

acid (*continued*)
carboxylic a.
carminic a.
catechinic a.
catechuic a.
a. cell
cerebronic a.
a. challenge test
chenodeoxycholic a. (CDC)
chloracetic a.
chloranilic a.
cholic a.
chromic a.
chromotropic a.
citric a.
a. clearance test (ACT)
conjugate a.
cytidylic a.
decanoic a.
dehydroascorbic a.
delta ALA a.
deoxyadenylic a.
deoxycholic a.
deoxycytidylic a.
deoxyguanylic a.
deoxyribonucleic a. (DNA)
deoxyuridylic a.
D-glucaric a.
diacetic a.
dibasic a.
dicarboxylic a.
dichlorophenoxy acetic a.
diethylenetriaminepentaacetic a.
dihomogammalinolenic a. (DGLA)
dihydrofolic a.
dihydroxymandelic a. (DHMA, DOMA)
dihydroxyphenylacetic a.
1-dimethylaminonaphthalene-5-sulfonic a. (DANS)
dimethylarsinic a. (DMA)
dinitrobenzoic a.
dipicolinic a.
docosahexaenoic a. (DHA)
a. dye
edetic a.
eicosapentaenoic a. (EPA)
elaidic a.
a. electrophoresis
a. elution test
epoxyeicosatrienoic a.
epsilon a.
essential fatty a. (EFA)
ethacrynic a. (ECA)
ethanoic a.
ethylenediaminetetraacetic a. (EDTA)
ethylene glycol tetraacetic a. (EGTA)

ethylene tetraacetic a.
fatty a.
ferric chloride, perchloric acid, nitric a. (FPN)
flavianic a.
folic a.
folinic a.
a. formaldehyde hematin
formic a.
formiminoglutamic a. (FIGLU)
free fatty a. (FFA)
a. fuchsin
fumaric a.
galacturonic a.
gamma-aminobutyric a. (GABA)
gastric a.
genomic deoxyribonucleic a. (gDNA)
Gerhardt test for acetoacetic a.
glacial acetic a.
a. gland
glucogenic amino a.
glucuronic a.
glutamic a. (E, Glu)
glutaric a.
glycochenodeoxycholic a.
glycocholic a.
glycodeoxycholic a.
glycolic a.
glycolithocholic a.
a. glycoprotein
guanidino-aminovaleric a.
guanylic a.
a. hemolysin test
a. hemolysis test
heparinic a.
hexanoic a.
hexuronic a.
hippuric a.
homogentisic a. (HGA)
homovanillic a. (HVA)
hyaluronic a. (HA)
hydrochloric a.
hydrocyanic a.
hydrofluoric a.
a. hydrolase
5-hydroxyindoleacetic a.
o-hydroxyphenylacetic a.
hydroxyphenylpyruvic a. (HPPA)
hypobromous a.
iduronic a.
imidazolepyruvic a.
imino a.
iminodiacetic a. (IDA)
indolacetic a.
indolaceturic a.
indolelactic a.
infectious nucleic a.
inorganic a.

inosinic a.
a. intoxication
iodic a.
a. ionization constant
isobutyric a.
isocitric a.
isolation of nucleic a.
isovaleric a.
keto a.
ketogenic amino a.
a. lability test
lactic a.
lauric a.
leukocyte ascorbic a. (LAA)
Lewis a.
lignoceric a.
linoleic a.
linolenic a.
linolic a.
lipoic a.
lithic a.
lithocholic a.
long-chain fatty a. (LCFA)
long-chain polyunsaturated fatty a.
 (LCPUFA)
lysergic a.
lysophosphatidic a. (LPA)
a. magenta
malic a.
Mallory phosphotungstic a.
malonic a.
a. maltase deficiency
medium-chain fatty a. (MCFA)
mercaptoacetic a.
messenger ribonucleic a. (mRNA)
metaphosphoric a.
methoxyhydroxymandelic a.
 (MOMA)
methylmalonic a.
modified amino a.
monoaminodicarboxylic a.
monoaminomonocarboxylic a.
monobasic a.
monoenoic fatty a.
monomethylarsonic a. (MMA)
a. mucopolysaccharide (AMP)
muramic a.
muriatic a.
mycolic a.
myristic a.
N-acetylaspartate a.
N-acetylmuramic a.

nalidixic a.
neuraminic a.
nicotinic a.
nitric a.
3-nitroproprionic a. (3NP)
nitrous a.
nonesterified fatty a.
n-tetracosanoic a.
a. number
octanoic a.
octulosonic a.
oleic a.
oleic a. I 125
a. orcein
organic a.
orotic a.
orthophosphoric a.
osmic a.
oxalic a.
oxaloacetic a.
oxo a.
oxobutyric a.
oxoglutaric a.
oxolinic a.
palmitic a.
palmitoleic a.
p-aminobenzoic a. (PAB, PABA)
p-aminohippuric a. (PAH, PAHA)
p-aminosalicylic a. (PAS)
pantothenic a.
paraaminobenzoic a. (PAB, PABA)
paraaminohippuric a. (PAH, PAHA)
para-aminosalicylic a. (PAS)
parahydroxyphenylpyruvic a.
 (PHPPA)
pentanoic a.
peptide nucleic a. (PNA)
peracetic a.
perchloric a.
performic a.
a. perfusion test
periodic a.
phenaceturic a.
phenylacetic a.
phenyllactic a.
phenylpyruvic a.
a. phosphatase (ACP)
a. phosphatase assay
a. phosphatase serum
a. phosphatase stain
a. phosphatase staining
a. phosphatase test

NOTES

11

acid *(continued)*
  a. phosphatase test for semen
  a. phosphate
  phosphatidic a.
  phosphogluconic a.
  phosphomevalonic a.
  phosphomolybdic a.
  phosphonoacetic a.
  phosphoric a.
  phosphotungstic a. (PTA)
  phthalic a.
  p-hydroxybenzoic a.
  p-hydroxyphenyllactic a.
  p-hydroxyphenylpyruvic a.
  phytanic a.
  phytic a.
  picramic a.
  picric a.
  p-nitrophenylic a.
  polyadenylic a. (polyA)
  polybasic a.
  polycytidylic a. (polyC)
  polyenoic a.
  polyphosphoric a.
  polysialic a.
  polyunsaturated fatty a. (PUFA)
  polyuridylic a. (polyU)
  pristanic a.
  propanoic a.
  propionic a.
  prostanoic a.
  proton a.
  prussic a.
  pteroic a.
  pteroylglutamic a.
  pyridoxic a.
  pyrophosphoric a.
  pyroracemic a.
  pyruvic a.
  quinolinic a.
  radioiodinated fatty a. (RIFA)
  a. reaction
  a. red 87, 91
  a. reflux test
  respiratory syncytial virus
    nucleic a.
  retinoic a.
  rhodanic a.
  ribonucleic a. (RNA)
  ribothymidylic a.
  ricinoleic a.
  rubeanic a.
  saccharic a.
  salicylic a.
  salicylsalicylic a.
  salicylsulfonic a.
  salicyluric a.
  saturated fatty a.
  a. secretion rate

  a. seromucoid
  serum uric a. (SUA)
  sialic a.
  silicic a.
  sodium *p*-aminohippuric a.
  soluble ribonucleic a. (sRNA)
  sorbic a.
  stearic a.
  succinic a.
  sugar a.
  sulfanilic a.
  sulfindigotic a.
  sulfinic a.
  sulfonic a.
  sulfosalicylic a. (SSA)
  sulfur-containing amino a.
  sulfuric a.
  sulfurous a.
  tannic a.
  tartaric a.
  taurochenodeoxycholic a.
  taurocholic a.
  taurodeoxycholic a.
  taurolithocholic a.
  ^{99m}Tc pentetic a.
  teichoic a.
  ternary a.
  tetrahydrofolic a.
  thioctic a.
  thioglycolic a.
  thiolaminopropionic a.
  thymidylic a.
  a. tide
  titratable a. (TA)
  toluic a.
  total fatty a. (TFA)
  tribasic a.
  tricarboxylic a. (TCA)
  trichloroacetic a.
  trichlorophenoxy acetic a.
  tuberculostearic a.
  tungstic a.
  UDP-glucuronic a.
  UDP-iduronic a.
  uncoded amino a.
  unesterified fatty a. (UFA)
  uric a. (UA)
  uridylic a.
  urine alpha hydroxybutyric a.
  urine amino a.
  urine argininosuccinic a.
  urine 2,5-dihydroxyphenylacetic a.
  urine homogentisic a.
  urine 5-hydroxyindoleacetic a.
  urine uric a.
  urine vanillylmandelic a.
  urobenzoic a.
  urocanic a.
  uronic a.

ursodeoxycholic a. (UDCA)
vaccenic a.
valeric a.
valproic a.
a. value
vanillic a.
vanillylmandelic a. (VMA)
vinegar a.
viral nucleic a.
a. wave
xanthurenic a.
xanthylic a.
acidristocetin
arachidonic a.
acidalbumin
acid-alcohol-formalin
acetic a.
acidaminiphila
Stenotrophomonas a.
Acidaminococcus fermentans
acidaminovorans
Dethiosulfovibrio a.
Thermanaerovibrio a.
Thermococcus a.
acidaminuria
acid-base
a.-b. balance
a.-b. diagram
a.-b. disorder
a.-b. indicator
a.-b. nomogram
a.-b. ratio (A:B)
acid-citrate-dextrose (ACD)
acid-concanavalin
periodic a.-c. A (PACONA)
acidemia
argininosuccinic a.
glutaric a.
hydroxy-3-methylglutaric a.
lactic a.
methylmalonic a.
propionic a.
acid-fast (AF)
a.-f. bacillus (AFB)
a.-f. bacterium
a.-f. culture (AFC)
a.-f. smear
a.-f. stain
a.-f. staining histopathology
a.-f. staining method
acid-forming
Acidianus

acidic
a. dye
a. isoferritin
acidifaciens
Bacteroides a.
acidifiable
acidified
a. phagolysosome
a. prelysosomal compartment
a. serum lysis test
acidifier
acidify
Acidilobus aceticus
acidimetry
Acidimicrobiaceae
Acidimicrobiales
Acidimicrobidae
acidiphilum
Ferroplasma a.
acidiphilus
Alicyclobacillus a.
acidipiscis
Lactobacillus a.
acidisoli
Clostridium a.
Acidisphaera rubrifaciens
Acidithiobacillus
A. albertensis
A. caldus
A. ferrooxidans
A. thiooxidans
aciditrophicus
Syntrophus a.
acidity
esophageal a.
a. reduction test
total a.
Acidobacteria
Acidobacteriales
acidocyte
acidocytopenia
acidocytosis
acidogenic
acidophil, acidophile
a. adenoma
alpha a.
a. cell
a. granule
acidophilic
a. adenoma
a. body
a. dye

NOTES

acidophilic *(continued)*
    a. index
    a. leukocyte
    a. necrosis
    a. normoblast
    a. yolk globule
acidophilum
    Hydrogenobaculum a.
    Thermoplasma a.
acidophilus
    Lactobacillus a.
    a. milk
    Rhodoblastus a.
acidosis
    carbon dioxide a.
    compensated a.
    diabetic a.
    D-lactic a.
    high anion gap a.
    hypercapnic a.
    hyperchloremic metabolic a.
    hypochloremic metabolic a.
    lactic a.
    metabolic a.
    normal-AG metabolic a.
    normal anion gap a.
    potassium a.
    primary renal tubular a.
    renal tubular a. (RTA)
    respiratory a.
    secondary renal tubular a.
    a. test
    uncompensated a.
Acidothermaceae
acidotic
acidovorans
    Delftia a.
    Pseudomonas a.
Acidovorax
    A. anthurii
    A. valerianellae
acid-Schiff
    diastase-periodic a.-S. (D-PAS, dPAS)
    performic a.-S. (PFAS)
    periodic a.-S. (PAS)
    a.-S. stain
acidulated
aciduria
    acetoacetic a.
    beta-aminoisobutyric a.
    glutamic a.
    glycolic a.
    hereditary orotic a.
    L-glyceric a.
    methylmalonic a.
    orotic a.
    paroxysmal a.

    propionic a.
    xanthurenic a.
aciduric
acificus
    Caldanaerobacter subterraneus subsp. *a.*
acinar
    a. adenocarcinoma
    a. cell
    a. cell carcinoma (ACC)
    a. cell tumor
    a. pattern
Acinetobacter
    A. baumannii
    A. baylyi
    A. bouvetii
    A. calcoaceticus
    A. calcoaceticus anitratus
    A. calcoaceticus lwoffi
    A. gerneri
    A. grimontii
    A. parapertussis
    A. parvus
    A. pneumonia
    A. radioresistens
    A. schindleri
    A. tandoii
    A. tjernbergiae
    A. towneri
    A. ursingii
acini (*pl. of* acinus)
acinic
    a. cell adenocarcinoma
    a. cell carcinoma
    a. cell tumor
    a. cell tumor of lung
    a. cell tumor of salivary gland
aciniform
acinitis
acinose carcinoma
acinotubular gland
acinous
    a. carcinoma
    a. cell
    a. gland
acinus, pl. **acini**
    hepatic a.
    liver a.
    mucous a.
    pulmonary a.
    Rappaport a.
    secretory a.
    serous a.
ACIS
    automated cellular imaging system
ACIT
    allogeneic cellular immune therapy
    ACIT system
ackee, akee

ACLA
American Clinical Laboratory
Association
Acladium
ACL 100, 1000, 7000, 8000, 9000, 10000 advance coagulation analyzer
aclasis
diaphysial a.
tarsoepiphyseal a.
AcLDL
acetylated low-density lipoprotein
ACM
albumin-calcium-magnesium
aCML
atypical chronic myeloid leukemia
acne
a. atrophia
a. conglobata
a. rosacea
a. rosacea keratitis
a. vulgaris
acneiform
acnes
Propionibacterium a.
aconitase
aconitate hydratase
aconitine
Aconitum
aconitus
Anopheles a.
acormus
holoacardius a.
Acosta disease
acoustic
a. cell
a. coupler
a. crest
a. micrograph
a. microscope
a. neurilemmoma
a. neurinoma
a. neuroma
a. papilla
a. schwannoma
a. spot
ACP
acid phosphatase
ACPA
anticytoplasmic antibody
ACPA test
acquired
a. agammaglobulinemia

a. atrophy
a. C1EInh deficiency
a. character
a. defect
a. deformity
a. dysplasia
a. fibrokeratoma
a. genetic factor
a. hemolytic anemia (AHA)
a. hemolytic icterus
a. hepatic porphyria
a. hypogammaglobulinemia
a. ichthyosis
a. immunity
a. immunodeficiency syndrome (AIDS)
a. leukoderma
a. leukopathia
a. methemoglobinemia
a. nevus
a. qualitative disorders of platelets
a. sensitivity
a. sideroblastic anemia
a. toxoplasmosis in adults
a. tufted angioma
a. von Willebrand disease
acquisita
epidermolysis bullosa a.
hypertrichosis lanuginosa acquisita
acral
a. lentiginous melanoma
a. nevus
acrania
Acrel ganglion
Acremoniella
Acremonium
acridine
a. dye
a. hydrochloride
a. orange (AO)
a. orange method
a. orange stain
tetramethyl a.
a. yellow
acridinium ester
acriflavine
acroasphyxia
acroblast
acrobrachycephaly
acrobystitis
Acrocarpospora
A. corrugata

NOTES

A

Acrocarpospora (continued)
    A. *macrocephala*
    A. *pleiomorpha*
acrocentric
acrocephalia (*var. of* acrocephaly)
acrocephalic
acrocephalosyndactyly
acrocephalous
acrocephaly, acrocephalia
acrochordon
acrocyanosis
Acrocylindrium
acrodermatitis
    a. chronica atrophicans
    a. continua
    a. enteropathica
    a. enteropathy
    a. perstans
acrodolichomelia
Acrodontium salmoneum
acroedema
acrofacial
    a. dysostosis
    a. syndrome
acrogenous
acrokeratoelastoidosis
acrokeratosis
    paraneoplastic a.
    a. verruciformis
acrolein
acromegalia (*var. of* acromegaly)
acromegalic
acromegalogigantism
acromegaloidism
acromegaly, acromegalia
acromelia
acromelic dwarfism
acromesomelia
acromicria
acroosteolysis
acroosteolytica
    osteopetrosis a.
acropachy
acropachyderma
acropathy
acropetal
Acrophialophora fusispora
acropleurogenous
acroposthitis
acroscleroderma
acrosclerosis
acrosomal
    a. cap
    a. complex
    a. granule
    a. vesicle
acrosome
    a. granule
    a. reaction

acrospiroma
    eccrine a.
Acrosporium
acrostealgia
acrosyringium
acroterica
    morphea a.
acrotheca
Acrotheca pedrosoi
Acrothesium floccosum
acrotrophoneurosis
acrylamide gel electrophoresis
acrylate
acrylic acid
acrylonitrile
ACS
    acute coronary syndrome
    American Chemical Society
    antireticular cytotoxic serum
        ACS grade
        ACS 180 SE automated
            chemiluminescent immunoassay
            system
ACS:180 CK/MB analyzer
ACT
    acid clearance test
    activated clotting time
    activated coagulation time
    alpha antichymotrypsin
    anticoagulant therapy
Ac·T
    Ac·T diff, Ac·T diff2 hematology
        analyzer
    Ac·T 5 diff AL auto loader
        hematology analyzer
    Ac·T 5 diff CP cap pierce
        hematology analyzer
    Ac·T 5 diff OV open vial
        hematology analyzer
    Ac·T series hematology analyzer
act
    Bayh-Dole A.
    Clinical Laboratory Improvement A.
        of 1988 (CLIA '88)
    Emergency Medical Treatment and
        Labor A. (EMTALA)
    Health Insurance Portability and
        Accountability A. (HIPAA)
    Resource Conservation and
        Recovery A.
Actaea
Actalyke test
ACTH
    adrenocorticotropic hormone
        ACTH stimulation test
ACTH-producing adenoma
ACTH-RF
    adrenocorticotropic hormone-releasing
        factor

actin
  alpha cardiac a.
  alpha skeletal a.
  alpha smooth muscle a. (ASMA)
  antisarcomeric a.
  antismooth muscle a.
  a. cytoskeleton
  a. distribution
  a. filament
  monomeric a.
  muscle a. (MA)
  muscle-specific a. (MSA)
  pan-muscle a.
  sarcomeric a.
  smooth muscle a. (SMA)
actin-filament polymerization
actinic
  a. dermatitis
  a. keratosis
  a. porokeratosis
  a. reticuloid
actinide
actinin
  alpha a.
actinium (Ac)
actin-myosin web
Actinoalloteichus cyanogriseus
Actinobacillus
  A. actinomycetemcomitans
  A. arthritidis
  A. equuli
  A. lignieresii
  A. mallei
  A. pseudomallei
Actinobacteria
Actinobacteridae
Actinobaculum urinale
Actinocorallia
  A. aurantiaca
  A. glomerata
  A. libanotica
  A. longicatena
actinohematin
actinoides
  Thysanosoma a.
Actinokineospora
  A. auranticolor
  A. enzanensis
Actinomadura
  A. africana
  A. catellatispora
  A. glauciflava

  A. latina
  A. madurae
  A. mexicana
  A. meyerae
  A. namibiensis
  A. pelletieri
  A. viridilutea
Actinomucor
Actinomyces
  A. bovis
  A. canis
  A. cardiffensis
  A. catuli
  A. coleocanis
  A. congolensis
  A. culture
  A. eriksonii
  A. funkei
  A. hongkongensis
  A. israelii
  Mallory stain for A.
  A. marimammalium
  A. muris
  A. muris-ratti
  A. naeslundii
  A. nasicola
  A. necrophorus
  A. odontolyticus
  A. oricola
  A. radicidentis
  A. rhusiopathiae
  A. suimastitidis
  A. urogenitalis
  A. vaccimaxillae
  A. vinaceus
  A. viscosus
  Weigert stain for A.
Actinomycetaceae
Actinomycetales
actinomycete
  nocardioform a.
  thermophilic a.
actinomycetemcomitans
  Actinobacillus a.
  Haemophilus a.
actinomycetic
actinomycetin
actinomycetoma
actinomycin
actinomycosis
  genital tract a.

NOTES

actinomycosis (*continued*)
    oral a.
    thoracic a.
actinomycotic
    a. appendicitis
    a. mycetoma
actinomyoma
Actinomyxidia
actinophage
actinophytosis
Actinoplanaceae
Actinoplanales
Actinoplanes
    A. capillaceus
    A. friuliensis
Actinopoda
Actinopolymorpha singaporensis
actinosclerus
    Hymenobacter a.
Actinosynnemataceae
action
    buffer a.
    calorigenic a.
    capillary a.
    cumulative a.
    diastasic a.
    law of mass a.
    opsonic a.
    a. potential synaptic cleft
    specific dynamic a.
    spectrum a.
    a. spectrum
    thermogenic a.
    vitaminoid a.
activated
    a. charcoal
    a. clotting factor
    a. clotting time (ACT)
    a. coagulation time (ACT)
    a. complex
    a. lymphocyte
    a. macrophage
    a. microglia
    a. partial thromboplastin substitution
       test
    a. partial thromboplastin time
       (APTT, aPTT)
    a. protein C (APC)
    a. protein C resistance (APCR)
activating
    a. agent
    a. enzyme
activation
    allosteric a.
    a. analysis
    cis a.
    a. of the coagulation pathways
    complement a.
    cross a.

    a. energy
    ergoreceptor a.
    lymphocyte a.
    oncofetal a.
    parthenogenetic a.
    plasma a.
    T-cell a.
    trans a.
    very late a. (VLA)
    washed platelet a.
activation-induced cell death (AICD)
activator
    glucokinase a. (GKA)
    plasminogen a.
    polyclonal a.
    a. protein 1 (AP1)
    urokinase plasminogen a. (uPA)
active
    a. anaphylaxis
    a. chronic hepatitis
    a. chronic inflammation
    a. electrode
    endocytotically a.
    a. immunity
    a. immunization
    a. medium
    a. prophylaxis
    a. protein expression
    a. rosette test
    a. sensitization
    a. total PSA ELISA kit
    a. transport
Activin AB free beta-HCG ELISA test
activity
    altered lipid-peroxidation a.
    antiatherogenic a.
    blood granulocyte-specific a.
      (BGSA)
    chemotactic a.
    c-kit a.
    Clinician Outreach and
      Communication a.'s (COCA)
    colony-stimulating a. (CSA)
    a. determination
    endogenous avidin-binding a.
      (EABA)
    erythrocyte aspartate
      aminotransferase a. (eAST)
    facilitation of sympathetic a.
    gelatinolytic a.
    general gonadotropic a. (GGA)
    a. index
    insulinlike a. (ILA)
    leukemia-associated inhibitory a.
      (LIA)
    mean dose per unit cumulated a.
    neutrophil killing a.
    nonsuppressible insulinlike a.
      (NSILA)

optical a.
plasma insulin a. (PIA)
plasma renin a. (PRA)
postheparin lipolytic a. (PHLA)
proliferative a.
protein tyrosine kinase a.
a. ratio
relative specific a. (RSA)
renal vein renin a. (RVRA)
rheumatoid factor-like a. (RFLA)
surface-oriented pinocytic a.
telomerase a.
thyroxine-specific a. (T$_4$SA)
total antitryptic a. (TAT)
tryptic a.
unit of luteinizing a.
unit of progestational a.
unit of thyrotrophic a.
actodigin
actomyosin
platelet a.
Actonia
ACTP
adrenocorticotropic polypeptide
actuate
Acuaria spiralis
aculeate
aculeatum
stratum a.
acuminata
verruca a.
acuminate
acuminatum
condyloma a.
giant anorectal condyloma a.
papilloma a.
acustica
tuba a.
acustici
dentes a.
acuta
parapsoriasis lichenoides et
varioliformis a.
pityriasis lichenoides et
varioliformis a. (PLEVA)
polyarthritis rheumatica a.
acute
a. abscess
a. anterior poliomyelitis
a. atrophic paralysis
a. bacterial endocarditis
a. biphenotypic leukemia

a. bleed
a. bronchitis
a. bronchitis/bronchiolitis (ABB)
a. bulbar poliomyelitis
a. cardiovascular disease (ACVD)
a. cellular rejection
a. or chronic cholecystitis
a. and chronic inflammation
a. compression triad
a. contagious conjunctivitis
a. coronary syndrome (ACS)
a. crescentic glomerulonephritis
a. cryptitis
a. diffuse peritonitis
a. disseminated encephalomyelitis
(ADEM)
a. disseminated lupus erythematosus
a. disseminated myositis
a. epidemic conjunctivitis
a. epidemic infectious adenitis
a. epidemic leukoencephalitis
a. erythroleukemia (M6)
a. exudative glomerulonephritis
a. fatty liver of pregnancy
a. febrile jaundice
a. fibrinous pleuritis
a. focal hepatitis
a. follicular conjunctivitis
a. fulminating meningococcal
septicemia
a. fulminating primary amebic
meningoencephalitis
a. gangrenous appendicitis
a. gelatinous pneumonia
a. glomerulonephritis (AGN)
a. goiter
a. granulocytic leukemia (AGL)
a. hemolytic transfusion reaction
a. hemorrhagic bronchopneumonia
a. hemorrhagic cholecystitis
a. hemorrhagic cystitis
a. hemorrhagic encephalitis
a. hemorrhagic erosive gastritis
a. hemorrhagic glomerulonephritis
a. hemorrhagic inflammation
a. hemorrhagic leukoencephalitis
(AHLE)
a. hemorrhagic pancreatitis
a. hemorrhagic ulcer
a. hemorrhagic ulceration
a. humoral rejection
a. hyperemia

NOTES

acute *(continued)*
  a. idiopathic polyneuritis
  a. infarct
  a. infectious disease (AID)
  a. infectious nonbacterial
    gastroenteritis
  a. infective endocarditis
  a. inflammatory exudate
  a. inflammatory infiltrate
  a. inflammatory membrane
  a. inflammatory necrosis
  a. inflammatory transudate
  a. intermittent porphyria (AIP)
  a. interstitial nephritis (AIN)
  a. interstitial pneumonia (AIP)
  a. isolated myocarditis
  a. lymphoblastic leukemia (ALL)
  a. lymphoblastic leukemia in older
    children
  a. lymphoblastic leukemia
    secondary to Burkitt lymphoma
  a. lymphocytic leukemia (ALL)
  a. massive liver necrosis
  a. mastitis
  a. megakaryoblastic leukemia
  a. megakaryocytic leukemia (M7)
  a. mesenteric adenitis
  a. miliary tuberculosis
  a. monoblastic leukemia (AMoL)
  a. monocytic leukemia (AMoL,
    M5)
  a. monocytic leukemia with
    differentiation (M5b)
  a. monocytic leukemia without
    differentiation (M5a)
  a. myeloblastic leukemia with
    maturation (M2)
  a. myeloblastic leukemia without
    localized differentiation (M0)
  a. myeloblastic leukemia without
    maturation (M1)
  a. myelocytic leukemia
  a. myelogenous leukemia
  a. myeloid leukemia (AML)
  a. myelomonocytic leukemia
    (AMML, M4)
  a. myocardial infarction (AMI)
  a. necrotizing encephalitis
  a. necrotizing enterocolitis
  a. necrotizing hemorrhagic
    encephalomyelitis
  a. necrotizing myelitis
  a. necrotizing ulcerative gingivitis
  a. necrotizing ulcerative tonsillitis
  a. nephrosis
  a. nonlymphocytic leukemia
    (ANLL)
  a. normovolemic hemodilution
    (ANH)

otitis media, purulent, a. (OMPA)
  a. parenchymatous hepatitis
  a. paroxysmal myoglobinuria
  a. phase protein
  a. phase reactant (APR)
  a. phase reaction
  a. physiology and chronic health
    evaluation (APACHE)
  a. posthemorrhagic anemia
  a. poststreptococcal
    glomerulonephritis
  a. primary hemorrhagic
    meningoencephalitis
  a. proliferative
  a. proliferative glomerulonephritis
  a. promyelocytic leukemia (APL,
    M3)
  a. pulmonary alveolitis
  a. pyelonephritis
  a. pyogenic membrane
  a. radiation syndrome (ARS)
  a. recurrent rhabdomyolysis
  a. renal failure (ARF)
  a. respiratory disease
  a. respiratory distress syndrome
    (ARDS)
  a. respiratory failure (ARF)
  a. rheumatic arthritis
  a. rheumatic fever (ARF)
  a. rhinitis
  a. rickets
  a. salivary adenitis
  a. self-limited hemolytic anemia
  a. serous synovitis
  a. splenic tumor
  a. splenitis
  a. suppurative appendicitis
  a. suppurative lymphadenitis
  a. thyroiditis
  a. transverse myelitis
  a. tubular necrosis (ATN)
  a. ulcerative colitis
  a. undifferentiated leukemia (AUL)
  a. urethral syndrome
  a. uric acid nephropathy
  a. vascular rejection
  a. viral hepatitis (AVH)
  a. yellow atrophy
  a. yellow atrophy of liver
ACVD
  acute cardiovascular disease
acyl
  a. carrier protein
  a. coenzyme A (acyl-CoA)
  a. enzyme
  a. peroxide
acylation
acyl-CoA
  acyl coenzyme A

a.-COA acyltransferase (ACAT)
a.-COA dehydrogenase
a.-COA desaturase
a.-COA synthetase
acyloxy group
acylsphingosine deacylase
acyltransferase
acetyl-CoA a.
acyl-CoA a. (ACAT)
cholesterol a.
lecithin-cholesterol a. (LCAT)
phosphatidylcholine-cholesterol a.
ADA
adenosine deaminase
ADA deficiency
AD 340 absorbance detector
adactyly
Adair-Dighton syndrome
ADAM
a disintegrin and metalloprotease
ADAM protein
1-adamantanamine sulfate
adamantina
prismata a.
substantia a.
adamantine prism
adamantinoma
a. of long bones
pituitary a.
adamantoblast
Adamkiewicz test
adamsite
Adams-Stokes
A.-S. attack (ASA)
A.-S. disease (AS)
ADAMTS 13
a disintegrin and metalloproteinase with
thrombospondin domain 13
ADAMTS 13 protein
Adansonia
adaptation
cellular a.
enzymatic a.
genetic a.
phenotypic a.
adapter
adaptive
a. enzyme
a. hormone
a. hypertrophy
AD7C Alzheimer test

ADD1
adipocyte determination and
differentiation factor 1
addiction
alcohol a.
drug a.
Addis
A. count
A. test
Addison
A. anemia
A. disease
A. keloid
Addison-Biermer disease
addisonian
a. anemia
a. crisis
a. syndrome
addisonism
addition
binary a.
a. polymer
a. reaction
addition-deletion mutation
additive
POES a.
addressin
vascular a.
addressing
indirect a.
a. ligand
adducin gene
adduct removal
adecarboxylata
Escherichia a.
adelomorphic
adelomorphous
ADEM
acute disseminated encephalomyelitis
adendritic, adendric
adenectopia
Aden fever
adenine (A)
a. arabinoside
a. deaminase
adenine-thymine/guanine-cytosine ratio
(AT:GC)
adeninivorans
Arxula a.
adenitis
acute epidemic infectious a.
acute mesenteric a.

NOTES

21

adenitis *(continued)*
    acute salivary a.
    cervical a.
    mesenteric a.
    phlegmonous a.
    a. tropicalis
adenoacanthoma
adenoameloblastoma
adeno-associated virus (AAV)
adenoblast
adenocarcinoma (AC, ACA)
    acinar a.
    acinic cell a.
    alveolar a.
    anaplastic a.
    Barrett a. (BCA)
    bronchial gland cell a.
    bronchial surface cell a.
    bronchiolar a.
    bronchioloalveolar a.
    Clara cell a.
    clear cell a.
    colloid a.
    dedifferentiated low-grade a.
    endometrial a.
    enteric-type a.
    fetal a.
    fungating a.
    gelatinous a.
    goblet cell a.
    indeterminate cell a.
    infiltrating duct a.
    inflammatory a.
    lobular a.
    Lucké a.
    medullary a.
    mesonephric a.
    metastatic a. (MA)
    mixed squamous cell carcinoma
      and a.
    a. of Moll
    mucinous a.
    mucoid a.
    nonmucinous a.
    oxyphilic endometrioid a.
    papillary a.
    a. phenotype
    polymorphous low-grade a. (PLGA)
    polypoid a.
    por1 a.
    por2 a.
    prostatic a. (PCA)
    renal a.
    scirrhous a.
    sebaceous a.
    signet ring a.
    a. in situ (AIS)
    solid a.
    sweat gland a.

    terminal duct a.
    trabecular a.
    tub1 a.
    tub2 a.
    tubular a.
    type II alveolar epithelial cell a.
    undifferentiated a.
    a. of the uterus with sarcomatous
      overgrowth
    vaginal clear cell a.
    villoglandular a. (VGA)
    well-differentiated fetal a. (WDFA)
adenocellulitis
adenochondroma
adenocystic carcinoma
adenocystoma lymphomatosum
adenocyte
adenodiastasis
adenoepithelioma
adenofibroma
    metanephric a. (MAF)
adenofibromyoma
adenofibrosis
adenohypophyseos
    pars distalis a.
adenohypophysial, adenohypophyseal
    a. hormone
adenohypophysis
adenohypophysitis
    lymphocytic a.
adenoid
    a. cystic carcinoma (ACC)
    a. face
    a. facies
    a. hyperplasia
    a. hypertrophy
    a. squamous cell carcinoma
    a. tissue
    a. tumor
adenoidal-pharyngeal-conjunctival (APC)
adenoleiomyofibroma
adenolipoma
adenolipomatosis
    symmetric a.
adenolymphocele
adenolymphoma
adenolysis
adenoma
    acidophil a.
    acidophilic a.
    ACTH-producing a.
    adnexal a.
    adrenal cortical a.
    adrenocortical a.
    adrenocorticotropic hormone-
      producing a.
    aldosterone-producing a. (APA)
    angioinvasive a.
    apocrine a.

basal cell a.
basophil a.
bile duct a.
black thyroid a.
bronchial a.
canalicular a.
carcinoma ex pleomorphic a.
ceruminous a.
chief cell a.
chromophil a.
chromophobe a.
chromophobic a.
clear cell a.
colloid a.
corticotrope a.
depressed a.
diploid a.
ductal a.
embryonal a.
eosinophil a.
fetal a.
fibroid a.
a. fibrosum
follicular a.
Fuchs a.
gastric tubular a.
gonadotrope a.
gonadotropin-producing a.
growth hormone-producing a.
hepatic a.
hepatocellular a. (HCA)
Hürthle cell a.
islet cell a.
lactating a.
lactotrope a.
Leydig cell a.
macrofollicular a.
malignant a.
mammosomatotropic a.
metanephric a.
microfollicular a.
middle ear a.
monomorphic a. (MA)
multiple a.
multiploid a.
nephrogenic a.
neuroendocrine-type feature in
  adrenal cortical a.
nipple a.
null cell a.
oncocytic a.
ovarian tubular a.

oxyphil a.
papillary cystic a.
papillary a. of large intestine
parathyroid a.
Pick tubular a.
pituitary a.
pleomorphic a. (PA)
Plummer a.
plurihormonal a.
polypoid a.
primary pulmonary a. (PPA)
prolactin-producing a.
prostatic a.
renal cortical a.
sebaceous a.
a. sebaceum
serrated a.
sessile serrated a.
somatotroph a.
somatotropic a.
sweat duct a.
sweat gland a.
syringomatous a.
testicular tubular a.
thyroid a.
thyrotrope a.
thyrotropin-producing a.
toxic a.
trabecular a.
tubovillous a.
tubular a.
undifferentiated cell a.
villous a.

adenomatoid
  a. cystic papillary nodule
  a. odontogenic tumor

adenomatosis
  endocrine a.
  familial multiple endocrine a., type
  1, 2
  fibrosing a.
  multiple endocrine a. (MEA)
  pluriglandular a.
  polyendocrine a.
  pulmonary a.

adenomatous
  a. crypt
  a. epithelium
  a. goiter
  a. hyperplasia
  a. polyp

adenomere

NOTES

adenomyoepithelial adenosis
adenomyoepithelioma
adenomyofibroma
    atypical polypoid a. (APA)
adenomyoma
    atypical polypoid a. (APA)
adenomyosarcoma
adenomyosis uteri
adenopathy
adenophlegmon
Adenophorasida
Adenophorea
adenophyma
adenosalpingitis
adenosarcoma
    metanephric a.
    müllerian a.
adenosatellite virus
adenosine
    a. 3′,5′-cyclic monophosphate (cAMP)
    a. 3′,5′-cyclic phosphate (cAMP)
    a. deaminase (ADA)
    a. deaminase assay
    a. deaminase deficiency
    a. diphosphate
    a. 5′-diphosphate (ADP)
    a. 5′-diphosphate/adenosine triphosphate
    a. 5′-diphosphate/adenosine triphosphate ratio (ADP:ATP)
    a. kinase
    a. monophosphate (AMP)
    a. triphosphatase (ATPase)
    a. triphosphate (ATP)
adenosis
    adenomyoepithelial a.
    apocrine a.
    blunt duct a.
    fibrosing a.
    microglandular a.
    nodular a.
    sclerosing polycystic a.
    sclerosis a.
    secretory a.
    simple a.
    tubular a.
    vaginal a.
adenotonsillar
adenoviral transduction
Adenoviridae
adenovirus
    alpha antigen of a.
    beta antigen of a.
    canine a. 1
    a. immunofluorescence
    porcine a.
    a. test kit

adenylate
    a. cyclase
    a. deaminase
    a. kinase
    a. kinase deficiency
adenyl cyclase
adenylic
    a. acid
    a. acid deaminase
adenylosuccinate lyase
adenylpyrophosphatase
adenylylation
adenylyl transferase
Adeza TLi fetal fibronectin analysis system
ADH
    alcohol dehydrogenase
    antidiuretic hormone
    atypical ductal hyperplasia
    ADH assay
    ADH deficiency
adhaerens
    Hyphomonas a.
adherence
    bacterial a.
    immune a.
    Treponema pallidum immobilization (immune) a. (TPIA)
adherens
    fascia a.
    a. junction-associated catenin
    macula a.
    zonula a.
adherent
    a. pericarditis
    a. pericardium
    a. plug
adhering junction
adhesin
adhesiolysis
adhesion
    amniotic a.
    a. assay
    fibrinous a.
    fibrous a.
    intraabdominal a.
    joint a.
    a. molecule
    a. phenomenon
    plaque a.
    sublabial a.
    a. test
    wispy a.
adhesive
    albumin slide a.
    a. arachnoiditis
    a. capsulitis
    a. chronic pachymeningitis
    a. extracellular domain

gelatin slide a.
a. inflammation
a. pericarditis
a. peritonitis
a. phlebitis
a. pleurisy
a. vaginitis
adiacens
    Granulicatella a.
adiadochokinesia
Adiantum
adiaspiromycosis
adiaspirosis
adiaspore
Adie
    A. pupil
    A. syndrome
Adinida
adiphenine hydrochloride
adipic
adipica
    Desulfovirga a.
adipocele
adipocellular
adipoceratous
adipocere
adipocyte
    a. determination and differentiation
      factor 1 (ADD1)
    a. differentiation
    mature a.
    necrotic a.
adipocytic neoplasm
adipoid
adipokinesis
adipokinetic hormone
adipolysis
adipolytic
adiponecrosis
adipose
    a. capsule
    a. cell
    a. degeneration
    a. fossa
    a. infiltration
    a. tissue
    a. tissue extract
    a. tumor
adiposis
    a. cardiaca
    a. cerebralis

    a. dolorosa
    a. hepatica
    a. orchica
    a. tuberosa simplex
    a. universalis
adiposity
adiposogenital dystrophy
adiposum
    cor a.
    sclerema a.
adiposuria
adiposus
    ascites a.
aditus
adjacent interstitial tissue
adjoining epithelial cell
adjunct
    anesthesia a.
adjusted rate
adjuvant
    a. chemotherapy
    Freund complete a.
    Freund incomplete a.
    mycobacterial a.
    a. vaccine
Adler test
admaxillary gland
administration
    Health Resources and Services A.
      (HRSA)
    Occupational Safety and Health A.
      (OSHA)
admix
admixture
ADN-B
    antideoxyribonuclease B
    ADN-B assay
adnexa (*pl. of* adnexum)
adnexal
    a. adenoma
    a. carcinoma
    a. neoplasm
adnexitis
adnexum, pl. **adnexa**
ADO2
    autosomal dominant osteopetrosis type 2
adolescent
    a. albuminuria
    a. round back
adolescentium
    apophysitis tibialis a.

NOTES

adoptive
    a. immunity
    a. immunotherapy
ADP
    adenosine 5′-diphosphate
ADP:ATP
    adenosine 5′-diphosphate/adenosine
    triphosphate ratio
adrenal
    accessory a.
    androgen-secreting a.
    a. antibody
    a. ascorbic acid depletion test
    a. body
    a. cancer
    a. capsule
    a. cortex
    a. cortex cell
    a. cortical adenoma
    a. cortical hyperplasia
    a. crisis
    a. disease
    a. epithelioid angiosarcoma
    a. failure
    a. feminizing syndrome
    a. function test
    a. gland
    a. gland virilizing syndrome
    a. hypofunction
    a. insufficiency
    Marchand a.'s
    a. medulla
    a. neoplasm
    a. rest
    a. tumor
    a. virilism
    a. virilization
adrenalectomized patient
adrenaline test
adrenalitis
adrenalopathy
adrenarche
    delayed a.
    precocious a.
adrenergic
    a. neuron blockade
    a. neuron blocking agent
adrenochrome
adrenocortical
    a. abnormality
    a. adenoma
    adrenocortical carcinoma
    adrenocortical hyperplasia
    a. extract (ACE)
    a. hormone (ACH)
    a. inhibition test
    a. insufficiency
    a. rest tumor
adrenocorticosteroid

adrenocorticotropic
    a. cell
    a. hormone (ACTH)
    a. hormone assay
    a. hormone-producing adenoma
    a. hormone-releasing factor (ACTH-RF)
    a. hormone suppression test
    a. polypeptide (ACTP)
adrenocorticotropin
adrenodoxin
adrenogenital syndrome (AGS)
adrenoleukodystrophy (ALD)
adrenomedullary
    a. catecholamine
    a. hormone
    a. triad
adrenomegaly
adrenomyeloneuropathy
adrenopathy
adrenoreceptor
ADS
    antibody deficiency syndrome
    antidiuretic substance
    autonomous detection system
adsorb
adsorbate
adsorbed plasma
adsorbent
    gastrointestinal a.
adsorption
    agglutinin a.
    chemical a.
    a. chromatography
    immune a.
    physical a.
ADSQC
    adenosquamous cell carcinoma
adult
    acquired toxoplasmosis in a.'s
    a. celiac disease
    a. cystic teratoma
    a. gonococcal conjunctivitis
    a. granulosa cell tumor (AGCT)
    a. hemoglobin
    a. medulloepithelioma
    a. polycystic kidney disease
    a. respiratory distress syndrome (ARDS)
    a. rickets
    a. stem cell
    a. stem cell plasticity
    a. T-cell leukemia (ATL)
    a. T-cell lymphoma (ATL)
    a. T-cell lymphoma/leukemia (ATLL)
    a. thymectomy
    a. tuberculosis
    a. worm

adulteration
adult-onset diabetes
adultorum
    blennorrhea a.
    scleredema a.
adult-type xanthogranuloma
advanced
    a. glycation end product (AGE)
    A. Instruments conductivity
    analyzer
adventitia
    aortic tunica a.
    membrana a.
    tunica a.
adventitial
    a. dermis
    a. neuritis
    a. reticular cell
adventitious
    a. albuminuria
    a. cyst
Advia
    A. 60, 120 automated cell
    counting instrument
    A. Centaur anti-HBs calibrator
    A. Centaur anti-HBs reagent
    A. Centaur HBc IgM control
    material
    A. Centaur HBc IgM reagent
    A. 1650 chemistry analyzer
    A. 120 hematology system
adynamia
    hereditary a.
adynamic ileus
AE
    antitoxin Einheit
AE1
    anion exchanger 1
    AE1 antibody
    AE1 immunoperoxidase stain
    AE1 plus CAM
AE1:AE3 antibody ratio
AE3 antibody
AEC
    3-amino-9-ethylcarbazole
    5-amino 9 ethyl carbazole
    AEC chromogen
    AEC detection system
Aedes
    A. aegypti
    A. albopictus
    A. atlanticus

    A. cinereus
    A. dorsalis
    A. flavescens
    A. leucocelaenus
    A. melanimon
    A. mitchellae
    A. nigromaculis
    A. polynesiensis
    A. scutellaris pseudoscutellaris
    A. sollicitans
    A. spencerii
    A. taeniorhynchus
    A. triseriatus
    A. trivittatus
    A. variegatus
    A. vexans
aegaeus
    Thermococcus a.
aegypti
    Aedes a.
aegyptia
    Natrialba a.
    Nocardiopsis a.
aegyptius
    Haemophilus a.
    Thermicanus a.
Aelurostrongylus
AEM
    analytical electron microscope
aeolius
    Bacillus a.
AEq
    age equivalent
aequorin
    photoprotein a.
    a. recombinant method
Aequorivita
    A. antarctica
    A. crocea
    A. lipolytica
    A. sublithincola
AER
    albumin excretion rate
    aldosterone excretion rate
aerated
aeration
aeria
    Rothia a.
aerial mycelium
aeriphila
    Aeriscardovia a.
Aeriscardovia aeriphila

NOTES

27

aerivorans
  Sporomusa a.
Aerobacter
  A. aerogenes
  A. cloacae
  A. liquefaciens
  A. subgroup A, B, C
aerobe
  obligate a.
aerobic
  a. and anaerobic blood culture
  a. bacterium
  a. coccobacillus
  a. diphtheroid
  a. metabolism
  a. respiration
aerobiological property
aerobiology
aerobiosis
aerobiotic
aerocele
Aerococcus
  A. urinaehominis
  A. viridans
aerodermectasia
aeroembolism
aerofaciens
  Collinsella a.
  Eubacterium a.
aerogen
aerogenes
  Aerobacter a.
  Enterobacter a.
  Pasteurella a.
  Peptococcus a.
  Vibrio a.
aerogenesis
aerogenic
aerogenoides
  Paracolobactrum a.
aerogenosum
  sputum a.
aerogenous
aerolata
  Promicromonospora a.
  Sphingomonas a.
Aeromicrobium marinum
Aeromonadaceae
Aeromonas
  A. culicicola
  A. hydrophila
  A. hydrophila subsp. *dhakensis*
  A. hydrophila subsp. *ranae*
  A. liquefaciens
  A. (Plesiomonas) shigelloides
  A. punctata
  A. salmonicida
  A. salmonicida subsp. *pectinolytica*

  A. simiae
  A. sobria
aerophil, aerophile
aerophila
  Caldilinea a.
aerophilic
aerophilous
aerophilum
  Thialkalimicrobium a.
aerophilus
  Hymenobacter a.
  Thominx a.
aeroplankton
Aeropyrum camini
Aeroset
  A. abused drugs/toxicology test
  A. clinical chemistry system
aerosis
aerosol
  a. generator
  lethal anthrax a.
  plague a.
  racemic a.
aerosolization
  secondary a.
aerosolized plague weapon
Aerosol Resistant Tips (ART)
Aerospray
  A. acid-fast bacteria slide
    stainer/cytocentrifuge
  A. cytocentrifuge
  A. hematology slide
    stainer/cytocentrifuge
aerotaxis
aerotitis media
aerotolerant
aerotonometer
aerotropism
aertrycke
  Bacillus a.
aeruginosa
  Microcystis a.
  Pseudomonas a.
aeschlimannii
  Rickettsia a.
Aessosporon
aestivalis
  prurigo a.
aestivoautumnal fever
aestuarianus
  Vibrio a.
aestuarii
  Nitrosomonas a.
Aestuariibacter
  A. halophilus
  A. salexigens
AET
  aminoethylisothiouronium bromide

aetherivorans
    Rhodococcus a.
aethiopica
    Leishmania a.
aethiopicum
    Plasmodium a.
AF
    acid-fast
    aldehyde fuchsin
AFA
    alcohol-formaldehyde-acetic acid
    AFA fixative
AFB
    acid-fast bacillus
    AFB smear
    AFB stain
AFC
    acid-fast culture
afebrile abortion
affected
    part a. (par. aff.)
afferens
    vas a.
affinis
    Shewanella a.
affinity
    a. antibody
    a. chromatography
    a. constant
    functional a.
    a. label
    A. multimode plate reader
    a. purified
    selective a.
    testosterone-binding a. (TBA)
Affymetrix
    A. GeneChip HU95 array
    A. GeneChip system
    A. human cancer chip
    A. U133A oligonucleotide
      microarray
afibrillar cementum
afibrinogenemia
    congenital a.
AFIP
    Armed Forces Institute of Pathology
Afipia
    A. *birgiae*
    A. *felis*
    A. *massiliensis*
aflatoxicosis
aflatoxin B

AFLH
AFM
    atomic force microscopy
AFP
    alpha fetoprotein
    AFP test
africae
    Rickettsia a.
African
    A. hemorrhagic fever
    A. histoplasmosis
    A. horse sickness
    A. horse sickness virus
    A. sleeping sickness
    A. swine fever
    A. swine fever virus
    A. tick-borne fever
    A. trypanosomiasis
africana
    Actinomadura a.
    Nocardia a.
    Taenia a.
africanum
    Mycobacterium a.
africanus
    Paragonimus a.
    Streptomyces a.
aftercataract
afterchroming
aftergilding
afterload-reducing drug
aftosa
AFX
    atypical fibroxanthoma
afzelii
    Borrelia a.
A:G
    albumin-globulin ratio
Ag
    antigen
    silver
AGA
    appropriate for gestational age
agalactiae
    Streptococcus a.
agamete
agamic
agammaglobulinemia
    acquired a.
    Bruton type a.
    congenital a.
    primary a.

NOTES

agammaglobulinemia *(continued)*
    secondary a.
    Swiss-type a.
    transient a.
    X-linked a. (XLA)
agamocytogeny
Agamodistomum ophthalmobium
Agamofilaria
agamogenesis
agamogenetic
agamogony
Agamomermis culicis
Agamonema
Agamonematodum migrans
agamont
agamous
aganglionic megacolon
aganglionosis
    congenital a.
    total colonic a. (TCA)
    zonal a.
agar
    a. agar
    ascitic a.
    bacteriostasis a.
    a. bead
    bile esculin a.
    bile salt a.
    birdseed a.
    bismuth-sulfite a. (BSA)
    blood a.
    Bordet-Gengou potato blood a.
    brain-heart infusion a.
    brilliant green bile salt a.
    Brucella a.
    Campylobacter selective a.
    casein a.
    CB a.
    cefsulodin-Irgasan-novobiocin a.
    cetrimide a.
    charcoal yeast extract a.
    chocolate blood a.
    Christensen urea a.
    CIN a.
    citrate a.
    clostrisel a.
    Columbia blood a.
    cornmeal a.
    a. cutter
    cycloserine cefoxitin fructose a.
    cycloserine mannitol a.
    cystine trypticase a.
    Czapek-Dox a.
    Czapek solution a.
    deep a.
    deoxycholate-citrate a. (DCA)
    deoxyribonuclease a.
    dextrose a.
    a. diffusion method

DNase a.
egg-yolk a.
EMB Levine a.
Emmon modification of Sabouraud dextrose a.
Endo a.
French proof a.
GC a.
gelatin a.
a. gel electrophoresis
heart infusion a.
Hektoen enteric a.
inhibitory mold a.
Kliger iron a. (KIA)
Krumwiede triple sugar a.
laked blood a.
Levine EMB a.
Löffler serum a.
Lowenstein-Jensen a.
lysine-iron a.
MacConkey a.
malt a.
Martin-Lester a.
Middlebrook a.
modified TM a.
Mueller-Hinton a.
mycobiotic a.
Mycoplasma a.
neomycin assay a.
nitrate a.
nutrient a.
nystatin assay a.
oatmeal-tomato paste a.
Pfeiffer blood a.
phenylalanine a.
phenylethyl alcohol blood a.
a. plate count
polymyxin test a.
potato-blood a.
potato dextrose a.
Pseudomonas selective a.
rabbit blood a.
rice-Tween a.
Russell double-sugar a.
Sabhi a.
Sabouraud dextrose and brain heart infusion a.
saccharose-mannitol a.
Salmonella-Shigella a.
Schaedler blood a.
seed a.
serum a.
sheep blood a.
Simmons citrate a.
standard method a.
sulfite a.
TCBS a.
tellurite glycine a.
Thayer-Martin a.

thistle seed a.
Trichophyton a.
triple sugar iron a.
trypticase soy a. (TSA)
tryptic soy a.
TSI a.
urea a.
Wilkins-Chilgren a.
XLD a.
yeast extract a.
Zein a.
Agarbacterium
agarexedens
    Paenibacillus a.
agaric
    a. acid
    deadly a.
    fly a.
Agaricus
agaridevorans
    Paenibacillus a.
Agar-IF
agariperforans
    Reibachia a.
agarivorans
    Pseudoalteromonas a.
    Vibrio a.
Agarivorans albus
agarose gel electrophoresis
Ag-AS
    silver-acidified serum
    Ag-AS stain
agassizii
    Mycoplasma a.
AGC
    absolute granulocyte count
AGCT
    adult granulosa cell tumor
AGE
    advanced glycation end product
age
    appropriate for gestational a. (AGA)
    bone a.
    chronological a. (CA)
    a. equivalent (AEq)
    gestational a. (GA)
    maternal a.
age-adjusted rate
aged serum
ageing (hippocampal region, patients over 75 years), tau pathology class I

agency
    Environmental Protection A. (EPA)
    A. for Toxic Substances & Disease Registry (ATSDR)
agenesis
    cerebellar a.
    gonadal a.
    ovarian a.
    pure red cell a.
    renal a.
    testicular a.
    thymic a.
    unilateral renal a.
agent
    A. 15
    activating a.
    adrenergic neuron blocking a.
    airborne a.
    alkylating a.
    androgenic anabolic a. (AAA)
    antibacterial a.
    antifungal a.
    antiretroviral a.
    antiviral a.
    bacteriostatic a.
    beta-adrenergic blocking a.
    biological alkylating a.
    Bittner a.
    blister a.
    blocking a.
    blood a.
    calmative a.
    category A, B, C a.
    caudalizing a.
    CDC category of biological a.
    chelating a.
    chemical a.
    chimpanzee coryza a. (CCA)
    choking a.
    cholinergic blocking a.
    convulsant antidote for nerve a. (CANA)
    Coulter Clenz cleaning a.
    CW a.
    delta a.
    disclosing a.
    droplet-borne a.
    drying a.
    Eaton a.
    embedding a.
    etiologic a.
    F a.

NOTES

agent *(continued)*
    fertility a.
    fluid-borne a.
    foamy a.
    G a.
    ganglionic blocking a. (GBA)
    gonadotropin-releasing a. (GRA)
    Gordon a.
    Hawaii a.
    immunomodulatory a.
    incapacitating chemical a.
    infectious a.
    initiating a.
    injurious a.
    lysing a.
    Marburg a.
    Marcy a.
    mechanical a.
    military nerve a.
    mobilizing a.
    MS-1 a.
    MS-2 a.
    NATO code for an extremely toxic persistent nerve a. (no common chemical name) (VX)
    NATO code for nonpersistent nerve a.
    NATO code for persistent nerve a.
    natriuretic a.
    nerve a.
    nitrosourea a.
    nonpersistent a.
    Norwalk a.
    oxidizing a.
    Panta antimicrobial a.
    persistent a.
    Pittsburgh pneumonia a.
    progestational a.
    promoting a.
    pulmonary a.
    a. in question
    radiological a.
    reducing a.
    reovirus-like a.
    riot control a.
    splatter-borne a.
    a., state, body site, effects, severity, time course, other (diagnoses), synergism (ASBESTOS)
    surface-active a.
    thermo a.
    thrombolytic a.
    tocolytic a.
    toxic chemical a.
    transforming a.
    urticating a.
    V a.
    vacuolating a.
    vesicating a.
    virus-inactivating a. (VIA)
    volatile nerve a.
    vomiting a.
    wetting a.
age-specific rate
agglomerate
agglomeration
agglutinable
agglutinant
agglutinate
agglutinating antibody
agglutination
    acid a.
    alpha a.
    bacterial a. (BA)
    bacteriogenic a.
    beta a.
    chick-cell a. (CCA)
    cold a.
    cross a.
    direct a.
    false a.
    febrile a.
    flagellar a.
    group a.
    H a.
    immune a.
    a. immunoassay
    indirect a.
    a. inhibition assay
    intravascular a.
    latex a. (LA)
    macroscopic a.
    mediate a.
    microscopic a.
    mixed a.
    nonimmune a.
    O a.
    passive a.
    platelet a.
    reverse a.
    reverse passive latex a. (RPLA)
    salt a.
    slide latex a. (SLA)
    spontaneous a.
    T a.
    a. test
    a. titer
    Treponema pallidum a. (TPA)
    tube a. (TA)
    Vi a.
    warm a.
agglutinative thrombus
agglutinator
    rheumatoid a.
agglutinin
    a. adsorption
    alpha a.

anti-A a.
anti-B a.
anti-M a.
anti-N a.
anti-P a.
anti-Rh a.
anti-S a.
beta a.
blood group a.
brucellosis a.
chief a.
cold a. (CA)
cross-reacting a.
febrile a.
flagellar a.
group a.
H a.
heterophil a.
immune a.
incomplete a.
latex a.
leukocyte a.
major a.
Mg a.
minor a.
natural a.
O a.
partial a.
plant a.
platelet a.
Rh a.
saline a.
salmonella a.
serum a.
somatic a.
tularemia a.
Ulex europaeus a.
warm a.
Weil-Felix a.
wheat germ a. (WGA)
agglutinogen
blood group a.
T a.
agglutinogenic
agglutinophilic
agglutinoscope
agglutogen
agglutogenic
aggregans
Eubacterium a.
aggregate
a. anaphylaxis

cytoplasmic crystalline a.
cytoplasmic lipid a.
cytoplasmic macromolecule a.
a. gland
insoluble complement-bound a.
lymphoid a.
lymphoreticular a.
nuclear crystalline a.
nuclear lipid a.
proteoglycan a.
sheetlike a.
transmural lymphoid a.
tubular a.
tubuloreticular a.
aggregated
a. albumin
a. human immunoglobulin G
(AHuG)
a. lymphatic follicle of small
intestine
a. lymphatic nodule
a. microsphere
aggregati
folliculi lymphatici a.
aggregation
cell a.
mitochondrial a.
platelet a.
aggregometer
aggregometry
turbidimetric a.
aggresome
aggressin
aggressive
a. angiomyxoma
a. follicular variant
a. infantile fibromatosis
agitata
Dechloromonas a.
agitation
AGL
acute granulocytic leukemia
aglandular
aglobuliosis
aglobulism
aglomerular
aglutition
aglycemia
aglycogenosis
aglycone
aglycosuria
aglycosuric

NOTES

agmen peyerianum
agminate
    a. gland
    a. nevus
agmination
AGN
    acute glomerulonephritis
agnathus
agnogenic myeloid metaplasia
AgNOR
    argyrophilic nucleolar organizer region
    silver-stained nucleolar organizer region
    silver-stained nucleolar organizing region
      AgNOR banding
      AgNOR method
agona
    Salmonella enteritidis serotype *a.*
agonadal
agonadism
agonal
    a. leukocytosis
    a. thrombosis
    a. thrombus
agonist
    calcium channel a.
    KOR a.
    NMDA receptor a.
agonist-induced activation of PLA2
agranular
    a. cell
    a. cortex
    a. endoplasmic reticulum
    a. leukocyte
agranulocyte
agranulocytic angina
agranulocytosis
    feline a.
    Kostmann a.
agranuloplasia
agranuloplastic
agreement
    level of a.
Agreia
    A. bicolorata
    A. pratensis
agretope
agria
    prurigo a.
agricultural terrorism
Agrobacterium
    A. larrymoorei
    A. meteori
Agrococcus baldri
Agrocybe
Agromyces
    A. albus
    A. aurantiacus
    A. bracchium
    A. hippuratus

    A. luteolus
    A. rhizospherae
agroterrorist
    a. attack
    a. event
AGS
    adrenogenital syndrome
AGT
    antiglobulin test
ague
AGUS
    atypical glandular cell of undetermined
      significance
    atypical glandular cell of unknown
      significance
AGV
    aniline gentian violet
aGVHD
    acute graft-versus-host disease
agyria
agyric
AH
    antihyaluronidase
      AH assay
      AH titer
AHA
    acquired hemolytic anemia
    autoimmune hemolytic anemia
ahangari
    Geoglobus a.
ahaptoglobinemia
    congenital a.
ahaustral
AHD
    arteriosclerotic heart disease
    atherosclerotic heart disease
AHF
    antihemophilic factor
AHG
    antihemophilic globulin
    antihuman globulin
      AHG factor
AHH
    analog of histidine
AHLE
    acute hemorrhagic leukoencephalitis
AHLS
    antihuman lymphocyte serum
Ahrensia kielensis
AHT
    antihyaluronidase titer
    augmented histamine test
AHuG
    aggregated human immunoglobulin G
Ahumada-Del Castillo syndrome
AI
    aortic incompetence
Aicardi syndrome

AICD
> activation-induced cell death

aichiensis
> *Gordonia a.*

AID
> acute infectious disease

aid
> cryostat frozen sectioning a.

AIDS
> acquired immunodeficiency syndrome
> AIDS serology

AIDS-KS
> AIDS-related Kaposi sarcoma

AIDS-related
> AIDS-r. complex (ARC)
> AIDS-r. Kaposi sarcoma (AIDS-KS)
> AIDS-r. virus (ARV)

AIH
> autoimmune hepatitis
> homologous artificial insemination

AIHA
> autoimmune hemolytic anemia

AIL
> angiocentric immunoproliferative lesion
> angioimmunoblastic lymphoma
> angioimmunoblastic T-cell lymphoma
> angioimmunoproliferative lesion

AILD
> angioimmunoblastic lymphadenopathy
>   with dysproteinemia

AIN
> acute interstitial nephritis
> allergic interstitial nephritis

ainhum
AIO
> amyloid of immunoglobulin origin

AIP
> acute intermittent porphyria
> acute interstitial pneumonia
> automated immunoprecipitation

AIPC
> androgen independent prostate cancer

air
> alveolar a.
> a. bleb assay
> a. bleb membrane
> a. cell
> a. cell of Mosher
> a. core
> a. dose
> a. embolism
> a. embolus

a. foil
high-efficiency particulate a.
> (HEPA)
intraperitoneal a.
a. monitor
a. powered forceps
a. quality standard
residual a.
a. sac
a. sampler
a. thermometer
tidal a.
a. vesicle

airborne
> a. agent
> a. infection

air-displacement pipette
air-dried smear
Aire
> autoimmune regulator
> Aire gene

air-filled tubular space
Airfuge ultracentrifuge
air-liquid interface
air-purifying respirator (APR)
airway
> a. obstruction disease
> a. resistance

AIS
> adenocarcinoma in situ
> androgen insensitivity syndrome
> antinsulin serum
> AIS of the cervix

AITT
> arginine insulin tolerance test

AIU
> absolute iodine uptake

AJCC
> American Joint Committee on Cancer
> AJCC classification
> AJCC staging modification on
>   prostate cancer

AJCCS
> American Joint Committee on Cancer
>   Staging

ajelloi
> *Trichophyton a.*

Ajellomyces
> *A. capsulatum*
> *A. dermatitidis*
> *A. dermatitis*

Akabane virus

NOTES

akagii
    Clostridium a.
akamushi
    a. disease
    Leptotrombidium a.
    Trombicula a.
akari
    Dermacentroxenus a.
    Rickettsia a.
akaryocyte
akaryote, acaryote
akee (*var. of* ackee)
akeratosis
Akkermansia muciniphila
AKT1 virus
AKT8 retrovirus
Akureyri disease
AL
    primary amyloidosis
ALA
    alpha-linolenic acid
    aminolevulinic acid
    ALA test
alactolyticus
    Pseudoramibacter a.
ALAD, ALA-D
    aminolevulinic acid dehydrase
Alagille syndrome
alanine
    a. aminotransferase (ALT)
    a. aminotransferase:aspartate
      aminotransferase ratio (ALT:AST)
    a. aminotransferase assay
    pantoyl-beta-a.
alaninemia
alaniniphila
    Pseudonocardia a.
alaninuria
alanyl
alanyl-ribonucleic acid synthetase
alanyl-RNA synthetase
alar chest
alaskensis
    Desulfovibrio a.
    Sphingomonas a.
    Sphingopyxis a.
AlaSTAT latex allergy test
alastrim
alata
    Ascaris a.
alba
    Brevundimonas a.
    morphea a.
    Nocardia a.
    pityriasis a.
    Prauserella a.
    Streptomonospora a.
    substantia a.
    Zimmermannella a.

Albarrán
    A. disease
    A. y Dominguez tubule
Albers-Schönberg disease
Albert
    A. diphtheria stain
    A. disease
albertensis
    Acidithiobacillus a.
albertii
    Escherichia a.
Albert-Linder bone sectioning
Albibacter methylovorans
albicans
    Candida a.
    corpus a.
    Monilia a.
    Saccharomyces a.
    Syringospora a.
albicantes
    lineae a.
albida
    Lentzea a.
    Longispora a.
    macula a.
albidocapillata
    Lentzea a.
    Saccharothrix a.
albidoflavus
    Amycolatopsis a.
Albidovulum inexpectatum
albidum
    atrophoderma a.
albiduria
albidus
    Cryptococcus a.
albimanus
    Anopheles a.
albinism
    oculocutaneous a.
albino
albinuria
albirubida
    Nocardiopsis dassonvillei subsp. *a.*
albitarsus
    Anopheles a.
alboatrum
    Verticillium a.
albopictus
    Aedes a.
    Dermacentor a.
alboprecipitans
    Pseudomonas a.
Albright
    A. disease
    A. hereditary osteodystrophy
    A. syndrome
Albright-McCune-Sternberg syndrome

albuginea
  tunica a.
albugineous
album
  Engyodontium a.
albumin
  a. A, B
  acetosoluble a.
  acid a.
  aggregated a.
  alkali a.
  a. assay
  Bence Jones a.
  blood a.
  bovine serum a. (BSA)
  cerebrospinal fluid a.
  a. clearance
  coagulated a.
  a. cobalt binding (ACB)
  a. cobalt binding test
  crystalline egg a. (CEA)
  delipidated a.
  derived a.
  a. excretion rate (AER)
  a. Ghent
  hematin a.
  human serum a. (HSA)
  I-125 iodinated human serum a.
  I-131 iodinated human serum a.
  iodinated human serum a. (IHSA)
  iodinated macroaggregated a.
   (IMAA)
  macroaggregated a. (MAA)
  a. Mexico
  a. Naskapi
  native a.
  normal human serum a.
  Patein a.
  a. quotient
  radioactive iodinated human
   serum a. (RIHSA)
  radioactive iodinated serum a.
   (RISA)
  radioiodinated serum a.
  a. reading
  serum a. (SA)
  a. slide adhesive
  a. suspension test
  a. tannate
  ^{99m}Tc labeled human serum a.
  thyroxine-binding a. (TBA)
  triphenyl a.

albumin-agglutinating antibody
albuminate
albuminaturia
albumin-calcium-magnesium (ACM)
albuminemia
  double a.
albumin-globulin ratio (A:G)
albuminiferous
albuminimeter
albuminimetry
albuminiparous
albuminocytologic dissociation
albuminogenous
albuminoid degeneration
albuminolysis
albuminoptysis
albuminoreaction
albuminorrhea
albuminous
  a. cell
  a. degeneration
  a. gland
  a. swelling
albuminuria
  adolescent a.
  adventitious a.
  a. of athletes
  Bamberger a.
  Bence Jones a.
  benign a.
  cardiac a.
  colliquative a.
  cyclic a.
  dietetic a.
  digestive a.
  essential a.
  false a.
  febrile a.
  functional a.
  intermittent a.
  lordotic a.
  march a.
  neuropathic a.
  orthostatic a.
  physiologic a.
  postrenal a.
  postural a.
  prerenal a.
  recurrent a.
  regulatory a.
  transient a.

NOTES

albuminuric
albumose-free tuberculin (TAF)
albumosuria
>Bence Jones a.

albus
>*Agarivorans a.*
>*Agromyces a.*
>*Bulleromyces a.*
>*Leucobacter a.*
>*Nocardioides a.*
>*Staphylococcus pyogenes a.*
>*Streptacidiphilus a.*
>*Streptomyces a.*
>*Thermocrinis a.*

Albustix reagent strip
ALC
>approximate lethal concentration

alcalescens
>*Veillonella alcalescens* subsp. *a.*

alcalifaciens
>*Providencia a.*

Alcaligenaceae
Alcaligenes
>*A. bookeri*
>*A. bronchisepticus*
>*A. denitrificans*
>*A. faecalis*
>*A. faecalis* subsp. *parafaecalis*
>*A. marshalli*
>*A. odorans*
>*A. recti*

alcaligenes
>*Bacillus faecalis A.*
>*Pseudomonas A.*

alcaliphila
>*Pseudomonas a.*

alcaliphilus
>*Thermococcus a.*

Alcanivorax
>*A. borkumensis*
>*A. jadensis*
>*A. venustensis*

alcaptonuria
Alcian
>A. blue (AB)
>A. blue stain

alcianophilic
ALCL
>anaplastic large cell lymphoma

alcohol
>absolute a.
>acid a.
>a. addiction
>aliphatic a.
>allyl a.
>anhydrous a.
>a. assay
>benzyl a.
>blood a.

>butyl a.
>a. consumption
>dehydrated a.
>a. dehydrogenase (ADH)
>dihydric a.
>ethyl a. (ETOH, EtOH)
>a. fixation
>a. fixed smear
>a. intoxication
>isobutyl a.
>isopropyl a. (IPA)
>monohydric a.
>polyhydric a.
>polyvinyl a. (PVA)
>propyl a.
>a. thermometer

alcohol-formaldehyde-acetic acid (AFA)
alcohol-glycerin fixative
alcoholic
>a. cardiomyopathy
>a. cirrhosis
>a. coma
>a. formalin
>a. hepatitis
>a. hyalin
>a. hyaline
>a. hyaline body
>a. ketoacidosis
>a. myopathy
>a. pneumonia
>a. polymyopathy
>severely malnourished a.

alcoholivorans
>*Desulfovibrio a.*

alcohol-soluble eosin
alcoholuria
AlcoSCRUB instant antiseptic hand cleanser
Alco-Sensor
ALD
>adrenoleukodystrophy

aldaric acid
aldehyde
>acetic a.
>a. dehydrogenase
>a. fixative
>formic a.
>a. fuchsin (AF)
>methyl a.
>a. oxidase

Alder
>A. anomaly
>A. body

Alder-Reilly
>A.-R. anomaly
>A.-R. body

aldicarb
aldimine
aldofuranose

aldohexose
aldolase
    alpha hydroxyprogesterone a.
    a. assay
    fructose-bisphosphate a.
    a. test
aldonic acid
aldopentose
aldopyranose
aldose
aldosterone
    a. assay
    a. excretion rate (AER)
    a. secretion
    a. secretion defect (ASD)
    a. secretion rate (ASR)
    a. secretory rate (ASR)
    a. stimulation test
    a. suppression test
aldosterone-producing adenoma (APA)
aldosteronism
    glucocorticoid suppressible a.
aldotriose
Aldrich syndrome
aldrin
Alectorobius talaje
alemmal
ALERT
    antibody-based lateral flow economical recognition ticket
alert check
Aletris
aleukemia
aleukemic
    a. granulocytic leukemia
    a. lymphocytic leukemia
    a. monocytic leukemia
    a. myelosis
aleukemoid
aleukia
aleukocytic
aleukocytosis
aleurioconidium
aleuriospore
Aleurodiscus
Aleurostrongylus
Aleutian
    A. mink disease
    A. mink disease virus
Alexander
    A. disease
    A. leukodystrophy

alexandrii
    Oceanicaulis a.
alexandrinus
    Haloferax a.
alexin unit
aleydigism
Alezzandrini syndrome
Alfamovirus
alfentanil
alfreddugesi
    Trombicula a.
ALG
    antilymphocyte globulin
alga, pl. **algae**
algae
    Formosa a.
algal
    a. filament
algens
    Gelidibacter a.
algeriensis
    Saccharothrix a.
algesidystrophy
Algibacter lectus
algicida
    Kordia a.
algicola
    Bacillus a.
    A. *bacteriolytica*
    Cellulophaga a.
    Ruegeria a.
algid
    a. malaria
    a. stage
algidixylanolyticum
    Clostridium a.
algidus
    Lactobacillus a.
algin
alginate
    sodium a.
alginic acid
alginolyticus
    Vibrio a.
Alginomonas
algodystrophy
algoid cell
Algoriphagus
    A. *aquimarinus*
    A. *chordae*
    A. *halophilus*

NOTES

Algoriphagus (continued)
   A. ratkowskyi
   A. winogradskyi
algorithm
   biopsy a.
   genetic a. (GA)
   linear discriminant a.
algoscopy
ALH
   atypical lobular hyperplasia
alicyclic hydrocarbon
Alicycliphilus denitrificans
Alicyclobacillus
   A. acidiphilus
   A. acidocaldarius subsp. *rittmannii*
   A. herbarius
   A. hesperidum
   A. pomorum
   A. sendaiensis
   A. vulcanalis
aliena
   Pseudoalteromonas a.
alienia
aliesterase
aligned grid
alignment chart
A-like antigen
alimentaria
   Halomonas a.
alimentarius
   Jeotgalibacillus a.
alimentary
   a. abstinence
   a. canal
   a. diabetes
   a. glycosuria
   a. hypoglycemia
   a. lipemia
   a. osteopathy
   a. pentosuria
   a. tract
   a. tract smear
alinjection
ALIP
   abnormally localized immature precursor
aliphatic
   a. acid
   a. alcohol
   a. saturated hydrocarbon
   a. unsaturated hydrocarbon
aliphaticivorans
   Desulfatibacillum a.
aliquant
aliquot
Alishewanella fetalis
Alistipes
   A. finegoldii
   A. putredinis
Alius-Grignaschi anomaly

alive
alizarin
   a. cyanin
   a. indicator
   a. purpurin
   a. red
   a. red S
   a. red stain
   a. test
   a. yellow
alizarinsulfonate
   sodium a.
ALK
   anaplastic lymphoma kinase
   ALK protein
ALK1 antibody
alkalemia
alkalescence
alkali
   a. albumin
   a. denaturation test
   a. metal
   a. tolerance test
Alkalibacterium olivapovliticus
Alkalilimnicola halodurans
alkalimeter
alkalimetry
alkaline
   a. earth metal
   a. intoxication
   a. phosphatase (alk phos, AP)
   a. phosphatase antialkaline phosphatase (APAAP)
   a. phosphatase antialkaline phosphatase antibody test
   a. phosphatase antialkaline phosphatase technique
   a. phosphatase assay
   a. phosphatase isoenzyme
   a. phosphatase isoenzyme electrophoresis
   a. phosphatase method
   a. phosphatase stain
   a. phosphatase staining
   a. phosphatase, tissue-nonspecific isozyme protein precursor (AP-TNAP)
   a. reaction
   a. RNase
   a. tide
   a. toluidine blue O
   a. tuberculin (TA)
   a. wave
alkalinization of urine
alkalinuria
alkaliphila
   Nocardiopsis a.
alkaliphilum
   Desulfotomaculum a.

alkaliphilus
> *A. crotonatoxidans*
> *Salinicoccus a.*
> *A. transvaalensis*

alkali-resistant hemoglobin
alkali-soluble nitrogen (ASN)
Alkalispirillum mobile
alkaloid test
alkalosis
> acapnial a.
> compensated a.
> hypokalemic a.
> metabolic a.
> nonrespiratory a.
> potassium a.
> respiratory a.
> uncompensated a.

alkalotic
alkaluria
alkane
alkanet
Alkanindiges illinoisensis
alkannin paper
alkanoclasticus
> *Planococcus a.*

alkapton body
alkaptonuria test
alkene
alkenivorans
> *Desulfatibacillum a.*

alkenyl
alkoxide ion
alkoxy
alk phos
> alkaline phosphatase

alkyl
> a. group
> a. peroxide

alkylate
alkylating agent
alkylation
alkylbenzene sulfonate (ABS)
alkyne
ALL
> acute lymphoblastic leukemia
> acute lymphocytic leukemia
> B-cell ALL
> CALLA-positive ALL
> T-cell ALL

allachesthesia
> optical a.

allantoic
> a. acid
> a. cyst
> a. duct remnant

allantoin
allantoinuria
allantois
Allegra
> A. 64R high-speed refrigerated benchtop centrifuge
> A. 25R refrigerated benchtop centrifuge
> A. X-12, X-15R, X-22 benchtop centrifuge

allele
> full-mutation a.
> HLA a.
> a. imbalance analysis
> multiple a.
> null a.
> premutation a.
> wild-type a.

allele-specific
> a.-s. loss
> a.-s. oligomer
> a.-s. oligonucleotide
> a.-s. PCR (A-PCR)

allelic
> a. exclusion
> a. gene
> a. imbalance
> a. loss

allelism
allelochemics
allelotyping
> molecular a.

Allen
> A. correction
> A. test

Allen-Doisy
> A.-D. test
> A.-D. unit

Allen-Masters syndrome
allergen
> atopic a.
> a. challenge test

allergenic
> a. extract
> a. protein preparation

allergen-specific IgE antibody
allergic
> a. airways disease

NOTES

allergic *(continued)*
- a. alveolitis
- a. asthma
- a. bronchopulmonary aspergillosis (ABPA)
- a. bronchopulmonary mycosis (ABPM)
- a. conjunctivitis
- a. coryza
- a. dermatitis
- a. eczema
- a. encephalitis
- a. encephalomyelitis
- a. extract
- a. fungal sinusitis
- a. granulomatosis
- a. granulomatosis of Churg and Strauss
- a. granulomatous angiitis
- a. granulomatous prostatitis
- a. inflammation
- a. interstitial nephritis (AIN)
- a. mucin
- a. neuritis
- a. proctitis
- a. pulmonary edema
- a. purpura
- a. rhinitis
- a. transfusion reaction

allergization
allergized
allergoid
allergosis
allergy
- atopic a.
- bacterial a.
- cold a.
- contact a.
- delayed a.
- drug a.
- food a.
- immediate a.
- latent a.
- latex a.
- physical a.
- polyvalent a.

Allescheria boydii
allescheriosis
Allexivirus
alligatoris
- *Mycoplasma a.*

alligator skin
Allisonella histaminiformans
alloagglutinin
alloalbuminemia
alloantibody
- anti-HLA a.
- a. inhibitor

alloantigen

alloantin-D antibody
allo-BMT
- allogeneic bone marrow transplantation

allocation
- dynamic storage a.
- static storage a.
- storage a.

allochroic
allochroism
Allodermanyssus sanguineus
alloepitope
Allofustis seminis
allogeneic, allogenic
- a. antigen
- a. bone marrow transplantation (allo-BMT)
- a. cellular immune therapy (ACIT)
- a. graft
- a. inhibition
- a. transplantation

allograft rejection
allogroup
alloimmune
- a. HDN
- a. hemolytic anemia
- a. hemolytic disease of newborn
- a. thrombocytopenia

alloimmunization
- leukocyte a.
- transfusion-related a.

Alloiococcus otitis
Allolevivirus
allometric
allometry
Allomonas
allomorphism
Allomyces
allophanamide
allophenic
allophore
allophycocyanin (APC)
alloplasia
alloplast
alloploidy
allopolyploidy
allopregnanediol
alloreactivity
allorecognition
allosensitization
allosome
- paired a.

allosteric
- a. activation
- a. effector
- a. enzyme
- a. inhibition
- a. site

allostery
allothreonine

allotope
allotopia
allotoxin
allotransplantation
allotrope
allotropic
allotropy
allotype
    InV a.
    Km a.
allotypic
    a. determinant
    a. marker
alloxan
alloxan-Schiff reaction
alloxuremia
alloxuria
alloy
all-*trans*-retinoic acid (ATRA)
allyl alcohol
Almeida disease
Almén test for blood
ALMI
    anterior lateral myocardial infarct
alni
    Pseudonocardia a.
Alocinma
alocis
    Filifactor a.
alopecia
    a. areatus
    congenital sutural a.
    a. mucinosa
    a. universalis
ALP
    antilymphocyte plasma
Alpers disease
alpha
    a. acid glycoprotein
    a. acidophil
    a. actinin
    a. adrenergic blockade
    a. adrenergic receptor
    a. agglutination
    a. agglutinin
    a. amino acid
    a. amino nitrogen
    a. amino nitrogen test
    a. amylose
    a. antichymotrypsin (ACT)
    a. antigen of adenovirus
    a. 2 antiplasmin

a. antitrypsin (AAT)
a. band
a. cardiac actin
a. cell
a. cell of anterior lobe of hypophysis
a. cell of hypophysis
a. cell of pancreas
a. chain
a. 3, 4, 5 chain collagen stain
a. chain disease
a. contamination
a. decay
A. Dx point-of-need test system
a. dystroglycan
estrogen receptor a.
a. fetoprotein (AFP)
a. fodrin protein
a. galactosidase A
a. galactosidase A deficiency
a. globin gene
a. globulin
a. globulin antibody
a. glucan-branching enzyme
a. glucan-branching glycosyltransferase
a. glucosidase
a. 1,4-glucosidase
a. granule
a. heavy-chain disease
a. helix
a. hemolysin
a. hemolysis
hepatocyte nuclear factor 1 a.
HIF-1 a.
a. hydrazine
a. hydroxyprogesterone
a. hydroxyprogesterone aldolase
a. interferon therapy
a. internexin
a. ketoglutarate
a. ketoglutaric acid
a. lipoprotein
a. macroglobulin
a. mannosidase
a. melanocytic-stimulating hormone
a. metachromasia
a. methyldopa
a. motor neuron
a. naphthol
NRG1 a.
NRG2 a.

NOTES

alpha *(continued)*
  a. particle
  a. particle detector
  a., PI
  a. porphyrin
  a. probe
  a. radiation
  retinoid X receptor a.
  RXR a.
  a. seromucoid
  a. skeletal actin
  a. source
  a. staphylolysin
  a. storage pool disease
  a. streptococcus
  a. substance
  a. synuclein
  TGF a.
  a. thalassemia
  a. thalassemia intermedia
  TNF a.
  a. tropomyosin
  tumor necrosis factor a.
  a. unit
alpha-1
  a. acid glycoprotein
  a. antichymotrypsin (A1AC)
  a. band
  a. fetoglobulin
  a. fetoprotein
  a. fetoprotein assay
  a. globulin
  a. protease inhibitor
  a. seromucoid
  a. trypsin inhibitor
alpha-2
  a. antiplasmin functional assay
  a. globulin
  a. macroglobulin
  a. macroglobulin inhibitor
  a. neuraminoglycoprotein
alpha$_1$
  a. antitrypsin (A1AT)
  a. antitrypsin deficiency
  a. antitrypsin deficiency panniculitis
  a. antitrypsin phenotyping
Alphabacteria
alpha1beta1
  integrin a.
alpha-beta variation
Alphacryptovirus
alpha-dextrinase
alpha-dinitrophenol
alpha-estradiol
alpha-fetoprotein
  amniotic fluid a.-f.
alpha-inhibin
alpha-keto acid dehydrogenase
alpha-L-fucosidase

alpha-L-iduronidase
alpha-linolenic acid (ALA)
alphalipoprotein deficiency
alpha-2-macroglobulin
alpha-methylacetoacetyl CoA thiolase
alpha-N-acetylgalactosaminidase
alpha-N-acetylglucosaminidase
alpha-naphthol thiourea
alpha-naphthyl acetate esterase (ANAE)
Alphanodavirus
Alpharetrovirus
Alphavirus
alpinus
  Microanthomyces a.
Alport
  A. hereditary nephropathy
  A. syndrome
AL protein
ALPS
  autologous leukapheresis, processing, and storage
  ALPS container
ALS
  amyotrophic lateral sclerosis
  antilymphocyte serum
Alsberg
  A. angle
  A. triangle
Alstonia
Alström syndrome
ALT
  alanine aminotransferase
  ALT test
ALT:AST
  alanine aminotransferase:aspartate aminotransferase ratio
alteplase
alteration
  bone matrix a.
  cartilage matrix a.
  chromosome a.
  crystalline macromolecule a.
  cyclic tissue a.
  cytologic a.
  cytoplasmic fiber a.
  cytoplasmic fibril a.
  cytoplasmic filament a.
  cytoplasmic lipid droplet a.
  cytoplasmic matrix a.
  decidual a.
  dentin crystal a.
  extracellular fibril a.
  extracellular matrix a.
  fibrocartilage matrix a.
  Golgi cavity a.
  Golgi membrane a.
  Golgi vacuole a.
  Golgi vesicle a.
  growth a.

A

hematopoietic maturation a.
keratohyaline a.
leukocytic maturation a.
mitochondrial crista a.
mitochondrial matrix a.
mitochondrial membrane a.
Nissl substance a.
nuclear-cytoplasmic ratio a.
nuclear membrane a.
nuclear pore a.
nuclear sap a.
nuclear shape a.
nuclear size a.
pH a.
predecidual a.
RB1 a.
syncytial a.
verrucopapillary a.
alterative inflammation
altered
a. intravascular hydrostatic pressure
a. intravascular osmotic pressure
a. lipid-peroxidation activity
alternant
trace a.
Alternaria tenuis
alternata
Psychoda a.
alternate host
alternating current
alternation of generations
alternative
a. complement pathway
a. hypothesis
a. inheritance
one-sided a.
two-sided a.
Alteromonadaceae
Alteromonas
A. litorea
A. marina
A. putrefaciens
A. stellipolaris
altitude
a. anoxia
a. disease
a. sickness
Altmann
A. anilin-acid fuchsin stain
A. fixative
A. fluid
A. granule

A. liquid
A. theory
Altmann-Gersh method
alum
a. carmine
chrome a.
Einarson gallocyanin-chrome a.
a. hematoxylin
potassium a.
a. precipitate
alumina
hydrated a.
aluminal tubule
aluminosis
aluminum
a. hydroxide
a. hydroxide gel
a. oxide
a. phosphate
alum-precipitated
a.-p. antigen
a.-p. pyridine (APP)
a.-p. toxoid (APT)
alvei
Bacillus a.
Enterobacter a.
Hafnia a.
alveolar
a. abscess
a. adenocarcinoma
a. air
a. air equation
a. asthma
a. bone resorption
a. bony crypt
a. cell
a. cell carcinoma
a. duct
a. edema
a. fenestra
a. gland
a. hydatid
a. hydatid cyst
a. hydatid disease
a. macrophage
a. periosteum
a. phagocyte
a. pneumocyte hyperplasia
a. pore
a. proteinosis
a. rhabdomyosarcoma (ARMS)
a. sac

NOTES

45

alveolar *(continued)*
    a. septum
    a. soft-part sarcoma (ASPS)
alveolar-arterial
    a.-a. carbon dioxide difference
    a.-a. oxygen
    a.-a. oxygen difference
alveolar-capillary interface
alveolaris
    ductulus a.
    sacculus a.
alveoli (*pl. of* alveolus)
alveolitis
    acute pulmonary a.
    allergic a.
    extrinsic allergic a. (EAA)
    fibrosing a.
alveoloclasia
alveolodental membrane
alveolus, pl. **alveoli**
    a. dentalis
    distal alveoli
    perfusion of alveoli
    pulmonary a.
    alveoli pulmonis
    tapetum alveoli
alveus
    a. hippocampi
    a. of hippocampus
alvinolith
ALW
    arch-loop-whorl
alymphia
alymphocytosis
alymphoplasia
    Nezelof type of thymic a.
    thymic a. (TAL)
Alzheimer
    A. cell
    A. disease
    A. disease familial and sporadic
    A. fibril
    A. fibrillary degeneration
    A. sclerosis
    A. stain
    A. type I, II astrocyte
Am
    americium
    arabinomannan
    Am antigen
AMA
    antimitochondrial antibody
amacrine cell
amalonatica
    Citrobacter a.
    Levinea a.
Amanita
    A. muscaria
    A. pantherina

    A. phalloides
    A. rubescens
    A. verna
    A. virosa
amanitiforme
    Angulomicrobium a.
amanitin
amarae
    Gordonia a.
    Rothia a.
amaranth
amaranthum
amastia
amastigote
Amauroascus
amaurosis fugax
amaurotic familial idiocy
amazia
amazonae
    Volucribacter a.
amazonensis
    Leishmania mexicana a.
Ambard
    A. constant
    A. laws
Amberlite
amber mutation
ambient
    a. temperature
    a. temperature and pressure, saturated (ATPS)
ambifaria
    Burkholderia a.
ambiguity
    ribosomal a.
    somatosexual a.
ambiguous external genitalia
ambiguus
    Bacillus a.
    Passalurus a.
amblychromasia
amblychromatic
Amblyomma
    A. americanum
    A. cajennense
    A. hebraeum
    A. maculatum
    A. variegatum
amblyopia
    a. neuropathy
    tobacco a.
amboceptor
    bacteriolytic a.
    Bordet a.
    hemolytic a.
    a. unit
ambroisiodes
    Chenopodium a.
Ambrosia

Ambrosiella
Ambrosiozyma cicatricosa
ambulans
    ulcus a.
ameba, pl. **amebae, amebas**
    coprozoic a.
amebacide
amebiasis, amoebiasis
    intestinal a.
amebic
    a. abscess of liver
    a. brain abscess
    a. colitis
    a. dysentery
    a. granuloma
    a. meningitis
    a. meningoencephalitis
    a. prevalence rate (APR)
    a. ulcer
amebicidal
amebicide
amebiform
amebiosis
amebism
amebocyte
ameboflagellate
ameboid
    a. cell
    a. movement
ameboididity
ameboidism
ameboma
amebula
amebule
ameburia
amegakaryocytic thrombocytopenia
amegakaryocytosis
amelanotic mucosal melanoma
amelia
ameloblast
ameloblastic
    a. adenomatoid tumor
    a. fibroma
    a. fibroodontoma
    a. fibrosarcoma
    a. hemangioma
    a. layer
    a. neurilemmoma
    a. odontoma
    a. sarcoma
ameloblastoma
    acanthomatous a.

    basal cell a.
    calcifying a.
    cystic a.
    desmoplastic a.
    extraosseous a.
    follicular a.
    granular cell a.
    malignant a.
    melanotic a.
    multicystic a.
    peripheral a.
    pigmented a.
    pituitary a.
    plexiform unicystic a.
    solid a.
    unicystic a.
ameloblastomatous craniopharyngioma
amelogenesis imperfecta
amelogenin
amendment
    Clinical Laboratory Improvement A.
    (CLIA)
amenorrhea
    a. and hirsutism
    primary a.
    secondary a. (SA)
amenorrhea-galactorrhea syndrome
amentia
    phenylpyruvic a.
amentoflavone
American
    A. Chemical Society (ACS)
    A. Clinical Laboratory Association
    (ACLA)
    A. hookworm
    A. Joint Committee on Cancer
    Staging (AJCCS)
    A. leech
    A. leishmaniasis
    A. National Standards Institute
    (ANSI)
    A. rat flea
    A. trypanosomiasis
    A. Type Culture Collection
    (ATCC)
    A. Urological Association (AUA)
americana
    Cochliomyia a.
    Scopulariopsis a.
    Spirochaeta a.
    Uncinaria a.

NOTES

americanum
> *Amblyomma a.*

americanus
> *Necator a.*

americium (Am)

amerism

ameristic

Amersham
> A. Biosciences
> A. International ECL gene detection system
> A. Life Science PCR product presequencing kit
> A. Life Science Thermo Sequenase sequencing kit

Ames
> A. assay
> A. Lab-Tek cryostat
> A. test

amethyst violet

AMeX
> acetone, methylbenzoate, xylene
> AMeX fixation
> AMeX processing and embedding method

AMF
> autocrine motility factor

AMFR
> autocrine motility factor receptor

AMG
> antimacrophage globulin
> autometallography

AMH
> antimüllerian hormone

AMI
> acute myocardial infarction

amiantacea

amianthoid collagen fibers

amicalis
> *Gordonia a.*

Amici
> A. disc
> A. line
> A. stria

amicrobic

amicroscopic

Amicus separator

amidase

amide

amidinotransferase

amidobenzene

amido black 10B

amidohydrolase method

amidonaphthol red

Amidostomum anseris

amiense
> *Sphingobium a.*

amine
> aromatic a.

> a. precursor uptake and decarboxylation (APUD)
> pressor a.

amino
> a. acid
> a. acid-activating enzyme
> a. acid analyzer
> a. acid disorder
> a. acid fractionation assay
> a. acid nitrogen (AAN)
> a. acid residue
> a. acid screen
> a. acid screening
> a. acid sequencer
> a. acid transporter E16 gene
> a. terminal

amino-9-ethyl carbazole

aminoacetic acid

aminoacidemia

aminoacidopathy

aminoaciduria
> branched-chain a.
> dibasic a.

aminoacridine hydrochloride

aminoacyl-histidine dipeptidase

aminoacyl-tRNA hydrolase

aminoalkylsilane (AAS)

aminoanthraquinone dye

aminoaromatica
> *Thauera a.*

Aminobacterium
> *A. colombiense*
> *A. mobile*

aminobenzene

aminobutyrate aminotransferase

aminocaproic acid

5-amino 9 ethyl carbazole (AEC)

3-amino-9-ethylcarbazole (AEC)
> 3-amino-9-ethylcarbazole stain

aminoethylcysteine ketimine

aminoethylisothiouronium bromide (AET)

aminoglutaric acid

aminoglycoside ototoxicity

aminoguanidine

aminoketone dye

aminolevulinic
> a. acid (ALA)
> a. acid dehydrase (ALAD, ALA-D)

aminomethane
> *tris*(hydroxymethyl) a.

aminopenicillanic acid (APA)

aminopeptidase (AP)
> a. cytosol
> leucine a. (LAP)

aminophenol

aminophilus
> *Desulfovibrio a.*

aminopropyltriethoxysilane (APES)

aminopropyltriethyoxysilane-coated glass slide
aminopurine
aminopyrine breath test
aminosuccinic acid
amino-terminal domain
aminoterminus
aminotransferase
    alanine a. (ALT)
    aminobutyrate a.
    aspartate a. (AST)
    ornithine a.
    ornithine-oxo-acid a.
    valine a.
aminoxidans
    Xanthobacter a.
aminuria
amitosis
amitotic
amitriptyline and nortriptyline assays
AML
    acute myeloid leukemia
    angiomyolipoma
AMLS
    antimouse lymphocyte serum
AMLV-RT
    avian myeloblastosis leukemia virus reverse transcriptase
AMM
    ammonia
ammeter, amperemeter
AMML
    acute myelomonocytic leukemia
Ammon
    A. filament
    A. fissure
    A. horn
ammonemia
ammonia (AMM)
    a. assay
    plasma a.
ammoniacal
    a. silver nitrate test
    a. silver solution
    a. urine
ammonia-lyase
    L-histidine a.
ammoniemia
ammonificans
    Thermovibrio a.
ammonium
    a. biurate crystal

    a. chloride
    a. chloride loading test
    a. magnesium phosphate
    a. magnesium phosphate stone
    a. molybdate
    a. nitrate bomb
    a. oxalate
    a. oxalate crystal violet
    a. peroxydisulfate
    a. silver carbonate stain
    a. sulfate
ammoniuria
AMN
    atypical melanocytic nevus
AMNGT
    atypical melanocytic nevi of genital type
amniocentesis
amniocyte
amniogenic cell
amnioma
amnion
    a. cell
    a. nodosum
    squamous metaplasia of a.
amnionic corpuscle
amnionitis
amniorrhea
amniotic
    a. adhesion
    a. band syndrome
    a. corpuscle
    a. fluid
    a. fluid alpha-fetoprotein
    a. fluid analysis
    a. fluid bilirubin
    a. fluid bilirubin optical density
    a. fluid color
    a. fluid creatinine
    a. fluid desaturated phosphatidylcholine
    a. fluid embolism
    a. fluid embolus
    a. fluid fern test
    a. fluid foam stability index
    a. fluid foam stability test
    a. fluid lecithin/sphingomyelin ratio
    a. fluid primary phospholipid
    a. fluid pulmonary surfactant
    a. fluid shake test
    a. fluid surfactant
    a. fluid total volume

NOTES

amniotic *(continued)*
  a. fluid unsaturated lecithin
  a. infection syndrome of Blane
amobarbital
  a. poisoning
  sodium a.
amodiaquine
Amoeba
  A. buccalis
  A. coli
  A. dentalis
  A. dysenteriae
  A. histolytica
  A. meleagridis
  A. proteus
  A. urogenitalis
  A. verrucosa
amoebiasis *(var. of* amebiasis*)*
Amoebotaenia
AMoL
  acute monoblastic leukemia
  acute monocytic leukemia
amorph
amorpha
  pars a.
amorphia
amorphic
amorphous
  a. eosinophilic appearance
  a. eosinophilic debris
  a. fraction of adrenal cortex
  a. phosphate crystal
amorphus
  holoacardius a.
Amoss sign
amount
  a. of insulin extractable from
    pancreas
  a. of substance
amoxapine
AMP
  acid mucopolysaccharide
  adenosine monophosphate
  cyclic AMP (cAMP)
  AMP deaminase
amp
  ampule
Ampelomyces
Ampelovirus
amperage
ampere (A)
  kilovolt a. (kVA)
amperemeter *(var. of* ammeter*)*
ampere-second per volt (As/V)
amperometric-coulometric titration
amperometry
amphetamine assay

Amphibacillus
  A. fermentum
  A. tropicus
amphibolic
  a. fistula
  a. pathway
amphibolous fistula
amphichroic
amphichromatic
amphicrine
  a. cell
  a. differentiation
amphicyte
amphigenous inheritance
amphikaryon
amphileukemic
Amphimerus
amphimicrobe
amphinucleolus
amphipath
amphipathic
amphiphile
amphiphilic
Amphiporthe
amphiprotic
amphistome
amphitrichate
amphitrichous
amphixenosis
amphochromatophil, amphochromatophile
amphochromophil, amphochromophile
amphocyte
ampholyte
amphophil, amphophile
  a. cell
  a. granule
amphophilic
  a. cytoplasm
  a. homogenization
amphophilous
amphoteric
  a. dye
  a. electrolyte
  a. reaction
amphotericin B
amphotropic virus
ampicillin
amplicon
Amplicor
  A. Chlamydia assay
  A. CMV Monitor
  A. CT/NG test
  A. HIV-1 monitor test
amplifiable DNA
amplification
  Chelex DNA a.
  c-myc a.
  a. factor
  gas a.

gene a.
group specific a. (GSA)
ligation-dependent a.
multiple biotin-avidin a.
multiple displacement a. (MDA)
N-myc a.
nucleic acid sequence based a.
  (NASBA)
polymerase chain reaction a.
polymerization-dependent a.
signal a.
strand displacement a. (SDA)
target a.
transcription-dependent a.
transcription-mediated a. (TMA)
tyramide signal a. (TSA)
whole genome a. (WGA)
amplified probe
amplifier
audio a.
buffer a.
complementary symmetry a.
Darlington a.
difference a.
direct-coupled a.
electrometer a.
a. host
linear a.
lock-in a.
logarithmic a.
operational a.
power a.
push-pull a.
amplitude
peak a.
peak-to-peak a.
wave a.
ampule (amp)
ampulla, pl. **ampullae**
a. tubae uterinae
a. of uterine tube
ampullar abortion
ampullaris
crista a.
cupula a.
ampullary
a. aneurysm
a. carcinoma
a. crest
a. cupula
a. tumor
ampullitis

ampullula
amputating ulcer
amputation
a. neuroma
spontaneous a.
AMS
antimacrophage serum
automated multiphasic screening
Amsterdam syndrome
amu
atomic mass unit
amurskyense
Salinibacterium a.
amurskyensis
Zobellia a.
Amussat
A. valve
A. valvula
AMV2
avian myelocytomatosis virus
Amycolatopsis
A. albidoflavus
A. balhimycina
A. decaplanina
A. eurytherma
A. fastidiosa
A. japonica
A. kentuckyensis
A. keratiniphila
A. keratiniphila subsp. keratiniphila
A. keratiniphila subsp. nogabecina
A. lexingtonensis
A. lurida
A. mediterranei
A. orientalis subsp. lurida
A. palatopharyngis
A. pretoriensis
A. rifamycinica
A. rubida
A. sacchari
A. tolypomycina
A. vancoresmycina
amycolatum
Corynebacterium a.
amyctic
amyelencephalia
amyelia
amyelinated
amyelination
amyelinic
amyeloic, amyelonic
amygdala

NOTES

amygdalase
amygdalin
amygdaline
amygdalinum
    Clostridium a.
amyl
    a. nitrite pearls
    a. nitrite perles
    a. nitrite popper
    a. nitrite, sodium nitrite, and
       sodium thiosulfate
amylaceous corpuscle
amylaceum, pl. **amylacea**
    corpus a. (CA)
amylase
    a. assay
    a. clearance (C_{Am})
    pancreatic a.
    salivary a.
    serum a.
    a. test
    urinary a.
    urine a.
amylase/creatinine
    a./c. clearance
    a./c. clearance ratio (A:C)
amylasuria
amylemia
amylin
amyloclast
amylo-1,6-glucosidase
amyloid
    a. A (AA)
    a. angiopathy
    a. beta protein
    a. body of prostate
    a. corpuscle
    a. degeneration
    a. fibril
    Highman method for a.
    a. of immunoglobulin origin (AIO)
    a. kidney
    a. nephrosis
    a. neuropathy
    a. P component
    a. plaque
    a. precursor protein (APP)
    a. protein A
    serum a. A (SAA)
    a. stain
    a. staining
    a. tumor
    a. of unknown origin (AUO)
amyloid-containing stroma
amyloidogenic potential
amyloidoma
    nodular a. (NA)
amyloidosis
    AA a.

    cardiac a.
    cutaneous a.
    a. cutis
    diffuse a.
    familial primary systemic a.
    focal a.
    lichen a.
    macular a.
    a. of multiple myeloma
    nodular a.
    primary a. (AL)
    renal a.
    secondary a.
    senile a.
    systemic familial primary a.
    tracheobronchial a.
amylolytic enzyme
amylolyticum
    Tenacibaculum a.
amylolyticus
    Desulfurococcus a.
    Lactobacillus a.
amylopectin
amylopectinosis
amylorrhea
amylose
    alpha a.
    crystalline a.
Amylostereum
amylosuria
amyluria
amyopathic dermatomyositis
amyoplasia congenita
amyotonia congenita
amyotrophia
amyotrophic
    a. lateral sclerosis (ALS)
    a. lateral
       sclerosis/parkinsonism±dementia
       complex of Guam
amyotrophy
    diabetic a.
    neuralgic a.
amyous
ANA
    antinuclear antibody
Anabaena
anabiotic cell
anabolic steroid
anabolism-promoting factor (APF)
anabolite
anacidity
anacmesis
anacrotism
anadenia ventriculi
ANAE
    alpha-naphthyl acetate esterase
Anaeroarcus burkinensis
Anaerobacter polyendosporus

Anaerobaculum
    A. *mobile*
    A. *thermoterrenum*
anaerobe
    facultative a.
    obligate a.
anaerobian
anaerobic
    a. bacteria culture
    a. bacterium
    a. chamber
    a. diphtheroid
    a. glycolysis
    a. jar
    a. metabolism
    a. *Neisseria*
    a. pneumonia
    a. respiration
    a. rod
    a. specimen collector
    a. streptococcus
anaerobiosis
Anaerobiospirillum
    A. *succiniciproducens*
    A. *thomasii*
anaerobius
    Peptococcus a.
    Peptostreptococcus a.
    Streptococcus a.
Anaerobranca
    A. *californiensis*
    A. *gottschalkii*
Anaerococcus
    A. *hydrogenalis*
    A. *lactolyticus*
    A. *octavius*
    A. *prevotii*
    A. *tetradius*
    A. *vaginalis*
Anaerofustis stercorihominis
anaerogenic
Anaeroglobus geminatus
Anaerolinea thermophila
Anaeromyxobacter dehalogenans
Anaerophaga thermohalophila
Anaeroplasmataceae
Anaeroplasmatales
Anaerostipes caccae
Anaerotruncus colihominis
Anaerovorax odorimutans
anagen
anagenesis

anagenetic
anákhré
anakmesis
anal
    a. atresia
    a. column
    a. duct
    a. fissure
    a. fistula
    a. gland
    a. gland carcinoma
    a. papillitis
    a. sinus
    a. skin tag
    a. verge
anal.
    analysis
analbuminemia
analeptic
anales
    columnae a.
analgesic
    a. nephritis
    a. nephropathy
analis
    linea pectinata canalis a.
anallergenic serum
anallergic
analog, analogue
    a. data
    a. of histidine (AHH)
    a. signal
analogous structure
analysis, pl. **analyses (anal.)**
    activation a.
    allele imbalance a.
    amniotic fluid a.
    antigenic a.
    arterial blood gas a.
    automated cell image a.
    blood acylcarnitine a.
    blood gas a.
    bloodstain pattern a.
    body fluid a.
    breakpoint a.
    breath hydrogen a.
    cell lineage a.
    cell sorting a.
    cerebrospinal fluid a.
    chemical a.
    chromosome a.
    clinicopathologic a.

NOTES

53

analysis *(continued)*
    compartmental a.
    computer-assisted image a.
    computer linkage a.
    Cox regression a.
    critical path a.
    cytofluorimetric a.
    cytogenetic a.
    cytometric image a.
    cytospin a.
    DDD a.
    discriminant function a.
    displacement a.
    DNA array a.
    Dpc4 immunohistochemical
        pancreatic cancer a.
    electroblot a.
    energy dispersed x-ray a. (EDS)
    fecal porphyrin a.
    fiber FISH a.
    flow cytometric reticulocyte a.
    Fourier a.
    gastric a.
    genetic abnormality a.
    genetic linkage a.
    graphic a.
    hair a.
    head space a.
    heteroduplex a. (HDA)
    hierarchical clustering a.
    image display and a. (IDA)
    immunohistochemical a.
    intracellular receptor a.
    kidney stone a.
    Ki-67 immunohistochemical well-
        differentiated gastric carcinoma a.
    leave-one-out cross-validation a.
    linkage a.
    membrane-bound receptor a.
    microanalytical EDS a.
    microdiffusion a.
    microsatellite a.
    molecular cytogenetic a.
    morphological a.
    morphometric a.
    multicolor FISH a.
    multilocus variable number (tandem
        repeat) a. (MLVA)
    multipixel spectral a.
    multivariate a.
    mutational a.
    Northern blot a.
    nucleic acid sequence based a.
        (NASBA)
    optimized robot for chemical a.
        (ORCA)
    pentagastrin stimulated a.
    phosphor image a.

    p53 immunohistochemical breast
        cancer a.
    ploidy a.
    proteome a.
    qualitative a.
    quantitative a.
    random amplified polymorphic
        DNA a. (RAPD)
    rapid microsatellite a.
    restriction endonuclease a. (REA)
    RFLP Southern hybridization a.
    saturation a.
    semen a.
    semiquantitative a.
    sequential a.
    simkin a.
    Southern blot a.
    stool a.
    sucrose density gradient a.
    tetramer a.
    transcriptome a.
    tubeless gastric a.
    univariate a.
    a. of variance (ANOVA)
    Western blot a.
    zymographic a.
analyte-specific reagent (ASR)
analytic
    a. cytology
    a. method
    a. ultracentrifuge
analytical
    a. balance
    a. chemistry
    a. electron microscope (AEM)
    a. immunofiltration
    a. reagent (AR)
    a. reagent grade
    a. sensitivity
    a. specificity
    a. toxicology
analyzer
    Abbott Cell-Dyn hematology a.
    ABI Prism 3100 Genetic A.
    Access AFP immunoassay a.
    ACL 100, 1000, 7000, 8000,
        9000, 10000 advance
        coagulation a.
    ACS:180 CK/MB a.
    Ac·T diff, Ac·T diff2
        hematology a.
    Ac·T 5 diff AL auto loader
        hematology a.
    Ac·T 5 diff CP cap pierce
        hematology a.
    Ac·T 5 diff OV open vial
        hematology a.
    Ac·T series hematology a.

Advanced Instruments
conductivity a.
Advia 1650 chemistry a.
amino acid a.
Apec glucose a.
Aution Max AX-4280 automated
urine chemistry a.
automatic clinical a.
automatic fluorescent image a.
AxSYM a.
batch a.
Bayer Technicon H-2 a.
Beckman Synchron CX-7
cholesterol a.
Careside a.
centrifugal fast a.
Cobas Fara H centrifugal a.
Cobas Helios differential a.
Cobra Amplicor a.
continuous flow a.
Coulter LH 500, 700, 750, 755,
1500 Series hematology analyzer
Coulter MAXM hematology a.
Coulter STKS hematology a.
Delsa 440 SX Zeta potential a.
discrete a.
Elecsys 2010 modular
immunoassay a.
enzyme a.
ESRA-10 erythrocyte sedimentation
rate a.
ESR-Auto Plus sedimentation
rate a.
FLx/TDx immunoassay a.
GenePhor DNA fragment a.
Gen-S hematology a.
HemoCue B-Glucose a.
Hitachi 704, 736, 911 a.
Hitachi 747-100 cholesterol a.
Hitachi 747 CK/MB a.
HmX hematology a.
Immulite 2000 chemiluminescent a.
Immulite Dynamic Duo a.
IMx a.
infrared CO_2 a.
KC1 Delta coagulation a.
kinetic a.
Kodak Ektachem DT-60
cholesterol a.
Kodak Ektachem Vitros 250, 750,
950 cholesterol a.

LH 500, 750, 1500 series
hematology a.
LS 100Q/200/230 series laser
diffraction particle size a.
LS 13 320 series laser diffraction
particle size a.
multichannel a. (MCA)
Nova Celltrak 12 hematology a.
N5 submicron particle size a.
Olympus AU5200 cholesterol a.
Oncometrics Imaging Cyto-Savant
image a.
oxygen a.
Paramax a.
Pentra 60C+ a.
Piccolo blood chemistry a.
platelet function a. (PFA)
PocketChem UA a.
pulse height a. (PHA)
RapidVUE particle shape and
size a.
SA 3100 surface area and pore
size a.
sequential multiple a. (SMA)
simultaneous multiple a. (SMA)
spectrum a.
Stat Profile pHOx blood gas a.
Stratus II automatic a.
SureStep Pro glucose a.
Sweat-Chek conductivity a.
Sysmex NE-8000 CBC a.
Sysmex XE-2100 hematology a.
Sysmex XT-2000i automated
hematology a.
TDxFlx a.
Urisys 2400 urine a.
Vi-CELL series cell viability a.
Vitros a.
wave a.
Wescor Sweat-Chek conductivity a.
YSI 2300 STAT glucose and
lactate a.
anamnesis
anamnestic
a. reaction
a. response
anamorph
ananaphylaxis
anangioplasia
anangioplastic
ANAP
anionic neutrophil activating peptide

NOTES

anaphase lag
anaphoresis
anaphylactic
    a. antibody
    a. intoxication
    a. shock
    a. transfusion reaction
anaphylactogen
anaphylactogenesis
anaphylactogenic
anaphylactoid
    a. crisis
    a. purpura
    a. reaction
    a. shock
anaphylatoxin
    C3a a.
    C4a a.
    C5a a.
    a. inactivator
anaphylaxis
    active a.
    aggregate a.
    antiserum a.
    chronic a.
    eosinophil chemotactic factor of a.
      (ECF-A)
    generalized a.
    inverse a.
    local a.
    passive cutaneous a. (PCA)
    pharmacologic mediators of a.
    reversed passive a.
    slow reacting factor of a. (SRF-A)
    slow reacting substance of a.
      (SRS-A, SRSA)
    systemic a.
anaphylotoxin
anaplasia
Anaplasma
    A. bovis
    A. phagocytophilum
    A. platys
Anaplasmataceae
anaplasmosis
anaplastic
    a. adenocarcinoma
    a. astrocytoma
    a. carcinoma
    a. cell
    a. large cell lymphoma (ALCL)
    a. large cell malignant lymphoma
    a. lymphoma kinase (ALK)
    a. malignant teratoma
    a. meningioma
    a. oligodendroglioma
    a. seminoma
anaplerotic
anapophysis

anarchic phenomenon
Ana-Sal HIV home test kit
anasarca
    fetoplacental a.
anasarcous
anastomosing fiber
anastomosis, pl. anastomoses
    arteriovenous a. (AVA)
    artery-to-artery a.
    artery-to-vein a.
    vein-to-vein a.
anastomoticus
    varix a.
anatina
    Coenonia a.
anatipester
    Pfeifferella a.
anatipestifer
    Moraxella a.
anatis
    Cochlosoma a.
    Gallibacterium a.
anatolicum
    Hyalomma a.
anatomic
    a. change
    a. pathology
    a. tubercle
    a. wart
anatomical
    a. element
    a. pathology
    a. tubercle
    a. wart
anatomically patent foramen ovale
anatomicopathologic
anatomicopathological
anatomy
    cross-section a.
    general a.
    microscopic a.
    pathologic a.
    pathological a.
    ultrastructural a.
anatoxic
anatoxin
Anatrichosoma
anaxon
anazoturia
ANC
    absolute neutrophil count
ANCA
    antineutrophil cytoplasmic antibody
    antineutrophil cytoplasmic autoantibody
anchorage
    cell a.
    a. dependence
    a. independence
anchoring fibril

anchovy sauce pus
anchusin
ancient schwannoma
anconitis
ancoratus
　　Pedicinus a.
ancrod
Ancylidae
Ancylobacter rudongensis
Ancylostoma
　　A. braziliense
　　A. caninum
　　A. ceylanicum
　　A. duodenale
　　A. tubaeforme
ancylostomatic
ancylostomiasis
Andernach ossicle
Andersch ganglion
Anders disease
Andersen
　　A. syndrome
　　A. triad
Anderson
　　A. and Goldberger test
　　A. phenomenon
Anderson-Collip test
andersoni
　　Dermacentor a.
Andes disease
Andrade
　　A. indicator
　　A. syndrome
André Thomas sign
Andrews
　　A. lymphocyte curve
　　A. nomogram
androblastoma
androgen
　　a. independent prostate cancer
　　　(AIPC)
　　a. receptor gene
　　a. unit
androgenesis
androgenic
　　a. anabolic agent (AAA)
　　a. arrhenoblastoma
　　a. hormone
　　a. zone
androgenization
androgen-normal epithelium
androgen-secreting adrenal

andropathy
androstanediol
androstene
androstenediol
androstenedione test
androsterone
anectasis
Anellaria
anemia
　　achlorhydric a.
　　achrestic a.
　　acquired hemolytic a. (AHA)
　　acquired sideroblastic a.
　　acute posthemorrhagic a.
　　acute self-limited hemolytic a.
　　Addison a.
　　addisonian a.
　　alloimmune hemolytic a.
　　angiopathic hemolytic a.
　　aplastic a.
　　aregenerative a.
　　asiderotic a.
　　a. associated with chronic renal
　　　failure
　　autoallergic hemolytic a.
　　autoimmune hemolytic a. (AHA,
　　　AIHA)
　　Belgian Congo a.
　　Biermer a.
　　blood loss a.
　　brickmaker's a.
　　cameloid a.
　　chlorotic a.
　　chronic autoimmune hemolytic a.
　　a. of chronic disease
　　chronic hemolytic a.
　　a. of chronic renal failure
　　cold autoimmune hemolytic a.
　　congenital aplastic a.
　　congenital aregenerative a.
　　congenital atransferrinemia
　　congenital dyserythropoietic a.
　　　(CDA)
　　congenital hypoplastic a. (CHA)
　　congenital nonregenerative a.
　　congenital nonspherocytic
　　　hemolytic a.
　　Cooley a.
　　cow's milk a.
　　crescent cell a.
　　deficiency a.
　　Diamond-Blackfan a.

NOTES

anemia *(continued)*
dilution a.
dimorphic a.
Diphyllobothrium a.
Dresbach a.
drug-induced autoimmune hemolytic a.
drug-induced immune hemolytic a.
dyserythropoietic congenital a.
dyshemopoietic a.
Ehrlich a.
elliptocytic a.
enzyme deficiency a.
enzyme-deficient a.
equine infectious a.
erythroblastic a.
Estren-Dameshek a.
Faber a.
factor deficiency a.
false a.
familial erythroblastic a.
familial hemolytic a.
familial hypoplastic a.
familial microcytic a.
familial pyridoxine-responsive a.
familial splenic a.
Fanconi a.
fish tapeworm a.
folic acid deficiency a.
frank megaloblastic a.
genetic a.
globe cell a.
glucose-6-phosphate dehydrogenase deficiency a.
goat's milk a.
G6PH deficiency a.
a. gravis
ground itch a.
Ham test for a.
Hayem-Widal a.
Heinz body hemolytic a.
hemolytic a.
hemorrhagic a.
hemotoxic a.
hereditary hemolytic a. (HHA)
hereditary nonspherocytic hemolytic a. (HNSHA)
hereditary sideroblastic a.
hookworm a.
hyperchromatic a.
hyperchromic a.
a. hypochromica sideroachrestica hereditaria
hypochromic microcytic a.
hypoferric a.
hypoplastic a.
hyporegenerative a.
iatrogenic a.
icterohemolytic a.

idiopathic refractory sideroblastic a. (IRSA)
idiopathic warm autoimmune hemolytic a.
immunohemolytic a.
a. infantum pseudoleukemica
infectious a.
intertropical a.
iron deficiency a. (IDA)
isochromic a.
isoimmune hemolytic a.
lead a.
Lederer a.
leukoerythroblastic a.
local a.
a. lymphatica
macrocytic achylic a.
malignant a.
march a.
Marchiafava-Micheli a.
Mediterranean a.
megaloblastic a.
megalocytic a.
metaplastic a.
microangiopathic hemolytic a. (MAHA, MHA)
microcytic hypochromic a.
microdrepanocytic a.
milk a.
mixed a.
molecular a.
myelofibrosis a.
myelopathic a.
myelophthisic a.
neonatal a.
a. neonatorum
nonimmune hemolytic a.
nonmegaloblastic a.
normochromic a.
normocytic a.
nosocomial a.
nutritional a.
osteosclerotic a.
ovalocytic a.
oxidase-induced acute hemolytic a.
pernicious a. (PA)
physiologic a.
polar a.
posthemorrhagic a.
primaquine-sensitive a.
primary erythroblastic a.
primary refractory a.
production-defect a.
protein deficiency a.
pure red cell a.
pyridoxine-responsive a.
radiation a.
a. refractoria sideroblastica
refractory sideroblastic a.

secondary refractory a.
severe hemolytic a.
sickle cell a.
sideroachrestic a.
sideroblastic a.
sideropenic a.
slaty a.
spastic a.
spherocytic a.
splenic a.
spur cell a.
target cell a.
thrombopenic a.
toxic a.
traumatic a.
tropical a.
unstable hemoglobin hemolytic a.
variant sickling hemoglobin a.
vitamin deficiency a.
warm-and-cold-type autoimmune
  hemolytic a.
warm autoimmune hemolytic a.
  (WAIHA)
anemic
a. anoxia
a. halo
a. hypoxia
a. infarct
anemicus
nevus a.
anemotrophy
anencephalia
anencephalic
anencephalous
anencephaly
anenterous
anenzymia catalasia
anephric
anergic leishmaniasis
anergy
cachectic a.
negative a.
nonspecific a.
positive a.
a. skin test battery
specific a.
anerythrogenesis
anerythroplasia
anerythroplastic
anerythroregenerative

anesthesia
a. adjunct
thalamic hyperesthetic a.
anesthetic leprosy
anetoderma
a. erythematosum
Schweninger-Buzzi a.
aneuploid
a. c. cell
a. c. tumor
aneuploidy
DNA a.
Aneurinibacillus danicus
aneurolemmic
aneurysm
abdominal aortic a. (AAA)
ampullary a.
aortic arch a.
arteriosclerotic aortic a.
arteriosclerotic thrombosed a.
arteriovenous a.
atherosclerotic a.
axial a.
bacterial a.
benign bone a.
Bérard a.
berry a.
cardiac a.
cirsoid a.
compound a.
congenital ruptured a.
consecutive a.
cylindroid a.
cystogenic a.
diffuse a.
dissecting a.
ectatic a.
embolic a.
embolomycotic a.
endogenous a.
erosive a.
exogenous a.
false a.
fusiform a.
hernial a.
intracavernous a.
intracranial a. (ICA)
luetic a.
miliary a.
mural a.
mycotic a.
nondissecting aortic a.

NOTES

59

aneurysm *(continued)*
Park a.
peripheral a.
popliteal a.
postoperative clipped a.
Pott a.
racemose a.
Rasmussen a.
Richet a.
Rodrigues a.
ruptured a.
saccular a.
sacculated a.
serpentine a.
sinus of Valsalva a.
syphilitic a.
thoracic a.
thrombosed arteriosclerotic a.
traction a.
traumatic a.
true a.
tubular a.
varicose a.
ventricular a.
aneurysmal
a. bone cyst (ABC)
a. dilatation
a. sac
a. varix
aneurysmatic
aneusomatic
aneusomy
AneuVysion prenatal test
ANF
antinuclear factor
angel of death mushroom
Angelman syndrome
Angelucci syndrome
Anger camera
angiectasia
congenital dysplastic a.
angiectasis
angiectatic
angiectopia
angiitic granulomatosis
angiitis, angitis
allergic granulomatous a.
Churg-Strauss a.
consecutive a.
cutaneous systemic a.
hypersensitivity a.
leukocytoclastic a.
a. livedo reticularis
necrotizing a.
angina
agranulocytic a.
Ludwig a.
lymphatic a.
a. lymphomatosa

monocytic a.
neutropenic a.
a. pectoris (AP)
Prinzmetal a.
Vincent a.
anginae
Saccharomyces a.
anginose scarlatina
anginosus
Streptococcus a.
anginosus-constellatus
Streptococcus a.-c.
angioblast
angioblastic cell
angioblastoma
angiocentric
a. immunoproliferative lesion (AIL)
a. lymphoproliferative lesion
a. pattern
a. T-cell lymphoma
angiocentricity
angiocholecystitis
angiocholitis
angiodermatitis
angiodestruction
angiodestructive pattern
angiodysgenetic myelomalacia
angiodystrophia, angiodystrophy
angioedema
angioelephantiasis
angioendothelioma
malignant endovascular papillary a.
papillary intralymphatic a.
angioendotheliomatosis
proliferating systematized a.
angiofibrolipoma
angiofibroma
juvenile a.
nasopharyngeal a. (NA)
angiofibrosis
angiofollicular mediastinal lymph node hyperplasia
angiogenesis
aberrant a.
a. factor
tumor a.
angiogenic switch
angioglioma
angiogliomatosis
angiogliosis
angiography
postmortem a.
angiohemophilia
angiohyalinosis
angiohypertonia
angiohypotonia
angioid streak
angioimmunoblastic
a. lymphadenopathy

a. lymphadenopathy with dysproteinemia (AILD)
a. lymphoma (AIL)
angioinvasion
angioinvasive adenoma
angiokeratoma
a. corporis diffusum
diffuse a.
Fordyce a.
Mibelli a.
angiokeratosis
angioleiomyoma
angioleucitis
angiolipofibroma
angiolipoma
angiolith
angiolithic
a. degeneration
a. sarcoma
angiolymphatic invasion
angiolymphoid hyperplasia with eosinophilia
angioma
acquired tufted a.
cavernous a.
cherry a.
littoral cell a.
a. lymphaticum
petechial a.
a. serpiginosum
spider a.
telangiectatic a.
a. venosum racemosum
angiomatodes
nevus a.
angiomatoid tumor
angiomatosis
bacillary a. (BA)
cephalotrigeminal a.
congenital dysplastic a.
cutaneomeningospinal a.
encephalotrigeminal a.
oculoencephalic a.
telangiectatic a.
angiomatous meningioma
angiomegaly
angiomyofibroblastoma
angiomyofibroma
angiomyolipoma (AML)
pulmonary a.
renal a.
angiomyoma

angiomyoneuroma
angiomyopathy
angiomyosarcoma
angiomyxoma
aggressive a.
angioneuromyoma
angioneurotica
purpura a.
angioneurotic edema
angioosteohypertrophy syndrome
angioparalysis
angioparesis
angiopathic hemolytic anemia
angiopathy
amyloid a.
British type amyloid a.
cerebral amyloid a.
congenital dysplastic a.
congophilic a.
diabetic a.
prion protein cerebral amyloid a.
angiophacomatosis
angioplany
angiopoietin
angioreninoma
angiorrhexis
angiosarcoma
adrenal epithelioid a.
low-grade a.
salivary gland a.
verrucous a.
angiosis
angiospasm
angiospastic
angiostaxis
angiostenosis
angiostrongylosis
Angiostrongylus
A. cantonensis
A. costaricensis
A. malaysiensis
angiotelectasia
angiotelectasis
angiotensin
a. 1 (A1)
a. 2 (A2)
a. 3 (A3)
a. I
a. I-converting enzyme
a. I, II test
angiotensin-converting enzyme
angiotensinogen

NOTES

angiotrophic lymphoma
angiotumoral complex
angiovascular
angitis (*var. of* angiitis)
angle
  Alsberg a.
  central collodiaphyseal a. (CCD)
  a. closure glaucoma
  critical a.
  a. head
  a. of incidence
  pectinate ligaments of
    iridocorneal a.
  a. of reflection
  a. of refraction
  solid a.
  space of iridocorneal a.
angled soot pattern
angstrom (Å)
Ångstrom law
Anguillula
angular
  a. acceleration
  a. aperture
  a. conjunctivitis
  a. frequency
  a. stomatitis
angularis
  incisura a.
angulate cell
angulated lysosome
Angulomicrobium amanitiforme
angulus, pl. **anguli**
  ligamentum pectinatum anguli
ANH
  acute normovolemic hemodilution
anhemolytic streptococcus
anhidrosis
anhidrotic ectodermal dysplasia
anhistic
anhydrase
  carbonic a.
anhydration
anhydride
  acetic a.
  basic a.
  cyclic lysine a. (CLA)
  heptafluorobutyric a. (HFBA)
  pentafluoropropionic a. (PFP)
  resorcinol phthalic a.
  trifluoroacetic a. (TFAA)
anhydrous
  a. alcohol
  a. sodium sulfite
ani (*gen. and pl. of* anus)
anicteric virus hepatitis
aniline
  a. blue
  a. blue modified trichrome stain

  a. dye
  a. fuchsin
  a. gentian violet (AGV)
  a., sulfur, formaldehyde (ASF)
anilinism
anilinophil, anilinophile
anilinophilous
animal
  anthrax-infected a.
  a. cell culture
  control a.
  conventional a.
  Houssay a.
  molluscous a.
  normal a.
  a. protein factor (APF)
  sentinel a.
  a. toxin
  a. virus
animalcule
animatum
  contagium a.
  virus a.
anion
  cyanide a.
  a. exchanger 1 (AE1)
  a. gap
  a. gap test
  a. interference
  superoxide a.
anion-exchange
  a.-e. chromatography
  a.-e. resin
anionic
  a. detergent
  a. dye
  a. neutrophil activating peptide
    (ANAP)
anionotropy
aniridia
anisakiasis
anisakid
Anisakidae
Anisakis marina
anise oil
anisochromasia
anisochromia
anisocytosis
anisohypercytosis
anisohypocytosis
anisokaryosis
anisoleukocytosis
anisonucleosis
anisopoikilocytosis
anisotropic
  a. disc
  a. lipid
anisotropy

anitrata
    Lingelsheimia a.
anitratus
    Acinetobacter calcoaceticus a.
Anitschkow
    A. cell
    A. myocyte
Anixiella
Anixiopsis
ankle-type fibrous histiocytoma
ankyloblepharon
ankylocolpos
ankyloglossia
ankyloproctia
ankylosing spondylitis
ankylosis
    bony a.
    cervical spine a.
    dorsal spine a.
    extracapsular a.
    fibrous a.
    intracapsular a.
    lumbosacral spine a.
    osseous a.
Ankylostoma
ankylostomiasis
ankyrin
anlage, pl. **anlagen**
ANLL
    acute nonlymphocytic leukemia
Ann
    A. Arbor staging classification
    A. Arbor staging system
    A. Arbor tumor classification
annatto, annotto
anneal
annealing temperature
annelid
Annelida
annelloconidium
annexin V
annexitis
annihilation
    positron a.
annotto (*var. of* annatto)
annua
    Artemisia a.
annulare
    granuloma a.
annularis
    Anopheles a.
    lichen a.

lipoatrophia a.
purpura a.
rachitis fetalis a.
annular pancreas
annulate lamellae
annulatus
    Boophilus a.
    Streptomyces a.
annulipes
    Anopheles a.
annulospiral
    a. ending
    a. organ
annulus (*var. of* anulus)
annum
    Capsicum a.
ano
    fissure in a.
    fistula in a.
anochromasia
anodal
anode voltage
anodontia
anogenital wart
anomalad
anomalous
    a. muscle band
    a. origin
    a. vascular distribution
    a. venous connection
    a. venous drainage
anomalus
    Hoplopsyllus a.
anomaly
    Alder a.
    Alder-Reilly a.
    Alius-Grignaschi a.
    cerebrovascular a.
    Chédiak-Steinbrinck-Higashi a.
    coloboma, heart disease, atresia choanae, retarded growth and development and ear a.'s (CHARGE)
    congenital a.
    developmental sequence a.
    dysraphic a.
    Ebstein a.
    Freund a.
    Hegglin a.
    Huët-Pelger nuclear a.
    Jordan a.
    May-Hegglin a.

NOTES

anomaly *(continued)*
  Pelger-Huët nuclear a.
  Shone a.
  Uhl a.
  Undritz a.
  vascular a.
  vertebral defects, anal atresia, tracheoesophageal fistula with esophageal atresia, and radial and renal a.'s (VATER)
anomer
anomeric
Anopheles
  A. aconitus
  A. albimanus
  A. albitarsus
  A. annularis
  A. annulipes
  A. aquasalis
  A. arabiensis
  A. aztecus
  A. balabacensis
  A. barbirostris
  A. bellator
  A. brunnipes
  A. campestris
  A. crucians
  A. cruzi
  A. culicifacies
  A. darlingi
  A. flavirostris
  A. fluviatilis
  A. freeborni
  A. funestus
  A. gambiae
  A. jeyporiensis
  A. karwari
  A. kweiyangensis
  A. labranchiae
  A. lesteri
  A. leucosphyrus
  A. maculatus
  A. maculipennis
  A. messeae
  A. minimus
  A. pseudopunctipennis
  A. quadrimaculatus
  A. stephensi
  A. sundaicus
  A. superpictus
anophelicide
anophelifuge
Anophelinae
anopheline
Anophelini
anophelism
anophthalmia
Anoplocephala perfoliata
Anoplocephalidae

Anoplura
anorchia
anorectal melanoma
anorectic, anoretic
anorexia nervosa
anosmia
anosteoplasia
anostosis
ANOVA
  analysis of variance
anovular ovarian follicle
anovulation
anovulatory
anoxemia
anoxemic
anoxia
  altitude a.
  anemic a.
  anoxic a.
  fulminating a.
  histotoxic a.
  hypoxic a.
  myocardial a.
  a. neonatorum
  oxygen affinity a.
  a. reaction
  stagnant a.
anoxic
  a. anoxia
  a. encephalopathy
Anoxybacillus
  A. ayderensis
  A. contaminans
  A. flavithermus
  A. gonensis
  A. kestanbolensis
  A. pushchinoensis
  A. voinovskiensis
Anoxynatronum sibiricum
Anoxyphotobacteria
Anoxyphotobacteriae
ANP
  atrial natriuretic peptide
ANS
  antineutrophilic serum
  arteriolonephrosclerosis
ansa
  Henle a.
anserina
  Borrelia a.
  cutis a.
anserine
anseris
  Amidostomum a.
ANSI
  American National Standards Institute
antagonism
  bacterial a.
  metabolic a.

microbial a.
salt a.
antagonist
    beta-adrenergic a.
    cholinergic a.
    competitive a.
    endothelin-1 receptor a.
    enzyme a.
    insulin a.
    metabolic a.
    narcotic a.
    NMDA receptor a.
    protein induced by vitamin K a.
    (PIVKA)
    sulfonamide a.
antarctica
    Aequorivita a.
    Oleispira a.
    Pseudonocardia a.
    Psychromonas a.
antarcticum
    Exiguobacterium a.
antarcticus
    Paenibacillus a.
    Planococcus a.
    Rhodoferax a.
antecedent
    plasma thromboplastin a. (PTA)
antegrade
antemortem
    a. clot
    a. thrombus
antenatal
antepartum hemorrhage (APH)
anterior
    a. acute poliomyelitis
    a. centriole
    a. complete dislocation
    a. displacement
    a. elastic layer
    a. epithelium of cornea
    a. ethmoidal air cell
    glandula lingualis a.
    a. horn cell
    a. incisural space
    lamina elastica a.
    a. lateral myocardial infarct
    (ALMI)
    a. limiting layer of cornea
    a. lingual gland
    a. lobe of hypophysis
    a. median fissure

a. part of septum
a. pituitary extract (APE)
a. pituitary hormone (APH)
a. pituitary hyperfunction
a. pituitary-like (APL)
a. pituitary-like substance
a. semicircular canal
a. wall
a. wall infarction (AWI)
a. wall myocardial infarction
    (AWMI)
anteriores
    cellulae ethmoidales a.
anterioris
    endothelium camerae a.
anterochoanal
anterofacial dysplasia
anterograde
anteroposterior facial dysplasia
anteroseptal myocardial infarct (ASMI)
anteverted/anteflexed (AV/AF)
anthelminthic, anthelmintic
anthelmycin
antheridium
anthina
    Burkholderia a.
anthocyanidin
anthocyanin
Anthomyia
    A. canicularis
    A. incisura
Anthomyiidae
Anthopsis deltoidea
anthracemia
anthracene blue
anthracic
anthracin
anthracis
    Bacillus a.
    encapsulated *Bacillus a.*
    veterinary vaccine Stern strain
    Bacillus a.
Anthracobia
anthracoid
anthracometer
anthracosilicosis
anthracosis linguae
anthracotic
    a. pigment
    a. tuberculosis
anthracycline cardiotoxicity
anthramucin

NOTES

anthranilic acid
anthrapurpurin
anthraquinone dye
anthrax
    abdominal a.
    a. as biological weapon
    a. bacillus
    a. belt
    black bane (a.)
    a. capsule
    cutaneous a.
    a. epizootic
    gastrointestinal a.
    inhalational a.
    a. malignant pustule
    a. meningitis
    oropharyngeal a.
    a. pneumonia
    pulmonary a.
    a. septicemia
    septicemic a.
    a. spore
    a. toxin
    a. vaccine absorbed
    woolsorter's disease (a.)
anthrax-containing chocolate
anthrax-contaminated animal product
anthrax-infected
    a.-i. animal
    a.-i. body fluid
anthrone
anthropoid
anthropology
    forensic a.
    hematological a.
    pathologic a.
    physical a.
anthropometric
anthropometry
    forensic a.
anthropomorphic table
anthroponosis, pl. anthroponoses
anthropophaga
    Cordylobia a.
    Ochromyia a.
anthropophilic
anthropozoonosis
anthurii
    Acidovorax a.
anti
    a. fas/APO-1 antibody
anti-A
    a.-A agglutinin
    a.-A antibody
antiadrenal antibody
antiagglutinin
antiaggregant
    platelet a.
antialexin

antialkaline phosphatase method
antiallergic
antiallotype
antialopecia factor
antianaphylaxis
antiandrogen
    pure a.
antianemic
    a. factor
    a. principle
antiantibody
antiantitoxin
antiapoptotic protein
antiarachnolysin
antiasialoglycoprotein receptor
antiatherogenic activity
antiautolysin
anti-B
    a.-B agglutinin
    a.-B antibody
antibacterial
    a. agent
    a. agent susceptibility testing
antibasement
    a. membrane antibody
    a. membrane glomerulonephritis
    a. membrane nephritis
antibiogram
antibiont
antibiosis
antibiotic
    a. antitumor drug
    bactericidal a.
    bacteriostatic a.
    broad-spectrum a.
    a. enterocolitis
    a. level
    macrolide a.
    oral a.
    peptide a.
    polyene a.
    a. sensitivity
    a. sensitivity test
antibiotica
    Kribbella a.
antibiotic-associated
    a.-a. colitis (AAC)
    a.-a. diarrhea (AAD)
antibiotic-resistant
antibody (Ab)
    A5B7 monoclonal a.
    ABO a.
    absorption of erythrocyte a.
    acetylcholine receptor a. (AChRAb)
    adrenal a.
    AE1 a.
    AE3 a.
    affinity a.
    a. affinity chromatography

agglutinating a.
albumin-agglutinating a.
ALK1 a.
allergen-specific IgE a.
alloantin-D a.
alpha globulin a.
anaphylactic a.
anti-A a.
antiadrenal a.
anti-B a.
antibasement membrane a.
anticardiolipin a. (ACA)
anti-CD11a humanized
  monoclonal a.
anti-CD18 humanized a.
anticentromere a.
anti-Chido a.
anticoilin a.
anticytokeratin a.
anticytoplasmic a. (ACPA)
anti-DAK a.
anti-DNA a.
anti-EA a.
anti-EGF-receptor a.
anti fas/APO-1 a.
antifibrin a.
antifibrinogen a.
anti-GBM a.
anti-Goa a.
antigranulocyte a.
antihistone a.
antiidiotype a.
antiinsulin a.
antiintrinsic factor a.
anti-Js a.
anti-kappa a.
anti-Kell a.
antikeratin AE1 a.
antikeratin AE3 a.
antikidney a.
anti-LA a.
antilambda a.
antileukocyte a.
antiliver-kidney microsomal a.
anti-LKM-1 a.
antilymphocytic a.
anti-M a.
antimetallothionein a. (MT)
antimicrosomal a.
antimitochondrial a. (AMA)
antineutrophil cytoplasmic a.
  (ANCA)

antinuclear a. (ANA)
anti-P a.
antiparietal cell a.
antiphospholipid a. (APA)
antiplatelet a.
antireceptor a.
anti-Rh a.
anti-RNA a.
anti-Ro a.
anti-Rodgers a.
anti-S a.
anti-*Saccharomyces cerevisiae* a.
  (ASCA)
antisera a.
anti-Sm a.
antismooth muscle a. (ASMA)
anti-T-cell a.
antithyroglobulin a.
antithyroid peroxidase a.
anti-*Toxoplasma* a. (ATA)
antitubular basement membrane a.
anti-VCA a.
anti-VS a.
APAAP a.
ASCA a.
autoantiidiotypic a.
autoimmune a.
autologous a.
avidity a.
B72.3 a.
basal cell carcinoma specific a.
basement membrane a.
B-cell a.
bcl-2 a.
bcl-6 a.
BE12 a.
Ber-EP4 a.
Ber-H2 a.
BG8 monoclonal a.
BH11 a.
bivalent a.
BLA 36 monoclonal a.
blocking a. (BA)
blood group a.
BrDu a.
C8/144 a.
C219 a.
C494 a.
CAM 5.2 a.
cA2 monoclonal a.
capture a.
a. capture ligand assay

NOTES

antibody *(continued)*
a. catabolism
cathepsin D a.
CB11 a.
CD a.
CD14 a.
CEJO65 monoclonal a.
cell-bound a.
CF a.
chimeric a.
CH/RG a.
circulatory antigliadin a.
Clonad monoclonal a.
CM1 a.
CMV a.
coccidioidomycosis a.
cold a.
cold-reacting a.
cold-reactive a.
a. combining site
complement-fixing a.
complete a.
coprecipitating a.
Coulter CLONE monoclonal a.
cross-reacting a.
cryptosporidiosis a.
cytomegalovirus a.
cytophilic a.
cytoplasmic antineutrophil
   cytoplasmic a. (cANCA)
Cyto-Stat/Coulter CLONE
   monoclonal a.
cytotoxic a.
cytotropic a.
a. deficiency disease
a. deficiency syndrome (ADS)
a. deficiency with near-normal
   immunoglobulins
desmin a.
a. detection
direct fluorescent a. (DFA)
DL a.
DO7 a.
donor-specific HLA a.
Duffy a.
dystrophin a.
EMA a.
endomysial a.
enhancing a.
erythrocyte a. (EA)
a. excess
a. excess zone
extractable nuclear antigen a.
   (ENA)
ferritin-conjugated a. (FCA)
ferritin-coupled a.
fluorescein-labeled a.
fluorescent a. (FA)
fluorescent antinuclear a. (FANA)

fluorescent treponemal a. (FTA)
Forssman a.
GB-7 a.
glomerular basement membrane a.
H a.
Ha-1A monoclonal a.
HAM 56 a.
HBME 1 a.
heat-labile a.
hemagglutinating antipenicillin a.
   (HAPA)
hemagglutination-inhibition a. (HIA)
hepatitis a.
hepatitis A a.
hepatitis B core a. (HB$_c$Ab)
a. to hepatitis B core antigen
   (HB$_c$Ab)
hepatitis Be a. (HB$_e$Ab)
hepatitis B surface a. (HB$_s$Ab)
a. to hepatitis B surface antigen
HepPar1 a.
herpes simplex a.
heteroclitic a.
heterocytotropic a.
heterogenetic a.
heteroligating a.
heterophil a.
HHF 35 a.
HMB 45 a.
HMFG-2 a.
homocytotropic a.
HTLV-I a.
human antichimeric a. (HACA)
human antimouse a. (HAMA)
human antimurine a. (HAMA)
humoral a.
hybrid a.
hybridoma a.
a. identification
idiotype a.
IgA-antigliadin a.
IgA endomysial a.
IgE a.
IgG desmoplakin a.
IgM a.
IgM-RF a.
immobilizing a.
immunosorbent a.
incomplete a.
inhibiting a.
IOTest monoclonal a.
islet cell a. (ICA)
isoimmune a.
isophil a.
Ki-1 a.
Ki-67 a.
kidney-fixing a. (KFAb)
Ki-FDC1p a.
Ki-M1p a.

Ki-M4p a.
Ki-S5 a.
KO89-kit a.
KP1 a.
KP1/CD68 monoclonal a.
L26 a.
LCA a.
Legionnaire's disease a.
LEMS a.
Leu 1–22 a.
LeuM1 a.
LeuM3 a.
LeuM5 a.
Lewis a.
LKM a.
LN1 a.
LN2 a.
LN3 monoclonal a.
lymphocytotoxic a.
lymphoid monoclonal a.
Mac387 a.
maternal a.
measles a.
MIB1 a.
MIC2 a.
microsomal thyroid a.
mirror-image complementary a.
  (MICA)
mitochondrial a.
MOC31 monoclonal a.
monoclonal a. (MAb, mAB)
MSA a.
MTI a.
natural a.
NCL-ARm monoclonal a.
NCL-ARp polyclonal a.
NCL-ER-LH2 monoclonal a.
NCL-PCR monoclonal a.
nephrotoxic a. (NTAB)
neutralizing a. (NA)
NK1-C3 a.
no demonstrable a.'s (NDA)
nonprecipitable a.
nonprecipitating a.
normal a.
nuclear a.
O a.
OKT-9 a.
OPD4 a.
opsonizing a.
OptiClone monoclonal a.
Orthomune a.

pan-B a.
panel-reactive a. (PRA)
panenteroviral a.
pankeratin a.
a. panning technique
PE-10 a.
pemphigus a.
phase II a.
phase I immunoglobulin A a.
platelet a.
p80NPM/ALK a.
polyclonal antiplacental a.
polyclonal prolactin a.
Prausnitz-Küstner a.
precipitating a.
a. producing plasma cell
reaginic a.
Rh a.
S-100 a.
saline-agglutinating a.
a. to SARS-CoV
scleroderma a.
a. screening
a. screening test
Sjögren a.
skeletal muscle a.
skin-sensitizing a. (SSA)
smooth muscle a. (SMA)
a. specificity prediction (ASP)
sperm agglutinating a.
a. stain
synaptophysin a.
T a.
TAB 250 a.
Thomsen a.
thyroglobulin a.
thyroid microsomal a. (TMAb)
TIA-1 a.
a. titer
treponema-immobilizing a.
treponemal a.
TSH displacing a. (TDA)
UCHL1 a.
UCHL1[a] a.
UCL3D3 a.
UJ127.11 a.
UJ13A monoclonal a.
ULCL4D12 a.
univalent a.
Vi a.
warm reactive a.
Wassermann a.

NOTES

antibody *(continued)*
    white blood cell a.
    xenocytophilic a.
    Yersinia enterocolitica a.
    Yersinia pestis a.
    ZB4 a.
antibody-absorption
    fluorescent treponemal a. (FTA-ABS, FTA-AB)
antibody/antigen
    CD14 a.
    CD117 a.
antibody-based lateral flow economical recognition ticket (ALERT)
antibody-coated microprobe technique
antibody-conjugate
    antidigoxigenin alkaline phosphatase a.-c.
antibody-dependent
    a.-d. cell-mediated cytotoxicity
    a.-d. immunity
antibody-forming cell
antibody-mediated
    a.-m. rejection
    a.-m. vascular damage
anti-BrdU
    anti-bromodeoxyuridine
anti-bromodeoxyuridine (anti-BrdU)
anticarcinoembryonic antigen
anticardiolipin antibody (ACA)
anticariensis
    Halomonas a.
anti-CD11a humanized monoclonal antibody
anti-CD18 humanized antibody
anticentromere antibody
anti-c-*erb*B-2
anti-Chido antibody
anti-*Chlamydia* antibody test
anticholera serum
anticholinergic delirium
anticholinesterase
antichromogranin
antichymotrypsin
    alpha a. (ACT)
    alpha-1 a. (A1AC)
    a. test
anticoagulant (AC)
    circulating a.
    a. heparin solution
    lupus a. (LA)
    partial thromboplastin time lupus anticoagulant (PTT-LA)
    pharmacology of a.
    phospholipid type a.
    a. therapy (ACT)
anticoagulant-citrate-dextrose
anticoagulant-citrate-phosphate-dextrose
anticoagulated blood

anticoagulative
anticoagulin
anticodon
anticoilin antibody
anticolibacillary serum
anticollagenase
anticommon leukocyte antigen
anticomplement
anticomplementary (AC)
    a. factor
    a. serum
anticontagious
anticytokeratin
    a. antibody
    a. immunohistochemistry
    a. stain
anticytoplasmic
    a. antibody (ACPA)
    a. autoantibody
anticytotoxin
anti-DAK antibody
antideoxyribonuclease
    a. B (ADN-B)
    a. B titer test
antidesmin
antidigoxigenin
    a. alkaline phosphatase antibody-conjugate
    a. antibody peroxidase conjugate
anti-D immunoglobulin
antidiphtheric serum
antidiphtheritic globulin
antidiuretic
    a. hormone (ADH)
    a. hormone deficiency
    a. substance (ADS)
anti-DNA
    a.-D. antibody
    a.-D. antibody assay
anti-DNaseB
    a.-DNaseB assay
    Immage a.-DNaseB
antidote
    oxime a.
antidromic
anti-EA antibody
anti-EGF-receptor antibody
antiendomysial antibody test
antienzyme
antiepithelial serum
anti-Epstein-Barr nuclear antigen
antiestrogen receptor
anti-F1 antigen titer
antifactor
    a. I–IX disorder
    a. Xa
antifibrin antibody
antifibrinogen antibody
antifibrinolysin

antifibrinolytic
antifol
antifolic
antifungal agent
anti-GBM
    antiglomerular basement membrane
      anti-GBM antibody
      anti-GBM disease
antigen (Ag)
    A a.
    ABH a.
    ABO a.
    accessible a.
    acetone-insoluble a.
    A-like a.
    allogeneic a.
    alum-precipitated a.
    Am a.
    antibody to hepatitis B core a.
      (HB$_c$Ab)
    antibody to hepatitis B surface a.
    anticarcinoembryonic a.
    anticommon leukocyte a.
    anti-Epstein-Barr nuclear a.
    Australia a. (AU Ag)
    autologous a.
    B a.
    B72.3 a.
    bacterial meningitis a.
    Be^a a.
    Becker a.
    Bi a.
    bile a.
    blood group a. (BGA)
    BR27.29 breast a.
    By a.
    C a.
    CA125 a.
    CA19-9 a.
    CA15-3 breast a.
    CAM 5.2 a.
    cancer a. (CA)
    cancer a. 125 (CA125)
    capsular a.
    a. capture ligand assay
    carbohydrate a.
    carcinoembryonic a. (CEA)
    Cartwright a.
    C carbohydrate a.
    CD a.
    chick embryo a.
    Chlamydia a.

    cholesterinized a.
    ChrA a.
    CH/RG a.
    class histocompatibility a.
    cluster 1 small-cell lung cancer a.
    Colton a.
    common acute lymphoblastic
      leukemia a. (CALLA, cALLA)
    common acute lymphocytic
      leukemia a.
    common enterobacterial a.
    complement-fixing a.
    complete a.
    complexed prostate-specific a.
      (cPSA)
    conjugated a.
    core a.
    cross-reacting a.
    cryptic T a.
    cryptococcal a.
    cyclin A a.
    cyclin E a.
    cytokeratin 1–20 a.
    D a.
    D10 a.
    delta a.
    DFA for capsular a.
    Dharmendra a.
    Di a.
    Diego a.
    differentiation a.
    Dombrock a.
    Duffy a.
    DU-PAN-2 pancreatic cancer-
      associated a.
    E a.
    early a. (EA)
    endogenous a.
    epithelial membrane a. (EMA)
    epsilon a.
    Epstein-Barr nuclear a. (EBNA)
    erythrocyte a.
    a. excess
    exogenous a.
    extractable nuclear a. (ENA)
    F a.
    1F6 a.
    fecal a.
    fetal a.
    fibrin-related a. (FRA)
    flagellar a.
    Forssman a.

NOTES

antigen *(continued)*
Frei a.
Fy a.
G a.
a. gain
gamma a.
Ge a.
Good a.
GPK a.
Gr a.
Gross virus a. (GSA)
group a.'s
group specific a.
guinea pig a.
H a.
H-2 a.
hapten X, Y a.
HBA71 a.
He a.
heart a.
heat-extracted a.
hepatitis-associated a. (HAA)
hepatitis B core a. (HB$_c$Ag)
hepatitis Be a. (HB$_e$Ag)
hepatitis B surface a. (HB$_s$Ag)
heterogeneic a.
heterogenetic a.
heterogenic enterobacterial a.
heterophil a.
hexon a.
HHV 8 a.
Hikojima a.
histo-blood group a.
histocompatibility a.
HLA-A a.
HLA-B a.
HLA BW 54 a.
HLA-D a.
HLA-DR a.
HMB 45 a.
Ho a.
homologous a.
Hu a.
human leukemia-associated a.
human leukocyte a. (HLA)
human lymphocyte a.
human progenitor cell a.
H-Y a.
I a.
Ia a.
idiotypic a.
I/i a.
I(Ma) a.
Inaba a.
incomplete a.
inhalant a.
a. interferon
InV group a.
isophile a.

Ja a.
Jaa a.
Jk a.
Jobbins a.
Js a.
K a.
KD a.
Kell a.
Ki-1 a.
Ki-67 a.
Kidd a.
K and k a.
Km a.
Kunin a.
Kveim a.
Kveim-Stilzbach a.
labeled a.
laminin a.
Lan a.
Le a.
Legionella urinary a. (LUA)
lens a.
Leu 1 a.
leukocyte common a. (LCA)
LeuM1 a.
Levay a.
Lewis a.
Lewis-X blood group a.
LP a.
Lu a.
Lw a.
Ly a.
Lyb a.
lymphocyte function associated a.
lymphogranuloma venereum a.
Lyt a.
M a.
M$_1$ a.
major histocompatibility a. (MHA)
merozoite a.
Mi-2 a.
MIB1 a.
Miltenberger a.
minor histocompatibility a.
Mitsuda a.
monoclonal antibody-specific
  immobilization of platelet a.
  (MAIPA)
monoclonal antiepithelial
  membrane a.
mouse-specific lymphocyte a.
  (MSLA)
mu a.
mumps skin test a.
N a.
non-heat-extracted a.
nonspecific cross-reacting a. (NCA)
normal fecal a. (NFA-I)
NP a.

O a.
Ogawa a.
oncofetal a.
oncoprotein a.
organ-specific a.
Ot a.
Oz a.
P a.
p27 a.
P54 a.
pan-B a.
pancreatic oncofetal a. (POA)
pan-T cell a.
parainfluenza virus a.
partial a.
penton a.
PHA a.
p24 HIV a.
plasma cell a.
pollen a.
polyclonal anticarcinoembryonic a.
polyclonal carcinoembryonic a.
  (pCEA)
a. presentation
private a.
a. processing
proliferating cell nuclear a. (PCHA,
  PCNA)
Pronase a.
prostate-specific a. (PSA)
prostate-specific membrane a.
  (PSMA)
prostate stem cell a. (PSCA)
protective a. (PA)
Proteus OX2 a.
Proteus OX19 a.
Proteus OXK a.
public a.
Qa a.
R a.
a. receptor activation motif
  (ARAM)
recognition of a.
a. recognition
respiratory syncytial virus a.
a. retrieval
Rh a.
Rhus toxicodendron a.
Rhus venenata a.
rose bengal a. (RBA)
S a.
SD a.

a. sensitivity
sensitized a.
sequestered a.
serologically defined a.
shock a.
Sialosyl-Tn a.
single human leukocyte a.
skin-specific histocompatibility a.
Sm a.
soluble human leukocyte a.
soluble liver a. (SLA)
somatic a.
species-specific a.
specific a.
S-100 protein a.
S and s a.
SS-A/Ro a.
SS-B/La a.
Stobo a.
Streptococcus M a.
surface a.
SV 40 T a.
Sw^a a.
Swann a.
synthetic a.
T a.
Tac a.
TAG-72 a.
T-cell a.
T-cell restricted intracellular a.
  (TIA)
T-dependent a.
theta a.
Thomas a.
Thomsen-Friedenreich a.
Thy-1 a.
thymus-dependent a.
thymus-independent a.
thymus-leukemia a.
tissue-specific a.
TL a.
Tn a.
TRA a.
TRA-1-60 human embryonal
  carcinoma marker a.
transplantation a.
tumor a.
tumor-associated rejection a.
  (TARA)
tumor-associated transplantation a.
  (TATA)

NOTES

antigen *(continued)*
    tumor-specific transplantation a. (TSTA)
    a. unit
    V a.
    Vel a.
    Ven a.
    Vi a.
    viral capsid a. (VCA)
    VLA a.
    Vw a.
    Wassermann a.
    Webb a.
    Wr^a a.
    Wr^b a.
    Wright a.
    Xg a.
    Yersinia pestis F1 capsular a.
    yolk sac a.
    Yta a.
antigen-antibody
    a.-a. complex
    a.-a. reaction
antigen-antiglobulin reaction
antigen-binding
    a.-b. capacity
    a.-b. region
    single-chain a.-b. (SCA)
    a.-b. site
antigen-combining site
antigenemia
antigenetic peptide
antigenic
    a. analysis
    a. assay
    a. competition
    a. complex
    a. deletion
    a. determinant
    a. difference
    a. distribution
    a. drift
    a. modulation
    a. shift
    a. similarity
    a. structural grouping
antigenicity
antigen-presenting cell (APC)
antigen-responsive cell
antigen-retrieval technique
antigen-sensitive cell
antigen-specific
    a.-s. helper factor
    a.-s. suppressor factor
antigen-transporting cell
antigen-triggered lymphocyte differentiation
antigenuria

anti-GFAP staining
antiglobulin test (AGT)
antiglomerular basement membrane (anti-GBM)
anti-glomerular basement membrane disease
anti-Goa antibody
antigranulocyte antibody
anti-HB$_c$
anti-HB$_e$
anti-HB$_s$
antihemagglutinin
antihemolysin
antihemolytic
antihemophilic
    a. factor (AHF)
    a. factor A, B
    a. globulin (AHG)
    a. globulin A, B
    a. plasma
    a. plasma human
antihemorrhagic
antiheparin factor
antihepatic serum
antiheterolysin
antihistamine
antihistaminic
antihistone antibody
anti-HLA alloantibody
antihormone
antihuman
    a. globulin (AHG)
    a. globulin test
    a. lymphocyte serum (AHLS)
antihyaluronidase (AH)
    a. assay
    a. titer (AHT)
antihypercholesterolemic
antihypertensive
antiidiotype
    a. antibody
    a. autoantibody
antiinfective
antiinflammatory
    a. corticoid (AC)
    nonsteroidal a. (NSAID)
antiinsulin antibody
antiintrinsic factor antibody
antiisolysin
anti-Js antibody
anti-kappa antibody
anti-Kell antibody
antikeratin
    a. AE1
    a. AE3
    a. AE1 antibody
    a. AE3 antibody

antikidney
a. antibody
a. serum nephritis
anti-LA antibody
antilambda antibody
anti-LA/SS-B test
antileukocidin
antileukocyte antibody
antileukotoxin
antilewisite
British a. (BAL)
antiliver-kidney microsomal antibody
anti-LKM-1 antibody
antilymphocyte
a. globulin (ALG)
a. plasma (ALP)
a. serum (ALS)
antilymphocytic
a. antibody
a. globulin
antilysin
anti-M
a.-M. agglutinin
a.-M. antibody
antimacrophage
a. globulin (AMG)
a. serum (AMS)
antimalarial
antimediated cytotoxicity
antimeningococcus serum
antimetabolite drug
antimetallothionein antibody (MT)
antimicrobial
a. spectrum
a. therapy
antimicrosomal antibody
antimitochondrial
a. antibody (AMA)
a. antibody assay
antimode
antimony
a. assay
butter of a.
a. chloride
a. hydride
a. pneumoconiosis
a. poisoning
a. stain
a. trichloride
antimonyltartrate
sodium a.

antimorph
antimorphic
antimouse
a. lymphocyte serum (AMLS)
a. thymocyte
antimüllerian hormone (AMH)
antimuscarinic effect
antimutagen
antimycotic
antimyoglobin
anti-N agglutinin
antineoplastic
antineurotoxin
antineutrophil
a. cytoplasmic antibody (ANCA)
a. cytoplasmic autoantibody (ANCA)
antineutrophilic serum (ANS)
antinsulin serum (AIS)
antinuclear
a. antibody (ANA)
a. antibody assay
a. factor (ANF)
antioncogene
antioxidant
anti-P
a.-P agglutinin
a.-P antibody
a.-P blood group specificity
anti-p53
antiparallel
antiparasitic
antiparietal
a. cell antibody
a. cell antibody assay
antiparticle
antipedicular
antipediculotic
antiperiodic
antipernicious anemia factor (APA)
antipertussis serum
antiphagocytic polypeptide capsule
antiphospholipid
a. antibody (APA)
a. antibody syndrome
a. syndrome (APS)
antiplague serum
antiplant pathogen
anti-PLAP
antiplasmin
alpha 2 a.

NOTES

antiplatelet
>a. antibody
>a. serum

antipneumococcic
antipneumococcus serum
antipodal cone
antiport
anti-Pr cold autoagglutinin
antiprecipitin
antiprogesterone receptor
antiprothrombin
anti-*Pseudomonas* human plasma
antipyogenic
antiqua
>*Hylemya a.*

antique weapon
antirabies serum (ARS)
antireceptor antibody
antireticular cytotoxic serum (ACS)
antiretroviral
>a. agent
>a. treatment (ART)

anti-Rh
>a.-Rh agglutinin
>a.-Rh antibody
>a.-Rh titer

anti-Rho-D titer test
antiricin
anti-RNA antibody
anti-Ro antibody
anti-Rodgers antibody
anti-Ro/SS-A test
anti-S
>a.-S agglutinin
>a.-S antibody

anti-S-100 protein
anti-*Saccharomyces cerevisiae* antibody (ASCA)
antisarcomeric actin
antiscarlatinal serum
antisense probe
antisepsis
antiseptic
antiserum, pl. **antisera**
>a. anaphylaxis
>antisera antibody
>blood group a.
>CALLA a.
>heterologous a.
>homologous a.
>human thymus a. (HUTHAS)
>monovalent a.
>nerve growth factor a.
>NGF a.
>polyvalent a.
>specific a.

anti-Sm
>anti-Smith

>a.-Sm antibody
>a.-Sm test

anti-Smith (anti-Sm)
antismooth
>a. muscle actin
>a. muscle antibody (ASMA)
>a. muscle antibody assay

antisnake venom (ASV)
antistaphylococcic
antistaphylococcus serum
antistaphylolysin
antisteapsin
antistreptococcic
antistreptococcus serum
antistreptokinase
antistreptolysin (AS)
>a. O (ASO)
>a. O titer

antisubstance
antisynthetase syndrome
anti-tac
anti-T-cell antibody
antitetanic serum (ATS)
antithoracic duct lymphocytic globulin (ATDLG)
antithrombin
>a. III (AT III)
>a. III test
>IL test liquid a.
>normal a.

antithromboplastin
antithymocyte
>a. globulin (ATG)
>a. serum (ATS)

antithyroglobulin (ATG)
>a. antibody

antithyroid peroxidase antibody
antitoxic serum
antitoxigen
antitoxin
>bivalent gas gangrene a.
>bothropic a.
>*Bothrops* a.
>botulinum a.
>botulism a.
>bovine a.
>*Crotalus* a.
>despeciated a.
>diphtheria a. (DAT)
>dysentery a.
>a. Einheit (AE)
>gas gangrene a.
>normal a.
>pentavalent gas gangrene a.
>plant a.
>a. rash
>scarlet fever a.
>staphylococcus a.
>tetanus a. (TAT)

tetanus and gas gangrene a.'s
tetanus-perfringens a.
a. unit (AU)
antitoxinogen
anti-*Toxoplasma* antibody (ATA)
antitrypsin
alpha a. (AAT)
alpha$_1$ a. (A1AT)
a. deficiency
a. test
antitryptic index
antitubular basement membrane antibody
antitumor enzyme
antitumorigenesis
antityphoid serum
antiuvomorulin Fab fragment
anti-VCA antibody
antivenin
antivenomous serum
antivimentin
antiviral
a. agent
a. immunity
a. protein
anti-VS antibody
anti-Xa assay
Anton
A. syndrome
A. test
Antoni type A, B neurilemmoma
Antopol-Goldman lesion
antra (*pl. of* antrum)
antral
a. follicle
a. gastritis
a. G-cell hyperplasia
antralization
antranikianii
Thermus a.
Antrodia
Antrodiella
antrum, pl. **antra**
antra ethmoidalia
follicular a.
anuclear
anucleated
anulus, annulus, pl. **anuli**
a. fibrosus
a. fibrosus of aorta
a. fibrosus disci intervertebralis
anuresis

anuria
anus, gen. and pl. **ani**
atresia ani
Bartholin a.
ectopic a.
imperforate a.
melanocarcinoma of a.
a. vesicalis
vestibular a.
vulvovaginal a.
AO
acridine orange
AOD
arterial occlusive disease
Aonchotheca
aorta, gen. and pl. **aortae**
anulus fibrosus of a.
coarctation of a.
cystic medial necrosis of ascending a. (CMN-AA)
medial necrosis of a.
medionecrosis of the a.
postductal coarctation of a.
preductal coarctation of a.
aortic
a. arch aneurysm
a. atresia
a. body
a. body tumor
a. dissection
a. explant assay
a. incompetence (AI)
a. knob
a. occlusion
a. regurgitation
a. septal defect
a. tunica adventitia
a. tunica intima
a. tunica media
a. valve replacement (AVR)
a. valvular insufficiency
a. valvular stenosis
aortica
glomera a.
aorticosympathetic paraganglioma
aorticum
corpus a.
aortitis
bacterial a.
Döhle-Heller a.
giant cell a.
luetic a.

NOTES

aortitis *(continued)*
    rheumatoid a.
    syphilitic a.
aortocaval
aortoiliac
    a. atherosclerosis
    a. occlusive disease
aortosclerosis
AP
    alkaline phosphatase
    aminopeptidase
    angina pectoris
AP1
    activator protein 1
APA
    aldosterone-producing adenoma
    aminopenicillanic acid
    antipernicious anemia factor
    antiphospholipid antibody
    atypical polypoid adenomyofibroma
    atypical polypoid adenomyoma
APAAP
    alkaline phosphatase antialkaline phosphatase
      APAAP antibody
      APAAP technique
      APAAP test
APACHE
    acute physiology and chronic health evaluation
apallic syndrome
APA-LMP
    atypical polypoid adenomyofibroma of low malignant potential
apatite calculus
APC
    activated protein C
    adenoidal-pharyngeal-conjunctival
    adenomatous polyposis coli
    allophycocyanin
    antigen-presenting cell
      APC gene
      APC gene stool test
      APC resistance
      APC virus
APCR
    activated protein C resistance
A-PCR
    allele-specific PCR
APE
    anterior pituitary extract
Apec glucose analyzer
apeidosis
aperistalsis
    esophageal a.
aperta
    spina bifida a.
Apert-Crouzon disease
Apert disease

aperture
    angular a.
    numerical a.
APES
    aminopropyltriethoxysilane
apeu virus
APF
    anabolism-promoting factor
    animal protein factor
APH
    antepartum hemorrhage
    anterior pituitary hormone
aphakia
Aphanoascus
Aphanocladium
aphasmid
Aphasmidia
apheresis platelet
aphrophilus
    Haemophilus a.
aphthosis
aphthous
    a. fever
    a. ileal ulcer
    a. stomatitis
    a. ulceration
Aphthovirus
aphylactic
aphylaxis
apical
    a. abscess
    a. dendrite
    a. gland
    a. granuloma
    a. process
    a. surface
apicitis
Apicomplexa
apiculate
apiculatus
    Saccharomyces a.
apiculus
apigenin
apii
    Cercospora a.
Apiocrea
Apiognomonia
Apiosordaria
apiospermum
    Monosporium a.
    Scedosporium a.
apiostomum
    Oesophagostomum a.
Apiotrichum
apista
    Pandoraea a.
API 20 Strep System
Apium

APL
    acute promyelocytic leukemia
    anterior pituitary-like
aplanatic
    a. lens
    a. objective
aplasia
    bone marrow a.
    congenital thymic a.
    erythroid a.
    germ cell a.
    germinal cell a. (GCA)
    gonadal a.
    granulocytic a.
    hematopoietic a.
    lymphoid a.
    megakaryocytic a.
    nuclear a.
    pure red cell a. (PRCA)
    red cell a.
    retinal a.
    thymic-parathyroid a.
aplasia-thrombocytopenia
    radial a.-t.
aplasmic
aplastic
    a. anemia
    a. anemia syndrome
    a. bone marrow
    a. crisis
    a. lymph
Aplitest
apnea
    Bedbugg system for at-home diagnosis of sleep a.
    neonatal a.
    obstructive sleep a.
Apo
    apolipoprotein
ApoA
    apolipoprotein A
ApoB
    apolipoprotein B
apobiosis
ApoC
    apolipoprotein C
apochromatic objective
apocrine
    a. adenoma
    a. adenosis
    a. carcinoma
    a. ductal carcinoma in situ

    a. hidrocystoma
    a. metaplasia
    a. miliaria
    a. nevus
    a. sweat gland
apocynin
Apocynum
ApoD
    apolipoprotein D
ApoE
    apolipoprotein E
apoenzyme
apoferritin
apogamia
ApoHyp
    apocrine hyperplasia
apolar cell
apolipoprotein (Apo)
    a. A (ApoA)
    a. A1
    a. B (ApoB)
    a. C (ApoC)
    a. C2
    a. D (ApoD)
    a. E (ApoE)
apomixia
apomorphine-induced hypermobility
apomucin
aponeurosis
aponeurositis
aponeurotic fibroma
apophylaxis
apophysial, apophyseal
apophysis, pl. **apophyses**
apophysitis
    a. tibialis
    a. tibialis adolescentium
Apophysomyces elegans
apoplasmia
apoplectic
    a. coma
    a. cyst
apoplexy
apoprotein
ApopTag Plus kit
apoptosis
    cellular inhibitor of a. (cIAP)
    epithelial a.
    a. gene
    lipoxygenase-induced a.
apoptotic
    a. body

NOTES

apoptotic *(continued)*
    a. cell
    a. index
    a. keratinocyte
    a. process
aposome
Aposphaeria fuscidula
apothecium
apotransferrin
APP
    alum-precipitated pyridine
    amyloid precursor protein
    capsase mediated cleavage of APP
apparatus
    Abbé-Zeiss a.
    achromatic a.
    Barcroft a.
    Beckman Paragon SPE-II gel a.
    Benedict-Roth a.
    chromatic a.
    chromidial a.
    Golgi a.
    juxtaglomerular a.
    Langendorff a.
    nuclear mitotic a. (NuMA)
    Roughton-Scholander a.
    self-contained breathing a. (SCBA)
    subneural a.
    a. suspensorius lentis
    Van Slyke a.
apparent power
appearance
    amorphous eosinophilic a.
    batwing a.
    blush a.
    chicken fat a.
    cobblestone a.
    cotton-wool a.
    currant jelly a.
    a. of external genitalia
    granular golden a.
    histologic a.
    immunoarchitectural a.
    jointed bamboo-rod cellular a.
    microscopic a.
    nutmeglike a.
    orange peel corneal a.
    owl eye a.
    plucked chicken a.
    pseudofollicular a.
    pseudoinvasive a.
    spike and dome a.
    starry-sky a.
    tram-track a.
    whorled a.
    window frame a.
    withering crypt a.
    wrinkled silk a.

appendage
    drumstick a.
appendiceal abscess
appendices (*pl. of* appendix)
appendicis
    Corynebacterium a.
appendicitis
    actinomycotic a.
    acute gangrenous a.
    acute suppurative a.
    catarrhal a.
    chronic a.
    focal a.
    gangrenous a.
    healed a.
    healing a.
    lumbar a.
    obstructive a.
    stercoral a.
    subperitoneal a.
    suppurative acute a.
appendicolithiasis
appendix, pl. **appendices**
    a. vermiformis
APPG
    aorticopulmonary paraganglioma
apple-green birefringence
apple jelly nodule
applied
    microiontophoretically a.
appliqué form
apposition
appositional growth
Appraise clinical densitometer
approach
    clinicogenetic a.
    per-operative a.
appropriate for gestational age (AGA)
approximate lethal concentration (ALC)
APR
    acute phase reactant
    air-purifying respirator
    amebic prevalence rate
apraxia
apri
    Metastrongylus a.
apron
    Hottentot a.
aprotic solvent
APS
    antiphospholipid syndrome
APS1
    autoimmune polyendocrine syndrome
    type 1
Apscaviroid
APT
    alum-precipitated toxoid

Apt
    A. test
    A. test for swallowed blood
Aptima Combo 2 assay
AP-TNAP
    alkaline phosphatase, tissue-nonspecific
    isozyme protein precursor
APTT, aPTT
    activated partial thromboplastin time
    APTT prolongation
    APTT STA assay
    APTT test
aptyalism
APUD
    amine precursor uptake and
    decarboxylation
    APUD cell
apudoma
    esophageal a.
apurinic acid
apyknomorphous
AQP
    aquaporin
AQP1
    aquaporin-1
Aquabacterium
    A. *citratiphilum*
    A. *commune*
    A. *parvum*
Aquabirnavirus
aquagenic urticaria
Aquamicrobium defluvii
Aquamount
aquaporin (AQP)
aquaporin-1 (AQP1)
aqua regia
Aquareovirus
aquasalis
    Anopheles a.
Aquaspirillum
aquatica
    Arcicella a.
    Comamonas a.
    Leifsonia a.
    Tepidimonas a.
aquaticus
    Gordius a.
    Nocardioides a.
    Thermus a.
aquatile
    Flavobacterium a.

aquatilis
    Sphingomonas a.
aqueduct
    cochlear a.
    Cotunnius a.
    a. veil
aqueductus
    a. cochleae
    a. cotunnii
    a. vestibuli
aqueous
    a. humor
    a. mounting medium
    a. phase
    a. solution
    a. uranyl acetate
    a. vaccine
aquibiodomus
    Nitratireductor a.
Aquicella
    A. *lusitana*
    A. *siphonis*
Aquificaceae
Aquificae
Aquificales
aquilae
    Corynebacterium a.
aquimarina
    Kangiella a.
    Sporosarcina a.
aquimarinus
    Algoriphagus a.
aquimaris
    Bacillus a.
aquiterrae
    Nocardioides a.
aquocobalamin
aquosa
    polyemia a.
aquosus
    humor a.
AR
    analytical reagent
    AR grade
arabiensis
    Anopheles a.
arabinomannan (Am)
arabinose operon
arabinoside
    adenine a.
    cytosine a. (CA)
arabinosuria

NOTES

arabinotarda
    Shigella a.
arabitol test
Arabobacteria
arachidonate
arachidonic
    a. acid (AA)
    a. acidristocetin
    a. containing phosphatidyl ethanolamine
Arachis hypogaea
Arachnia propionica
Arachnida
arachnidism
Arachniotus
arachnodactyly
arachnoid
    a. cyst
    a. granulation
    a. trabeculae
    a. villus
arachnoideae
    granulationes a.
arachnoideus
    nevus a.
arachnoidism
arachnoiditis
    adhesive a.
    neoplastic a.
    obliterative a.
arachnolysin
Arachnomyces nodososetosus
araguata
    Stenella a.
Araldite
ARAM
    antigen receptor activation motif
Aran-Duchenne disease
araneism
araneosa
    Lentisphaera a.
araneus
    nevus a.
Arantius
    A. body
    A. canal
    A. duct
    A. ligament
    A. nodule
arborescence
arborescens
    lipoma a.
arborescent
arboris
    Ensifer a.
    Propionispira a.
arborization
arborize

arborizing pattern
arboroid
arboviral virus disease
arbovirus, arborvirus
    a. group A, B, C
    a. group unclassified
ARC
    AIDS-related complex
arcade
    Flint a.
Arcanobacterium
    A. haemolyticum
    A. hippocoleae
    A. pluranimalium
ARCD
    acquired renal cystic disease
arch
    Corti a.
Archaebacteria
Archaeobacteria
Archaeoglobaceae
Archaeoglobales
Archaeoglobea
Archaeoglobi
archamphiaster
Archangiaceae
archibaldi
    Leishmania donovani a.
archil
architectonics
architectural
    a. pattern
    a. sheeting
architecture
    bone a.
    crypt a.
    diagram of normal splenic a.
    effacement of lymph node a.
    loculated a.
    papillary/verrucous a.
archival brain tissue
arch-loop-whorl (ALW)
archnoid sheath
Arcicella aquatica
Arcobacter butzleri
arctation
arctica
    Desulfotalea a.
    Psychromonas a.
arcuata
    zona a.
arcuate
    a. nucleus
    a. zone
arcuatus uterus
arcus senilis
arc-welder's disease
ardor urinae

ARDS
    acute respiratory distress syndrome
    adult respiratory distress syndrome
area, pl. **areae**
    Betz cell a.
    body surface areas (BSA)
    Broca a.
    carcinoma with adenomatous areas
    (CWA)
    a. centralis
    clinical laboratory maximum a.
    Cohnheim a.
    congested centrilobular a.
    a. cribrosa
    a. cribrosa papillae renalis
    gray a.
    mean nuclear a. (MNA)
    paucicellular a.
    peak a.
    a. postrema
    radiation emergency a. (REA)
    regulated a.
    skip areae
    a. striata
areatus, pl. **areata**
    alopecia a.
arecoline
areflexia
areflexic quadriplegia
aregenerative anemia
arenacea
    corpora a.
arenaceous
Arenaviridae
Arenavirus
Arenibacter
    A. certesii
    A. latericius
    A. troitsensis
arenosus
    Psychrobacter a.
areola, pl. **areolae**
    Chaussier a.
areolar
    a. connective tissue
    a. gland
areolares
    glandulae a.
ARF
    acute renal failure
    acute respiratory failure
    acute rheumatic fever

Argas
    A. persicus
    A. reflexus
argasid
Argasidae
argentaffin, argentaffine
    a. cell
    a. granule
    a. reaction
    a. stain
argentaffinoma
argentation
Argentinean hemorrhagic fever
Argentine hemorrhagic fever virus
argentinense
    Clostridium a.
argentipes
    Phlebotomus a.
argentophil, argentophile
argentum (silver)
arginase
arginine
    a. deiminase
    a. glutamate
    a. hydrochloride
    a. insulin tolerance test (AITT)
    a. monohydrochloride
    a. stimulation test
    suberyl a.
    a. tolerance test (ATT)
    a. vasopressin (AVP)
argininemia
argininosuccinate
    a. lyase
    a. lyase assay
    a. synthetase
    a. synthetase deficiency
argininosuccinic
    a. acid
    a. acidemia
argininosuccinicaciduria
arginyl
Argo corn starch test
argon
Argonz-Del Castillo syndrome
Argyll
    A. Robertson pupil
    A. Robertson pupil sign
argyremia
argyria
argyrophil, argyrophile
    a. stain

NOTES

argyrophilic
    a. ductal carcinoma in situ
    a. enterochromaffin-like cell
    a. fiber
    a. grain dementia
    a. nucleolar organizer region
    (AgNOR)
argyrosis
arhinencephaly
Arias-Stella
    A.-S. cell
    A.-S. effect
    A.-S. phenomenon
    A.-S. reaction (ASR)
Arias syndrome
ariboflavinosis
aristata
    Tetraploa a.
Arizona
    A. hinshawii
    A. organism
arizonae
    Paracolobactrum a.
    Salmonella a.
arizonensis
    Lactobacillus a.
ARM
    artificial rupture of membranes
arm
    dynein a.
armamentarium
Armanni-Ebstein
    A.-E. cell
    A.-E. change
    A.-E. disease
    A.-E. kidney
    A.-E. lesion
armata
    Taenia a.
armchair immunology
armed
    A. Forces Institute of Pathology
    (AFIP)
    a. macrophage
Armigeres obturbans
Armillaria
armillatus
    Armillifer a.
    Porocephalus a.
Armillifer
    A. armillatus
    A. moniliformis
armored heart
ARMS
    alveolar rhabdomyosarcoma
Armstrong disease
Arndt-Gottron syndrome
Arneth
    A. classification

    A. count
    A. formula
    A. index
    A. stage
Arnium leporinum
Arnold
    A. body
    A. bundle
    A. canal
    A. ganglion
    A. nerve reflex cough syndrome
    A. tract
Arnold-Chiari
    A.-C. deformity
    A.-C. malformation
    A.-C. syndrome
aromatase
aromatic
    a. amine
    a. amino acid
    a. compound
    a. hydrocarbon
    a. ring
aromaticity
aromaticivorans
    Novosphingobium a.
aromatization
AR-PKD
    autosomal recessive polycystic kidney
    disease
arranged in series
arrangement
    bcl-2 gene a.
    organoid a.
array
    Affymetrix GeneChip HU95 a.
    A. 360, 360CE/CE-AL
      protein/drug/serology system
    oligonucleotide genomic a.
    whorl-like a.
array-based comparative genomic
  hybridization (aCGH)
arrector pili muscle
arrest
    cell cycle a.
    complete maturation a. (CMA)
    developmental a.
    epiphysial a.
    growth a.
    hematopoietic maturation a.
    maturation a.
    mitotic a.
    spermatogenic maturation a.
    a. of tumor emboli
arrested tuberculosis
arrhaphia
Arrhenius
    A. doctrine
    A. equation

A. formula
A. theory
Arrhenius-Madsen theory
arrhenoblastoma
androgenic a.
arrhinencephaly
arrhizus
Rhizopus a.
arrhythmogenicity
arrhythmogenic right ventricular dysplasia
arrival
dead on a. (DOA)
arrowhead
Arroyo sign
ARS
acute radiation syndrome
antirabies serum
ARS A
arylsulfatase A
arsenate
sodium a.
arsenaticum
Pyrobaculum a.
arsenazo III dye
arsenic
a. assay
a. hydride
a. keratosis
a. pigmentation
a. poisoning
a. stain
a. trihydride
arsenical keratosis
arsenic-fast
Arsenicicoccus bolidensis
arseniciselenatis
Bacillus a.
arsenide
hydrogen a.
arsenious hydride
arseniuretted hydrogen
arsenophilum
Sulfurospirillum a.
arsenoxide
arsine
a. gas
NATO code for a. (SA)
ART
absolute retention time
Aerosol Resistant Tips

antiretroviral treatment
automated reagin test
Artemisia annua
arteria, gen. and pl. **arteriae**
arteriae arcuatae renis
arterial
a. blood
a. blood collection
a. blood gas (ABG)
a. blood gas analysis
a. blood oximetry
a. cannulation
a. capillary
a. embolism
a. hemangioma
a. hypertension
a. insufficiency
a. line culture
a. nephrosclerosis
a. occlusive disease (AOD)
a. oxygen saturation
a. pCO_2
a. pO_2
a. pressure
a. sclerosis
a. spider
a. thrombosis
arterialization of vein
arterialized blood
arteries (*pl. of* artery)
arterioatony
arteriocapillary sclerosis
arteriococcygeal gland
arteriola, gen. and pl. **arteriolae**
arteriolae rectae
arteriolar
a. nephrosclerosis
a. sclerosis
a. thrombonecrosis
arteriole
hepatic a.
tunica media of a.
arteriolith
arteriolitis
necrotizing a.
arteriolization of venous blood
arteriolonecrosis
arteriolonephrosclerosis (ANS)
arteriolosclerosis
hyaline a.
arteriolosclerotic kidney
arteriolovenular bridge

NOTES

arteriomalacia
arteriomyomatosis
arterionephrosclerosis
arteriopathy
    hypertensive a.
    plexogenic pulmonary a.
arterioplania
arteriorrhexis
arteriosclerosis (AS, ATS)
    hyperplastic a.
    hypertensive a.
    medial a.
    Mönckeberg a.
    nodular a.
    a. obliterans
    renal artery a.
    senile a.
arteriosclerotic
    a. aortic aneurysm
    a. cardiovascular disease (ASCVD)
    a. gangrene
    a. heart disease (AHD)
    a. kidney
    a. thrombosed aneurysm
arteriostenosis
arteriosus
    double ductus a.
    patent ductus a.
    persistent truncus a. (PTA)
    pseudotruncus a.
    truncus a.
arteriovenous
    a. anastomosis (AVA)
    a. aneurysm
    a. carbon dioxide
    a. carbon dioxide difference
    a. fistula (AVF)
    a. malformation (AVM)
    a. oxygen difference
arteritica
    polymyalgia a.
arteritis
    cranial a.
    equine viral a.
    giant cell a.
    a. nodosa
    a. obliterans
    obliterating a.
    rheumatic a.
    rheumatoid a.
    Takayasu a.
    temporal a.
Arterivirus
artery, pl. **arteries**
    branches of the carotid a.
    branches of the mesenteric a.
    copper-wire a.
    distributing a.
    dolichoectatic a.

elastic laminae of a.
elastic layer of a.
end a.
medium a.
muscular a.
obturator a.
occlusion of arteries
a. of the penis
pipestem a.
a. of pulp
screw a.
sheathed a.
small a.
spiral a.
supernumerary segmental a.
transposition of great arteries
    (TGA)
uninvolved a.
artery-to-artery anastomosis
artery-to-vein anastomosis
Arthobotrys oligospora
arthragra
arthralgia
    rheumatic a.
    a. saturnina
Arthrinium
arthritic calculus
arthriticum
    tuberculum a.
arthritidis
    Actinobacillus a.
arthritis, pl. **arthritides**
    acute rheumatic a.
    atrophic a.
    chronic absorptive a.
    chronic proliferative a.
    chronic villous a.
    chylous a.
    crystal-induced a.
    a. deformans
    degenerative a.
    exudative a.
    filarial a.
    gonococcal a.
    gouty a.
    hypertrophic a.
    infectious a.
    inflammatory a.
    Jaccoud a.
    juvenile rheumatoid a. (JRA)
    a. mutilans
    navicular a.
    neuropathic a.
    a. nodosa
    ochronotic a.
    a. of probable autoimmune origin
    proliferative chronic a.
    psoriatic a.
    rheumatoid a. (RA)

septic a.
suppurative a.
a. uratica
vertebral a.
arthritis-dermatitis syndrome
Arthrobacter
    A. *chlorophenolicus*
    A. *flavus*
    A. *gandavensis*
    A. *koreensis*
    A. *luteolus*
    A. *methylotrophus*
    A. *nasiphocae*
    A. *nitroguajacolicus*
    A. *roseus*
    A. *russicus*
    A. *sulfonivorans*
Arthrobacteria
Arthrobotrys
arthrocentesis
arthrochondritis
arthroconidium
Arthroderma
arthrogram
Arthrographis langeroni
arthrography
    facet joint a.
arthrokatadysis
arthrolith
arthrolithiasis
arthroonychodysplasia
arthroophthalmopathy
    hereditary progressive a.
arthropathy
    Charcot a.
    hemophilic a.
    Jaccoud a.
    neurogenic a.
    osteopulmonary a.
arthrophyma
arthropica
    psoriasis a.
Arthropoda
arthropod-borne
    a.-b. viral disease
    a.-b. virus encephalitis
arthropodiasis
arthropodic
arthropod identification
Arthropsis hispanica
arthrosis
arthrospore

arthrosynovitis
arthrotropic
Arthus
    A. phenomenon
    A. reaction
articular
    a. calculus
    a. capsule
    a. chondrocalcinosis
    a. corpuscle
    a. gout
    a. lamella
    a. leprosy
    a. rheumatism
articularia
    corpuscula a.
articularis
    capsula a.
    membrana fibrosa capsulae a.
    stratum fibrosum capsulae a.
articulated
articuli
    empyema a.
artifact
    bubble a.
    cautery a.
    crush a.
    electrical a.
    fixation a.
    iatrogenic a.
    movement a.
    perimortem a.
    retraction a.
    shock a.
    tissue a.
    xylene a.
artifactitious
artifactual
artificial
    a. abortion
    a. active immunity
    a. kidney
    a. leech
    a. melanin
    a. passive immunity
    a. rupture of membranes (ARM)
Artyfechinostomum
arupensis
    Bartonella vinsonii subsp. *a.*
ARV
    AIDS-related virus
Arxiozyma

NOTES

Arxula adeninivorans
arylaminopeptidase
arylesterase
aryl-ester hydrolase
aryl group
arylsulfatase
    a. A (ARS A)
    a. test
arytenoid gland
arytenoiditis
AS
    Adams-Stokes disease
    antistreptolysin
    arteriosclerosis
    atherosclerosis
ASA
    acetylsalicylic acid
    Adams-Stokes attack
asaccharolytica
    Porphyromonas a.
asaccharolyticus
    Peptococcus a.
    Peptoniphilus a.
    Peptostreptococcus a.
asahii
    Trichosporon a.
Asaia
    A. bogorensis
    A. krungthepensis
    A. siamensis
Asanoa
    A. ferruginea
    A. ishikariensis
ASAP biopsy system
asbestoid
ASBESTOS
    agent, state, body site, effects, severity,
    time course, other (diagnoses),
    synergism
asbestos
    a. body (AB)
    a. transformation
asbestosis
ASCA
    anti-*Saccharomyces cerevisiae* antibody
    ASCA antibody
ascariasis, ascaridiasis
    a. serological test
ascaricidal
ascaricide
ascarid, pl. ascarides
Ascaridae
Ascaridata
ascarides (*pl. of* ascarid)
Ascaridia
ascaridiasis (*var. of* ascariasis)
Ascaridida
Ascarididae
Ascaridoidea

Ascaridorida
Ascaris
    A. alata
    A. canis
    A. equorum
    A. lumbricoides
    A. mystax
    A. pneumonitis
    A. suum
ascaron
Ascarops strongylina
ascending
    a. cholangitis
    a. chromatography
    a. degeneration
    a. myelitis
    a. pyelonephritis
Aschelminthes
Ascher syndrome
Aschheim-Zondek (A-Z)
    A.-Z. hormone
    A.-Z. pregnancy test
Aschoff
    A. body
    A. cell
    A. nodule
Aschoff-Rokitansky sinus
asci (*pl. of* ascus)
ascites
    a. adiposus
    cardiac a.
    chyliform a.
    a. chylosus
    chylous a.
    cirrhotic a.
    fatty a.
    gelatinous a.
    hemorrhagic a.
    malignancy-related a.
    milky a.
    nephrogenous a.
    pancreatic a.
    pseudochylous a.
ascitic
    a. agar
    a. fluid
ascitogenous
Ascobolus
ascocarp
Ascochyta
Ascocoryne
Ascodesmis
Ascodichaena
ascogenous
ascogonium
Ascoidea
Ascoli
    A. reaction
    A. test

ascomycete
Ascomycetes
ascomycetous
Ascomycota
Ascomycotina
ascorbate
    sodium a.
ascorbate-cyanide test
ascorbic
    a. acid
    a. acid assay
    a. acid test
Ascosphaera
Ascospora campanulae
ascospore
ascospore-forming fungus
Ascotricha novae-caledoniae
Ascovirus
ASCUS
    atypical squamous cells of undetermined
        significance
    ASM subset of ASCUS
ascus, pl. asci
ASCVD
    arteriosclerotic cardiovascular disease
    atherosclerotic cardiovascular disease
ASD
    aldosterone secretion defect
    atrial septal defect
asepsis
aseptate
aseptic
    a. meningitis
    a. necrosis
asexual reproduction
ASF
    aniline, sulfur, formaldehyde
Asfivirus
ASGPR
    asialoglycoprotein receptor
ASH
    asymmetric septal hypertrophy
Ashbya
Ashby differential agglutination method
Asherman syndrome
ashfordi
    Parasaccharomyces a.
ash-leaf spot
asialoglycoprotein receptor (ASGPR)
asiatica
    Nocardia a.
Asiatic cholera

asiaticus
    Streptomyces a.
asiderosis
asiderotic anemia
asini
    Strongylus a.
asinigenitalis
    Taylorella a.
Askanazy cell
Askin tumor
Ask-Upmark kidney
ASM
    atypical squamous metaplasia
    ASM subset of ASCUS
ASMA
    alpha smooth muscle actin
    antismooth muscle antibody
ASMI
    anteroseptal myocardial infarct
ASN
    alkali-soluble nitrogen
Asn
    asparagine
ASO
    antistreptolysin O
    ASO probe
    ASO test
    ASO titer
As_2O_3
    arsenic trioxide
ASP
    antibody specificity prediction
Asp
    aspartic acid
asparaginase
asparagine (Asn, N)
asparaginic acid
asparaginyl
aspartate
    a. aminotransferase (AST)
    a. aminotransferase assay
    a. kinase
    potassium aspartate and
        magnesium a.
    a. transaminase
aspartic
    a. acid (Asp)
    a. proteinase
aspartokinase
aspartyl
aspartylglycosaminuria
aspergilloma

NOTES

aspergillosis
    allergic bronchopulmonary a.
      (ABPA)
    bronchopulmonary a.
    disseminated a.
    invasive a.
    pulmonary a.
    rhinocerebral a.
Aspergillus
    A. antibody test
    A. *auricularis*
    A. *barbae*
    A. *bouffardi*
    A. *candidus*
    A. *clavatus*
    A. *concentricus*
    A. *fisherii*
    A. *flavus*
    A. *fumigatus*
    A. fungus ball
    A. *giganteus*
    A. *glaucus*
    A. *gliocladium*
    A. *mucoroides*
    A. *nidulans*
    A. *niger*
    A. *ochraceus*
    A. *parasiticus*
    A. *pictor*
    A. *repens*
    A. serology
    A. *terreus*
    A. *versicolor*
aspermatism
aspermatogenesis
    induced a.
aspermia
asperum
    Trichocladium a.
aspheric
asphyxia
    autoerotic a.
    intrauterine a.
    mechanical a.
    positional a.
asphyxial
asphyxiant
    chemical a.
    simple a.
asphyxiating
    a. thoracic chondrodystrophy
    a. thoracic dysplasia
    a. thoracic dystrophy (ATD)
asphyxiation
Aspiculuris tetraptera
aspidium oleoresin
aspirate
    bronchotracheal a.
    nasopharyngeal a.

aspiration
    a. biopsy
    a. biopsy cytology (ABC)
    bone marrow a.
    a. of endometrium
    fine-needle a. (FNA)
    foreign body a.
    lung a.
    meconium a.
    microsurgical epididymal sperm a.
      (MESA)
    mineral oil a.
    newborn a.
    a. pneumonia
    a. pneumonitis
    suprapubic needle a.
    tracheal a.
    transbronchial needle a. (TBNA)
    uterine a. (UA)
    vacuum a. (VA)
    wound a.
aspirator
    water a.
aspirin
    long-term treatment with a.
    a. poisoning
    a. tolerance
    a. tolerance test
    a. toxicity
ASPIRINcheck urine test
asplenia
asplenic
asporogenic
asporogenous
asporous
asporulate
ASPS
    alveolar soft-part sarcoma
ASR
    aldosterone secretion rate
    aldosterone secretory rate
    analyte-specific reagent
    Arias-Stella reaction
assassin bug
assay (*See also* test, kit)
    Abbott AxSYM Prizm HCV a.
    Access testosterone a.
    acetaminophen a.
    acetylcholinesterase a.
    acid phosphatase a.
    adenosine deaminase a.
    ADH a.
    adhesion a.
    ADN-B a.
    adrenocorticotropic hormone a.
    agglutination inhibition a.
    AH a.
    air bleb a.
    alanine aminotransferase a.

albumin a.
alcohol a.
aldolase a.
aldosterone a.
alkaline phosphatase a.
alpha-2 antiplasmin functional a.
alpha-1 fetoprotein a.
Ames a.
amino acid fractionation a.
amitriptyline and nortriptyline a.'s
ammonia a.
amphetamine a.
Amplicor Chlamydia a.
amylase a.
antibody capture ligand a.
anti-DNA antibody a.
anti-DNaseB a.
antigen capture ligand a.
antigenic a.
antihyaluronidase a.
antimitochondrial antibody a.
antimony a.
antinuclear antibody a.
antiparietal cell antibody a.
antismooth muscle antibody a.
anti-Xa a.
aortic explant a.
Aptima Combo 2 a.
APTT STA a.
argininosuccinate lyase a.
arsenic a.
ascorbic acid a.
aspartate aminotransferase a.
Auto Dimer a.
Aware Rapid HIV a.
bacterial inhibition a.
bacterial killing a.
barbiturate a.
Bayer Immuno 1 HER-2/neu a.
Bayer Versant HCV RNA 3.0 a.
Beckman a.
benzene a.
benzodiazepine a.
beta-hydroxybutyrate a.
bile acid a.
bilirubin a.
Bioclot protein S a.
biologic a.
biological a.
Bio-Rad protein a.
biotin a.
bismuth a.

blastogenesis a.
blood spot screening a.
B-lymphocyte a.
boron a.
branched DNA signal
  amplification a.
Breslow malignant melanoma a.
bromide a.
butanol-extractable iodine a.
CA19-9 a.
CA125 a.
cadmium a.
caffeine a.
calcitonin a.
calcium ionized a.
CALLA a.
camphor a.
capture a.
carbamazepine a.
carbaryl a.
carbon dioxide concentration a.
carbon disulfide a.
carbon monoxide a.
carbon tetrachloride a.
carboxyhemoglobin a.
Cardiac STATus rapid a.
Cardiac T rapid a.
carotene a.
catecholamine a.
^{13}C bicarbonate a.
CEA a.
CEDIA sirolimus a.
cell-mediated lympholysis a.
CellProbe HT caspase-3/7 whole
  cell a.
cerebrospinal fluid a.
ceruloplasmin a.
chemiluminescence a.
chemiluminescent a. (CLIA)
chemotaxis a.
Chlamydiazyme EIA a.
chloral hydrate a.
chloranil a.
chlorate a.
chlordiazepoxide a.
chlorinated hydrocarbon pesticide a.
chloroform a.
chlorohydrocarbon a.
chlorpromazine a.
cholesterol a.
cholinesterase a.
chorionic gonadotropin a.

NOTES

assay *(continued)*
  chromatographic a.
  chromium a.
  chromogenic Xa inhibition a.
  citric acid a.
  clonogenic a.
  Clostridium difficile toxin a.
  coagulation factor a.
  cobalt a.
  cocaine metabolite a.
  codeine a.
  collagen gel invasion a.
  4-color PCR a.
  competitive binding a.
  competitive protein-binding a.
  complement binding a.
  compressed spectral a. (CSA)
  copper a.
  coproporphyrin a.
  cortisol a.
  CPB a.
  C-reactive protein a.
  creatine kinase a.
  creatinine a.
  cresol a.
  C-terminal a.
  cyanide a.
  cytochrome b5 reductase a.
  cytolytic T-cell lysis a.
  cytotoxicity a.
  DCC a.
  D-dimer a.
  DDT a.
  DeBakey aortic a.
  delta aminolevulinic acid a.
  depramine a.
  desipramine a.
  DHPLC a.
  diazepam a.
  dihydroxycholecalciferol a.
  dimeric inhibin-A a.
  diquat a.
  direct fluorescence a. (DFA)
  direct fluorescent a. (DFA)
  disulfiram a.
  double antibody
    immunoenzymometric a.
  double antibody sandwich a.
  doxepin hydrochloride a.
  drug screening a.
  EAC rosette a.
  E erythrocyte rosette a.
  Elecsys Anti-HBe a.
  electrophoretic mobility shift a.
  ELISA titer a.
  ELISPOT enzymatic test a.
  endorphin a.
  endotoxin activity a. (EAA)
  enzyme a.
  enzyme-linked immunosorbent a.
    (ELISA)
  epinephrine and norepinephrine a.'s
  Epstein-Barr virus antibody a.
  Erlanger and Gasser peripheral
    nerve a.
  erythrocyte antibody complement
    rosette a.
  erythroid colony a.
  ESR a.
  estradiol a.
  estriol a.
  estrogen receptor a. (ERA)
  ethanol a.
  ethchlorvynol a.
  ethosuximide a.
  ethylene glycol a.
  factor III multimer a.
  fat a.
  fatty acid a.
  ferritin a.
  fibrin clot retraction a.
  fibrinogen a.
  FiF a.
  flow cytometric a.
  fluorescent cytoprint a.
  fluorescent protection a.
  fluoride a.
  fluoroacetate a.
  fluorocarbon a.
  folic acid a.
  follicle-stimulating hormone a.
  fructose a.
  FSH a.
  FSH-RH a.
  galactose a.
  gastrin a.
  GGT a.
  glucose a.
  glucosephosphate isomerase a.
  glucosylceramidase a.
  glutathione reductase a.
  glutethimide a.
  glycine a.
  glycosylated hemoglobin a.
  gold a.
  Groome a.
  guanine deaminase a.
  Guthrie bacterial inhibition a.
    (GBIA)
  halogenated hydrocarbon a.
  haloperidol a.
  halothane a.
  hamster egg penetration a.
  haptoglobin a.
  HDL cholesterol a.
  hemagglutination inhibition a.
  Hemochron Jr. Citrate PT a.
  hemoglobin F, H a.

hemolytic plaque a.
hemolytic tube a.
heparin-induced platelet
  activation a. (HIPA)
HercepTest breast cancer
  immunohistochemical a.
heterogeneous a.
hexachlorophene a.
Hexaplex a.
histocompatibility a.
histoculture drug response a.
  (HDRA)
Histoplasma antibody a.
homogeneous ligand a.
hybridization protection a. (HPA)
hydroxyapatite a.
17-hydroxycorticosteroid a.
5-hydroxyindoleacetic acid a.
hydroxyproline a.
25-hydroxyvitamin D a.
iditol dehydrogenase a.
imipramine and desipramine a.'s
ImmuKnow immune cell
  function a.
Immulite free PSA a.
Immulite 2000 PSA a.
Immulite third-generation PSA a.
immune adherence
  hemagglutination a. (IAHA)
immunochemical a.
immunoconcentration a.
immunocytochemical a. (ICA)
Immuno 1 DPD a.
immunoenzymometric a.
immunofluorescence a. (IFA)
immunofluorescent a.
immunoluminometric a.
immunometric a. (IMA)
immunoradiometric a. (IRMA)
indirect a.
inhibitor a.
iodide a.
ionized calcium a.
iron a.
isocitrate dehydrogenase a.
isoniazid a.
isopropanol a.
IVTT a.
Jaffe a.
Jerne plaque a.
17-ketogenic steroids a.
17-ketosteroid a.

lactate dehydrogenase a.
lactic acid a.
LATS a.
LDL cholesterol a.
lead a.
leukotactic a.
lidocaine a.
ligand a.
limulus amebocyte lysate a.
lipase a.
lipid a.
Lipi+Plus direct HDL a.
Lipi+Plus direct LDL a.
lipoprotein a.
liquid-phase hybridization
  protection a.
lithium a.
LMC a.
LOH a.
LRP a.
luteinizing hormone a.
lymphocyte marker a.
lymphocyte microcytotoxicity a.
lysergic acid diethylamide a.
lysozyme a.
macroglobulin a.
magnesium a.
manganese a.
MBP a.
meprobamate a.
mercury a.
mersalyl exchange a.
metanephrine a.
methadone a.
methanol a.
methaqualone a.
methemalbumin a.
3,4-methylenedioxyamphetamine a.
methylphenidate
methyprylon a.
metronidazole a.
microalbumin
  immunoturbidimetric a.
microarray expression profiling a.
microbiologic a.
microbiological a. (MB)
microhemagglutination a. (MHA)
microlymphocytotoxicity a.
microtoxicity a.
mitogen a.
mixed lymphocyte culture a.
MLC a.

NOTES

assay *(continued)*
  molecular a.
  morphine a.
  MUC1 gene derived
    glycoprotein a.
  mucoprotein a.
  multiplex reverse transcription PCR
    enzyme hybridization a.
  NAP modified LRP a.
  NaSCN exchange a.
  NBT reduction a.
  nephelometric inhibition a. (NIA)
  nitroblue tetrazolium dye
    reduction a.
  noncompetitive a.
  NucliSens CMV a.
  NucliSens HIV-1 QT a.
  one-stage factor a.
  opiate a.
  Opus cardiac troponin I a.
  organothiophosphate compound a.
  ornithine carbamoyltransferase a.
  osteoblast proliferation
    fluorometric a.
  osteoclastic factor a.
  oxalic acid a.
  pantothenic acid a.
  paraldehyde a.
  paraquat a.
  pentose a.
  pepsinogen a.
  phagocytosis a.
  phencyclidine a.
  phenobarbital a.
  phenol a.
  phenothiazine tranquilizers a.
  phenylalanine a.
  phenylbutazone a.
  phenytoin a.
  phosphate a.
  phosphogluconate dehydrogenase a.
  phospholipid a.
  phosphorus a.
  phytohemagglutinin a.
  plaque-forming cell a.
  plasma clot solubility a.
  plasminogen activator inhibitor a.
  p-methoxyamphetamine a.
  polychlorinated biphenyl a.
  polyethylene glycol precipitation a.
  porphobilinogen synthase a.
  porphyrin a.
  potassium a.
  PP-CAP H. pylori IgA a.
  ^{32}P-postlabeling a.
  PRA-Stat enzyme linked
    immunosorbent a.
  pregnanediol a.

  PreVue *Borrelia burgdorferi*
    antibody detection a.
  primidone a.
  procainamide a.
  Procleix HIV-1/HCV A.
  progesterone receptor a. (PRA)
  properdin a.
  propoxyphene a.
  propranolol a.
  ProSpecT *Clostridium difficile* toxin
    A microplate a.
  protamine sulfate a.
  protein-bound iodine a.
  protein-protein binding a.
  protein truncation a.
  protoporphyrin a.
  protriptyline a.
  PSFR a.
  PTH a.
  pyrimethamine a.
  pyruvate kinase a.
  pyruvic acid a.
  quinidine a.
  quinine a.
  radioallergosorbent a.
  radioenzymatic a. (REA)
  radioimmunoprecipitation a. (RIPA)
  radioligand a.
  radioreceptor a. (RRA)
  Raji cell radioimmune a.
  rapid susceptibility a. (RSA)
  receptor a.
  recombinant immunoblot a. (RIBA)
  renal venous renin a. (RVRA)
  renin a.
  Retic-Chex linearity a.
  reverse hemolytic plaque a.
  riboflavin a.
  ribonuclease protection a.
  RID a.
  saccharogenic a.
  salicylate a.
  sandwich nucleic acid
    hybridization a.
  saturation and displacement a.
  selenium a.
  serial cardiac isoenzyme a.
  serotonin a.
  serotonin release a. (SRA)
  Simplify D-dimer a.
  single-agent kinetic enzyme a.
  single-analyte immunologic a.
  single-analyte molecular a.
  slide immunoenzymatic a. (SIA)
  sodium and potassium a.'s
  spectrophotometric a.
  sperm penetration a.
  SPIFE acid hemoglobin a.
  SPIFE alkaline hemoglobin a.

SSCP a.
Stamper-Woodruff a.
staphylococcal protein A binding a.
stem cell a.
stool toxin a.
strychnine a.
sucrose pad nuclear exchange a.
sugar assimilation a.
sugar fermentation a.
sulfonamide a.
sulfonylurea a.
superoxide a.
Syva EMIT-II a.
TBG a.
T and B lymphocyte subset a.
tellurium a.
telomeric repeat amplification
 protocol a.
thallium a.
theophylline a.
thiamine a.
thiamphenicol a.
thioridazine a.
thyroid-stimulating hormone a.
thyroxine a.
thyroxine-binding globulin a.
tissue culture cytotoxin a. (TCCA)
total calcium a.
TPI a.
transferrin a.
transketolase a.
TRAP a.
Treponema pallidum
 hemagglutination a. (TPHA)
Treponema pallidum
 immobilization a.
triglyceride a.
triiodothyronine a.
triosephosphate isomerase a.
trypsin a.
TSH a.
TUNEL a.
two-site immunoenzymometric a.
tyrosine a.
UDP-glucose-hexose-1-phosphate
 uridylyltransferase a.
urea nitrogen a.
uric acid a.
urobilin a.
urobilinogen a.
uromucoid a.
uropepsinogen a.

uroporphyrin a.
vancomycin-resistant enterococci a.
Versant HCV RNA 3.0 a.
vitamin A and carotene a.'s
vitamin B_6 a.
vitamin B_{12} a.
vitamin D a.
vitamin E a.
vitamin K a.
in vitro invasion a.
Vitros anti-HBs a.
Vitros HBsAg a.
volatile organic substances a.
von Kossa calcium a.
warfarin a.
zinc a.
Asserachrom
 A. APA immunoassay
 A. D-Dimer kit
assessment
 cancer risk a.
 histocompatibility a.
 purinergic receptor translocation a.
assignment statement
assimilation limit
assistant
 Certified Laboratory A.
Assmann tuberculous infiltrate
associate
 microbial a.
associated macrophage
association
 American Clinical Laboratory A.
 (ACLA)
 American Urological A. (AUA)
 CHARGE a.
 a. constant
 independent practice a.
 a. system
 a. tract
associative reaction
assortative mating
assortment
 independent a.
assurance
 quality a. (QA)
AST
 aspartate aminotransferase
 AST test
astacoid rash
astasia
astatine

NOTES

asteatosis
aster
asterixis
Asterococcus
asteroid body
asteroides
    Nocardia a.
    Trichophyton a.
    Trichosporon a.
Asterophora
asthma
    allergic a.
    alveolar a.
    atopic a.
    bronchial a. (BA)
    chronic bronchitis with a. (CBA)
    cotton dust a.
    a. crystal
    emphysematous a.
    essential a.
    exercise-induced a.
    extrinsic a.
    grinder's a.
    hay a.
    intrinsic a.
    miller's a.
    miner's a.
    potter's a.
    steam-fitter's a.
    stone-stripper's a.
    summer a.
asthmatic bronchitis (AB)
asthmaticus
    status a.
asthmogenic
Astler-Coller modification of Dukes classification
astomatous
Astra blood chemistry profile
astral fiber
astringent
astroblastoma
astrocele
astrocyte
    Alzheimer type I, II a.
    atypical a.
    fibrillar a.
    fibrillary a.
    fibrous a.
    gemistocytic a.
    perivascular fibrous a.
    protoplasmic a.
    reactive a.
    a. stain
    a. staining
astrocytic
    a. foot process
    a. neoplasm
    a. tumor

astrocytoma
    anaplastic a.
    cerebellar a.
    desmoplastic cerebral a.
    fibrillary a.
    fibrous a.
    gemistocytic a.
    grade I–IV a.
    juvenile cerebellar a.
    juvenile pilocytic a.
    low grade a.
    pigmented pilocytic a.
    pilocytic a.
    piloid a.
    protoplasmic a.
    subependymal giant cell a.
astrocytosis cerebri
astroependymoma
astroglia cell
astrokinetic
astronyxis
    Acanthamoeba a.
astrosphere
Astrup method
Astwood test
ASV
    antisnake venom
As/V
    ampere-second per volt
asymmetric
    a. carbon atom
    a. chondrodystrophy
    a. septal hypertrophy (ASH)
    a. unit membrane
    a. uterus
asymmetry
asymptomatic
    a. carrier
    a. coccidioidomycosis
    a. interval
    a. viremia
asymptote
asynapsis
asynchronism
asynchronous data transmission
asynchrony
asynechia
asystematic
AT III
    antithrombin III
ATA
    anti-*Toxoplasma* antibody
atabrine hydrochloride
Atadenovirus
atavistic phenomenon
ataxia
    a. telangiectasia
    a. telangiectasia syndrome
ataxia-telangiectasia

ataxin gene
ATC
    aggressive thyroid carcinoma
ATCC
    American Type Culture Collection
ATD
    asphyxiating thoracic dystrophy
ATDLG
    antithoracic duct lymphocytic globulin
atelectasis
    a. neonatorum
    obstructive a.
    primary a.
    round a.
    rounded a.
    secondary a.
atelia
ateliosis
ateliotic
Atelosaccharomyces
ATG
    antithymocyte globulin
    antithyroglobulin
AT:GC
    adenine-thymine/guanine-cytosine ratio
Athelia
atheroembolism
atherogenesis
atherogenic
atherogenicity
atheroma embolism
atheromatosis
atheromatous
    a. degeneration
    a. embolism
    a. embolus
    a. plaque
atherosclerosis (AS)
    aortoiliac a.
atherosclerotic
    a. aneurysm
    a. cardiovascular disease (ASCVD)
    a. heart disease (AHD)
atherosis
atherothromboembolism
atherothrombosis
atherothrombotic
athetoid
athetosis
athetotic
athletes
    albuminuria of a.

athlete's foot
athletic heart
athrepsia
athrocytosis
athrombia
ATL
    adult T-cell leukemia
    adult T-cell lymphoma
atlantica
    Ruegeria a.
atlanticus
    Aedes a.
    Croceibacter a.
    Thermococcus a.
atlantoaxial subluxation
ATLL
    adult T-cell leukemia/lymphoma
    adult T-cell lymphoma/leukemia
    smoldering form of ATLL
atmosphere
    a. absolute
    explosive a.
atmospheric monitoring
ATN
    acute tubular necrosis
atom
    asymmetric carbon a.
atomic
    a. absorption
    a. absorption spectrophotometer (AAS)
    a. absorption spectrophotometry (AAS)
    a. absorption spectroscopy
    a. force microscopy (AFM)
    a. mass
    a. mass unit (amu)
    a. number
    a. spectrum
    a. weight
    a. weight unit (awu)
atomization
atomizer
atony
atopen
atopic
    a. allergen
    a. allergy
    a. asthma
    a. dermatitis
    a. disease
    a. reagin

NOTES

Atopobacter phocae
Atopobium
Atopostipes suicloacalis
atopy
ATP
  adenosine triphosphate
    extracellular ATP
    ATP pyrophosphohydrolase
ATP7B gene
ATPase
  adenosine triphosphatase
    calcium-activated ATPase
    magnesium-activated ATPase
    Padykula-Herman stain for myosin
      ATPase
    ATPase stain
ATP-binding cassette (ABC)
ATPS
  ambient temperature and pressure,
    saturated
ATRA
  all-*trans*-retinoic acid
atrabiliaris
  glandula a.
atrabiliary capsule
atransferrinemia
Atrax robustus
atrepsy
atresia
  anal a.
  a. ani
  aortic a.
  biliary a.
  choanal a.
  colon a.
  congenital a.
  duodenal a.
  esophageal a.
  extrahepatic biliary a. (EHBA)
  follicular a.
  intestinal a.
  mitral a.
  prepyloric a.
  pulmonary a.
  tricuspid a.
  ureteral a.
  vaginal a.
  valvular a.
atresic
atretic
  a. corpus luteum
  a. ovarian follicle
atreticum
  corpus a.
atretocystia
atretogastria
atria (*pl. of* atrium)
atrial
  a. infarction

  a. myxoma
  a. natriuretic factor
  a. natriuretic peptide (ANP)
  a. septal defect (ASD)
  a. septum
atrichous
atriodigital dysplasia
atriomegaly
atriopeptin
atrioventricular (AV)
  a. block
  a. bundle
  a. valve
atrioventricularis
  fasciculus a.
  truncus fascicularis a.
atrium, pl. **atria**
  accessory a.
  epicardium of a.
Atropa
atrophedema
atrophia
  acne a.
  a. blanche
  a. maculosa varioliformis cutis
atrophic
  a. arthritis
  a. chronic gastritis
  a. endometrium
  a. fenestration
  a. glossitis
  a. inflammation
  a. kidney
  a. lichen planus
  a. microcrypt
  a. pharyngitis
  a. rhinitis
  a. rhinitis of swine
  a. thrombosis
atrophica, pl. **atrophicae**
  hyperkeratosis figurata centrifuga a.
  lineae atrophicae
  macula a.
  striae atrophicae
atrophicans
  acrodermatitis chronica a.
  dermatitis a.
atrophicus
  lichen sclerosus et a.
atrophied
atrophin gene
atrophoderma
  a. albidum
  a. maculatum
  a. neuriticum
  a. of Pasini and Pierini
  a. pigmentosum
  a. reticulatum

atrophy
acquired a.
acute yellow a.
brain a.
brown a.
cerebral a.
Charcot-Marie-Tooth muscular a.
circumscribed a.
compensatory a.
cyanotic a.
cystic a.
dentatorubral pallidoluysian a.
  (DRPLA)
disuse a.
essential a.
exhaustion a.
fatty a.
focal a.
gelatinous a.
granular a.
Gudden a.
gyrate a.
hypertrophic polyneuritic-type
  muscular a.
infantile muscular a.
ischemic muscular a.
Kienböck a.
Leber optic a.
lobar cerebral a.
macular a.
marantic a.
mucinous a.
multiple system a.
muscular a.
neuritic a.
neurogenic muscular a. (NMA)
neurotrophic a.
olivocerebellar a.
olivopontocerebellar a.
optic a.
peroneal muscular a.
Pick a.
polyneuritic-type hypertrophic
  muscular a.
postmenopausal a.
pressure a.
progressive spinal muscular a.
red a.
senile a.
serous a.
simple a.
small muscle a. (SMA)

spinal muscular a. (SMA)
subtotal villous a. (STVA)
Sudeck a.
traction a.
traumatic a.
villous a.
atropine
a. autoinjector
a. suppression test
atrosepticum
  Pectobacterium a.
Atroxin solution
AT/RT
atypical teratoid/rhabdoid tumor
ATRT-CNS
atypical teratoid/rhabdoid tumor of the
  CNS
ATS
antitetanic serum
antithymocyte serum
arteriosclerosis
ATSDR
Agency for Toxic Substances & Disease
  Registry
ATT
arginine tolerance test
atypical teratoid tumor
attached cranial section
attachment
epithelial a.
muscle-tendon a.
pericemental a.
a. plaques
spindle a.
attack
Adams-Stokes a. (ASA)
agroterrorist a.
a. rate
transient ischemic a. (TIA)
vasovagal a.
attenuant
attenuate
attenuated
a. culture
a. familial adenomatous polyposis
a. strain
a. tuberculosis
a. vaccine
a. viral form
a. virus
attenuation
ground glass a.

NOTES

attenuator
AttoFluor RatioVision
attracted
> chemotactically a.

attraction sphere
atypia
> cellular a.
> condylomatous a.
> cytologic a.
> cytonuclear a.
> koilocytotic a.

atypica
> *Veillonella parvula* subsp. *a.*

atypical
> a. adenomatous hyperplasia (AAH)
> a. apocrine hyperplasia
> a. astrocyte
> a. carcinoid
> a. carcinoid tumor
> a. cell
> a. chronic myeloid leukemia (aCML)
> a. ductal hyperplasia (ADH)
> a. endometrial hyperplasia
> a. favor reactive
> a. fibrous histiocytoma
> a. fibroxanthoma (AFX)
> a. glandular cell of undetermined significance (AGUS)
> a. glandular cell of unknown significance (AGUS)
> a. insulin
> a. lipoma
> a. lymphocyte
> a. measles
> a. medullary carcinoma
> a. melanocytic hyperplasia
> a. melanocytic nevi of genital type (AMNGT)
> a. melanocytic nevus (AMN)
> a. mycobacteria
> a. mycobacteria infection
> a. polypoid adenomyofibroma (APA)
> a. polypoid adenomyofibroma of low malignant potential (APA-LMP)
> a. polypoid adenomyoma (APA)
> a. primary pneumonia
> a. regeneration
> a. squamous cells of undetermined significance (ASCUS)
> a. squamous metaplasia (ASM)
> a. verrucous endocarditis

atypicum
> *Corynebacterium a.*

atypism

AU
> antitoxin unit
> Australia

AUA
> American Urological Association
> AUA bladder cancer staging classification

AU Ag
> Australia antigen

Auchmeromyia luteola
AuCN
> gold cyanide

audio amplifier
auditiva
> tuba a.

auditivae
> cellulae pneumaticae tubae a.
> lamina lateralis cartilaginis tubae a.
> lamina medialis cartilaginis tubae a.
> lamina membranacea cartilaginis tubae a.
> tunica mucosa tubae a.

auditoria
> tuba a.

auditoriae
> lamina lateralis cartilaginis tubae a.
> lamina medialis cartilaginis tubae a.

auditory
> a. blast injury
> a. hair
> a. receptor cell
> a. string
> a. teeth
> a. tube

audouinii
> *Microsporum a.*

Audouin microsporon
Auer
> A. body
> A. rod

Auerbach
> A. ganglia
> A. nerve
> A. node
> A. plexus

Auger
> A. effect
> A. electron

augmented histamine test (AHT)
Aujeszky
> A. disease
> A. disease virus

AUL
> acute undifferentiated leukemia

Aulographina
AUO
> amyloid of unknown origin

aural polyp
auramine O fluorescent stain
auramine-rhodamine stain
auramine-stained buffy coat smear
aurantiaca
    Actinocorallia a.
    Brevundimonas a.
    Gemmatimonas a.
    Pseudonocardia a.
    Sphingomonas a.
aurantiacum
    Cryptosporangium a.
    Virgisporangium a.
aurantiacus
    Agromyces a.
    Thermoascus a.
aurantiasis
auranticolor
    Actinokineospora a.
Aurantimonas coralicida
Aurantiporus
aurati
    Helicobacter a.
aurea
    Leifsonia a.
Aureobasidium pullulans
aureus
    glycopeptide-insensitive
      Staphylococcus a. (GISA)
    lichen a.
    methicillin-resistant
      Staphylococcus a. (MRSA)
    Scopulariopsis a.
    Staphylococcus pyogenes a.
    Streptomyces a.
    vancomycin-insensitive
      Staphylococcus a. (VISA)
Aureusvirus
auricular docimasia
Auricularia
auricularis
    Aspergillus a.
aurimucosum
    Corynebacterium a.
aurin tricarboxylic acid
auripigmenti
    Desulfosporosinus a.
auripigmentum
    Desulfotomaculum a.
auriscanis
    Corynebacterium a.
aurochromoderma

Aurococcus
aurothiomalate
    sodium a.
aurothiosuccinate
    sodium a.
aurothiosulfate
    sodium a.
auscultatory gap
austeni
    Culicoides a.
Australia (AU)
    A. antigen (AU Ag)
Australian
    A. X disease
    A. X disease virus
    A. X encephalitis
    A. X encephalitis virus
australiense
    Propionibacterium a.
australiensis
    Bipolaris a.
    Quadricoccus a.
    Tetrasphaera a.
australis
    Dermacentroxenus a.
    Photorhabdus asymbiotica subsp. *a.*
    Rickettsia a.
    Streptococcus a.
Austrobilharzia variglandis
autecic
Aution Max AX-4280 automated urine
  chemistry analyzer
autoabsorption
    cold a.
autoadhesive cellulose nitrate filter
autoadsorption
autoagglutination
autoagglutinin
    anti-Pr cold a.
    cold a.
autoallergic hemolytic anemia
autoallergization
autoallergy
autoanalyzer
    sequential multichannel a. (SMA,
      SMAC)
autoanaphylaxis
autoantibody
    anticytoplasmic a.
    antiidiotype a.
    antineutrophil cytoplasmic a.
    (ANCA)

NOTES

autoantibody *(continued)*
    cold a.
    cytoplasmic antineutrophil
      cytoplasmic a. (cANCA)
    Donath-Landsteiner cold a.
    hemagglutinating cold a.
    idiotype a.
    perinuclear antineutrophil
      cytoplasmic a. (pANCA)
    platelet a.
    specific a.
    thymocytotoxic a.
    warm a.
autoanticomplement
autoantigen
autoantiidiotypic antibody
autoanti-P
autoantitoxin
autoassay
autoblast
autocatalysis
autochthonous
autoclasia
autoclasis
autoclave (AC)
autocoid
autocorrelation function
autocrine
    a. growth factor
    a. hypothesis
    a. motility factor (AMF)
    a. motility factor of the bladder
    a. motility factor receptor (AMFR)
autocrine-paracrine growth regulator
AutoCyte PREP system
autocytolysin
autocytolysis
autocytotoxin
autodigestion
Auto Dimer assay
autoerotic
    a. asphyxia
    a. death
autoerythrocyte
    a. sensitization
    a. sensitization syndrome
autoerythrophagocytosis
autofluorescence
autofluoroscope
autogamous
autogamy
autogeneic, autogenetic, autogenic
    a. graft
autogenesis
autogenous vaccine
autograft
autografting
autohemagglutination
autohemagglutinin

autohemolysin
autohemolysis test
autohemotherapy
autoimmune
    a. antibody
    a. encephalomyelitis
    a. enteropathy
    a. gastritis
    a. hemolytic anemia (AHA, AIHA)
    a. hepatitis (AIH)
    a. leukopenia
    a. mechanism
    a. mucocutaneous disease
    a. neonatal thrombocytopenia
    a. orchitis
    a. pancytopenia
    a. polyendocrine syndrome type 1
      (APS1)
    a. reaction
    a. regulator (Aire)
    a. thrombocytopenic purpura
    a. thyroiditis
autoimmunity
autoimmunization
autoimmunocytopenia
autoimplant
autoinfection
autoinjector
    atropine a.
autoinoculable
autoinoculation
autoisolysin
Autolet blood glucose test
autologous
    a. antibody
    a. antigen
    a. bone marrow transplantation
      (ABMT)
    a. graft
    a. hemagglutinin
    a. leukapheresis, processing, and
      storage (ALPS)
    a. lymphokine activated killer cell
    a. peripheral blood stem cell
      (Auto-PBSC)
    a. transfusion
autolyse
autolysin
autolysis
    postmortem a.
autolysosome
autolytic enzyme
autolyze
automated
    a. activated partial thromboplastin
    a. assay optimization (AAO)
    a. bacteriology
    a. cell-counter technology
    a. cell image analysis

a. cellular imaging system (ACIS)
a. coagulation time
a. differential leukocyte counter
a. immunoprecipitation (AIP)
a. motility factor
a. multiphasic screening (AMS)
a. reagin
a. reagin test (ART)
a. reticulocyte counting
a. slide staining

automatic
a. clinical analyzer
a. fluorescent image analyzer
a. hone
a. tissue processing

automation
blood cell count a.
clinical chemistry a.
differential leukocyte count a.
a. initiative in laboratory
   management
microbiology a.
radioimmunoassay a.
total laboratory a. (TLA)

Automeris io
autometallographic silver enhancement
autometallography (AMG)
automixis
autonomic
a. dysfunction
a. motor neuron

autonomous
a. detection system (ADS)
a. growth

autooxidation
autooxidative degradation
autoparenchymatous metaplasia
Autopath QC test
Auto-PBSC
autologous peripheral blood stem cell
Auto-PBSC BMT

autophagia
autophagic
a. granule
a. vacuole

autophagocytosis
autophagolysosome
autophagosome
autophagy
autophosphorylation
autoplast
autoplastic graft

autoplasty
autoploidy
autopsy
digital a.
endoscopic a.
forensic a.
medicolegal a.
psychological a.
virtual a.

autoradiography
storage phosphor a.

autoradiolysis
autoregulation
autoreinfection
autoreproduction
autosensitization
autosensitize
autosepticemia
autoserotherapy
autoserum therapy
autosomal
a. dominant disorder
a. dominant hemochromatosis
a. dominant inheritance
a. dominant osteopetrosis type 2
   (ADO2)
a. gene
a. heredity
a. recessive
a. recessive disorder
a. recessive inheritance

autosome translocation
Autostainer
Dako A.
Jung A. XL

autotemnous
autotherapy
autotomy
autotoxemia
autotoxicus
horror a.

autotransformer
variable a.

autotransfusion
autotransplant
autotransplantation
autotroph
facultative a.
obligate a.

autotrophic
a. bacterium
a. fixation

NOTES

autotrophica
    Sulfurimonas a.
autotrophicum
    Trichophyton equinum var. *a.*
autovaccination
autumnalis
    Galerina a.
    Neotrombicula a.
auxanography
Auxarthron
auxesis
auxetic growth
auxilytic
auxochrome
auxocyte
auxotroph
auxotrophic mutation
AV
    atrioventricular
    AV block
Av
    avoirdupois
AVA
    arteriovenous anastomosis
AV/AF
    anteverted/anteflexed
available
    no data a. (NDA)
avalanche ionization
Avanti J-20XP, J-25, J-30I, J-HC, J-E centrifuge
avascular necrosis
Avastrovirus
Avellis syndrome
Avenavirus
average
    a. deviation
    a. gradient
    a. life
    Walsh a.
    weighted a.
averaging
    signal a.
avermectinius
    Streptomyces a.
avermitilis
    Streptomyces a.
AVF
    arteriovenous fistula
AVH
    acute viral hepatitis
avian
    a. diphtheria
    a. encephalomyelitis virus
    a. erythroblastosis virus
    a. infectious encephalomyelitis
    a. infectious laryngotracheitis
    a. infectious laryngotracheitis virus
    a. influenza

    a. influenza virus
    a. leukosis
    a. leukosis-sarcoma complex
    a. leukosis-sarcoma virus
    a. lymphomatosis
    a. lymphomatosis virus
    a. monocytosis
    a. myeloblastosis
    a. myeloblastosis leukemia virus reverse transcriptase (AMLV-RT)
    a. myeloblastosis virus
    a. myelocytomatosis virus (AMV2)
    a. neurolymphomatosis virus
    a. pneumoencephalitis virus
    a. reticuloendotheliosis
    a. sarcoma
    a. sarcoma virus
    a. tubercle bacillus
    a. viral arthritis virus
Avibirnavirus
Avicenna gland
avidin
avidin-biotin
    a.-b. based detection system
    a.-b. complex
    a.-b. complex immunodetection system
    a.-b. immunoperoxidase technique
    a.-b. peroxidase complex (ABC)
avidity
    a. antibody
    a. testing
avidum
    Propionibacterium a.
Avihepadnavirus
Avipoxvirus
avipoxvirus
avirulence
avirulent strain
avitaminosis
avium
    Mycobacterium a.
    Trypanosoma a.
avium-intracellulare
    Mycobacterium a.-i. (MAI)
AVM
    arteriovenous malformation
Avogadro
    A. law
    A. number
avoirdupois (Av)
AvoSure INR test device
AVOXimeter 4000 CO oximeter
AVP
    arginine vasopressin
AVR
    aortic valve replacement
Avsunviroid
Avulavirus

avulsed wound
avulsion
    a. fracture
    a. injury
A&W
    alive and well
Aware Rapid HIV assay
AWD
    alive with disease
AWI
    anterior wall infarction
AWMI
    anterior wall myocardial infarction
AWOD
    alive without disease
awu
    atomic weight unit
axanthum
    Acholeplasma a.
axei
    Trichostrongylus a.
Axenfeld syndrome
axenic
axes (*pl. of* axis)
axial
    a. aneurysm
    a. chordoma
    a. filament
axialensis
    Halomonas a.
axifugal
axillare
    hygroma a.
axillares
    nodi lymphoidei a.
axillary sweat gland
axioplasm
axiopodium
axis, pl. **axes**
    brain-hair follicle a. (BHA)
    cell a.
    a. corpuscle
    a. cylinder
    hypothalamic-pituitary-testicular a.
    renin-aldosterone a.
    a. of rotation
    a. of symmetry
axoaxonic synapse
axodendritic synapse
axofugal
axolemma

axolysis
    terminal a.
axon
    a. of anterior root
    bundle of a.
    cervix of the a.
    a. containing microtubule
    a. hillock
    motor a.
    a. of neuroglial cell
    a. of pyramidal cell
    a. staining method
    a. terminal
    unmyelinated a.
axonal
    a. degeneration
    a. demyelination
    a. process
    a. terminal bouton
axoneme
axonotmesis
axopetal
axoplasm
axoplasmic transport
axopodium
axosomatic synapse
axostyle
AxSYM
    A. analyzer
    A. free PSA test
ayderensis
    Anoxybacillus a.
Ayerza
    A. disease
    A. syndrome
Ayoub-Shklar method
Ayre spatula
ayr phenotype
ayw phenotype
A-Z
    Aschheim-Zondek
    A-Z pregnancy test
azacytidine
azan stain
azar
    kala a.
azathioprine
azeotrope
azeotropic solution
azeotropy
azide
    sodium a.

NOTES

azidothymidine
azin dye
azinphosmethyl
azo
    a. coupling reaction
    a. dye
Azoarcus
    A. buckelii
    A. toluvorans
azobenzene
azobilirubin
azocarmine
    a. B
    a. dye
    a. G
azoic dye
azolitmin paper
Azonexus fungiphilus
azoospermia
azophloxin
azoprotein
azoreducens
    Paenibacillus a.
azorense
    Sulfurihydrogenibium a.
azorensis
    Caloranaerobacter a.
Azospira oryzae
Azospirillum doebereinerae
azote
azotemia
    chloropenic a.
    extrarenal a.
    hypochloremic a.

    nonrenal a.
    postrenal a.
    prerenal a.
    renal a.
azotemic
Azotobacter
Azotobacteraceae
azotonutricium
    Treponema a.
azotorrhea
azoturia
azovan blue
Azovibrio restrictus
aztecus
    Anopheles a.
azure
    a. I, II
    a. A
    a. B
    a. C
    a. II-methylene blue stain
    methylene a.
azure-eosin stain
azuresin
azurophil, azurophile
    a. granule
azurophilia
azurophilic granule
azymia
Azymoprocandida
Azzopardi
    A. criteria
    A. phenomenon

B
Baumé scale
Benoist scale
whole blood
   aflatoxin B
   amphotericin B
   B antigen
   azocarmine B
   azure B
   celestine blue B
   B cell
   B cell lymphoma of MALT type
   B cell lymphopoiesis
   B lymphocyte
   B lymphocyte stimulator (BLyS)
   plasma thromboplastin factor B
   rhodamine B

2B
   Uvitex 2B

4B
   benzopurpurin 4B

B4
   isolectin B4

B5
   B5 fixative
   B5 sodium acetate-sublimate
     formalin

B19
   human parvovirus B19

B72.3
   B72.3 antibody
   B72.3 antigen
   B72.3 stain

B$_2$
   Sherman-Bourquin unit of vitamin
     B$_2$

B12^a
   vitamin B12^a

b
   bis
   blood

BA
   bacillary angiomatosis
   bacterial agglutination
   blocking antibody
   bronchial asthma

Baastrup syndrome
Babcock tube
Babès
   B. node
   B. nodule
   B. tubercle
Babès-Ernst
   B.-E. body

   B.-E. corpuscle
   B.-E. granule
Babesia
   B. divergens
   B. microti
Babesiella
Babesiidae
babesiosis serological test
Babinski-Fröhlich syndrome
Babinski-Nageotte syndrome
Babinski syndrome
Babinski-Vaquez syndrome
Babuvirus
baby
   blue b.
   collodion b.
   giant b.
BabyBIG
Babystart
   B. fertility test kit
   B. ovulation test
BAC
   blood alcohol concentration
   bronchioloalveolar carcinoma
BACA
   bronchioalveolar carcinoma
BACE
   beta site APP cleaving enzyme
Bachmann bundle
Bachman-Pettit test
Bachman test
Bacillaceae
Bacillales
bacillary
   b. angiomatosis (BA)
   b. body
   b. dysentery
   b. embolism
   b. emulsion (tuberculin) (BE)
   b. hemoglobinuria
   b. layer
bacille bilié de Calmette-Guérin (BCG)
bacillemia
bacilli (*pl. of* bacillus)
bacilliform
bacilliformis
   Bartonella b.
bacillosis
bacilluria
Bacillus
   B. aeolius
   B. aerogenes capsulatus
   B. aertrycke
   B. algicola
   B. alvei

B

Bacillus (continued)
B. *ambiguus*
B. *anthracis*
B. *anthracis* toxin
B. *aquimaris*
B. *arseniciselenatis*
B. *barbaricus*
B. *bataviensis*
B. *botulinus*
B. *brevis*
B. *bronchisepticus*
B. *cereus*
B. *circulans*
B. *coli*
B. *decolorationis*
B. *diphtheriae*
B. *drentensis*
B. *dysenteriae*
B. *endophyticus*
B. *enteritidis*
B. *faecalis alcaligenes*
B. *farraginis*
B. *fordii*
B. *fortis*
B. *fumarioli*
B. *funiculus*
B. *galactosidilyticus*
B. *gelatini*
B. *hemolyticus*
B. *histolyticus*
B. *hwajinpoensis*
B. *indicus*
B. *influenzae*
B. *jeotgali*
B. *krulwichiae*
B. *larvae*
B. *leprae*
B. *licheniformis*
B. *luciferensis*
B. *mallei*
B. *marisflavi*
B. *megaterium*
B. *nealsonii*
B. *necrophorus*
B. *neidei*
B. *novalis*
B. *odysseyi*
B. *oedematiens*
B. *oedematis maligni*
B. *okuhidensis*
B. *pertussis*
B. *pestis*
B. *pneumoniae*
B. *polymyxa*
B. *proteus*
B. *pseudomallei*
B. *psychrodurans*
B. *psychrotolerans*
B. *pumilus*

B. *pycnus*
B. *pyocyaneus*
B. *selenitireducens*
B. *shackletonii*
B. *siralis*
B. *soli*
B. *sonorensis*
B. *sphaericus*
B. *stearothermophilus*
B. *subterraneus*
B. *subtilis*
B. *suipestifer*
B. *tetani*
B. *thermantarcticus*
B. *thermodenitrificans*
B. *thuringiensis*
B. *tuberculosis*
B. *tularense*
B. *typhi*
B. *typhosus*
B. *vireti*
B. *vulcani*
B. *weihenstephanensis*
B. *welchii*
B. *whitmori*

bacillus, pl. **bacilli**
acid-fast b. (AFB)
anthrax b.
avian tubercle b.
Bang b.
Battey b.
Boas-Oppler b.
Bordet-Gengou b.
bovine tubercle b.
b. Calmette-Guérin (BCG)
Calmette-Guérin b.
cholera b.
coliform b.
colon b.
comma b.
diphtheria b.
diphtheroid bacilli
Döderlein b.
Ducrey b.
dysentery bacilli
enteric b.
Escherich b.
Fick b.
Flexner b.
Flexner-Strong b.
Friedländer b.
fusiform b.
Gärtner b.
Ghon-Sachs b.
glanders b.
gram-negative b.
gram-positive b.
Hansen b.
hay b.

B

Hofmann b.
human tubercle b.
Johne b.
Klebs-Löffler b.
Klein b.
Koch b.
Koch-Weeks b.
leprosy b.
Morax-Axenfeld b.
Morgan b.
Mott bacilli
Newcastle-Manchester b.
Nocard b.
nonfermentative b. (NFB)
paracolon b.
Park-Williams b.
Pfeiffer b.
plague b.
Preisz-Nocard b.
pseudotuberculosis b.
rhinoscleroma b.
Schmitz b.
Schmorl b.
Shiga b.
smegma b.
Sonne-Duval b.
Strong b.
swine rotlauf b.
tetanus b.
timothy b.
tubercle b. (TB)
typhoid b.
vegetative b.
vegetative anthrax bacilli
Vincent b.
vole b.
Weeks b.
Welch b.
Whitmore b.
bacitracin disc test
back
  adolescent round b.
  b. splatter
backbone
backcross
background
  b. count
  flame b.
  b. interference
  pathoanatomic b.
  b. radiation
  smear b.

backlash
backpropagation
backscatter
Backusia
backward failure
backwash ileitis
bacoti
  Bdellonyssus b.
bact
  bacterium
BacT/Alert
  B. automated microbial detection
  system
Bactec
  B. blood culture system
  B. 9000 MB system
  B. MGIT 960
bacteremia
  clostridial b.
  platelet-associated b.
bacteria (*pl. of* bacterium)
bacteria-free stage of bacterial endocarditis
bacterial
  b. adherence
  b. agar method
  b. agglutination (BA)
  b. allergy
  b. aneurysm
  b. antagonism
  b. antigen detection method
  b. aortitis
  b. capsule
  b. classification
  b. culture
  b. culturing
  b. dissociation
  b. encephalitis
  b. endaortitis
  b. endarteritis
  b. endocarditis (BE)
  b. enzyme
  b. filter
  b. genetics
  b. hemolysin
  b. infection
  b. inhibition assay
  b. interference
  b. killing assay
  b. lipochitooligosaccharide
  compound elicitor
  b. meningitis

NOTES

bacterial *(continued)*
- b. meningitis antigen
- b. myocarditis
- b. nephritis
- b. opsonin
- b. opsonization
- b. overgrowth syndrome
- b. pathogenicity
- b. pericarditis
- b. permeability-inducing (BPI)
- b. plaque
- b. prostatitis
- b. serology
- b. spore
- b. stain
- b. staining
- b. susceptibility testing
- b. toxin
- b. transformation
- b. transfusion reaction
- b. urinary cast
- b. vaginitis
- b. vegetation
- b. virus
- b. zoonosis

bacterial-fungal interaction
bactericholia
bactericidal
- b. antibiotic
- b. concentration (BC)

bactericide
- specific b.

bacterid
- pustular b.

bacteriform
bacterioagglutinin
bacteriocide
bacteriocidin
bacteriocin factor
bacteriocinogen
bacteriocinogenic plasmid
bacterioclasis
bacteriogenic agglutination
bacterioid
bacteriological index (BI)
bacteriologic specimen
bacteriologist
bacteriology
- automated b.
- clinical diagnostic b.
- b. laboratory
- medical b.
- public health b.
- sanitary b.
- systematic b.

bacteriolysin
bacteriolysis

bacteriolytic
- b. amboceptor
- b. serum

bacteriolytica
- *Algicola b.*

bacteriolyze
bacterioopsonin
bacteriopexy
bacteriophage
- defective b.
- filamentous b.
- b. genetics
- b. immunity
- mature b.
- b. resistance
- temperate b.
- typhoid b.
- b. typing
- vegetative b.
- virulent b.

bacteriophagia
bacteriophagology
bacteriopsonic
bacteriopsonin
bacteriosis
bacteriostasis agar
bacteriostat
bacteriostatic
- b. agent
- b. antibiotic

bacteriotoxic
bacteriotropic substance
bacteriotropin
Bacteriovoracaceae
Bacteriovorax
- *B. litoralis*
- *B. marinus*
- *B. starrii*
- *B. stolpii*

bacteriovorus
- *Bdellovibrio b.*

bacterium, pl. bacteria (bact)
- acid-fast b.
- aerobic b.
- anaerobic b.
- autotrophic b.
- beaded b.
- bifid b.
- *Campylobacter b.*
- chemoautotrophic b.
- chemoheterotrophic b.
- chromogenic b.
- commensal bacteria
- corkscrew-like bacteria
- denitrifying b.
- endogenous b.
- enterotoxigenic bacteria
- exogenous b.
- exotoxin product of bacteria

facultative b.
fastidious b.
gram-negative b.
gram-positive b.
heterotrophic b.
higher bacteria
hydrogen b.
indigenous b.
intermediate coliform bacteria
lactic acid bacteria
lysogenic b.
mesophilic b.
monocytogenes b.
nitrifying b.
nonlactose-fermenting b.
nonmotile bacteria
nonspore-forming b.
organotropic b.
ovoid b.
psychrophilic b.
pyogenic b.
rod shaped b.
rough b.
smooth b.
sulfur b.
thermophilic b.
toxigenic b.
water b.
bacteriuria
significant asymptomatic b. (SAB)
bacteroid
Bacteroidaceae
Bacteroideae
Bacteroides
B. acidifaciens
B. bivius
B. capillosus
B. corrodens
B. disiens
B. distasonis
B. fragilis
B. funduliformis
B. furcosus
B. fusiformis
B. melaninogenicus
B. nodosus
B. ochraceus
B. oralis
B. oris
B. pneumonia
B. pneumosintes
B. praeacutus

B. putredinis
B. ruminicola
B. serpens
B. splanchnicus
B. thetaiotamicron
B. ureolyticus
bacteroides
Brevundimonas b.
Bactigen
BactiSwab
B. II
B. NPG
Bactoderma
Bactometer
Bacto Middlebrook
Bactrol Plus quality control culture
Bactron 1.5 anaerobic chamber
baculata
Heliorestis b.
Baculoviridae
Badhamia utricularis
Badnavirus
Baehr-Lohlein lesion
Baelz disease
Baermann concentration
Baer vesicle
BAFF
B-cell activating factor
Bäfverstedt syndrome
bag
biohazard b.
nuclear b.
Speci-Gard specimen transport b.
bagassosis
Baggenstoss change in pancreas
bag-valve-mask device
baikonurensis
Rhodococcus b.
Baillarger
B. band
B. line
B. stria
B. stripe
Bairnsdale ulcer
bajacaliforniensis
Spirochaeta b.
Bakamjian deltopectoral flap
Baker
B. acid hematein
B. acid hematein test
B. cyst
B. formol calcium

B

NOTES

Baker *(continued)*
    B. pyridine extraction
    B. pyridine extraction test
    B. Sudan black method
baker's
    b. eczema
    b. yeast
BAL
    British antilewisite
    bronchoalveolar lavage
    BAL ointment
balabacensis
    Anopheles b.
balaenopterae
    Granulicatella b.
Balamuth
    B. aqueous egg yolk infusion medium
    B. buffer solution
    B. culture medium
Balamuthia mandrillaris
balance
    acid-base b.
    analytical b.
    calcium b.
    enzyme b.
    fluid b.
    genic b.
    microchemical b.
    nitrogen b.
    b. translocation
    water b.
balanced
    b. polymorphism
    b. salt solution (BSS)
balanitis
    keratotic micaceous b.
    b. xerotica obliterans
    Zoon b.
balanoposthitis
balantidial
    b. colitis
    b. dysentery
balantidiasis
Balantidium
    B. coli
    B. suis
Balbiani
    B. body
    B. chromosome
    B. nucleus
    B. ring
baldri
    Agrococcus b.
BALF
    bronchoalveolar lavage fluid
Balfour disease
balhimycina
    Amycolatopsis b.

baliensis
    Kozakia b.
Balint syndrome
Balkan
    B. grippe
    B. nephropathy
B-ALL
    B-cell acute lymphoblastic leukemia
ball
    Aspergillus fungus b.
    chondrin b.
    food b.
    fungus b.
    hair b.
    pleural fibrin b.
    b. thrombus
Baller-Gerold syndrome
Ballet disease
Ballingall disease
balloon
    b. cell
    b. cell nevus
    b. cytology
    b. dilatation
    b. neuron
    b. scraping
ballooning
    b. colliquation
    b. degeneration
ball-valve
    b.-v. obstruction
    b.-v. thrombus
Balnearium lithotrophicum
balnei
    Mycobacterium b.
Balneimonas flocculans
Baló disease
BALT
    bronchus-associated lymphoid tissue
baltica
    Belliella b.
    Cellulophaga b.
    Idiomarina b.
    Rheinheimera b.
    Rhodopirellula b.
balticum
    Desulfotignum b.
Bamberger
    B. albuminuria
    B. disease
Bamberger-Marie
    B.-M. disease
    B.-M. syndrome
BamH1 enzyme
Bamle disease
banal cystitis
Bancroft
    B. filarial worm
    B. filariasis

B

bancrofti
>   *Filaria b.*
>   *Wuchereria b.*
bancroftiasis
band
>   A b.
>   alpha b.
>   alpha-1 b.
>   anomalous muscle b.
>   Baillarger b.
>   birefringent collagen b.
>   b. cell
>   centromeric b.
>   cerebrospinal fluid oligoclonal b.'s
>   chromosomal b.
>   chromosome b.
>   contraction b.
>   creatine phosphokinase-
>   myocardial b. (CPK-MB)
>   b. form
>   b. form granulocyte
>   ghost b.'s
>   giant b.
>   H b.
>   Hunter-Schreger b.
>   I b.
>   Kaes-Bekhterev b.
>   b. keratopathy
>   Ladd b.
>   light b.
>   M b.
>   MB b.
>   MM b.
>   moderator b.
>   monoclonal b.
>   b. neutrophil
>   nondiscrete b.'s
>   nongermline b.
>   oligoclonal b.
>   b. 3 protein
>   Q b.
>   Securline blood b.
>   b. shaped nucleus
>   Soret b.
>   b. spectrum
>   stromal collagen b.
>   subepithelial collagen b.
>   theta b.
>   thick fibrous b.
>   Z b.
banding
>   AgNOR b.

>   BrDu b.
>   C b.
>   chromosome b.
>   G b.
>   high-resolution b.
>   NOR b.
>   oligoclonal b.
>   prometaphase b.
>   Q b.
>   quinacrine b.
>   R b.
>   reverse b.
>   T b.
>   telomere b.
>   terminal b.
Bandl ring
bandpass
bandwidth
Banff classification
Bang
>   B. bacillus
>   B. disease
>   B. method
>   B. test
bank
>   blood b. (BB)
>   gene b.
Bannister disease
Banti
>   B. disease
>   B. spleen
>   B. syndrome
bantianum
>   *Cladosporium (Xylohypha) b.*
BAO
>   basal acid output
BAP
>   blood agar plate
bar
>   median b. of Mercier
>   terminal b.
baragnosis
Barany caloric test
baratii
>   *Clostridium b.*
Barbados leg
barbae
>   *Aspergillus b.*
>   folliculitis b.
>   *Penicillium b.*
>   tinea b.
>   trichophytosis b.

NOTES

barbaricus
    Bacillus b.
Barber psoriasis
barber's itch
barbiero
barbirostris
    Anopheles b.
barbital
barbiturate
    b. assay
    b. level
    b. spindle
Barclay-Baron disease
Barcoo
    B. disease
    B. rot
Barcroft apparatus
Bardet-Biedl syndrome
Bard needle
bare lymphocyte syndrome
Bargen streptococcus
bariatric surgery
barium
    b. granuloma
    b. test
Barlow
    B. disease
    B. syndrome
Barnavirus
barnesae
    Gallicola b.
Barnett-Bourne acetic alcohol-silver nitrate method
barometer
barometric
    b. bomb
    b. pressure (Pb)
barophilus
    Thermococcus b.
barosinusitis
barotrauma
Barr
    B. body scoring
    B. body test
    B. chromatin body
Barraquer disease
Barré-Guillain syndrome
barrel chest
barreling distortion
Barrett
    B. epithelium
    B. esophagus
    B. metaplasia
    B. syndrome
    B. ulcer
barrier
    blood-air b.
    blood-aqueous b.
    blood-brain b. (BBB)

blood-cerebral b.
blood-testis b.
blood-thymus b.
b. filter
glomerular b.
immune b.
b. isolation precaution
placental b.
protective osmatic b.
barrier-layer cell
barrier-sustained
    cesarean-obtained b.-s. (COBS)
Barrnett-Seligman
    B.-S. dihydroxydinaphthyl disulfide method
    B.-S. indoxyl esterase method
Barroso-Moguel and Costero silver method
Bartholin
    B. abscess
    B. anus
    B. cyst
    B. duct
    B., urethral, Skene (BUS)
bartholinitis
bartlettii
    Clostridium b.
Bartonella
    B. bacilliformis
    B. birtlesii
    B. bovis
    B. capreoli
    B. chomelii
    B. elizabethae
    B. henselae
    B. koehlerae
    B. quintana
    B. schoenbuchensis
    B. vinsonii
    B. vinsonii subsp. arupensis
Bartonellaceae
bartonellosis
Bart syndrome
Bartter syndrome
baruria
basal
    b. acid output (BAO)
    b. apoptotic rate
    b. body
    b. cell
    b. cell acanthoma
    b. cell adenoma
    b. cell ameloblastoma
    b. cell carcinoma specific antibody
    b. cell epithelioma
    b. cell hyperplasia
    b. cell layer
    b. cell nevus
    b. cell nevus syndrome

b. cell papilloma
b. corpuscle
b. feet
b. gastric secretion test
b. granule
b. hemosiderosis
b. lamina
b. lamina of choroid
b. layer of choroid
b. metabolic rate (BMR)
b. metabolism
b. nucleus of Ganser
b. secretory flow rate (BSFR)
b. secretory flow rate test
b. squamous cell carcinoma
b. striation
b. tuberculosis

basale
stratum b.
basalis
decidua b.
basaloid
b. blastema
b. cell
b. growth pattern
b. hyperplasia
b. invasive squamous cell
carcinoma (BISCC)
b. squamous cell carcinoma
(BSCC)
b. tumor
basaloma
base
blood buffer b. (BB)
Brönsted-Lowry b.
buffer b. (BB)
complementary b.
conjugate b.
b. deficit (BD)
delta b.
b. excess (BE)
b. ionization constant
Lewis b.
b. lymphocyte syndrome (BLS)
National Cancer Data B. (NCDB)
b. pair (bp)
b. pairing
pressor b.
purine and pyrimidine b.'s
pyrimidine b.
b. ratio

Schiff b.
b. unit
Basedow disease
baseline steady state
basement
b. lamina
b. membrane
b. membrane antibody
b. membrane component
b. membrane zone
basic
Acceava hCG B.
b. amino acid
b. anhydride
b. calcium phosphate (BCP)
b. calcium phosphate crystal
b. dye
b. fuchsin
b. fuchsin-methylene blue stain
b. helix-loop-helix transcription
factor (bHLH)
b. magenta
b. metabolic panel (BMP)
basicaryoplastin
basichromatin
basichromiole
basicity
basicytoparaplastin
basidiobolomycosis
Basidiobolus
B. haptosporus
B. ranarum
Basidiomycetes
Basidiomycota
basidiospore
basidium
basilar
b. artery ischemia
b. cell
b. crest of cochlear duct
b. lamina
b. leptomeningitis
b. membrane
b. membrane of cochlear duct
b. meningitis
basilaris
glandula b.
membrana b.
basilemma
basilensis
Wautersia b.
basiparaplastin

NOTES

basipetal
Basipetospora rubra
basis pontis
basisquamous (*var. of* basosquamous)
basket
    b. cell
    fibrillar b.
basket-weave pattern
baso
    basophil
    basophilic leukocyte
basocyte
basocytopenia
basocytosis
basoerythrocyte
basoerythrocytosis
basolateral membrane
basometachromophil,
  basometachromophile
basopenia
basophil, basophile (baso)
    b. adenoma
    beta b.
    b. cell
    b. cell of anterior lobe of
      hypophysis
    b. chemotactic factor (BCF)
    b. degranulation test
    b. granule
    polymorphonuclear b. (PMB)
    b. substance
    tissue b.
basophilia
    Grawitz b.
    peripheral b.
    pituitary b.
    punctate b.
    substantia b.
basophilic
    b. cell of anterior lobe of
      hypophysis
    b. cytoplasm
    b. deposit
    b. erythroblast
    b. granular degeneration
    b. granule
    b. hyperplasia
    b. leukemia
    b. leukocyte (baso)
    b. leukocytosis
    b. leukopenia
    b. marrow
    b. megakaryocyte
    b. megaloblast
    b. metamyelocyte
    b. myelocyte
    b. normoblast
    b. promyelocyte
    b. stippling

basophilism
    Cushing b.
    pituitary b.
basophilocyte
basophilocytic leukemia
basoplasm
basosquamous, basisquamous
    b. carcinoma
Bassen-Kornzweig syndrome
bassiana
    Beauveria b.
bastinii
    Desulfovibrio b.
BAT
    biliary acid transporter
bataviensis
    Bacillus b.
batch analyzer
Bateman syndrome
bath
    flotation b.
    isopentane-dry ice b.
    water b.
bathing trunk nevus
bathochromic shift
bathophenanthroline
bathycardia
batsensis
    Oceanicola b.
Batson
    B. plexus
    B. system
Batten disease
Batten-Mayou syndrome
battered child
battery
    anergy skin test b.
Battey bacillus
Battey-type mycobacterium
battledore
    b. insertion
    b. placenta
batwing appearance
Bauer
    B. chromic acid leucofuchsin stain
    B. reaction
Bauer-Kirby test
Bauermeister scale
Bauhin gland
baumannii
    Acinetobacter b.
    Oceanimonas b.
Baumé
    B. law
    B. scale (B)
baumgartneri
    Caulochora b.
Baumgartner method

B

bauxite
b. pneumoconiosis
b. worker's disease
Bax
B. apoptosis gene
B. protein
Bayer
B. AG II chemistry analyzer system
B. Immuno 1 HER-2/neu assay
B. Technicon H-2 analyzer
B. Technicon H1 automated flow cytometer
B. Versant HCV RNA 3.0 assay
Bayes theorem
Bayh-Dole Act
Bayle
B. disease
B. granulation
Baylisascaris procyonis
baylyi
Acinetobacter b.
Bazex syndrome
Bazin disease
BB
blood bank
blood buffer base
blue bloater
breakthrough bleeding
breast biopsy
buffer base
creatine kinase BB (CK-BB)
glycogen phosphorylase isoenzyme BB (GPBB)
orseillin BB
BBB
blood-brain barrier
bundle branch block
BC
bactericidal concentration
BCA
Barrett adenocarcinoma
bicinchoninic acid method
BCAA
branched-chain amino acid
BCB
brilliant cresyl blue
BCC
basal cell carcinoma
B-cell
B-c. activating factor (BAFF)
B-c. ALL

B-c. antibody
B-c. antigen receptor
B-c. chronic lymphoproliferative disorder (BCLPD)
B-c. CLL/SLL
B-c. count
B-c. deficiency
B-c. differentiating factor
B-c. differentiation/growth factor
B-c. growth factor I, II
B-c. immunodeficiency
B-c. lymphoma (BCL)
B-c. malignancy
B-c. marker
B-c. neoplasm
B-c. non-Hodgkin lymphoma (B-NHL)
B-c. prolymphocytic leukemia (B-PLL)
B-c. stimulating factor
BCF
basophil chemotactic factor
BCG
bacille bilié de Calmette-Guérin
bacillus Calmette-Guérin
bicolor guaiac test
bronchocentric granulomatosis
BCG vaccine
BChE
butyrylcholinesterase
BCKA
branched-chain keto acid
BCL
B-cell lymphoma
bcl-2
b. antibody
b. gene arrangement
b. gene rearrangement
b. oncogene
b. protein
b. protooncogene
bcl-1 gene
bcl-6 antibody
BCLL
B-cell chronic lymphocytic leukemia
BCLPD
B-cell chronic lymphoproliferative disorder
bcl-X$_L$ protein
BCP
basic calcium phosphate
BCP crystal

NOTES

BCP-D
 bromocresol purple desoxycholate
BCP-LBL
 B-cell precursor lymphoblastic leukemia
BCR-ABL
 breakpoint cluster region-Abelson murine
  leukemia virus
  BCR-ABL hybrid protein
  BCR-ABL protein test
  BCR-ABL transcript
BD
 base deficit
  BD BBL CultureSwab Plus
   collection and transport system
  BD BeAware test
  BD Phoenix automated
   microbiology system
BD/BS
 bile duct-to-portal space ratio
BD-CHEK intestinal inflammation kit
Bdellomicrovirus
Bdellonyssus bacoti
Bdellovibrio bacteriovorus
BDG
 buffered desoxycholate glucose
b-DNA
 branched DNA
BDNF
 brain-derived neurotrophic factor
B-domain-deleted
  B.-d.-d. factor VIII concentrate
  B.-d.-d. rFVIII product
BDS
 biohazard detection system
BE
 bacillary emulsion (tuberculin)
 bacterial endocarditis
 base excess
 bovine enteritis
BE12 antibody
bead
  agar b.
  controlled pore glass b.
  glutathione agarose b.'s
  IOBeads magnetic b.'s
beaded
  b. bacterium
  b. hair
beading of ribs
beaked pelvis
beaker
  b. cell
  Griffin b.
Beale ganglion cell
beam
  electron b.
  b. splitting
bean
  castor b.

Be^a antigen
Beard
  B. disease
  B. test
beaten egg white appearance colony
Beau
  B. disease
  B. line
  B. syndrome
Beauvais disease
Beauveria bassiana
Beaver direct smear method
Bechterew disease
Beck
  B. disease
  B. triad
Becker
  B. antigen
  B. disease
  B. muscular dystrophy (BMD)
  B. nevus
  B. stain for spirochetes
Beckman
  B. assay
  B. Paragon SPE-II gel apparatus
  B. Synchron CX-7 cholesterol
   analyzer
Beckmann thermometer
Beckwith syndrome
Beckwith-Wiedemann syndrome
becquerel (Bq)
Becton-Dickinson needle
bed
  microcapillary b.
bedbug
Bedbugg system for at-home diagnosis
 of sleep apnea
Bednar tumor
Bedsonia
bedtime salivary cortisol test
beef tapeworm
beer
  b. drinker's cardiomyopathy
  b. drinker's potomania
  b. heart
  B. law
Beer-Boguer law
beeturia
bee venom toxin
Begbie disease
Beggiatoaceae
Beggiatoales
Begomovirus
Béguez César disease
behavior
  dementia pugilistica/autism with
   self-injury b.
  b. genetics
  neoplasm of uncertain b.

Behçet
    B. disease
    B. syndrome
behenic acid
Behnken unit (R)
Behr disease
Behring law
BEI
    butanol-extractable iodine
    BEI test
Beigel disease
beijiangensis
    Streptomyces b.
beijingensis
    Nocardia b.
bejel
Bekhterev
    B. disease
    B. nucleus
bel
Belascaris
Belgian Congo anemia
beliardensis
    Legionella b.
belladonna
belladonnine
bellator
    Anopheles b.
bell-clapper abnormality
Bell disease
belli
    Isospora b.
Belliella baltica
Bellini
    B. duct
    B. duct carcinoma
    medullary ducts of B.
Bell-Magendie law
belly
    prune b.
belt
    anthrax b.
Belzer solution
Bence
    B. Jones (BJ)
    B. Jones albumin
    B. Jones albuminuria
    B. Jones albumosuria
    B. Jones body
    B. Jones cast nephropathy
    B. Jones cylinder
    B. Jones globulin

    B. Jones myeloma
    B. Jones protein
    B. Jones proteinemia
    B. Jones protein method
    B. Jones protein test
    B. Jones proteinuria
    B. Jones reaction
bench
    b. method
    B. needle biopsy
benchmark
Benditt hypothesis
benedeni
    Moniezia b.
Benedict
    B. method
    B. solution
    B. test
    B. test for glucose
Benedict-Hopkins-Cole reagent
Benedict-Roth apparatus
Benedikt syndrome
bengal
    rose b.
Bengston method
benign
    b. albuminuria
    b. bone aneurysm
    b. chronic bullous dermatosis of childhood
    b. cystic teratoma
    b. dry pleurisy
    b. dyskeratosis
    b. epithelial breast tumor
    b. epithelioma
    b. familial hematuria
    b. familial icterus
    b. familial pemphigus
    b. florid lymphoid hyperplasia
    b. giant lymph node hyperplasia
    b. glycosuria
    b. inoculation lymphoreticulosis
    b. inoculation reticulosis
    b. intracranial hypertension (BIH)
    b. juvenile melanoma
    b. lymphadenosis
    b. lymphocytic angiitis and granulomatosis
    b. lymphocytoma cutis
    b. lymphoepithelial lesion
    b. lymphoma
    b. lymphoma of rectum

B

NOTES

benign *(continued)*
  b. mediastinal lymph node hyperplasia
  b. mesenchymoma
  b. mesothelioma
  b. mesothelioma of genital tract
  b. metastasizing leiomyoma (BML)
  b. monoclonal gammopathy (BMG)
  b. mucosal pemphigoid
  b. mucous membrane pemphigus
  b. myalgic encephalomyelitis
  b. neoplasm
  b. nephrosclerosis (BNS)
  b. paroxysmal peritonitis
  b. proliferative lesion
  b. prostatic hyperplasia
  b. prostatic hypertrophy (BPH)
  b. tertian malaria
benigna
  variola b.
benignum
  empyema b.
  lymphogranuloma b.
Bennet corpuscle
Bennett
  B. disease
  B. sulfhydryl method
Bennhold
  B. Congo red method
  B. Congo red stain
Benoist scale (B)
Bensley
  B. aniline-acid fuchsin-methyl green method
  B. osmic dichromate fluid
  B. safranin acid violet
  B. specific granule
Benson disease
bentiromide test
bentonite flocculation test (BFT)
Benyvirus
benzalkonium chloride
benzanthracene
benzene
  b. assay
  b. derivative
  b. hexachloride (BHC)
  b. poisoning
benzeneamine
benzenivorans
  Pseudonocardia b.
benzenoid
benzidine
  b. method for myoglobin peroxidase
  b. test
benzilate
  3-quinuclidinyl b. (QNB)

benzimidazole
  budding uninhibited by b. (BUB)
benzine, benzin
benzoate
  caffeine sodium b.
  estradiol b. (EB)
  sodium b.
benzodiazepine assay
benzoic acid
benzol
benzopurpurin 4B
benzopyrene
benzoquinone
benzo sky blue method
benzosulfimide
  sodium b.
benzoxiquine
benzoylaminoacetic acid
benzoylation
benzoylecgonine
benzoylglycine
benzoyl phenylcarbinol
3,4-benzpyrene
benzyl alcohol
benzylamine
Beradinelli syndrome
Bérard aneurysm
berbera
  Borrelia b.
Ber-EP4
  Ber-EP4 antibody
  Ber-EP4 immunoperoxidase stain
Berg
  B. chelate removal method
  B. stain
bergamot oil
Berger
  B. cell
  B. disease
  B. focal glomerulonephritis
Bergeron
  B. chorea
  B. disease
Bergey classification
berghei
  Plasmodium b.
Bergmann
  B. cord
  B. fiber
  B. glia
Ber-H2 antibody
beriberi
  cardinal manifestation of wet b.
  dry b.
  b. heart
  wet b.
Berkefeld filter
berkelium

Berlin
 B. blue
 B. breakage syndrome
 B. disease
bermudensis
 Parvularcula b.
Bernard
 B. canal
 B. duct
 B. syndrome
Bernard-Horner syndrome
Bernard-Sergent syndrome
Bernard-Soulier syndrome (BSS)
Bernatz classification
Bernhardt disease
Bernhardt-Roth syndrome
Bernheim syndrome
Bernoulli
 B. law
 B. principle
 B. theorem
Bernstein test
Bernthsen methylene violet
berrensis
 Thermohalobacter b.
berry
 b. aneurysm
 b. cell
Berson test
Berthelot reaction
Bertiella studeri
bertiellosis
Bertin
 B. column
 columns of B.
Bertolotti syndrome
berylliosis
beryllium granuloma
Besnier-Boeck disease
Besnier-Boeck-Schaumann
 B.-B.-S. disease
 B.-B.-S. syndrome
Besnier prurigo
Besnoitia
Besnoitiidae
besnoitiosis, besnoitiasis
Bessey-Lowry (BL)
 B.-L. unit (BLU)
Bessey, Lowry, Bock (BLB)
Bessman anemia classification

Best
 B. carmine stain
 B. disease
beta
 b. adrenergic blockade
 b. agglutination
 b. agglutinin
 b. amyloid precursor protein
 immunohistochemical stain
 b. antigen of adenovirus
 b. basophil
 b. blocker
 b. burn
 b. cell
 b. cell of anterior lobe of
 hypophysis
 b. cell of hypophysis
 b. cell of pancreas
 b. corynebacteriophage
 b. decay
 b. emitter
 b. endorphin
 b. erythroidine
 17 b. estradiol
 estrogen receptor b.
 b. fetoprotein
 b. galactosidase test
 b. globin gene
 b. globulin
 b. granule
 b. hCG
 b. hemolysin
 b. hemolysis
 b. hydroxybutyrate (BHBA)
 b. isoform
 b. lactoglobulin (BLG)
 b. lipoprotein
 b. lysin
 b. metachromasia
 b. monooxygenase
 b. myosin heavy chain
 b. naphthol
 NRG1 b.
 NRG2 b.
 b. oxidation
 b. particle
 b. phage
 b. quick strep test
 b. radiation
 b. ray
 b. ray microscope

B

NOTES

beta *(continued)*
    b. site APP cleaving enzyme (BACE)
    b. sitosterolemia
    b. staphylolysin
    b. streptococcus
    b. substance
    TGF b.
    b. thalassemia major
    b. thalassemia minor
    b. thromboglobulin
    TNF b.
    transcription factor b.
    b. tubulin
    tumor necrosis factor b.
beta-1A globulin
beta-1C globulin
beta-1E globulin
beta-1F globulin
beta-2 microglobulin
beta-adrenergic
    b.-a. antagonist
    b.-a. blocking agent
beta-aminoisobutyric aciduria
beta-amyloid
    b.-a. compound
    b.-a. fibril
    b.-a. plaque
beta-catenin
    b.-c. gene
Betacryptovirus
betacyaninuria
beta-delta thalassemia
betae
    Bradyrhizobium b.
beta-enolase
beta-galactosidase
    cerebroside b.-g.
betaglobulin
    steroid-binding b.
beta-glucosidase
    cerebroside b-g.
beta-glucuronidase
beta-D-glucuronidase deficiency
beta-glycoprotein
    glycine-rich b-g.
beta-hCG test
beta-hemolytic streptococcus (BHS)
beta-hydroxybutyrate assay
beta-hydroxy-delta-5-steroid dehydrogenase
betaine
beta-lactamase
    b.-l. negative
    b.-l. positive
    b.-l. test
beta-lipoprotein
beta-methylcrotonylglycinuria
beta-microglobulin

beta-N-acetylgalactosaminidase
beta-nicotyrine
Betanodavirus
beta-pleated sheet
Betaretrovirus
Betatetravirus
beta-tubulin
    neuron-associated class III b-t.
betavasculorum
    Pectobacterium b.
beta-VLDL
betel cancer
Bethesda
    B. Pap smear
    B. Pap smear rating scale
    B. system
    B. 2001 system diagnosis
    B. 2001 terminology for reporting results of cervical cytology
    B. unit (BU)
Bethesda-Ballerup group of *Citrobacter* (CBB)
Betke-Kleihauer
    B.-K. stain
    B.-K. test
Betke stain
Bettendorff test
Betula
betulina
    Lenzites b.
Betz
    B. cell
    B. cell area
beurmanni
    Sporotrichum b.
Beutler test
Bevan-Lewis cell
BeWo choriocarcinoma cell line
bezoar
Bezold
    B. abscess
    B. ganglion
BF
    blastogenetic factor
B:F
    bound-free ratio
bf
    bouillon filtrate
bFGF
    basic fibroblast growth factor
BFP
    biologic false-positive
BFR
    biologic false-positive reactor
    bone formation rate
BFT
    bentonite flocculation test
    blunt force trauma

BFU-E
  burst-forming unit-erythroid
BG
  blood glucose
  bone graft
  Bordet-Gengou
    BG test
BG8
  BG8 immunostain
  BG8 monoclonal antibody
BGA
  blood group antigen
BGG
  bovine gamma globulin
BGH
  bovine growth hormone
BGP
  biliary glycoprotein
  bone GLA-protein
BGSA
  blood granulocyte-specific activity
BGTT
  borderline glucose tolerance test
BH11 antibody
BHA
  brain-hair follicle axis
BHBA
  beta hydroxybutyrate
BHC
  benzene hexachloride
BHI
  brain-heart infusion
bHLH
  basic helix-loop-helix transcription factor
BHS
  beta-hemolytic streptococcus
BHTU microscope
BH:VH
  body hematocrit-venous hematocrit ratio
BI
  bacteriological index
  burn index
Bial
  B. pentosetest
  B. reagent
  B. test
biallelic
Bianchi
  B. syndrome
  B. valve
Bi antigen

bias
  forward b.
  reverse b.
biased estimate
biatriatum
  cor pseudotriloculare b.
  cor triloculare b.
Biber-Haab-Dimmer corneal lattice dystrophy
bibulous
bicameral abscess
bicapsular
bicarb
  bicarbonate
  carbon dioxide
bicarbonate (bicarb, HCO$_3$)
  blood b.
  b. buffer
  b. buffer system
  b. ion
  plasma b.
  potassium b.
  serum b.
  sodium b.
  standard b.
  b. titration test
bicellular
Bichat
  B. canal
  B. fissure
  B. foramen
  B. membrane
  B. tunic
bichromate
  potassium b.
biciliate
bicinchoninic acid method (BCA)
biclonal
  b. gammopathy
  b. peak
biclonality
bicolorata
  Agreia b.
bicolor guaiac test (BCG)
biconcave
biconvex
bicornuate uterus
bicytopenia
bidirectional information exchange
BIDLB
  block in posteroinferior division of left branch

NOTES

Biebrich
  B. scarlet
  B. scarlet-picroaniline blue
  B. scarlet red
Biedl disease
Bielschowsky
  B. disease
  B. method
  B. stain
Bielschowsky-Jansky disease
Biemond syndrome
bieneusi
  Enterocytozoon b.
Biermer
  B. anemia
  B. disease
bifemoral
bifermentans
  Clostridium b.
bifid
  b. bacterium
  b. tongue
  b. ureter
  b. uterus
bifida
  spina b.
  Zimmermannella b.
Bifidobacteriaceae
Bifidobacteriales
Bifidobacterium
  B. bifidum
  B. dentium
  B. eriksonii
  B. infantis
  B. psychraerophilum
  B. scardovii
  B. thermacidophilum subsp. porcinum
  B. thermacidophilum subsp. thermacidophilum
bifidum
  Bifidobacterium b.
  cranium b.
bifidus
  Lactobacillus b.
biflorus
  Dolichos b.
biformata
  Robiginitalea b.
bifurcation
bifurcum
  Oesophagostomum b.
bigemina
  Isospora b.
bigeminal
bigeminy
  ventricular b.

BIG-IV
  botulism immune globulin intravenous (human)
biglycan
BIH
  benign intracranial hypertension
bilat
  bilateral
bilateral (bilat)
  b. left-sidedness
  b. micronodular adrenal hyperplasia
  b. otitis media (BOM)
  b., symmetrical, and equal (BSE)
  b. symmetry
Bilderbeck disease
bile
  b. acid
  b. acid assay
  b. acid tolerance test
  b. antigen
  b. canaliculi
  b. capillary
  b. cast
  b. duct
  b. duct adenoma
  b. duct canaliculus
  b. duct carcinoma
  b. duct necrosis
  b. duct-to-portal space ratio (BD/BS)
  b. esculin agar
  b. esculin hydrolysis test
  b. extravasation
  b. fluid examination
  b. infarct
  b. lake
  b. nephrosis
  b. peritonitis
  b. pigment
  b. pigment demonstration in tissue
  b. pigment hemoglobin
  b. pigment test
  b. salt agar
  b. salt breath test
  b. salt deficiency syndrome
  b. salts
  b. solubility test
  b. stasis
  b. thrombus
  white b.
Bilharzia
bilharzial
  b. deposition pigment
  b. dysentery
  b. granuloma
  b. pigment deposition
bilharziasis, bilharziosis
Bilharziella polonica

biliaris
    tunica mucosa vesicae b.
    tunica muscularis vesicae b.
    tunica serosa vesicae b.
biliary
    b. achalasia
    b. acid transporter (BAT)
    b. atresia
    b. calculus
    b. canaliculus
    b. cirrhosis
    b. colic
    b. disorder
    b. drainage
    b. duct
    b. ductule
    b. dyssynergia
    b. fistula
    b. glycoprotein (BGP)
    b. obstruction
    b. progenitor marker
    b. reflux
    b. scan
    b. stricture
    b. tract disease
    b. tract infection
    b. xanthomatosis
biliferi
    ductuli b.
    ductus b.
    tubuli b.
Bili-Labstix
biliosae
    glandulae mucosae b.
biliousness
bilious remittent malaria
bilirubin
    amniotic fluid b.
    b. assay
    conjugated b.
    b. demonstration in tissues
    direct reacting b.
    b. encephalopathy
    indirect reacting b.
    minimum concentration of b. (MCBR)
    neonatal b.
    b. scan
    serum b. (SB)
    b. tolerance test
    total serum b. (TSB)
    unconjugated b.

    volume of distribution of b. (VDBR)
bilirubinemia
    hereditary nonhemolytic b.
bilirubinometer
    Unistat b.
bilirubinuria
biliuria
biliverdin
biliverdinglobin
Billheimer method
Billroth
    B. cord
    B. disease
    B. venae cavernosae
bilobalide
bilobate placenta
bilobed right lung
biloculare
    cor b.
bilocular stomach
biloma
Bilopaque
Bilophila wadsworthia
bimetal thermometer
bimodal manner
bimolecular
bimorphic
bimucosa
    fistula b.
binary
    b. acid
    b. addition
    b. cytotoxin
    b. fission
    b. nomenclature
    b. variate
binasal hemianopsia
Binax
    B. Now *Legionella* urine antigen test
    B. Now *Streptococcus pneumoniae* antigen test
    B. Now urinary antigen test
Bindazyme ANA Screening ELISA kit
binding
    albumin cobalt b. (ACB)
    b. constant
    cortisol b.
    b. energy
    patchy b.
    protein b. (PB)

NOTES

Binet chronic lymphocytic leukemia classification
binocular microscope
binomial
    b. coefficient
    b. distribution
    b. nomenclature
Binswanger
    B. disease
    B. encephalopathy
binuclear
binucleate
    b. cell
    b. fiber
binucleated lymphocyte
binucleation disproportionate
binucleolate
Binz test
bioaccumulation
bioactive
bioanalysis
bioanalyst
bioassay
bioavailability
biocenosis
biochemical
    b. energetics
    b. fuel cell
    b. genetics
    b. metastasis
    b. profile
    b. sequestration
    b. testing
biochemically mediated effect
biochemistry
biochemorphic
biochemorphology
biocidal
bioclimatology
Bioclot protein S assay
bioconversion
biodefense
    Working Group on Civilian B.
biodegradability
biodegradable
bioelectronic sensor technology
bioenergetics
bioequivalence
bioethicist
biofidelic human surrogate
biogenesis
biogenetic
biogenic amine hypothesis
biographer
    GlucoWatch B.
biohazard
    b. bag
    b. detection system (BDS)
bioinjectable

biologic
    b. assay
    b. false-positive (BFP)
    b. false-positive reactor (BFR)
    b. half-life
    b. WMD
biological
    b. alkylating agent
    b. assay
    b. clock
    b. half-life
    b. immunotherapy
    b. matrix reference materials
    b. safety cabinet (BSC)
    B. Stain Commission
    b. standard unit
    b. terrorism
    b. vector
    b. warfare (BW)
    b. weapon
    B. Weapons and Toxins Convention
biologist
biology
    cellular b.
    molecular b.
    population b.
bioluminescence
bioluminescent method
biomarker
    ovarian cancer b.
biomass
biomechanical preparation
biomechanician
biomechanics
biomedical
    b. engineering
    b. scientist
Biomek 2000, 3000, FX, FX assay, NX laboratory automation workstation
biometrician
biometric identifier
biometry
biomicroscopy
biomonitor
Biomphalaria glabrata
Biondi-Heidenhain stain
Biondi ring
bionecrosis
bionics
biophage
biophagism
biophagous
biophagy
biophylactic
biophylaxis
biophysical profile
biophysics
bioplasm

B

bioplasmic
biopolitics
Biopore membrane device
Biopreparat
biopsy
abdominal fat pad b.
b. algorithm
aspiration b.
Bench needle b.
blind punch b.
bone b.
breast b. (BB)
bronchial brush b.
cervical punch b.
cone b.
conventional core b. (CCB)
core needle b. (CNB)
CT-guided stereotactic b.
deep wedge b.
embryo b.
endometrial b.
endomyocardial b.
excisional b.
fine-needle aspiration b. (FNAB)
formalin-fixed skin b.
full-series b.
image-guided breast b.
image-guided core b.
incisional b.
jumbo b.
labial salivary gland b.
large-needle aspiration b. (LNB)
LSG b.
lung b.
minimally invasive breast b. (MIBB)
minor salivary gland b.
muscle b.
needle core length in sextant b.
open lung b. (OLB)
passive epithelial displacement by needle b.
percutaneous liver b.
percutaneous renal b.
placental b.
plasmacytoma on tissue b.
pleural b.
prostate gland b.
prostate needle core b.
punch b.
4 quadrant b.
scalene node b. (SNB)
sentinel lymph node b.
sextant b.
shave b.
skin shave b.
small bowel b.
b. specimen
stereotactic brain b.
stereotactic breast b.
stereotactic core-needle b. (SCNB)
suction-type b.
synovial membrane b.
thin-needle b.
thyroid b.
transbronchial lung b. (TBBx, TBLB)
transrectal ultrasound-guided sextant b. (TRUS)
trephine b.
Tru-Cut b.
urinary tract brush b.
vacuum-assisted core b. (VACB)
biopterin
biopyoculture
Bio-Rad
B.-R. H2500 microwave oven
B.-R. protein assay
bioreagent
Biosafe TSH test
biosafety
b. containment
b. level (BSL)
b. level 1 (BSL1)
b. level 2 (BSL2)
b. level 3 (BSL3)
b. level 4 (BSL4)
biosampler
Accelon Combi b.
biosciences
Amersham B.
Bioshaf automated one-step fertility kit
biospectrometry
biospectroscopy
biospeleology
BioStar Strep A OIA MAX
Streptococcus **A test**
biosynthesis
biosynthetic pathway
biotaxis
Bio-Tek EIx800 plate reader
bioterrorism
food-based b.

NOTES

bioterrorism *(continued)*
    B. Preparedness and Response Program
    B. Readiness Plan
BioThrax
biotin
    b. assay
    labeled streptavidin b. (LSAB)
biotin-labeled probe
biotin-streptavidin-alkaline phosphatase method
biotin-streptavidin detection method
biotin-streptavidin-peroxidase method
biotinylated DNA probe
biotinylation
biotope
biotoxin
biotransformation
Biot respiration
biotype
biowarfare
BioWatch
BIP
    bismuth iodoform paraffin
biparasitism
biparental inheritance
biphasic
    b. blastoma
    b. helical CT
    b. pattern
    b. response
    b. tumor
biphenotypic
    b. differentiation
    b. lymphoma
biphenotypy
biphenyl
    polychlorinated b. (PCB)
biphosphate
    sodium b.
bipolar
    b. cell
    b. depression disorder
    b. needle electrode
    b. neuron
    b. spindle
    b. stain
    b. staining
    b. uptake
Bipolaris
    B. *australiensis*
    B. *hawaiiensis*
    B. *spicifera*
bipotential cell
bipulmonary
bipunctata
    Macromonas b.
bipyridyl
Birbeck granule

Birch-Hirschfeld stain
bird
    B. disease
    B. formula
    B. Nest filter
    b. unit
bird-breeder's
    b.-b. disease
    b.-b. lung
bird-fancier's lung
birdseed agar
bird's nest lesion
birefringence
    apple-green b.
    crystalline b.
    flow b.
    form b.
    strain b.
birefringent
    b. collagen band
    b. crystal
    b. crystalline cleft
birgiae
    Afipia b.
Birnaviridae
Birnavirus
birth injury
birthmark (bmk)
    strawberry b.
    vascular b.
Birt-Hogg-Dube syndrome
birtlesii
    Bartonella b.
bis (b)
bisalbuminemia
BISCC
    basaloid invasive squamous cell carcinoma
bis(2-chloroethyl)sulfide
bischloromethyl ether
bisection
Bismarck
    B. brown
    B. brown R, Y
bismuth
    b. assay
    B. cholangiocarcinoma classification
    b. iodide
    b. iodoform paraffin (BIP)
    b. pigmentation
    b. subnitrate
    b. triiodide
Bismuth-Corlette perihilar tumor classification
bismuth-sulfite agar (BSA)
bisonis
    Cooperia b.
bisphosphate
    fructose b.

bisphosphatidylglycerol
2,3-bisphosphoglycerate
bisphosphoglycerate phosphatase
bisphosphoglyceromutase
bistratal
bis-trimethylsilylacetamide
bis-trimethylsilyltrifluoroacetamide (BSTFA)
bisulfate
bisulfide
    carbon b.
bisulfite
bit
    check b.
    parity b.
bitartrate
    potassium b.
bite cell
bitemporal hemianopsia
Bithynia
Bitot spot
bitropic
bitten colony
Bittner
    B. agent
    B. milk factor
    B. virus
biundulant
    b. meningoencephalitis
    b. milk fever virus
biurate
biuret
    b. reaction
    b. test
biuret-reactive material (BRM)
bivalent
    b. antibody
    b. gas gangrene antitoxin
    heteromorphic b.
    homomorphic b.
biventriculare
    cor triloculare b.
bivia
    Prevotella b.
bivius
    Bacteroides b.
bixin
bizarre
    b. leiomyoma
    b. megakaryocyte
    b. parosteal osteochondromatous proliferation (BPOP)

Bizzozero
    B. corpuscle
    B. platelet
    B. red cell
    Sudan black B.
BJ
    Bence Jones
    BJ protein
Bjerkandera
Bjork-Shiley mitral prosthesis
Björnstad syndrome
BK virus
BL
    Bessey-Lowry
    bleeding
    blood loss
    Burkitt lymphoma
black
    amido b. 10B
    b. bane (anthrax)
    b. Bizzozero, Sudan
    b. currant rash
    b. death
    b. fly
    b. hairy tongue
    b. house rat
    b. jaundice
    b. lead
    b. light
    b. lung
    b. lung disease
    b. periodic acid method
    b. piedra
    b. plague
    b. powder
    Sudan b.
    Sudan b. B (SBB)
    b. thyroid adenoma
    b. thyroid syndrome
    b. urine
    b. widow spider
black-dot ringworm
Blackfan-Diamond syndrome
blackhead
blackwater fever
bladder
    autocrine motility factor of the b.
    b. carcinoma
    b. disorder
    b. dysfunction
    exstrophy of the b.
    fasciculate b.

B

NOTES

129

bladder *(continued)*
    low-compliance b.
    b. neck margin involvement
    b. neck margin of the prostate
    b. neck obstruction (BNO)
    neurogenic b.
    b. polyp
    poorly compliant b.
    b. spasm
    b. tumor (BT)
bladderworm
Blakeslea
BLA 36 monoclonal antibody
blanch
blanche
    atrophia b.
    tache b.
blanching
    tongue b.
bland
    b. embolism
    b. embolus
    b. infarct
Blandin gland
Blane
    amniotic infection syndrome of B.
Blaschko line
Blasius duct
blast
    b. cell
    b. cell leukemia
    b. chest
    b. crisis
    b. effect
    b. injury
    b. lung
    refractory anemia with excess
      of b.'s (RAEB)
    rice b.
    b. wind
blastema
    basaloid b.
    b. cell
    nodular b.
    serpentine b.
blastemal cell
blastemic
blastic
    b. phase
    b. transformation
blast-induced
    b.-i. cognitive defect
    b.-i. memory defect
Blastobotrys
Blastococcus saxobsidens
Blastoconidium
Blastocystis hominis
blastocyte
blastocytoma

blastogenesis assay
blastogenetic, blastogenic
    b. factor (BF)
blastoid
    b. variant
    b. variant of mantel cell
      lymphoma (BMCL)
blastoma
    biphasic b.
    epithelial predominant b.
    b. mantel cell lymphoma (BMCL)
    pleuropulmonary b.
    pluricentric b.
    pulmonary b.
    unicentric b.
blastomere
blastomogenic
Blastomonas ursincola
Blastomyces
    B. brasiliensis
    B. coccidioides
    B. dermatitidis
blastomycete
blastomycin
Blastomycoides
blastomycosis
    European b.
    North American b.
    pulmonary b.
    b. serology
    South American b.
blastophore
Blastopirellula marina
Blastoschizomyces capitatus
blastospore
blastula, pl. **blastulae**
blastulation
Blatin syndrome
Blatta
blattae
    Escherichia b.
Blattella
Blattidae
blauseare (Berlin blue acid)
BLB
    Bessey, Lowry, Bock
    Boothby, Lovelace, Bulbulian
    BLB mask
    BLB unit
bleb
    blunt b.
    cytoplasmic b.
    emphysematous b.
    plasma membrane b.
    subpleural b.
bleed
    acute b.
bleeder
bleeding (BL)

breakthrough b. (BB, BTB)
dysfunctional uterine b.
estrogen withdrawal b. (EWB)
functional b.
gastrointestinal b.
implantation b.
occult b.
placentation b.
b. polyp
postmenopausal b.
postmortem b.
rectal b.
b. time (BT)
b. time test

blennadenitis
blennogenic
blennogenous
blennoid
blennorrhagia
blennorrhagica
keratoderma b.
keratosis b.

blennorrhagic inflammation
blennorrhea
b. adultorum
b. inclusion
inclusion b.
b. neonatorum

blennorrheal conjunctivitis
blennuria
blepharitis ulcerosa
blepharoplast
blepharoptosis
Blessig
B. groove
B. space

BLG
beta lactoglobulin

blighted ovum
blind
b. fistula
b. loop syndrome
b. passage
b. punch biopsy
b. test

blindness
hysterical b.
river b.

B-lineage
blister
b. agent
blood b.

b. cell
cutaneous b.
fever b.
subepidermal b.

Blitz nevi
bloated cell
bloater
blue b. (BB)

bloc
en b.

Bloch
B. method
B. reaction

blochi
Scopulariopsis b.

Bloch-Sulzberger
B.-S. disease
B.-S. syndrome

block
b. in anterosuperior division of left branch (BSDLB)
atrioventricular b.
AV b.
bundle branch b. (BBB)
complete heart b. (CHB)
complete left bundle-branch b. (CLBBB)
complete right bundle-branch b. (CRBBB)
b. diagram
first-degree heart b.
horse serum b.
incomplete right bundle branch b.
left bundle branch b.
paraffin b.
b. in posteroinferior division of left branch (BIDLB)
second-degree heart b.
third-degree heart b.

blockade
adrenergic neuron b.
alpha adrenergic b.
beta adrenergic b.
cholinergic b.
combined androgen b.
narcotic b.
renal b.
virus b.

blocker
beta b.
histamine receptor b.

B

NOTES

blocking
  b. agent
  b. antibody (BA)
  b. antibody reaction
  b. filter
  b. solution
block-like chromatin condensation
Blocq disease
blood (b)
  b. acylcarnitine analysis
  b. agar
  b. agar plate (BAP)
  b. agent
  b. albumin
  b. alcohol
  b. alcohol concentration (BAC)
  Almén test for b.
  anticoagulated b.
  Apt test for swallowed b.
  arterial b.
  arterialized b.
  arteriolization of venous b.
  b. bank (BB)
  b. bank technology specialist
  b. bicarbonate
  b. blister
  b. buffer base (BB)
  b. buffering capacity
  buffer value of the b.
  b. calcium level
  b. calculus
  b. capillary
  b. cast
  b. cell
  b. cell count
  b. cell count automation
  b. chemistry study
  chocolate b. (CB)
  b. cholesterol level
  citrated b.
  b. clot
  CMV-seronegative b.
  b. coagulation disorder
  b. coagulation factor
  b. component
  connective tissue supply b.
  cord b.
  b. corpuscle
  b. crisis
  b. crystal
  b. culture
  b. cyst
  b. cytolysate
  defibrinated b.
  b. disc
  b. donation
  b. dust
  b. dyscrasia
  b. extravasation

  b. film
  b. filter
  b. fluke
  fragility of the b.
  b. gas
  b. gas analysis
  b. ghost
  b. glucose (BG)
  b. granulocyte-specific activity
    (BGSA)
  b. group
  b. group agglutinin
  b. group agglutinogen
  b. group antibody
  b. group antigen (BGA)
  b. group antigen SLex
  b. group antiserum
  b. group chimera
  b. grouping
  b. grouping serum
  b. group-specific substances A, B
  b. group substance
  b. group systems
  b. incompatibility
  b. indices
  intravascular coagulation of b.
  irradiated CPD b.
  b. island
  laky b.
  b. loss (BL)
  b. loss anemia
  b. lymph
  b. microvessel density
  mixed venous b.
  b. mole
  b. mote
  occult b.
  oxygen capacity of b.
  oxygen content of b.
  peripheral b.
  b. pH
  b. plasma
  b. plasma fraction
  b. plastid
  platelet-poor b. (PPB)
  b. poisoning
  b. pressure (BP)
  b. puzzles
  b. quotient
  red venous b. (RVB)
  b. salvage
  b. sinusoid
  sludged b.
  b. smear
  b. smear morphology
  b. spot
  b. spot screening assay
  stool occult b.
  strawberry-cream b.

b. substitute
b. sugar (BS)
b. trematode
b. tumor
b. type
b. typing
unspun peripheral b.
b. urea clearance
b. urea nitrogen (BUN)
b. urea nitrogen test
venous b.
b. vessel
b. vessel fibrosis
b. volume (BV)
b. volume measurement
b. volume nomogram
b. warming
whole b. (B, WB)
blood-air barrier
blood-aqueous barrier
blood-brain barrier (BBB)
blood-cerebral barrier
blood-clot lysis time (BLT)
Bloodgood disease
bloodless glomeruli
bloodstain pattern analysis
blood-testis barrier
blood-thymus barrier
bloodworm
bloody
b. feces
b. inflammatory exudate
b. stool
Bloom
B. and Richardson classification
B. syndrome
Bloom-Richardson scale
Bloor test
blot
Southern b. (SB)
b. test
Western b.
Blount
B. disease
B. test
Blount-Barber disease
blowback
blowfly
blowout pipette
Bloxam test
BLPD
B-cell lymphoproliferative disorder

BLS
base lymphocyte syndrome
BLT
blood-clot lysis time
BLU
Bessey-Lowry unit
blue
Alcian b. (AB)
aniline b.
anthracene b.
azovan b.
b. baby
Berlin b.
Biebrich scarlet-picroaniline b.
b. bloater (BB)
brilliant cresyl b. (BCB)
bromphenol b.
bromthymol b.
carbolic methylene b. (CMB)
b. cell pattern
b. cell tumor
cresyl b.
b. cytoplasm
dextran b. (DB)
Diagnex B.
b. diaper syndrome
b. dome cyst
b. edema
eosin-methylene b. (EMB)
Evans b.
b. formazan
indigo b.
insoluble Prussian b.
Isamine b.
isosulfan b.
Kühne methylene b.
leucomethylene b.
leuco patent b.
b. litmus paper
Löffler methylene b.
martius scarlet b. (MSB)
methyl b.
methylene b. (MB)
methylthymol b.
new methylene b.
Nile b.
Nile b. A
patent b. V
polychrome methylene b.
Prussian b.
b. pus
pyrrol b.

B

NOTES

blue *(continued)*
    rhodanile b.
    b. rubber bleb nevus
    sky b.
    b. spot
    thymol b.
    toluidine b. (TB)
    trypan b.
    Turnbull b.
    Victoria b.
bluecomb
    b. disease of chickens
    b. disease of turkeys
    b. virus
bluetongue virus
bluish
    eosin I b.
Blumenthal disease
Blum syndrome
blunt
    b. bleb
    b. duct adenosis
    b. end
    b. force trauma (BFT)
    b. head injury
    b. trauma
blush
    b. appearance
    tumor b.
BLV
    bovine leukemia virus
B-lymphocyte
    B.-l. assay
    B.-l. stimulatory factor (BSF)
BLyS
    B lymphocyte stimulator
BM
    body mass
    bone marrow
BMCL
    blastoid variant of mantel cell lymphoma
    blastoma mantel cell lymphoma
BMD
    Becker muscular dystrophy
BMG
    benign monoclonal gammopathy
BMI
    body mass index
bmk
    birthmark
BML
    benign metastasizing leiomyoma
B-mode
BMP
    basic metabolic panel
BMR
    basal metabolic rate

BMT
    bone marrow transplantation
        Auto-PBSC BMT
BN
    branchial neuritis
        BN ProSpec
B-NHL
    B-cell non-Hodgkin lymphoma
BNO
    bladder neck obstruction
BNS
    benign nephrosclerosis
Boas
    B. point
    B. test
Boas-Oppler
    B.-O. bacillus
    B.-O. lactobacillus
boat clinger
boat-shaped heart
Bodansky unit (BU)
Bodian
    B. copper-PROTARGOL stain
    B. histochemical stain
    B. method
Bodo
    B. caudatus
    B. saltans
    B. urinaria
    B. urinarius
body
    acetone b.
    acidophilic b.
    adrenal b.
    alcoholic hyaline b.
    Alder b.
    Alder-Reilly b.
    alkapton b.
    aortic b.
    apoptotic b.
    Arantius b.
    Arnold b.
    asbestos b. (AB)
    Aschoff b.
    asteroid b.
    Auer b.
    Babès-Ernst b.
    bacillary b.
    Balbiani b.
    Barr chromatin b.
    basal b.
    Bence Jones b.
    Bollinger b.
    Borrel b.
    brassy b.
    bronchial obstruction by
      foreign b.
    Cabot ring b.
    Call-Exner b.

cancer b.
b. cavity
cell b.
central b.
chromaffin b.
chromatin b.
chromatinic b.
Civatte b.
coccygeal b.
colloid b.
conchoidal b.
Councilman hyaline b.
Cowdry type A, B inclusion b.
creola b.
curvilinear b.
cytoid b.
cytoplasmic inclusion b.
Deetjen b.
demilune b.
dense b.
Döhle inclusion b.
Donné b.
Donovan b.
Dutcher b.
Ehrlich inner b.
elementary b.
embryoid b.
eosinophilic viral inclusion b.
F b.
ferruginous b.
fibrin b.
fibrous b.
b. fluid
b. fluid analysis
b. fluid loss
foreign b. (FB)
fruiting b.
fuchsin b.
gall b.
Gamna-Favre b.
Gamna-Gandy b.
glass b.
glomus b.
Gordon b.
Guarnieri b.
Halberstaedter-Prowazek b.
Hassall b.
Heinz b.
Heinz-Ehrlich b.
b. hematocrit-venous hematocrit
   ratio (BH:VH)
hematoxylin b.

Herring b.
Hirano b.
HJ b.
hyaline Civatte b.
hyaloid b.
immune b. (IB)
inclusion b. (IB)
intercarotid b.
intraocular foreign b. (IOFB)
intrauterine foreign b. (IUFB)
Jaworski b.
Joest b.
Jolly b.
juxtaglomerular b.
Kamino b.
ketone b. (KB)
Lafora b.
Lallemand b.
lamellar b.
lateral geniculate b.
LCL b.'s
LE b.
Leishman-Donovan b.
Lewy b.
Lindner b.
Lipschütz b.
b. louse
Luse b.
b. of Luys syndrome
Mallory b.
malpighian b.
Maragiliano b.
b. mass (BM)
b. mass index (BMI)
Masson b.
May-Hegglin b.
Medlar b.
melon seed b.
membranous cytoplasmic b. (MCB)
metachromatic b.
metallic foreign b. (MFB)
Michaelis-Gutmann b.
mineral oil foreign b.
Miyagawa b.
molluscum b.
multilamellar b.
multivesicular b.
myelin b.
Negri b.
nerve cell b.
neuroepithelial b.
Nissl b.

B

NOTES

body *(continued)*
nodular b.
nuclear inclusion b.
Odland b.
onion b.
oval fat b. (OFB)
oxyphil inclusion b.
pacchionian b.
Pappenheimer b.
paraaortic b.
paranephric b.
paranuclear b.
Paschen b.
pectinate b.
Pick inclusion b.
pigmented layer of ciliary b.
pineal b.
Plimmer b.
polar b.
polyhedral b.
Prowazek-Greeff b.
psammoma b.
psittacosis inclusion b.
Renaut b.
residual b.
retained foreign b. (RFB)
reticulate b.
rice b.
Rushton b.
Russell b.
sand b.
Sandström b.
Schaumann b.
Schiller-Duval b.
Schmorl b.
sclerotic b.
selenoid b.
b. snatching
spiculated b.
striate b.
b. substance isolation (BSI)
suprarenal b.
b. surface areas (BSA)
b. surface burned (BSB)
tactoid b.
b. temperature
b. temperature, ambient pressure, saturated (BTPS)
thermostable b.
threshold b.
thyroid b.
tigroid b.
tingible b.
Todd b.
trachoma b.
Trousseau-Lallemand b.
tuffstone b.
tympanic b.
ultimobranchial b.

Verocay b.
Virchow-Hassall b.
vitreous b.
Weibel-Palade b.
Wesenberg-Hamazaki b.
Wolf-Orton b.
X chromatin b.
Y b.
yellow b.
zebra b.
Zuckerkandl b.
bodypacker syndrome
body-section radiography
Boeck
B. disease
B. sarcoid
Boeck-Drbohlav-Locke egg-serum medium
Boehmer hematoxylin
Boehringer
B. Mannheim DIG-Nucleic Detection kit
B. Mannheim DIG-Oligonucleotide Tailing kit
B. Mannheim Kermix cytokeratin cocktail
B. in vitro transcription kit
boenickei
Mycobacterium b.
Boerhaave syndrome
Boettcher cell
Bogaert disease
bogorensis
Asaia b.
Bogoriellaceae
bogoriensis
Rhodobaca b.
bohemica
Verpa b.
Bohr
B. effect
B. equation
boil
Madura b.
boiling point (bp)
Bolande tumor
Boletus piperatus
bolidensis
Arsenicicoccus b.
Boling burner
Bolivian hemorrhagic fever
boliviensis
Halomonas b.
Boll cell
Bollinger
B. body
B. granule
bolteae
Clostridium b.

Boltzmann constant
BOM
    bilateral otitis media
bomb
    ammonium nitrate b.
    barometric b.
    dirty b. (radiation dispersal device)
    fertilizer truck b.
    letter b.
    nail b.
    parcel b.
    pipe b.
    remotely controlled b.
Bombardia
bombardment
Bombay
    B. blood group
    B. phenotype
bombesin receptor
Bombidae
Bonanno test
bond
    chemical b.
    coordinate covalent b.
    covalent b.
    disulfide b.
    electron pair b.
    b. energy
    high-energy b.
    hydrogen b.
    intrachain disulphide b.
    ionic b.
    metallic b.
    peptide b.
    pi b.
    sigma b.
    triple b.
bone
    b. abscess
    adamantinoma of long b.'s
    b. age
    b. architecture
    b. aseptic necrosis
    b. biopsy
    brittle b.
    bundle b.
    b. canaliculus
    cancellous b.
    cartilage b.
    b. chip
    compact b.
    b. corpuscle

cortical b.
creeping substitution of b.
cribriform plate of ethmoid b.
b. cyst
decalcified b.
dermal b.
developing b.
b. disease
endochondral b.
epihyal b.
fibrous dysplasia of b.
b. formation rate (BFR)
giant cell tumor of b. (GCTB)
b. GLA-protein (BGP)
b. graft (BG)
heterologous b.
hyperlucency of b.
b. infarct
lamella of b.
lamellar b.
malignant giant cell tumor of b.
marble b.
b. marrow (BM)
b. marrow abnormality
b. marrow aplasia
b. marrow aspiration
b. marrow aspiration and biopsy
b. marrow carcinoma
b. marrow depression
b. marrow differential count
b. marrow disorder
b. marrow embolism
b. marrow embolus
b. marrow failure
b. marrow iron stores
b. marrow lesion
b. marrow macrophage
b. marrow particle
b. marrow precursor cell
b. marrow scan
b. marrow suppression
b. marrow transplant
b. marrow transplantation (BMT)
b. matrix
b. matrix alteration
membrane b.
b. morphogenetic protein 7 gene
nonlamellar b.
nonneoplastic disease of b.
Paget disease of b.
b. pain
painful b.

B

NOTES

bone *(continued)*
    perforating fiber of periodontal
      ligament and b.
    perichondral b.
    periosteal b.
    ping-pong b.
    b. rarefaction
    Recklinghausen disease of b.
    replacement b.
    b. resorption
    reticulated b.
    b. sawing
    b. sclerosis
    septal b.
    b. sialoprotein
    sieve b.
    solitary plasmacytoma of b. (SPB)
    spicule of b.
    spongy b.
    tibial cortical b.
    b. tissue
    trabecular b.
    b. tumor
    b. turnover
    b. weapon
    b. whorl
    woven b.
bone-resorbing osteoclast
bongori
    Salmonella b.
bonnei
    Phaneropsolus b.
Bonnet-Dechaume-Blanc syndrome
Bonnevie-Ullrich syndrome
Bonnier syndrome
bony
    b. ankylosis
    b. callus
    b. heart
    b. island
    b. semicircular canal
bookeri
    Alcaligenes b.
Böök syndrome
Boolean function
BOOP
    bronchiolitis obliterans organizing
    pneumonia
Boophilus annulatus
booster
    b. dose
    b. effect
    b. response
Boothby, Lovelace, Bulbulian (BLB)
borate
    sodium b.
Borchgrevink method
border
    brush b.

    b. cell
    striated brush b.
    vermilion b.
borderline
    b. glucose tolerance test (BGTT)
    b. leprosy
    b. malignancy
    b. ovarian tumor
Bordet amboceptor
Bordetella
    B. bronchiseptica
    B. hinzii
    B. holmesii
    B. parapertussis
    B. pertussis
    B. pertussis indirect fluorescent
    B. petrii
Bordet-Gengou (BG)
    B.-G. bacillus
    B.-G. culture medium
    B.-G. phenomenon
    B.-G. potato blood agar
    B.-G. reaction
    B.-G. test
borealis
    Paenibacillus b.
boreus
    Subtercola b.
boric
    b. acid
    b. acid broth
borism
Börjeson-Forssman-Lehmann syndrome
Börjeson syndrome
borkumensis
    Alcanivorax b.
Born
    B. method
    B. method of wax plate
      reconstruction
Borna
    B. disease
    B. disease virus
Bornavirus
Bornholm
    B. disease
    B. disease virus
boron
    b. assay
    b. trifluoride-methanol
Borrel
    B. blue stain
    B. body
Borrelia
    B. afzelii
    B. anserina
    B. berbera
    B. burgdorferi
    B. burgdorferi sensu lato

B. *burgdorferi* sensu stricto
B. *carteri*
B. *caucasica*
B. *crocidurae*
B. *duttonii*
B. *garinii*
B. *hermsii*
B. *hispanica*
B. *kochii*
B. *latyschewii*
B. *mazzottii*
B. *parkeri*
B. *persica*
B. *recurrentis*
B. *refringens*
B. *sinica*
B. *turcica*
B. *turicatae*
B. *venezuelensis*
B. *vincentii*
borreliosis
Lyme b.
Borrmann classification
Borst-Jadassohn type intraepidermal epithelioma
Bosea
B. *eneae*
B. *massiliensis*
B. *minatitlanensis*
B. *vestrisii*
bosselated
bosselation
Bostock disease
Boston exanthema
botfly
bothria
bothridium
bothriocephaliasis
Bothriocephalus
B. *cordatus*
B. *latus*
B. *mansoni*
B. *mansonoides*
bothrium
bothropic antitoxin
Bothrops
B. antitoxin
B. *atrox* serine proteinase
botniense
Mycobacterium b.
Botryoascus
Botryobasidium

Botryodiplodia theobromae
botryoid
b. odontogenic cyst
b. rhabdomyosarcoma
b. sarcoma
botryoides
pseudosarcoma b.
sarcoma b.
Botryomyces caespitosus
botryomycosis
botryomycotic
botryosa
Veronaea b.
Botryosphaeria rhodina
Botryotinia
Botryotrichum
Botrytis
bots
Böttcher
B. cell
B. crystal
bottle
Nalgene PETG media b.
Roux b.
botulin
botulinum
b. antitoxin
Clostridium b.
b. toxin
botulinus
Bacillus b.
b. toxin
botulism
b. antitoxin
foodborne b.
b. immune globulin intravenous (human) (BIG-IV)
infant b.
inhalational b.
intestinal b.
b. intoxication
wound b.
Bouchard
B. coefficient
B. disease
B. node
Bouchardat test
Boudierella
Bouffardi
B. black mycetoma
B. white mycetoma

B

NOTES

139

bouffardi
    Aspergillus b.
    Penicillium b.
Bouguer law
Bouillaud
    B. disease
    B. syndrome
bouillon filtrate (bf)
Bouin
    B. fluid
    B. picroformol-acetic fixative
    B. solution
boundary lamina
bound-free ratio (B:F)
bound serum iron (BSI)
bouquet fever
Bourneville disease
Bourneville-Pringle disease
bouton
    axonal terminal b.
    b. en passage
    synaptic b.
    terminal b.
boutonneuse fever
Bouveret
    B. disease
    B. syndrome
bouvetii
    Acinetobacter b.
Bovicola
bovihominis
    Sarcocystis b.
bovine
    b. antitoxin
    b. colloid
    b. enteritis (BE)
    b. ephemeral fever
    b. gamma globulin (BGG)
    b. growth hormone (BGH)
    b. herpes mammillitis
    b. leukemia virus (BLV)
    b. leukosis virus
    b. malaria
    b. mastitis
    b. papular stomatitis
    b. papular stomatitis virus
    b. red blood cell (BRBC)
    b. rhinovirus
    b. serum albumin (BSA)
    b. smooth muscle cytosol
    b. spongiform encephalopathy
    b. tubercle bacillus
    b. ulcerative mammillitis
    b. vaccinia mammillitis
    b. virus diarrhea
bovinum
    cor b.
bovis
    Actinomyces b.

    Anaplasma b.
    Bartonella b.
    Cysticercus b.
    Haemophilus b.
    Lachnobacterium b.
    Moraxella b.
    Mycobacterium b.
    Streptococcus b.
bowel
    b. bypass syndrome
    b. infarction
    b. perforation
Bowen
    B. disease
    B. precancerous dermatosis
bowenoid papulosis (BP)
Bowers-McComb unit
Bowie stain
Bowman
    B. capsule
    B. disc
    B. gland
    B. layer
    B. membrane
    B. space
bowmanii
    Clostridium b.
boxcar organism
Boyden
    B. chamber
    B. chamber assay device
boydii
    Allescheria b.
    Petriellidium b.
    Pseudallescheria b.
    Shigella b.
Boyle law
bozemanii
    Legionella b.
BP
    blood pressure
    bowenoid papulosis
    bypass
bp
    base pair
    boiling point
BPC
    benign pheochromocytoma
BPCHI
    benign pheochromocytoma with
      histological invasion
BPD
    bronchopulmonary dysplasia
BPG
    benign paraganglioma
BPH
    benign prostatic hypertrophy

BPI
bacterial permeability-inducing
BPI protein
B-PLL
B-cell prolymphocytic leukemia
B-plus Fix
BPOP
bizarre parosteal osteochondromatous
proliferation
BPP
binding protein protease
Bq
becquerel
BR27.29 breast antigen
Braak neurofibrillary tangle staging
BRACAnalysis genetic susceptibility breast and ovarian cancer test
bracchium
Agromyces b.
brachial
b. dance
b. gland
b. plexitis
Brachiola
Brachmann-de Lange syndrome
Brachybacterium
B. fresconis
B. muris
B. sacelli
brachycephalic
Brachycladium
brachydactyly
brachymesomelia-renal syndrome
Brachysporium
Brackiella oedipodis
Bracovirus
Bradford microassay procedure
Bradley disease
Bradshaw test
bradykinin
Bradyrhizobium
B. betae
B. yuanmingense
bradyzoite
Brailsford-Morquio disease
brain
b. abscess
b. atrophy
b. cicatrix
compression of b.
b. concussion
b. congestion

b. contusion
b. death
b. death syndrome
b. edema
b. lesion
b. oxytocin
primary Ki-1 lymphoma of b.
respirator b.
b. sand
b. swelling
b. tumor (BT)
brain-derived neurotrophic factor (BDNF)
Brainerd diarrhea
brain-hair follicle axis (BHA)
brain-heart
b.-h. infusion (BHI)
b.-h. infusion agar
b.-h. infusion broth
b.-h. infusion broth medium
brainstem
b. disease
b. glioma
b. tumor
braking radiation
branch
block in anterosuperior division of left b. (BSDLB)
block in posteroinferior division of left b. (BIDLB)
b.'s of the carotid artery
b.'s of the mesenteric artery
b.'s of the renal cortex
branched
b. calculus
b. chain
b. DNA (b-DNA)
b. DNA signal amplification assay
branched-chain
b.-c. alpha keto acid decarboxylase
b.-c. alpha keto acid dehydrogenase
b.-c. amino acid (BCAA)
b.-c. aminoaciduria
b.-c. keto acid (BCKA)
b.-c. ketoaciduria
b.-c. ketonuria
brancher
b. deficiency
b. enzyme
branchial
b. cleft cyst

NOTES

branchial *(continued)*
    b. fistula
    b. neuritis (BN)
branching
    b. cardiac fiber
    b. decay
    b. enzyme
    b. fraction
    b. glycogen storage disease
    b. ratio
branchioma
Branhamaceae
Branhamella catarrhalis
brasilensis
    Paenibacillus b.
Brasil fixative
brasiliensis
    Blastomyces b.
    Nocardia b.
    Paracoccidioides b.
    Vibrio b.
    Xenopsylla b.
brassicacearum
    Pseudomonas b.
brassicae
    Hylemya b.
brassy
    b. body
    b. cough
brauni
    Digramma b.
    Diplogonoporus b.
brazilein
Brazilian trypanosomiasis
brazilianum
    Plasmodium b.
braziliense
    Ancylostoma b.
braziliensis
    Leishmania braziliensis b.
brazilin
BRBC
    bovine red blood cell
BRCA1 gene
BRCA2 gene
BrDu, BrdU
    5-bromodeoxyuridine
    BrDu antibody
    BrDu banding
bread-and-butter pericardium
bread-loaf method
break
    DNA b.
    isochromatid b.
breakbone fever
breakdown
    protein b.
    starvation-induced protein b.

breaker
    circuit b.
    vacuum b.
breakpoint
    b. analysis
    b. cluster region-Abelson murine leukemia virus (BCR-ABL)
    b. cluster region rearrangement
    b. region
breakthrough bleeding (BB, BTB)
breast
    b. biopsy (BB)
    b. cancer
    b. carcinoma
    b. cyst
    cystic disease of the b.
    cystic hyperplasia of the b.
    b. duct
    fibroadenoma of b.
    fibrocystic condition of b.
    fibrocystic disease of b.
    funnel b.
    intracystic papillary lesion of the b.
    medullary carcinoma of b.
    Paget disease of b.
    papillomatosis of b.
    pigeon b.
    pleomorphic lobular carcinoma in situ of the b. (PLCIS)
    shotty b.
    b. specimen radiography
    tension cyst of b.
    b. tumor
breath
    b. analysis test
    b. hydrogen analysis
BreathTek UBT *H. pylori* **test**
Brecher-Cronkite method
Brecher new methylene blue technique
Breda disease
Breed smear
Breen and Tullis method
bregma
Breisky disease
bremensis
    Geobacter b.
Bremsstrahlung radiation
Brennemann syndrome
brenneri
    Pseudomonas b.
Brenner tumor
Breslow
    B. malignant melanoma assay
    B. malignant melanoma classification
    B. thickness
    B. tumor index
Bretonneau disease

Brettanomyces
Breus mole
breve
>*Flavobacterium b.*
>*Gymnodinium b.*

Brevibacillus
>*B. invocatus*
>*B. limnophilus*

Brevibacteriaceae
Brevibacterieae
Brevibacterium
>*B. luteolum*
>*B. paucivorans*
>*B. picturae*
>*B. sanguinis*

brevicaeca
>*Heterophyes b.*

brevicaudum
>*Oesophagostomum b.*

brevicaulis
>*Scopulariopsis b.*

brevicollis
>dystrophia b.

Brevidensovirus
brevis
>Bacillus b.
>Janibacter b.
>Lactobacillus b.
>Sulfitobacter b.
>Thermomonas b.

Brevundimonas
>*B. alba*
>*B. aurantiaca*
>*B. bacteroides*
>*B. diminuta*
>*B. intermedia*
>*B. nasdae*
>*B. subvibrioides*
>*B. variabilis*
>*B. vesicularis*

Brewer infarct
brickdust deposit
brickmaker's anemia
brick-shaped virus
bridge
>arteriolovenular b.
>cell b.
>conjugation b.
>b. corpuscle
>cytoplasmic b.
>fibrinogen b.
>Gaskell b.

intercellular b.
myocardial b.
b. rectifier
salt b.
Wheatstone b.
bridging
>b. fibrosis
>b. hepatic necrosis
>internuclear b. (INB)

bright
>b. contrast
>B. disease

bright-field microscopy
Brill disease
brilliant
>b. cresyl blue (BCB)
>b. crocein
>b. green
>b. green bile salt agar
>b. vital red
>b. yellow

Brill-Symmers disease
Brill-Zinsser disease
Brinton disease
Brion-Kayser disease
Briosia
Briquet syndrome
brisance
brisk infiltrate
Brissaud disease
Brissaud-Marie syndrome
Brissaud-Sicard syndrome
bristle cell
Bristowe syndrome
British
>B. antilewisite (BAL)
>B. thermal unit (BTU)
>B. type amyloid angiopathy

brittle bone
BRM
>biuret-reactive material

broad
>b. fish tapeworm
>b. smear
>b. spectrum
>b. urinary cast

broad-beta disease
broad-betalipoproteinemia
broadening
>peak b.

broad-spectrum antibiotic
Broca area

NOTES

Brock syndrome
Brocq disease
Broders
    B. classification
    B. tumor index
Brodie
    B. abscess
    B. disease
    B. knee
broegbernensis
    Pseudoxanthomonas b.
broken
    b. cell preparation
    b. compensation
bromate
bromcresol
    b. green
    b. purple
bromelain
bromide
    aminoethylisothiouronium b. (AET)
    b. assay
    cetyltrimethylammonium b.
    ethidium b.
    glycopyrronium b.
    hexamethonium b.
    methyl b.
    potassium b.
    sodium b.
bromination
bromine
bromobenzylcyanide
    NATO code for riot control
    agent b. (CA)
bromocresol purple desoxycholate (BCP-D)
bromocriptine suppression test
bromodeoxyuridine
5-bromodeoxyuridine (BrDu, BrdU)
bromoderma
bromoiodism
bromomethane
Bromovirus
bromphenol, bromophenol
    b. blue
    b. test
bromsulphalein (BSP)
    b. test
bromthymol blue
bronchi (*pl. of* bronchus)
bronchial
    b. adenoma
    b. aspirate anaerobic culture
    b. asthma (BA)
    b. brush biopsy
    b. calculus
    b. carcinoid
    b. carcinoma
    b. challenge test

    b. cyst
    b. gland
    b. gland cell adenocarcinoma
    b. hyperreactivity
    b. lymphocyte
    b. obstruction by foreign body
    b. pneumonia
    b. polyp
    b. surface cell adenocarcinoma
    b. wall abnormality
    b. washing
    b. washing cytology
bronchialis
    Cyathostoma b.
    Gordonia b.
bronchic cell
bronchiectasia sicca
bronchiectasis
    cylindrical b.
    cystic b.
    dry b.
    fusiform b.
    saccular b.
bronchiectatic
bronchiolar
    b. adenocarcinoma
    b. carcinoma
    b. exocrine cell
    b. lymphocyte
    b. metaplasia
bronchiole
    b. obstruction
    respiratory b.
    terminal b.
bronchiolectasis
bronchioli (*pl. of* bronchiolus)
bronchiolitis
    exudative b.
    b. fibrosa obliterans
    b. obliterans organizing pneumonia (BOOP)
    b. obliterans syndrome
    obliterative b.
    proliferative b.
    respiratory b.
bronchioloalveolar
    b. adenocarcinoma
    b. carcinoma (BAC)
bronchiolus, pl. bronchioli
    bronchioli respiratorii
bronchiorum
    tunica muscularis b.
bronchiostenosis
bronchiseptica
    Bordetella b.
    Brucella b.
bronchisepticus
    Alcaligenes b.

Bacillus b.
Haemophilus b.
bronchitic
bronchitis
 acute b.
 asthmatic b. (AB)
 chronic b. (CB)
 croupous b.
 fibrinous b.
 infectious avian b.
 b. obliterans
 obliterative b.
 plastic b.
 pseudomembranous b.
bronchitis/bronchiolitis
 acute b./b. (ABB)
bronchoalveolar lavage (BAL)
bronchoaspergillosis
bronchoblastomycosis
bronchocandidiasis
bronchocavernous
bronchocentric granulomatosis (BCG)
bronchoconstriction
bronchoconstrictor
bronchodilatation
bronchodilator
bronchoedema
bronchoesophageal fistula
bronchofiberscopy
bronchogenic
 b. carcinoma
 b. cyst
 b. tumor
broncholith
broncholithiasis
bronchomalacia
bronchomycosis
bronchopathy
bronchopleural fistula
bronchopneumonia
 acute hemorrhagic b.
 confluent b.
 diffuse b.
 focal b.
 hemorrhagic b.
 necrotizing b.
 sequestration b.
 subacute b.
 tuberculous b.
 virus b.
bronchopneumopathy
bronchoprovocation

bronchopulmonary
 b. aspergillosis
 b. dysplasia (BPD)
 b. histoplasmosis
 b. lavage
 b. sequestration
bronchoscopic smear
bronchospasm
bronchostenosis
bronchotracheal aspirate
bronchovesicular
bronchus, pl. **bronchi**
 mucous gland adenoma of b.
 (MGAB)
 tunica mucosa bronchi
bronchus-associated lymphoid tissue (BALT)
Brönsted-Lowry
 B.-L. acid
 B.-L. base
bronzed disease
bronze diabetes
bronzinum
 chloasma b.
brood cell
Brooke
 B. disease
 B. tumor
Brooker heterotopic ossification classification
broomstick extremity
broth
 Bacto Middlebrook 7H9 b.
 boric acid b.
 brain-heart infusion b.
 carbohydrate b.
 Casman b.
 chopped meat b.
 decarboxylase b.
 Eijkman lactose b.
 ethyl violet azide b.
 glucose-format b.
 glycerin b.
 glycerin-potato b.
 GN b.
 gram-negative b.
 haricot b.
 hippurate b.
 Imago b.
 indole-nitrate b.
 inosite-free b.
 iron b.

B

NOTES

broth *(continued)*
    Kitasato b.
    Koser citrate b.
    lactose-litmus b.
    lauryl sulfate b.
    lead b.
    MacConkey b.
    malachite green b.
    malt extract b.
    Martin b.
    methyl red, Voges-Proskauer b.
    Middlebrook b.
    MR-VP b.
    Mueller-Hinton b.
    nitrate b.
    nutrient b.
    b. OADC Enrichment b.
    Parietti b.
    Pike streptococcal b.
    Rosenow veal-brain b.
    selenite b.
    selenite-cystine b.
    serum b.
    sodium chloride b.
    Spirolate b.
    sterility test b.
    Stuart b.
    sugar b.
    tetrathionate enrichment b.
    thioglycolate b.
    Todd-Hewitt b.
    trypticase soy with agar b.
    urease test b.
    Voges-Proskauer b.
    wheat b.
    wort b.
brown
    b. adipose tissue
    b. atrophy
    Bismarck b.
    Bismarck b. R, Y
    b. bowel syndrome
    b. edema
    b. fat
    b. hemoglobin-derived pigment
    b. induration of the lung
    b. layer
    b. recluse spider
    b. striae
    Sudan b.
    b. tumor
Brown-Brenn
    B.-B. stain
    B.-B. technique
Brown-Hopp tissue Gram stain
brownian
    b. motion
    b. movement
Brown-Pearce tumor

Brown-Sequard paralysis
Brown-Symmers disease
brucei
    Trypanosoma brucei b.
Brucella
    B. abortus
    B. agar
    B. agglutination test
    B. bronchiseptica
    B. canis
    B. melitensis
    B. strain 19 vaccine
    B. suis
Brucellaceae
Brucelleae
brucellergin
brucellin
brucellosis agglutinin
Bruch
    B. gland
    B. membrane
Bruck disease
Brücke tunic
Brudzinski meningeal sign
Brugia
    B. malayi
    B. microfilariae
Brugsch syndrome
bruit
    flank b.
Brumimicrobium glaciale
brumpti
    Oesophagostomum b.
Brumpt white mycetoma
Brunchorstia
brunescens
    cataracta b.
Brunhilde virus
Brunn
    B. epithelial nest
    B. membrane
Brunner gland
brunneroma
brunnerosis
brunnipes
    Anopheles b.
Bruns
    B. glucose medium
    B. syndrome
Brunsting-Perry pemphigoid
Brunsting syndrome
brush
    b. bipolar cell
    b. border
    b. border enzyme
    endometrial b.
    protected catheter b.
    b. specimen
brush-border microvillus

brushings
    cytologic b.
    b. cytology
Bruton
    B. disease
    B. type agammaglobulinemia
    B. tyrosine kinase (BTK)
    X-linked agammaglobulinemia of B.
Bryantella formatexigens
BS
    blood sugar
BSA
    bismuth-sulfite agar
    body surface areas
    bovine serum albumin
BSB
    body surface burned
BSC
    biological safety cabinet
BSCC
    basaloid squamous cell carcinoma
BSDLB
    block in anterosuperior division of left
    branch
BSE
    bilateral, symmetrical, and equal
BSF
    B-lymphocyte stimulatory factor
BSFR
    basal secretory flow rate
    BSFR test
BSI
    body substance isolation
    bound serum iron
BSL
    biosafety level
BSL1
    biosafety level 1
BSL2
    biosafety level 2
BSL3
    biosafety level 3
BSL4
    biosafety level 4
BSP
    bromsulphalein
    BSP excretion test
BSS
    balanced salt solution
    Bernard-Soulier syndrome
    buffered saline solution

BSTFA
    bis-trimethylsilyltrifluoroacetamide
BT
    bladder tumor
    bleeding time
    brain tumor
BTB
    breakthrough bleeding
BTK
    Bruton tyrosine kinase
BTPS
    body temperature, ambient pressure,
    saturated
      BTPS conditions of gas
BTTP
    British Testicular Tumour Panel
BTU
    British thermal unit
BU
    Bethesda unit
    Bodansky unit
    busulfan
BUB
    budding uninhibited by benzimidazole
    cancer gene BUB
bubas
bubble
    b. artifact
    b. boy disease
    replication b.
bubo
    cervical b.
    climatic b.
    malignant b.
    primary b.
    tropical b.
bubonic plague
bubonulus
buccal
    b. gland
    b. psoriasis
    b. smear
    b. smear for sex chromatin
    evaluation
buccale
    Mycoplasma b.
buccales
    glandulae b.
buccalis
    Amoeba b.
    Entamoeba b.

NOTES

B

buccalis (continued)
    Leptotrichia b.
    Trichomonas b.
Büchner
    B. extract
    B. tuberculin
buchneri
    Lactobacillus b.
buckelii
    Azoarcus b.
Buckley syndrome
Bucky grid
bud
    gustatory b.
    taste b.
    vascular b.
Budd
    B. cirrhosis
    B. disease
    B. syndrome
Budd-Chiari syndrome
budding
    glandular b.
    b. uninhibited by benzimidazole (BUB)
Buerger disease
buetschlii
    Entamoeba b.
buffalo neck
buffalopox
buffer
    b. action
    b. amplifier
    b. base (BB)
    bicarbonate b.
    cacodylate b.
    b. capacity
    citrate b.
    diluent b.
    HEPES b.
    Holmes alkaline b.
    Joklik b.
    Krebs-Ringer bicarbonate b. (KRB)
    loading b.
    LST b.
    lysis b.
    Millonig phosphate b.
    phosphate b.
    protein b.
    proteinase K b.
    secondary b.
    Supre-Heme b.
    b. system
    Tris-HCl b.
    b. value
    b. value of the blood
    Vector Laboratories VectaShield antifading b.
    veronal b.

buffered
    b. desoxycholate glucose (BDG)
    b. formalin fixative
    b. implant
    b. neutral formalin
    b. saline solution (BSS)
buffy
    b. coat
    b. coat micromethod
    b. coat smear
    b. coat smear study
    b. coat smear test
    b. crust
buffy-coated cell
bug
    assassin b.
    cone-nose b.
    harvest b.
Bugula
Buhl disease
bulb
    conjunctival layer of b.
    end b.
    glomerular layer of olfactory b.
    hair b.
    Krause end b.
    molecular layer of olfactory b.
    olfactory b.
    taste b.
bulbar
    b. conjunctiva
    b. myelitis
    b. palsy
bulbi (*gen. and pl. of* bulbus)
bulbitis
bulboid corpuscle
bulboidea
    corpuscula b.
bulbourethral gland
bulbourethralis
    glandula b.
bulbous pemphigoid
bulbus, gen. and pl. **bulbi**
    ligamentum anulare bulbi
    b. olfactorius
    b. pili
    stratum pigmenti bulbi
    tunica conjunctiva bulbi
    tunica fibrosa bulbi
    tunica vasculosa bulbi
bulgaricus
    Lactobacillus b.
bulimia
bulla, gen. and pl. **bullae**
    intraepidermic b.
    pulmonary b.
    subepidermic b.
bullata
    Mycoplana b.

bulldog head
Bulleidia extructa
Bullera
Bulleromyces albus
bullet
    migrating b.
    b. wipe
bulliform cell
Bullis fever
bull neck
bullosa
    epidermolysis b. (EB)
    junctional epidermolysis b.
    Pseudostertagia b.
bullosis diabeticorum
bullosum
    erythema multiforme b.
bullous
    b. disease
    b. edema
    b. edema vesicae
    b. emphysema
    b. eruption
    b. granulomatous inflammation
    b. impetigo
    b. impetigo of newborn
    b. lichen planus
    b. myringitis
    b. pemphigoid
    b. syphilid
bull's
    b. eye granule
    b. eye lesion
bump
BUN
    blood urea nitrogen
BUN/creatinine ratio
bundle
    Arnold b.
    atrioventricular b.
    b. of axon
    Bachmann b.
    b. bone
    b. branch block (BBB)
    Bürdach b.
    Clarke collateral b.
    collagen b.
    Helie b.
    His b.
    Keith b.
    Kent b.
    Kent-His b.

    Monakow b.
    muscle b.
    Pick b.
    Rathke b.
    tendon b.
    trunk of atrioventricular b.
bungpagga
bunion
Bunostomum
    B. phlebotomum
    B. trigonocephalum
Bunsen
    B. burner
    B. coefficient
Bunyamwera
    B. fever
    B. virus
Bunyaviridae
Bunyavirus
buoyant density
buphthalmos
Burchard-Liebermann reaction
Bürdach
    B. bundle
    B. column
    B. cuneate fasciculus
    B. fissure
    B. tract
Burdach fiber
burden
    mutation b.
    radionuclide body b.
    tumor b.
buret, burette
burgdorferi
    Borrelia b.
Bürger-Grütz syndrome
Burkholderia
    B. ambifaria
    B. anthina
    B. caledonica
    B. cenocepacia
    B. cepacia
    B. dolosa
    B. fungorum
    B. hospita
    B. kururiensis
    B. mallei
    B. phymatum
    B. pseudomallei
    B. sacchari
    B. sordidicola

B

NOTES

Burkholderia (continued)
    B. stabilis
    B. terricola
    B. tuberum
    B. ubonensis
    B. unamae
    B. xenovorans
burkinensis
    Anaeroarcus b.
    Desulfovibrio b.
Burkitt
    B. lymphoma (BL)
    B. tumor
Burkitt-like lymphoma
burn
    beta b.
    b. culture
    first-degree b.
    flash b.
    fourth-degree b.
    full-thickness b.
    b. index (BI)
    mustard-induced b.
    partial-thickness b.
    screen b.
    second-degree b.
    superficial b.
    third-degree b.
    ultraviolet b.
burned
    body surface b. (BSB)
burner
    Boling b.
    Bunsen b.
    Fischer b.
    laminar flow b.
burnetii
    Coxiella b.
Burnett
    B. disinfecting fluid
    B. syndrome
burn-in
burnt-out germ cell tumor
Burow solution
burr cell
burrow
burrowing pus
bursa-equivalent tissue
bursal
    b. abscess
    b. cyst
bursata
    exostosis b.
bursitis
    radiohumeral b.
    xanthogranulomatous b.
burst
    respiratory b.
burst-forming unit-erythroid (BFU-E)

Buruli ulcer
Bury disease
BUS
    Bartholin, urethral, Skene
    BUS glands
busanensis
    Legionella b.
Buschke disease
Buschke-Löwenstein
    giant condyloma of B.-L.
    B.-L. giant condyloma
    B.-L. tumor
Buschke-Ollendorf syndrome
buski
    Fasciolopsis b.
    Glyciphagus b.
Busquet disease
Buss disease
Busse-Buschke disease
Busse saccharomyces
busulfan, busulphan (BU)
    b. lung
busy dermis
butabarbital
    sodium b.
butane
butanoic acid
butanol-extractable
    b.-e. iodine (BEI)
    b.-e. iodine assay
    b.-e. iodine test
butanone
Butchart tumor staging
bütschlii
    Iodamoeba b.
butter
    b. of antimony
    b. yellow
butterfly
    b. lung
    b. pattern on chest x-ray
    b. rash
button
    cell b.
    corneoscleral b.
buttonhole stenosis
butyl
    b. alcohol
    b. 2-cyanoacrylate
    b. methacrylate
butyraceous
butyrate esterase stain
butyric acid
butyricum
    Clostridium b.
    Mycobacterium b.
Butyrivibrio hungatei
butyrous colony
butyrylcholinesterase (BChE)

butzleri
> *Arcobacter b.*

buyo cheek cancer

BV
> blood volume

BW
> biological warfare

Bwamba
> B. fever
> B. fever virus

By antigen

Byler disease

Bymovirus

bypass (BP)

> b. capacitor
> cardiopulmonary b.

byssina
> *Dendrostilbella b.*

byssinosis

Byssoascus

Byssochlamys

bystander
> b. hemolysis
> b. lysis
> b. suppression

Bywaters syndrome

BZ
> NATO code for QNB

NOTES

B

C
calculus
Celsius temperature scale
centigrade temperature scale
coulomb
large calorie
    activated protein C (APC)
    C antigen
    azure C
    C banding
    C carbohydrate antigen
    C cell
    C group virus
    C lactose test
    C peptide
    C region
    C virus

C1
    C1 esterase
    C1 esterase inhibitor (C1EInh)

C2
    Clostridium botulinum cytotoxin type C2

C3
    C3 Nef factor
    C3 proactivator
    C3 proactivator convertase

C_{Am}
amylase clearance

C_{in}
insulin clearance

C_{pah}
p-aminohippurate clearance

c
contact
small calorie

C219 antibody
"c2-like viruses"
C3a anaphylatoxin
C494 antibody
C4a anaphylatoxin
C5a anaphylatoxin
C5B-9 complex
C8/144 antibody
CA
cancer
cancer antigen
carcinoma
chronological age
cold agglutinin
corpus amylaceum
croup-associated
cytosine arabinoside

NATO code for riot control agent bromobenzylcyanide
    CA virus
CA15-3
    C. breast antigen
    C. RIA
CA19-9
    C. antigen
    C. assay
CA72-4
Ca
calcium
cancer
Ca2+
calcium ion
CA125
cancer antigen 125
    CA125 antigen
    CA125 assay
Ca2+-free perfusion
cA2 monoclonal antibody
CABG
coronary artery bypass graft
cabinet
    biological safety c. (BSC)
c-abl oncogene
Cabot ring body
caccae
    Anaerostipes c.
Cacchi-Ricci syndrome
cache
    c. memory
    C. Valley virus
cachectic
    c. anergy
    c. endocarditis
    c. purpura
cachectin
cachexia
cancerous c.
c. exophthalmica
malarial c.
c. strumipriva
thyroid c.
uremic c.
CaCN
calcium cyanide
cacocholia
cacodylate
    c. buffer
    sodium c.
cacodylic acid
cactinomycin
cacumen

C

CAD
compound absorption device
coronary artery disease
CaD
caldesmon
CADASIL
cerebral autosomal dominant arteriopathy
with subcortical infarcts and
leukoencephalopathy
cadaver donor
cadaveric
c. ecchymoses
c. spasm
cadaverine
cadaveris
Clostridium c.
cadence
counting c.
cadherin
epithelial c. (E-cadherin)
vascular endothelial c. (VE-
cadherin)
cadherin/catenin complex
cadmium
c. assay
c. telluride detector
Ca-DTPA
calcium diethylenetriaminepentaacetate
caduca
CAE
chloroacetate esterase
caecutiens
Chrysops c.
Onchocerca c.
Ca-EDTA
calcium ethylenediaminetetraacetic
Caenibacterium
C. thermophilum
caerulea
cataracta c.
caesar
Lucilia c.
caespitosus
Botryomyces c.
café au lait spot
caffeine
c. assay
c. sodium benzoate
Caffey
C. disease
C. syndrome
Caffey-Silverman syndrome
CAG
chronic atrophic gastritis
cagA toxin
CAH
chronic active hepatitis
congenital adrenal hyperplasia

CAHD
coronary atherosclerotic heart disease
CAHM
complex atypical hyperplasia/metaplasia
CAIS
complete androgen insensitivity
syndrome
caishijiensis
Nocardia c.
caisson disease
Cajal
C. astrocyte stain
C. cell
C. formol ammonium bromide
solution
C. gold sublimate method
C. gold sublimate stain
horizontal cell of C.
C. interstitial nucleus
C. uranium silver method
cajennense
Amblyomma c.
cake kidney
Cal
large calorie
cal
small calorie
Calabar swelling
calbindin protein
calcaneonavicular
calcaneus
calcar
calcarea
Nocardia c.
peritendinitis c.
calcareous
c. cystitis
c. degeneration
c. infiltration
c. metastasis
calcarine
Calcarisporium
calcariuria
calcemia
calcergy
**Cal-Chex for Cell-Dyn whole blood
calibrator**
calcicosis
calcific
c. bicuspid aortic valve stenosis
c. concretion
c. nodular aortic stenosis
calcificans
chondrodysplasia c.
calcification
dystrophic c.
egg-shell c.
focal c.
indeterminate c.

c. line of Retzius
medial c.
metastatic c.
mitral valve c.
Mönckeberg medial c.
pathologic c.
presenile dementia with tangles
and c.'s
psammomatous c.
soft tissue c. (STC)

calcified
c. cartilage
c. gallbladder
c. granuloma
c. granulomatous inflammation

calcifying
c. ameloblastoma
c. epithelial odontogenic tumor
(CEOT)
c. epithelioma of Malherbe
c. fibrous pseudotumor
c. odontogenic cyst
c. pancreatitis

calcigerous
calcineurin (CN)
calcinosis
c. circumscripta
c. cutis
c. cutis, Raynaud phenomenon,
sclerodactyly, and telangiectasia
(CRST)
dystrophic c.
c. intervertebralis
c., Raynaud phenomenon,
esophageal motility disorders,
sclerodactyly, and telangiectasia
(CREST)
reversible c.
tumoral c.
c. universalis

calciokinesis
calciokinetic
calciorrhachia
calciotropism
calcipenia
calcipexic
calcipexis
calcipexy
calciphilia
calciphylaxis (CPX)
systemic c.
topical c.

calcite
calcitonin
c. assay
c. gene-related peptide (CGRP)
plasma c.
c. receptor-like receptor
c. testing

calcitrans
Stomoxys c.

calcium (Ca)
c. acetate formalin
Baker formol c.
c. balance
c. channel agonist
c. chloride
c. cyanide (CaCN)
c. deposit demonstration
c. deposition
c. diethylenetriaminepentaacetate
(Ca-DTPA)
c. disodium edetate
endogenous fecal c. (EFC)
c. ethylenediaminetetraacetic (Ca-
EDTA)
c. gout
c. imbalance
c. ion (Ca2+)
c. ionized assay
leucovorin c.
c. oxalate (CO)
c. oxalate calculus
c. oxalate crystal
c. oxalate test
c. phosphate
c. phosphate calculus
c. pyrophosphate deposition disease
(CPPD)
c. pyrophosphate dihydrate (CPD)
c. red
c. time
urine c.

calcium-45
calcium-activated
c.-a. ATPase
c.-a. neutral protease

calcium-magnesium-ATPase
calcium-sensing
c.-s. receptor
c.-s. receptor protein (CASR)

calciuria
calcoaceticus
Acinetobacter c.

NOTES

calcofluor white stain
calcospherite
calculated
    c. mean organism (CMO)
    c. serum osmolality
calculi (*pl. of* calculus)
calculosis
calculous pigment
calculus, pl. **calculi (C)**
    apatite c.
    arthritic c.
    articular c.
    biliary c.
    blood c.
    branched c.
    bronchial c.
    calcium oxalate c.
    calcium phosphate c.
    cardiac c.
    cerebral c.
    cholesterol c.
    combination c.
    coral c.
    cystine c.
    decubitus c.
    dendritic c.
    dental c.
    encysted c.
    fibrin c.
    fusible c.
    gastric c.
    hemic c.
    indigo c.
    intestinal c.
    joint c.
    lacrimal c.
    mammary c.
    matrix c.
    mixed c.
    mulberry c.
    nephritic c.
    oxalate c.
    pancreatic c.
    pharyngeal c.
    pigment c.
    pleural c.
    pocketed c.
    preputial c.
    primary renal c.
    prostatic c.
    renal c.
    salivary c.
    secondary renal c.
    staghorn c.
    struvite c.
    urate c.
    ureteral c.
    uric acid c.
    urinary c.

    uterine c.
    vesical c.
    weddellite c.
    whewellite c.
Caldanaerobacter
    C. subterraneus
    C. subterraneus subsp. *acificus*
    C. subterraneus subsp. *subterraneus*
    C. subterraneus subsp. *tengcongensis*
    C. subterraneus subsp. *yonseiensis*
Caldariomyces
caldesmon (CaD)
    C. cell protein
Caldilinea aerophila
Caldimonas manganoxidans
Caldisphaera lagunensis
Caldithrix abyssi
Caldivirga maquilingensis
caldoxylosilyticus
    Geobacillus c.
caldus
    Acidithiobacillus c.
Caldwell-Moloy
    C.-M. classification
    C.-M. method
caledonica
    Burkholderia c.
calefacient
caliber
calibrate
calibration
    c. curve
    film density c.
    c. interval
    c. material
calibrator
    Advia Centaur anti-HBs c.
    Cal-Chex for Cell-Dyn whole
     blood c.
    dose c.
    Vitros Immunodiagnostic Products
     anti-HBc c.
calicectasis
caliciform, calyciform
    c. cell
    c. ending
Caliciviridae
Calicivirus
calicivirus
calicoblast cell
calicoblastic epithelium
caliculus gustatorius
caliectasis, calyectasis
caliensis
    Paragonimus c.
California
    C. encephalitis (CE)
    C. encephalitis virus

C. encephalitis virus titer
C. myxoma virus
californiensis
    Anaerobranca c.
    Lentzea c.
    Thelazia c.
    Tindallia c.
californium (Cf)
caliper
    vernier dial c.
caliper micrometer
CALLA, cALLA
    common acute lymphoblastic leukemia
    antigen
        CALLA antiserum
        CALLA assay
CALLA-positive ALL
Calleja
    islands of C.
    islets of C.
Call-Exner body
callipaeda
    Thelazia c.
Calliphora vomitoria
Calliphoridae
Callison fluid
Callitroga
callosity
callus
    bony c.
    central c.
    definitive c.
    ensheathing c.
    fracture c.
    myelogenous c.
    provisional c.
calmagite
calmative agent
Calmette-Guérin
    bacille bilié de C.-G. (BCG)
    C.-G. bacillus
    bacillus C.-G. (BCG)
    C.-G. vaccine
Calmette test
calmodulin
calnexin
Calocera
Calodium
calomel electrode
Calomys colossus
Calonectria

calor
    c. febrilis
    c. fervens
    c. innatus
Caloramator
    C. coolhaasii
    C. viterbiensis
Caloranaerobacter azorensis
caloric
    c. disease
    c. quotient
calorie
    large c. (C, Cal)
    small c. (c, cal)
calorigenesis
calorigenic action
calorimeter
calorimetry
Calospora
CALP
    calponin
calpain family of protease
calponin (CALP)
calretinin expression
calsequestrin
calvaria, pl. **calvariae**
Calvatia gigantea
Calvé-Perthes disease
Calvé-Perthes-Legg disease
calviensis
    Vibrio c.
calyciform (*var. of* caliciform)
calyectasis (*var. of* caliectasis)
Calymmatobacterium
    C. donovania
    C. granulomatis
CAM
    cell adhesion molecule
    chemical agent monitor
        AE1 plus CAM
        CAM 5.2 antibody
        CAM 5.2 antigen
cambium layer
Cambridge
    C. Biotech HIV-1 urine Western
    blot test
    factor V C.
cambriense
    Varibaculum c.
cameloid anemia
camelpox

C

NOTES

camera
    Anger c.
    gamma c.
    Ikegami video c.
    Insight digital c.
    Nikon microprocessor-controlled c.
    scintillation c.
    Spot RT Monochrome Kodak KAI-2000 CCD digital c.
camera/microscope
    Coolscope digital c.
Cameron lesion
camerostome
camini
    Aeropyrum c.
Caminibacter
    C. hydrogeniphilus
    C. profundus
Caminicella sporogenes
caminithermale
    Clostridium c.
CAMP
    Christie-Atkins-Munch-Petersen
    CAMP factor
    CAMP test
cAMP
    adenosine 3′,5′-cyclic monophosphate
    adenosine 3′,5′-cyclic phosphate
    cyclic adenosine monophosphate
    cyclic AMP
        cAMP response element binding activation transcription factor (CREB/ATF)
        cAMP response element binding protein (CREB)
Campanacci
    osteofibrous dysplasia of C.
campanulae
    Ascospora c.
cAMP-dependent protein kinase
campestris
    Anopheles c.
camp fever
Camp-Gianturco method
camphor assay
camphorism
campinensis
    Ralstonia c.
    Wautersia c.
campisalis
    Halomonas c.
camptobactrum
    Leptodontium c.
camptocormia
camptothecin
Campylobacter
    C. bacterium
    C. cinaedi
    C. coli

    C. concisus
    C. curvus
    C. fennelliae
    C. fetus subsp. fetus
    C. fetus subsp. venerealis
    C. (Helicobacter) pylori
    C. hominis
    C. hyointestinalis
    C. jejuni
    C. lanienae
    C. lari
    C. rectus
    C. selective agar
    C. showae
    C. sputorum
Campylobacteraceae
Campylobacter-**like organism (CLO)**
Camurati-Engelmann disease
CANA
    convulsant antidote for nerve agent
Canada-Cronkhite syndrome
canadensis
    Chromohalobacter c.
    Helicobacter c.
    Onychocola c.
canal
    alimentary c.
    anterior semicircular c.
    Arantius c.
    Arnold c.
    Bernard c.
    Bichat c.
    bony semicircular c.
    central c.
    ciliary c.
    Cloquet c.
    Corti c.
    deferent c.
    dentinal c.
    Dorello c.
    haversian c.
    Hensen c.
    c. of Hering
    Holmgren-Golgi c.
    Hoyer c.
    hyaloid c.
    interfacial c.
    Kovalevsky c.
    Lambert c.
    lateral semicircular c.
    Leeuwenhoek c.
    Löwenberg c.
    lower anal c.
    nutrient c.
    obturator c.
    Petit c.
    portal c.
    posterior semicircular c.
    Santorini c.

c. of Schlemm
semicircular c.
Stilling c.
Sucquet c.
Sucquet-Hoyer c.
uniting c.
upper anal c.
vestibular c.
Volkmann c.
Walther c.
Wirsung c.
canales (*pl. of* canalis)
canalicular
c. adenoma
c. duct
c. membrane
c. organic anion transplant
c. pattern
c. phase of lung development
c. space
canaliculi (*pl. of* canaliculus)
canaliculization
canaliculum
papilloma c.
canaliculus, pl. **canaliculi**
bile canaliculi
bile duct c.
biliary c.
bone c.
canaliculi dentales
intracellular c.
pseudobile c.
c. reuniens
secretory c.
Thiersch c.
tiny canaliculi
canalis, pl. **canales**
c. hyaloideus
c. nutricius
c. reuniens
canales semicircularis ossei
canalization
canalized thrombus
canariasense
Mycobacterium c.
canarypox virus
Canavalia
Canavan
C. disease
C. sclerosis

cANCA
cytoplasmic antineutrophil cytoplasmic antibody
cytoplasmic antineutrophil cytoplasmic autoantibody
cancellated
cancellous
c. bone
c. tissue
cancellus
cancer (CA, Ca)
adrenal c.
AJCC staging modification on prostate c.
American Joint Committee on C. (AJCC)
androgen independent prostate c. (AIPC)
c. antigen (CA)
c. antigen 125 (CA125)
betel c.
c. body
breast c.
buyo cheek c.
c. chemotherapy
chimney-sweep's c.
colloid c.
colorectal c. (CRC)
conjugal c.
encephaloid c.
c. en cuirasse
endocervical c.
epidermoid c.
epithelial c.
fallopian tube c.
familial c.
c. family
foamy gland prostate c.
c. free white mouse (CFWM)
gastrointestinal c.
c. gene BUB
glandular c.
green c.
hereditary diffuse gastric c. (HDGC)
hereditary nonpolyposis colon c. (HNPCC)
hereditary nonpolyposis colorectal c. (HNPCC)
inherited c.
c. juice
kangri c.

NOTES

159

cancer *(continued)*
    kidney c.
    laryngeal c.
    liver c.
    lung c.
    lymphatic c.
    lymph node c.
    lymphoreticular c.
    c. management therapy
    mule-spinner's c.
    mutated in colon c. (MCC)
    nonsmall cell c. (NSCC)
    nonsmall cell lung c. (NSCLC)
    ovarian c.
    pancreatic c.
    paraffin c.
    PathVysion HER-2 DNA probe for breast c.
    penile c.
    peritoneal c.
    pipe-smoker's c.
    pitch-worker's c.
    c. promoter
    prostate c.
    qualitative staging of breast c.
    c. risk assessment
    scar c.
    small cell c. (SCC)
    somatic mutation theory of c.
    spider c.
    c. staging
    stomach c.
    stump c.
    synchronous c.
    synovial c.
    telangiectatic c.
    testicular c.
    uterine c.
    vaginal c.
    vulvar c.
canceration
cancericidal
cancerigenic
cancerization
    lobular c.
cancerocidal
cancerous cachexia
cancra (*pl. of* cancrum)
cancriform
cancroid
cancrum, pl. **cancra**
    c. nasi
    c. oris
candela (cd)
candicans
    corpus c.
Candida
    C. albicans
    C. dubliniensis

    C. endocarditis
    C. esophagitis
    C. glabrata
    C. guilliermondi
    C. krusei
    C. meningitis
    C. parapsilosis
    C. pneumonia
    C. precipitin test
    C. pseudotropicalis
    C. tropicalis
    C. vulvovaginitis
candidal
candidate
    c. tumor marker
    c. tumor suppressor gene
candidemia
candidiasis
    chronic mucocutaneous c. (CMC)
    disseminated c.
    c. serologic test
    vulvovaginal c.
candidid
candidosis
candidum
    Geotrichum c.
candidus
    Aspergillus c.
    Thermoactinomyces c.
cangkringensis
    Streptomyces c.
canicularis
    Anthomyia c.
canicular multispecific organic anion transporter (CMOAT)
canimorsus
    Capnocytophaga c.
canine
    c. adenovirus 1
    c. carcinoma 1
    c. distemper virus
    c. herpesvirus
    c. herpetovirus
    c. oral papilloma
caninum
    Ancylostoma c.
    Dipylidium c.
    Episthmium c.
    Neospora c.
canis
    Actinomyces c.
    Ascaris c.
    Brucella c.
    Ctenocephalides c.
    Ehrlichia c.
    Enterococcus c.
    Isospora c.
    Microsporum c.

Streptococcus c.
Toxocara c.
canities
canker sore
cannabina
   Pseudomonas c.
cannabinoid
cannabinol
Cannabis
cannabism
canning
   home c.
Cannizzaro reaction
cannulation
   arterial c.
Cantharellula
cantharidin
cantonensis
   Angiostrongylus c.
CAO
   chronic airway obstruction
caoutchouc pelvis
CAP
   College of American Pathologists
    CAP sweat analysis proficiency
    testing program
cap
   acrosomal c.
   c. cell
   cradle c.
   fibrin c.
   head c.
   phrygian c.
   TBG c.
capability
   morgue c.
capacitance
   membrane c.
capacitation
capacitive reactance
capacitor
   bypass c.
   ceramic c.
   coupling c.
   disc c.
   electrolytic c.
   filter c.
   junction c.
   Mylar c.
   output c.
   paper c.

resistor c. (RC)
variable c.
capacity
   antigen-binding c.
   blood buffering c.
   buffer c.
   dye-binding c. (DBC)
   forced vital c. (FVC)
   functional reserve c. (FRC)
   functional residual c. (FRC)
   inspiratory reserve c. (IRC)
   iron-binding c. (IBC)
   latent iron-binding c. (LIBC)
   maximal sustained ventilatory c. (MSVC)
   molar heat c.
   proatherogenic c.
   residual lung c. (RLC)
   single breath carbon monoxide diffusing c.
   slow vital c. (SVC)
   specific heat c.
   storage c.
   total iron-binding c. (TIBC)
   total lung c. (TLC)
   trypsin-inhibitory c. (TIC)
   unsaturated vitamin B_{12}-binding c. (UBBC)
Capdepont disease
Capella
   tumor of C.
Capetown
   hemoglobin J C.
Capgras syndrome
capillaceus
   Actinoplanes c.
capillare
   vas c.
capillarectasia
Capillaria
   C. hepatica
   C. philippinensis
capillariasis
capillarioscopy
capillaris
   Muellerius c.
capillaritis
capillarity
capillaron
capillaropathy
capillaroscopy

NOTES

capillary
    c. action
    arterial c.
    bile c.
    blood c.
    c. blood sugar (CBS)
    continuous c.
    distention of alveolar c.
    c. electrophoresis
    c. electrophoresis electropherogram
    c. embolism
    erythrocyte in c.
    fenestrated c.
    c. flame
    c. fragility
    c. fragility test
    c. hemangioma
    c. loop
    lymph c.
    c. microscope
    c. nevus
    sinusoidal c.
    c. tube
    c. vein
    venous c.
    c. vessel
    c. zone electrophoresis (CE)
capillary-like space
capillatus
    Solenopotes c.
capillitii
    Saccharomyces c.
capillosus
    Bacteroides c.
Capillovirus
capillus
Capim virus
capistration
capita (*pl. of* caput)
capitation
capitatus
    Blastoschizomyces c.
    Dipodascus c.
capitis
    tinea c.
capitovis
    Corynebacterium c.
capitular
capitulum
Caplan
    C. nodule
    C. syndrome
capneic
Capnocytophaga canimorsus
capnocytophagoides
    Dysgonomonas c.
capnohepatography
capon-comb-growth test

capping
    patching c.
caprae
    Mycobacterium c.
    Mycobacterium bovis subsp. *c.*
caprate
    cellulose c.
capreoli
    Bartonella c.
capricola
    Trichostrongylus c.
caprine
    c. herpesvirus
    c. herpetovirus
caprinus
    Streptococcus c.
Capripoxvirus
Capronia pulcherrima
caprylate
    sodium c.
capsaicin
capsase mediated cleavage of APP
Capsicum
    C. annum
    C. frutescens
capsicum
    oleoresin c. (OC)
capsid
capsomer
    c. capsular space
    c. capsule
capsula, pl. **capsulae**
    c. adiposa renis
    c. articularis
    c. cordis
    c. glomeruli
capsular
    c. antigen
    c. cell
    c. cirrhosis of liver
    c. drop
    c. lipochondral degeneration
    c. precipitation reaction
    c. space
    c. synovial-like hyperplasia (CSH)
    c. tissue
capsulare
    lipoma c.
capsularis
    decidua c.
capsulata
    Emmonsiella c.
capsulatum
    Ajellomyces c.
    Histoplasma c. var. *capsulatum*
    Novosphingobium c.
capsulatus
    Bacillus aerogenes c.

Endomyces c.
Torula c.
capsule
adipose c.
adrenal c.
anthrax c.
antiphagocytic polypeptide c.
articular c.
atrabiliary c.
bacterial c.
Bowman c.
capsomer c.
cartilage c.
c. cell
connective tissue c.
extreme c.
fibrous articular c.
fibrous membrane of joint c.
Friedländer stain for c.'s
Gerota c.
hyaline c.
joint c.
malpighian c.
Müller c.
Nicolle stain for c.'s
renal c.
sooty c.
suprarenal c.
tumor c.
capsulitis
adhesive c.
hepatic c.
capture
c. antibody
c. assay
c. cross section
electron c. (EC)
radiative c.
viral hybrid c.
caput, gen. **capitis**, pl. **capita**
c. medusae
pityriasis capitis
c. quadratum
Caraparu virus
carateum
Treponema c.
Caraway method
Carazzi hematoxylin
carbamate
carbamazepine assay
carbamide
carbamino-carbon dioxide

carbamino compound
carbaminohemoglobin
carbamoyl
c. phosphate synthetase (CPS)
c. phosphate synthetase I deficiency
carbamoyltransferase
ornithine c. (OCT)
carbamyl
c. phosphate
c. phosphate synthetase (CPS)
carbamylurea
carbanion
carbaprostacyclin
carbaryl assay
carbazole
5-amino 9 ethyl c. (AEC)
amino-9-ethyl c.
carbenicillin indanyl sodium
carbhemoglobin
carbinol
Carbitol
carbohemoglobin
carbohydrate (CHO)
accumulation of c.'s
c. antigen
c. broth
fecal c.
c. fermentation test
c. identification test
c. inversion
c. metabolism index (CMI)
stool c.
c. tolerance test
c. utilization test
carbohydrate-induced hyperlipidemia
carbohydraturia
carbolfuchsin (CF)
c. stain
Ziehl-Neelsen c.
carbolfuchsin-methylene blue staining method
carbolic
c. acid
c. methylene blue (CMB)
carbolism
carbol-thionin stain
carboluria
carbomycin
carbon
c. bisulfide
c. dioxide (bicarb, CO_2)

NOTES

carbon *(continued)*
  c. dioxide absorbent
  c. dioxide acidosis
  c. dioxide challenge test
  c. dioxide combining power
  c. dioxide combining power measurement
  c. dioxide combining power test
  c. dioxide concentration
  c. dioxide concentration assay
  c. dioxide content
  c. dioxide dissociation curve
  c. dioxide electrode
  c. dioxide fixation
  c. dioxide myoglobin (MbCO)
  c. dioxide narcosis
  c. dioxide output ($\overset{\circ}{V}_{CO_2}$)
  c. dioxide production
  c. dioxide response curve
  c. dioxide tension
  c. disulfide
  c. disulfide assay
  c. disulfide poisoning
  c. gelatin mass
  c. inorganic compound
  c. 13-labeled ketoisocaproate breath test
  c. monoxide (CO)
  c. monoxide assay
  c. monoxide hemoglobin
  c. monoxide oximeter (CO-oximeter)
  c. monoxide poisoning
  c. monoxide test
  c. oxychloride
  c. resistor
  c. tetrachloride (CCl4)
  c. tetrachloride assay
  c. tetrachloride poisoning
carbon-11, -12, -13, -14
carbonaceous residue of combustion
carbonate
  c. dehydratase
  potassium c.
  sodium c.
carbon-film resistor
carbon-hydrogen (C-H)
carbonic
  c. acid
  c. acid chloride
  c. anhydrase
  c. anhydrase inhibitor
  c. anhydrase-related protein (CA-RP)
carbonis
  Streptacidiphilus c.
carbonium ion
carbonized

carbonuria
  dysoxidative c.
carbonyl
  c. chloride
  c. cyanide p-(trifluoromethoxy)phenylhydrazone (FCCP)
carbonylhemoglobin
carbophenothion
Carborundum
Carbowax
Carboxydibrachium pacificum
Carboxydocella thermautotrophica
carboxyhemoglobin (COHB, COHb, HbCO, HbCo)
  c. assay
carboxyhemoglobinemia
carboxyhemoglobinuria
carboxylase
  acetyl-CoA c.
  propionate c.
  propionyl-CoA c.
  pyruvate c.
carboxylate
  c. ion
  pyrrolidone c.
carboxylesterase
carboxylic acid
carboxyl terminal
carboxymethylcellulose (CM-cellulose)
carboxypeptidase
carbuncle
  kidney c.
  malignant c.
  renal c.
carbuncular
carbunculosis
carcinemia
carcinoembryonic
  c. antigen (CEA)
  c. antigen-related cell adhesion molecule 1 (CEACAM1)
  c. antigen test
carcinogen
  complete c.
  direct-reacting c.
  group 1 c.
carcinogenesis
  viral c.
carcinogenic hydrocarbon
carcinoid
  atypical c.
  bronchial c.
  foregut c.
  goblet cell c.
  c. heart disease
  intestinal tract c.
  lung c.
  mucous c.

strumal c.
c. syndrome
c. tumor
carcinoides
papillomatosis cutis c.
carcinoid-like architectural pattern
carcinolytic
carcinoma, pl. **carcinomas, carcinomata**
  (CA)
acinar cell c. (ACC)
acinic cell c.
acinose c.
acinous c.
adenocystic c.
adenoid cystic c. (ACC)
adenoid squamous cell c.
adenosquamous cell c. (ADSQC)
adnexal c.
adrenocortical c.
aggressive thyroid c. (ATC)
alveolar cell c.
ampullary c.
anal gland c.
anaplastic c.
apocrine c.
atypical medullary c.
basal cell c. (BCC)
basaloid invasive squamous cell c.
  (BISCC)
basaloid squamous cell c. (BSCC)
basal squamous cell c.
basosquamous c.
Bellini duct c.
bile duct c.
bladder c.
bone marrow c.
breast c.
bronchial c.
bronchioalveolar c. (BACA)
bronchiolar c.
bronchioloalveolar c. (BAC)
bronchogenic c.
canine c. 1
CD44v6 staining in prostate c.
cecal c.
ceruminous c.
cervical c.
chorionic c.
chromophobe c.
chromophobe renal cell c. (CRCC)
clear cell c. (CCC)

clear cell hepatocellular c. (HCC-
  CC)
clear cell myoepithelial c.
  (CCMEC)
clear cell odontogenic c.
clear cell renal cell c. (RCC-CC)
clinging c.
cloacogenic c.
collecting duct c. (CDC)
colloid c.
colon c.
colorectal c.
contralateral infiltrating duct c.
conventional papillary c. (CPC)
cribriform c.
cribriform-morular variant of
  papillary thyroid c.
crypt cell c.
cuboidal c.
c. cutaneum
cylindromatous c.
cystic c.
duct c.
ductal c.
duodenal c.
Ehrlich ascites c.
embryonal cell c.
endocervical c.
endometrial c.
endometrial intraepithelial c. (EIC)
endometrioid c.
endometrioid endometrial c. (EEC)
epidermoid c.
epimyoepithelial c.
epithelial-myoepithelial c. (EMEC)
esophageal c.
c. ex pleomorphic adenoma
fibrolamellar liver cell c.
follicular variant of papillary
  thyroid c. (FVPTC)
gallbladder c.
gastric c.
gastrointestinal tract c.
gelatinous c.
giant cell c.
glandular c.
glassy cell c. (GCC)
glycogen-rich squamous cell c.
grade 1, 2 neuroendocrine c.
granulosa cell c.
head and neck squamous cell c.
  (HNSCC)

C

NOTES

carcinoma *(continued)*

hepatocellular c. (HCC)
hepatocellular bile duct c.
hereditary papillary renal cell c.
  (HPRC)
histiocytoid c.
Hürthle cell c.
hyalinizing clear cell c. (HCCC)
hypervascular hepatocellular c.
incidence of hepatocellular c.
infiltrating cribriform c.
infiltrating ductal c. (IDC)
infiltrating lobular c. (ILC)
infiltrating papillary c.
inflammatory c.
insular c.
intermediate c.
intracystic papillary c.
intraductal papillary c. (IPC)
intraepidermal squamous cell c.
intraepithelial c.
invasive ductal c.
invasive lobular c.
invasive papillary c.
invasive squamous cell c. (ISCC)
ipsilateral intraductal c.
islet cell c.
Jewett bladder c.
juvenile c.
kangri burn c.
keratinizing invasive squamous
  cell c. (KISCC)
keratinizing squamous cell c.
  (KSCC)
Krompecher c.
large-cell neuroendocrine c.
  (LCNEC)
laryngeal c.
lateral aberrant thyroid c.
leptomeningeal c.
liver cell c.
lobular c.
Lucké c.
lung c.
lymphoepithelioma-like c. (LELC)
lymphoepithelioma-like thymic c.
  (LETC)
matrix-producing c.
medullary c. (MC)
medullary renal c. (MRC)
medullary thyroid c. (MTC)
melanotic c.
meningeal c.
mesometanephric c.
metaplastic c.
metastatic c.
metastatic hepatocellular c. (HCC)
metatypical c.
microinvasive c.

micropapillary serous c. (MPSC)
minimally invasive follicular c.
  (MIFC)
mixed hepatocellular c.
mucin-depleted mucoepidermoid c.
mucinous bronchioloalveolar c.
mucoepidermoid c. (MEC)
myoblastoid c.
myoblastomatoid c.
myoepithelial c.
c. myxomatodes
nasopharyngeal c. (NPC)
noncystic mucinous c.
noninfiltrating lobular c.
oat cell c.
occult c.
oncocytic c.
oncoplastic c.
ovarian c.
oxyphilic papillary c.
pancreatic c.
papillary renal cell c. (PRCC)
papillary thyroid c. (PTC)
papillary transitional cell c.
peritoneal mucinous c. (PMC)
pilomatrix c.
piriform sinus c.
pleomorphic lobular c. (PLC)
poorly differentiated c.
primary thymic c. (PTC)
pseudoangiosarcomatous c.
pseudosarcomatous c.
pseudovascular adenoid squamous
  cell c. (PASCC)
recurrent c.
renal cell c. (RCC)
renal clear cell c.
reserve cell c.
residual c.
rhabdoid phenotype of large-cell c.
Robson stage I, II renal c.
Sakamoto poorly differentiated c.
salivary gland c.
sarcomatoid c.
sarcomatoid thymic c. (STC)
scar c.
schneiderian c.
scirrhous c.
sclerosing bronchioloalveolar c.
sclerosing sarcomatoid transitional
  cell c.
sebaceous c.
secondary c.
secretory c.
serous c.
serous epithelial ovarian c. (SEOC)
sertoliform endometrioid c. (SEC)
signet ring cell c.
c. simplex

sinonasal undifferentiated c. (SNUC)
c. in situ (CIS)
c. in situ/intratubular germ cell neoplasia unclassified (CIS/ITGCNU)
skin c.
small cell lung c. (SCLC)
small cell neuroendocrine c. (SCNC)
small cell undifferentiated neuroendocrine c. (SCUNC)
solid c.
spindle cell c.
sporadic papillary renal cell c.
squamous cell c. (SCC, SQC)
stomach c.
stump c.
superficial multicentric basal cell c.
sweat gland c. (SGC)
terminal duct c.
testis c.
thymic c.
thyroid c.
trabecular c.
transitional cell c. (TCC)
trichilemmal cystic squamous cell c.
tubular c.
tubulopapillary c.
undifferentiated epidermoid c.
undifferentiated squamous cell c.
urachal c.
ureteral c.
urothelial c. (UcA)
usual type papillary c. (UTPC)
uterine endometrial c. (UEC)
uterine serous c. (USC)
uterine surface c.
vaginal c.
verrucous c.
villous c.
Walker c.
warty c.
well-differentiated c. (WDCA)
Wolfe breast c.
wolffian duct c.
yolk sac c.
carcinomatoid
carcinomatosa
lymphangitis c.

carcinomatosis
leptomeningeal c.
meningeal c.
peritoneal c.
carcinomatous
c. component
c. encephalomyelopathy
c. epithelium
c. implant
c. meningoencephalopathy
c. micrometastasis
c. myelopathy
c. myopathy
c. neuromyopathy
c. pericarditis
carcinosarcoma
embryonal c.
female genital tract c. (FGTCS)
renal c.
Walker c.
carcinosis
carcinostatic
carcoma
CARD
catalyzed reporter deposition
card
CloneSaver c.
ecarin clotting time test c.
Guthrie c.
card-amplified
c.-a. nanogold-gold staining
c.-a. nanogold-silver staining
cardiac
c. albuminuria
c. amyloidosis
c. aneurysm
c. ascites
c. calculus
c. catheterization
c. cell necrosis
c. cirrhosis
c. concussion
c. decompensation
c. dilation
c. disease
c. diuretic
c. edema
c. enlargement (CE)
c. enzymes/isoenzymes
c. failure (CF)
c. failure cell
c. fibrosis of the liver

NOTES

cardiac *(continued)*
    c. gland
    c. gland of esophagus
    c. glycoside
    c. hemoptysis
    c. heterotaxia
    c. histiocyte
    c. index
    c. muscle
    c. muscle in longitudinal section
    c. muscle tissue
    c. myocyte
    c. myxoma (CM)
    c. polyp
    C. Reader
    C. Reader D-Dimer test
    C. Reader IQC test strip
    C. Reader M myoglobin test
    C. Reader T quantitative troponin-
      T test
    c. remodeling after acute
      myocardial infarction
    c. sclerosis
    c. shunt detection
    c. silhouette
    c. standstill
    C. STATus CK-MB/myoglobin
      panel test
    C. STATus CK-MB test
    C. STATus controls for troponin I
    C. STATus myoglobin/troponin I
      test
    C. STATus rapid assay
    C. STATus rapid format troponin
      I panel test
    c. tamponade
    c. thrombosis
    C. T rapid assay
    C. T rapid assay for troponin T
    c. valve myxomatosis
    c. valvular malformation
    c. valvular regurgitation
cardiaca
    adiposis c.
cardiasthenia
Cardiasure cardiac markers control
cardiectasis
cardiffensis
    Actinomyces c.
cardinal manifestation of wet beriberi
cardioauditory
Cardiobacteriaceae
Cardiobacterium
    C. hominis
    C. valvarum
    C. violaceum
cardiocentesis
cardiochalasia
cardiogenic shock

CardioGram
Cardio-Green (CG)
cardioid condenser
cardiolipin
    c. antibody syndrome
    c. test
cardiolith
cardiomalacia
cardiomegaly
cardiomyoliposis
cardiomyopathy (CMP)
    alcoholic c.
    beer drinker's c.
    cardiotoxic
    congestive c.
    dilated c.
    familial c.
    hypertrophic obstructive c. (HOCM)
    idiopathic c.
    peripartum c.
    periportal c.
    primary c.
    restrictive c.
    uremic c.
cardionecrosis
cardionector hypothesis
cardiopathy
cardioplegia
cardioptosia
cardiopulmonary (CP)
    c. bypass
    c. exercise testing
    c. function
    c. sleep study
    c. stress test
cardiotocography
cardiotoxicity
    anthracycline c.
    hydroxychloroquine c.
cardiotoxic myolysis
cardiovascular (CV)
    c. disease (CVD)
    c. malformation
    c. renal disease (CVRD)
    c. system and central nervous
      system (CVS/CNS)
Cardiovirus
carditis
    rheumatic c.
    streptococcal c.
    verrucous c.
care
    episode of c.
    point of c. (POC)
Careside analyzer
caretaker gene
Carey Ranvier technique
carfentanil
Carica papaya

caricis
  Rathayibacter c.
caries
  dental c.
carinate
carinatum
  pectus c.
carinii
  Pneumocystis c.
cariogenesis
carious
Carlavirus
carlsbadense
  Halosimplex c.
carlsbergensis
  Saccharomyces c.
carmalum
carminate
  Nonomuraea roseoviolacea subsp. *c.*
carmine
  alum c.
  chrome alum c.
  indigo c.
  lithium c.
  Schneider c.
carminic acid
carminophil, carminophile
carminophilous
carmonensis
  Virgibacillus c.
Carmovirus
carnaria
  Sarcophaga c.
carnea
  tunica c.
carneae
  columnae c.
carneous
  c. degeneration
  c. mole
Carney
  C. complex
  C. syndrome
carnification
carniphilus
  Vagococcus c.
carnis
  Clostridium c.
carnitine
  c. palmitoyltransferase 2 (CPT2)
  c. palmitoyltransferase 2 deficiency

Carnobacterium
  C. inhibens
  C. maltaromaticum
  C. viridans
carnosa
  membrana c.
carnosinase
carnosine
carnosinemia
carnosinuria
carnosity
carnosus
  panniculus c.
Carnoy fixative
Caroli disease
carolinense
  Solanum c.
carotene assay
carotenemia
carotenoid
caroticum
  glomus c.
caroticus
  nodulus c.
carotid
  c. artery occlusion
  c. artery stenosis
  c. body tumor
  c. cavernous fistula
  c. disease
  c. endarterectomy
  c. sinus syndrome
carotovorum
  Pectobacterium c.
CA-RP
  carbonic anhydrase-related protein
carpal
  c. tunnel decompression (CTD)
  c. tunnel syndrome
Carpenter syndrome
carpet tack follicular keratotic plug
Carpoglyphus passularum
carrageenin
  lambda c.
  c. solution
Carrell test
carrier
  asymptomatic c.
  c. cell
  convalescent c.
  female c.
  c. gas

C

NOTES

carrier *(continued)*
> incubatory c.
> c. protein
> c. state
> c. strain

carrier-free (CF)
carrier-mediated transport
Carrión disease
carrionii
> *Cladosporium c.*
> *Hormodendrum c.*

Carr-Price
> C.-P. reaction
> C.-P. test

carry-over effect
Carson formalin
Carswell grape
cart
> Reach & Roll c.

Carter black mycetoma
carteri
> *Borrelia c.*

cartesian
> c. coordinates
> c. nomogram

cartilage
> c. bone
> c. and bone comparison
> calcified c.
> c. capsule
> c. cell
> cellular c.
> connecting c.
> elastic c.
> hyaline c.
> hypsiloid c.
> interosseous c.
> c. lacuna
> c. matrix
> c. matrix alteration
> precursory c.
> reticular c.
> c. space
> spicule of calcified c.
> temporary c.
> uniting c.
> Y c.
> yellow c.

cartilage-hair hypoplasia (CHH)
cartilaginea
> exostosis c.

cartilagines
cartilaginoid
cartilaginous
> c. abnormality
> c. metaplasia
> c. rest
> c. tissue

cartilago

cartridge
> HDL direct test prefilled c.
> LDL direct test prefilled c.

Cartwright antigen
caruncle
> Santorini major c.
> Santorini minor c.
> urethral c.

Caryophanaceae
Caryophanales
caryotheca, gen. and pl. **caryothecae**
> cisterna caryothecae

Cary 100 UV-Vis spectrophotometer
CAS
> cold agglutinin syndrome
> CAS DNA staining kit
> CAS 200 Image Analysis system
> CAS 200 image cytometer

cascade
> chain-reaction c.
> coagulation c.
> c. filtration
> metastatic c.
> ras c.

case
> c. fatality rate
> c. history
> index c.
> c. management
> sentinel c.

caseating
> c. granuloma
> c. granulomatous inflammation

caseation necrosis
case-control study
casei
> *Corynebacterium c.*
> *Lactobacillus c.*
> *Philopia c.*
> *Piophila c.*
> *Staphylococcus succinus* subsp. *c.*

casein
> c. agar
> c. hydrolysate

caseinate
> sodium c.

caseosa
> vernix c.

caseous
> c. abscess
> c. degeneration
> c. inflammation
> c. necrosis
> c. osteitis
> c. pneumonia
> c. tubercle

CaSki cell
Casman broth
Casoni intradermal test

caspase
c. immunoreactivity
c. protein
caspase-14
caspium
Corynebacterium c.
CASR
calcium-sensing receptor protein
cassette
ATP-binding c. (ABC)
cassiicola
Corynespora c.
cast
bacterial urinary c.
bile c.
blood c.
broad urinary c.
coma c.
corrosion c.
crystal urinary c.
decidual c.
endometrial c.
epithelial cell urinary c.
false c.
fatty urinary c.
fibrinous c.
fungal c.
granular urinary c.
hemoglobin c.
hyaline urinary c.
mucous c.
muddy brown urinary c.
OFB c.
pigment c.
pigmented c.
red blood cell c.
renal c.
RTE cell c.
spurious c.
tube c.
urinary c.
vascular corrosion c.
waxy urinary c.
WBC urinary c.
white blood cell c.
Castellanella castellani
Castellani
C. disease
C. test
castellani
Castellanella c.

castellanii
Acanthamoeba c.
castenholzii
Roseiflexus c.
casting
CASTLE
carcinoma showing thymus-like differentiation
Castle factor
Castleman
C. disease
C. syndrome
castor bean
castration
c. cell
female c.
male c.
parasitic c.
casualty
irradiated c.
CAT
chlormerodrin accumulation test
cat
c. distemper virus
c. liver fluke
c. unit
catabolic
c. enzyme
c. flow phase
catabolism
antibody c.
protein c.
catabolite
c. activator protein
c. repression
cataclysm
catagen
catagenesis
catalase
catalase-negative organism
catalase-positive organism
catalasia
anenzymia c.
catalasitica
Crocinitomix c.
Catalpa
catalysis
contact c.
catalyst
negative c.
catalytic
catalyze

NOTES

catalyzed signal amplification system
catalyzer
catanella
    Gonyaulax c.
cataphoresis
cataphoretic
cataphylaxis
cataplasia
catapulting
    pressure c.
cataract
    poikiloderma atrophicans and c.
    posterior subcapsular c. (PSC)
    progeria with c.
cataracta
    c. brunescens
    c. caerulea
    c. centralis pulverulenta
    c. complicata
    c. nigra
catarrh
    dry c.
catarrhal
    c. appendicitis
    c. conjunctivitis
    c. dysentery
    c. gastritis
    c. inflammation
    c. jaundice
catarrhalis
    Branhamella c.
    Moraxella c.
catastrophe
    obstetric c.
catastrophic complication
catatorulin test
catatrichy
cat-bite fever
catechin
catechinic acid
catechol
catecholamine
    adrenomedullary c.
    c. assay
    c. fraction
    c. test
    urinary c.
    urine c.'s
catechol-O-methyl transferase (COMT)
catechuic acid
categorical data
category A, B, C agent
catellatispora
    Actinomadura c.
Catellatospora koreensis
Catellibacterium nectariphilum
Catenabacterium
catenaformis
    Lactobacillus c.

catenating
catenatus
    Phaeococcomyces c.
Catenibacterium mitsuokai
cateniformis
    Coprobacillus c.
catenin
    adherens junction-associated c.
catenoid
catenulate
caterpillar
    c. cell
    urticating c.
Cathaemasia
cathartic colon
cathemoglobin
cathepsin
    c. B, D, E, K, L, S
    c. D antibody
    c. D enzyme
cathepsin-mediated disease
catheptic enzyme
catheterization
    cardiac c.
cathode
    c. ray
    c. ray tube
cati
    Notoedres c.
cation
    c. channel
    c. exchange resin
    c. interference
    organic c.
cation-anion difference
cationic
    c. charge
    c. dye
    c. trypsinogen gene
catoniae
    Porphyromonas c.
cat's
    c. cry syndrome
    c. eye syndrome
cat-scratch disease (CSD)
cattle
    ephemeral fever of c.
    infectious papilloma of c.
    c. plague
    c. plague virus
    c. wart
    winter dysentery of c.
Cattoretti technique
catuli
    Actinomyces c.
Catu virus
caucasica
    Borrelia c.
    Physaloptera c.

caudal
  c. dipygus duplication
  c. sheath
caudalizing agent
caudate nucleus
caudati
  corpus nuclei c.
caudatus
  Bodo c.
cauliflower ear
Caulimovirus
Caulobacter
Caulobacteraceae
Caulobacterales
Caulobacterineae
Caulochora baumgartneri
causative
cause
  constitutional c.
  c. of death (COD)
  death of other c. (DOC)
  predisposing c.
  proximate c.
cause-specific death rate
caustic
cauterant
cauterization
cautery artifact
CAV
  congenital absence of vagina
  congenital adrenal virilism
CAV1 gene
CAV2 gene
Cavare disease
cave
  c. fever
  Meckel c.
Cavemovirus
caveola, pl. **caveolae**
caveolin
Cavernicola pilosa
cavernitis
  fibrous c.
cavernosae
  Billroth venae c.
cavernositis
cavernosorum
  trabeculae corporum c.
  tunica albuginea corporum c.
cavernosum
  lipoma c.
  lymphangioma c.

cavernosus
  nevus c.
cavernous
  c. angioma
  c. hemangioma
  c. lymphangiectasis
  c. malformation (CM)
  c. sinus
  c. sinus thrombosis
  c. space
  c. tissue
caviae
  Chlamydophila c.
  Neisseria c.
cavitary lesion
cavitating inflammation
cavitation
  temporary c.
cavity
  absorption c.
  body c.
  chorionic c.
  idiopathic bone c.
  inflammatory c.
  internal c.
  marrow c.
  maxillectomy c.
  oral c.
  synovial c.
  vitreous c.
cayenne
  mal de C.
  c. pepper spot
cayetanensis
  Cyclospora c.
Cazenave disease
CB
  centroblastic
  chocolate blood
  chondroblastoma
  chronic bronchitis
    CB agar
CB11 antibody
CBA
  chronic bronchitis with asthma
C-banding stain
CBB
  Bethesda-Ballerup group of *Citrobacter*
CBC
  complete blood count
CBCL
  cutaneous B-cell lymphoma

C

NOTES

173

CBF
    cerebral blood flow
    coronary blood flow
Cbfa1/Runx2
      Cbfal/Runx2 isoform
      transcription factor Cbfa1/Runx2
CBG
    corticosteroid-binding globulin
    cortisol-binding globulin
^{13}C bicarbonate assay
CBIRF
    Chemical Biological Incident Response
    Force (of the U.S. Marine Corps)
CBN
    cellular blue nevus
CBP
    CREB binding protein
CBR
    chemical, biological, and radiological
CBRN
    chemical, biological, radiological or
    nuclear
      CBRN weapon
CBRNE
    chemical, biological, radiological,
    nuclear, explosive
CBS
    capillary blood sugar
    chronic brain syndrome
    citrate-buffered saline
CBV
    central blood volume
    circulating blood volume
    corrected blood volume
CBW
    chemical and biological warfare
CC
    cholangiocarcinoma
    cord compression
    creatinine clearance
CCA
    chick-cell agglutination
    chimpanzee coryza agent
CCAT
    conglutinating complement absorption
    test
CCB
    conventional core biopsy
CCC
    chronic calculous cholecystitis
    clear cell carcinoma
      primary salivary CCC
C_3, C_4 complement
CCD
    central collodiaphyseal angle
C-cell hyperplasia
CCF
    cephalin-cholesterol flocculation
    compound comminuted fracture
    congestive cardiac failure
CCFH
    cellular cutaneous fibrous histiocytoma
CCH
    circumscribed choroidal hemangioma
CCK
    cholecystokinin
CCl4
    carbon tetrachloride
CCl$_2$NOH
    dichloroformoxime CCl$_2$NOH
CC/MCL
    centrocytic/mantle-cell lymphoma
CCMEC
    clear cell myoepithelial carcinoma
CCP
    ciliocytophthoria
    cyclic citrullinated peptide
C/cr/
    creatinine clearance
CCSK
    clear cell sarcoma of the kidney
CCV
    columnar cell variant
    conductivity cell volume
CD
    cluster of differentiation
      CD antibody
      CD antigen
      CD2AP
      CD$^+$
      CD1a
      CD1b
      CD1c
      CD2
      CD3
      CD4 lymphopenia
      CD5
      CD6
      CD7
      CD9
      CD11a
      CD11b
      CD11c
      CDw12
      CD13
      CD14 antibody
      CD14 antibody/antigen
      CD16b
      CDw17
      CD18
      CD19
      CD20
      CD23
      CD24
      CD25
      CD26
      CD27

CD28
CD29
CD30
CD31
CD32
CD33
CD34
CD34 staining
CD35
CD36
CD37
CD38
CD39
CD40
CD41
CD42
CD42b
CD43
CD44
CD45
CD46
CD47
CD48
CD49a
CD49b
CD49c
CD49d
CD49e
CD49f
CD50
CD51
CD52
CD53
CD54
CD55
CD56
CD57
CD58
CD59
CDw60
CD61
CD63
CD64
CDw65
CD66a
CD66b
CD66c
CD66d
CD66e
CD68
CD69
CD70

CD71
CD72
CD73
CD74
CDw76
CD77
CDw78
CD79a
CD79b
CD80
CD81
CD82
CD83
CDw84
CD85
CD86
CD87
CD88
CD89
CDw90
CD91
CDw92
CD93
CD94
CD95
CD96
CD97
CD98
CD99
CD100
CDw101
CD102
CD103
CD104
CD105
CD106
CD107a
CD107b
CDw108
CDw109
CD115
CD116
CDw116
CD117
CD117 antibody/antigen
CD120a
CD120b
CDw121a
CDw121b
CDw122
CD123
CDw124

C

NOTES

CD (*continued*)
    CD126
    CDw127
    CDw128
    CD129
    CDw130
    CD138
    CDw75
    CD99 immunostain
    CD44H
    CD molecule
    CD protease
    CD protein
    CD white blood cell
cd
    candela
CD11/CD18 deficiency
CD$_{50}$
    median curative dose
CDA
    congenital dyserythropoietic anemia
    CDA type I–III
2-CDA
    2-chlorodeoxyadenosine
CDC
    cell-dependent cytotoxicity
    Centers for Disease Control
    chenodeoxycholic acid
    collecting duct carcinoma
    CDC Category A biological agents (the highest risk)
    CDC Category B biological agents (next highest risk)
    CDC category of biological agent
    CDC Category C biological agents (third highest risk)
    CDC test
CD55/CD59
    Cellquant CD38/CD8-PE, CD55/CD59
CD-Chex
    CD-C. C34 control for flow cytometry
    CD-C. Plus control for flow cytometry
CDH
    congenital dislocation of hip
CDH1 gene
CDK
    cyclin-dependent kinase
CDK5
    cyclin-dependent kinase 5
Cdk1
    cyclin-dependent protein kinase 1
CDK4 gene
CDKI
    cyclin-dependent kinase inhibitor
cDNA
    complementary DNA

    cDNA clone
    cDNA library
CDP
    continuous distending pressure
    cytidine diphosphate
CDP-choline
CDP-diglyceride
CDP-ethanolamine
CDR
    complementarity determining region
CdTOX A OIA
CD44v6
    C. score
    C. staining in prostate carcinoma
CDX1 intestine-specific transcription factor
CDX2
    C. immunohistochemical marker
    C. intestine-specific transcription factor
CE
    California encephalitis
    capillary zone electrophoresis
    cardiac enlargement
CEA
    carcinoembryonic antigen
    crystalline egg albumin
    CEA assay
    CEA Gold-5 stain
    CEA immunoperoxidase stain
    CEA test
CEACAM1
    carcinoembryonic antigen-related cell adhesion molecule 1
    CEACAM1 expression
ceanothus extract
CEAP
    clinical manifestations, etiologic factors, anatomic involvement, pathophysiologic features
    CEAP classification of venous disorders
cebocephalus
cebocephaly
ceca (*pl. of* cecum)
cecal carcinoma
cecitis
cecum, pl. **ceca**
cedar oil
Cedecea
CEDIA
    cloned enzyme donor immunoassay
    CEDIA drug of abuse test
    CEDIA sirolimus assay
cedrina
    Pseudomonas c.
Ceelen-Gellerstedt syndrome
CEEV
    Central European encephalitis virus

CEF
chick embryo fibroblast
cefaclor
cefamandole
cefoperazone
cefotaxime
cefoxitin
cefsulodin-Irgasan-novobiocin (CIN)
    c.-i.-n. agar
C1EInh
C1 esterase inhibitor
CEJO65 monoclonal antibody
CEL
chronic eosinophilic leukemia
celebensis
    Raillietina c.
Celebes vibrio
celestine blue B
celiac
    c. crisis
    c. disease
    c. rickets
    c. sprue
celiocentesis
celioma
celiomyositis
celioparacentesis
celiopathy
celitis
cell
    A c.
    absorption c.
    absorptive c.
    acanthoid c.
    accessory c.
    acid c.
    acidophil c.
    acinar c.
    acinous c.
    acoustic c.
    c. adhesion molecule (CAM)
    adipose c.
    adjoining epithelial c.
    adrenal cortex c.
    adrenocorticotropic c.
    adult stem c.
    adventitial reticular c.
    c. aggregation
    agranular c.
    A549 human lung carcinoma c.
    air c.
    albuminous c.

algoid c.
alpha c.
alveolar c.
Alzheimer c.
amacrine c.
ameboid c.
amniogenic c.
amnion c.
amphicrine c.
amphophil c.
anabiotic c.
anaplastic c.
c. anchorage
aneuploid c.
angioblastic c.
angulate c.
Anitschkow c.
anterior ethmoidal air c.
anterior horn c.
antibody-forming c.
antibody producing plasma c.
antigen-presenting c. (APC)
antigen-responsive c.
antigen-sensitive c.
antigen-transporting c.
apolar c.
apoptotic c.
APUD c.
argentaffin c.
argyrophilic enterochromaffin-like c.
Arias-Stella c.
Armanni-Ebstein c.
Aschoff c.
Askanazy c.
astroglia c.
atypical c.
auditory receptor c.
autologous lymphokine activated killer c.
autologous peripheral blood stem c. (Auto-PBSC)
c. axis
axon of neuroglial c.
axon of pyramidal c.
B c.
balloon c.
band c.
barrier-layer c.
basal c.
basaloid c.
basilar c.
basket c.

NOTES

cell *(continued)*

    basophil c.
    beaker c.
    Beale ganglion c.
    Berger c.
    berry c.
    beta c.
    beta c. of pancreas
    Betz c.
    Bevan-Lewis c.
    binucleate c.
    biochemical fuel c.
    bipolar c.
    bipotential c.
    bite c.
    Bizzozero red c.
    blast c.
    blastema c.
    blastemal c.
    blister c.
    bloated c.
    c. block preparation
    blood c.
    c. body
    Boettcher c.
    Boll c.
    bone marrow precursor c.
    border c.
    Böttcher c.
    bovine red blood c. (BRBC)
    c. bridge
    bristle c.
    bronchic c.
    bronchiolar exocrine c.
    brood c.
    brush bipolar c.
    buffy-coated c.
    bulliform c.
    burr c.
    c. button
    C c.
    Cajal c.
    caliciform c.
    calicoblast c.
    cap c.
    capsular c.
    capsule c.
    cardiac failure c.
    carrier c.
    cartilage c.
    CaSki c.
    castration c.
    caterpillar c.
    CD white blood c.
    c. center
    centrifugal bipolar c.
    centroacinar c.
    centrocytelike c. (CLL)
    centrofollicular c.

chalice c.
chief c.
chromaffin c.
chromophobe c.
chronic cell leukemia
chronic lymphosarcoma c.
ciliated c.
circulating reticuloendothelial c.
Clara c.
Claudius c.
clear c.
cleaved follicular center c.
clonal proliferated c.
clonogenic c.
clue c.
CMV-negative allogeneic c.
c. coat
cochlear hair c.
coelenterazine-treated c.
column c.
columnar absorptive c.
comet c.
commissural c.
committed c.
companion c.
compound granule c.
cone bipolar c.
conjunctival c.
connective tissue c.
contrasuppressor c.
control c.
Conway c.
cornified c.
Corti c.
c. count
c. counter
c. coupling
crenated c.
crescent c.
crystal c.
cuboidal c.
c. cycle
c. cycle arrest
c. cycle S phase
c. cycle time
cytomegalic c.
cytotoxic T c.
cytotrophoblastic c.
D c.
dark c.
daughter c.
Davidoff c.
c. death
c. death gene
decidual c.
decoy c.
deep c.
degenerating secretory c.
Deiters c.

delta c.
dendrite of pyramidal c.
dendritic c. (DC)
dendritic clear c.
dendritic epidermal c.
deposit of amyloid in islet c.
dermal dendritic c.
destruction of pancreatic beta c.
c. differentiation
diffuse ganglion c.
diploid c.
displaced ganglion c.
dissociated islet c.
c. division
DNA-aneuploid tumor c.
Dogiel c.
dome c.
Dorothy Reed c.
Downey c.
ductular reactive c.
dust c.
early B c.
early myeloid progenitor c.
eating c.
ectoblastic c.
ectodermal c.
effector c.
electrochemical c.
electrolytic c.
electromotive force c.
elongated c.
embryonic germ c.
embryonic stem c.
emigration of white c.'s
enamel c.
end c.
endocervical c.
endocrine c.
endodermal c.
endometrial c.
endothelial c.
c. engraftment
enterochromaffin c.
enteroendocrine c.
entodermal c.
enumeration of hematopoietic
  stem c.'s
c. envelope
ependymal c.
epidermic c.
epithelial reticular c.
epithelioid c.

epulis c.
E rosette-forming c.
erythrocytic blood c.
erythroid precursor c.
erythropoietin-responsive c. (ERC)
established c. line
eta c.
ethmoidal c.
exocrine c.
exploding crypt c.
external pillar c.
exudation c.
faggot c.
c. of Fañanás
fasciculata c.
fat c.
fat-storing c.
FCL c.
Ferrata c.
Ficoll-Paque purified c.
fixed c.
flame c.
flat bipolar c.
flattened c.
floor c.
foam c.
follicular cell lymphoma c.
follicular center c. (FCC)
follicular dendritic c. (FDC)
follicular epithelial c.
follicular ovarian c.
foreign body giant c.
formative c.
free c.
frozen red blood c.'s
fuchsinophil c.
c. fusion
G c.
galvanic c.
gamma c.
ganglion c.
gastrointestinal mucosal c.
gastrointestinal pacemaker c.
Gaucher c.
Gegenbaur c.
gemistocytic c.
generative c.
genetically abnormal c.
Gerbich-negative red c.
germ c.
germinal c.
ghost c.

NOTES

cell (continued)
giant c.
Gierke c.
gitter c.
glandular c.
Gley c.
glia c.
glial c.
glitter c.
glomerulosa c.
glomus c.
glucose, age, lactate dehydrogenase,
  aspartate aminotransferase, white
  blood c.'s (GA LAW)
goblet c.
Golgi c.
Goormaghtigh c.
granule c.
granulocytic blood c.
granulocytic precursor c.
granulosa lutein c.
grape c.
great alveolar c.
ground glass c.
guanine c.
guard c.
gustatory c.
gyrochrome c.
hair c. (HC)
hairy c.
hallmark of protein-secreting c.
hallmark of steroid-secreting c.
Hanseman c.
haploid c.
Hargraves c.
heart failure c.
HEK c.
HEL c.
HeLa c.
helmet c.
helper T c.
hematopoietic cord blood c.
hematopoietic progenitor c. (HPC)
hematopoietic stem c. (HSC)
HEMPAS c.
Hensen c.
hepatic progenitor c.
hepatic stellate c.
heteromeric c.
HGPRT-deficient c.
hilar c.
hilus c.
hobnail c.
Hodgkin and Reed-Sternberg c.
Hofbauer c.
homozygous typing c.
c. honeycombing
horny c.
horse red blood c. (HRBC)

Hortega c.
HOSE c.
hot c.
HPRT-deficient c.
HRS c.
human dermal microvascular
  endothelial c. (HDMEC)
human umbilical vein endothelial c.
  (HUVEC)
Hürthle c.
hyaline c.
hybrid c.
c. hybridization
hyperchromatic c.
hyperdiploid c. (HDC)
hypotetraploid c.
hypoxic c.
I c.
immunocompetent c. (ICC)
immunohistochemical stain for T c.
immunologically activated c.
immunologically competent c.
Immuno-trol c.
inclusion c.
c. inclusion
indifferent c.
inducer c.
infiltration of leukemic c.
inflammatory c.
c. injury
inner hair c.
inner phalangeal c.
innocent bystander c.
c. interaction (CI)
intercalary c.
intercapillary c.
intercellular canaliculus of
  parietal c.
interdigitating dendritic c. (IDC)
interdigitating reticulum c.
intermediate c.
internal pillar c.
internuncial c.
intestinal crypt c.
intimal c.
intracytoplasmic inclusion c.
intrasinusoidal cytokeratin-positive
  mesothelial c.
irreversibly sickled c. (ISC)
irritation c.
islet alpha c.
islet beta c.
islet delta c.
Ito c.
c. junction
juvenile c.
juxtaglomerular c.
K c.
karyochrome c.

keratinized c.
killer c.
c. kinetics
Ki-67-positive c.
koilocytotic c.
Kulchitsky c.
Kupffer c.
C. Lab IC 100 image cytometer
labile c.
lacis c.
lactate dehydrogenase, aspartate
  aminotransferase, white blood c.'s
  (LAW)
lacunar c.
lacZ-tagged c.
Langhans giant c.
large c. (LC)
large unstained c. (LUC)
late cortical T c.
LE c.
Leclanché c.
Leishman chrome c.
lepra c.
leukocyte-poor packed red
  blood c.'s
leukocyte-reduced red blood c.'s
Leydig interstitial c.
L-H c.
light chain class-restricted B c.
c. line
c. lineage analysis
lining c.
lipid-rich neoplastic c.
Lipschütz c.
littoral c.
locomotive c.
Loevit c.
lupus erythematosus c.
luteal c.
lutein c.
luteum c.
lymph c.
lymphoblastic plasma c.
lymphocytic blood c.
lymphoid progenitor c.
lymphoid stem c.
lymphokine-activated killer c.
  (LAK)
lymphoplasmacytoid c.
M c.
macroglia c.

malignant Hodgkin and Reed-
  Sternberg c.
malpighian c.
mammosomatotroph c.
Marchand wandering c.
marrow c.
Martinotti c.
mast c.
c. matrix
maturation B c.
mature B c.
mediator c.
medium sized pyramidal c.
medullary carcinoma c.
medullary interstitial c.
medullary T c.
medulloepithelial c.
megakaryocytic blood c.
melanotropic c.
c. membrane
c. membrane interdigitation
memory B, T c.
Merkel-Ranvier c.
Merkel tactile c.
mesangial c.
mesenchymal c.
mesoderm c.
mesoglial c.
mesothelial c.
metallophil c.
metaphase c.
metaplastic c.
Mexican hat c.
Meynert c.
microdissected chief c.
microfold c.
microglia c.
microglial c.
middle c.
midget bipolar c.
migratory c.
Mikulicz c.
mirror-image c.
mitral c.
modified red blood c.
monocytic blood c.
monocytic precursor c.
monocytoid c.
c. monolayer
mononuclear c.
monosomic c.
monosynaptic bipolar c.

NOTES

C

cell *(continued)*
    mop bipolar c.
    Mosher air c.
    mossy c.
    mother c.
    motile c.
    motor c.
    Mott c.
    MRC-5 human diploid fibroblast c.
    mucoalbuminous c.
    mucoserous c.
    mucous neck c.
    Müller radial c.
    multinucleated c.
    multinucleated giant c. (MGC)
    multipolar c.
    mummified c.
    mural c.
    myeloid stem c.
    myeloma c.
    myocardial endocrine c.
    myoepithelial c.
    myogenic c.
    myoid c.
    Nageotte c.
    naive c.
    natural killer c. (NK)
    navicular c.
    neoplastic epidermal c.
    nerve c.
    c. nest
    Neumann c.
    neural crest c.
    neurilemma c.
    neuroectoderm-derived c.
    neuroendocrine transducer c.
    neuroepithelial c.
    neuroglia c.
    neuroglial c.
    neurological c.
    neuroprogenitor c.
    neurosecretory c.
    nevus c.
    Niemann-Pick c.
    no lymph nodes containing cancer c.'s (N0)
    nonadherent c.
    noncleaved follicular center c.
    nonflagellated vegetative c.
    nonfollicular center c. (non-FCC)
    nonleukoreduced red c.
    nonreplicating c.
    normal complement of c.'s
    nuclear wreath c.
    nucleated red blood c. (NRBC)
    null c.
    nurse c.
    oat c.
    olfactory receptor c.

    oligodendrogenic c.
    oligodendroglia c.
    oligodendroglia-like c. (OLC)
    oncocytic c.
    Opalski c.
    c. organelle
    Ortho-Kung T c. (OKT)
    osseous c.
    osteochondrogenic c.
    osteoclast-like giant c. (OLGC)
    osteogenic c.
    osteoprogenitor c.
    outer hair c.
    outer phalangeal c.
    oval-shaped goblet c.
    oxyntic c.
    oxyphil c.
    oxyphilic c.
    P c.
    packed human blood c.'s
    packed red blood c.'s
    Paget c.
    palisading c.
    pancreaticoduodenal endocrine c.
    Paneth granular c.
    parabasal c.
    parafollicular c.
    paraganglionic c.
    paraimmunoblast c.
    paraluteal c.
    parathyroid chief c.
    parathyroid oxyphil c.
    parathyroid transitional c.
    parathyroid wasserhelle c.
    parenchymal c.
    parent c.
    parietal c.
    passenger c.
    pathologic c.
    pearl c.
    Pelger-Huët c.
    pencil c.
    peptic c.
    pericapillary c.
    perineurial c.
    perineuronal satellite c.
    peripheral blood mononuclear c. (PBMC)
    peripheral blood progenitor c. (PBPC)
    peripolar c.
    perithelial c.
    peritoneal exudate c.
    peritubular contractile c.
    perivascular epithelioid c.
    perivenular c.
    permanent c.
    pessary c.
    phagocytic c.

phalangeal c.
phantom c.
pheochrome c.
photoconductive c.
photoreceptor c.
photovoltaic c.
physaliphorous c.
pi c.
Pick c.
picket c.
pigment c.
pillar c.
pineal c.
plaque-forming c. (PFC)
plasma c. (PC)
plasma blood c.
plasmacytic blood c.
pleomorphic binucleated giant c.
pleomorphic mononucleated giant c.
plump c.
pluripotent hematopoietic stem c.
pluripotential basal c.
pluripotential hemopoietic stem c.
pluripotential stromal c.
pluripotent myeloid stem c.
pluripotent primitive mesodermal c.
polar c.
c. polarity
polychromatic c.
polychromatophil c.
polygonal c.
polyhedral c.
popcorn c.
Portland c.
positive c.
posterior c.
postmitotic c.
pre-B c.
preconfluent c.
precornified c.
precursor c.
predominant c.
pregnancy c.
pregranulosa c.
prickle c.
primary embryonic c.
primitive-looking c.
primitive neuroblastic c.
primitive reticular c.
primordial germ c.
primordial sex c.
principal c.

prismatic follicular c.
progenitor c.
prolactin c.
c. proliferation
prolymphocyte c.
pseudo-Gaucher c.
pseudosarcomatous c.
pseudounipolar c.
pseudoxanthoma c.
pulmonary neuroendocrine c.
 (PNEC)
pulpar c.
Purkinje c.
pus c.
pyknotic c.
pyramidal c.
pyroninophilic blast c.
pyrrol c.
RA c.
RACE c.
radiosensitivity of specialized c.
ragocyte c.
Raji c.
reactive c.
reagent red blood c.
red blood c. (RBC)
Reed c.
Reed-Sternberg c. (RS)
Reed-variant c.
regeneration c.
renal tubular epithelial c.
Renshaw c.
reproductive c.
reserve c.
resident c.
responder c.
resting B c.
resting wandering c.
restructured c.
reticular c.
reticularis c.
reticuloendothelial c.
reticulum c.
rhabdoid c.
rhagiocrine c.
Rieder c.
Rindfleisch c.
rod nuclear c.
rod photoreceptor c.
Rolando c.
rosette-forming c.
Rouget c.

NOTES

cell *(continued)*
round c.
rounded mononuclear c.
RTE c.
Russell-Crooke c.
Sala c.
c. salvage
c. sap
sarcogenic c.
satellite c.
scavenger c.
Schilling band c.
Schultze c.
Schwann c.
secretory c.
sedimented red c. (SRC)
c. seeding
segmented c.
self-renewing c.
sensitized c.
c. separation method
septal c.
seromucous c.
serous c.
Sertoli c.
sex c.
Sézary c.
shadow c.
sheep red blood c. (SRBC)
sickle c. (SC)
sickled c.
signet ring c.
SiHa c.
silver c.
singe-to-multiple layers of
  follicular c.
sinusoidal endothelial c.
skein c.
small cleaved c.
small noncleaved c. (SNCC)
smooth muscle c.
smudge c.
smudged c.
solid masses of epithelial c.
somatic c.
somatostatin-producing small c.
c. sorting analysis
sperm c.
spider c.
spindle c.
spindle-shaped neoplastic stromal c.
spindly squamoid c.
spine c.
splenic c.
spur c.
squamous alveolar c.
squamous epithelial c.
stab c.
stable c.

staff c.
static balance receptor c.
stellate c.
stem c.
Stem-Trol control c.
Sternberg giant c.
Sternberg-Reed c.
Sternheimer-Malbin positive c.
stichochrome c.
stimulator c.
stipple c.
c. strain
strap c.
stroma c.
subnuclear vacuolated c.
superficial c.
supporting c.
suppressor c.
surface absorptive c.
c. surface glycoprotein
c. surface immunophenotyping
c. surface marker
surface mucous c.
c. surface receptor
survival of cancer c.
suspicious c.
sustentacular c.
sympathetic formative c.
sympathicotropic c.
sympathochromaffin c.
sympathotropic c.
syncytiotrophoblastic c.
synovial c.
tactile c.
tadpole c.
tailed red c.
tanned red c. (TRC)
tapetal c.
target c.
tart c.
taste c.
^{99m}Tc labeled red blood c.
T cytotoxic c.
TDTH c.
teardrop red c.
tendon c.
tennis racket c.
tetracarcinoma c.
Tg c.
theca interna c.
theca lutein c.
T helper c.
thymic epithelial c.
thymic reticulum c.
thymus-dependent c.
thymus-derived c.
thymus nurse c.
Tiselius electrophoresis c.
Tm c.

T-natural killer c. (TNK)
Toker clear c.
totipotent c.
totipotential stem c.
touch c.
Touton giant c.
c. traffic
transducer c.
c. transformation
transitional c.
transport of cancer c.
trisomic c.
trophoblast c.
T-suppressor c.
tube c.
tufted c.
tumor c.
tunnel c.
Türk c.
tympanic c.
type C nevus c.
type I c.
type II alveolar epithelial c.
typical smooth muscle c.
Tzanck c.
umbrella c.
undifferentiated c.
unipolar c.
unit c.
Unna c.
vacuolated c.
van Hansemann c.
vascular smooth muscle c. (VSMC)
vasoformative c.
vegetative c.
veil c.
veiled c.
Vero c.
vestibular hair c.
Vignal c.
Virchow c.
virgin B c.
virus-transformed c.
visual receptor c.
vitreous c.
c. volume (CV)
volume of packed c.'s (VPC)
volume of packed red c.'s (VPRC)
c. volume profile (CVP)
c. wall
c. wall defective bacteria culture

c. wall-deficient bacterial form (CWDF)
Walthard c.
wandering c.
Warthin-Finkeldey multinucleate giant c.
washed red c. (WRC)
washed red blood c.
wasserhelle c.
water-clear c.
c. web
white blood c. (WBC)
whorling c.
WI-38 c.
wing c.
xanthoma c.
yolk c.
Zeiss counting c.
zombie c.
zymogenic c.
cell-bound antibody
cell-cell
    c.-c. adhesion molecule
    c.-c. contact region
    c.-c. interaction
Cell-Chex body fluid procedural control
cell-cycle
    c.-c. inhibitor
    c.-c. inhibitory protein
    c.-c. perturbation
    c.-c. regulator
cell-dependent cytotoxicity (CDC)
Cell-Dyn
    C.-D. 1200, 3200, 4000 automated cell counting instrument
Cellfalcicula
cell-fat ratio
cell-free system
cellicolous
cell-mediated
    c.-m. immunity (CMI)
    c.-m. lympholysis assay
    c.-m. reaction
cellobiase
cellobiose
celloidin section
cellophane tape method
Cellosolve
CellPrep sample preparation system
CellProbe
    C. cytoenzymology reagent

C

NOTES

CellProbe *(continued)*
 C. HT caspase-3/7 whole cell
 assay
Cellquant
 C. CD38/CD8-PE, CD55/CD59
 C. Kit
**CellQuest Pro 4.0 flow cytometry
 software**
cell-substrate adhesion molecule
cell-surface
 c.-s. carbohydrate chain
 c.-s. protein
cell-suspension flow cytometry
cell-to-cell adherent protein
cellula, pl. **cellulae**
 cellulae ethmoidales
 cellulae ethmoidales anteriores
 cellulae ethmoidales mediae
 cellulae ethmoidales posteriores
 cellulae pneumaticae tubae auditivae
 cellulae tympanicae
cellulans
 Cellulosimicrobium c.
cellular
 c. adaptation
 c. atypia
 c. biology
 c. blue nevus (CBN)
 c. cartilage
 c. cloning
 c. cutaneous fibrous histiocytoma
 (CCFH)
 c. debris
 c. debris centrifuge polarizing
 microscope
 c. degeneration
 c. dyscohesion
 c. embolism
 c. fibronectin
 c. hybridization
 c. immune theory
 c. immunity
 c. immunity deficiency syndrome
 (CIDS)
 c. immunodeficiency with abnormal
 immunoglobulin synthesis
 c. infiltration
 c. inhibitor of apoptosis (cIAP)
 c. kinetics
 c. neurothekeoma
 c. pathology
 c. polyp
 c. respiration
 c. schwannoma
 c. senescence
 c. spill
 c. swelling
 c. tenacity
 c. tumor

cellularity
 mixed c. (MC)
cellulase
cellulicidal
cellulifugal
cellulipetal
cellulite
cellulitic phlegmasia
cellulitis
 eosinophilic c.
 epizootic c.
 orbital c.
 pelvic c.
 phlegmonous c.
 streptococcal c.
cellulocutaneous plague
Cellulomonadaceae
Cellulomonas
 C. humilata
 C. iranensis
 C. persica
 C. xylanilytica
Cellulophaga
 C. algicola
 C. baltica
 C. fucicola
 C. lytica
 C. pacifica
 C. uliginosa
cellulosa
 vagina c.
cellulosae
 Cysticercus c.
cellulose
 c. acetate
 c. caprate
 DEAE c.
 diethylaminoethyl c.
 c. tape technique
cellulosilytica
 Xylanimonas c.
Cellulosimicrobium
 C. cellulans
 C. variabile
cellulosity
Cellvibrio
 C. fibrivorans
 C. fulvus
 C. gandavensis
 C. japonicus
 C. mixtus
 C. ostraviensis
 C. vulgaris
CELO
 chicken embryo lethal orphan
 CELO virus
celom *(var. of* coelom)
celomic metaplasia
celoschisis

celosomia
celozoic
Celsior solution
Celsius
    C. temperature scale (C)
    C. thermometer
Celsus kerion
cement
    c. corpuscle
    intercellular c.
    c. line
    polymethylmethacrylate c.
    c. substance
    tooth c.
cementification
cementifying fibroma
cementing substance
cementoblast
cementoblastoma
cementoclast
cementocyte
cementoma
    familial gigantiform c. (FGC)
cementoosseous dysphasia (COD)
cementoossifying fibroma (COF)
cementum
    afibrillar c.
    primary c.
    secondary c.
Cenangium
Cenarchaeales
cenobium
cenocepacia
    Burkholderia c.
Cenococcum
cenocyte, coenocyte
cenocytic
CenSlide 2000 urinalysis system
censored observation
census tract (CT)
center
    cell c.
    chiral c.
    chondrification c.
    diaphysial c.
    C.'s for Disease Control (CDC)
    epiotic c.
    follicular cell c.
    germinal c. (GC)
    ossific c.
    c. of ossification
    Poison Control C.

    primary ossification c.
    progressive transformation of
      germinal c. (PTGC)
    proliferation c.
    pseudofollicular growth c. (PFGC)
    pseudofollicular proliferation c.
    ratty edge of germinal c.
    reaction c.
    regressively transformed germinal c.
center-fire rifle wound
centigrade
    c. temperature scale (C)
    c. thermometer
centigram (cg)
centiliter (cL)
centimeter (cm)
    cubic c. (cm^3, cu cm)
centimeter-gram-second (CGS)
    c. system
centimorgan (cMo)
centipede
centipoise (cP)
centistoke (cSt)
central
    c. achromia
    c. blood volume (CBV)
    c. body
    c. callus
    c. canal
    c. chemoreceptor
    c. chromatolysis
    c. clonal deletion
    c. collodiaphyseal angle (CCD)
    c. core disease
    c. diabetes insipidus
    C. European encephalitis virus
      (CEEV)
    C. European tick-borne encephalitis
      virus
    C. European tick-borne fever
    c. excitatory state (CES)
    c. ganglioneuroma
    c. hemorrhagic necrosis (CHN)
    c. hyaline sclerosis
    c. inhibitory state (CIS)
    c. lacteal
    c. lesion
    c. limit theorem
    c. necrosis
    c. nervous system disorder
    c. nervous system involvement
    c. nervous system tuberculosis

C

NOTES

central *(continued)*
>c. nervous system tumor
>c. neurocytoma
>c. obesity
>c. osteitis
>c. osteocarcinoma
>c. osteosarcoma
>c. pit
>c. pneumonia
>c. pontine myelinolysis
>c. pontine myelinosis
>c. processing unit
>c. radiolucency
>c. Recklinghausen disease type II
>c. spindle
>c. spore
>c. tendency
>c. type neurofibromatosis
>c. venous pressure

centralis
>area c.
>fovea c.
>substantia gelatinosa c.
>substantia intermedia c.

central-patch infiltrate
centriacinar emphysema
centric fusion
Centriflo filter
centrifugal
>c. bipolar cell
>c. fast analyzer
>c. flotation
>c. force

centrifugalization
centrifugalize
centrifugation
>cesium chloride gradient c.
>density gradient c.
>microhematocrit c.
>zonal c.

centrifuge
>Allegra 64R high-speed refrigerated benchtop c.
>Allegra 25R refrigerated benchtop c.
>Allegra X-12, X-15R, X-22 benchtop c.
>Avanti J-20XP, J-25, J-30I, J-HC, J-E c.
>CritSpin microhematocrit c.
>CytoFuge 2 c.
>Eppendorf 5702 c.
>HemataSTAT Easy Read c.
>J6-HC, J6-MC, J6-MI high capacity c.
>c. microscope
>PK110 c.
>Spinchron DLX, 15 series c.
>Stat-60 c.

>StatSpin Express 2 c.
>StatSpin MP c.

centrifugum
>leukoderma acquisitum c.

centrilobar steatosis
centrilobular
>c. dilatation
>c. emphysema
>c. fibrosis
>c. necrosis
>c. necrosis of the liver
>c. zone

centriole
>anterior c.
>distal c.
>posterior c.
>proximal c.

centripetal force
centroacinar cell
centroblast
centroblastic (CB)
>c. lymphoma

Centrocestus
centrocyte
centrocytic lymphoma
centrocytic/mantle-cell lymphoma (CC/MCL)
centrofollicular cell
centrolecithal
centromere
>c. banding stain
>c. enumeration probe (CEP)
>c. interference

centromere/kinetochore antibody
centromeric
>c. band
>c. region

centronuclear myopathy
centroplasm
centrosome
centrosphere
Centrospora acerina
Centruroides suffusus suffusus
cenuris
cenurosis
CEOT
>calcifying epithelial odontogenic tumor

CEP
>centromere enumeration probe
>chronic eosinophilic pneumonia
>congenital erythropoietic porphyria
>counterelectrophoresis
>>CEP 12 SpectrumOrange DNA probe kit
>>CEP X, Y SpectrumOrange DNA probe kit

cepacia
>*Burkholderia c.*
>*Pseudomonas c.*

Cephaelis
cephalalgia, cephalgia
cephaledema
cephalemia
cephalgia (*var. of* cephalalgia)
cephalhematocele
cephalhematoma
cephalhydrocele
cephalic index
cephalin
      c. flocculation
      c. flocculation test
cephalin-cholesterol
      c.-c. flocculation (CCF)
      c.-c. flocculation test
cephaline
Cephaliophora irregularis
cephalitis
Cephaloascus
cephalocele
cephalocentesis
cephaloglycin
cephalohematocele
cephalohematoma
cephalohemometer
cephalomegaly
cephalomeningitis
Cephalomyia
cephalont
cephalooculocutaneous telangiectasia
cephalopathy
cephalopelvic disproportion (CPD)
Cephalopoda
cephaloridine
cephalosporin
Cephalosporium
      C. falciforme
      C. granulomatis
cephalothin
cephalothoracopagus
Cephalotrichum
cephalotrigeminal angiomatosis
cephamycin
Ceprate SC stem cell concentration system
CEQ 8000, 8800 genetic analysis system
cera
ceramic capacitor
ceramidase
ceramide
      c. dihexoside

glycosyl c.
c. lactoside
lactosyl c.
c. moiety
c. trihexosidase
c. trihexoside (CTH)
Cerasibacillus quisquiliarum
Ceratocystiopsis
Ceratocystis
Ceratophyllidae
Ceratophyllus punjatensis
Ceratopogonidae
c-erb-B2
      c-erb-B2 oncoprotein
      c-erb-B2 protooncogene
cercaria
cercaria-hullen reaction schistosomiasis test
cercarien-hullen-reaktion test
cerci (*pl. of* cercus)
cercocystis
cercomer
cercomonad
Cercomonas
Cercopithecus
Cercospora apii
cercus, pl. cerci
cerealis
      Oidiodendron c.
cerebella (*pl. of* cerebellum)
cerebellar
      c. agenesis
      c. amyloid plaque
      c. astrocytoma
      c. cortex
      c. cyst
      c. degeneration
      c. fissure
      c. pontine
      c. sarcoma
      c. tumor
cerebelli
      cortex c.
      fissurae c.
      stratum granulosum corticis c.
      stratum moleculare corticis c.
cerebellin
cerebellitis
cerebellomedullary malformation syndrome

NOTES

cerebellopontine angle tumor
cerebellum, pl. **cerebella**
  molecular layer of c.
cerebral
  c. amyloid angiopathy
  c. atrophy
  c. blood flow (CBF)
  c. calculus
  c. cladosporiosis
  c. compression
  c. cortex
  c. cortex perfusion rate (CPR)
  c. death
  c. dysplasia
  c. edema
  c. embolism
  c. epidural abscess
  c. glucose oxygen quotient
    (CG:OQ)
  c. hemorrhage
  c. hernia
  c. herniation
  c. infarct
  c. infarction (CI)
  c. layer of retina
  c. lupus
  c. metabolic rate (CMR)
  c. metabolic rate of glucose
    (CMRG)
  c. metabolic rate of oxygen
    (CMRO)
  c. palsy (CP)
  c. porosis
  c. salt-washing syndrome
  c. sphingolipidosis
  c. thrombosis (CT)
  c. tuberculosis
cerebralis
  adiposis c.
  Coenurus c.
  mycetism c.
cerebri
  astrocytosis c.
  commotio c.
  cortex c.
  epiphysis c.
  falx c.
  fungus c.
  gliomatosis c.
  hypophysis c.
  c. pseudotumor
cerebriform nucleus
cerebritis
  suppurative c.
cerebrocuprein
cerebrohepatorenal syndrome
cerebromalacia
cerebromeningitis
cerebronic acid

cerebropathia
cerebropathy
cerebrosclerosis
cerebroside
  c. beta-galactosidase
  c. beta-glucosidase
  c. lipidosis
  c. sulfatide
cerebrosidosis
cerebrospinal
  c. fever
  c. fluid (CSF)
  c. fluid albumin
  c. fluid albumin index
  c. fluid analysis
  c. fluid assay
  c. fluid culture
  c. fluid cytology
  c. fluid glucose
  c. fluid glutamine
  c. fluid IgG index
  c. fluid IgG synthesis rate
  c. fluid immunoglobulin
  c. fluid lactate
  c. fluid lactate dehydrogenase
    fractions
  c. fluid lactate dehydrogenase
    isoenzymes
  c. fluid leukocyte count
  c. fluid myelin basic protein
  c. fluid oligoclonal bands
  c. fluid pressure
  c. fluid protein electrophoresis
  c. fluid-to-serum albumin index
  c. fluid total protein
  c. meningitis (CSM)
cerebrospinalis
  liquor c.
cerebrospinant
cerebrosus
  Morococcus c.
cerebrotendinous
  c. cholesterinosis
  c. xanthomatosis
cerebrovascular
  c. accident (CVA)
  c. anomaly
  c. disease (CVD)
  c. malformation (CVM)
  c. obstructive disease (CVOD)
  c. resistance (CVR)
cereus
  Bacillus c.
cerevisiae
  Acetobacter c.
  Saccharomyces c.
Cerinosterus cyanescens
Cerithidea
cerium

ceroid
    c. lipofuscin
    c. pigment
    c. storage disease
ceroidosis
ceroplasty
cerradoensis
    Nocardia c.
CERT
certesii
    Arenibacter c.
certification
    operator c.
certified
    C. Laboratory Assistant
    c. reference material
    c. stain
    c. standard
cerulea
    macula c.
cerulein
ceruleus
    locus c.
ceruloplasmin
    c. assay
    c. level
    c. test
cerumen
ceruminal
ceruminoma
ceruminosae
    glandulae c.
ceruminous
    c. adenoma
    c. carcinoma
    c. gland
cervi
    Lipotena c.
    Setaria c.
cervical
    c. abortion
    c. adenitis
    c. bubo
    c. canal stenosis
    c. carcinoma
    c. culture
    c. disk syndrome
    c. diverticulum
    c. dysplasia
    c. fistula
    c. fracture
    c. gland

    c. gland of uterus
    c. Gram stain
    c. hygroma
    c. intraepithelial neoplasia (CIN)
    c. mucus sperm penetration test
    c. myalgia
    c. myelopathy
    c. polyp
    c. punch biopsy
    c. radiculitis
    c. rib syndrome
    c. scraper
    c. secretion
    c. smear
    c. somatosensory evoked potential
    c. spine ankylosis
    c. spondylosis
cervicalis
    Onchocerca c.
cervical-vaginal
    c.-v. cytology
    c.-v. junction
cervices (*pl. of* cervix)
cervicitis
    cystic chronic c.
cervicovaginal
    c. lavage
    c. smear preparation
cervix, pl. **cervices**
    AIS of the c.
    c. of the axon
    epidermidization of c.
    GCC of the uterine c.
    incompetent c.
CES
    central excitatory state
cesarean-obtained barrier-sustained (COBS)
cesium (Cs)
    c. chloride gradient centrifugation
Cestan-Chenais syndrome
Cestan-Raymond syndrome
Cestan syndrome
Cestoda
Cestodaria
cestode
cestodiasis
Cestoidea
Cetobacterium somerae
Cetraria
cetrimide agar
cetyl

NOTES

cetylpyridium chloride test
cetyltrimethylammonium bromide
Ceuthospora
ceylanicum
    Ancylostoma c.
ceylonica
    Haemadipsa c.
Ceylon mouth sore
CF
    carbolfuchsin
    cardiac failure
    carrier-free
    chemotactic factor
    Christmas factor
    citrovorum factor
    complement fixation
    complement-fixing
    cystic fibrosis
        CF antibody
        CF antibody titer
        CF indicator system chloride patch
        CF test
Cf
    californium
CFF
    critical flicker fusion
        CFF test
CFIDS
    chronic fatigue immune dysfunction
    syndrome
CFLP
    cleavase fragment length polymorphism
c-fos oncogene
CFP
    chronic false-positive
    cystic fibrosis of pancreas
CFS
    congenital fibrosarcoma
CFT
    complement-fixation test
CFTR
    cystic fibrosis transmembrane
    conductance regulator
        CFTR gene
CFU
    colony-forming unit
CFU-C
    colony-forming unit-culture
CFU-E
    colony-forming unit-erythroid
CFU-GEMM
    colony-forming unit granulocyte,
    erythrocyte, monocyte, and
    megakaryocyte
CFU-GM
    colony-forming unit granulocyte-
    macrophage
CFU-Meg
    colony-forming unit-megakaryocyte

CFU/mL
    colony-forming units/mL
CFU-S
    colony-forming unit-spleen
CFWM
    cancer free white mouse
CG
    Cardio-Green
    chorionic gonadotropin
    colloidal gold
    NATO code for phosgene (choking gas)
        chrome violet CG
cg
    centigram
CgA
    chromogranin A
        CgA marker for CHF
CGD
    chronic granulomatous disease
CGG
    cytosine-guanine-guanine
CGH
    comparative genomic hybridization
CGL
    chronic granulocytic leukemia
C-glycocholic acid breath test
CGN
    chronic glomerulonephritis
CG:OQ
    cerebral glucose oxygen quotient
CGP
    chorionic growth hormone prolactin
    circulating granulocyte pool
CGRP
    calcitonin gene-related peptide
CGS
    centimeter-gram-second
        CGS system
        CGS unit
CGT
    chorionic gonadotropin
CGTT
    cortisone-glucose tolerance test
CH
    cholesterol
    crown-heel
C-H
    carbon-hydrogen
        C-H stretch
CHA
    congenital hypoplastic anemia
Chabert disease
Chabertia
chaeta
Chaetocladium
Chaetoconidium
Chaetomidium
Chaetomium
Chaetophoma dermo-unguis

Chaetosphaeronema
chaffeensis
    Ehrlichia c.
Chagas
    C. disease
    C. disease serological test
Chagas-Cruz disease
chagasi
    Leishmania donovani c.
chagasii
    Vibrio c.
chagoma
Chagres virus
chahannaoensis
    Natrialba c.
chain
    alpha c.
    beta myosin heavy c.
    branched c.
    cell-surface carbohydrate c.
    c. of custody
    electron transport c.
    H c.
    heavy c.
    hemolytic c.
    invariant c.
    c. isomerism
    J c.
    kappa light c.
    L c.
    lambda light c.
    laminin c.
    light c.
    monoclonal free light c.
    nuclear c.
    pearl c.
    c. reaction
    respiratory c.
    restricted light c.
    ricin A, B c.
    sympathetic c.
chaining
chain-reaction cascade
Chalara
chalasia
chalazion, chalaza, pl. **chalazia**
Chalciporus
chalcogen
chalcogenide
chalcone
chalcosis
chalice cell

chalicosis
challenge
    radioactive c.
    sulfite c.
chalone
chamber
    Abbé-Zeiss counting c.
    anaerobic c.
    Bactron 1.5 anaerobic c.
    Boyden c.
    counting c.
    endothelium of anterior c.
    hyperbaric c.
    ionization c.
    multiwire proportional c.
    Petroff-Hauser counting c.
    Sandison-Clark c.
    Shandon Cytospin c.
    Thoma counting c.
    Zappert counting c.
Chamberland filter
chamecephaly
Chameleon Cooler
Championnière disease
Champy fixative
chancre
    hard c.
    mixed c.
    monorecidive c.
    c. redux
    soft c.
    sporotrichositic c.
    tularemic c.
chancriform
    c. pyoderma
    c. syndrome
chancroid
chancroidal ulcer
chancrous
chandelier
    favic c.
Chang aniline-acid fuchsin method
change
    anatomic c.
    Armanni-Ebstein c.
    Crooke hyaline c.
    decidual c.
    degenerative c.
    desmoplastic c.
    DNA sequence copy number c.
    fatty c.
    harlequin color c.

C

NOTES

change *(continued)*
    hyperplastic-like mucosal c. (HPC)
    myxoid c.
    onionskin c.
    Paneth cell-like c.
    polycystic c.
    polyneuropathy, organomegaly, endocrinopathy, monoclonal gammopathy, and skin c.'s (POEMS)
    postcurettage reparative c.
    progestagenic c.
    pseudobowenoid c.
    pseudocarcinomatous c.
    pseudoepitheliomatous c.
    pseudo-Pelger-Huët c.
    reactive c.
    reversible c.
    single nucleotide c.
    Tenney c.
channel
    cation c.
    epithelial sodium c. (ENaC)
    ion c.
    ligand-gated c.
    transmitter-gated ion c.
    transnexus c.
    voltage-gated c.
channel-forming integral protein (CHIP-1)
channelopathy
Chantemesse reaction
chaotic heart
Chapel Hill Consensus Conference classification
chapellei
    Geobacter c.
chaperone
    molecular c.
character
    acquired c.
    c. density
    dominant c.
    mendelian c.
    monogenic c.
    primary sex c.
    recessive c.
    secondary sex c.
    sex-conditioned c.
    sex-limited c.
    sex-linked c.
    X-linked c.
    Y-linked c.
characteristic
    c. curve
    c.'s of hepatocyte
    organism c.
    c. pathologic

    receiver operating c. (ROC)
    ultrastructural c.
characterization
    definitive c.
    molecular c.
charcoal
    activated c.
    coelenterazine dextran-coated c.
    dextran-coated c. (DCC)
    c. yeast extract agar
Charcot
    C. arthropathy
    C. disease
    C. syndrome
    C. triad
Charcot-Böttcher crystalloid
Charcot-Leyden
    C.-L. crystal
    C.-L. crystalloid
Charcot-Marie-Tooth
    C.-M.-T. disease
    C.-M.-T. muscular atrophy
Charcot-Neumann crystal
Charcot-Robin crystal
Charcot-Weiss-Baker syndrome
CHARGE
    coloboma, heart disease, atresia choanae, retarded growth and development and ear anomalies
    CHARGE association
    CHARGE syndrome
charge
    cationic c.
    elementary c.
    ionic c.
    space c.
charged particle
charge-transfer complex
Charles law
Charlin syndrome
Charlouis disease
chart
    alignment c.
    flow c.
    Levey-Jennings c.
    pedigree c.
    quality control c.
chartarum
    Ulocladium c.
chattoni
    Entamoeba c.
Chauffard-Still syndrome
Chauffard syndrome
Chaussier areola
chauvoei
    Clostridium c.
CHB
    complete heart block

CHD
    congestive heart disease
ChE
    cholesterol ester
    cholinesterase
Cheadle disease
check
    alert c.
    c. bit
    delta c.
    c. digit
    limit c.
    linearity c.
    pacemaker c.
    parity c.
    previous value c.
checkerboard microdilution test
checkpoint
    mitotic spindle assembly c.
Chédiak-Higashi
    C.-H. disease
    C.-H. syndrome (CHS)
Chédiak-Steinbrinck-Higashi
    C.-S.-H. anomaly
    C.-S.-H. syndrome
Chédiak test
cheek
    cleft c.
cheese
    c. washer's disease
    c. worker's lung
cheesy
    c. necrosis
    c. pus
cheilitis
cheilosis
Cheilospirura hamulosa
cheiragra
cheirarthritis
chejuensis
    Hahella c.
chelate
    Sequestrene iron c.
chelating agent
chelation therapy
chelerythrine
Chelex
    C. DNA amplification
    C. resin
chelicera
cheloid
chelonae

chem
    chemistry panel
    chemistry profile
chemical
    c. adsorption
    c. agent
    c. agent detector paper
    c. agent detector tape
    c. agent monitor (CAM)
    c. analysis
    c. asphyxiant
    C. Biological Incident Response Force (of the U.S. Marine Corps) (CBIRF)
    c., biological, and radiological (CBR)
    c., biological, radiological or nuclear (CBRN)
    c., biological, radiological, nuclear, explosive (CBRNE)
    c. bond
    c. environment
    c. equation
    c. equilibrium
    c. examination of feces
    c. examination of stool
    c. gastritis
    c. incompatibility
    incompatible c.
    c. inhibition isoamylase test
    c. interference
    c. mediator
    nuclear, biological, and c.
    c. peritonitis
    c. pneumonia
    c. pneumonitis
    c. porphyria
    c. prophylaxis
    c. reaction
    c. shift
    c. spectrum
    c. splash suit
    c. styptic
    c. warfare (CW)
    c. waste
    c. WMD
chemically pure (CP)
chemical-resistant
    c.-r. inner gloves
    c.-r. outer gloves
chemiluminescence, chemoluminescence
    c. assay

C

NOTES

195

chemiluminescence *(continued)*
    electrogenerated c. (ECL)
    c. test
chemiluminescent
    c. assay (CLIA)
    c. immunoassay
    c. probe
chemiosmotic hypothesis
chemiotaxis *(var. of* chemotaxis)
chemisorption
chemistry
    analytical c.
    clinical c.
    histological c.
    inorganic c.
    organic c.
    c. panel (chem)
    physical c.
    physiologic c.
    c. profile (chem)
ChemMate
    C. capillary gap slide
    C. multistep detection system
chemoattractant
chemoautotroph
chemoautotrophic bacterium
chemoceptor
chemocoagulation
chemodectoma
chemodectomatosis
chemodifferentiation
chemoheterotroph
chemoheterotrophic bacterium
chemoimmunology
chemoimmunotherapy (CI)
chemokine
    Duffy antigen receptor for c.
    (DARC)
chemokinesis
chemolithotroph
chemoluminescence *(var. of*
  chemiluminescence)
chemoorganotroph
chemopreventive
chemoradioresistance
chemoreceptor
    central c.
    medullary c.
    peripheral c.
    c. tumor
chemoresistance
chemosensitive
chemostat
chemosterilant
chemosynthesis
chemotactic
    c. activity
    c. cytokine

    c. factor (CF)
    c. gradient
chemotactically attracted
chemotactin
chemotaxin
chemotaxis, chemiotaxis
    c. assay
chemotherapeutic index (CI)
chemotherapy
    ablative c.
    adjuvant c.
    cancer c.
    cytotoxic c.
    c. gastritis
    high-dose c. (HDCT)
    preoperative c. (preChx)
    c. resistance
chemotransmitter
chemotroph
chemotropism
Chempack Project
chemrad
    chemotherapy and radiotherapy
Chemstrip
    C. BG test
    C. dipstick
chemstrip
    Micral c.
chemTRAK liquid chemistry control
CHEMXpress system
Cheney syndrome
chenodeoxycholate
chenodeoxycholic
    c. acid (CDC)
    c. acid test
Chenopodium ambroisiodes
chenopodium oil
Chen test
cheopis
    Pulex c.
    Xenopsylla c.
Cherchevski disease
Chernobyl nuclear plant accident
cherry
    c. angioma
    c. red spot
Cherry-Crandall
    C.-C. procedure
    C.-C. serum lipase test
cherubic facies
cherubism
Chesapeake
    Hb C.
chest
    alar c.
    barrel c.
    blast c.
    cobbler's c.
    flail c.

foveated c.
pterygoid c.
c. radiography
tetrahedron c.

Chester disease
Cheyletiella parasitovorax
CHF
congestive heart failure
CgA marker for CHF
CHH
cartilage-hair hypoplasia
CHI
creatinine height index
Chiari
C. disease
C. II syndrome
C. net
Chiari-Arnold syndrome
Chiari-Budd syndrome
Chiari-Frommel syndrome
chiasm
glioma of optic c.
chiasma
chiasmal tumor
chick
c. embryo antigen
c. embryo fibroblast (CEF)
chick-cell agglutination (CCA)
chicken
bluecomb disease of c.'s
c. embryo lethal orphan (CELO)
c. embryo lethal orphan virus
c. fat appearance
c. fat clot
c. louse
chickenpox
hemorrhagic c.
c. immune globulin (human)
c. immunoglobulin
c. virus
chicken-wire pattern
Chick-Martin test
chiclero ulcer
Chido/Rodgers (CH/RG)
chief
c. agglutinin
c. cell
c. cell adenoma
c. cell of corpus pineale
c. cell of parathyroid gland
c. cell of stomach

Chievitz
juxtaoral organ of C.
C. layer
C. organ
Chiffelle and Putt method
chigger
chigoe
chikungunya
c. fever virus
c. hemorrhagic fever
Chilaiditi syndrome
chilblain lupus
CHILD
congenital hemidysplasia with
ichthyosiform erythroderma and limb
defects
CHILD syndrome
child
battered c.
C. hepatic risk criteria
childbed fever
childhood
benign chronic bullous dermatosis
of c.
chronic bullous dermatosis of c.
granulomatous disease of c.
c. hemolytic uremic syndrome
plexiform fibrohistiocytic tumor
of c.
recurring digital fibroma of c.
transient erythroblastopenia of c.
(TEC)
c. type tuberculosis
children
acute lymphoblastic leukemia in
older c.
linear IgA bullous disease in c.
Child-Turcotte-Pugh score
chilensis
Sphingopyxis c.
chill-fever reaction
chilomastigiasis
Chilomastix mesnili
chilomastosis
chilopod
Chilopoda
chilopodiasis
chimaera
Mycobacterium c.
chimera
blood group c.
dispermic c.

NOTES

C

chimera *(continued)*
    heterologous c.
    homologous c.
    isologous c.
    radiation c.
chimeric
    c. antibody
    c. gene
chimerism
    hematolymphoid c.
chimney-sweep's cancer
chimpanzee coryza agent (CCA)
chin
    galoche c.
chinensis
    Phlebotomus c.
Chinese
    C. liver fluke
    C. restaurant syndrome (CRS)
chinjuensis
    Paenibacillus c.
CHIP-1
    channel-forming integral protein
chip
    Affymetrix human cancer c.
    bone c.
    DNA c.
    c. fracture
    TURP c.
chiral
    c. center
    c. crystal
chirality
Chiroptera
chi squared distribution
chitin
Chitinibacter tainanensis
Chitinimonas taiwanensis
chitinolyticus
    Paenibacillus c.
CHL
    classic Hodgkin lymphoma
Chlamydia
    C. antigen
    C. culture
    C. group titer
    C. infection
    C. oculogenitalis
    C. OIA
    C. pneumoniae
    C. psittaci
    C. sepsis
    C. trachomatis
    C. trachomatis direct FA test
Chlamydiaceae
Chlamydiae
chlamydial
    c. disease
    c. pneumonia

Chlamydiales
Chlamydiamicrovirus
Chlamydiazyme
    C. EIA assay
    C. test
chlamydiosis
Chlamydoabsidia padenii
Chlamydobacteriaceae
Chlamydobacteriales
chlamydoconidium
Chlamydophila
    C. abortus
    C. caviae
    C. felis
    C. pecorum
    C. pneumoniae
    C. psittaci
Chlamydophrys
chlamydospore
Chlamydozoon
chloasma bronzinum
chloracetate
    c. esterase
    c. esterase histochemical stain
    naphthol AS-D c. (NASDCA)
chloracetic acid
chloracetophenone
    NATO code for c. (CS)
chloracne
chloral
    c. hydrate
    c. hydrate assay
chloramine-T
chloramphenicol
chloranil assay
chloranilate method
chloranilic acid
chlorate
    c. assay
    potassium c.
chlorazol
    c. black E
    c. black E stain
chlorbenside
chlordane
chlordiazepoxide assay
chloremia
chlorfenthion insecticide
chloride
    ammonium c.
    antimony c.
    benzalkonium c.
    calcium c.
    carbonic acid c.
    carbonyl c.
    c. channel 7 (ClCN7)
    cobaltous c.
    dansyl c.
    edrophonium c.

fecal c.
gold c.
hydrogen c.
c. imbalance
indium 111 c.
c. method
methylene c.
methylrosaniline c.
NATO code for cyanogen c.
  (CNCl$_2$) (CK)
Orion skin electrode for c.
polyvinyl c.
potassium c. (KCl)
pralidoxime c.
Schales and Schales method for c.
c. shield
c. shift
sodium c.
stool c.
urine c.
vinyl c.
chloridimetry
Chloridium
chloridometer
  coulometric c.
chloriduria
chlorinated
  c. hydrocarbon pesticide
  c. hydrocarbon pesticide assay
chlorine (Cl)
Chloriridovirus
chloritidismutans
  Pseudomonas c.
chlormerodrin accumulation test (CAT)
chloroacetate
  c. esterase (CAE)
  c. esterase reaction
1-chloroacetophenone
  NATO code for 1-c. (CN)
chloroanemia
chloroarsine
  organic c.
Chlorobacteria
Chlorobacteriaceae
Chlorobacterium
Chlorobaculum
  C. limnaeum
  C. parvum
  C. tepidum
  C. thiosulfatiphilum
Chlorobea
chlorobenzilate

chlorobenzoica
  Thauera c.
chlorobenzylidene malonitrile
Chlorobiaceae
Chlorobiales
Chlorobium
  C. clathratiforme
  C. luteolum
Chlorochromatium
2-chlorodeoxyadenosine (2-CDA)
chloroethenivorans
  Pseudonocardia c.
Chloroflexi
chlorofluorocarbon
chloroform
  c. assay
  methyl c.
  c. poisoning
chloroform-methanol
chloroguanide hydrochloride
chlorohydrin
  ethylene c.
chlorohydrocarbon assay
chloroleukemia
chlorolymphosarcoma
chloroma
chloromatous
chloromethanicum
  Hyphomicrobium c.
Chloromycetin
chloromyeloma
chloro-naphthol
chloropenia
chloropenic azotemia
chlorophenolicum
  Herbaspirillum c.
  Sphingobium c.
chlorophenolicus
  Arthrobacter c.
chlorophenol red
chlorophenoxy herbicide
Chlorophyllum molybdites
chlorophyll unit
chloropicrin
Chloropidae
chloroplast
chloropsia
chloroquine pump
chlororespirans
  Desulfitobacterium c.
chlorosis
Chlorothion

NOTES

chlorotic anemia
chlorous acid reagent
Chlorovirus
chlorpromazine assay
chlortetracycline
chloruresis
chloruria
CHN
    central hemorrhagic necrosis
CHO
    carbohydrate
choanal
    c. atresia
    c. polyp
Choanephora
choanoflagellate
choanomastigote
Choanotaenia infundibulum
chocolate
    anthrax-containing c.
    c. blood (CB)
    c. blood agar
    c. cyst
chocolatization
    c. of blood culture medium
    medium c.
choke
    ophthalmovascular c.
choking agent
chol.
    cholesterol
cholagogue
cholaneresis
cholangeitis
cholangiectasis
cholangiocarcinoma (CC)
cholangiocyte
cholangiofibrosis
cholangiogram
cholangiolar proliferation
cholangiole
cholangiolitic
    c. cirrhosis
    c. hepatitis
cholangiolitis
cholangioma
cholangiopancreatography
    endoscopic retrograde c.
cholangitic abscess
cholangitis
    ascending c.
    primary sclerosing c. (PSC)
    pyogenic c.
    sclerosing c.
    suppurative c.
cholate
cholecalciferol
cholecyst
cholecystagogue

cholecystectasia
cholecystitis
    acalculous c.
    acute or chronic c.
    acute hemorrhagic c.
    chronic calculous c. (CCC)
    emphysematous c.
    follicular c.
    glandularis proliferans c.
    xanthogranulomatous c.
cholecystoduodenal fistula
cholecystogram
    oral c. (OCG)
cholecystokinin (CCK)
    c. test
cholecystokinin-pancreozymin
cholecystolithiasis
cholecystosis
    hyperplastic c.
choledochal cyst
choledoch duct
choledochitis
choledochocele
choledochoduodenal junction
choledocholith
choledocholithiasis
choledochus
    ductus c.
choleglobin
cholehemia
cholelith, chololith
cholelithiasis, chololithiasis
cholelithic, chololithic
cholemia
cholemic nephrosis
cholepathia
choleperitoneum
choleperitonitis
cholera
    Asiatic c.
    c. bacillus
    hog c.
    pancreatic c.
    c. sicca
    c. toxin (CTX)
    typhoid c.
    c. vaccine
    c. vibrio
cholerae
    Vibrio c.
    Vibrio c. biotype El Tor (El Tor
    vibrio)
choleraesuis
    Salmonella c. subsp. *arizona*
choleragen
choleraic
choleraphage
cholera-red reaction
cholestasia

cholestasis
chronic c.
cholestatic
c. hepatitis
c. jaundice
cholesteatoma
cholesteatomatous
cholesteremia
cholesterinemia
cholesterinized antigen
cholesterinosis
cerebrotendinous c.
cholesterinuria
cholesterol (CH, chol.)
c. acyltransferase
c. assay
c. calculus
c. cleft
c. crystal
c. deposition
c. emboli
c. embolism
c. ester (ChE)
c. esterase
c. ester storage disease
intracellular free c.
C. Manager
c. 1,2,3 noninvasive testing device
c. polyp
remnantlike lipoprotein particles-c. (RLP-C)
c. side-chain cleavage enzyme deficiency
c. staining method
c. test
total c. (TC)
cholesterolemia
cholesterol-free medium
cholesterol-lecithin flocculation test
cholesterolosis
extracellular c.
cholesterol/phospholipid ratio (C:P)
cholesteroluria
CholesTrak
cholestyramine resin
choleuria (*var. of* choluria)
cholic acid
cholicele
choliformis
mycetism C.

choline
c. acetyltransferase
lysophosphatidyl c.
cholinergic
c. antagonist
c. blockade
c. blocking agent
c. crisis
c. urticaria
cholinesterase (ChE, CHS)
c. assay
c. blood test
c. enzyme
c. inhibitor
red blood cell c. (RBC-ChE)
chololith (*var. of* cholelith)
chololithiasis (*var. of* cholelithiasis)
chololithic (*var. of* cholelithic)
choloplania
cholothorax
choluria, choleuria
cholylglycine
14C-cholylglycine breath excretion test
chomelii
    Bartonella c.
Chondodendron
chondral
chondralloplasia
chondrification center
chondrify
chondrin ball
chondritis
chondroblast
differentiating c.
chondroblastic subtype
chondroblastoma (CB)
chondroblastoma-like osteosarcoma
chondrocalcinosis
articular c.
chondroclast
chondrocyte
hypertrophied c.
isogenous c.
c. lacuna
nuclei of c.
chondrodermatitis nodularis chronica helicis
chondrodysplasia
c. calcificans
hereditary deforming c.
c. punctata

C

NOTES

chondrodystrophia
    c. calcificans congenita
    c. congenita punctata
chondrodystrophic dwarfism
chondrodystrophy
    asphyxiating thoracic c.
    asymmetric c.
    hereditary deforming c.
chondroectodermal dysplasia
chondrofibroma
chondrogenic
chondrohypoplasia
chondroid
    c. chordoma
    c. lipoma
    c. metaplasia
    c. syringoma
    c. tissue
chondroitin
    c. sulfate
    c. sulfate proteoglycan (CSPG)
    c. sulfate stain
    c. sulfate staining
chondrology
chondroma
    extraskeletal c.
    juxtacortical c.
    periosteal c.
chondromalacia
    c. fetalis
    generalized c.
    c. of larynx
    c. patellae
    systemic c.
chondromatosis
    synovial c.
chondromatous
    c. exostosis
    c. giant cell tumor
chondrometaplasia
chondromucoprotein
chondromyxoid fibroma (CMF)
chondromyxoma
chondronectin
chondroosseous
chondroosteodystrophy
chondropathy
chondrophila
    Waddlia c.
chondrophyte
chondroplast
chondroporosis
chondrosarcoma
    dedifferentiated c.
    extraskeletal myxoid c. (EMC)
    mesenchymal c. (MC)
    skeletal myxoid c. (SMC)
chondrosis
Chondrostereum

chondrotrophic hormone
chondrus
chopped
    c. meat broth
    c. meat medium
chorangiosis
chorda, pl. **chordae**
    chordae willisii
chordae
    Algoriphagus c.
chordalis
    endocarditis c.
chordee
chorditis
chordoblastoma
Chordodes morgani
chordoid features
chordoma
    axial c.
    chondroid c.
    familial clival c.
    sacrococcygeal c.
chorea
    Bergeron c.
    Huntington c. (HC)
    Sydenham c.
choreic
choreiform
choreoathetosis
chorioadenoma destruens
chorioallantoic culture
chorioamnionic hemorrhage
chorioamnionitis
chorioangioma
chorioangiomatosis
chorioangiosis
choriocapillaris
    lamina c.
    membrana c.
choriocapillary layer
choriocarcinoma
    gestational c.
    monophasic c.
choriodecidual inflammatory response syndrome
choriodeciduitis
chorioepithelioma
chorioma
choriomeningitis
    lymphatic c. (LCM)
    lymphocytic c. (LCM)
chorion
    abnormal c.
    c. frondosum
    c. laeve
    mature abnormal c.
chorionic
    c. carcinoma
    c. cavity

c. epithelioma
c. gonadotropin (CG, CGT)
c. gonadotropin-alpha subunit
c. gonadotropin assay
c. gonadotropin-beta subunit
c. gonadotropin test
c. gonadotropin unit
c. growth hormone prolactin (CGP)
c. plate
c. somatomammotropin (CS)
c. villus
c. villus embolism
c. villus sampling (CVS)
Chorioptes
chorista
choristoblastoma
choristoma
neuromuscular c.
neuronal c.
choroid
basal lamina of c.
basal layer of c.
c. plexus
c. plexus papilloma
choroidal
c. hemangioma
c. neovascularization (CNV)
choroidea, pl. **choroideae**
lamina basalis choroideae
lamina vasculosa choroideae
tela c.
choroideremia
choroiditis
choroidocapillaris
lamina c.
Chotzen syndrome
CHR
chromogranin
CHR reaction
ChrA
chromogranin A
ChrA antigen
ChrA immunoperoxidase stain
CH/RG
Chido/Rodgers
CH/RG antibody
CH/RG antigen
CH/RG blood group
Christeller reaction
Christensen-Krabbe disease
Christensen urea agar

Christian
C. disease
C. syndrome
Christian-Hand-Schüller disease
Christian-Weber disease
Christie-Atkins-Munch-Petersen (CAMP)
Christison formula
Christmas
C. disease
C. factor (CF)
Christopherson nuclear grading system
Christopher spot
Christ-Siemens syndrome
Christ-Siemens-Touraine syndrome
chromaffin
c. body
c. cell
Gomori method for c.
c. hormone
c. paraganglioma
c. reaction
c. reaction test
c. system
c. tissue
c. tumor
chromaffinoma
medullary c.
chromaffinopathy
chromaphil
chromate
lead c.
c. method
c. stain for lead
Chromatiaceae
Chromatibacteria
chromatic
c. aberration
c. apparatus
c. fiber
c. granule
chromatica
trichomycosis c.
chromatid
c. gap
c. interference
nonsister c.
sister c.
chromatin
c. body
c. dust
heteropyknotic c.

NOTES

C

chromatin *(continued)*
    Klinger-Ludwig acid-thionin stain for sex c.
    marginated c.
    c. material
    c. network
    nucleolar-associated c.
    oxyphil c.
    c. particle
    c. reservoir
    sex c.
    c. spot
    X c.
    Y c.
chromatinic body
chromatin-negative
chromatinolysis
chromatinorrhexis
chromatin-positive
chromation
chromatism
chromatofocusing
    high-performance c. (HPCF)
chromatogram
chromatograph
    gas c.
chromatographic assay
chromatography
    adsorption c.
    affinity c.
    anion-exchange c.
    antibody affinity c.
    ascending c.
    DEAE anion exchange c.
    denaturing high-performance liquid c. (DHPLC)
    electric c.
    filter paper c.
    gas c. (GC)
    gas-liquid c. (GLC)
    gas-solid c. (GSC)
    gel-filtration c.
    gel-permeation c.
    high-performance ion exchange c. (HPIEC)
    high-performance liquid c. (HPLC)
    high-performance size exclusion c. (HPSEC)
    high-pressure liquid c. (HPLC)
    immunoaffinity c.
    instant thin-layer c. (ITLC)
    ion-exchange c.
    liquid-liquid c.
    liquid-solid c.
    microcolumn c.
    molecular exclusion c.
    molecular sieve c.
    paper c.
    SDS gel filtration c.

    serum thyroxine measured by column c. (T_4(C))
    size-exclusion c.
    thin-layer c. (TLC)
    two-dimensional c.
    vapor-phase c. (VPC)
chromatoid
chromatokinesis
chromatolysis
    central c.
    neuronal c.
    retrograde c.
    transsynaptic c.
chromatolytic
chromatometer
chromatopectic
chromatopexis
chromatophil, chromatophile
chromatophilia
chromatophilic granule
chromatophilous
chromatophobia
chromatophore
chromatophorotropic hormone
chromatoplasm
chromatotaxis
chromatotropism
chromaturia
chrome
    c. alum
    c. alum carmine
    c. alum hematoxylin-phloxine method
    c. alum hematoxylin-phloxine stain
    c. hematoxylin
    c. red
    c. violet
    c. violet CG
    c. yellow
chromic
    c. acid
    c. acid fixative
chromidia (*pl. of* chromidium)
chromidial
    c. apparatus
    c. net
    c. substance
chromidiation
chromidiosis
chromidium, pl. **chromidia**
chromium (Cr)
    c. assay
chromium-51 red cell survival
Chromobacterieae
Chromobacterium violaceum
chromoblastomycosis
chromocenter
chromocyte

chromogen
    AEC c.
    Porter-Silber c. (PSC)
    tetramethylbenzidine c.
chromogenesis
chromogenic
    c. bacterium
    c. cephalosporin test
    c. enzyme substrate test
    c. Xa inhibition assay
chromogranin (CHR)
    c. A (CgA, ChrA)
Chromohalobacter
    C. canadensis
    C. israelensis
    C. marismortui
    C. salexigens
chromolipid
chromolysis
chromolytic method
chromomere
chromometer
chromomycin A3
chromomycosis
chromonema, pl. **chromonemata**
chromopectic
chromopexis
chromophage
chromophil, chromophile
    c. adenoma
    c. granule
    c. substance
chromophilia
chromophilic
chromophilous
chromophobe
    c. adenoma
    c. carcinoma
    c. cell
    c. cell of anterior lobe of
      hypophysis
    c. granule
    c. tumor
chromophobia
chromophobic adenoma
chromophore
chromophoric
chromophorous
chromoplastid
chromoprotein
chromoscopy
    gastric c.

chromosomal
    c. aberration
    c. abnormality
    c. band
    c. breakage syndrome
    c. deletion
    c. deletion syndrome
    c. derangement
    c. disorder
    c. endoreduplication
    c. instability (CIN)
    c. inversion
    c. linkage
    c. malformation syndrome
    c. marker
    c. mutagen
    nonhistone c. (NHC)
    c. RNA (cRNA)
chromosomally mediated resistant
Neisseria gonorrhoeae
chromosome
    c. aberration
    accessory c.
    c. alteration
    c. analysis
    Balbiani c.
    c. band
    c. banding
    c. breakage syndrome
    c. complement
    derivative c. (der)
    c. dicentric malformation
    double minute c.
    fragile X c.
    gametic c.
    heteromorphic c.
    homologous c.
    i(12p) marker c.
    long arm of c.
    c. map
    marker c.
    metaphase c.
    mitotic c.
    c. nomenclature
    c. painting
    phage 1 artificial c.
    Philadelphia c. (Ph1)
    polytene c.
    c. 14q tumor marker
    reduplication of meiotic c.
    ring c.
    sex c.

C

NOTES

chromosome *(continued)*
    somatic c.
    surnumerary c.
    c. translocation
    c. trisomy
    X c.
    Y c.
    yeast artificial c. (YAC)
Chromotorula
chromotoxic
chromotrope 2R
chromotropic acid
chronic
    c. abscess
    c. absorptive arthritis
    c. acholuric jaundice
    c. active hepatitis (CAH)
    c. active inflammation
    c. active liver disease
    c. adhesive pachymeningitis
    c. airway obstruction (CAO)
    c. allograft rejection
    c. anaphylaxis
    c. anterior poliomyelitis
    c. appendicitis
    c. atrophic gastritis (CAG)
    c. atrophic polychondritis
    c. atrophic thyroiditis
    c. atrophic vulvitis
    c. autoimmune hemolytic anemia
    c. brain syndrome (CBS)
    c. bronchitis (CB)
    c. bronchitis with asthma (CBA)
    c. bullous dermatosis of childhood
    c. calculous cholecystitis (CCC)
    c. carrier state
    c. cell leukemia
    c. cholestasis
    c. cicatrizing enteritis
    c. constrictive pericarditis
    c. cystic mastitis
    c. decubitus ulcer zone I, II
    c. discoid lupus
    c. discoid lupus erythematosus
    c. eczema
    c. eosinophilic leukemia (CEL)
    c. false-positive (CFP)
    c. familial icterus
    c. familial jaundice
    c. fatigue immune dysfunction
    syndrome (CFIDS)
    c. fibrosing pancreatitis
    c. follicular keratoconjunctivitis
    c. glomerulonephritis (CGN)
    c. granulocytic leukemia (CGL)
    c. granulomatous disease (CGD)
    c. hemolytic anemia
    c. hypertrophic gastritis
    c. hypertrophic vulvitis

    c. idiopathic jaundice
    c. idiopathic megacolon
    c. idiopathic myelofibrosis (CIMF)
    c. inflammatory demyelinating
    polyneuropathy (CIDP)
    c. inflammatory disease
    c. interstitial cystitis
    c. interstitial hepatitis
    c. interstitial nephritis (CIN)
    c. interstitial salpingitis
    c. intervillositis
    c. intestinal pseudoobstructive
    syndrome (CIPS)
    c. lingual papillitis
    c. lobular hepatitis (CLH)
    c. lymphatic leukemia (CLL)
    c. lymphocytic leukemia (CLL)
    c. lymphoproliferative disorder
    (CLPD)
    c. lymphosarcoma cell
    c. lymphosarcoma leukemia (CLSL)
    c. membranous glomerulonephritis
    (CMGN)
    c. monoblastic leukemia (CMoL)
    c. monocytic leukemia (CMoL)
    c. mucocutaneous candidiasis
    (CMC)
    c. myelocytic leukemia (CML)
    c. myelogenous leukemia (CML)
    c. myeloid leukemia
    c. myelomonocytic leukemia
    (CMML)
    c. myeloproliferative disorder
    (CMPD)
    c. neutrophilic leukemia
    c. nonleukemic myelosis
    c. nonspecific inflammation
    c. obstructive lung disease (COLD)
    c. obstructive pulmonary disease
    (COPD)
    c. passive congestion (CPC)
    c. persistent hepatitis (CPH)
    c. pneumonitis of infancy (CPI)
    c. proliferative arthritis
    c. prolymphocytic leukemia
    c. pulmonary emphysema (CPE)
    c. pulmonary vascular occlusive
    disease
    c. pyelonephritis (CPN)
    c. pyelonephritis/reflux nephropathy
    c. renal disease (CRD)
    c. renal failure (CRF)
    c. respiratory failure
    c. rheumatism
    c. specific endometritis
    c. subdural hematoma (CSH)
    c. ulcer
    c. ulcerative colitis (CUC)
    c. ulcerative proctitis

c. villous arthritis
c. viral hepatitis
chronica
mycosis cutis c.
pityriasis lichenoides c.
polyarthritis c.
chronicity index
chronological age (CA)
chronooncology
chronotropic
chronotropism
Chroobacteria
Chroococcales
chrotoplast
Chryseobacterium
C. defluvii
C. joostei
C. meningosepticum
C. miricola
chrysiasis
Chrysiogenaceae
Chrysiogenales
Chrysiogenetes
chrysocyanosis
chrysoidin
Chrysomyia
Chrysonilia sitophila
Chrysops
C. caecutiens
C. dimidiata
C. discalis
C. silacea
chrysorrhoea
Euproctis c.
chrysosporium
Phanerochaete c.
Chrysosporium parvum
chrysotile
Chrysovirus
CHS
Chédiak-Higashi syndrome
cholinesterase
CHUK
conserved helix-loop-helix ubiquitous
kinase
chungbukensis
Sphingomonas c.
church spire papillomatosis
Churg-Strauss
C.-S. angiitis
C.-S. granuloma

C.-S. syndrome
C.-S. vasculitis
Churukian-Schenck stain
chutta
Chvostek sign
Chvostek-Weiss sign
chylangioma
chylaqueous
chyle
c. corpuscle
c. cyst
c. peritonitis
c. vessel
chylemia
chyli
cisterna c.
chyliform ascites
chylocele
parasitic c.
chyloderma
chylomediastinum
chylomicrograph
chylomicron, pl. **chylomicra,**
chylomicrons
c. composition
lipoprotein c.
chylomicronemia
chylopericarditis
chylopericardium
chyloperitoneum
chylopleura
chylopneumothorax
chylorrhea
chylosus
ascites c.
chylothorax
congenital c.
filarial c.
nonfilarial c.
traumatic c.
chylous
c. arthritis
c. ascites
c. effusion
c. hydrothorax
c. urine
chyluria
chymase
mast cell positive tryptase and c.
(MCTC)
mast cell tryptase positive c.
negative (MCT)

NOTES

chyme
chymosin
chymotrypsin
  fecal c.
  c. stain
CI
  cell interaction
  cerebral infarction
  chemoimmunotherapy
  chemotherapeutic index
  confidence interval
  coronary insufficiency
  crystalline insulin
    CI molecule
    CI number
C.I.
  Colour Index
Ci
  curie
Ciaccio
  C. fluid
  C. gland
  C. method
  C. stain
Ciaccio-positive lipid
cIAP
  cellular inhibitor of apoptosis
Ciarrocchi disease
cibaria
  Weissella c.
cibinongensis
  Acetobacter c.
cicatrices (*pl. of* cicatrix)
cicatricial
  c. horn
  c. pemphigoid
cicatricosa
  Ambrosiozyma c.
cicatrix, pl. cicatrices
  brain c.
  meningocerebral c.
cicatrizant
cicatrization
cicatrizing enterocolitis
Cicuta
cicutoxin
CID
  cytomegalic inclusion disease
cidal level
CIDP
  chronic inflammatory demyelinating
    polyneuropathy
CIDS
  cellular immunity deficiency syndrome
  combined immunodeficiency syndrome
CIE
  countercurrent immunoelectrophoresis

CIEP
  countercurrent immunoelectrophoresis
  counterimmunoelectrophoresis
CIF
  clone-inhibiting factor
  congenital infantile fibrosarcoma
ciferii
  Stephanoascus c.
ciferrii
  Prototheca c.
cigarette-paper scar
cigar-shaped nucleus
ciguatera
ciguatoxin
Ci-hr
  curie-hour
cilia (*pl. of* cilium)
ciliares
  glandulae c.
  plicae c.
ciliaris
  fibrae meridionales muscularis c.
  stratum pigmenti corporis c.
  zona c.
  zonula c.
ciliary
  c. canal
  c. dysentery
  c. fold
  c. gland
  c. zone
  c. zonule
Ciliata
ciliated
  c. cell
  c. epithelium
  c. hepatic foregut cyst
  c. metaplasia
ciliate dysentery
ciliocytophthoria (CCP)
ciliogenesis
Ciliophora
ciliorum
  pediculosis c.
cilium, pl. cilia
  microtubule in cilia
  motile cilia
Cillobacterium
CIM
  cardia intestinal metaplasia
Cimex
  C. hemipterus
  C. lectularius
CIMF
  chronic idiopathic myelofibrosis
cimicosis
CIN
  cefsulodin-Irgasan-novobiocin
  cervical intraepithelial neoplasia

chromosomal instability
chronic interstitial nephritis
CIN agar
cinaedi
    Campylobacter c.
    Helicobacter c.
cinchonism
cinemicrography
cinephotomicrography
cinereus
    Aedes c.
    Scopulariopsis c.
cinetoplasm
cingulate gyrus
cinnabarina
    Haemaphysalis c.
cinnamivorans
    Papillibacter c.
cinocentrum
cintus
    Paragordius c.
CIP
    critical infrastructure protection
CipherGen Express software biomarker analysis system
CIPS
    chronic intestinal pseudoobstructive syndrome
circadian
    c. cycle
    c. quotient (CQ)
    c. rhythm
circinata
circinate retinopathy
Circinella
circle of confusion
circling disease
Circovirus
circuit
    c. breaker
    delay c.
    open c.
    parallel c.
    printed c.
    RC c.
    series c.
    short c.
circuitry
circulans
    Bacillus c.
circular
    c. dichroism
    c. fiber
    c. fold of small intestine
    c. layer of muscular tunic
    c. layer of tympanic membrane
circulares
    fibrae c.
    plicae c.
circulating
    c. anticoagulant
    c. antithromboplastin disorder
    c. atypical lymphocyte
    c. blood volume (CBV)
    c. granulocyte pool (CGP)
    c. reticuloendothelial cell
circulation
    introduction of air into c.
    c. rate
    c. time (CT)
circulatory
    c. antigliadin antibody
    c. collapse
    c. disease
    c. failure
    c. insufficiency
    c. overload
circumanal gland
circumferential
    c. implantation
    c. lamella
circumgemmal
circummarginata
    placenta c.
circummarginate placenta
circumnevic vitiligo
circumnuclear
circumscribed
    c. atrophy
    c. choroidal hemangioma (CCH)
    c. craniomalacia
    c. edema
    c. inflammation
    c. mass
    c. peritonitis
    c. pyocephalus
circumscripta
    calcinosis c.
    lipoatrophia c.
    myositis ossificans c.
    osteitis fibrosa c.
    osteoporosis c.
circumscription

NOTES

circumscriptum
> lymphangioma c.

circumscriptus
> keratoconus posticus c.

circumvallate
> c. papillae
> c. placenta
> c. placentation

circumvallation
cirrhogenic
cirrhogenous
cirrhonosus
cirrhosis
> alcoholic c.
> biliary c.
> Budd c.
> cardiac c.
> cholangiolitic c.
> congestive c.
> cryptogenic c.
> diffuse septal c.
> fatty c.
> Glisson c.
> Hanot c.
> Indian childhood c. (ICC)
> juvenile c.
> Laënnec c.
> necrotic c.
> nutritional c.
> obstructive c.
> c. pigment
> pigmentary c.
> pipestem c.
> portal c.
> posthepatitic c.
> postnecrotic c.
> primary biliary c. (PBC)
> stasis c.
> toxic c.

cirrhotic
> c. ascites
> c. glomerulosclerosis

cirrose
cirrus, pl. **cirri**
cirsocele
cirsoid
> c. aneurysm
> c. varix

cirsomphalos
CIS
> carcinoma in situ
> central inhibitory state

cis
> c. activation
> c. configuration

cis-acting locus
CIS/ITGCNU
> carcinoma in situ/intratubular germ cell
> neoplasia unclassified

CISM
> critical incident stress management

cisplatin
cistern
> c. of cytoplasmic reticulum
> c. of nuclear envelope

cisterna, pl. **cisternae**
> c. caryothecae
> c. chyli
> membranous cisternae
> perinuclear c.
> sacroplasmic cisternae
> subsurface c.
> terminal c.

cisternal
cisternogram
cis/trans test
cistron
CIT
> corneal impression test

Citelli syndrome
Citellus
Citeromyces matritensis
citrate
> c. agar
> c. agar gel electrophoresis
> c. buffer
> c. condensing enzyme
> indole, methyl red, Voges-
> Proskauer, and c. (IMViC)
> c. intoxication
> lead c.
> c. phosphate dextrose (CPD)
> potassium c.
> Reynolds lead c.
> sodium acid c.
> standard saline c. (SSC)
> c. test

citrated blood
citrate-phosphate-dextrose-adenine (CPD adenine)
citratiphilum
> *Aquabacterium c.*

citreus
> *Erythrobacter c.*

citric
> c. acid
> c. acid assay
> c. acid cycle

Citricoccus muralis
Citrobacter
> *C. amalonatica*
> Bethesda-Ballerup group of *C.*
> (CBB)
> *C. diversus*
> *C. freundii*
> *C. koseri*
> *C. murliniae*

Citroclear
citrovorum factor (CF)
citrulline
    urine c.
citrullinemia
citrullinuria
Civatte
    C. body
    C. disease
    poikiloderma of C.
CJD
    Creutzfeldt-Jakob disease
CK
    creatine kinase
    cytokeratin
    NATO code for cyanogen chloride
      $(CNCl_2)$
CK20 reactivity
CK-BB
    creatine kinase BB
c-Ki-ras gene
c-kit
    c.-k. activity
    c.-k. oncogene
    c.-k. protooncogene
    c.-k. receptor
CK-MB tandem test
Cl
    chlorine
cL
    centiliter
CLA
    cyclic lysine anhydride
Cladobotryum
Cladophialophora
Cladorchis watsoni
Cladorrhinum
cladosporioides
    Hormodendrum c.
cladosporiosis
    cerebral c.
    c. epidermica
Cladosporium
    C. carrionii
    C. mansonii
    C. trichoides
    C. werneckii
    C. (Xylohypha) bantianum
Cladothrix
clamp connection
clandestine aerosol release

Clara
    C. cell
    C. cell adenocarcinoma
    C. cell secretory protein gene
    C. hematoxylin
clarificant
Clark
    C. level
    C. malignant melanoma
     classification
    C. malignant melanoma staging
    C. nevus
    C. oxygen electrode
    C. rule
    C. test
Clark-Collip method
Clarke
    C. collateral bundle
    C. column
    C. dorsal nucleus
    C. fluid
Clarke-Hadfield syndrome
Clark-Elder malignant melanoma
  classification
CLAS
    congenital localized absence of skin
CLASH
    cryoglobulinemia, leukemia, arthritis,
     Sjögren syndrome, and hepatitis B
clasmatocyte
clasmatosis
class
    c. A, B, C, D pathogen
    Hallervorden-Spatz disease, tau
     pathology c.
    c. histocompatibility antigen
    immunoglobulin c.
    c. switch
    c. switching
classic
    c. hemophilia
    c. liver lobule
    c. RTA
classical
    c. complement pathway
    c. hemophilia
    c. swine fever
classification
    AJCC c.
    Ann Arbor staging c.
    Ann Arbor tumor c.
    Arneth c.

NOTES

C

classification *(continued)*

    Astler-Coller modification of Dukes c.
    AUA bladder cancer staging c.
    bacterial c.
    Banff c.
    Bergey c.
    Bernatz c.
    Bessman anemia c.
    Binet chronic lymphocytic leukemia c.
    Bismuth cholangiocarcinoma c.
    Bismuth-Corlette perihilar tumor c.
    Bloom and Richardson c.
    Borrmann c.
    Breslow malignant melanoma c.
    Broders c.
    Brooker heterotopic ossification c.
    Caldwell-Moloy c.
    Chapel Hill Consensus Conference c.
    Clark-Elder malignant melanoma c.
    Clark malignant melanoma c.
    Denver c.
    Dukes-Astler-Coller adenocarcinoma c.
    Dukes carcinoma c.
    Dutch c.
    Edmondson-Steiner hepatocellular carcinoma grading c.
    Eggel tumor c.
    Elder malignant melanoma c.
    Enzinger tumor c.
    c. of epithelium
    FAB leukemia c.
    Fredrickson dyslipoproteinemia c.
    Gell and Coombs c.
    Griffith c.
    Horie tumor c.
    Hyams esthesioneuroblastoma c.
    Isaacson c.
    Jansky human blood group c.
    Jensen c.
    Jewett bladder carcinoma c.
    Kauffman-White c.
    Keith-Wagener c.
    Keith-Wagener-Barker c.
    Kiel non-Hodgkin lymphoma c.
    Klatskin tumor c.
    Lancefield c.
    Landsteiner c.
    Lauren c.
    Lennert c.
    Levine-Rosai tumor c.
    Ljubljana c.
    Lukes-Butler Hodgkin disease c.
    Lukes-Butler non-Hodgkin lymphoma c.
    Lukes-Collins non-Hodgkin lymphoma c.
    Masaoka c.
    McNeer c.
    MMH osteogenic c.
    Moss c.
    Paris c.
    Portmann c.
    Rappaport c.
    REAL c.
    Revised European-American Lymphoma c.
    Runyon c.
    Rye histopathologic Hodgkin disease c.
    Sakamoto c.
    c. scheme
    Schilling c.
    Seattle c.
    Shimada c.
    Shimosato-Mukai c.
    Skinner c.
    Sydney c.
    Talerman c.
    WHO/ISUP c.

clastic

clastothrix

clathrate

clathratiforme
    Chlorobium c.

clathrin

clathrin-coated vesicle

Clathrochloris

Clathrocystis

Clauberg
    C. test
    C. unit

Claude Bernard-Horner syndrome

claudication
    intermittent c. (IC)
    venous c.

claudin 4 gene

Claudius cell

clause
    Delaney c.

claustrum

clausura

clavate papilla

clavatus
    Aspergillus c.
    Porocephalus c.

clavi (*pl. of* clavus)

Claviceps purpurea

claviculus

Clavispora lusitaniae

clavus, pl. **clavi**

claw
    griffin c.

clawfoot

clawhand
clay shoveler's fracture
CLBBB
   complete left bundle-branch block
ClCN7
   chloride channel 7
   ClCN7 gene
clean area (contamination-free)
clean-catch
   c.-c. collection method
   c.-c. urine culture
   c.-c. urine specimen
cleaning solution
cleanser
   AlcoSCRUB instant antiseptic
   hand c.
cleanup
   Wizard MagneSil PCR c.
   Wizard MagneSil sequencing c.
clean-voided specimen (CVS)
clear
   c. cell
   c. cell acanthoma
   c. cell adenocarcinoma
   c. cell adenoma
   c. cell borderline tumor
   c. cell carcinoma (CCC)
   c. cell carcinoma of salivary gland
   c. cell cribriforming hyperplasia
   c. cell hidradenoma
   c. cell hyperplasia of parathyroid
   gland
   c. cell lciomyoma
   c. cell meningioma
   c. cell morphology
   c. cell myoepithelial carcinoma
   (CCMEC)
   c. cell neoplasm
   c. cell odontogenic carcinoma
   c. cell pattern
   c. cell sarcoma
   c. cell sugar tumor
   c. layer of epidermis
   c. plaque mutation
clearance
   albumin c.
   amylase c. (C_{Am})
   amylase/creatinine c.
   blood urea c.
   creatinine c. (CC, C/cr/)
   decreased creatine c.
   endogenous creatinine c.

exogenous creatinine c.
free water c.
immune c.
insulin c. (C_{in})
interocclusal c.
inulin c.
iron plasma c.
maximum urea c.
osmolal c.
osmolar c. (Cosm)
osmotic c.
p-aminohippurate c. (C_{pah})
paraaminohippurate c.
plasma c.
serum creatinine c.
sodium c.
standard urea c.
thyroidal c.
total body c. (Q_B)
urea c.
ClearCRIT microhematocrit tube
clearing
   c. factor
   c. factor lipase
   c. medium
ClearView C. Diff A test
Cleary
   method of C.
cleavage
   heterolytic c.
   homolytic c.
   c. line
   c. of ovum
   c. plane
   c. product
   progressive c.
   c. spindle
cleaved follicular center cell
cleft
   action potential synaptic c.
   birefringent crystalline c.
   c. cheek
   cholesterol c.
   c. face
   Larrey c.
   c. lip
   Maurer c.
   c. nose
   c. palate
   residual c.
   Schmidt-Lanterman c.
   c. spine

NOTES

cleft *(continued)*
    synaptic c.
    c. tongue
clefting
    suprabasal c.
cleidocranial, clidocranial
    c. dysostosis
    c. dysplasia
cleistothecium
Cleland reagent
cleptoparasite
CLH
    chronic lobular hepatitis
    cutaneous lymphoid hyperplasia
CLIA
    chemiluminescent assay
    Clinical Laboratory Improvement
    Amendment
CLIA '88
    Clinical Laboratory Improvement Act of
    1988
click
    systolic murmur with a
    midsystolic c.
clidocranial *(var. of* cleidocranial*)*
cliftonensis
    Rubrimonas c.
Climacocystis
Climacodon
climacteric
    delayed c.
climatic bubo
climbing fiber
clindamycin
cline
clinger
    boat c.
clinging
    c. carcinoma
    c. ductal carcinoma in situ
clinical
    c. bacteriologic specimen
    c. chemistry
    c. chemistry automation
    c. chemistry quality control
    c. consideration
    c. cytogenetics
    c. diagnosis
    c. diagnostic bacteriology
    c. end point
    c. genetics
    c. indicator
    c. laboratory
    C. Laboratory Improvement Act of
    1988 (CLIA '88)
    C. Laboratory Improvement
    Amendment (CLIA)
    C. Laboratory Management
    Association (CLMA)

    c. laboratory maximum area
    c. manifestations, etiologic factors,
    anatomic involvement,
    pathophysiologic features (CEAP)
    c. medicine
    c. microbiology quality control
    c. microscopy
    c. pathology
    c. response
    c. sample
    c. sensitivity
    c. spectrometry
    c. spectroscopy
    c. spectrum
    c. toxicology
    c. trial
    c. variant of malignant melanoma
**Clinician Outreach and Communication
    Activity (COCA)**
clinicogenetic approach
clinicopathologic
    c. analysis
    c. conference (CPC)
    c. study
Clinistix
Clinitest stool test
clinodactyly
clinoscope
    exogenous creatinine c.
Clinostomum marginatum
Clitocybe dealbata
Clitocybula
Clitopilus
clitoridauxe
clitoridis
    smegma c.
clivus, pl. **clivi**
CLL
    centrocytelike cell
    chronic lymphatic leukemia
    chronic lymphocytic leukemia
    Rai classification of CLL
CLL/SLL
    B-cell C.
CLMA
    Clinical Laboratory Management
    Association
CLO
    Campylobacter-like organism
    CLO test
cloacae
    Aerobacter c.
    ectopia c.
    Enterobacter c.
    Sphingomonas c.
cloacal exstrophy
cloacogenic
    c. carcinoma
    c. polyp

clock
>biological c.
>real-time c.

clomiphene test
Clonad monoclonal antibody
clonal
>c. deletion theory
>c. disorder
>c. eosinophilia
>c. expansion
>c. gene rearrangement
>c. hematological nonmast cell lineage disease
>c. proliferated cell
>c. seborrheic keratosis
>c. selection theory
>c. thrombocytosis

clonality study
clone
>cDNA c.
>complementary DNA c.
>forbidden c.
>genomic DNA c. (chromosomal)

cloned enzyme donor immunoassay (CEDIA)
clone-inhibiting factor (CIF)
CloneSaver card
clonic
clonidine suppression test
cloning
>cellular c.
>gene c.
>c. inhibitory factor
>molecular c.
>therapeutic c.
>c. vector

clonogenic
>c. assay
>c. cell

clonorchiasis
Clonorchis endemicus
Clontech gene expression profiling procedure
clonus
Cloquet
>C. canal
>C. canal remnant
>node of C.

closed
>c. dislocation
>c. fracture

closed-loop obstruction

close range entrance wound
Closterovirus
Clostridiaceae
clostridial
>c. bacteremia
>c. collagenase
>c. myonecrosis
>c. myositis
>c. strain

Clostridiales
clostridioforme
>*Clostridium c.*

clostridiopeptidase A
Clostridium
>*C. acetobutylicum*
>*C. acidisoli*
>*C. akagii*
>*C. algidixylanolyticum*
>*C. amygdalinum*
>*C. argentinense*
>*C. baratii*
>*C. bartlettii*
>*C. bifermentans*
>*C. bolteae*
>*C. botulinum*
>*C. botulinum* cytotoxin type C2
>*C. botulinum* neurotoxin type A, B, C1, D, E, F, G
>*C. bowmanii*
>*C. butyricum*
>*C. cadaveris*
>*C. caminithermale*
>*C. carnis*
>*C. chauvoei*
>*C. clostridioforme*
>*C. cochlearium*
>*C. colicanis*
>*C. difficile*
>*C. difficile* toxin
>*C. difficile* toxin assay
>*C. diolis*
>*C. estertheticum* subsp. *laramiense*
>*C. fallax*
>*C. frigoris*
>*C. gasigenes*
>*C. haemolyticum*
>*C. hathewayi*
>*C. hiranonis*
>*C. histolyticum*
>*C. histolyticum* collagenase
>*C. hungatei*
>*C. hylemonae*

NOTES

215

Clostridium (continued)
    C. innocuum
    C. jejuense
    C. kluyveri
    C. lactatifermentans
    C. lacusfryxellense
    C. novyi
    C. paraputrificum
    C. pasteurianum
    C. peptidivorans
    C. perfringens
    C. perfringens alpha toxin
    C. perfringens beta toxin
    C. perfringens enterotoxin
    C. perfringens enterotoxin iota
    (CPI)
    C. perfringens epsilon toxin
    C. perfringens iota toxin
    C. phytofermentans
    C. psychrophilum
    C. ramosum
    rare clostridial strain of *C.*
      argentinense
    rare clostridial strain of *C. baratii*
    C. saccharobutylicum
    C. septicum
    C. sordellii
    C. sphenoides
    C. sporogenes
    C. stercorarium subsp.
      thermolacticum
    C. sticklandii
    C. tertium
    C. tetani
    C. tetanomorphum
    C. thermosaccharolyticum
    C. thiosulfatireducens
    C. uliginosum
    C. xylanovorans
clostrisel agar
closure
    delayed primary c. (DPC)
clot
    antemortem c.
    blood c.
    chicken fat c.
    currant jelly c.
    c. lysis
    c. lysis time (CLT)
    postmortem c.
    c. reaction
    c. retraction
    c. retraction time
CLOtest
clothing
    disposable chemical-resistant c.
    hooded chemical-resistant c.
clottage

clotting
    c. factor
    c. factor deficiency
    c. time (CT)
Cloudman melanoma
cloudy
    c. swelling
    c. swelling degeneration
    c. urine
Clough-Richter syndrome
Clouston syndrome
clove oil
cloverleaf skull
CLPD
    chronic lymphoproliferative disorder
CLSL
    chronic lymphosarcoma leukemia
CLSM
    confocal laser scan microscopy
CLT
    clot lysis time
clubbed
    c. digit
    c. finger
    c. toe
clubbing
    digital c.
    hereditary c.
clubfoot
club hair
clubhand
clue cell
clump
clumping
    ex vivo platelet c.
cluster
    c. of differentiation (CD)
    epithelioid cell c.
    glomerular-like c.
    metastatic c.
    sinusoidal foam cell c.
    c. 1 small-cell lung cancer antigen
    temporal c.
clusterin
    c. immunostaining
    c. marker
clustering
    hierarchical c.
Clutton joint
CM
    cardiac myxoma
    cavernous malformation
cm
    centimeter
cm^3, cu cm
    cubic centimeter
CM1 antibody
CMA
    complete maturation arrest

CMB
carbolic methylene blue
CMC
chronic mucocutaneous candidiasis
critical micelle concentration
CM-cellulose
carboxymethylcellulose
CMF
chondromyxoid fibroma
CMGN
chronic membranous glomerulonephritis
CMI
carbohydrate metabolism index
cell-mediated immunity
CMID
cytomegalic inclusion disease
c/min
cycle per minute
CML
chronic myelocytic leukemia
chronic myelogenous leukemia
CMM
cutaneous malignant melanoma
cmm, cu mm
cubic millimeter
CMML
chronic myelomonocytic leukemia
CMN
congenital melanocytic nevi
congenital mesoblastic nephroma
cystic medial necrosis
CMN-AA
cystic medial necrosis of ascending aorta
CMO
calculated mean organism
cMo
centimorgan
CMOAT
canicular multispecific organic anion
transporter
CMoL
chronic monoblastic leukemia
chronic monocytic leukemia
CMP
cardiomyopathy
colorimetric microtiter plate
cytidine monophosphate
c-mp1 receptor
CMP-*N*-acetyl-ᴅ-neuraminate
CMPD
chronic myeloproliferative disorder

CMR
cerebral metabolic rate
crude mortality ratio
CMRG
cerebral metabolic rate of glucose
CMRO
cerebral metabolic rate of oxygen
CMRR
common mode rejection ratio
CMV
cytomegalovirus
CMV antibody
CMV culture
CMV isolation
CMV-negative allogeneic cell
CMV-seronegative blood
CMXRos
MitoTracker Red CMXRos
c-myc
c-myc amplification
c-myc gene
c-myc oncoprotein
CN
calcineurin
NATO code for 1-chloroacetophenone
CN-
cyanide radical
CNB
core needle biopsy
Cnephia
CNHD
congenital nonspherocytic hemolytic
disease
Cnidospora
Cnidosporidia
CNS
central nervous system
atypical teratoid/rhabdoid tumor of
the CNS (ATRT-CNS)
CNT
cutaneous neural tumor
CNV
choroidal neovascularization
contingent negative variation
interindividual CNV
CO
calcium oxalate
carbon monoxide
corneal opacity
CO₂
carbon dioxide

NOTES

CO$_2$ *(continued)*
    CO$_2$ output
    CO$_2$ production
CoA
  coenzyme A
coacervate
coacervation
coactivator
coactosinlike 1
coag
  coagulation
Coag-a-mate prothrombin device
coagglutinin
CoaguChek
    C. Pro/DM coagulometer
    C. Pro/DM system
coagula (*pl. of* coagulum)
coagulable
coagulant complex
coagulase test
coagulate
coagulated albumin
coagulating enzyme
coagulation (coag)
    c. cascade
    diffuse intravascular c. (DIC)
    disseminated intravascular c. (DIC)
    exogenous anticoagulant c.
    c. factor assay
    c. factor inhibitor
    c. factor I–XIII
    c. factor transfusion
    fibrinolysin c.
    c. necrosis
    c. pathway
    plasmin c.
    spontaneous c.
    c. time (CT)
    c. time test
coagulative necrosis
coagulin-B
coagulogram
coagulometer
    CoaguChek Pro/DM c.
coagulopathy
    consumption c.
    dilutional c.
    intravascular consumption c. (IVCC)
    c. of liver disease
coagulum, pl. coagula
    seminal c.
coal
    c. tar
    c. tar naphtha
    c. worker's pneumoconiosis (CWP)
coalescence
coalition
    tarsal c.

coarctate
coarctation of aorta
coarse
    c. gravel
    c. marking
    c. material
coarsening
coat
    buffy c.
    cell c.
    C. disease
    fuzzy c.
    sclerotic c.
    serous c.
coated electron-lucent vesicle
coating fixative
cobalamin
cobalt assay
cobalticyanide (CoCN6)
cobaltinitrite method
cobaltous chloride
Cobas
    C. Amplicor HIV-1 monitor test
    C. Fara H centrifugal analyzer
    C. Helios differential analyzer
    C. Integra Cyclosporine Immunoassay
cobbler's chest
cobblestone appearance
cobblestoning
Cobetia marina
Coblentz test method
cobra
    C. Amplicor analyzer
    c. hemotoxin
    c. venom
    c. venom cofactor
    c. venom factor
COBS
  cesarean-obtained barrier-sustained
COCA
  Clinician Outreach and Communication Activity
coca
    Erythroxylon c.
cocacinogen
Cocadviroid
cocaethylene
cocaine
    c. hydrochloride
    c. metabolite assay
    tetracaine, Adrenalin (epinephrine), and c. (TAC)
cocarboxylase
cocarcinogen
cocarcinogenesis
cocarde reaction
coccal
cocci (*pl. of* coccus)

Coccidia
coccidia (*pl. of* coccidium)
coccidial
Coccidiasina
coccidioidal granuloma
coccidioides
    Blastomyces c.
Coccidioides immitis
coccidioidin test
coccidioidoma
coccidioidomycosis
    c. antibody
    asymptomatic c.
    disseminate c.
    latent c.
    primary c.
    secondary c.
    subclinical c.
coccidiosis
coccidium, pl. **coccidia**
Coccidium hominis
coccinella
coccinellin
coccobacillus
    aerobic c.
    facultative c.
    intracellular c.
    obligate c.
    safety pin shaped c.
coccobacteria
coccoid *Helicobacter pylori*
coccus, pl. **cocci**
    gram-negative cocci
    gram-positive cocci
coccygeal
    c. body
    c. fistula
    c. gland
coccygeum
    corpus c.
    glomus c.
Cochin China diarrhea
cochineal
cochlea, pl. **cochleae**
    aqueductus cochleae
    fenestra cochleae
    lamina basilaris cochleae
    ligamentum spirale cochleae
    membranous c.
    spiral ligament of c.
cochlear
    c. aqueduct

    c. duct
    c. hair cell
    c. hydrops
    c. otosclerosis
    c. window
cochleariform
cochlearis
    crista basilaris ductus c.
    ductus c.
    membrana tectoria ductus c.
    membrana vestibularis ductus c.
    paries tympanicus ductus c.
    paries vestibularis ductus c.
    stria vascularis ductus c.
cochlearium
    Clostridium c.
cochleate
Cochliobolus
Cochliomyia
    C. americana
    C. hominivorax
Cochlosoma anatis
$^{14}CO_2$-cholyl-glycine breath test
Cockayne
    C. disease
    C. syndrome
Cockcroft-Gault equation
cockscomb
    c. polyp
    c. ulcer
cocktail
    Boehringer Mannheim Kermix
      cytokeratin c.
    DIG c.
    keratin c.
    Molotov c.
CoCN6
    cobalticyanide
coctoprecipitin
cocultivation
cocurrent
COD
    cause of death
    cementoosseous dysphasia
code
    degenerate c.
    gene c.
    genetic c.
    Hollerith c.
    mnemonic c.
    NATO c.
    object c.

C

NOTES

code *(continued)*
    OP c.
    operation c.
    resistor color c.
    triplet c.
codeine assay
Code-On Immunoslide stainer
coding
    color c.
    polypeptide c.
    c. triplet
CODIS
    combined DNA index system
Codman tumor
codocyte
codominance
codominant
    c. gene
    c. inheritance
codon
    initiation c.
    start c.
    stop c.
    termination c.
coefficient
    absorption c.
    binomial c.
    Bouchard c.
    Bunsen c.
    conversion c.
    correlation c.
    creatinine c.
    decay c.
    diffusion c.
    dilution c.
    distribution c.
    extinction c.
    extraction c.
    hygienic laboratory c.
    inbreeding c.
    c. of inbreeding
    isotonic c.
    lethal c.
    Long c.
    mass attenuation c.
    osmotic c.
    oxygen utilization c.
    partition c.
    phenol c.
    rank correlation c.
    regression c. (R)
    Rideal-Walker c.
    sedimentation c.
    c. of selection
    solubility c.
    Spearman rank correlation c.
    Svedberg unit of sedimentation c.
    (S)
    temperature c. (Q_{10})

    urohemolytic c.
    urotoxic c.
    c. of variation (CV)
    velocity c.
    volume c.
Coelenterata
coelenterate
coelenterazine dextran-coated charcoal
coelenterazine-treated cell
coeliaci
    nodi lymphoidei c.
coeloblastula
coelom, celom
coelomic granulocyte
Coemansia
coenocyte (*var. of* cenocyte)
coenocytic
Coenonia anatina
coenurosis
Coenurus
    C. cerebralis
    C. serialis
coenzyme
    c. A (CoA)
    acyl c. A (acyl-CoA)
    D-3-hydroxyacyl c. A
    L-hydroxyacyl c. A
    malonyl c. A
    c. Q (CoQ)
    c. thiamine pyrophosphate
coenzyme-labeled immunoassay
coeur en sabot
Coe virus
coexpression
COF
    cementoossifying fibroma
cofactor
    cobra venom c.
    heparin c.
    platelet c.
    ristocetin c. (RcoF)
    c. of thromboplastin
coffee-bean groove
coffin formation
Coffin-Lowry syndrome
Coffin-Siris syndrome
Cogan syndrome
COGTT
    cortisone-primed oral glucose tolerance
    test
COHB, COHb
    carboxyhemoglobin
coherent smallpox
cohesion
cohesiveness
Cohn fractionation
Cohnheim
    C. area

C. field
C. theory
cohort
    c. labeling
    c. study
coil
    c. gland
    Macroduct c.
    plectonemic c.
    primary c.
    random c.
    secondary c.
coiled artery of the uterus
coincidence
    c. correction
    c. error
    c. sum peak
coinfection
coin lesion
coinlike
cokeri
    Septobasidium c.
Cokeromyces
COL4A5 gene
Colcemid
Colcher-Sussman method
colchicine
COLD
    chronic obstructive lung disease
cold
    c. abscess
    c. agglutination
    c. agglutinin (CA)
    c. agglutinin disease
    c. agglutinin screen
    c. agglutinin syndrome (CAS)
    c. agglutinin test
    c. agglutinin titer
    c. allergy
    c. antibody
    c. autoabsorption
    c. autoagglutinin
    c. autoantibody
    c. autoimmune hemolytic anemia
    c. gangrene
    c. hemagglutinin
    c. hemagglutinin disease
    c. hemoglobinuria
    c. hemolysin
    c. hemolysin test
    c. injury
    c. intolerance

c. lesion
c. microtome
c. nodule
c. rigor point
c. room
rose c.
c. silver nitrate
c. sore
c. spot
c. stage
c. ulcer
c. urticaria
c. virus
cold-agglutination phenomenon
cold-knife conization
cold-reacting antibody
cold-reactive antibody
cold-sensitive mutation
colectasia
Cole hematoxylin
Coleman Feulgen solution
Coleman-Schiff reagent
coleocanis
    Actinomyces c.
coleohominis
    Lactobacillus c.
Coleophoma
Coleoptera
coleoptosis
colestipol hydrochloride
Coleviroid
Coley toxin
coli
    adenomatous polyposis c. (APC)
    Amoeba c.
    Bacillus c.
    Balantidium c.
    Campylobacter c.
    diarrheagenic *E. c.*
    Entamoeba c.
    enteroaggregative *Escherichia c.* (EaggEC)
    enteroinvasive *Escherichia c.* (EIEC)
    enteropathogenic *Escherichia c.* (EEC, EPEC)
    enterotoxic *Escherichia c.* (ETEC)
    enterotoxigenic *Escherichia c.* (ETEC)
    Escherichia c.
    Escherichia c. 0157:h7

NOTES

221

coli *(continued)*
   extraintestinal pathogenic
     Escherichia c. (ExPEC)
   familial adenomatous polyposis c.
   familial polyposis c.
   Holophyra c.
   juvenile polyposis c.
   melanosis c.
   Paramecium c.
   polyposis c.
   pseudomelanosis c.
   stratum longitudinale tunicae
     muscularis c.
   Streptococcus infantarius subsp. *c.*
   teniae c.
   tunica mucosa c.
   tunica muscularis c.
   tunica serosa c.
colibacillary
colibacillemia
colibacilluria
colibacillus
colic
   biliary c.
   endemic c.
   intestinal c.
   c. intussusception
   lead c.
   menstrual c.
   pancreatic c.
   renal c.
   uterine c.
   verminous c.
colicanis
   Clostridium c.
colicin
colicinogeny
coliform bacillus
coliforme
   Paracolobactrum c.
colihominis
   Anaerotruncus c.
colinearity
colipase
   pancreatic c.
coliphage
colistimethate sodium
colistin sulfate
colitis, pl. colitides
   acute ulcerative c.
   amebic c.
   antibiotic-associated c. (AAC)
   balantidial c.
   chronic ulcerative c. (CUC)
   collagenous c.
   c. cystica profunda
   c. cystica superficialis
   diversion c.
   eosinophilic c.

fulminant c.
granulomatous c.
c. gravis
hemorrhagic c.
indeterminate c.
infectious c.
ischemic c.
lymphocytic c. (LC)
metachronous collagenous c.
microscopic c.
mucous c.
nonrelapsing c.
nontyphoidal infectious c.
pseudomembranous c. (PMC)
radiation c.
regional c.
self-limited c.
spastic c.
toxic c.
ulcerative c. (UC)
uremic c.
colitose
colitoxicosis
colitoxin
coliuria
collacin
collagen
   c. bundle
   c. degeneration
   c. deposition
   c. disease
   c. disorder
   endomysial c.
   c. fiber
   c. fibril
   fibrous long-spacing c. (FLS)
   c. flower
   c. gel invasion assay
   hyaluronidase c.
   lack of c.
   lamellar c.
   c. marker
   paucicellular c.
   c. receptor deficiency
   ropey c.
   SLS c.
   c. staining method
   subepithelial c.
   c. type IX alpha 2 gene
   type I–XX c.
   wire-like c.
   c. X, XVIII
   Zyderm c.
collagenase
   clostridial c.
   Clostridium histolyticum c.
   c. synthesis
collagenation
collagenic

collagenization
collagenoblast
collagenocyte
collagenoma
    giant cell c. (GCC)
collagenosis
    reactive perforating c. (RPC)
collagenous
    c. colitis
    c. fiber
    c. fibroma
    c. spherulosis
    c. sprue
collagen-vascular disease
collapse
    circulatory c.
    hemodynamic c.
    c. induration
    massive c.
    structural c.
    structure c.
collar
    abrasion c.
    c. button abscess
    c. button lesion
    false abrasion c.
collarette
collaring
    periglandular c.
collastin
collateral
    periumbilical venous c.
collecting
    c. duct
    c. duct carcinoma (CDC)
collection
    American Type Culture C. (ATCC)
    arterial blood c.
    c. of forensic evidence
    GLOB c.
    Macroduct system for sweat
      stimulation and c.
    stool c.
    urine specimen c.
collector
    anaerobic specimen c.
College of American Pathologists (CAP)
Colletotrichum
Collet-Sicard syndrome
Collet syndrome
colli
    cystitis c.

    fibromatosis c.
    lipoma annulare c.
colliculitis
colliculus
    seminal c.
collidine
collier's lung
colligative
colligin
collimate
collimator
Collimonas fungivorans
Collinsella
    C. aerofaciens
    C. intestinalis
    C. stercoris
collinsii
    Trichococcus c.
colliquation
    ballooning c.
    reticulating c.
colliquative
    c. albuminuria
    c. degeneration
    c. necrosis
collision tumor
collodion
    c. baby
    c. filter
colloid
    c. adenocarcinoma
    c. adenoma
    c. body
    bovine c.
    c. cancer
    c. carcinoma
    c. corpuscle
    c. cyst
    c. degeneration
    extrafollicular c.
    c. goiter
    c. milium
    c. oncotic pressure (COP)
    c. osmotic hemolysis
    c. shift
    c. shock
    thyroid c.
colloidal
    c. dispersion
    c. electrolyte
    c. gold (CG)
    c. gold reaction

NOTES

colloidal *(continued)*
    c. gold test
    c. iron stain
    c. osmotic pressure (COP)
    c. silica gradient
    c. silicon dioxide
colloides
    struma c.
colloidin
colloidoclasia
colloid-osmotic lysis
collum folliculi pili
Collybia
Collyriclum
coloboma, pl. **colobomas, colobomata**
    c., heart disease, atresia choanae,
      retarded growth and development
      and ear anomalies, pl. colobomas,
      colobomata (CHARGE)
    c. syndrome
colocalization
colocutaneous fistula
coloenteric
coloileal fistula
colombiense
    Aminobacterium c.
colon
    c. atresia
    c. bacillus
    c. carcinoma
    cathartic c.
    giant c.
    c. glandular tissue
    irritable c. (IC)
    lead-pipe c.
    c. polyp
    sigmoid c.
    spastic c.
    c. tumor
colonic
    c. fistula
    c. smear
    c. vomitus
colonization infection
colony
    beaten egg white appearance c.
    bitten c.
    butyrous c.
    c. count
    curled hair c.
    D c.
    daughter c.
    dwarf c.
    effuse c.
    fried egg c.
    grayish-white c.
    ground glass appearance c.
    H c.

    hammered copper c.
    irregular border c.
    irregularly round c.
    M c.
    c. morphology
    mucoid c.
    O c.
    opaque c.
    R c.
    raised c.
    rough c.
    S c.
    satellite c.
    shiny surface c.
    slightly yellow c.
    smooth c.
    c. stands up
    swirling comet tail c.
    tenacious consistency c.
    undulating edges c.
    wavy border c.
colony-forming
    c.-f. unit (CFU)
    c.-f. unit-culture (CFU-C)
    c.-f. unit-erythroid (CFU-E)
    c.-f. unit granulocyte, erythrocyte,
      monocyte, and megakaryocyte
      (CFU-GEMM)
    c.-f. unit granulocyte-macrophage
      (CFU-GM)
    c.-f. unit-megakaryocyte (CFU-Meg)
    c.-f. units/mL (CFU/mL)
    c.-f. unit-spleen (CFU-S)
colony-stimulating
    c.-s. activity (CSA)
    c.-s. factor (CSF)
coloproctitis
    cryptal lymphocytic c.
coloptosia
coloptosis
color
    amniotic fluid c.
    c. coding
    complementary c.
    fecal c.
    primary c.
    spectral c.
    stool c.
Colorado
    C. tick fever
    C. tick fever virus
color-contrast microscope
colorectal
    c. carcinoma
    c. polyp
colorectitis
Colorfrost disposable microscope slide
colorimeter

colorimetric
    c. antibody detection
    c. microtiter plate (CMP)
colorimetry
Colormark slide
Colormate Tlc.BiliTest system
ColorPAC toxin A test
4-color PCR assay
Coloscreen Self test
colossus
    Calomys c.
colostrum corpuscle
Colour Index (C.I.)
colovaginal fistula
colovesical fistula
colpatresia
colpectasia
colpitis
colpocystitis
colpocytology
colpohyperplasia
    c. cystica
    c. emphysematosa
Colpoma
Coltivirus
Colton antigen
colubriformis
    Trichostrongylus c.
Columbia
    C. blood agar
    C. medium
    C. SK virus
columbianum
    Oesophagostomum c.
columbium
columella
column
    anal c.
    Bertin c.
    c.'s of Bertin
    Bürdach c.
    c. cell
    Clarke c.
    DEAE-Sephacel ion exchange c.
    ion-exchange c.
    Morgagni c.
    rectal c.
    renal c.
    Sertoli c.
columna, pl. **columnae**
    columnae anales

    columnae carneae
    columnae renales
columnar
    c. absorptive cell
    c. cell hyperplasia
    c. cuff
    c. epithelium
    c. layer
    c. metaplasia
Colwelliaceae
Colwellia piezophila
coma
    alcoholic c.
    apoplectic c.
    c. cast
    c. dépassé
    diabetic c.
    Harvard criteria of irreversible c.
    hepatic c.
    hyperosmolar diabetic c.
    irreversible c.
    metabolic c.
    uremic c.
Comamonadaceae
Comamonas
    C. aquatica
    C. denitrificans
    C. kerstersii
    C. koreensis
    C. nitrativorans
comatose
combesi
    Eubacterium c.
comb-growth test
combination calculus
combinatorial immunity
combined
    c. androgen blockade
    c. DNA index system (CODIS)
    c. immunodeficiency
    c. immunodeficiency disease
    c. immunodeficiency syndrome (CIDS)
    c. pituitary function test
    c. sclerosis
    c. systems disease
    c. ventricular hypertrophy (CVH)
combining site
Combo
    Acceava hCG C.
    QuickVue+ One-Step hCG C.

NOTES

225

combustible
 c. gas
 c. gas detector
 c. liquid
 c. vapor
combustion
 carbonaceous residue of c.
 heat of c.
comedo, pl. comedones
 c. ductal carcinoma in situ
 c. necrosis
 c. nevus
comedocarcinoma
comedomastitis
comedonecrosis
comedones (*pl. of* comedo)
comedonicus
 nevus c.
comet cell
comma bacillus
commensal bacteria
commensalism
commercial insulin preparation
commingled remains
comminuted fracture
commission
 Biological Stain C.
commissura anterior grisea
commissural cell
commissure
 Ganser c.
 gray c.
committed cell
committee
 transfusion adult c.
common
 c. acute lymphoblastic leukemia antigen (CALLA, cALLA)
 c. acute lymphocytic leukemia antigen
 c. bile duct
 c. bile duct obstruction
 c. cold virus
 c. enterobacterial antigen
 c. logarithm
 c. mode rejection ratio (CMRR)
 c. mode signal
 c. opsonin
 c. reference
 c. storage
 c. variable
 c. variable hypogammaglobulinemia (CVH)
 c. variable immunodeficiency (CVID)
 c. variable immunodeficiency syndrome
 c. viral etiology
 c. wart

commotio cerebri
commune
 Aquabacterium c.
 integumentum c.
communicable disease
communicans
 macula c.
communicate
 esophagus c.
communicating
 c. hydrocephalus
 c. junction
communication
 gap junction intercellular c.
communis
 macula c.
 Ricinus c.
 sacculus c.
 Sericopelma c.
commutator
Comovirus
compacta
 pars c.
 substantia c.
compact bone
compactum
 Hormodendrum c.
 stratum c.
companion cell
comparascope
comparative
 c. genome hybridization
 c. genomic hybridization (CGH)
 c. pathology
comparator microscope
comparison
 cartilage and bone c.
 c. eyepiece
 c. microscope
 c. operation
compartment
 acidified prelysosomal c.
 panstromal c.
 peptide-loading c.
 c. syndrome
compartmental
 c. analysis
 c. syndrome
compatibility
 ABO c.
 c. test
compatible
compensated
 c. acidosis
 c. alkalosis
 c. eyepiece
compensating ocular
compensation
 broken c.

dosage c.
temperature c. (TC)
compensatory
  c. atrophy
  c. emphysema
  c. hypertrophy
  c. hypertrophy of the heart
  c. mechanism
  c. polycythemia
  c. regeneration
competence
  embryonic c.
  c. gene
  immunologic c.
  immunological c.
competition
  antigenic c.
  c. hybridization
competitive
  c. antagonist
  c. binding assay
  c. heterogeneous enzyme
    immunoassay
  c. inhibition
  c. protein-binding (CPB)
  c. protein-binding assay
  c. protein-binding test
  c. reverse transcription polymerase
    chain reaction (cRT-PCR)
competitor DNA
compiler
  optimizing c.
compile time
complement
  c. activation
  c. binding assay
  C_3, C_4 c.
  c. chemotactic factor
  chromosome c.
  component of c.
  c. component
  c. deficiency state
  c. direct Coombs test
  dominant c.
  endocellular c.
  erythrocyte antibody c. (EAC)
  c. fixation (CF)
  c. inactivation
  c. lysis sensitivity test
  c. receptor (CR)
  c. receptor 3 (CR3)
  c. system

c. total
two's c.
c. unit
whole c. (WC)
complemental inheritance
complementarity
  c. determining region (CDR)
  dominant c.
complementary
  c. base
  c. color
  c. DNA (cDNA)
  c. DNA clone
  c. gene
  c. groove
  c. hypertrophy
  c. strand
  c. symmetry amplifier
complementation
complement-fixation
  c.-f. reaction
  Reiter protein c.-f. (RPCF)
  c.-f. test (CFT)
complement-fixing (CF)
  c. antibody
  c. antigen
complement-mediated cytotoxicity
complementophil
complete
  c. abortion
  c. androgen insensitivity syndrome
    (CAIS)
  c. anterior dislocation
  c. antibody
  c. antigen
  c. blood count (CBC)
  c. carcinogen
  c. fistula
  c. heart block (CHB)
  c. inferior dislocation
  c. left bundle-branch block
    (CLBBB)
  c. mole
  c. obstruction
  c. penetrance
  c. posterior dislocation
  c. reaction of degeneration (CRD)
  c. right bundle-branch block
    (CRBBB)
  c. superior dislocation
  c. transduction
  c. trisomy

C

NOTES

complex
    acrosomal c.
    activated c.
    c. adrenal endocrine disorder
    AIDS-related c. (ARC)
    angiotumoral c.
    antigen-antibody c.
    antigenic c.
    c. atypical hyperplasia/metaplasia
      (CAHM)
    avian leukosis-sarcoma c.
    avidin-biotin c.
    avidin-biotin peroxidase c. (ABC)
    cadherin/catenin c.
    Carney c.
    C5B-9 c.
    charge-transfer c.
    coagulant c.
    cytochrome bc1 c.
    electron transport chain c. I–IV
    c. endometrial hyperplasia
    feline leukemia-sarcoma virus c.
    FN-MCD c.
    gene c.
    Ghon c.
    Ghon-Sachs c.
    glucocorticoid-glucocorticoid
      receptor c.
    glucocorticoid-GR c.
    Golgi c.
    c. gonadal endocrine disorder
    H-2 c.
    healed Ghon c.
    histocompatibility c.
    HLA c.
    homotetrameric c.
    horseradish peroxidase conjugated
      streptavidin-biotin c.
    immune c.
    immune-stimulating c. (ISCOM)
    junctional c.
    juxtaglomerular c.
    major histocompatibility c. (MHC)
    membrane attack c. (MAC)
    Meyenburg c.
    MHC I/calreticulin c.
    minor histocompatibility c.
    mitochondrial c. II
    Mycobacterium avium-
      intracellulare c. (MAC)
    Mycobacterium phlei cell wall
      DNA c. (MCC)
    nuclear pore c.
    c. number
    c. odontoma
    Ornithodoros moubata c.
    orthocresolphthalein c. (OPCP)
    ostiomeatal c.
    PAG c.

    PAP c.
    peroxidase-antiperoxidase c.
    c. pituitary endocrine disorder
    platelet phospholipid c.
    primary c.
    prothrombin c.
    pyruvate dehydrogenase c. (PDC)
    renal dysplasia c.
    ribonucleoprotein c.
    ribosome-lamella c.
    RNP c.
    c. sclerosing lesion
    sicca c.
    steroid-receptor c.
    SWI/SNF c.
    synaptinemal c.
    synaptonemal c.
    T-cell receptor c.
    TCR c.
    tenase c.
    c. thyroid endocrine disorder
    triple symptom c.
    tuberous sclerosis c. (TSC)
    VATER c.
    vitamin B c.
    von Meyenburg c.

complexed
    c. prostate-specific antigen (cPSA)
    c. PSA

complexity
    DNA c.

compliance
    dynamic pulmonary c.
    static pulmonary c.

complicata
    cataracta c.

complication
    catastrophic c.
    c. of silicosis

component
    amyloid P c.
    c. A of prothrombin
    basement membrane c.
    blood c.
    carcinomatous c.
    c. of complement
    complement c.
    dense fibrillar c.
    epsilon c.
    extensive intraductal c. (EIC)
    Immunotech immunoassay c.
    inorganic c.
    late positive c. (LPC)
    M c.
    c. management
    micropapillary c. (MPC)
    no mineral c.
    plasma thromboplastin c. (PTC)
    sarcomatous c.

secretory c.
sertoliform c.
spindle cell c.
thromboplastic plasma c. (TPC)
composite lymphoma
composition
chylomicron c.
c. resistor
three dimensional c.
composta
Nocardiopsis c.
compound
c. absorption device (CAD)
acetone c.
c. aneurysm
aromatic c.
beta-amyloid c.
carbamino c.
carbon inorganic c.
c. comminuted fracture (CCF)
condensation c.
c. cyst
c. dislocation
c. exocrine gland
gossypol c.
c. granular corpuscle
c. granule cell
heterocyclic c.
c. heterozygote
c. leukemia
meso c.
c. microscope
c. multiple fractures
c. nevus
c. odontoma
organometallic c.
organophosphate c.
organosilicon c.
polar c.
c. presentation
c. tumor
volatile organic c. (VOC)
c. X
compransoris
Zavarzinia c.
compressed
c. fracture
c. gas storage
c. spectral assay (CSA)
compression
c. of brain
cerebral c.

cord c. (CC)
extrinsic c.
c. fracture
c. injury
spinal cord c.
c. of tissue
compressive myelopathy
computer
c. graphics visualization
c. linkage analysis
computer-assisted image analysis
COMT
catechol-O-methyl transferase
Con A
concanavalin A
conarium
conc
concentrated
concentration
concameration
concanavalin
c. A (Con A)
c. A-horseradish peroxidase
concatenate
concatenation
Concato disease
concentrate
B-domain-deleted factor VIII c.
granulocyte c.
intrinsic factor c. (IFC)
malondialdehyde c.
marine protein c. (MPC)
metallothionein c.
platelet c.
random-donor platelet c.
Trizma buffer c.
concentrated (conc)
concentration (conc)
c. of adenosine monophosphate
approximate lethal c. (ALC)
bactericidal c. (BC)
Baermann c.
blood alcohol c. (BAC)
carbon dioxide c.
cotinine urinary c.
c. of creatinine in serum (Scr)
c. of creatinine in urine (Ucr)
critical micelle c. (CMC)
c. and dilution test
fecal c.
formalin-ether sedimentation c.

NOTES

229

concentration *(continued)*
    formalin-ethyl acetate
      sedimentation c.
    gravity c.
    hazardous c.
    HCO_3 c.
    hepatic iron c. (HIC)
    high trough c.
    hydrogen ion c. (pH)
    hydroxyl c. (pOH)
    ion c.
    ionic c.
    lethal c. (LC, LCt)
    limiting isorrheic c. (LIC)
    M c.
    mass c.
    maximum permissible c. (MPC)
    maximum urinary c. (MUC)
    mean cell hemoglobin c. (MCHC)
    mean corpuscular hemoglobin c.
      (MCHC)
    microhematocrit c.
    micromolar c.
    minimal bactericidal c. (MBC)
    minimal inhibitory c. (MIC)
    minimal isorrheic c. (MIC)
    minimal lethal c.
    minimum bactericidal c.
    minimum complete-killing c.
      (MCC)
    minimum detectable c. (MDC)
    minimum inhibitory c. (MIC)
    minimum lethal c. (MLC)
    minimum mycoplasmacidal c.
      (MPC)
    molar c.
    c. procedure
    prothrombin complex c. (PCC)
    radioactive c.
    renal vein renin c. (RVRC)
    serum p24 antigen c.
    c. of sodium in serum (SNa)
    c. of sodium in urine (UNa)
    substance c.
    time of maximum c. (T_{max})
    total L-chain c. (TLC)
    c. of total oxygen (CtO_2)
    zinc sulfate flotation c.
concentration-dependent nanomolar
  response
concentration-time
    c.-t. product (Ct)
    c.-t. product for 50% of exposed
      group (Ct_{50})
concentrator
    speed vacuum c.
concentric
    c. fibroma
    c. hypertrophy
    c. intimal thickening
    c. lamella
concentricum
    Trichophyton c.
concentricus
    Aspergillus c.
conception
    retained products of c.
conchoidal body
concinna
    Haemaphysalis c.
concisus
    Campylobacter c.
concomitant immunity
concordance
concrement
concrescence
concretio
    c. cordis
    c. pericardii
concretion
    calcific c.
concurrent infection
concussion
    brain c.
    cardiac c.
    c. myelitis
    spinal cord c.
condensans
    osteitis c.
    osteopathia c.
condensation
    block-like chromatin c.
    c. compound
    c. fibrosis
    c. polymer
condenser
    Abbé c.
    cardioid c.
    dark-field c.
    paraboloid c.
condensing
    c. osteitis
    c. vacuole
condition
    RNase-free c.
    steady-state c.
    sufficient c.
conditional
    c. jump
    c. lethal mutation
    c. probability
conditional-lethal mutant
conditionally lethal mutant
conductance
conducting system of heart
conduction
    c. electron

saltatory c.
volume c.
conductive hearing loss
conductivity
c. cell volume (CCV)
thermal c. (TC)
water c.
conductometry
conductor
conduit
conduplicate
condyloma, pl. **condylomata**
c. acuminatum
Buschke-Löwenstein giant c.
flat c.
genital c.
giant c.
c. latum
pointed c.
condylomatous atypia
cone
antipodal c.
c. biopsy
c. bipolar cell
c. cell of retina
c. disc
c. fiber
c. granule
Haller c.
implantation c.
layer of rods and c.'s
retinal c.
theca interna c.
twin c.
vascular c.
cone-nose bug
Conexibacter woesei
conexus
conference
clinicopathologic c. (CPC)
confertus
confidence
c. interval (CI)
c. level
confidential unit exclusion (CUE)
configuration
cis c.
germline c.
villiform c.
confined
organ c. (OC)
c. placental mosaicism (CPM)

confinement
expected date of c. (EDC)
confirmatory
c. test
c. testing
confirmed diagnosis
confluent
c. bronchopneumonia
c. hepatic necrosis
c. inflammation
c. pneumonia
c. and reticulate papillomatosis
c. smallpox
confocal
c. image
c. laser scan microscopy (CLSM)
c. microscopy
confocal laser scan microscopy (CLSM)
conformation
conformer
confusion
circle of c.
congelans
Pseudomonas c.
congelation urticaria
congener
congenita
amyoplasia c.
amyotonia c.
chondrodystrophia calcificans congenita
dyskeratosis c.
hyperkeratosis c.
osteogenesis imperfecta c.
osteosclerosis c.
pachyonychia c.
paramyotonia c.
congenital
c. absence
c. absence of vagina (CAV)
c. achromia
c. adrenal hyperplasia (CAH)
c. adrenal virilism (CAV)
c. afibrinogenemia
c. agammaglobulinemia
c. aganglionosis
c. ahaptoglobinemia
c. anomaly
c. aplasia of thymus
c. aplastic anemia
c. aregenerative anemia
c. atransferrinemia

NOTES

C

congenital *(continued)*
   c. atresia
   c. biliary ectasia
   c. cardiovascular malformation
   c. chylothorax
   c. contracture
   c. cyst
   c. dislocation
   c. dislocation of hip (CDH)
   c. duplication
   c. dyserythropoietic anemia (CDA)
   c. dysphagocytosis
   c. dysplastic angiectasia
   c. dysplastic angiomatosis
   c. dysplastic angiopathy
   c. ectodermal defect
   c. ectodermal dysplasia
   c. elephantiasis
   c. erythropoietic porphyria (CEP)
   c. familial icterus
   c. familial nonhemolytic jaundice
   c. generalized fibromatosis
   c. glaucoma
   c. goiter
   c. hemidysplasia with ichthyosiform erythroderma and limb defects (CHILD)
   c. hemolytic icterus
   c. hemolytic jaundice
   c. hepatic fibrosis
   c. hyperbilirubinemia
   c. hypophosphatasia
   c. hypoplastic anemia (CHA)
   c. lactase deficiency
   c. leukemia
   c. lobar emphysema
   c. localized absence of skin (CLAS)
   c. lymphedema
   c. megacolon
   c. melanocytic nevi (CMN)
   c. methemoglobinemia
   c. muscular dystrophy
   c. musculoskeletal deformity
   c. myopathy
   c. nonregenerative anemia
   c. nonspherocytic hemolytic anemia
   c. nonspherocytic hemolytic disease (CNHD)
   c. pancytopenia
   c. pectus excavatum
   c. pterygium
   c. pyloric stenosis
   c. rest
   c. rubella syndrome
   c. ruptured aneurysm
   c. sebaceous hyperplasia
   c. spherocytosis

   c. sucrase-isomaltase deficiency (CSID)
   c. sutural alopecia
   c. thymic aplasia
   c. thymic dysplasia (CTD)
   c. torticollis
   c. total lipodystrophy
   c. toxoplasmosis
   c. valve
   c. valvular heart disease
   c. vascular weakness
   c. X-linked infantile hypogammaglobulinemia

congenitale
   poikiloderma c.

congenitum
   megacolon c.

congested centrilobular area

congestion
   brain c.
   chronic passive c. (CPC)
   hypostatic c.
   passive c.
   postoperative c.
   pulmonary venous c. (PVC)
   venous c.

congestive
   c. cardiac failure (CCF)
   c. cardiomyopathy
   c. cirrhosis
   c. edema
   c. heart disease (CHD)
   c. heart failure (CHF)
   c. splenomegaly

conglobata
   acne c.

conglobate

conglobation

conglomerata
   elastosis colloidalis c.

conglomerate

conglomeratus
   Micrococcus c.

conglutinating complement absorption test (CCAT)

conglutination

conglutinin

conglutinogen-activating factor

Congo
   C. Corinth
   C. floor maggot
   C. red
   C. red paper
   C. red stain
   C. red test
   rubrum C.

congolense
   Trypanosoma c.

congolensis
  Actinomyces c.
  Dermatophilus c.
  Thysanotaenia c.
congophilic angiopathy
coni
  c. epididymidis
  c. vasculosi
conicae
  papillae c.
conical shaped filiform papillae
conidia (*pl. of* conidium)
conidial
Conidiobolus
  C. coronatus
  C. incongruus
conidiogenous
conidiophore
  Phialophore-type c.
conidiospore
conidium, pl. **conidia**
coniine
Coniochaeta
coniofibrosis
coniolymphstasis
coniophage
Coniophora
coniosis
Coniosporium
Coniothecium
Coniothyrium
Conium
conization
  cold-knife c.
conjoined twins
conjugal cancer
conjugant
conjugate
  c. acid
  c. acid-base pairs
  antidigoxigenin antibody
    peroxidase c.
  c. base
  c. division
  fluorochrome-avidin/streptavidin c.
  c. focus
  mercuric c.
  c. redox pair
conjugated
  c. antigen
  c. bilirubin
  c. estriol

  c. hapten
  c. hyperbilirubinemia I–III
  c. protein
conjugation bridge
conjugative plasmid
conjunctional
conjunctiva, pl. **conjunctivae**
  bulbar c.
  Dirofilaria conjunctivae
  lithiasis conjunctivae
  tela c.
  tunica c.
conjunctival
  c. cell
  c. fungus culture
  c. gland
  c. layer of bulb
  c. layer of eyelid
conjunctivales
  glandulae c.
conjunctive
conjunctivitis
  acute contagious c.
  acute epidemic c.
  acute follicular c.
  adult gonococcal c.
  allergic c.
  angular c.
  blennorrheal c.
  catarrhal c.
  follicular c.
  gonococcal c.
  granular c.
  inclusion c.
  infantile purulent c.
  lymphogranuloma venereum-trachoma
    inclusion c. (LGV-TRIC)
  meningococcus c.
  Moraxella c.
  c. neonatorum
  phlyctenular c.
  spring catarrhal c.
  swimming pool c.
  toxicogenic c.
  trachoma-inclusion c. (TRIC)
  tularemic c.
  vernal c.
  welder's c.
conjunctivoma
connectin
connecting
  c. cartilage

C

NOTES

connecting *(continued)*
    c. ring
    c. tubule
connection
    anomalous venous c.
    clamp c.
    fetoscopic laser coagulation of vascular c.
    partial anomalous pulmonary venous c. (PAPVC)
connective
    c. tissue
    c. tissue capsule
    c. tissue cell
    c. tissue disease (CTD)
    c. tissue disorder
    c. tissue fiber
    c. tissue group
    c. tissue growth factor
    c. tissue nevus
    c. tissue septa
    c. tissue stroma
    c. tissue supply blood
    c. tissue trabecula
    c. tumor
connexin
connexus intertendinei musculi extensoris digitorum
conniventes
    valvulae c.
Conn syndrome
Conocybe cyanopus
conoid
conoideum
    Hypoderaeum c.
conomyoidin
Conor and Bruch disease
conorii
    Rickettsia c.
Conradi disease
consanguineous
    c. donor
    c. mating
consanguinity
consecutive
    c. aneurysm
    c. angiitis
consensus pathology opinion
consent
    informed c.
consequences of intrahepatic scarring
conservatrix
    Desulforegula c.
conserved helix-loop-helix ubiquitous kinase (CHUK)
consideration
    clinical c.
    differential diagnostic c.

consistency
    fecal c.
    stool c.
consistent estimate
consolidation
conspecific
conspicuous amyloid deposition
Conspicuum conspicuum
constant (k)
    absorption c.
    acid ionization c.
    affinity c.
    Ambard c.
    association c.
    base ionization c.
    binding c.
    Boltzmann c.
    decay c.
    dielectric c.
    diffusion c.
    disintegration c.
    dissociation c.
    equilibrium c.
    Faraday c.
    gas c.
    ionization c.
    Planck c. (h)
    radioactive c.
    rate c.
    c. region
    C. Spring mutation of hemoglobin
constellatus
    Diplococcus c.
    Peptococcus c.
    Streptococcus c.
constipation
    functional c.
constituent
    endocrine granule c. (EGC)
constitution
constitutional
    c. cause
    c. disease
    c. dwarf
    c. hepatic dysfunction
    c. hyperbilirubinemia
    c. reaction
    c. thrombopathy
    c. ulcer
constitutive
    c. enzyme
    c. expression
    c. heterochromatin
    c. heterochromatin method
    c. mutation
    c. protein
constriction
    primary c.
    secondary c.

constrictive
    c. endocarditis
    c. pericarditis
constrictum
    Pentastoma c.
constrictus
    Porocephalus c.
constructible
construction
constructive
    c. interference
    c. proof
consultation
    in-house c.
    intradepartmental c.
    undiagnosing c.
consumption
    alcohol c.
    c. coagulopathy
    oxygen c.
contact (c)
    c. activation product
    c. allergy
    c. catalysis
    c. dermatitis
    c. entrance wound
    hospital-acquired penetration c.
    c. hypersensitivity
    c. inhibition
    metal-to-metal c.
    c. sensitivity
contactant
contagion
    immediate c.
    mediate c.
contagiosum
    molluscum c.
contagious
    c. bovine pleuropneumonia
    c. disease
    c. ecthyma
    c. ecthyma (pustular dermatitis) virus of sheep
    c. pustular dermatitis
    c. pustular stomatitis virus
contagiousness
contagium
    c. animatum
    c. vivum
contain
    to c. (TC)
contained criticality

container
    ALPS c.
    screw-cup c.
    c. size limitations
containment
    biosafety c.
contaminans
    Anoxybacillus c.
contaminant
contaminate
contaminated
    dirty area (c.)
    c. patient
contamination
    alpha c.
    c. irradiation
    primary c.
    secondary c.
contamination-free
    clean area (c.-f.)
content
    carbon dioxide c.
    dye c.
    gastrointestinal c.'s
    heat c.
    supranormal venous oxygen c.
    total carbon dioxide c.
contiguum
continence
continent
contingency table
contingent negative variation (CNV)
continua
    acrodermatitis c.
    epilepsia partialis c. (EPC)
    Heterophyopsis c.
continued fever
continuous
    c. capillary
    c. distending pressure (CDP)
    c. endothelium
    c. flow analyzer
    c. flow culture
    c. function
    c. phase
    c. spectrum
continuum
contorti
    tubuli c.
contortum
    Eubacterium c.

NOTES

contortus
    tubulus renalis c.
contour line of Owen
contracted kidney
contractile
    c. ring
    c. vacuole
contraction
    c. band
    c. band necrosis
    isovolumic c. (IC)
    c. stress test
contracture
    congenital c.
    Dupuytren c.
    ischemic c.
    organic c.
    Volkmann c.
contrafissura
contraindication
contralateral
    c. axillary metastasis
    c. infiltrating duct carcinoma
contrast
    bright c.
    c. media reaction
    c. medium
    c. stain
contrasuppressor cell
contrecoup
contributory cause of death
control
    c. animal
    Cardiasure cardiac markers c.
    c. cell
    Cell-Chex body fluid procedural c.
    Centers for Disease C. (CDC)
    chemTRAK liquid chemistry c.
    clinical chemistry quality c.
    clinical microbiology quality c.
    Elecsys PreciControl Anti-HBe c.
    ESR-Chex hematology c.
    c. experiment
    c. group
    healthy c.
    HemataCHEK hematology
      reference c.
    HepCheck whole blood c.
    ignition source c.
    infection c. (IC)
    Liquichek hematology-16 c.
    Liquichek hematology c. (A)
    Liquichek hematology c. (C)
    Liquichek immunology c.
    Liquichek qualitative urine
      toxicology c.
    Liquichek sedimentation rate c.
    Liquichek ToRCH Plus c.
    lupus anticoagulant positive c.

    Lyphochek anemia c.
    Lyphochek fertility c.
    Lyphochek hypertension markers c.
    Lyphochek maternal serum c.
    Lyphochek tumor marker c.
    Lyphochek whole blood c.
    c. material
    Para 12 Plus Retics c.
    process c.
    quality c. (QC)
    riot c.
    Sed-Chek 2 bilevel whole blood
      reference c.
    spill c.
    Sugar-Chex II glucose c.
    Virotrol syphilis total c.
controlled
    c. access laboratory
    c. pore glass bead
    c. substance
contused wound
contusion
    brain c.
    incomplete muzzle c.
    muzzle c.
    scalp c.
    wind c.
conular
convalescent
    c. carrier
    c. serum
convection
convention
    Biological Weapons and Toxins C.
conventional animal
convergence
conversational mode
conversion
    c. coefficient
    c. electron
    c. of glucose
    internal c.
    Mantoux c.
    mediated c.
    c. ratio
    serum prothrombin c.
convertase
    C3 proactivator c.
converter
    D/A c.
    digital-to-analog c. (DAC)
    voltage-to-frequency c.
convertin
converting enzyme
convexobasia
convoluted
    c. endometrial gland
    c. part of kidney lobule

c. seminiferous tubule
c. tubule of kidney
convulsant antidote for nerve agent (CANA)
convulsion
Conway cell
COOH-terminal tagging
cookei
    Ixodes c.
cookii
    Paenibacillus c.
cooled-knife method
Cooler
    Chameleon C.
Cooley
    C. anemia
    C. disease
coolhaasii
    Caloramator c.
Coolscope digital camera/microscope
Coomassie
    C. blue-stained gel
    C. brilliant blue R-250
Coombs
    C. serum
    C. test (CT)
Cooperative Human Tissue Network
Cooper disease
Cooperia
    C. bisonis
    C. curticei
    C. fieldingi
    C. oncophora
    C. pectinata
    C. punctata
    C. spatulata
Coopernail sign
coordinate
    cartesian c.'s
    c. covalent bond
    polar c.'s
    spherical polar c.'s
    X-Y-Z beam scanning method c.'s
coossification
coossify
CO-oximeter
    carbon monoxide oximeter
COP
    colloidal osmotic pressure
    colloid oncotic pressure
    cryptogenic organizing pneumonia

COPD
    chronic obstructive pulmonary disease
Copelandia
copepod
Copepoda
Coplin jar
copolymer
copper (Cu)
    c. assay
    c. cyanide (CuCN)
    c. deposit demonstration
    c. grid
    c. metabolism
    c. reduction test
    c. storage protein
    c. sulfate
    c. sulfate method
    c. sulfate test
    urine c.
    c. wire effect
copper-binding protein test
copper-wire artery
coprecipitating antibody
coprecipitation
coprecipitin
copremesis
Coprinus
coproantibody
Coprobacillus cateniformis
coprogenus
    Saccharomyces c.
coprolith
coprology
coproma
Copromastix prowazeki
Copromonas subtilis
coprophagous
coprophagy
coprophil
coprophilia
coproporphyria
    erythropoietic c. (ECP)
    hereditary c. (HCP)
coproporphyrin (CP)
    c. assay
    free erythrocyte c. (FEC)
    c. test
    urinary c. (UCP)
    urine c.
coproporphyrinogen oxidase
coproporphyrinuria
coprostanol

NOTES

coprostasis
coprosterol
coprozoa
coprozoic ameba
CoQ
    coenzyme Q
cor
    c. adiposum
    c. biloculare
    c. bovinum
    c. mobile
    c. pendulum
    c. pseudotriloculare biatriatum
    c. pulmonale
    c. triatriatum
    c. triloculare biatriatum
    c. triloculare biventriculare
coracidium
coral calculus
coralicida
    Aurantimonas c.
coralliilyticus
    Vibrio c.
corallin
    yellow c.
Corallobothrium
Corbin technique
Corbus disease
cord
    Bergmann c.
    Billroth c.
    c. blood
    c. blood screen
    c. compression (CC)
    dental c.
    c. factor
    glioma of the spinal c.
    hepatic c.
    lymph c.
    marginal insertion of umbilical c.
    medullary c.
    prolapsed umbilical c.
    psalterial c.
    red pulp c.
    rete c.
    ruptured umbilical c.
    sex c.
    splenic c.
    subacute combined degeneration of spinal c.
    two-cell wide vertical c.
    velamentous c.
    Willis c.
Cordana
cordatum
    Diphyllobothrium c.
cordatus
    Bothriocephalus c.

cordis
    capsula c.
    concretio c.
    ectasia c.
    membrana c.
    mucro c.
    myofibrosis c.
    steatosis c.
    theca c.
cordocentesis
Cordyceps
Cordylobia anthropophaga
cordylobiasis
core
    air c.
    c. antigen
    hyaline c.
    hyalinized c.
    magnetic c.
    c. memory
    c. pneumonia
    c. promoter mutant
corectasis
coremium
corepressor
Cori
    C. cycle
    C. disease
    C. ester
coria (*pl. of* corium)
coriaceus
    Ornithodoros c.
corii
    papillae c.
    rete cutaneum c.
    sclerosis c.
    stratum papillare c.
    stratum reticulare c.
    tunica propria c.
Corinth
    Congo C.
Coriobacteriaceae
Coriobacteriales
Coriobacteridae
Coriolopsis
Coriolus
coriphosphine O
corium, pl. **coria**
    papillae of c.
    reticular layer of c.
corkscrew hair
corkscrew-like bacteria
cornea
    anterior epithelium of c.
    anterior limiting layer of c.
    elastic layer of c.
    ichthyosis sebacea c.
    limiting layer of c.

posterior limiting layer of c.
substantia propria of c.

corneae
epithelium anterius c.
herpes c.
lamina limitans anterior c.
lamina limitans posterior c.
limbus c.
substantia propria c.

corneal
c. corpuscle
c. impression test (CIT)
c. layer of epidermis
c. margin
c. opacity (CO)
c. space
c. ulcer
c. vascularization

Cornelia de Lange syndrome
corneocyte envelope
corneoscleral
c. button
c. junction
c. part of trabecular tissue of
sclera
c. tunic

corneous
Corner-Allen
C.-A. test
C.-A. unit

corn ergot
corneum
Nosema c.
stratum c.

cornification
cornified
c. cell
c. layer of nail

cornifying form
cornmeal agar
cornoid lamella
cornu, gen. **cornus**, pl. **cornua**
c. cutaneum

cornual pregnancy
corona, pl. **coronae**
c. radiata
c. veneris

coronal section
coronary
c. artery bypass graft (CABG)
c. artery disease (CAD)

c. atherosclerotic heart disease
(CAHD)
c. blood flow (CBF)
c. embolism
c. insufficiency (CI)
c. insufficiency syndrome
c. occlusion
c. ostial stenosis
c. prognostic index (CPI)
c. risk factor
c. sinus
c. tendon
c. thrombosis (CT)

coronata
Delacroixia c.
Diploscapter c.
Entomophthora c.

coronatum
Cyathostomum c.

coronatus
Conidiobolus c.

Coronaviridae
Coronavirus
coronavirus (CoV)
novel c.
severe acute respiratory
syndrome c. (SARS-CoV)

coroner
coronoidectomy
coronoid process fracture
corpora (*pl. of* corpus)
corporis
corps
c. grains
c. ronds

corpse temperature
corpulence
corpulency
corpus, pl. **corpora**
c. albicans
c. amylaceum (CA)
c. aorticum
c. atreticum
c. candicans
c. cavernosum urethrae
c. coccygeum
corpora arenacea
c. delicti
c. glandulae sudoriferae
c. hemorrhagicum
c. hemorrhagicum cyst
corpora lutea cyst

NOTES

C

corpus *(continued)*
   corpora lutea twins
   c. luteum
   c. luteum cyst
   c. luteum hematoma
   c. luteum hormone
   c. luteum hormone unit
   c. luteum of pregnancy
   c. nuclei caudati
   c. papillare
   corpora paraaortica
   c. pineale
   c. spongiosum
   c. spongiosum penis
   c. spongiosum urethrae muliebris
   c. striatum
   c. vitreum
corpuscle
   amnionic c.
   amniotic c.
   amylaceous c.
   amyloid c.
   articular c.
   axis c.
   Babès-Ernst c.
   basal c.
   Bennet c.
   Bizzozero c.
   blood c.
   bone c.
   bridge c.
   bulboid c.
   cement c.
   chyle c.
   colloid c.
   colostrum c.
   compound granular c.
   corneal c.
   Dogiel c.
   Donné c.
   Drysdale c.
   dust c.
   Eichhorst c.
   exudation c.
   genital c.
   ghost c.
   Gierke c.
   Gluge c.
   Golgi-Mazzoni c.
   Grandry c.
   Hassall concentric c.
   Herbst c.
   inflammatory c.
   Jaworski c.
   lamellated c.
   lymph c.
   lymphatic c.
   lymphoid c.
   malpighian c.

   Mazzoni c.
   Meissner c.
   Merkel c.
   Mexican hat c.
   molluscum c.
   Negri c.
   Norris c.
   oval c.
   pacchionian c.
   pacinian c.
   pessary c.
   phantom c.
   plastic c.
   Purkinje c.
   pus c.
   red c.
   renal c.
   reticulated c.
   Ruffini c.
   Russell c.
   salivary c.
   Schwalbe c.
   shadow c.
   splenic c.
   tactile c.
   taste c.
   terminal nerve c.
   third c.
   thymic c.
   touch c.
   Toynbee c.
   Traube c.
   Tröltsch c.
   Valentin c.
   Vater c.
   Vater-Pacini c.
   Virchow c.
   Wagner-Meissner c.
   white c.
   Zimmermann c.
corpuscular
   c. lymph
   c. volume (CV)
corpusculum, pl. **corpuscula**
   corpuscula articularia
   corpuscula bulboidea
   corpuscula genitalia
   corpuscula lamellosa
   corpuscula nervosa terminalia
   c. renis
   c. tactus
corralin yellow
corrected
   c. blood volume (CBV)
   c. dextrocardia
   c. retention time
   c. reticulocyte count
   c. sedimentation rate (CSR)
   c. transposition (CT)

correction
Allen c.
coincidence c.
c. factor
correlation
c. coefficient
functional c.
structural c.
corresponding ray
Corrigan disease
corrin ring
corrodens
Bacteroides c.
Eikenella c.
corrosion
c. cast
c. preparation
corrosive
c. esophagitis
c. gastric secretions
corrosivity
corrugata
Acrocarpospora c.
cortex, pl. **cortices**
adrenal c.
agranular c.
amorphous fraction of adrenal c.
branches of the renal c.
cerebellar c.
c. cerebelli
cerebral c.
c. cerebri
deep c.
fetal adrenal c.
fusiform cell of cerebral c.
ganglionic layer of cerebellar c.
ganglionic layer of cerebral c.
c. glandulae suprarenalis
granular layer of cerebellar c.
granular layer of cerebral c.
c. of hair shaft
intercalated cell of the renal c.
kidney c.
layer of cerebellar c.
layer of cerebral c.
c. of lens
c. lentis
c. of lymph node
molecular layer of cerebral c.
multiform layer of cerebral c.
c. nodi lymphatici
c. ovarii

plexiform layer of cerebral c.
provisional c.
renal c.
c. renalis
stained c.
stellate cell of cerebral c.
suprarenal c.
tertiary c.
thymic c.
c. of thymus
Corti
C. arch
C. auditory teeth
C. canal
C. cell
C. ganglion
C. membrane
C. organ
C. pillar
pillar cell of C.
C. rod
C. tunnel
corti
Mesocestoides c.
cortical
c. achromia
c. bone
c. defect
c. dysplasia
c. hormone
c. necrosis
c. osteitis
c. stromal hyperplasia (CSH)
c. substance
c. thumb
c. thymoma
c. U-fiber
corticale
Cryptostroma c.
corticalis
substantia c.
corticalization
cortices (*pl. of* cortex)
Corticium
corticobasal degeneration
corticoid
antiinflammatory c. (AC)
corticola
Griphosphaeria c.
corticoliberin
corticomedullary junction
corticosteroid (CS)

NOTES

corticosteroid *(continued)*
    c. crystal
    inhalant c.
    c. myopathy
    rectal c.
    c. therapy
    topical c.
corticosteroid-binding
    c.-b. globulin (CBG)
    c.-b. protein
corticosterone
corticotrope adenoma
corticotroph cell hyperplasia
corticotropin
    hyperproduction of pituitary c.
corticotropin-releasing
    c.-r. factor (CRF)
    c.-r. hormone (CRH)
Corticoviridae
Corticovirus
Cortinarius orellanus
cortisol
    c. assay
    c. binding
    c. production rate (CPR)
    c. secretion rate (CSR)
    c. synthesis pathway
    urinary free c.
cortisol-binding globulin (CBG)
cortisone
cortisone-glucose tolerance test (CGTT)
cortisone-primed oral glucose tolerance test (COGTT)
cortol
cortolone
Cortrosyn
Corvac integrated serum separator tube
Corvisart disease
corymbifera
    Absidia c.
    Lechtheimia c.
corymbiform
Coryne
Corynebacteriaceae
Corynebacterineae
corynebacteriophage
    beta c.
Corynebacterium
    C. amycolatum
    C. appendicis
    C. aquilae
    C. atypicum
    C. aurimucosum
    C. auriscanis
    C. capitovis
    C. casei
    C. caspium
    C. diphtheriae
    C. diphtheriae throat culture

C. efficiens
C. equi
C. felinum
C. freneyi
C. glaucum
C. glucuronolyticum
C. halotolerans
C. hoagii
C. jeikeium
C. matruchotii
C. minutissimum
C. mooreparkense
C. mycetoides
C. nigricans
C. parvum
C. pseudodiphtheriticum
C. pseudotuberculosis
C. pyogenes
C. renale
C. simulans
C. sphenisci
C. spheniscorum
C. striatum
C. suicordis
C. testudinoris
C. tuberculostearicum
C. ulcerans
C. xerosis
coryneform group
Corynespora cassiicola
coryza
    allergic c.
    c. virus
coryzavirus
cosine
Cosm
    osmolar clearance
cosmid
Cosmocephalus obvelatus
Cosmocerella
cosmopolitan
costa
costal pleurisy
costantinii
    Pseudomonas c.
costaricensis
    Angiostrongylus c.
    Morerastrongylus c.
Costello syndrome
Costen syndrome
costimulatory molecule
cosynthase
    uroporphyrinogen III c.
cosyntropin test
Cotard syndrome
Cotasil silicone slide coating material
cothromboplastin
cotinine urinary concentration
Cotlove titrator

cotransport
cotton dust asthma
cotton-fiber embolism
cotton-wool appearance
Cotugno disease
cotunnii
    aqueductus c.
    liquor c.
Cotunnius
    C. aqueduct
    C. disease
    C. liquid
cot value
Cotylaspis
cotyledon
    fetal c.
    maternal c.
Cotylogonimus
Cotylurus
cough
    brassy c.
    c. plate
    whooping c.
coulomb (C)
    C. law
coulometer
coulometric
    c. chloridometer
    c. titration
coulometry
Coulter
    C. Clenz cleaning agent
    C. CLONE monoclonal antibody
    C. counter
    C. Gen-S Cell hematology
    workstation
    C. LH 500, 700, 750, 755, 1500
    Series hematology analyzer
    C. Manual CD4 Kit
    C. MAXM hematology analyzer
    C. reticONE system
    C. STKS hematology analyzer
    C. tetraONE system
    C. TQ-Prep workstation
coumachlor
coumarin
Coumatrak prothrombin time device
Councilman
    C. hyaline body
    C. lesion
Councilmania

counseling
    genetic c.
count
    absolute eosinophil c.
    absolute granulocyte c. (AGC)
    absolute neutrophil c. (ANC)
    Addis c.
    agar plate c.
    Arneth c.
    background c.
    B-cell c.
    blood cell c.
    bone marrow differential c.
    CD4/CD8 c.
    cell c.
    cerebrospinal fluid leukocyte c.
    colony c.
    complete blood c. (CBC)
    corrected reticulocyte c.
    differential leukocyte c. (DLC)
    differential white blood c.
    egg c.
    eosinophil c.
    erythrocyte c.
    fecal leukocyte c.
    filament-nonfilament c.
    c. information density
    leukocyte c.
    microvessel c. (MVC)
    mitotic c.
    peripheral white c.
    c. per minute (cpm)
    platelet c. (PC)
    proportional c.
    c. rate
    c. rate meter
    red blood cell c.
    reticulocyte c.
    Schilling blood c.
    scintillation c.
    Sézary c.
    spinal fluid leukocyte c.
    stool leukocyte c.
    too numerous to c. (TNTC)
    total cell c.
    total ridge c. (TRC)
    viable cell c.
    white blood cell c.
    white cell c. (WCC)
counter
    automated differential leukocyte c.
    cell c.

NOTES

C

counter *(continued)*
- Coulter c.
- decade c.
- electronic cell c.
- frequency c.
- gamma well c.
- Geiger-Müller c.
- ion c.
- liquid scintillation c.
- Multisizer 3 Coulter c.
- proportional c.
- radiation c.
- ring c.
- ripple c.
- scintillation c.
- shift c.
- synchronous c.
- Sysmex R-1000 reticulocyte c.
- Z1, Z2 series Coulter c.
- Z2 Coulter C.

counterclockwise
countercurrent
- c. extraction
- c. immunoelectrophoresis (CIE, CIEP)
- c. mechanism
- c. multiplier system

counterelectrophoresis (CEP)
counterflow centrifugal elutriation
counterimmunoelectrophoresis (CIEP)
counterstain
counterstaining technique
counting
- automated reticulocyte c.
- c. cadence
- c. chamber
- liquid scintillation c.
- photon c.
- c. plate

couple
- redox c.

coupler
- acoustic c.

coupling
- c. capacitor
- cell c.
- c. defect

Courvoisier
- C. law
- C. sign

Courvoisier-Terrier syndrome
CoV
- coronavirus

covalent bond
Covalink MicroElisa culture plate
covariance
covariate
coverglass
cover glass

coverslip
Coverslipper
- Jung CV 5000 Robotic C.

cowanii
- *Enterobacter c.*

Cowden
- C. disease
- C. syndrome

Cowdria ruminantium
Cowdry type A, B inclusion body
cow kidney
Cowper
- C. cyst
- C. gland

cowperitis
cowpox virus
cow's milk anemia
COX-1
- cyclooxygenase-1

COX-2
- cyclooxygenase-2

Cox
- C. proportional hazards regression model
- C. regression analysis
- C. vaccine

coxa, pl. **coxae**
- c. magna
- c. plana

Coxiella burnetii
coxitis
coxsackievirus encephalitis
CP
- cardiopulmonary
- cerebral palsy
- chemically pure
- coproporphyrin
- cystosarcoma phyllodes

C:P
- cholesterol/phospholipid ratio

cP
- centipoise

CPB
- competitive protein-binding
- CPB assay

CPC
- chronic passive congestion
- clinicopathologic conference
- conventional papillary carcinoma

CPD
- calcium pyrophosphate dihydrate
- cephalopelvic disproportion
- citrate phosphate dextrose
- CPD adenine
- citrate-phosphate-dextrose-adenine

CPDN
- cystic partially differentiated nephroblastoma

CPE
  chronic pulmonary emphysema
C-peptide test
CpG
  cytosine phosphate guanine
    CpG island
CPH
  chronic persistent hepatitis
CPI
  chronic pneumonitis of infancy
  Clostridium perfringens enterotoxin iota
  coronary prognostic index
CPK
  creatine phosphokinase
CPK-MB
  creatine phosphokinase-myocardial band
CPL
  congenital pulmonary lymphangiectasis
cPLA2
  cytosol phospholipase A2
CPM
  confined placental mosaicism
cpm
  count per minute
CPN
  chronic pyelonephritis
CPPD
  calcium pyrophosphate deposition disease
CPR
  cerebral cortex perfusion rate
  cortisol production rate
CPS
  carbamoyl phosphate synthetase
  carbamyl phosphate synthetase
    CPS deficiency
cps
  cycle per second
cPSA
  complexed prostate-specific antigen
CPT2
  carnitine palmitoyltransferase 2
    CPT2 deficiency
CPX
  calciphylaxis
CQ
  circadian quotient
C1q
  C. immune complex detection
  C. nephropathy
  C. radioassay
CR
  complement receptor

  crown rump
  NATO code for dibenz(b,f)-1:4-
    oxazepine
CR3
  complement receptor 3
    CR3 deficiency
Cr
  chromium
^{51}Cr
  ^{51}Cr red cell survival test
crab
  c. hand
  c. louse
  c. yaws
Crabtree effect
cracked heel
cradle cap
Craigia
Craigie
  C. tube
  C. tube method
Crandall syndrome
craniad
cranial
  c. arteritis
  c. gunshot wound
  c. insufflation
  c. monocephalus duplication
cranii
  osteoporosis circumscripta c.
craniocarpotarsal
  c. dysplasia
  c. dystrophy
craniocele
craniocleidodysostosis
craniodiaphysial dysplasia
craniofacial
  c. dysostosis
  c. fracture
craniomalacia
  circumscribed c.
craniomeningocele
craniometaphysial dysplasia
craniopagus
craniopathy
  metabolic c.
craniopharyngioma
  ameloblastomatous c.
  cystic papillomatous c.
craniorachischisis
cranioschisis
craniosclerosis

NOTES

craniostenosis
craniosynostosis
craniotabes
craniotrypesis
cranium bifidum
Cranston hemoglobin
crapulent
crassamentum
Crassicauda grampicola
crassicollis
    Taenia c.
crateriform ulceration
craw-craw
CRBBB
    complete right bundle-branch block
CRC
    colorectal cancer
CRCC
    chromophobe renal cell carcinoma
CRD
    chronic renal disease
    complete reaction of degeneration
C-reactive
    C-r. protein (CRP)
    C-r. protein assay
    C-r. protein test
cream
    leukocyte c.
    SoftGUARD hand c.
crease
    palmar c.
    simian c.
creatine
    c. kinase (CK)
    c. kinase assay
    c. kinase isoenzyme
    c. kinase isoenzyme electrophoresis
    c. kinase test
    c. phosphate
    c. phosphokinase (CPK)
    c. phosphokinase-myocardial band
    (CPK-MB)
creatinemia
creatinine
    amniotic fluid c.
    c. assay
    c. clearance (CC, C/cr/)
    c. clearance test
    c. coefficient
    c. height index (CHI)
    urine c.
creatinuria
CREB
    cAMP response element binding protein
    CREB binding protein (CBP)
CREB/ATF
    cAMP response element binding
    activation transcription factor
Credé method

credentialing
creeping
    c. disease
    c. eruption
    c. substitution of bone
    c. ulcer
CREG
    cross-reactive group
    CREG matching
cremoricolorata
    Pseudomonas c.
cremoris
    Streptococcus c.
Crenarchaeota
crenate
crenated cell
crenation
crenocyte
crenocytosis
Crenosoma vulpis
Crenotrichaceae
crenulate
creola body
crepitans
    tenosynovitis c.
crescens
    Emmonsia parva var. *c.*
crescent
    c. cell
    c. cell anemia
    c. formation
    Giannuzzi c.
    glomerular c.
    Heidenhain c.
    c. sign
crescentic
    c. anti-GBM glomerulonephritis
    c. histiocyte
    c. nephritis
cresol
    c. assay
    c. red
cresol-ammonia spot test
CREST
    calcinosis, Raynaud phenomenon,
    esophageal motility disorders,
    sclerodactyly, and telangiectasia
    CREST syndrome
crest
    acoustic c.
    ampullary c.
    embryonic neural c.
    neural c. (NC)
    neuroepithelium of ampullary c.
    obturator c.
    spiral c.
cresta
cresyl
    c. blue

c. blue brilliant
c. blue brilliant stain
c. echt
c. fast violet
c. violet (CV)
c. violet acetate
c. violet stain
cresylecht violet
cretinism
Creutzfeldt-Jakob disease (CJD)
crevicular
c. epithelium
c. fluid
CRF
chronic renal failure
corticotropin-releasing factor
CRH
corticotropin-releasing hormone
crib death
cribra (*pl. of* cribrum)
cribrate
cribration
cribriform
c. area of renal papilla
c. carcinoma
c. field of vision
c. growth pattern
c. nest
c. plate of ethmoid bone
cribriform-morular
c.-m. variant
c.-m. variant of papillary thyroid carcinoma
cribrosa
area c.
macula c.
cribrum, pl. **cribra**
Crichton-Browne sign
cricothyroid
cri du chat syndrome
Crigler-Najjar
C.-N. disease
C.-N. syndrome
Crimean-Congo
C.-C. hemorrhagic fever
C.-C. hemorrhagic fever virus
Crimean hemorrhagic fever virus
crime scene investigation
criminal abortion
Crinipellis
Crinivirus
crinophagy

Cripavirus
Crippa lead tetraacetate method
crisis, pl. **crises**
addisonian c.
adrenal c.
anaphylactoid c.
aplastic c.
blast c.
blood c.
celiac c.
cholinergic c.
hypercalcemic c.
myasthenic c.
myelocytic c.
parvovirus B19 aplastic c.
salt-losing c.
scleroderma renal c.
sequestration c.
sickle cell c.
thyroid c.
c. value
vasoocclusive c.
crispatum
Eubacterium c.
crispatus
Lactobacillus c.
crista, pl. **cristae**
c. ampullaris
c. basilaris ductus cochlearis
c. cutis
c. of mitochondrion
c. quarta
c. spiralis
swollen c.
tubular cristae
criteria, sing. **criterion**
Azzopardi c.
Child hepatic risk c.
Dallas myocarditis c.
Katzenstein and Peiper c.
Krauss and Neubecker morphologic c.
Laurén c.
Masaoka staging c.
morphologic c.
Muller-Hermelink histological c.
prognostic c.
Ranson acute pancreatitis c.
Van Diest c.
Weiss c.
Crithidia **immunofluorescence testing**

NOTES

247

critical
- c. angle
- c. flicker fusion (CFF)
- c. flicker fusion test
- c. illumination
- c. incident stress management (CISM)
- c. limit
- c. mass
- c. micelle concentration (CMC)
- c. path analysis
- c. pathway
- c. region
- c. staining level
- c. temperature

criticality
- contained c.
- c. incident
- c. locket dosimeter
- c. lockout
- uncontained c.

Crit-Line
- C.-L. fluid monitor
- C.-L. III TQA fluid management and access device

CritSpin microhematocrit centrifuge

CRM
- cross-reacting material

cRNA
- chromosomal RNA

crocea
- *Aequorivita c.*

Croceibacter atlanticus

crocein
- brilliant c.

Crocicreas

crocidolite

crocidurae
- *Borrelia c.*

Crocinitomix catalasitica

Crocker silver impregnation technique

Crocq disease

Crohn
- C. disease
- C. ileitis

Cronkhite-Canada
- C.-C. polyp
- C.-C. syndrome

Crooke
- C. granule
- C. hyaline change
- C. hyaline degeneration

cross
- c. activation
- c. agglutination
- hair c.
- c. hybridization
- c. infection
- Maltese c.

- c. product
- Ranvier c.
- c. reaction
- c. striation
- c. striation pattern
- three-point c.
- c. wall

cross-assembler

cross-bridge
- myosin c.-b.

cross-compiler

crossed
- c. grid
- c. immunoelectrophoresis

Crossiella
- *C. cryophila*
- *C. equi*

cross-link
- urine pyridinoline c.-l.

cross-linked N-telopeptide

cross-linking

crossmatch (XM)
- flow cytometric c.
- immediate-spin c.
- newborn c.

crossmatching
- donor-specific c.

crossover
- c. frequency
- c. hemoglobin

cross-protective immunity

cross-reacting
- c.-r. agglutinin
- c.-r. antibody
- c.-r. antigen
- c.-r. material (CRM)

cross-reactive group (CREG)

cross-reactivity

cross-sectional survey

cross-section anatomy

cross-striation

crossway
- sensory c.

crotalariae
- *Phaeotrichoconis c.*

crotalin

Crotalus **antitoxin**

crotonatoxidans
- *Alkaliphilus c.*

croton oil

croup

croup-associated (CA)
- c.-a. virus

crouposus
- pemphigus c.

croupous
- c. bronchitis
- c. inflammation
- c. lymph

c. membrane
c. pharyngitis
Crouzon
    C. craniofacial dysostosis
    C. disease
    C. syndrome
crowded cell index
crowding
    c. effect
    gland c.
Crow-Fukase syndrome
crown
    C. needle
    radiate c.
    c. rump (CR)
crown-heel (CH)
CRP
    C-reactive protein
CRPH high-sensitivity C-reactive protein reagent
CRS
    Chinese restaurant syndrome
CRST
    calcinosis cutis, Raynaud phenomenon, sclerodactyly, and telangiectasia
    CRST syndrome
cRT-PCR
    competitive reverse transcription polymerase chain reaction
cruces pilorum
crucians
    Anopheles c.
cruciate ligament tear
Crucibulum
crude
    c. mortality ratio (CMR)
    c. rate
    c. urine
cruor
crura (*pl. of* crus)
crural diaphragm
cruris
    Trichophyton c.
crus, pl. **crura**
    crura of the penis
crush
    c. artifact
    c. injury
    c. kidney
    c. syndrome

crushing
    c. chest pain
    c. of tissue
crust
    buffy c.
    scale c.
crusta, pl. **crustae**
    c. inflammatoria
    c. phlogistica
Crustacea
crusted ringworm
Cruveilhier
    C. disease
    C. paralysis
    C. ulcer
Cruveilhier-Baumgarten
    C.-B. disease
    C.-B. syndrome
Cruz-Chagas disease
cruzi
    Anopheles c.
    Schizotrypanum c.
    Trypanosoma c.
cryalgesia
crymophilic
crymophylactic
cryoablation
Cryobacterium psychrophilum
cryobank
cryobiology
cryocrit
CryoCults culture
cryoelectron microscopy
cryofibrinogen
cryofibrinogenemia
cryofracture
cryogammaglobulin
Cryo-Gel embedding medium
cryogenic spray
cryoglobulin
cryoglobulinemia
    crystal c.
    c., leukemia, arthritis, Sjögren syndrome, and hepatitis B (CLASH)
    mixed c.
cryoglobulinemic
    c. glomerulonephritis
    c. vasculitis
cryohydrocytosis
Cryokwik
cryolysis

C

NOTES

249

CryoMed freezer
Cryomorphaceae
Cryomorpha ignava
cryopathic hemolytic syndrome
cryophila
    Crossiella c.
cryophile
cryophilic
cryophylactic
cryoprecipitated
    c. antihemophilic factor
    c. fibrinogen
cryoprecipitate-depleted plasma
cryoprecipitate transfusion
cryoprecipitation
cryopreservation
cryopreservative
    Microbank c.
cryoprobe
cryoprotectant
cryoprotein
Cryo rubber mold
cryoscope
cryoscopy
cryostat
    Ames Lab-Tek c.
    c. frozen sectioning aid
    quick-cool option on the c.
    c. section
cryotolerant
Cryo-Vac-A cryostat vacuum system
Cryphonectria
crypt
    c. abscess
    adenomatous c.
    alveolar bony c.
    c. architecture
    c. cell carcinoma
    dental c.
    c. dilatation
    c. disarray
    c. distortion
    enamel c.
    c. epithelium
    c. hypoplasia
    c. of iris
    c. isolation technique
    c.'s of Lieberkühn
    lingual c.
    mutated c.
    numbers of unique patterns per c.
    regenerative c.
    synovial c.
    tonsillar c.
cryptal lymphocytic coloproctitis
crypta tonsillaris
cryptic
    c. enzyme
    c. T antigen

cryptitis
    acute c.
    neutrophilic c.
Cryptobacterium curtum
Cryptobia salmositica
Cryptococcaceae
cryptococcal
    c. antigen
    c. antigen titer
    c. meningitis
    c. polysaccharide
cryptococcemia
cryptococci (*pl. of* cryptococcus)
cryptococcoma
cryptococcosis
Cryptococcus
    C. albidus
    C. antibody titer
    C. neoformans
cryptococcus, pl. cryptococci
cryptocrystalline
Cryptocystis trichodectis
Cryptodiaporthe
Cryptogamia
cryptogenic
    c. cirrhosis
    c. infection
    c. organizing pneumonia (COP)
    c. pyemia
    c. septicemia
cryptolith
cryptolytic lesion
cryptomenorrhea
cryptomere
Cryptomyces pleomorpha
cryptophthalmos
cryptophthalmus syndrome
cryptoplasmic
cryptorchidism
cryptorchid testis
Cryptosporangium
    C. aurantiacum
    C. minutisporangium
cryptosporidia
cryptosporidiosis antibody
Cryptosporidium
    C. diagnostic procedure
    C. parvum
Cryptosporiopsis
Cryptostroma corticale
cryptostromosis
cryptoxanthin
cryptozoite
cryptus
    Porphyrobacter c.
crystal
    ammonium biurate c.
    amorphous phosphate c.
    asthma c.

basic calcium phosphate c.
BCP c.
birefringent c.
blood c.
Böttcher c.
calcium oxalate c.
c. cell
Charcot-Leyden c.
Charcot-Neumann c.
Charcot-Robin c.
chiral c.
cholesterol c.
corticosteroid c.
c. cryoglobulinemia
cystine c.
c. deposition disease
ear c.
Florence c.
hematoidin c.
hippuric acid c.
intracytoplasmic c.
knife-rest c.
leukocytic c.
Leyden c.
liquid c.
Lubarsch c.
c. of Lubarsch
mineral c.
monosodium urate c.
MSU c.
Reinke c.
scintillation c.
sperm c.
spermine c.
talc c.
thorn apple c.
triple phosphate c.
twin c.
tyrosine c.
urate c.
uric acid c.
c. urinary cast
urine c.'s
c.'s in urine sediment
urine sediment c.
c. violet
c. violet stain
c. violet vaccine
Virchow c.
whetstone c.

crystal-induced
    c.-i. arthritis
    c.-i. chemotactic factor
crystalline
    c. amylose
    c. birefringence
    c. egg albumin (CEA)
    c. insulin (CI)
    c. macromolecule alteration
    c. zinc insulin
crystallization
    intraglomerular c.
crystallography
    x-ray c.
crystalloid
    Charcot-Böttcher c.
    Charcot-Leyden c.
    Reinke c.
crystalluria
CS
    chorionic somatomammotropin
    corticosteroid
    NATO code for chloracetophenone
    NATO code for o-chlorobenzylidene
    malononitrile
        CS gas
C&S
    culture and sensitivity
        C&S test
Cs
    cesium
CSA
    colony-stimulating activity
    compressed spectral assay
CSD
    cat-scratch disease
CSF
    cerebrospinal fluid
    colony-stimulating factor
        CSF glutamine test
        CSF morphologic investigation
CSH
    capsular synovial-like hyperplasia
    chronic subdural hematoma
    cortical stromal hyperplasia
CSID
    congenital sucrase-isomaltase deficiency
Csillag disease
CSM
    cerebrospinal meningitis
CSPG
    chondroitin sulfate proteoglycan

NOTES

C

CSR
corrected sedimentation rate
cortisol secretion rate
cSt
centistoke
CT
census tract
cerebral thrombosis
circulation time
clotting time
coagulation time
Coombs test
coronary thrombosis
corrected transposition
cytotechnologist
biphasic helical CT
high-resolution CT
CT number
Ct
concentration-time product
Ct$_{50}$
concentration-time product for 50% of
exposed group
effective Ct$_{50}$ (ECt$_{50}$)
incapacitating Ct$_{50}$ (ICt$_{50}$)
lethal Ct$_{50}$ (LCt$_{50}$)
Ct0$_2$
concentration of total oxygen
CTCL
cutaneous T-cell lymphoma
CTD
carpal tunnel decompression
congenital thymic dysplasia
connective tissue disease
Ctenocephalides canis
C-terminal
C-t. assay
C-t. fragment
C-terminus region
CT-guided stereotactic biopsy
CTH
ceramide trihexoside
CTL
cytologic T lymphocyte
CTLA-4 interaction
CTP
cytidine triphosphate
cytosine triphosphate
CTX
cholera toxin
Cu
copper
cu
cubic
Cuban itch
cubic (cu)
c. centimeter (cm^3, cu cm)
c. millimeter (cmm, cu mm, mm^3)

cuboidal
c. carcinoma
c. cell
c. epithelium
simple ciliated c.
cuboidalization
CUC
chronic ulcerative colitis
cu cm (*var. of* cm^3)
CuCN
copper cyanide
cucumerina
Plectosphaerella c.
Trichosanthes c.
cucumerinum
Tracheophilus c.
Typhlocoelum c.
Cucumovirus
cucurbitina
Taenia c.
CUE
confidential unit exclusion
cuff
columnar c.
perivascular c.
cuffing
lymphocytic c.
lymphoid c.
peribronchial c.
perivascular c.
cuffitis
cuirasse
cancer en c.
culbertsoni
Acanthamoeba c.
cul-de-sac
c.-d.-s. mass
c.-d.-s. smear
Culex
C. nigripalpus
C. pipiens
C. quinquefasciatus
C. restuans
C. salinarius
C. tarsalis
culicicola
Aeromonas c.
Culicidae
culicifacies
Anopheles c.
culicis
Agamomermis c.
Culicoides
C. austeni
C. furens
C. milnei
culicosis

Culiseta
   C. inornata
   C. melanura
Cullen sign
cullin family protein
Cult-Dip Plus bacteriologic culture
cultivation
culture
   abscess aerobic c.
   acid-fast c. (AFC)
   Actinomyces c.
   adenovirus c.
   aerobic and anaerobic blood c.
   anaerobic bacteria c.
   animal cell c.
   arterial line c.
   attenuated c.
   bacterial c.
   Bactrol Plus quality control c.
   blood c.
   bronchial aspirate anaerobic c.
   burn c.
   cell wall defective bacteria c.
   cerebrospinal fluid c.
   cervical c.
   Chlamydia c.
   chorioallantoic c.
   clean-catch urine c.
   CMV c.
   colony-forming unit-c. (CFU-C)
   conjunctival fungus c.
   continuous flow c.
   Corynebacterium diphtheriae
    throat c.
   CryoCults c.
   Cult-Dip Plus bacteriologic c.
   cytomegalovirus c.
   direct c.
   duodenal contents c.
   ear c.
   EBV c.
   elective c.
   endometrium anaerobic c.
   enrichment c.
   enterovirus c.
   Epstein-Barr virus c.
   fibroblast c.
   flask c.
   fluid c.
   c. fluid supernatant
   fungus c.
   gastric c.

   genital c.
   gonorrhea c. (GC)
   gravity-settling c. (GSC)
   group A beta hemolytic
    streptococci throat c.
   hanging-block c.
   hanging-drop c.
   Harada-Mori filter paper strip c.
   Helicobacter pylori urease test
    and c.
   herpes simplex virus c.
   HIV c.
   HSV c.
   human immunodeficiency virus c.
   influenza virus c.
   Legionella pneumophila c.
   Leptospira c.
   c. medium
   mixed leukocyte c. (MLC)
   mixed lymphocyte c. (MLC)
   mixed lymphocyte-tumor c.
    (MLTC)
   monoxenic c.
   mumps virus c.
   mycobacteria c.
   nasopharyngeal c.
   needle c.
   Neisseria gonorrhoeae c.
   Nocardia c.
   organ c.
   parainfluenza virus c.
   Petri dish c.
   plate c.
   polymicrobial c.
   pouch c.
   primary explant c.
   print c.
   pure c.
   radioisotopic c.
   RSV c.
   rubella virus c.
   secondary c.
   semiquantitative viral c.
   c. and sensitivity (C&S)
   sensitized c.
   shake c.
   skin fungus c.
   skin mycobacteria c.
   slant c.
   slope c.
   smear c.
   spinal fluid c.

C

NOTES

culture *(continued)*
    sputum fungus c.
    sputum mycobacteria c.
    stab c.
    Staphylococcus aureus
      nasopharyngeal c.
    sterility c.
    stock c.
    stool fungus c.
    stool mycobacteria c.
    streak c.
    synchronized c.
    throat c.
    thrust c.
    tissue c. (TC)
    tube c.
    type c.
    Ureaplasma urealyticum genital c.
    urine fungus c.
    urine mycobacteria c.
    c. of vesicular fluid
    viral c.
    VZV c.
    wound c.
    xenic c.
cultured autologous melanocyte
culturing
    bacterial c.
cu mm *(var. of* cmm)
cummidelens
    Nocardia c.
cumulated activity ratio
cumulative
    c. action
    c. distribution
cumulative-frequency histogram
cumulative-summation technique (cusum)
cumulus
    c. oophorus
    c. ovaricus
cuneate
cuneiform
cuniculatum
    epithelioma c.
cuniculi
    Encephalitozoon c.
    Gemella c.
    Spilopsyllus c.
    Treponema c.
cuniculus
Cunninghamella elegans
cup
    cytospin c.
cupremia
cupric ion-inhibited acid phosphatase
cupriuresis
cuprizone model of chronic demyelination

cuprous
cupula, pl. **cupulae**
    c. ampullaris
    ampullary c.
curare
curariform paralysis
curative dose
curdy pus
curet, curette
curettage
    endocervical c. (ECC)
    endometrial c.
curetting
curie (Ci)
curie-hour (Ci-hr)
curiosum eroticum
curium
curled hair colony
Curling ulcer
currant
    c. jelly appearance
    c. jelly clot
currens
    larva c.
current
    alternating c.
    dark c.
    diffusion c.
    direct c.
    eddy c.
    c. gain
    c. regulator
    saturation c.
    three-phase c.
Curschmann
    C. disease
    C. spiral
curticei
    Cooperia c.
Curtis-Fitz-Hugh syndrome
Curtius syndrome
Curtobacterium herbarum
Curtovirus
curtum
    Cryptobacterium c.
curvata
    Syntrophomonas c.
curvatus
    Lactobacillus c.
curve
    Andrews lymphocyte c.
    calibration c.
    carbon dioxide dissociation c.
    carbon dioxide response c.
    characteristic c.
    distribution c.
    dye-dilution c.
    epidemic c.
    c. fitting

indicator-dilution c.
logarithmic c.
multiple event c.
oxygen-hemoglobin dissociation c.
precipitin c.
pressure-volume c.
Price-Jones c.
regression c.
ROC c.
sigmoid shape of the c.
standard c.
whole-body titration c.
curvilinear body
Curvularia
    C. geniculata
    C. lunata
    C. pallescens
    C. senagalensis
    C. verruculosa
curvus
    Campylobacter c.
Cushing
    C. basophilism
    C. disease
    C. syndrome
    C. ulcer
cushingoid facies
cushion
    muscular c.
custody
    chain of c.
customary temperature scale
cusum
    cumulative-summation technique
cutanea
    sclerosis c.
cutaneomandibular polyoncosis
cutaneomeningospinal angiomatosis
cutaneomucouveal syndrome
cutaneous
    c. amyloidosis
    c. anthrax
    c. anthrax infection
    c. blister
    c. deciduosis
    c. dermal mucinosis
    c. emphysema
    c. extravascular necrotizing granuloma
    c. focal mucinosis
    c. fungus
    c. hemorrhoid

c. horn
c. larva migrans
c. layer of tympanic membrane
c. leishmaniasis
c. leprosy
c. lymphoid hyperplasia (CLH)
c. lymphoma
c. malformation
c. malignant melanoma (CMM)
c. meningioma
c. myiasis
c. necrotizing venulitis
c. perifollicular
c. pseudolymphoma
c. reaction
c. systemic angiitis
c. systemic sclerosis
c. T-cell lymphoma (CTCL)
c. tissue
c. tuberculin test
c. tuberculosis
c. vasculitis
cutaneum
    carcinoma c.
    cornu c.
cutdown
Cuterebra
cuticle
    c. of hair
    c. of root sheath
cuticula, pl. cuticulae
    c. vaginae folliculi pili
cutireaction test
cutis
    amyloidosis c.
    c. anserina
    atrophia maculosa varioliformis c.
    benign lymphocytoma c.
    calcinosis c.
    crista c.
    c. elastica
    glandulae c.
    c. hyperelastica
    hyperelastosis c.
    c. laxa
    leiomyoma c.
    leukemia c.
    neuroma c.
    osteoma c.
    osteosis c.
    stratum reticulare c.
    sulci c.

NOTES

cutis *(continued)*
    tuberculosis c.
    c. vera
    c. verticis gyrata
cutization
cutoff frequency
cut surface
cutter
    agar c.
    rare base c.'s
cutting
    section c.
cuvet, cuvette
CV
    cardiovascular
    cell volume
    coefficient of variation
    corpuscular volume
    cresyl violet
CVA
    cerebrovascular accident
      neonatal CVA
CVD
    cardiovascular disease
    cerebrovascular disease
CVH
    combined ventricular hypertrophy
    common variable
      hypogammaglobulinemia
CVID
    common variable immunodeficiency
      CVID syndrome
CVM
    cerebrovascular malformation
CVOD
    cerebrovascular obstructive disease
CVP
    cell volume profile
CVR
    cerebrovascular resistance
CVRD
    cardiovascular renal disease
CVS
    chorionic villus sampling
    clean-voided specimen
      transabdominal CVS
      transcervical CVS
CVS/CNS
    cardiovascular system and central
      nervous system
CW
    chemical warfare
      CW agent
CWA
    carcinoma with adenomatous areas
CWDF
    cell wall-deficient bacterial form
CWP
    coal worker's pneumoconiosis

CX
    NATO code for phosgene oxime
CX4, CX5, CX9, CX500, CX1000
  PRO clinical system
CX9 ALX clinical system
CX3, CX4, CX5 Delta clinical system
CX4, CX5, CX7 super clinical system
^{14}C-xylose breath test
cyanemia
cyanescens
    Cerinosterus c.
cyanhemoglobin
cyanide
    c. anion
    c. antidote kit
    c. assay
    calcium c. (CaCN)
    copper c. (CuCN)
    diphenylarsine c. (DC)
    ethyl c.
    gold c. (AuCN)
    hydrogen c. (HCN)
    mercuric c.
    mercury c. (HgCN)
    c. poisoning
    potassium c. (KCN)
    c. radical (CN-)
    sodium c. (NaCN)
cyanide-ascorbate test
cyanide-nitroprusside test
cyanidol
cyanin
    alizarin c.
cyaniventris
    Dermatobia c.
cyanmethemoglobin
cyanoacrylate
2-cyanoacrylate
    butyl 2-c.
Cyanobacteria
cyanochroic
cyanochrous
cyanocobalamin Co 57
cyanogen
cyanogriseus
    Actinoalloteichus c.
cyanohydrin metabolite
cyanophil, cyanophile
cyanophilia
    cytoplasmic c.
cyanophilous
cyanophoric glycoside
cyanopus
    Conocybe c.
cyanosed
cyanosis
    enterogenous c.
    false c.

hereditary methemoglobinemic c.
toxic c.
cyanotic
  c. atrophy
  c. atrophy of liver
  c. induration
cyanuria
Cyathostoma bronchialis
Cyathostomum coronatum
Cyathus
cyberattack
cyberterrorism
cybrid
cyclamate
  sodium c.
cyclase
  adenyl c.
  adenylate c.
cycle
  cell c.
  circadian c.
  citric acid c.
  Cori c.
  eukaryotic cell c.
  futile c.
  hair c.
  Krebs c.
  Krebs-Henseleit c.
  menstrual c.
  mitotic c.
  operating c.
  c. per minute (c/min)
  c. per second (cps)
  pregnancy c.
  RANTES c.
  replication c.
  schizogonic c.
  suppression of cell c.
  TCA c.
  tricarboxylic acid c.
  urea c.
cycler
  Perkin-Elmer DNA Thermal C. 480
cyclic
  c. adenosine monophosphate (cAMP)
  c. albuminuria
  c. AMP (cAMP)
  c. AMP test
  c. citrullinated peptide (CCP)
  c. endoperoxide
  c. GMP

c. guanosine monophosphate
c. hydrocarbon
c. neutropenia
c. nucleotide
c. tissue alteration
cyclicum
  Thialkalimicrobium c.
cyclin
  c. A antigen
  c. D1 gene
  c. D1 oncogene
  c. D1 protein
  c. D stain
  c. E antigen
cyclin-dependent
  c.-d. kinase 5 (CDK5)
  c.-d. protein
  c.-d. protein kinase 1 (Cdk1)
cycling probe
cyclitis
cyclitol
cyclitrophicus
  Vibrio c.
cyclization
cycloalkane
cycloalkene
cyclocreatine
cyclodiene hydrocarbon pesticide
cyclodimerization
Cyclodontostomum purvisi
cyclogeny
cyclohexane
cyclohexatriene
cycloheximide
cyclohexylamine
cyclonite
cyclooxygenase-1 (COX-1)
cyclooxygenase-2 (COX-2)
cyclooxygenase enzyme
cyclopentane
cyclopentanoperhydrophenanthrene
cyclophilin A (CypA)
Cyclophyllidea
cyclopia
Cyclops
cyclosarin
  NATO code for c. (GF)
cycloserine
  c. cefoxitin fructose agar
  c. mannitol agar
cyclosis
Cyclospora cayetanensis

NOTES

cyclosporiasis
cyclosporine
cyclotron
cyclozoonosis
cylinder
    axis c.
    Bence Jones c.
    graduated c.
    Külz c.
cylinderization
cylindraxis
cylindrical
    c. bronchiectasis
    c. embryo
    c. epithelium
cylindricum
    stratum c.
cylindroadenoma
Cylindrocarpon
Cylindrocephalum
Cylindrocladium
cylindroid aneurysm
cylindroma
    dermal eccrine c.
cylindromatous carcinoma
cylindrosarcoma
cylindruria
Cymatoderma
cynanche
    c. maligna
    c. tonsillaris
CYNAP
    cytotoxicity negative, absorption positive
cynarae
    Xanthomonas c.
cynodontis
    Leifsonia c.
    Leifsonia xyli subsp. *c.*
cynomolgi
    Plasmodium c.
CYP2D6 drug screen test
CypA
    cyclophilin A
Cyphellopsis
Cypovirus
cypricasei
    Lactobacillus c.
cyproheptadine hydrochloride
cyriacigeorgica
    Nocardia c.
Cyriax syndrome
cyrtometer
cyst
    adventitious c.
    allantoic c.
    alveolar hydatid c.
    aneurysmal bone c. (ABC)
    apoplectic c.
    arachnoid c.

Baker c.
Bartholin c.
blood c.
blue dome c.
bone c.
botryoid odontogenic c.
branchial cleft c.
breast c.
bronchial c.
bronchogenic c.
bursal c.
calcifying odontogenic c.
cerebellar c.
chocolate c.
choledochal c.
chyle c.
ciliated hepatic foregut c.
colloid c.
compound c.
congenital c.
corpus hemorrhagicum c.
corpus luteum c.
Cowper c.
Dandy-Walker c.
daughter c.
dental follicular c.
dentigerous c.
dermoid c.
dermoid c. of ovary
developmental jaw c.
distention c.
duplication c.
echinococcus c.
embryonal duct c.
endometrial c.
endothelial c.
enterogenous c.
ependymal c.
epidermal inclusion c. (EIC)
epidermoid inclusion c.
epididymal c.
epithelial inclusion c.
extravasation c.
exudation c.
false c.
fissural c.
c. fluid cytology
follicle c.
follicular c.
foregut c.
ganglion c.
Gartner c.
gas c.
germinal epithelial inclusion c.
gingival c.
glandular odontogenic c.
globulomaxillary c.
glomerular c.
granddaughter c.

hemorrhagic c.
hepatic c.
hydatid c.
implantation c.
inclusion c.
inflammatory odontogenic c.
involution c.
iodine c.
c. of Jadassohn
junctional c.
keratinous c.
Kobelt c.
lacteal c.
leptomeningeal c.
liver c.
luteal c.
luteinized follicular c.
meibomian c.
mesonephric c.
mesothelial c.
milium c.
milk c.
mixed multilocular thymic c.
Morgagni c.
mother c.
mucinous c.
mucous c.
multilocular hydatid c.
multiloculate hydatid c.
myxoid c.
nabothian c.
nasolabial c.
nasopalatine duct c.
necrotic c.
neural c.
nonodontogenic c.
odontogenic c.
oil c.
oophoritic c.
orbital c.
orthokeratinized odontogenic c.
  (OOC)
osseous hydatid c.
ovarian c.
palatal c.
pancreatic c.
paradental c.
paraphysial c.
parasitic c.
parathyroid c.
parent c.
paroophoritic c.

parvilocular c.
pericardial c.
periodontal c.
phaeohyphomycotic c.
phaeomycotic c.
pilar c.
piliferous c.
pilonidal c.
pineal c.
posttraumatic leptomeningeal c.
primordial c.
proliferating trichilemmal c.
proliferation c.
proliferative c.
proliferous c.
pseudomucinous c.
radicular c.
ranular c.
Rathke cleft c.
renal c.
retention c.
sanguineous c.
sebaceous c.
secretory c.
seminal vesical c.
sequestration c.
serous c.
simple bone c.
simple renal c.
simple solitary c.
sinus c.
smooth-walled c.
solitary bone c.
sterile c.
sublingual c.
suprasellar c.
surgical ciliated c.
synovial c.
Tarlov c.
tarry c.
tarsal c.
tension c.
teratomatous c.
theca lutein c.
third pharyngeal pouch c.
thyroglossal duct c.
thyroid c.
thyrolingual c.
traumatic bone c.
trichilemmal c.
tubular c.
umbilical c.

C

NOTES

cyst *(continued)*
    unicameral bone c.
    unilocular hydatid c.
    urachal c.
    urinary c.
    utricular c.
    vellus hair c.
    vitellointestinal c.
    wolffian c.
cystacanth
cystadenocarcinoma
    mucinous c.
    papillary serous c.
    primary mammary mucinous c.
    pseudomucinous c.
    serous c.
cystadenofibroma
    serous c.
cystadenoma
    hepatobiliary c.
    c. lymphomatosum
    mucinous c.
    oncocytic papillary c.
    papillary c.
    pseudomucinous c.
    serous c.
cystathionase
cystathionine
    urine c.
cystathionine-beta-synthase
cystathionine-gamma-lyase
cystathioninuria
cystauchenitis
cystaugens
    Jannaschia c.
cysteamine
cystectasia
cystectasy
cysteic acid method
cysteine test
cysteinyl
cystic
    c. acute inflammation
    c. adenomatoid malformation
    c. ameloblastoma
    c. atrophy
    c. bronchiectasis
    c. carcinoma
    c. chronic cervicitis
    c. chronic inflammation
    c. corpus hemorrhagicum
    c. corpus luteum
    c. degeneration
    c. dermoid teratoma
    c. diathesis
    c. disease
    c. disease of the breast
    c. disease of lung
    c. disease of renal medulla

    c. duct
    c. endometrial hyperplasia
    c. fibrosis (CF)
    c. fibrosis of pancreas (CFP)
    c. fibrosis test
    c. fibrosis transmembrane
      conductance regulator (CFTR)
    c. fibrosis transmembrane
      conductance regulator gene
    c. goiter
    c. granulomatous inflammation
    c. hamartoma
    c. hygroma
    c. hyperplasia of the breast
    c. hyperplasia of endometrium
    c. hypersecretory ductal carcinoma
      in situ
    c. hypersecretory hyperplasia
    c. kidney
    c. lymphangiectasis
    c. mastitis
    c. mastopathy
    c. medial necrosis (CMN)
    c. medial necrosis of ascending
      aorta (CMN-AA)
    c. medionecrosis
    c. mole
    c. myxoma
    c. nephroma
    c. ovarian follicle
    c. papillomatous craniopharyngioma
    c. partially differentiated
      nephroblastoma (CPDN)
    c. polyp
    c. prostatic hyperplasia
    c. struma
cystica
    colpohyperplasia c.
    cystitis c.
    medionecrosis aortae idiopathica c.
    osteitis fibrosa c.
    osteitis tuberculosa multiplex c.
    pachyvaginitis c.
    pneumatosis intestinalis c.
    pyelitis c.
    spina bifida c.
    ureteritis c.
    vaginitis c.
cysticerci *(pl. of* cysticercus)
cysticercoid
cysticercosis titer
Cysticercus
    C. bovis
    C. cellulosae
    C. fasciolaris
    C. ovis
    C. tenuicollis
cysticercus, pl. **cysticerci**

cysticum
  acanthoma adenoides c.
  epithelioma adenoides c.
  hygroma colli c.
  lymphangioma c.
cysticus
  ductus c.
cystides (*pl. of* cystis)
cystification
cystiform
cystigerous
cystine
  c. calculus
  c. crystal
  c. stone
  c. storage disease
  c. trypticase agar
  urine c.
cystinemia
cystinosis
cystinotic leukocyte
cystinuria
  familial c.
  c. test
cystiphorous
cystis, pl. **cystides**
cystitis
  acute hemorrhagic c.
  banal c.
  calcareous c.
  chronic interstitial c.
  c. colli
  c. cystica
  eosinophilic c.
  erosive c.
  follicular c.
  c. follicularis
  c. glandularis
  hemorrhagic c.
  Hunner c.
  interstitial c. (IC)
  c. pneumatoides
  polypoid c.
  radiation c.
  schistosomal c.
  tuberculous c.
  ulcerative c.
cystoadenoma
cystocarcinoma
cystocele
Cystoderma
cystodiverticulum

cystoepithelioma
cystofibroma
Cystofilobasidium
cystogenic aneurysm
cystoid macular degeneration
cystolith
cystolithiasis
cystolithic
cystoma
  parvilocular c.
  serous c.
cystomorphous
cystomyoma
cystomyxoadenoma
cystomyxoma
Cystoopsis scomber
cystopherous
cystoprostatectomy
cystoptosia
cystoptosis
cystopyelitis
cystopyelonephritis
cystosarcoma phyllodes (CP)
cystoureteritis
cystourethritis
cystourethrocele
cystous
Cystoviridae
Cystovirus
cystyl
cytapheresis
  therapeutic c.
cytase
Cytauxzoon
cytauxzoonosis
cythemolytic icterus
cytidine
  c. diphosphate (CDP)
  c. monophosphate (CMP)
  c. triphosphate (CTP)
cytidine-5'-phosphate
cytidylic acid
cytidylyl
cytoadhesin
cytoanalyzer
cytoarchitectonics
cytoarchitectural
cytoarchitecture
cytobiology
cytobiotaxis
cytoblast
cytoblastema

C

NOTES

cytoblock technique
cytocentrifugation
cytocentrifuge
    Aerospray c.
    CytoFuge 2 c.
    Cytopro c.
    Cyto-Tek c.
cytocentrum
cytochalasin B, D
cytochemical probe
cytochemistry
cytochrome
    c. bc1 complex
    c. b5 reductase
    c. b5 reductase assay
    c. b5 reductase gene
    c. C protein
    c. oxidase
    c. oxidase test
cytochylema
cytocidal
cytocide
cytoclasis
cytoclastic
cytoclesis
cytocrine secretion
cytocyst
cytode
cytodegenerative necrosis
cytodiagnosis
    exfoliative c.
cytodieresis
cytodifferentiation
cytofluorimetric analysis
cytofluorography
cytofluorometer
cytofluorometry
CytoFuge
    C. 2 centrifuge
    C. 2 cytocentrifuge
cytogene
cytogenetic
    c. analysis
    clinical c.'s
    c. disorder
    c. map
    population c.'s
    c. study
cytogenous
cytoglucopenia
cytohyaloplasm
cytoid body
cytokeratin (CK)
    c. 1–20
    c. 1–20 antigen
    c. antigen-antibody reaction
    c. expression
    c. filament

high molecular weight c. (HMW-CK)
    c. immunoreactivity
    c. neoepitope
cytokine
    chemotactic c.
    c. formation
    multiplexed fluorescent microsphere immunoassay for TH1, TH2 c.'s
    c. network
    proinflammatory c.
cytokines
cytokinesis
cytolemma
cytolipin H
CytoLite luminescence assay system
cytologic
    c. abnormality
    c. alteration
    c. atypia
    c. brushings
    c. degeneration
    c. diagnosis
    c. engulfment
    c. examination
    c. filter preparation
    c. nuclear grading
    c. screening
    c. smear
    c. specimen
    c. T lymphocyte (CTL)
cytologist
cytology
    abrasive c.
    analytic c.
    aspiration biopsy c. (ABC)
    balloon c.
    Bethesda 2001 terminology for reporting results of cervical c.
    bronchial washing c.
    brushings c.
    cerebrospinal fluid c.
    cervical-vaginal c.
    cyst fluid c.
    cytomegalic inclusion disease c.
    effusion c.
    endometrial c.
    exfoliative c.
    fine-needle aspiration c. (FNAC)
    herpes c.
    image c.
    impression c.
    intraoperative c.
    nasal c.
    needle aspiration c.
    nipple discharge c.
    ocular c.
    oral cavity c.
    sputum c.

thin-layer c.
ThinPrep c.
touch imprint c.
urine c.
washing c.
cytolymph
cytolysate
blood c.
cytolysin
cytolysis
immune c.
cytolysosome
CytoLyt fixative
cytolytic
T (cell) c. (Tc)
c. T-cell lysis assay
cytoma
cytomatrix
cytomegalic
c. cell
c. inclusion disease (CID, CMID)
c. inclusion disease cytology
c. inclusion disease virus
Cytomegalovirus
cytomegalovirus (CMV)
c. antibody
c. culture
c. disease
c. esophagitis
c. infection
c. isolation
c. lymphadenitis
cytomegaly
cytomembrane
cytomere
cytometaplasia
cytometer
Bayer Technicon H1 automated
flow c.
CAS 200 image c.
Cell Lab IC 100 image c.
Epics C flow c.
Epics Profile flow c.
FACScalibur flow c.
FACScan flow c.
FACSort flow c.
FACStar Plus flow c.
FACSVantage flow c.
flow c.
MAXM hematology flow c.
cytometric image analysis

cytometry
CD-Chex C34 control for flow c.
CD-Chex Plus control for flow c.
cell-suspension flow c.
DNA flow c.
Feulgen c.
flow c. (FC, FCM)
gel and flow c.
image c.
multiparameter flow c.
cytomicrosome
Cytomics FC 500 series flow cytometry system
cytomorphology
cytomorphosis
cyton
cytonuclear
c. atypia
c. pleomorphism
cytopathic effect
cytopathogenesis
cytopathogenic virus
cytopathologic, cytopathological
cytopathologist
cytopathology
nongynecologic c. (NGC)
cytopathy
cytopenia
Cytophagaceae
Cytophagales
cytophagic histiocytic panniculitis
cytophagous
cytophagy
cytophanere
cytopharynx
cytophil group
cytophilic antibody
cytophotometer
cytophotometry
DNA c.
flow c.
cytophylactic
cytophylaxis
cytophyletic
cytopipette
cytoplasm
abundant c.
amphophilic c.
basophilic c.
blue c.
eosinophilic c.
foamy c.

NOTES

cytoplasm *(continued)*
  glassy c.
  ground glass c.
  intensely basophilic c.
  lavender c.
  light-staining apical c.
  neurofibril in c.
  c. of neuron
  paranuclear c.
  pink c.
  rim of scant c.
  c. of smooth muscle
  vacuolated c.
  water clear c.
cytoplasmic
  c. antineutrophil cytoplasmic antibody (cANCA)
  c. antineutrophil cytoplasmic autoantibody (cANCA)
  c. bleb
  c. bridge
  c. crystalline aggregate
  c. cyanophilia
  c. extension
  c. fiber alteration
  c. fibril alteration
  c. filament alteration
  c. glycogen
  c. granulation
  c. immunoreactivity
  c. inclusion
  c. inclusion body
  c. inheritance
  c. lipid aggregate
  c. lipid droplet alteration
  c. macromolecule aggregate
  c. matrix
  c. matrix alteration
  c. membrane
  c. organelle
  c. pattern
  c. process
  c. projection
  c. ratio
  c. snout
  c. staining
  c. striation
  c. tail
  c. vacuole
  c. vacuolization
cytoplast
cytopoiesis
cytopreparation
Cytopro cytocentrifuge
cytopuncture
  fine-needle c.
  c. smear
cytopyge
cytoreductive therapy

Cytorhabdovirus
CytoRich
  C. cervical cytology monolayer system
  C. Red fixative
cytorrhyctes
cytoryctes
cytoscopy
cytoscreener
cytosine
  c. arabinoside (CA)
  guanine c. (GC)
  c. phosphate guanine (CpG)
  c. triphosphate (CTP)
cytosine-guanine-guanine (CGG)
cytosis
cytoskeletal
  c. filament
  c. polymerization
  c. protein
  c. protein hyperphosphorylation disease
cytoskeleton
  actin c.
cytoskeleton-associated protein
cytosmear
cytosol
  aminopeptidase c.
  bovine smooth muscle c.
cytosolic concentration of calcium ions
cytosome
cytospin
  c. analysis
  c. cup
  c. slide centrifuge gram-stained smear
Cytospora
cytospray fixation
cytostasis
Cyto-Stat/Coulter CLONE monoclonal antibody
cytostatic
cytostome
cytotactic
cytotaxia
cytotaxis
  negative c.
  positive c.
cytotechnologist (CT)
Cyto-Tek cytocentrifuge
cytothesis
cytotoxic
  c. antibody
  c. chemotherapy
  c. edema
  c. hypersensitivity reaction
  c. necrosis
  c. protein

T (cell) c. (Tc)
c. T cell
cytotoxicity
antibody-dependent cell-mediated c.
antimediated c.
c. assay
cell-dependent c. (CDC)
complement-mediated c.
lymphocyte-mediated c. (LMC)
c. negative, absorption positive
(CYNAP)
cytotoxin
binary c.
vero c.
cytotrophic (*var. of* cytotropic)
cytotrophoblast
cytotrophoblastic cell
cytotropic, cytotrophic
c. antibody
c. antibody test

cytotropism
cytozoic
cytozoon
cytozyme
cyturia
Cytyc
C. CytoLyt preservative solution
C. PreservCyt preservative solution
Czapek-Dox
C.-D. agar
C.-D. medium
Czapek solution agar
Czermak
globular space of C.
C. space
Czerny disease

C

NOTES

D

    D antigen
    D cell
    D colony
    D line
    D value

2D

    two-dimensional

D_{CO}

    diffusing capacity for carbon monoxide

D^u

    D. negative
    D. positive

d

    decigram

D-

    sterically related to D-glyceraldehyde

D10 antigen
Daae disease
Daae-Finsen disease
DAB

    diaminobenzidine
    dimethylaminoazobenzene
        DAB reaction

Dabska tumor
DAC

    diazacholesterol
    digital-to-analog converter

dacarbazine
Dacie method
D/A converter
DaCosta

    D. disease
    D. syndrome

dacrocyte
Dacron patch
Dacrymyces
dacryoadenitis
dacryoblennorrhea
dacryocyst
dacryocystitis
dacryocyte
dacryolith

    Desmarres d.
    Nocardia d.

dacryoma
dacryosolenitis
Dactylaria gallopava
dactylitis
Dactylium dendroides
Dactylogyrus
dactylolysis spontanea
DAD

    diffuse alveolar damage

Daedalea

Daedaleopsis
daejeonensis

    Paenibacillus d.

DAF

    decay accelerating factor

Da Fano stain
DAG

    diacylglycerol
    diffuse antral gastritis

DAGT

    direct antiglobulin test

DAH

    disordered action of heart

Dakin solution
Dako

    D. Autostainer
    D. Envision system peroxidase
    D. Fast Red Substrate System
    D. hepatocyte immunostain
    D. HercepTest
    D. large volume LSAB2 alkaline phosphatase kit
    D. target retrieval solution

DakoCytomation EGFR pharmDx colorectal cancer diagnostic kit
dalapon
Dale-Laidlaw clotting time method
Dalen-Fuchs nodule
Dale reaction
Dallas myocarditis criteria
DALM

    dysplasia-associated lesion or mass

Dalrymple disease
Dalton law
damage

    antibody-mediated vascular d.
    diffuse alveolar d. (DAD)
    end-organ d.
    irradiation d.
    irreversible d.
    minimal brain d. (MBD)
    myocardial d.
    ossicular d.
    radiation d.

damaged

    d. during passage
    d. fibrotic valve

Damalina
Damalinia
D-amino acid oxidase
dammar
dammini

    Ixodes d.

damnosum

    Simulium d.

D

dAMP
  deoxyadenosine monophosphate
damping
Dam unit
Danbolt-Closs syndrome
dance
  brachial d.
  hilar d.
  hilus d.
  St. Anthony d.
  St. Guy d.
  St. John d.
dandy fever
Dandy-Walker
  D.-W. cyst
  D.-W. malformation
  D.-W. syndrome
Dane
  D. and Herman keratin stain
  D. method
  D. particle
danicus
  Aneurinibacillus d.
Danielssen-Boeck disease
Danielssen disease
dankaliense
  Trichophyton a.
dankaliensis
  Gymnoascus d.
Danlos syndrome
DANS
  1-dimethylaminonaphthalene-5-sulfonic
    acid
dansyl chloride
Danubian endemic familial nephropathy
Danysz phenomenon
DAOS
  N-ethyl-N-(2-hydroxy-3-sulfopropyl)-3,
    5-dimethoxyaniline
DAP
  death-associated protein
  dihydroxyacetone phosphate
DAPI
  4,6-diamidino-2-phenylindole-2-HCl
  DAPI dye
  DAPI stain
DAPT
  direct agglutination pregnancy test
D-arabitol dehydrogenase
DARC
  Duffy antigen receptor for chemokine
Darier disease
Darier-Roussy sarcoid
dark
  d. cell
  d. current
  d. reaction
  d. reactivation

dark-field
  d.-f. condenser
  d.-f. examination
  fluorescent antibody d.-f. (FADF)
  d.-f. microscope
  d.-f. microscopy
dark-ground microscope
Darling disease
darlingi
  Anopheles d.
Darlington amplifier
Darrow
  D. red
  D. red stain
d'Arsonval meter
dartoic tissue
dartos
  d. muliebris
  d. muscle
  tunica d.
dashboard knee
dassonvillei
  Nocardiopsis d.
Dasyprocta
DAT
  differential agglutination titer
  diphtheria antitoxin
  direct agglutination test
  direct antiglobulin test
data, sing. **datum**
  analog d.
  categorical d.
  metric d.
  ranked d.
database
  GenBank d.
  unigene d.
date fever
Datronia
datum (*sing. of* data)
Datura stramonium
daughter
  d. cell
  d. colony
  d. cyst
daurensis
  Heliorestis d.
Davainea
Davaineidae
Davenport graph
David disease
Davidoff cell
Davidsohn
  D. differential absorption test
  D. modification of Paul-Bunnell
    heterophile antibody test
Davies disease
davtiani
  Teladorsagia d.

dawn phenomenon
Dawson encephalitis
Day test
DB
dextran blue
DBA
dibenzanthracene
DBC
dye-binding capacity
DBCL
dilute blood clot lysis
DBI
development-at-birth index
DC
dendritic cell
diphenylarsine cyanide
DCA
deoxycholate-citrate agar
DCC
dextran-coated charcoal
DCC assay
DCF
direct centrifugal flotation
DCIS
ductal carcinoma in situ
DCO
diffusing capacity for carbon monoxide
DCT
direct Coombs test
DCTMA
desoxycorticosterone trimethylacetate
DCTPA
desoxycorticosterone triphenylacetate
DDD
dense-deposit disease
dichlorodiphenyldichloroethane
digital differential display
dihydroxydinaphthyl disulfide
DDD analysis
DDGE
denaturing density gradient
electrophoresis
D-dimer
D-d. assay
D-d. test
DDR
discoidin domain receptor
DDS
dystrophy-dystocia syndrome
DDT
dichlorodiphenyltrichloroethane
DDT assay

DDVP
dimethyldichlorovinyl phosphate
de
de Castro fluid
de Clerambault syndrome
de Galantha method for urates
de Lange syndrome
de Morgan spot
de novo tissue formation
de Quervain disease
de Quervain tenosynovitis
de Quervain thyroiditis
de Ritis ratio
de Sanctis-Cacchione syndrome
de Toni-Fanconi syndrome
deacetylase
histone d. (HDAC)
deactivation
deacylase
acylsphingosine d.
deacylate
dead
d. of disease (DOD)
d. fetus in utero (DFU)
d. finger
d. on arrival (DOA)
d. time
dead-end host
deadly agaric
dead-space hyponatremia
DEAE
diethylaminoethyl
DEAE anion exchange
chromatography
DEAE cellulose
DEAE-Sephacel ion exchange column
dealbata
Clitocybe d.
dealbation
dealcoholization
deallergization
deallergize
deaminase
adenine d.
adenosine d. (ADA)
adenylate d.
adenylic acid d.
AMP d.
guanine d.
histidine alpha d.
myoadenylate d.
porphobilinogen d.

D

NOTES

deaquation
dearterialization
death
    activation-induced cell d. (AICD)
    autoerotic d.
    black d.
    brain d.
    cause of d. (COD)
    cell d.
    cerebral d.
    contributory cause of d.
    crib d.
    early neonatal d.
    d. effector domain
    fetal d.
    d. fever
    functional d.
    indirect maternal d.
    infant d.
    infectious cause of d. (ICOD)
    intrauterine fetal d. (IUFD)
    d. investigation resources
    late neonatal d.
    local d.
    manner of d.
    maternal d.
    natural d.
    neonatal d. (ND, NND)
    nonrenal d. (NRD)
    d. notification
    perinatal d.
    programmed cell d.
    somatic d.
    sports-related sudden d.
    sudden cardiac d. (SCD)
    sudden coronary d. (SCD)
    sudden intrauterine unexplained d. (SIUD)
    sudden unexpected d. (SUD)
    sudden unexpected, unexplained d. (SUUD)
    sudden unexplained d. (SUD)
    sudden unexplained infant d. (SUID)
    d. trance
    underlying cause of d.
death-associated protein (DAP)
DeBakey aortic assay
Debaromyces japonicus
Debaryomyces
    D. hansenii
    D. hominis
    D. neoformans
Debove membrane
debrancher deficiency limit dextrinosis
debranching enzyme
Debré phenomenon
Debré-Semelaigne syndrome
débridement

debris
    amorphous eosinophilic d.
    cellular d.
    inflammatory cell d.
    karyorrhectic nuclear d.
    lamellated collection of inspissated inflammatory d.
    purulent d.
    stonelike d.
debubbling
debug
debye
DEC1
    differentiated embryo-chondrocyte expressed gene 1
decade counter
decagram
decalcification
    AB d.
decalcified bone
Decalcifier
    Surgipath D. I, II
decalcify
decalcifying
decaliter
Decal Plus
decameter
decanoic acid
decanoyl-Arg-Val-Lys-Arg-chloromethylketone (dec-RVKR-cmk)
decant
decantation
decaplanina
    Amycolatopsis d.
decarboxylase
    aromatic l-amino acid d. (AADC)
    branched-chain alpha keto acid d.
    d. broth
    glutamate d.
    glutamic acid d. (GAD)
    histidine d. (HDC)
    hydroxytryptophan d.
    methylmalonyl-CoA d.
    ornithine d.
    orotidine-5′-phosphate d.
    orotidylate d.
    oxaloacetate d.
    uroporphyrinogen d. (UROD)
decarboxylation
    amine precursor uptake and d. (APUD)
decay (DK)
    d. accelerating factor (DAF)
    alpha d.
    d. antibody-accelerating factor
    beta d.
    branching d.
    d. coefficient
    d. constant

exponential d.
d. mode
positron beta d.
d. product
radioactive d.
d. rate
d. scheme
deceleration of head
decentration
decerebrate rigidity
dechloracetivorans
    Desulfovibrio d.
Dechloromonas agitata
Dechlorosoma suillum
decibel
decidua
d. basalis
d. capsularis
ectopic d.
membrana d.
d. vera
decidual
d. alteration
d. cast
d. cell
d. change
d. endometritis
d. membrane
d. metaplasia
d. microvessel
d. plate
d. polyp
d. reaction
decidualis
periappendicitis d.
decidualized endometrium
deciduitis
membranous d.
deciduoid
deciduoma
Loeb d.
deciduosis
cutaneous d.
deciduous
d. membrane
d. skin
decigram (d)
decile
deciliter (dL)
milligram per d. (mg/dL)
decimal reduction time
decimeter (dm)

decipiens
    Phocanema d.
    Pseudoterranova d.
    Terranova d.
decision
d. table
warfarin dosing d.
decoagulant
decode
decoder
decolorationis
    Bacillus d.
decolorize
decolorizer
decompensation
cardiac d.
d. injury
d. sickness
decomposition potential
decompression
carpal tunnel d. (CTD)
d. injury
d. sickness
decontaminating room
decontamination
dry d.
external d.
internal d.
d. wipe
d. zone
deconvolution fluorescence microscopy
decora
    Macrobdella d.
decorin
decorporate
decortication
decoy cell
decrease in bone mass
decreased
d. cardiac output
d. creatine clearance
d. serum iron
decrement
dec-RVKR-cmk
decanoyl-Arg-Val-Lys-Arg-
chloromethylketone
decubation
decubitus
d. calculus
d. ulcer
decurrent

D

NOTES

decussate
decussatio, pl. **decussationes**
decussation
dedifferentiated
    d. chondrosarcoma
    d. liposarcoma
    d. low-grade adenocarcinoma
dedifferentiation phenomenon
deefferentation
deep
    d. agar
    d. cell
    d. cortex
    d. fascia
    d. penetrating nevus (DPN)
    rapture of the d.
    d. vein thrombosis (DVT)
    d. wedge biopsy
deer
    epizootic hemorrhagic disease of d.
    hemorrhagic disease of d.
deerfly
    d. disease
    d. fever (tularemia)
Deetjen body
de-expression
def
    deficiency
defect
    acquired d.
    aldosterone secretion d. (ASD)
    aortic septal d.
    atrial septal d. (ASD)
    blast-induced cognitive d.
    blast-induced memory d.
    congenital ectodermal d.
    congenital hemidysplasia with
      ichthyosiform erythroderma and
      limb d.'s (CHILD)
    cortical d.
    coupling d.
    diffusion d.
    dual hemostatic d.
    ectodermal d.
    endocardial cushion d.
    fibrous cortical d.
    filling d.
    focal bone marrow d.
    Gerbode d.
    hydrogen-detected ventricular
      septal d. (HVSD)
    interatrial septal d. (IASD)
    interventricular septal d. (IVSD)
    intraventricular conduction d.
      (IVCD)
    iodide transport d.
    iodotyrosine deiodinase d.
    isolated conotruncal heart d.
    labyrinthine d. (LD)

    lingual mandibular salivary
      gland d.
    mitotic spindle d.
    neural tube d.
    no significant d. (NSD)
    organification d.
    perfusion d.
    plasma d. (PD)
    platelet d. (PLD)
    protein d.
    red cell membrane protein d.
    septal d. (SD)
    serum d. (SD)
    solubilization d.
    surgical d.
    transport protein d.
    ventilation d.
    ventricular septal d. (VSD)
    zero d.'s (Z/D)
defective
    d. bacteriophage
    d. formation of mesenchymal tissue
    d. interfering (DI)
    d. interfering particle
    d. phage
    d. probacteriophage
    d. prophage
    d. virus
defense
    host d.'s
    d. mechanism
defensin
deferens
    ductus d.
    vas d.
deferent
    d. canal
    d. duct
deferentis
    tunica mucosa ductus d.
    tunica muscularis ductus d.
deferentitis
deferoxamine
    d. challenge test
    d. mesylate
    d. mesylate infusion test
Deferribacter
    D. abyssi
    D. desulfuricans
    D. thermophilus
Deferribacteraceae
Deferribacterales
Deferribacteres
defervescent stage
defibrinated blood
defibrination syndrome
defibrinogenating effect
deficiency (def)
    A1AT d.

acid maltase d.
acquired C1EInh d.
ADA d.
adenosine deaminase d.
adenylate kinase d.
ADH d.
alpha₁ antitrypsin d.
alpha galactosidase A d.
alphalipoprotein d.
d. anemia
antidiuretic hormone d.
antitrypsin d.
argininosuccinate synthetase d.
B-cell d.
beta-ᴅ-glucuronidase d.
brancher d.
carbamoyl phosphate synthetase
  I d.
carnitine palmitoyltransferase 2 d.
CD11/CD18 d.
cholesterol side-chain cleavage
  enzyme d.
clotting factor d.
collagen receptor d.
congenital lactase d.
congenital sucrase-isomaltase d.
  (CSID)
CPS d.
CPT2 d.
CR3 d.
desmolase d.
dihydropteridine reductase d.
disaccharidase d.
d. disease
duplication d.
factor I, II, V, VII, VIII, IX, X,
  XI d.
ferrochelatase d.
folic acid d.
fructose 1,6-diphosphatase d.
galactokinase d.
GALT d.
glucose-6-phosphate
  dehydrogenase d.
glucosephosphate isomerase d.
glutathione reductase d.
glutathione synthetase d.
d. of gonadotropin
growth hormone d. (GHD)
heparin cofactor II d.
hepatic lipase d.

hereditary plasmathromboplastin
  component d.
hexosaminidase A d.
HLA class I d.
human growth hormone d.
IL-2 receptor alpha-chain d.
immune d.
immunity d.
immunological d.
iodine d.
lactase d.
LCAT d.
leukocyte adhesion d. (LAD)
lipoprotein lipase d.
medullary serotonergic network d.
mineralocorticoid d.
multiple carboxylase d. (MCD)
myeloperoxidase d.
myoadenylate deaminase d.
ornithine carbamoyltransferase d.
ornithine transcarbamoylase d.
OTC d.
d. of pancreatic enzyme
phosphofructokinase d.
phosphohexose isomerase d.
phosphorylase d.
PK d.
placental steroid sulfatase d.
d. of plasma clotting factor
plasma thromboplastin antecedent d.
plasminogen activator d.
PNP d.
porphobilinogen deaminase d.
porphobilinogen synthase d.
prothrombin d.
protoporphyrinogen oxidase d.
pseudocholinesterase d.
PTA d.
PTC d.
purine nucleoside phosphorylase d.
pyruvate kinase d.
red blood cell enzyme d.
secondary antibody d.
selective d.
SPCA d.
specific antibody d.
specific coagulation factor d.
stable factor d.
sulfite oxidase d.
systemic ʟ-carnitine d.
tenascin-X d.
thiamine d.

D

NOTES

deficiency *(continued)*
thromboplastin antecedent d.
triosephosphate isomerase d.
tuftsin d.
tyrosinase d.
uroporphyrinogen decarboxylase d.
uroporphyrinogen III cosynthase d.
uroporphyrinogen synthase d.
vitamin B_{12} d.
vitamin K d.
ZAP-70 d.
zinc d.
ZPI d.

deficit
base d. (BD)

defined
d. culture medium
serologically d. (SD)
d. substrate (DS)

definition
recursive d.

definitive
d. callus
d. characterization
d. erythroblast
d. host
d. lysosome
d. method
d. organism identification

deflagration
deflection signal
deflorescence
Defluvibacter
D. lusatiensis
defluvii
Aquamicrobium d.
Chryseobacterium d.
Pseudaminobacter d.

defoliant
deformability
deformans
arthritis d.
endarteritis d.
hyperostosis corticalis d.
osteitis d.
osteochondrodystrophia d.
peritonitis d.

deformation
deforming
deformity
acquired d.
Arnold-Chiari d.
congenital musculoskeletal d.
Erlenmeyer flask d.
gibbus d.
J-sella d.
Klippel-Feil d.
lobster-claw d.
Michel d.

pigeon-breast d.
swan-neck d.
valgus d.
varus d.

deg
degeneration
degree

degeneracy
degenerate
d. code
d. oligonucleotide-primed (DOP)
d. oligonucleotide primed
polymerase chain reaction (DOP-PCR)

degenerated
d. intervertebral disc
d. intervertebral fibrocartilage
d. meniscus

degenerating
d. myelin demonstration
d. secretory cell

degeneratio
degeneration (deg)
adipose d.
albuminoid d.
albuminous d.
Alzheimer fibrillary d.
amyloid d.
angiolithic d.
ascending d.
atheromatous d.
axonal d.
ballooning d.
basophilic granular d.
calcareous d.
capsular lipochondral d.
carneous d.
caseous d.
cellular d.
cerebellar d.
cloudy swelling d.
collagen d.
colliquative d.
colloid d.
complete reaction of d. (CRD)
corticobasal d.
Crooke hyaline d.
cystic d.
cystoid macular d.
cytologic d.
descending d.
elastoid d.
elastotic d.
fatty d.
feathery d.
fibrinoid d.
fibrinous d.
fibrous d.
floccular d.

foamy d.
granular d.
granulovacuolar d.
gray d.
hepatolenticular d.
hyaline d.
hydatid d.
hydropic d.
lateral collateral ligament d.
lenticular progressive d.
lipid d.
lipochondral d. (LCD)
lipoid d.
liquefaction d.
liquefactive d.
medial collateral ligament d.
meniscal d.
Mönckeberg d.
mucinoid d.
mucinous d.
mucoid medial d.
myelin d.
myelinic d.
myxohyaline d.
myxoid d.
myxomatous d.
neurofibrillary d. (tau)
Nissl d.
parenchymatous d.
partial reaction of d. (PRD)
pigmentary d.
pseudomucinous d.
pseudotubular d.
reaction of d. (DeR, DR)
red d.
reticular d.
retrograde d.
Schnabel cavernous d.
secondary d.
senile d.
spongiform d.
striatonigral d.
subacute combined d. (SACD, SCD)
transsynaptic d.
Türck d.
vacuolar d.
wallerian d. (WD)
waxy d.
Zenker d.
degenerativa
melanosis corii d.

degenerative
d. arthritis
d. change
d. index
d. inflammation
d. joint disease (DJD)
d. pannus
degenerativus
pannus d.
degerlachei
Flavobacterium d.
deglycerolization
Degos
D. disease
D. syndrome
degradation
autooxidative d.
glycogen d.
proteolytic d.
degranulation
degree (deg)
degrees of freedom (df)
Dehalobacter restrictus
dehalogenans
Anaeromyxobacter d.
Dehalospirillum multivorans
dehiscence
dehydrase
aminolevulinic acid d. (ALAD, ALA-D)
dehydratase
carbonate d.
dehydrate
dehydrated alcohol
dehydration
dehydroascorbic acid
dehydrobilirubin
dehydroepiandrosterone (DHEA)
d. sulfate (DHEAS)
dehydrogenase
acyl-CoA d.
alcohol d. (ADH)
aldehyde d.
alpha-keto acid d.
beta-hydroxy-delta-5-steroid d.
branched-chain alpha keto acid d.
D-arabitol d.
flipped pattern of lactate d.
formaldehyde d.
glucose-6-phosphate d. (G6PD)
glutamate d.

D

NOTES

dehydrogenase *(continued)*
glyceraldehyde phosphate d. (GAPDH)
heat-stable lactic d. (HLDH)
hexosephosphate d.
hydroxybutyrate d. (HBD, HBDH)
hydroxybutyric d.
iditol d.
isocitrate d.
isocitric d.
isovaleryl-CoA d.
lactate d. (LD)
lactic d. (LD)
L-arabinose d.
L-arabitol d.
L-xylulose d.
lysine d.
malate d.
malic d. (MDH)
NADH d.
oxoglutarate d.
oxoisovalerate d.
phosphate d. (PDH)
phosphogluconate d.
polyol d.
proline d.
pyrroline-5-carboxylate d.
saccharopine d.
sarcosine d.
serum hydroxybutyrate d. (SHBD)
serum isocitric d. (SICD)
serum lactate d. (SLD, SLDH)
Shikimate d.
sorbitol d.
succinate d.
tetrahydrofolate d.
triosephosphate d.
xylitol d.
dehydrogenate
dehydrogenation
dehydroisoandrosterone (DHIA)
DEIA
DNA-enzyme immunoassay
deiminase
arginine d.
Deinococcaceae
Deinococcales
Deinococci
Deinococcus indicus
deiodinase
deiodinate
deionization
deionized formamide
Deiters
D. cell
phalangeal cell of D.
D. terminal frame

Dejerine
D. disease
D. syndrome
Dejerine-Klumpke
D.-K. paralysis
D.-K. syndrome
Dejerine-Roussy syndrome
Dejerine-Sottas
D.-S. disease
D.-S. syndrome
Dekkera
DEL1
developmental endothelial locus 1
DEL1 gene
Delacroixia coronata
Delafield
D. fixative solution
D. fluid
D. hematoxylin
D. hematoxylin stain
Delaney clause
delay
d. circuit
d. line
delayed
d. adrenarche
d. allergy
d. climacteric
d. development
d. graft function
d. hemolytic transfusion reaction
d. hypersensitivity
d. hypersensitivity reaction
d. menopause
d. primary closure (DPC)
d. puberty
d. radiation toxicity
d. traumatic intracerebral hematoma (DTICH)
triage d.
delayed-phase skin response
delayed-type hypersensitivity (DTH)
delbrueckii
Lactobacillus d.
deletion
antigenic d.
central clonal d.
chromosomal d.
gene d.
gross d.
hemizygous d.
intercalary d.
interstitial d.
large d.
d. mutation
4p d. syndrome
terminal d.
d. theory
X d.

DELFIA
  dissociation enhanced lanthanide
  fluoroimmunoassay
Delftia
  D. acidovorans
  D. tsuruhatensis
delicatus
  Sulfitobacter d.
delicti
  corpus d.
deliensis
  Trombicula d.
delipidated albumin
deliquescence
deliquescent
delirium
  anticholinergic d.
  excited d.
  d. tremens (DT)
delitescence
deliver
  to d. (TD)
delivery
  spontaneous d. (SD)
delle
delomorphous
delphian node
del Rio Hortega stain
Delsa 440 SX Zeta potential analyzer
delta
  d. agent
  d. ALA acid
  d. aminolevulinic acid assay
  d. antigen
  d. base
  d. cell
  d. cell of anterior lobe of
    hypophysis
  d. cell islet
  d. cell of pancreas
  d. check
  d. fiber
  d. granule
  d. hepatitis
  d. ray
  d. staphylolysin
  d. storage pool disease
  d. thalassemia
  d. virus
delta-5 desaturase enzyme
Deltabacteria
delta^2-isopentenyl diphosphate

delta^3-isopentenyl diphosphate
deltalike 1 homolog (DLK1)
Deltaretrovirus
Deltavirus
deltoidea
  Anthopsis d.
demarcated raised papule
demarcation
  line of d.
demargination
demarquayi
  Mansonella d.
Dematiaceae
dematiaceous fungus
dematioides
  Hormonema d.
  Phaeosclera d.
Dematium
d'emblée
  mycosis fungoides d.
demeclocycline
dementia
  argyrophilic grain d.
  multiinfarct d.
  non-Alzheimer d.
  d. praecox
  d. pugilistica/autism with self-injury
    behavior
  tangle only d.
  transmissible d.
  vascular d.
demerariensis
  Raillietina d.
  Taenia d.
demethylchlortetracycline
demeton
  methyl d.
Demetria terragena
demilune
  d. body
  Giannuzzi d.
  Heidenhain d.
  serous d.
demineralization
deminutus
  Ternidens d.
demobilization
Demodex folliculorum
demonstration
  calcium deposit d.
  copper deposit d.
  degenerating myelin d.

D

NOTES

demonstration *(continued)*
    iron-positive pigment d.
    d. of organism
demyelinate
demyelinated myelitis
demyelinating
    d. disease
    d. encephalopathy
demyelination
    axonal d.
    cuprizone model of chronic d.
demyelinization
    spinal cord d.
denaturation
    protein d.
denatured hemoglobin
denaturing
    d. density gradient electrophoresis (DDGE)
    d. gel
    d. gradient gel electrophoresis (DGGE)
    d. high-performance liquid chromatography (DHPLC)
dendraxon
dendriform
dendrite
    apical d.
    d. of pyramidal cell
dendritic
    d. calculus
    d. cell tumor
    d. clear cell
    d. cytoplasmic process
    d. epidermal cell
    d. spine
    d. synovitis
    d. thorn
dendriticum
    Diphyllobothrium d.
dendrocyte
    dermal d.
dendroid
dendroides
    Dactylium d.
dendron
Dendrosporobacter quercicolus
Dendrostilbella byssina
Dendryphion
dengue
    hemorrhagic d.
    d. hemorrhagic fever
    d. shock syndrome
    d. virus, types 1–4
denhamense
    Roseibium d.
Denhardt solution
denitrificans
    Achromobacter d.

    Alcaligenes d.
    Alicycliphilus d.
    Comamonas d.
    Listeria d.
    Shewanella d.
    Sterolibacterium d.
    Thialkalivibrio d.
denitrifying bacterium
Denitrobacterium detoxificans
Denitrovibrio acetiphilus
Dennie-Marfan syndrome
Dennis technique
Denonvilliers fascia
dens
densa
    lamina d.
    macula d.
dense
    d. body
    d. deposit
    d. fibrillar component
    d. irregular connective tissue
    d. regular connective tissue
    d. secondary granule
dense-core neurosecretory granule
dense-deposit disease (DDD)
densimeter
densitometer
    Appraise clinical d.
densitometry
density
    amniotic fluid bilirubin optical d.
    blood microvessel d.
    buoyant d.
    character d.
    count information d.
    extra electron d.
    fiber d.
    d. function
    d. gradient centrifugation
    intratumoral lymph vessel d.
    intratumor microvessel d.
    luminous flux d.
    macrophage d.
    microvessel d. (MVD)
    optical d. (OD)
    plating d.
    PSA d. (PSAD)
    scan information d.
    stellate d.
    subplasmalemmal d.
    total body d. (TBD)
    vascular d.
density-dependent repair
Densovirus
dental
    d. amalgam tattoo
    d. calculus
    d. caries

d. cord
d. crypt
d. fluorosis
d. follicle
d. follicular cyst
d. granuloma
d. identification record
d. lymph
d. overexposure
d. pathology
d. plaque
d. pulp
d. sac
d. tubule

dentales
canaliculi d.
tubuli d.

dentalis
alveolus d.
Amoeba d.

dentata
lamina d.
Taenia d.

dentate
d. line
d. nucleus

dentatorubral pallidoluysian atrophy (DRPLA)

dentatum
Oesophagostomum d.

dentatus
Stephanurus d.

dentes acustici

denticola
Prevotella d.
Treponema d.

denticolens
Parascardovia d.

denticulate
denticulated

denticulatum
Pentastoma d.

denticulatus
Porocephalus d.

dentigerous
d. cyst
d. mixed tumor

dentin, dentine
d. crystal alteration
d. dysplasia
d. globule
d. tubule

dentinal
d. canal
d. fiber
d. fluid
d. pulp
d. sheath
d. tubule

dentinogenesis imperfecta
dentinoma
fibroameloblastic d.

dentinum
dentis
ebur d.
pulpa d.
substantia ossea d.

dentistry
forensic d.

dentium
Bifidobacterium d.

dentocariosa
Rothia d.

dentrificans
Jonesia d.

dentriticum
Dicrocoelium d.

denucleated
denudation
surface d.

Denver classification
Denys-Drash syndrome
Denys-Leclef phenomenon
deontology
deossification
deoxyadenosine monophosphate (dAMP)
deoxyadenosine 5′-phosphate
deoxyadenylic acid
6-deoxy-beta-L-mannose
deoxycholate
deoxycholate-citrate agar (DCA)
deoxycholic acid
deoxycorticoid (DOC)
deoxycorticosterone (DOC)
d. acetate (DOCA)
d. test

deoxycortisol test
deoxycytidine monophosphate
deoxycytidine 5′-phosphate
deoxycytidylic acid
6-deoxy-L-galactose
deoxygenated hemoglobin

NOTES

D

deoxyguanosine
    d. monophosphate (dGMP)
    d. phosphate
deoxyguanosine 5′-phosphate
2-deoxyguanosine 5′-triphosphate (dGTP)
deoxyguanylic acid
deoxyhemoglobin (MbO₂)
deoxynivalenol (DON)
deoxynucleotidyltransferase
    terminal d. (TdT)
deoxypyridinoline (DPD)
deoxyribonuclease (DNase, DNAse)
    d. agar
    d. digestion
    d. I, II
    d. test
deoxyribonucleic
    d. acid (DNA)
    d. acid stain
    d. acid staining
    competitor DNA
deoxyribonucleoprotein (DNP)
deoxyribonucleoside
deoxyribonucleotide
deoxyribose
deoxysugar
deoxythymidine triphosphate (dTTP)
deoxyuridine
    d. monophosphate (dUMP)
    d. phosphate
    d. 5′-phosphate
    d. suppression test
deoxyuridylic acid
deoxyvirus
deparaffinization
department
    D. of Health and Human Services (DHHS)
    Joint Task Force for Civil Support (of the Defense D.) (JTF-CS)
    D. of Public Health (DPH)
dépassé
    coma d.
DEPC
    diethyl pyrocarbonate
DEPC-treated water
dependence
    anchorage d.
    drug d.
dependent
    d. edema
    d. variable
Dependovirus
depigmentation
deplasmolysis
depleted
    d. uranium (DU)
    d. uranium-containing explosion

depletion
    d. layer
    lipid d.
    mucin d.
    ovarian ascorbic acid d. (OAAD)
    plasma d.
    volume d.
depolarization
deposit
    d. of amyloid in islet cell
    basophilic d.
    brickdust d.
    dense d.
    endogenous pigments and d.'s
    fingerprint d.
    hump d.
    iron d.
    lumpy-bumpy d.
    mesangial d.
    micrometastatic vascular d.
    posterior corneal d. (PCD)
    properdin d.
    washed out d.
deposition
    bilharzial pigment d.
    calcium d.
    catalyzed reporter d. (CARD)
    cholesterol d.
    collagen d.
    conspicuous amyloid d.
    diffuse membrane hemosiderin d.
    diffuse perivillous fibrin d.
    fatty d.
    fibrin d.
    foreign material d.
    granular d.
    hemosiderin d.
    intestinal ceroid d.
    Kupffer cell iron d.
    linear d.
    malarial pigment d.
    particulate crystalline material d.
    perivillous fibrin d.
    subendothelial immune complex d.
    xanthomatous d.
depot
    fat d.
    d. reaction
depramine assay
depressant
depressed
    d. adenoma
    d. fracture
depression
    bone marrow d.
    myeloid d.
    respiratory d.

deprivation
    d. disease
    severe protein d.
deproteinization
depth
    d. dose
    d. of field
    d. of focus
    relative sagittal d. (RSD)
depulization
depurination
DER
    desmin ensheathment ratio
DeR
    reaction of degeneration
der
    derivative chromosome
deradelphus
derangement
    chromosomal d.
Dercum disease
derepressed gene
derepression
    transient d.
derivation
derivative
    benzene d.
    d. chromosome (der)
    purified protein d. (PPD)
derivative-standard
    purified protein d. (PPD-S)
derived
    d. albumin
    d. protein
Dermabacteraceae
Dermacentor
    D. albopictus
    D. andersoni
    D. occidentalis
    D. reticulatus
    D. variabilis
Dermacentroxenus
    D. akari
    D. australis
    D. orientalis
    D. rickettsi
    D. sibericus
Dermacoccaceae
Dermacoccus nishinomiyaensis
dermal
    d. bone
    d. dendritic cell

    d. dendrocyte
    d. duct tumor
    d. eccrine cylindroma
    d. epidermal junction
    d. nevus
    d. papilla
    d. sinus
    d. tuberculosis
Dermanyssus avium et gallinae
dermatan sulfate
dermatis
    papilla d.
dermatitidis
    Ajellomyces d.
    Blastomyces d.
    Fonsecaea d.
    Wangiella d.
dermatitis, pl. **dermatitides**
    actinic d.
    allergic d.
    atopic d.
    d. atrophicans
    d. atrophicans diffusa
    d. atrophicans maculosa
    d. chronica atrophicans idiopathica
    contact d.
    contagious pustular d.
    eczematoid d.
    eczematous d.
    d. escharotica
    d. exfoliativa
    d. exfoliativa infantum
    d. exfoliativa neonatorum
    exfoliative d.
    factitious d.
    flaky paint d.
    d. gangrenosa infantum
    d. herpetiformis
    infectious eczematoid d.
    lichenoid interface d.
    d. medicamentosa
    myositis sine dermatitides
    nickel d.
    nummular d.
    photocontact d.
    phototoxic contact d.
    pigmented purpuric lichenoid d.
    polymorphous d.
    psoriasiform d.
    radiation d.
    d. repens
    Schamberg d.

D

NOTES

dermatitis *(continued)*
   seborrheic d.
   spongiotic d.
   stasis d.
   subcorneal pustular d.
   toxic d.
   vacuolar interface d.
   d. venenata
   d. verrucosa
dermatoarthritis
   lipoid d.
Dermatobia
   D. cyaniventris
   D. hominis
dermatobiasis
dermatocele
dermatocellulitis
dermatochalasis
dermatocyst
dermatofibroma (DF)
dermatofibrosarcoma
   pigmented d.
   d. protuberans (DFSP)
dermatofibrosis
   d. lenticularis
   d. lenticularis disseminata
dermatogen
dermatographism
dermatolysis
dermatoma
dermatomegaly
dermatomycosis pedis
dermatomyoma
dermatomyositis
   amyopathic d.
dermatopathia
   d. pigmentosa
   d. pigmentosa reticularis
dermatopathic
   d. lymphadenitis
   d. lymphadenopathy
dermatopathology
Dermatophagoides pteronyssinus
Dermatophilaceae
dermatophilosis
Dermatophilus
   D. congolensis
   D. penetrans
dermatophylaxis
dermatophyte test medium (DTM)
dermatophytid
dermatophytosis
dermatorrhagia
dermatorrhexis
dermatosclerosis
dermatosis, pl. **dermatoses**
   acantholytic d.
   Bowen precancerous d.

   dermolytic bullous d.
   inflammatory d.
   neutrophilic d.
   d. papulosa nigra
   pigmentary d.
   progressive pigmentary d.
   radiation d.
   rheumatoid neutrophilic d.
   subcorneal pustular d.
   transient acantholytic d.
   ulcerative d.
dermatozoon
dermatozoonosis, dermatozoiasis
dermatrophia
dermatrophy
Dermea
dermis
   adventitial d.
   busy d.
   reticular d.
   tombstone-like d.
Dermobacter
dermoepidermal interface
dermographia
dermoid
   d. cyst
   d. cyst of ovary
   implantation d.
   inclusion d.
   sequestration d.
   d. tumor
dermolysis
dermolytic bullous dermatosis
dermonecrotic
dermopathy
   diabetic d.
dermophlebitis
dermostenosis
dermostosis
dermosyphilopathy
dermotoxin
dermotuberculin reaction
dermo-unguis
   Chaetophoma d.-u.
derodidymus
derotation
DES
   diethylstilbestrol
des-Arg9-bradykinin
desaturase
   acyl-CoA d.
desaturated phosphatidylcholine (DSPC)
desaturation
Descemet membrane
descemetocele
descending
   d. degeneration
   d. flaccid paralysis

descensus
    uterine d.
    d. ventriculi
description
    figure d.
    gross d.
desensitization
    drug d.
    heterologous d.
    homologous d.
    d. therapy
desensitize
desert fever
desetope
desferrioxamine
deshydremia
desiccant
desiccate
desiccation
desiccative
desiccator
designated blood donation
desipramine assay
Desmarres dacryolith
desmectasia
desmectasis
desmin
    d. antibody
    d. ensheathment ratio (DER)
desmitis
desmocollin
Desmodus
desmogenous
desmoglein
desmoid
    extraabdominal d.
    d. fibromatosis
    d. tumor
desmolase
    17,20 d.
    20,22 d.
    d. deficiency
    mitochondrial enzyme d.
desmon
desmoplakin I
desmoplasia
    stromal d.
desmoplastic
    d. ameloblastoma
    d. cerebral astrocytoma
    d. change
    d. fibroblastoma

    d. fibroma
    d. infantile ganglioglioma
    d. medulloblastoma
    d. melanoma
    d. plaque
    d. small round cell tumor
    (DSRCT)
    d. stroma
    d. subtype
    d. trichoblastoma
    d. trichoepithelioma
desmosine
desmosome
desmosterol
desolvation
desoxycholate
    bromocresol purple d. (BCP-D)
desoxycorticosterone
    d. trimethylacetate (DCTMA)
    d. triphenylacetate (DCTPA)
11-desoxycorticosterone
despeciate
despeciated antitoxin
despeciation
despumation
desquamate
desquamation
    dry d.
    moist d.
desquamativa
    otitis d.
desquamative
    d. inflammatory vaginitis
    d. interstitial pneumonia (DIP)
    d. interstitial pneumonitis (DIP)
    d. interstitial poisoning
destruction
    immune-mediated d.
    d. of pancreatic beta cell
    red cell d.
    weapon of mass d. (WMD)
destructiva
    Ramularia d.
destructive
    d. distillation
    d. interference
destruens
    chorioadenoma d.
    Hyphomyces d.
Desulfacinum
    D. hydrothermale
    D. infernum

D

NOTES

Desulfatibacillum
  D. aliphaticivorans
  D. alkenivorans
desulfhydrase
  homocysteine d.
Desulfitobacterium
  D. chlororespirans
  D. metallireducens
Desulfobacca acetoxidans
Desulfobacula
  D. phenolica
  D. toluolica
Desulfobulbus mediterraneus
Desulfocapsa sulfexigens
Desulfocella halophila
Desulfofaba
  D. fastidiosa
  D. gelida
  D. hansenii
Desulfofrigus
  D. fragile
  D. oceanense
Desulfomicrobium
  D. macestii
  D. orale
Desulfomonile
  D. limimaris
  D. tiedjei
Desulfomusa hansenii
Desulfonatronum thiodismutans
Desulfonauticus submarinus
Desulfonispora thiosulfatigenes
Desulforegula conservatrix
Desulforhopalus
  D. singaporensis
  D. vacuolatus
Desulfosporosinus
  D. auripigmenti
  D. meridiei
  D. orientis
Desulfotalea
  D. arctica
  D. psychrophila
Desulfotignum
  D. balticum
  D. phosphitoxidans
Desulfotomaculum
  D. alkaliphilum
  D. auripigmentum
  D. gibsoniae
  D. nigrificans
  D. solfataricum
  D. thermobenzoicum subsp.
    thermosyntrophicum
Desulfovibrio
  D. alaskensis
  D. alcoholivorans
  D. aminophilus
  D. bastinii

  D. burkinensis
  D. dechloracetivorans
  D. gracilis
  D. hydrothermalis
  D. indonesiensis
  D. magneticus
  D. mexicanus
  D. oxyclinae
  D. piger
  D. vietnamensis
  D. zosterae
Desulfovirga adipica
desulfurans
  Oceanithermus d.
desulfuricans
  Deferribacter d.
  Gordonia d.
Desulfurococcaceae
Desulfurococcales
Desulfurococcus amylolyticus
Desulfuromonas palmitatis
desynapsis
desynchronization
detached cranial section
detachment
  retinal d.
detect, incident command, scene safety and security, assess hazard, support required, triage and treatment, evacuation, recovery (DISASTER)
detection
  antibody d.
  cardiac shunt d.
  colorimetric antibody d.
  C1q immune complex d.
  digoxigenin-mediated d.
  direct antigen d.
  Filtracheck-UTI disposable colormetric bacteriuria d.
  nucleic acid d.
  radiometric antibody d.
detector
  AD 340 absorbance d.
  alpha particle d.
  cadmium telluride d.
  combustible gas d.
  DTX series multimode d.
  EC d.
  electron capture d.
  error d.
  flame ionization d. (FID)
  forward fluorescence d. (FED)
  LD 400 luminescence d.
  lithium-drifted d.
  paralyzable d.
  surface-barrier d.
  TC d.
  thermal conductivity d.

thermoluminescent d.
d. transfer function (DTF)
detergent
anionic d.
nonionic d.
oxidizing d.
determinant
allotypic d.
antigenic d.
genetic d.
d. group
idiotypic antigenic d.
immunogenic d.
isoallotypic d.
R d.
resistance d. (RD)
rough d.
determination
activity d.
fetal activity-acceleration d.
lactate dehydrogenase isoenzyme d.
sex d.
Shimadzu hemoglobin d.
shunt d.
deterministic
detersive
Dethiosulfovibrio
D. acidaminovorans
D. marinus
D. russensis
detonation
detoxicate
detoxication
detoxificans
Denitrobacterium d.
detoxification
drug d.
metabolic d.
detoxify
detrition
detritus
detrusor-external sphincter dyssynergia
detrusor-sphincter dyssynergia
detumescence
deuteranomaly
deuteranopia
deuterium
deuterohemophilia
deuteromycetes
Deuteromycota
deuteron
deuteroplasm

deuterosome
deuterotocia, deuterotoky
deutomerite
deutoplasm
deutoplasmic
deutoplasmigenon
deutoplasmolysis
Deutschländer disease
developing bone
development
canalicular phase of lung d.
delayed d.
pseudoglandular phase of lung d.
developmental
d. arrest
d. endothelial locus 1 (DEL1)
d. jaw cyst
d. mixoploid
d. sequence anomaly
d. synchronism
development-at-birth index (DBI)
Devergie disease
deviant
deviate
deviated septum
deviation
average d.
immune d.
d. to the left
mean square d.
no significant d. (NSD)
relative standard d. (RSD)
d. to the right
right axis d. (RAD)
standard d. (SD)
sum of square d.'s (SSD)
Devic disease
device
AvoSure INR test d.
bag-valve-mask d.
Biopore membrane d.
Boyden chamber assay d.
cholesterol 1,2,3 noninvasive testing d.
Coag-a-mate prothrombin d.
compound absorption d. (CAD)
Coumatrak prothrombin time d.
Crit-Line III TQA fluid management and access d.
EMP d.
HERF d.

D

NOTES

device *(continued)*
Hybrid Capture 2 (cervical cancer screening) d.
improvised explosive d. (IED)
intrauterine contraceptive d. (IUD)
I/O d.
IsoCode Stix d.
OnTrak TestTcard drug testing d.
OralScreen rapid oral fluid screening and test d.
OraSure HIV-1 oral specimen collection d.
Osteomark NTx point-of-care d.
Profile-II ER drug screening d.
ProTime INR test d.
Qualitative Platform Immunoassay D. (QuPID)
radiation dispersal d. (RDD)
Rheolog d.
Riechert-Mundiger stereotactic d.
semiconductor d.
Sepacell RZ-2000 d.
simple radiological d.
Status Cup Plus drug testing d.
Stratagene CastAway sequencing d.
stretch d.
Surgicutt d.
Tenderlett Plus finger-stick blood collection d.
thromboelastographic monitor d. (TEG)
Verdict-II drug screening d.
devil's
d. grip
d. pinch
devolution
Devon polyposis syndrome
Devosia neptuniae
devriesei
Streptococcus d.
Dewar flask
dexamethasone
d., insulin, and glucose (DIG)
d. suppression test (DST)
dexiocardia *(var. of* dextrocardia)
dextra
pericolitis d.
dextran
d. blue (DB)
low molecular weight d. (LMD, LMWD)
dextran-coated charcoal (DCC)
dextrin
limit d.
dextrinosis
debrancher deficiency limit d.
limit d.
dextrinuria

dextrocardia, dexiocardia
corrected d.
false d.
isolated d.
secondary d.
type 1–4 d.
d. with situs inversus
dextrogastria
dextroposition of the heart
dextrorotatory
dextrose
d. agar
citrate phosphate d. (CPD)
d. nitrogen ratio (DN)
d. solution mixture (DSM)
d. test
d. in water (percent) (D/W)
yeast peptone d.
dextrose-saline (DS)
dextrosuria
dextrothyroxine sodium
dextroversion of the heart
DF
dermatofibroma
disseminated foci
df
degrees of freedom
DFA
direct fluorescence assay
direct fluorescent antibody
direct fluorescent assay
DFA for capsular antigen
DFA test
DFA-TP
direct fluorescent antibody-*Treponema pallidum* test
DFA-TP test
DFDT
difluorodiphenyltrichloroethane
D-FISH
double-fusion FISH
DFL
dense fibrous lamina
DFS
disease-free survival
DFSP
dermatofibrosarcoma protuberans
DFU
dead fetus in utero
DGGE
denaturing gradient gel electrophoresis
DGGE technique
DGLA
dihomogammalinolenic acid
D-glucaric acid
dGMP
deoxyguanosine monophosphate
dGTP
2-deoxyguanosine 5′-triphosphate

DHA
  docosahexaenoic acid
dhakensis
  Aeromonas hydrophila subsp. *d.*
Dharmendra antigen
DHE
  dihydroergotamine
DHEA
  dehydroepiandrosterone
    DHEA test
DHEAS
  dehydroepiandrosterone sulfate
d'Herelle phenomenon
DHFR
  dihydrofolate reductase
DHHS
  Department of Health and Human
    Services
DHIA
  dehydroisoandrosterone
DHL
  diffuse histocytic lymphoma
DHMA
  dihydroxymandelic acid
dhobie itch
DHPLC
  denaturing high-performance liquid
    chromatography
    DHPLC assay
DHT
  dihydrotachysterol
  dihydrotestosterone
    DHT test
D-3-hydroxyacyl coenzyme A
DI
  defective interfering
  DNA index
    DI particle
Di
    Di antigen
    Di Guglielmo disease
    Di Guglielmo syndrome
diabetes
    adult-onset d.
    alimentary d.
    bronze d.
    d. innocens
    d. insipidus
    insulin-dependent d. mellitus
      (IDDM)
    juvenile-onset d.
    lipoatrophic d.

    maturity-onset d.
    d. mellitus
    Mosler d.
    noninsulin-dependent d. mellitus
      (NIDDM)
    phloridzin d.
    renal d.
diabetic
    d. acidosis
    d. amyotrophy
    d. angiopathy
    d. coma
    d. dermopathy
    d. gangrene
    d. glomerulosclerosis
    d. ketoacidosis (DKA)
    d. lipemia
    d. mastopathy
    d. microangiopathy
    d. myelopathy
    d. nephropathy
    d. neuropathy
    d. retinopathy (DR)
    d. ulcer
    d. urine
diabeticorum
    bullosis d.
    necrobiosis lipoidica d.
diabetogenic hormone
diacetemia
diacetic acid
diacetonuria
diaceturia
diacetyl monoxime
diaclasia
diaclasis
diacrinous
diacylglycerol (DAG)
diadenosine oligophosphate hydrolase
diag
    diagnosis
Diagnex
    D. Blue
    D. Blue test
diagnosis, pl. **diagnoses (diag)**
    Bethesda 2001 system d.
    clinical d.
    confirmed d.
    cytologic d.
    differential d.
    histologic d. (Histo-Dx)
    laboratory d.

D

NOTES

diagnosis (*continued*)
    number of add-on tests needed to obtain a d.
    pathologic d.
    physical d.
    preimplantation genetic d. (PGD)
    prenatal d.
    presumptive d.
    provocative d.
    serum d.
    specific virologic d.
    suspected d.
    tumor stage at d.
diagnostic
    d. diphtheria toxin
    d. sensitivity
    d. serology
    d. specificity
    virtually d.
diagram
    acid-base d.
    block d.
    d. of the hypophysis
    d. of normal splenic architecture
    scatter d.
diakinesis
Dialister
    D. invisus
    D. pneumosintes
dial unit
dialysance
dialysate
dialysis dysequilibrium syndrome
diamagnetic
Diamanus montanus
diameter
    Mantoux d. (MD)
    mean cell d. (MCD)
    mean corpuscular d. (MCD)
    mean tubular d. (MTD)
    nuclear profile d.
    outside d. (OD)
diamide
4,6-diamidino-2-phenylindole-2-HCl (DAPI)
diamine
    high iron d. (HID)
    low-iron d. (LID)
diaminobenzidine (DAB)
    d. reaction
    d. stain
    d. tetrahydrochloride
diamniotic
diamond
    diamond fuchsin
    D. TYM medium
Diamond-Blackfan
    D.-B. anemia
    D.-B. syndrome

Diamyl
Dianthovirus
diapause
diapedesis
Diaphane solution
diaphanometer
diaphanoscope
Diaphorobacter nitroreducens
diaphragm
    crural d.
    eventration of d.
    d. paralysis
diaphragmatic
    d. hernia
    d. peritonitis
    d. pleurisy
diaphysial, diaphyseal
    d. aclasis
    d. center
    d. dysplasia
    d. juxtaepiphysial exostosis
diaphysitis
Diaporthe
Diaptomus
diarrhea
    antibiotic-associated d. (AAD)
    bovine virus d.
    Brainerd d.
    Cochin China d.
    hypokalemic d.
    medication-related d.
    opsoclonus-myoclonus d.
    traveler's d.
    tropical d.
diarrheagenic *E. coli*
diarrheogenic bacterial enterocolitis
diastase digestion
diastase-resistant material
diastasic action
diastasis
diastasuria
diastatic
diastematocrania
diastematomyelia
diastereoisomer
diastereoisomerism
diastereomer
Diastix
diastolic hypertension
Diatest
    D. diabetes breath test
    D. diabetes breath test kit
diathermy
diathesis, pl. diatheses
    cystic d.
    hemorrhagic d.
diathetic
diatom
diatomaceous earth

diauxic
diauxie
diazacholesterol (DAC)
diazepam
    d. assay
    d. breath test
diazinon
diazo
    d. reaction
    d. reagent
    d. stain for argentaffin granules
    d. staining method
diazomethane generator
diazonium salt
diazotize
dibasic
    d. acid
    d. aminoaciduria
    d. potassium phosphate
dibenz[*a,h*]anthracene
dibenzanthracene (DBA)
dibenz(b,f)-1:4-oxazepine
    NATO code for d.-o. (CR)
dibenzopyridine
diborane
dibothriocephaliasis
Dibothriocephalus latus
dibrachius
    dicephalus dipus d.
    monocephalus tetrapus d.
    monocephalus tripus d.
1,2-dibromethane
dibromide
    ethylene d.
dibucaine number (DN)
DIC
    diffuse intravascular coagulation
    disseminated intravascular coagulation
dicarboxylic acid
dicelous
dicentric malformation
dicephalus
    d. dipus dibrachius
    d. dipus tetrabrachius
    d. dipus tribrachius
    d. dipygus
    d. tripus tribrachius
dicheirus
Dichelobacter nodosus
dichlobenil
dichloride
    ethylene d.

    ethylidene d.
    methylene d.
dichloroarisine
dichlorodiethyl sulfide
dichlorodiphenyldichloroethane (DDD)
dichlorodiphenyltrichloroethane (DDT)
1,1-dichloroethane
1,2-dichloroethane
dichloroformoxime
    d. CCl$_2$NOH
2,6-dichloroindophenol
dichloromethane
2,6-dichlorophenol-indophenol
dichlorophenoxy acetic acid
dichloropropene-dichloropropane mixture
dichlorvos
Dichomitus
dichorionic
    d. diamniotic placenta
    d. placenta twins
dichotic
Dichotomophthora portulacae
Dichotomophthoropsis nymphearum
dichotomous variable
dichotomy
dichroic filter system
dichroism
    circular d.
dichromate
    potassium d.
dichromatic erythrocyte
dichromophil, dichromophile
Dick
    D. method
    D. test
    D. test toxin
dicobalt edentate
dicofol
dicrocoeliosis
Dicrocoelium dentriticum
Dictyocaulus viviparus
Dictyonella
Dictyopanus
Dictyosporium
Dictyostelium
dictyotene
dicumarol
didelphis
    Streptococcus d.
dideoxy terminator
Didymella phacidiomorpha
didymitis

NOTES

D

Diego
- D. antigen
- D. blood group system

diel

dieldrin

dielectric
- d. constant
- d. strength

diener

Dientamoeba fragilis

dieretic

diet
- elimination d.
- gluten-free d.
- low-fiber d.
- phenylalanine-free d.

dietary protein

Dieterle
- D. method
- D. stain

dietetic albuminuria

diethyl
- d. pyrocarbonate (DEPC)
- d. sulfate

diethylamide
- lysergic acid d. (LSD)

diethylamine

diethylaminoethyl (DEAE)
- d. cellulose

diethylcarbamazine

diethyldithiocarbamate

diethylene dioxide

diethylenetriaminepentaacetate
- calcium d. (Ca-DTPA)

diethylenetriaminepentaacetic acid

diethylstilbestrol (DES)

Dietzia
- D. natronolimnaea
- D. psychralcaliphila

Dietziaceae

dietziae
- Nonomuraea d.

Dieulafoy malformation

Difco ESP testing system

difference
- alveolar-arterial carbon dioxide d.
- alveolar-arterial oxygen d.
- d. amplifier
- antigenic d.
- arteriovenous carbon dioxide d.
- arteriovenous oxygen d.
- cation-anion d.
- electric potential d.
- fluorescence decay d.
- d. limen (DL)
- mean of consecutive d.'s (MCD)
- no significant d. (NSD)
- ultrastructural d.

differential
- d. agglutination titer (DAT)
- d. cell lysis
- d. diagnosis
- d. diagnostic consideration
- d. extraction
- left shift (increased band forms on WBC d.)
- d. leukocyte count (DLC)
- d. leukocyte count automation
- pressure d.
- d. renal function test
- d. stain
- d. test for infectious mononucleosis
- d. thermometer
- d. ureteral catheterization test
- d. white blood count

differentiated
- moderately d. (MD)
- poorly d. (PD)
- d. teratoma
- teratoma d. (TD)
- well d.

differentiated embryo-chondrocyte expressed gene 1 (DEC1)

differentiating chondroblast

differentiation
- acute monocytic leukemia with d. (M5b)
- acute monocytic leukemia without d. (M5a)
- acute myeloblastic leukemia without localized d. (M0)
- adipocyte d.
- amphicrine d.
- d. antigen
- antigen-triggered lymphocyte d.
- biphenotypic d.
- carcinoma showing thymus-like d. (CASTLE)
- cell d.
- cluster of d. (CD)
- endothelial d.
- epithelial d.
- invisible d.
- leukotriene-dependent erythroid d.
- meissnerian d.
- mesenchymal d.
- myofibroblastic d.
- neuroendocrine d.
- plasmacytoid d.
- rhabdomyoblastic d.
- sex d.
- spindle cell epithelial tumor with thymus-like d. (SETTLE)
- terminal d.

differentiator

difficile
- Clostridium d.

Diff-Quik
    D.-Q. histochemical stain
    D.-Q. smear
diffraction grating
DiffSpin slide spinner
diffusa
    dermatitis atrophicans d.
    leishmaniasis tegumentaria d.
diffusate
diffuse
    d. abscess
    d. acute inflammation
    d. acute peritonitis
    d. alveolar damage (DAD)
    d. amyloidosis
    d. aneurysm
    d. angiokeratoma
    d. arterial ectasia
    d. axonal injury
    d. bronchopneumonia
    d. chronic inflammation
    d. emphysema
    d. enlargement
    d. esophageal spasm
    d. extracapillary proliferative glomerulonephritis
    d. follicular variant
    d. ganglion
    d. ganglion cell
    d. histocytic lymphoma (DHL)
    d. hyperplasia
    d. hypertrophy
    d. idiopathic skeletal hyperostosis
    d. illumination
    d. infantile familial sclerosis
    d. infiltrative lung disease (DILD)
    d. interstitial fibrosis
    d. interstitial pneumonia
    d. interstitial pulmonary disease
    d. intramural calcification of the gallbladder
    d. intravascular coagulation (DIC)
    d. large B-cell lymphoma (DLBCL)
    d. lesion
    d. lymphatic tissue
    d. membrane hemosiderin deposition
    d. meningiomatosis
    d. mesangial proliferation
    d. necrosis
    d. neuroendocrine system

    d. nontoxic goiter
    d. panbronchiolitis (DPB)
    d. pattern
    d. perivillous fibrin deposition
    d. phlegmon
    d. poorly differentiated lymphoma (DPDL)
    d. proliferative form
    d. proliferative lupus nephritis
    d. pyelonephritis
    d. reflection
    d. septal cirrhosis
    d. small cleaved cell lymphoma
    d. ulceration
    d. waxy spleen
diffusible
diffusing
    d. capacity for carbon monoxide (D_{CO}, DCO)
    d. capacity of lung
    d. capacity of lung for carbon monoxide (DLCO)
diffusion
    d. coefficient
    d. constant
    d. current
    d. defect
    double d.
    facilitated d.
    gel d.
    d. method
    Ouchterlony double d.
    d. potential
    radial d.
    d. shell
    single d.
diffusivity
diffusum
    angiokeratoma corporis d.
    papilloma d.
difluorodiphenyltrichloroethane (DFDT)
DIG
    dexamethasone, insulin, and glucose
    DIG cocktail
Digenea
Digene hc2 high-risk HPV DNA test
digenesis
digenetic
DiGeorge syndrome
digest
    TaqI restriction d.

NOTES

D

digestion
    deoxyribonuclease d.
    diastase d.
    enzymatic d.
    glycogen d.
    hyaluronidase d.
    neuraminidase d.
    proteinase K d. (PKD)
    proteolytic d.
    sialidase d.
    d. vacuole
digestive
    d. albuminuria
    d. disorder
    d. glycosuria
    d. leukocytosis
    d. organ
    d. tract
    d. tube
digestorius
    tubus d.
digit
    check d.
    clubbed d.
    significant d.
digital
    d. autopsy
    d. clubbing
    d. differential display (DDD)
    d. fibrokeratoma
    d. infarct
    d. karyotyping
    d. macrophotography
    d. photomicrography
    d. rectal examination (DRE)
    d. voltmeter
digitalis
    d. glycoside
    d. unit
Digitalis purpurea
digital-to-analog converter (DAC)
digitata
    verruca d.
digitate wart
digitation
digiti (*pl. of* digitus)
digitize
digitizer
digitonin
    d. method
    d. reaction
digitopalmar
digitorum
    connexus intertendinei musculi
      extensoris d.
digitoxin
digitus, pl. **digiti**
    digiti hippocratici
diglyceride

diglycosylated
digoxigenin-labeled riboprobe
digoxigenin-mediated detection
digoxigenin-UTP
digoxin
Digramma brauni
Diheterospora
dihexoside
    ceramide d.
dihomogammalinolenic acid (DGLA)
dihydrate
    calcium pyrophosphate d. (CPD)
dihydric alcohol
dihydrobiopterin
dihydroergotamine (DHE)
dihydroethidine
dihydrofolate reductase (DHFR)
dihydrofolic acid
dihydrofolliculin
dihydropteridine
    d. reductase
    d. reductase deficiency
dihydropyrimidinase
dihydropyrimidine
dihydropyrimidinuria
dihydrorhodamine
dihydrosphingosine
dihydrotachysterol (DHT)
dihydrotestosterone (DHT)
dihydroubiquinone
dihydrouridine
dihydroxyacetone phosphate (DAP)
dihydroxycholecalciferol assay
dihydroxydinaphthyl disulfide (DDD)
dihydroxymandelic acid (DHMA, DOMA)
dihydroxyphenylacetic acid
dihydroxyphenylalanine (DOPA)
diiodothyronine
diiodotyrosine (DIT)
diisocyanate
    toluene d.
diisopropyl
    d. phosphate (DIP)
    d. phosphofluoridate
dikaryon
diktyoma
Dilantin
dilatation
    aneurysmal d.
    balloon d.
    centrilobular d.
    crypt d.
    poststenotic d.
    sinusoidal d.
    d. thrombosis
dilate
dilated cardiomyopathy

dilation
  cardiac d.
  localized arteriolar d.
dilator
  d. pupillae
  d. pupillae muscle
DILD
  diffuse infiltrative lung disease
diluent buffer
dilute
  d. blood clot lysis (DBCL)
  d. blood clot lysis method
diluted
  d. whole blood clot lysis
  d. whole blood clot lysis test
dilution
  d. anemia
  d. coefficient
  doubling d.
  isotopic d.
  log d.
  maximum inhibiting d. (MID)
  nitrogen d.
  routine test d. (RTD)
  serial d.
  d. test
dilutional
  d. coagulopathy
  d. hypochloremia
  d. thrombocytopenia
dilution-filtration technique
DIM
  divalent ion metabolism
Dimastigamoeba
dimefox
dimension
  single (gel) diffusion precipitin test
    in one d.
  single (gel) diffusion precipitin test
    in two d.'s
dimer
  thymine d.
dimercaprol
dimercaptopropanol
dimeric inhibin-A assay
dimerization
  ligand-dependent d.
  pyrimidine d.
dimerous
dimethoate

5-dimethoxyaniline
  N-ethyl-N-(2-hydroxy-3-sulfopropyl)-
    3, 5-d. (DAOS)
dimethoxyphenylethylamine (DMPE)
dimethyl
  d. ether
  d. ketone
  d. sulfate
  d. sulfoxide
dimethyladenosine (DMA)
dimethylallyl diphosphate
1-dimethylaminonaphthalene-5-sulfonic
  acid (DANS)
dimethylaminoazobenzene (DAB)
dimethylaminobenzaldehyde (DMAB)
4-dimethylaminophenol (DMAP)
dimethylarsinic acid (DMA)
7,12-dimethylbenz[a]anthracene
dimethylbenzanthracene (DMBA)
dimethylbenzene
dimethyldichlorovinyl phosphate (DDVP)
dimethylguanosine
dimethylisopropylsilyl (DMIPS)
dimethyl ketone
dimethylnitrosamine
5,5-dimethyl-2,4-oxazolidinedione
dimethylsulfoxide (DMSO)
dimidiata
  Chrysops d.
diminazene aceturate
diminuta
  Brevundimonas d.
  Hymenolepis d.
  Pseudomonas d.
dimorpha
  Mycoplana d.
dimorphic
  d. anemia
  d. pathogenic fungus
dimorphism
dimorphon
  Trypanosoma d.
dimorphous leprosy
dimple sign
DIN
  ductal intraepithelial neoplasia
dinitrate
  ethylene glycol d.
dinitrobenzene

D

NOTES

dinitrobenzoic acid
dinitrocarbanilide (DNC)
dinitrochlorobenzene (DNCB)
dinitrofluorobenzene (DNFB)
dinitrogen tetroxide
dinitroorthocresol (DNOC)
dinitrophenol
dinitrophenylhydrazine (DNPH)
    d. test
Dinobdella ferox
dinoflagellate toxin
dinormocytosis
dinucleotide
    flavin adenine d. (FAD)
    nicotinamide adenine d. (NADH, NAD)
    reduced nicotinamide-adenine d.
    d. repeat
Dioctophyma renale
dioctophymiasis
diolis
    Clostridium d.
diolivorans
    Lactobacillus d.
dioxane
    dioxane 1,4-d.
dioxathion
dioxide
    arteriovenous carbon d.
    carbamino-carbon d.
    carbon d. (bicarb, CO_2)
    colloidal silicon d.
    diethylene d.
    partial pressure of carbon d. (PCO_2, pCO_2)
    silicone d. (SiO_2)
    solid carbon d.
    thorium d.
dioxin
dioxygenase
    p-hydroxyphenylpyruvate d.
    proline-2-oxoglutarate d.
1,2-dioxygenase
    homogentisate d.
DIP
    desquamative interstitial pneumonia
    desquamative interstitial pneumonitis
    diisopropyl phosphate
dipalmitoylphosphatidylcholine
dipeptidase
    aminoacyl-histidine d.
    glycyl-glycine d.
    glycyl-leucine d.
dipeptidyl peptidase IV protein (DPPIV)
Dipetalonema
    D. perstans
    D. reconditum
    D. streptocerca

dipetalonemiasis
diphacinone
diphasic
    d. meningoencephalitis virus
    d. milk fever
    d. milk fever virus
    d. wave
diphenadione
diphenhydramine (DPH)
    d. hydrochloride
diphenyl
diphenylaminearsine
    NATO code for d. (adamsite) (DM)
diphenylaminochloroarsine
    NATO code for d. (adamsite) (DM)
diphenylarsine cyanide (DC)
diphenyleneiodonium (DPI)
diphenylhexatriene (DPH)
diphenylhydantoin (DPH)
    d. gingivitis
    sodium d.
diphenylmethane dye
diphosphate
    adenosine d.
    adenosine 5′-d. (ADP)
    cytidine d. (CDP)
    delta^2-isopentenyl d.
    delta^3-isopentenyl d.
    dimethylallyl d.
    fructose d.
    geranylgeranyl d.
    guanosine d.
    hexose d.
    inosine d.
    thiamine d. (TDP)
    thymidine d. (dTDP)
    uridine d. (UDP)
diphosphatidylglycerol
diphosphoglycerate
    d. mutase
    d. phosphatase
2,3-diphosphoglycerate mutase
diphosphoinositide
diphosphonate
diphosphopyridine nucleotide (DPN, DPNH)
diphosphosulfate
    phosphoadenosine d.
diphtheria
    d. antitoxin (DAT)
    d. antitoxin unit
    avian d.
    d. bacillus
    false d.
    fowl d.
    d. test

d., tetanus, and pertussis vaccine (DTP)
d. toxin
d. toxin immunization reaction
d. toxin normal (DTN)
d. toxoid, tetanus toxoid, and pertussis vaccine
diphtheriae
    Bacillus d.
    Corynebacterium d.
diphtheritic
    d. enteritis
    d. membrane
    d. ulcer
diphtheritica
    otitis d.
diphtheroid
    aerobic d.
    anaerobic d.
    d. bacilli
diphtherotoxin
diphyllobothriasis
Diphyllobothrium
    D. anemia
    D. cordatum
    D. dendriticum
    D. hians
    D. houghtoni
    D. latum
    D. linguloides
    D. mansoni
    D. mansonoides
    D. nihonkaiense
    D. orcini
    D. pacificum
    D. parvum
    D. scoticum
    D. taenioides
dipicolinic acid
diploalbuminuria
diplobacillus
diplobacterium
diploblastic
diplochromosome
diplococcemia
diplococci (*pl. of* diplococcus)
diplococcin
Diplococcus
    D. constellatus
    D. magnus
    D. morbillorum
    D. mucosus

    D. paleopneumoniae
    D. plagarumbelli
    D. pneumoniae
diplococcus, pl. **diplococci**
    gram-negative intracellular diplococci (GNID)
    Morax-Axenfeld d.
    d. of Morax-Axenfeld
    d. of Neisser
    Weichselbaum d.
Diplodia
diploë
Diplogaster
Diplogonoporus
    D. brauni
    D. grandis
diploic
diploid
    d. adenoma
    d. cell
    d. merogony
    d. mosaicism
    d. nucleus
    d. number
    d. tumor
diploidea
    Sappinea d.
diploidy
diplokaryon
Diplomate of the National Board of Medical Examiners
diplomelituria
diplomyelia
diplonema
diplont
diplopia, dysphagia, dysarthria, dysphonia (4Ds)
diplopod
Diplopoda
Diploscapter coronata
diplosome
Diplosporium
diplotene
Dipodascus capitatus
dipodomis
    Pterygodermatites d.
dipolar
    d. ion
    d. structure
dipole moment
dipsosauri
    Gracilibacillus d.

D

NOTES

dipstick
    Chemstrip d.
    Rapid One single drug screen d.
    screening d.
Diptera
dipteran
dipterous
Dipus sagitta
dipygus
    dicephalus d.
    d. parasiticus
dipylidiasis
Dipylidium caninum
diquat assay
direct
    d. agglutination
    d. agglutination pregnancy test
    (DAPT)
    d. agglutination test (DAT)
    d. antigen detection
    d. antiglobulin test (DAGT, DAT)
    d. bilirubin test
    d. centrifugal flotation (DCF)
    d. Coombs test (DCT)
    d. culture
    d. current
    d. fluorescence assay (DFA)
    d. fluorescent antibody (DFA)
    d. fluorescent antibody stain
    d. fluorescent antibody technique
    d. fluorescent antibody test
    d. fluorescent antibody-*Treponema*
    pallidum test (DFA-TP)
    d. fluorescent assay (DFA)
    d. hernia
    d. immunofluorescence
    d. immunofluorescence testing
    d. maternal death
    d. probe
    d. quenching fluorescent
    immunoassay
    d. reacting bilirubin
    d. sequencing
    d. transport
    d. vision spectroscope
    d. wet mount examination
direct-coupled amplifier
directed donor transfusion
Directigen Flu A + B test kit
directional selection
direct-reacting carcinogen
direct-reading potentiometer
Dirofilaria
    D. conjunctivae
    D. immitis
    D. repens
    D. tenuis
dirofilariasis
    pulmonary d.

dirty
    d. area (contaminated)
    d. bomb (radiation dispersal
    device)
    d. necrosis
disaccharidase deficiency
disaccharide tolerance test
disaggregated ribosome
disaggregation of membrane-bound
    polyribosomes
disappearance
    plasma iron d. (PID)
disappearing bone disease
disarray
    crypt d.
    lobular d.
    myocyte d.
DISASTER
    detect, incident command, scene safety
    and security, assess hazard, support
    required, triage and treatment,
    evacuation, recovery
disaster
disc, disk
    A d.
    Amici d.
    anisotropic d.
    d. approximation synergy test
    blood d.
    Bowman d.
    d. capacitor
    cone d.
    degenerated intervertebral d.
    d. diffusion test
    d. electrophoresis
    excavation of optic d.
    H d.
    hair d.
    Hensen d.
    I d.
    intercalated d.
    intermediate d.
    isotropic d.
    d. kidney
    Merkel tactile d.
    Miller ocular d.
    proligerous d.
    Q d.
    Ranvier d.
    rod d.
    d. sensitivity method
    tactile d.
    transverse d.
    Z d.
discalis
    Chrysops d.
Discella
discharge
    double d.

epileptiform d. (ED)
exit d.
d. frequency
d. tube
urethral d. (UD)
discharging tubule
disci (*pl. of* discus)
disciform, diskiform
disciformis
　Thiothrix d.
Disciotis
discitis, diskitis
disclosing
　d. agent
　d. solution
discocyte, diskocyte
discohesive
discoid
　d. lupus erythematosus (DLE)
　d. ulcer
discoidin domain receptor (DDR)
discontinuous
　d. endothelium
　d. epitope
　d. sterilization
discordance
discordant lymphoma
Discovery SE ultracentrifuge
discrete
　d. analyzer
　d. lesion
　d. nodule
　d. smallpox
　d. subaortic stenosis
discriminant
　d. function
　d. function analysis
discriminator
Discula
discus, pl. **disci**
　excavatio disci
　d. proligerus
discussive
discutient
disdiaclast
disease
　ABO hemolytic d. of the newborn
　abortive viral d.
　accumulation d.
　Acosta d.
　acquired renal cystic d. (ARCD)
　acquired von Willebrand d.

acute cardiovascular d. (ACVD)
acute graft-versus-host d. (aGVHD)
acute infectious d. (AID)
acute respiratory d.
Adams-Stokes d. (AS)
Addison d.
Addison-Biermer d.
adrenal d.
adult celiac d.
adult polycystic kidney d.
airway obstruction d.
akamushi d.
Akureyri d.
Albarrán d.
Albers-Schönberg d.
Albert d.
Albright d.
Aleutian mink d.
Alexander d.
alive with d. (AWD)
alive without d. (AWOD)
allergic airways d.
Almeida d.
Alpers d.
alpha chain d.
alpha heavy-chain d.
alpha hydrazine
alpha storage pool d.
altitude d.
Alzheimer d.
Anders d.
Andes d.
anemia of chronic d.
antibody deficiency d.
anti-GBM d.
anti-glomerular basement
　membrane d.
aortoiliac occlusive d.
Apert d.
Apert-Crouzon d.
Aran-Duchenne d.
arboviral virus d.
arc-welder's d.
Armanni-Ebstein d.
Armstrong d.
arterial occlusive d. (AOD)
arteriosclerotic cardiovascular d.
　(ASCVD)
arteriosclerotic heart d. (AHD)
arthropod-borne viral d.
atherosclerotic cardiovascular d.
　(ASCVD)

D

NOTES

disease *(continued)*

atherosclerotic heart d. (AHD)
atopic d.
Aujeszky d.
Australian X d.
autoimmune mucocutaneous d.
autosomal recessive polycystic
  kidney d. (AR-PKD)
Ayerza d.
Baelz d.
Balfour d.
Ballet d.
Ballingall d.
Baló d.
Bamberger d.
Bamberger-Marie d.
Bamle d.
Bang d.
Bannister d.
Banti d.
Barclay-Baron d.
Barcoo d.
Barlow d.
Barraquer d.
Basedow d.
Batten d.
bauxite worker's d.
Bayle d.
Bazin d.
Beard d.
Beau d.
Beauvais d.
Bechterew d.
Beck d.
Becker d.
Begbie d.
Béguez César d.
Behçet d.
Behr d.
Beigel d.
Bekhterev d.
Bell d.
Bennett d.
Benson d.
Berger d.
Bergeron d.
Berlin d.
Bernhardt d.
Besnier-Boeck d.
Besnier-Boeck-Schaumann d.
Best d.
Biedl d.
Bielschowsky d.
Bielschowsky-Jansky d.
Biermer d.
Bilderbeck d.
biliary tract d.
Billroth d.
Binswanger d.

Bird d.
bird-breeder's d.
black lung d.
Bloch-Sulzberger d.
Blocq d.
Bloodgood d.
Blount d.
Blount-Barber d.
Blumenthal d.
Boeck d.
Bogaert d.
bone d.
Borna d.
Bornholm d.
Bostock d.
Bouchard d.
Bouillaud d.
Bourneville d.
Bourneville-Pringle d.
Bouveret d.
Bowen d.
Bradley d.
Brailsford-Morquio d.
brainstem d.
branching glycogen storage d.
Breda d.
Breisky d.
Bretonneau d.
Bright d.
Brill d.
Brill-Symmers d.
Brill-Zinsser d.
Brinton d.
Brion-Kayser d.
Brissaud d.
broad-beta d.
Brocq d.
Brodie d.
bronzed d.
Brooke d.
Brown-Symmers d.
Bruck d.
Bruton d.
bubble boy d.
Budd d.
Buerger d.
Buhl d.
bullous d.
Bury d.
Buschke d.
Busquet d.
Buss d.
Busse-Buschke d.
Byler d.
Caffey d.
caisson d.
calcium pyrophosphate deposition d.
  (CPPD)
caloric d.

Calvé-Perthes d.
Calvé-Perthes-Legg d.
Camurati-Engelmann d.
Canavan d.
Capdepont d.
carcinoid heart d.
cardiac d.
cardiovascular d. (CVD)
cardiovascular renal d. (CVRD)
Caroli d.
carotid d.
Carrión d.
Castellani d.
Castleman d.
cathepsin-mediated d.
cat-scratch d. (CSD)
Cavare d.
Cazenave d.
celiac d.
central core d.
central Recklinghausen d. type II
cerebrovascular d. (CVD)
cerebrovascular obstructive d.
  (CVOD)
ceroid storage d.
Chabert d.
Chagas d.
Chagas-Cruz d.
Championnière d.
Charcot d.
Charcot-Marie-Tooth d.
Charlouis d.
Cheadle d.
Chédiak-Higashi d.
cheese washer's d.
Cherchevski d.
Chester d.
Chiari d.
chlamydial d.
cholesterol ester storage d.
Christensen-Krabbe d.
Christian d.
Christian-Hand-Schüller d.
Christian-Weber d.
Christmas d.
chronic active liver d.
chronic granulomatous d. (CGD)
chronic inflammatory d.
chronic obstructive lung d. (COLD)
chronic obstructive pulmonary d.
  (COPD)

chronic pulmonary vascular
  occlusive d.
chronic renal d. (CRD)
Ciarrocchi d.
circling d.
circulatory d.
Civatte d.
clonal hematological nonmast cell
  lineage d.
coagulopathy of liver d.
Coat d.
Cockayne d.
cold agglutinin d.
cold hemagglutinin d.
collagen d.
collagen-vascular d.
combined immunodeficiency d.
combined systems d.
communicable d.
Concato d.
congenital nonspherocytic
  hemolytic d. (CNHD)
congenital valvular heart d.
congestive heart d. (CHD)
connective tissue d. (CTD)
Conor and Bruch d.
Conradi d.
constitutional d.
contagious d.
Cooley d.
Cooper d.
Corbus d.
Cori d.
coronary artery d. (CAD)
coronary atherosclerotic heart d.
  (CAHD)
Corrigan d.
Corvisart d.
Cotugno d.
Cotunnius d.
Cowden d.
creeping d.
Creutzfeldt-Jakob d. (CJD)
Crigler-Najjar d.
Crocq d.
Crohn d.
Crouzon d.
Cruveilhier d.
Cruveilhier-Baumgarten d.
Cruz-Chagas d.
crystal deposition d.
Csillag d.

D

NOTES

disease *(continued)*

Curschmann d.
Cushing d.
cystic d.
cystine storage d.
cytomegalic inclusion d. (CID, CMID)
cytomegalovirus d.
cytoskeletal protein hyperphosphorylation d.
Czerny d.
Daae d.
Daae-Finsen d.
DaCosta d.
Dalrymple d.
Danielssen d.
Danielssen-Boeck d.
Darier d.
Darling d.
David d.
Davies d.
dead of d. (DOD)
deerfly d.
deficiency d.
degenerative joint d. (DJD)
Degos d.
Dejerine d.
Dejerine-Sottas d.
delta storage pool d.
demyelinating d.
dense-deposit d. (DDD)
deprivation d.
de Quervain d.
Dercum d.
Deutschländer d.
Devergie d.
Devic d.
diffuse infiltrative lung d. (DILD)
diffuse interstitial pulmonary d.
Di Guglielmo d.
disappearing bone d.
diverticular d.
dog d.
Döhle d.
dominantly inherited Lévi d.
Dubini d.
Dubois d.
Duchenne d.
Duchenne-Aran d.
Duchenne-Griesinger d.
Duhring d.
Dukes d.
Duncan d.
Durand d.
Durand-Nicolas-Favre d.
Durante d.
Duroziez d.
Dutton d.
Eales d.

Ebola virus d.
Ebstein d.
echinococcus d.
Economo d.
Edsall d.
endemic d.
endocrine d.
Engelmann d.
Engel-von Recklinghausen d.
English d.
Engman d.
eosinophilic endomyocardial d.
epidemic d.
epithelial cell d.
Epstein d.
Erb d.
Erb-Charcot d.
Erb-Goldflam d.
Erdheim d.
Erdheim-Chester d. (ECD)
Eulenburg d.
exanthematous d.
extramammary Paget d. (EPD)
extrapyramidal d.
Fabry d.
Fahr d.
familial nephronophthisis-medullary cystic d. (FN-MCD)
Farber d.
farmer's lung d.
fatal granulomatous d. (FGD)
fat-deficiency d.
Fauchard d.
Favre-Racouchot d.
Fede d.
Feer d.
femoropopliteal occlusive d.
Fenwick d.
fibrocontractive d.
fibrocystic d.
Fiedler d.
fifth d.
Filatov d.
fish-slime d.
Flajani d.
Flatau-Schilder d.
Flegel d.
flint d.
floating beta d.
focal d.
Folling d.
foot-and-mouth d. (FMD)
Forbes d.
Fordyce d.
Forestier d.
Förster d.
Fothergill d.
Fournier d.
fourth venereal d.

Fox-Fordyce d.
Francis d.
Frankl-Hochwart d.
Franklin d.
Frei d.
Freiberg d.
Friedländer d.
Friedmann d.
Friedreich d.
Friend d.
Frommel d.
functional d.
Furstner d.
Gairdner d.
Gaisböck d.
gametic d.
gamma chain d.
gamma heavy-chain d.
Gamna d.
Gandy-Nanta d.
gannister's d.
Garré d.
gasping d.
gastroesophageal reflux d. (GERD)
gastrointestinal d.
Gaucher d.
gay-related immunodeficiency d.
Gee d.
Gee-Herter d.
Gee-Herter-Heubner d.
Gee-Thaysen d.
Gensoul d.
Gerhardt d.
Gerlier d.
gestational trophoblastic d. (GTD)
giant platelet d.
Gibney d.
Gierke d.
Gilbert d.
Gilchrist d.
Glanzmann d.
Glénard d.
Glisson d.
glomerular basement membrane d.
glomerulocystic kidney d. (GCKD)
glycogen storage d. (GSD)
Goldflam d.
Goldflam-Erb d.
Goldscheider d.
Goldstein d.
Gorham d.
Gougerot-Blum d.

Gougerot-Ruiter d.
Gougerot-Sjögren d.
Graefe d.
graft versus host d. (GVHD)
granulomatous d.
Graves d.
Greenfield d.
Greenhow d.
Griesinger d.
Gross d.
Grover d.
Guinon d.
Gull d.
Günther d.
Habermann d.
Haff d.
Haglund d.
Hagner d.
Hailey-Hailey d.
Hall d.
Hallervorden-Spatz d.
Hallopeau d.
Hamman d.
Hamman-Rich d.
Hammond d.
Hand d.
hand-foot-and-mouth d.
Hand-Schüller-Christian d.
Hanot d.
Hansen d.
d. of Hapsburg
hard pad d.
Harley d.
Hartnup d.
Hashimoto d.
heavy chain d.
Heberden d.
Hebra d.
Heckathorn d.
Heerfordt d.
Heine-Medin d.
Heller-Döhle d.
helminthic d.
hemoglobin C d.
hemoglobin E-thalassemia d.
hemoglobin H d.
hemoglobin SO Arab sickle cell d.
Henderson-Jones d.
hepatic venoocclusive d.
hepatolenticular d.
hepatorenal glycogen storage d.
hereditary d.

D

NOTES

disease *(continued)*
  heredodegenerative d.
  herpetic viral d.
  herring-worm d.
  Hers d.
  Herter d.
  Herter-Heubner d.
  Heubner d.
  hidebound d.
  Hildenbrand d.
  Hippel d.
  Hippel-Lindau d.
  Hirschfeld d.
  Hirschsprung d. (HD)
  His d.
  His-Werner d.
  Hjärre d.
  hock d.
  Hodara d.
  Hodgkin d. (HD)
  Hodgson d.
  Hoffa d.
  holoendemic d.
  hoof-and-mouth d.
  hookworm d.
  Hoppe-Goldflam d.
  Horton d.
  Huchard d.
  Hunt d.
  Huntington d. (HD)
  Hurler d.
  Hutchinson d.
  Hutchinson-Boeck d.
  Hutchinson-Gilford d.
  Hutinel d.
  hyaline membrane d. (HMD)
  hydatid d. (HD)
  Hyde d.
  hydrocephaloid d.
  hyperendemic d.
  hypertensive arteriosclerotic heart d. (HASHD)
  hypertensive cardiovascular d. (HCVD)
  hypertensive pulmonary vascular d. (HPVD)
  hypopigmentation-immunodeficiency d.
  iatrogenic d.
  I-cell d.
  idiopathic Bamberger-Marie d.
  idiopathic Parkinson d.
  IgE-mediated d.
  immune complex d.
  immune-deposit d.
  immunodeficiency d.
  immunoproliferative small intestinal d. (IPSID)
  inborn lysosomal d.

inclusion body d.
inclusion cell d.
incompatible hemolytic blood transfusion d. (IHBTD)
infantile celiac d.
infantile polycystic kidney d.
infectious d.
infiltrative d.
inflammatory bowel d. (IBD)
inflammatory pelvic d. (IPD)
inherited d.
intercurrent d.
International Classification of D.'s (ICD)
interstitial lung d.
intestinal chronic graft-versus-host d.
iron-storage d.
Isambert d.
ischemic bowel d.
ischemic heart d. (IHD)
ischemic leg d. (ILD)
ischemic limb d. (ILD)
island d.
itai-itai d.
Jaffe-Lichtenstein d.
Jakob d.
Jakob-Creutzfeldt d.
Jaksch d.
Janet d.
Jansen d.
Jansky-Bielschowsky d.
Jensen d.
Johne d.
Johnson-Steven d.
joint d.
Jourdain d.
jumping d.
Jüngling d.
Kahlbaum d.
Kahler d.
Kalischer d.
Kashin-Bek d.
Kawasaki d.
Kayser d.
kedani d.
Keshan d.
Kienböck d.
Kikuchi d.
Kikuchi-Fujimoto d. (KFD)
Kimmelstiel-Wilson d.
Kimura d.
kinky hair d.
Kinnier Wilson d.
Kirkland d.
kissing d.
Klebs d.
Klemperer d.
Klippel d.

knight d.
Köhler d.
Köhlmeier-Degos d.
Koshevnikoff d.
Krabbe d.
Krishaber d.
Kufs d.
Kugelberg-Welander d.
Kuhnt-Junius d.
Kümmell d.
Kümmell-Verneuil d.
Kussmaul d.
Kussmaul-Maier d.
Kyasanur Forest d.
Kyrle d.
Laënnec d.
Lafora d.
Lancereaux-Mathieu d.
Landouzy d.
Landry d.
Lane d.
Langdon-Down d.
Larrey-Weil d.
Larsen d.
Larsen-Johansson d.
Lasègue d.
Lauber d.
L-chain d.
Leber d.
Ledderhose d.
Legal d.
Legg d.
Legg-Calvé-Perthes d.
Legg-Perthes d.
Legionnaire's d. (LD)
Leigh d.
Leiner d.
Leloir d.
Lenègre d.
Leri-Weill d.
Leroy d.
Letterer-Siwe d.
Lev d.
Lévi d.
Lewandowski-Lutz d.
Leyden d.
Libman-Sacks d.
Lichtheim d.
light chain deposition d.
Lignac d.
Lindau d.
Lindau-von Hippel d.

linear IgA bullous d. in children
lipid storage d.
Lipschütz d.
Little d.
Lobo d.
Lobstein d.
Löffler d.
long-segment Hirschsprung d.
Lorain d.
Lou Gehrig d.
Lowe d.
Lucas-Championnière d.
Luft d.
lumpy skin d.
lunger d.
Lutz-Splendore-Almeida d.
Lyell d.
Lyme d.
lymphocyte-depleted Hodgkin d.
 (LDHD)
lymphocyte-predominant Hodgkin d.
 (LPHD)
lymphoproliferative d. (LPD)
lymphoreticular d.
lysosomal storage d.
Madelung d.
Maffucci d.
Magitot d.
Maher d.
Majocchi d.
malabsorption d.
Malassez d.
maldigestive d.
Malherbe d.
Malibu d.
mammary Paget d.
Manson d.
maple bark stripper's d.
maple syrup urine d. (MSUD)
marble bone d.
Marburg virus d.
March d.
Marchiafava-Bignami d.
Marek d.
Marek herpesvirus d. (MDHV)
Marfan d.
Marie d.
Marie-Bamberger d.
Marie-Strümpell d.
Marie-Tooth d.
Marion d.
Marsh d.

D

NOTES

disease *(continued)*
    Martin d.
    mast cell d.
    Mathieu d.
    Maunier-Kuhn d.
    Maxcy d.
    McArdle d.
    McArdle-Schmid-Pearson d.
    McLean-Maxwell d.
    Medin d.
    Mediterranean hemoglobin E d.
    medullary cystic d. (MCD)
    Meige d.
    Meleda d.
    Ménétrier d.
    Ménière d.
    Merzbacher-Pelizaeus d.
    metabolic bone d.
    metabolic stone d.
    metabolic storage d.
    Meyenburg d.
    Meyer d.
    Mibelli d.
    microdrepanocytic d.
    micrometastatic d.
    microvillus inclusion d.
    Mikulicz d.
    Mills d.
    Milroy d.
    Milton d.
    Minamata d.
    minimal-change d.
    minimal residual d. (MRD)
    Minor d.
    Mitchell d.
    mixed-cellularity Hodgkin d.
      (MCHD)
    mixed connective tissue d.
      (MCTD)
    Miyasato d.
    Möbius d.
    molecular d.
    Möller-Barlow d.
    Molten d.
    Mondor d.
    Monge d.
    Morel-Kraepelin d.
    Morgagni d.
    Morquio d.
    Morquio-Ullrich d.
    Morton d.
    Morvan d.
    Moschcowitz d.
    motor neuron d.
    moyamoya d.
    Mucha d.
    Mucha-Habermann d.
    mucopolysaccharide storage d.
    mucosal d.

    mu heavy chain d.
    multicore d.
    multifactorial inherited d.
    Munchmeyer d.
    Myá d.
    myeloproliferative d.
    myocardial d.
    Nairobi sheep d.
    Neftel d.
    neoautoimmune d.
    neoplastic d.
    Neumann d.
    neuromuscular system d.
    neuronal intermediate filament
      inclusion d. (NIFID)
    neutral lipid storage d.
    newborn hemolytic d.
    newborn hemorrhagic d.
    Newcastle d.
    Newcastle virus d. (NVD)
    Nicolas-Favre d.
    Nidoko d.
    Nieden d.
    Niemann d.
    Niemann-Pick d. (NPD)
    nil d.
    nodular lymphocyte-rich Hodgkin d.
    nodular sclerosing Hodgkin d.
      (NSHD)
    no evidence of d. (NED)
    nonalcoholic fatty liver d.
      (NAFLD)
    Nonne-Milroy d.
    nonrelapsing d.
    Nordau d.
    Norwalk d.
    no significant d. (NSD)
    Notch3 gene polymorphism in
      ischemic cerebrovascular d.
    Novy rat d.
    oasthouse urine d.
    obstructive airway d. (OAD)
    obstructive lung d.
    occupational lung d.
    ocular inflammatory d. (OID)
    Ofuji d.
    Oguchi d.
    Ohara d.
    oid-oid d.
    Ollier d.
    Olmer d.
    Opitz d.
    Oppenheim d.
    Oppenheim-Urbach d.
    optic nerve d.
    organic d.
    Oriental lung fluke d.
    Ormond d.
    Osgood-Schlatter d.

Osler d.
Osler-Vaquez d.
Osler-Weber-Rendu d.
Otto d.
Owren d.
ox-warble d.
Paas d.
Paget d.
Panner d.
paper mill worker's d.
Parkinson d. (PD)
Parrot d.
Parry d.
Parson d.
Patella d.
Pauzat d.
Pavy d.
Payr d.
pearl-worker's d.
Pel-Ebstein d.
Pelizaeus-Merzbacher d.
Pellegrini d.
Pellegrini-Stieda d.
pelvic inflammatory d. (PID)
periodic d.
periodontal d.
peripheral arterial occlusive d. (PAOD)
peripheral arteriosclerotic occlusive d. (PAOD)
peripheral vascular d. (PVD)
Perrin-Ferraton d.
Perthes d.
Pette-Döring d.
Peyronie d.
Pfeiffer d.
Phocas d.
Pick d.
pickwickian d.
pigeon breeder d.
Pinkus d.
platelet-type von Willebrand d.
Plummer d.
polycystic kidney d. (PKD)
polycystic liver d.
polycystic ovary d.
polycystic renal d.
polyendocrine autoimmune d.
polyglutamine d.
Pompe d.
Poncet d.
Posada d.

Posada-Wernicke d.
posttransplant lymphoproliferative d. (PTLD)
Pott d.
Potter d.
Poulet d.
poultry handler's d.
Preiser d.
primary cold agglutinin d.
primary myocardial d. (PMD)
primary ovarian gestational trophoblastic d. (POGTD)
primary pigmented nodular adrenocortical d. (PPNAD)
Pringle d.
prion d.
prion-transmitted d.
Profichet d.
proliferative breast d. (PBD)
pseudo-von Willebrand d.
pulmonary heart d.
pulmonary thromboembolic d. (PTED)
pulmonary vascular d.
pulmonary veno-occlusive d. (PVOD)
pulseless d.
Purtscher d.
Pyle d.
pyramidal d.
quiet hip d.
Quincke d.
Quinquaud d.
Rangoon beggar's d.
Ranikhet d.
rat-bite d.
Rayer d.
Raynaud d. (RD)
Recklinghausen d.
Reclus d.
redwater d.
Reed-Hodgkin d.
Refsum d.
Reichmann d.
Reiter d.
relapsing d.
renal atheroembolic d.
renal cystic d.
Rendu-Osler-Weber d.
respiratory viral d.
restrictive lung d.
Rh_{null} d.

D

NOTES

disease *(continued)*
rheumatic heart d. (RHD)
rheumatic lung d.
rheumatoid heart d.
rhinocerebral d.
Ribas-Torres d.
Riedel d.
Riga-Fede d.
Rigg d.
Ritter d.
Robinson d.
Roble d.
Roger d.
Rokitansky d.
Romberg d.
Rosai-Dorfman d. (RDD)
Rosenbach d.
Rossbach d.
Roth d.
Roth-Bernhardt d.
Rougnon-Heberden d.
Roussy-Lévy d.
Rubarth d.
Rummo d.
runt d.
Rust d.
Ruysch d.
Rye classification of Hodgkin d.
Sachs d.
salivary gland virus d.
Sanders d.
Sandhoff d.
Saunders d.
Savill d.
Schamberg d.
Schanz d.
Schaumann d.
Schenck d.
Scheuermann d.
Schilder d.
Schimmelbusch d.
Schlatter d.
Schlatter-Osgood d.
Schmorl d.
Scholz d.
Schönlein d.
Schottmüller d.
Schroeder d.
Schüller d.
Schüller-Christian d.
Schultz d.
Schweninger-Buzzi d.
sea-blue histiocyte d.
secondary cold agglutinin d.
Seitelberger d.
self-limited d.
Selter d.
Senear-Usher d.
senile hip d.

septic d.
serum d.
sexually transmitted d. (STD)
Shaver d.
Shichito d.
shimamushi d.
sickle cell hemoglobin C, D d.
sickle cell thalassemia d.
silo-filler's d.
Simmonds d.
Simons d.
Siwe-Letterer d.
sixth venereal d.
Sjögren d.
skeletal d.
Skevas-Zerfus d.
skinbound d.
skip-segment Hirschsprung d.
slow virus d.
Sly d.
Smith d.
Smith-Strang d.
Sneddon-Wilkinson d.
specific d.
Spencer d.
sphingolipid storage d.
Spielmeyer-Stock d.
Spielmeyer-Vogt d.
spinal cord d.
sponge d.
stable d. (SD)
Stanton d.
Stargardt d.
Steinert d.
Sternberg d.
Sticker d.
Stieda d.
Still d.
Stokes-Adams d.
storage pool d.
Strümpell d.
Strümpell-Leichtenstern d.
Strümpell-Lorrain d.
Strümpell-Marie d.
Strümpell-Westphal d.
Sudeck d.
d. susceptibility
Sutton d.
Swediaur d.
Sweet d.
Swift d.
Swift-Feer d.
swine vesicular d.
Sydenham d.
Sylvest d.
Symmers d.
systemic autoimmune d.
systemic febrile d.
systemic mast cell d. (SMCD)

Takahara d.
Takayasu d.
Talfan d.
Talma d.
Tangier d.
Tarui d.
Taussig-Bing d.
Tay d.
Taylor d.
Tay-Sachs d. (TSD)
T-cell mediated d.
Teschen d.
thalassemia-sickle cell d.
Thaysen d.
Theiler d.
Thiemann d.
thin basement membrane d.
third d.
Thomsen d.
thromboembolic d. (TED)
Thygeson d.
thyrocardiac d.
thyrotoxic heart d.
Tillaux d.
Tommaselli d.
Tooth d.
Tornwaldt d.
Tourette d.
transfusion-associated graft-versus-host d. (TAGVHD)
transmissible d.
transplant vascular d.
transport d.
Trevor d.
trophoblastic d.
tropical d.
tsutsugamushi d.
tuberculosis-respiratory d. (TB-RD)
Tyzzer d.
ultrashort-segment Hirschsprung d.
Underwood d.
United States Army Medical Research Institute of Infectious D. (USAMRIID)
Unna d.
unstable hemoglobin d.
Unverricht d.
upper respiratory d. (URD)
Urbach-Oppenheim d.
Urbach-Wiethe d.
urinary tract d.
vagabond's d.

van Bogaert d.
van Buren d.
Vaquez d.
Vaquez-Osler d.
velogenic Newcastle d.
venereal d. (VD)
venereal d. gonorrhea (VDG)
Verneuil d.
Verse d.
Vidal d.
Vincent d.
vinyl chloride d.
viral hematodepressive d. (VHD)
Virchow d.
virus X d.
vocal cord d.
Vogt-Spielmeyer d.
Volkmann d.
Voltolini d.
von Bechterew d.
von Economo d.
von Gierke d.
von Hippel d.
von Hippel-Lindau d.
von Jaksch d.
von Meyenburg d.
von Recklinghausen d.
von Willebrand d. (VW)
Voorhoeve d.
Vrolik d.
Wagner d.
Waldenström d.
Wardrop d.
Wartenberg d.
Wassilieff d.
wasting d.
Weber-Christian d.
Weber-Rendu-Osler d.
Wegner d.
Weil d.
Weir Mitchell d.
Wenckebach d.
Werdnig-Hoffmann d.
Werlhof d.
Werner-His d.
Werner-Schultz d.
Wesselsbron d.
Westphal d.
Westphal-Strümpell d.
Whipple d.
White d.
white muscle d.

D

NOTES

disease *(continued)*
    white spot d.
    Whitmore d.
    Whytt d.
    Wilkie d.
    Willis d.
    Wilson d. (WD)
    Winckel d.
    Windscheid d.
    Winiwarter-Buerger d.
    Winkler d.
    Winton d.
    Witkop d.
    Wohlfart-Kugelberg-Welander d.
    Wolman d.
    Woringer-Kolopp d.
    X-linked lymphoproliferative d.
    Zahorsky d.
    Ziehen-Oppenheim d.
    Zinsser-Brill d.
    zoonotic d.
disease-associated bacterial toxin
disease-free survival (DFS)
disease-specific survival
disfigurative
disgerminoma
dish
    Petri d.
    Stender d.
disiens
    Bacteroides d.
    Prevotella d.
disinfect
disinfectant
    nonoemulsion d.
disinfection
disinsection
disintegration constant
disjunction
disjunctive absorption
disjunctum
    stratum d.
disk *(var. of* disc)
diskiform *(var. of* disciform)
diskitis *(var. of* discitis)
diskocyte *(var. of* discocyte)
dislocation
    anterior complete d.
    closed d.
    complete anterior d.
    complete inferior d.
    complete posterior d.
    complete superior d.
    compound d.
    congenital d.
    fracture d.
    lens d.
    pathologic d.

dismutase
    extracellular superoxide d. (EC-SOD)
    superoxide d.
disomic population
disomy
    uniparental d. (UPD)
disopyramide
disorder
    absorptive d.
    acid-base d.
    amino acid d.
    antifactor I–IX d.
    autosomal dominant d.
    autosomal recessive d.
    B-cell chronic lymphoproliferative d. (BCLPD)
    B-cell lymphoproliferative d. (BLPD)
    biliary d.
    bipolar depression d.
    bladder d.
    blood coagulation d.
    bone marrow d.
    CEAP classification of venous d.'s
    central nervous system d.
    chromosomal d.
    chronic lymphoproliferative d. (CLPD)
    chronic myeloproliferative d. (CMPD)
    circulating antithromboplastin d.
    clonal d.
    collagen d.
    complex adrenal endocrine d.
    complex gonadal endocrine d.
    complex pituitary endocrine d.
    complex thyroid endocrine d.
    connective tissue d.
    cytogenetic d.
    digestive d.
    element d.
    fatty acid oxidation d. (FOD)
    fibrinolytic d.
    functional d.
    glomerular d.
    glycogen storage d. (GSD)
    gonadal endocrine d.
    growth d.
    hemolytic d.
    hemorrhagic d.
    homozygous-type hemoglobin d.
    immune complex d.
    immunoglobulin d.
    immunoproliferative d.
    infectious d.
    inflammatory d.
    inherited giant platelet d. (IGPD)
    intestinal flow d.

ion d.
lipid transport d.
lymphoproliferative d.
lymphoreticular d.
malabsorption d.
metabolic d.
mitochondrially inherited d.
myeloproliferative d.
nasal allergic d.
neurodegenerative d.
neurovisceral storage d.
neutrophil functional d.
paraneoplastic d.
parathyroid d.
Paris-Trousseau platelet d.
peristalsis d.
phagocytic function d.
pharyngeal muscle d.
pituitary endocrine d.
plasma iodoprotein d.
polyglutamine expansion d.
posttransplant lymphoproliferative d.
  (PTLD)
proliferative d.
Quebec platelet d.
respiratory acid-base d.
retinal d.
sickling d.
single gene d. (SGD)
sleep d.
T-cell d.
thyroid endocrine d.
tic d.
transient myeloproliferative d.
trinucleotide repeat d.
uncommon developmental d.
ureteral peristalsis d.
urogenital d.
vascular d.
X-linked recessive d.
XXX d.
XXXX d.
XXXXY d.
XXXY d.
XXYY d.
disordered
d. action of heart (DAH)
d. epithelial growth
d. immunoregulation
d. proliferative endometrium
disorganization

dispar
  Entamoeba d.
  Veillonella alcalescens subsp. *d.*
disparate
disparity
dispermic chimera
dispermy
disperse phase
dispersion
colloidal d.
d. medium
molecular d.
optical rotary d. (ORD)
population d.
dispersive medium
Dispira
displaceability
tissue d.
displaced ganglion cell
displacement
d. analysis
anterior d.
epithelial d.
d. of epithelium
mechanical d.
tissue d.
display
digital differential d. (DDD)
seven-segment d.
Disporotrichum
disposable chemical-resistant clothing
disposition of victim remains
disproportion
cephalopelvic d. (CPD)
disproportionate
binucleation d.
disrupter
ultrasonic cell d.
disruption
ossicular chain d.
dissecans
endometritis d.
osteochondritis d.
pneumonia d.
dissect
dissecting
d. aneurysm
d. microscope
d. osteitis
dissection
aortic d.
d. resorption

D

NOTES

dissection *(continued)*
    retroperitoneal lymph node d. (RPLND)
    spontaneous coronary artery d. (SCAD)
    d. tubercle
    vascular d.
disseminata
    dermatofibrosis lenticularis d.
    leiomyomatosis peritonealis d.
    osteitis fibrosa d.
disseminate coccidioidomycosis
disseminated
    d. acute lupus erythematosus
    d. aspergillosis
    d. candidiasis
    d. condensing osteopathy
    d. foci (DF)
    d. inflammation
    d. intravascular coagulation (DIC)
    d. lipogranulomatosis
    d. sclerosis
    d. superficial actinic porokeratosis (DSAP)
    d. tuberculosis
dissemination
    hematogenous d.
disseminatum
    keratoma d.
    xanthoma d. (XD)
disseminatus
    lupus erythematosus d. (LED)
Disse space
dissociated islet cell
dissociation
    albuminocytologic d.
    bacterial d.
    d. constant
    d. enhanced lanthanide fluoroimmunoassay (DELFIA)
    microbic d.
dissolution
Dissolve-A-Way tape
dissymmetry
distal
    d. alveoli
    d. centriole
    d. ileitis
    d. latency
    d. metastases
    d. muscular dystrophy
    d. myopathy
    d. RTA
distal-type progressive muscular dystrophy
distance
    focal d.
    interelectrode d.
    d. learning

    skin-to-tumor d. (STD)
    working d.
distant
    d. organ metastasis
    d. range entrance wound
distantly vaccinated
distasonis
    Bacteroides d.
distemper
    feline d.
    d. virus
distended bursa, shoulder
distensae
    striae cutis d.
distention, distension
    d. of alveolar capillary
    d. cyst
    d. ulcer
distill
distillate
distillation
    destructive d.
    fractional d.
    molecular d.
    vacuum d.
distilled oil
distincta
    Pseudoalteromonas d.
distinctive
    d. epithelium
    d. form
Distoma
distome
distomiasis
    pulmonary d.
Distomum
distortion
    barreling d.
    crypt d.
distortum
    Microsporum canis var. *d.*
distress
    fetal d.
distributa
    Vulcanisaeta d.
distributing artery
distribution
    actin d.
    anomalous vascular d.
    antigenic d.
    binomial d.
    chi squared d.
    d. coefficient
    cumulative d.
    d. curve
    dose d.
    extracellular in d.
    F d.
    fetal-maternal erythrocyte d.

focal segmental d.
frequency d.
d. function
gaussian d.
intron-exon d.
d. leukocytosis
lognormal d.
nitrogen d.
patchy d.
Poisson d.
probability d.
reference d.
sample d.
skewed d.
symmetric d.
t d.
disulfide
d. bond
carbon d.
dihydroxydinaphthyl d. (DDD)
glutathione d. (GSSG)
disulfiram assay
disulfonate
sodium indigotin d.
disulfoton
disuse atrophy
DIT
diiodotyrosine
drug-induced thrombocytopenia
dithionate
sodium d.
dithionite test
dithiothreitol (DTT)
Dittrich
D. plug
D. stenosis
diuresis, pl. **diureses**
postobstructive d.
diuretic
cardiac d.
hemopoiesic d.
loop d.
mechanical d.
osmotic d.
potassium-sparing d.
thiazide d.
diurna
microfilaria d.
diurnal
diuron
divalent ion metabolism (DIM)
divarication

divergence
divergens
Babesia d.
divergent
diversion
d. colitis
d. pouchitis
d. proctocolitis
diversity
methylation pattern d.
NK clonal d.
viral genomic d.
diversum
Mogibacterium d.
diversus
Citrobacter d.
Levinea d.
diverticula (*pl. of* diverticulum)
diverticular disease
diverticulitis
hemorrhagic d.
obstructive d.
perforated d.
diverticuloma
diverticulosis
segmental colitis associated with d.
(SCAD)
diverticulum, pl. **diverticula**
cervical d.
duodenal d.
epiphrenic d.
false d.
hypopharyngeal d.
Meckel d.
Pertik d.
pharyngoesophageal d.
pulsion d.
traction d.
true d.
urethral d.
ventricular d.
vesical d.
Zenker d.
divided dose
divider
voltage d.
diving goiter
divisio
division
cell d.
conjugate d.
equational d.

D

NOTES

division (*continued*)
    maturation d.
    parasympathetic d.
    reduction d.
Dixon test
dizygotic twins
DJD
    degenerative joint disease
DK
    decay
DKA
    diabetic ketoacidosis
DL
    difference limen
    Donath-Landsteiner
        DL antibody
        DL biphasic hemolysis
        DL hemolysin
dL
    deciliter
D-lactic acidosis
DLBCL
    diffuse large B-cell lymphoma
DLC
    differential leukocyte count
DLCL
    diffuse large cell lymphoma
DLCO
    diffusing capacity of lung for carbon
      monoxide
DL2000 data management system
DLE
    discoid lupus erythematosus
DLK1
    deltalike 1 homolog
        DLK1 gene
D-loop region
DM
    myotonic dystrophy
    NATO code for diphenylaminearsine
      (adamsite)
    NATO code for
      diphenylaminochloroarsine (adamsite)
dm
    decimeter
DMA
    dimethyladenosine
    dimethylarsinic acid
DMAB
    dimethylaminobenzaldehyde
DMAP
    4-dimethylaminophenol
DMAT
    Disaster Medical Assistance Team
DMBA
    dimethylbenzanthracene
DMD
    Duchenne muscular dystrophy

DME
    drug metabolizing enzyme
DMH
    diffuse mesangial hypercellularity
DMIPS
    dimethylisopropylsilyl
DMORT
    Disaster Mortuary Team
DMPE
    dimethoxyphenylethylamine
DMPH
    dysgenetic male pseudohermaphroditism
DMSO
    dimethylsulfoxide
DN
    dextrose nitrogen ratio
    dibucaine number
DNA
    deoxyribonucleic acid
    DNA adduct level
    amplifiable DNA
    DNA aneuploidy
    DNA array analysis
    branched DNA (b-DNA)
    DNA break
    DNA chip
    complementary DNA (cDNA)
    DNA complexity
    DNA copy number
    DNA cytophotometry
    double-stranded DNA (DS-DNA)
    DNA fingerprint
    DNA fingerprinting
    DNA flow cytometry
    fluorochrome-conjugated DNA
    DNA gel electrophoresis
    hairpin DNA
    DNA homology
    DNA hybridization
    DNA ligase
    DNA marker
    DNA microarray
    DNA microarray technology
    mouthwash method collection of
      genomic DNA
    DNA multiploidy
    DNA nucleotidylexotransferase
    DNA nucleotidyltransferase
    plasma DNA
    DNA ploidy
    DNA polymerase
    DNA probe
    DNA reassociation
    recombinant DNA (rDNA)
    DNA renaturation
    DNA repair
    ribosomal DNA (rDNA)
    self-complementary DNA

DNA sequence copy number change
DNA sequencing
single-stranded DNA (SS-DNA)
DNA slot blot technique
DNA synthesis
DNA synthesis reagent
DNA template
DNA transfer
DNA virus
DNA-aneuploid tumor cell
DNA-DNA hybridization
DNA-enzyme immunoassay (DEIA)
DNA-Prep workstation & reagent system
DNA-RNA hybridization
DNA/RNA Protect
DNase, DNAse
deoxyribonuclease
DNase agar
DNase test
DNAzole cell suspension
DNC
dinitrocarbanilide
DNCB
dinitrochlorobenzene
DNET
dysplastic neuroepithelial tumor
DNFB
dinitrofluorobenzene
DNOC
dinitroorthocresol
DNP
deoxyribonucleoprotein
DNPH
dinitrophenylhydrazine
DNPH test
DO7 antibody
DOA
dead on arrival
drugs of abuse
DOC
death of other cause
deoxycorticoid
deoxycorticosterone
DOCA
deoxycorticosterone acetate
docimasia
auricular d.
hepatic d.
pulmonary d.
docosahexaenoic acid (DHA)

doctrine
Arrhenius d.
documentation
forensic d.
DOD
dead of disease
Döderlein bacillus
doebereinerae
Azospirillum d.
dog
d. disease
d. distemper virus
d. flea
d. fly
d. hookworm
d. louse
d. nose
d. unit
Dogiel
D. cell
D. corpuscle
Döhle
D. disease
D. inclusion
D. inclusion body
Döhle-Heller aortitis
Dold
D. reaction
D. test
dolens
leukophlegmasia d.
phlegmasia alba d.
phlegmasia cerulea d.
dolichocolon
dolichoectatic artery
dolichol phosphate
Dolichos biflorus
dolipore
doll's
d. eye movement
d. kidney
dolor
doloresi
Gnathostoma d.
dolorosa
adiposis d.
tubercula d.
dolosa
Burkholderia d.
Dolosicoccus paucivorans
DOMA
dihydroxymandelic acid

NOTES

D

domain
> adhesive extracellular d.
> amino-terminal d.
> death effector d.
> a disintegrin and metalloproteinase with thrombospondin d. 13 (ADAMTS 13)

Dombrock antigen
dombrowskii
> *Halococcus d.*

dome cell
dome-shaped
domestica
> *Musca d.*

domesticus
> *Glyciphagus d.*

domiciliated
dominance
> incomplete d.

dominant
> d. character
> d. complement
> d. complementarity
> d. gene
> d. inheritance
> d. negative mutation

dominantly inherited Lévi disease
DON
> deoxynivalenol

Donath-Landsteiner (DL)
> D.-L. antibody
> D.-L. biphasic hemolysin
> D.-L. cold autoantibody
> D.-L. phenomenon
> D.-L. syndrome
> D.-L. test

donation
> blood d.
> designated blood d.
> NAT for HCV and HIV-1 in blood d.

donensis
> *Superstitionia d.*

Donkioporia
Donnan potential
Donné
> D. body
> D. corpuscle
> D. test

Donohue syndrome
donor
> cadaver d.
> consanguineous d.
> F d.
> living d. (LD)
> d. neocyte
> proton d.
> d. tissue
> universal d.

donor-specific
> d.-s. crossmatching
> d.-s. HLA antibody

Donovan body
donovani
> *Leishmania donovani d.*

donovania
> *Calymmatobacterium d.*

Donovania granulomatis
DOP
> degenerate oligonucleotide-primed
> DOP PCR

DOPA
> dihydroxyphenylalanine
> DOPA stain

dopamine
> d. hydroxylase
> d. monooxygenase
> urine d.

dopaminergic neuron
dopaquinone
dopa reaction
DOP-PCR
> degenerate oligonucleotide primed polymerase chain reaction

doppel protein
Doppler effect
Dora
> hemoglobin Koya D.

d'orange
> peau d.

Doratomyces stemonitis
Dorea
> *D. formicigenerans*
> *D. longicatena*

Dorello canal
doricum
> *Mycobacterium d.*

Doriden
dormancy
dormant
Dorner stain
Dorothy Reed cell
dorsal
> d. nerve root
> d. spine ankylosis

dorsalis
> *Aedes d.*
> tabes d.

dorsi
> elastofibroma d.
> osteochondritis deformans juvenilis d.

dorsopancreaticus
> ductus d.

dosage
> d. compensation
> gene d.
> high d. (HD)

dose
absorbed d.
d. account
air d.
booster d.
d. calibrator
curative d.
depth d.
d. distribution
divided d.
effective d. (ED)
epilating d.
erythema d.
d. estimate
exit d.
fatal d. (FD)
genetically significant d. (GSD)
guinea pig intraperitoneal
  infectious d. (GPIPID)
incapacitating d.
infecting d. (ID)
infective d. (ID)
integral d.
L d.
L^+ d.
L_0 d.
lethal d. (LD)
Lf d.
loading d.
Lr d.
maximal permissible d. (MPD)
mean hemolytic d. (MHD)
median curative d. (CD_{50})
median effective d. (ED_{50})
median fatal d. (FD_{50})
median infectious d. (ID_{50})
median lethal d. (LD_{50})
median tissue culture d. (TCD_{50})
median tissue culture infective d.
  ($TCID_{50}$)
medical internal radiation d.
  (MIRD)
minimal erythema d. (MED)
minimal infecting d. (MID)
minimal lethal d.
minimal morbidostatic d. (MMD)
minimal reacting d. (MRD)
minimum hemolytic d. (MHD)
minimum infective d. (MID)
minimum lethal d. (MLD)
normal single d. (NSD)
organ tolerance d. (OTD)

radiation absorbed d. (rad)
d. rate
sensitizing d.
shocking d.
skin test d. (STD)
threshold erythema d. (TED)
tissue culture d. (TCD)
tissue culture infective d. (TCID)
tissue tolerance d. (TTD)
titrated initial d. (TID)
tumor lethal d. (TLD)
dose-rate/meter
dose-reduction factor (DRF)
dosimeter
criticality locket d.
neutron personnel d.
pencil d.
pocket d.
quartz fiber d. (QFD)
thermoluminescent d. (TLD)
ultraviolet fluorescent d.
dosimetry
dot
d. blot test
Maurer d.
Mittendorf d.
d. product
d. scan
Schüffner d.
Ziemann d.
dot-blot
forward d.-b.
reverse d.-b.
Dothichiza
Dothiorella mangiferae
double
d. albuminemia
d. antibody immunoassay
d. antibody immunoenzymometric
  assay
d. antibody method
d. antibody precipitation
d. antibody sandwich assay
d. antibody technique
d. blood supply
d. diffusion
d. diffusion test
d. discharge
d. ductus arteriosus
d. fluorescence labeling
d. (gel) diffusion precipitin test in
  one dimension

D

NOTES

double *(continued)*
    d. (gel) diffusion precipitin test in two dimensions
    d. helix
    d. immunodiffusion
    d. immunolabeling
    d. intussusception
    d. minute chromosome
    d. oxalate
    d. phenotypic pattern
    d. pneumonia
    d. refraction
    d. stain
    d. staining technique
    d. tertian malaria
    d. trisomy
double-beam photometer
double-blind
    double-blind experiment
    d.-b. study
double-contrast
    d.-c. examination
    d.-c. study
doublecortin
double-crossed immunoelectrophoresis
double-fluorescence microlymphocytotoxicity
double-fusion FISH (D-FISH)
double-layer fluorescent antibody technique
double-masked experiment
double-pole
    d.-p. double-throw switch
    d.-p. single-throw switch
double-precision variable
double-stranded
    d.-s. DNA (DS-DNA)
    d.-s. DNA virus
double-voided urine specimen
doubling
    d. dilution
    d. time
Doucas
    purpura of D.
doudoroffii
    Oceanimonas d.
Douglas
    D. abscess
    pouch of D.
dourine
Dowex
Down
    D. syndrome (DS)
    D. syndrome tau pathology
Downey cell
Downey-type lymphocyte
down-regulation
downstream

doxepin
    d. hydrochloride
    d. hydrochloride assay
Doyère eminence
D-PAS, dPAS
    diastase-periodic acid-Schiff
        D-PAS stain
DPB
    diffuse panbronchiolitis
DPC
    delayed primary closure
Dpc4 immunohistochemical pancreatic cancer analysis
DPC4 gene
DPD
    deoxypyridinoline
DPDL
    diffuse poorly differentiated lymphoma
DPH
    Department of Public Health
    diphenhydramine
    diphenylhexatriene
    diphenylhydantoin
DPI
    diphenyleneiodonium
DPN
    deep penetrating nevus
    diphosphopyridine nucleotide
DPNH
    diphosphopyridine nucleotide
DPPIV
    dipeptidyl peptidase IV protein
DPX
    ER-Tracker blue-white D.
DR
    diabetic retinopathy
    reaction of degeneration
DR-70 tumor marker test
Drabkin reagent
dracontiasis
dracunculiasis, dracunculosis
Dracunculus
    D. lova
    D. medinensis
    D. oculi
    D. persarum
Dragendorff
    D. solution
    D. test
dragon
    d. worm
    d. worm infection
drainage
    anomalous venous d.
    biliary d.
    percutaneous transhepatic biliary d.
drain-trap stomach
dramatic response

drancourtii
: *Legionella d.*

DRE
: digital rectal examination

Drechslera hawaiiensis
drench hose
drentensis
: *Bacillus d.*

drepanidium
Drepanidotaenia lanceolata
drepanocyte
drepanocythemia
drepanocytic
drepanocytosis
Drepanopeziza
Dresbach
: D. anemia
: D. syndrome

Dressler syndrome
DRF
: dose-reduction factor

dried
: d. blood spot
: d. human serum
: d. smear
: d. sodium phosphate
: d. yeast

drift
: antigenic d.
: genetic d.
: nosologic d.
: random genetic d.

drip-arm hyponatremia
drop
: capsular d.
: d. heart
: voltage d.

droplet
: electron-dense d.
: fat d.
: d. infection
: macrovesicular fat d.
: d. nuclei
: d. precautions

droplet-borne agent
dropsical
dropsy
: abdominal d.

Drosophila
: wingless signaling pathway in *D.*

drozanskii
: *Legionella d.*

drozdowiczii
: *Streptomyces d.*

DRPLA
: dentatorubral pallidoluysian atrophy

drug
: d.'s of abuse (DOA)
: d. abuse screen
: d. addiction
: afterload-reducing d.
: d. allergy
: antibiotic antitumor d.
: antimetabolite d.
: d. dependence
: d. desensitization
: d. detoxification
: d. interaction
: d. interference
: d. metabolism
: d. metabolizing enzyme (DME)
: ototoxic d.
: pharmacology of immunosuppressive d.
: radioactive d.
: d. screening assay
: sulfa d.
: d. tolerance
: d. utilization review

drug-fast
drug-induced
: d.-i. autoimmune hemolytic anemia
: d.-i. hepatitis
: d.-i. immune hemolytic anemia
: d.-i. myocarditis
: d.-i. neutropenia
: d.-i. thrombocytopenia (DIT)

drug-resistant
drum membrane
drumstick
: d. appendage
: d. finger
: d. spore

drusen
DRx quantitative hCG patient monitor test
dry
: d. abscess
: d. beriberi
: d. bronchiectasis
: d. catarrh
: d. decontamination
: d. desquamation
: d. gangrene

D

NOTES

dry *(continued)*
    d. leprosy
    d. objective
    d. pleurisy
    d. tap
drying agent
Drysdale corpuscle
DS
    defined substrate
    dextrose-saline
    Down syndrome
4Ds
    diplopia, dysphagia, dysarthria,
      dysphonia
DSAP
    disseminated superficial actinic
      porokeratosis
DS-DNA
    double-stranded DNA
DSM
    dextrose solution mixture
DSPC
    desaturated phosphatidylcholine
DSRCT
    desmoplastic small round cell tumor
DST
    dexamethasone suppression test
D-Stoff (phosgene gas)
DSX automated ELISA system
DT
    delirium tremens
dTDP
    thymidine diphosphate
DTF
    desmoid-type fibromatosis
    detector transfer function
DTH
    delayed-type hypersensitivity
DTICH
    delayed traumatic intracerebral hematoma
DTM
    dermatophyte test medium
DTN
    diphtheria toxin normal
DTP
    diphtheria, tetanus, and pertussis vaccine
DTT
    dithiothreitol
dTTP
    deoxythymidine triphosphate
DTX series multimode detector
DU
    depleted uranium
      DU Series 500, DU 800 UV/Vis
        spectrophotometer
dual
    d. color probe
    d. hemostatic defect
dual-color fluorescence

dual-contrast study
dual-in-line package
dualism
Duane-Hunt relation
Duane syndrome
Dubini disease
Dubin-Johnson syndrome
Dubin-Sprinz syndrome
dubius
    Sulfitobacter d.
dubliniensis
    Candida d.
Dubois
    D. abscess
    D. disease
Duboisia myoporoides
duboisii
    Histoplasma capsulatum var. *d.*
Dubreuil-Chambardel syndrome
Dubreuilh
    precancerous melanosis of D.
Duchenne
    D. disease
    D. muscular dystrophy (DMD)
    D. syndrome
Duchenne-Aran disease
Duchenne-Erb syndrome
Duchenne-Griesinger disease
duck
    d. embryo origin vaccine
    d. hepatitis virus
    d. influenza virus
    d. plague
    d. plague virus
Ducrey
    D. bacillus
    D. test
ducreyi
    Haemophilus d.
duct
    aberrant d.
    accessory pancreatic d.
    alveolar d.
    anal d.
    Arantius d.
    Bartholin d.
    basilar crest of cochlear d.
    basilar membrane of cochlear d.
    Bellini d.
    Bernard d.
    bile d.
    biliary d.
    Blasius d.
    breast d.
    canalicular d.
    d. carcinoma
    choledoch d.
    cochlear d.
    collecting d.

common bile d.
cystic d.
deferent d.
efferent d.
ejaculatory d.
endolymphatic d.
d. of epididymis
excretory d.
galactophorous d.
gall d.
guttural d.
hemithoracic d.
Hensen d.
Hoffmann d.
intercalated d.
interlobar d.
interlobular d.
intralobular d.
lactiferous d.
Luschka d.
lymphatic d.
major sublingual d.
mamillary d.
mammary d.
milk d.
minor sublingual d.
pancreatic d.
papillary d.
d. papilloma
paraurethral d.
parotid d.
perilymphatic d.
prostatic d.
Rivinus d.
salivary d.
Santorini d.
Schüller d.
secretory d.
semicircular d.
d. of Skene gland
spermatic d.
Stensen d.
striated d.
submandibular d.
submaxillary d.
sudoriferous d.
sweat d.
tectorial membrane of cochlear d.
testicular d.
tympanic wall of cochlear d.
uniting d.
utriculosaccular d.

vestibular wall of cochlear d.
Walther d.
Wharton d.
Wirsung d.
ductal
  d. adenoma
  d. carcinoma
  d. carcinoma in situ (DCIS)
  d. hyperplasia
  d. intraepithelial neoplasia (DIN)
  d. lavage
  d. papilloma
  d. plate
ductectatic-type mucinous cystic tumor
ductibus
  glandulae sine d.
ductless gland
ductography
ductopenia
ductoscopy
ductular
  d. piecemeal necrosis
  d. reactive cell
ductule
  aberrant d.
  biliary d.
  efferent d.
  interlobular d.
  intralobular d.
  perilesional d.
  proliferating bile d.'s (PBD)
  prostatic d.
ductulus, pl. **ductuli**
  d. aberrans inferior
  d. aberrans superior
  ductuli aberrantes
  d. alveolaris
  ductuli biliferi
  ductuli efferentes testis
  ductuli excretorii glandula
  ductuli interlobulares
  ductuli paroophori
  ductuli prostatici
ductus, gen. and pl. **ductus**
  d. aberrantes
  d. biliferi
  d. choledochus
  d. cochlearis
  d. cysticus
  d. deferens
  d. deferens tumor
  d. dorsopancreaticus

NOTES

319

ductus *(continued)*
    d. ejaculatorius
    d. endolymphaticus
    d. epididymidis
    d. excretorius
    d. excretorius vesiculae seminalis
    d. hemithoracicus
    d. lactiferi
    d. pancreaticus
    d. pancreaticus accessorius
    d. paraurethrales
    d. parotideus
    d. perilymphaticus
    d. prostatici
    d. reuniens
    d. semicirculares
    d. sublinguales minores
    d. sublingualis major
    d. submandibularis
    d. submaxillaris
    d. sudoriferus
    d. utriculosaccularis
Duddell membrane
Duffy
    D. antibody
    D. antibody Fya
    D. antibody Fyb
    D. antigen
    D. antigen receptor for chemokine (DARC)
    D. blood antibody type
    D. blood group system
Duganella violaceinigra
Duhamel technique
Duhring disease
Duke
    D. bleeding time test
    D. method
    D. method of bleeding time
Dukes
    D. A, B, C tumor stage
    D. carcinoma classification
    D. disease
    D. staging
Dukes-Astler-Coller adenocarcinoma classification
dullness
    Gerhardt d.
    relative hepatic d. (RHD)
dumbbell ganglioneuroma
Dumdum fever
dummy variable
dumoffii
    Legionella d.
dUMP
    deoxyuridine monophosphate
dumping syndrome
Duncan
    D. disease

    D. multiple-range test
    D. syndrome
Dunnett multiple component test
duodenal
    d. atresia
    d. carcinoma
    d. contents culture
    d. contents examination
    d. diverticulum
    d. fistula
    d. gland
    d. gland in submucosa
    d. parasite
    d. smear
    d. ulcer
    d. ulcer perforation (DUP)
duodenale
    Ancylostoma d.
duodenales
    glandulae d.
duodeni
    pseudomelanosis d.
duodenitis
duodenocholangitis
duovirus
DUP
    duodenal ulcer perforation
DU-PAN-2 pancreatic cancer-associated antigen
Duplay syndrome
duplex
    Haemophilus d.
    ileum d.
    d. ileum
    d. kidney
    d. placenta
    d. scan
duplication
    caudal dipygus d.
    congenital d.
    cranial monocephalus d.
    d. cyst
    d. deficiency
    facial diprosopus d.
    fetal d.
    trunk d.
Dupré syndrome
Dupuytren
    D. contracture
    D. disease of the foot
    D. fibromatosis
dural sheath
dura mater
Durand disease
Durand-Nicolas-Favre disease
Duran-Reynals permeability factor
durans
    Streptococcus d.
Durante disease

Dura-Temp specimen transporter
Dürck node
Durella
Duret hemorrhage
Durham tube
durianis
    Lactobacillus d.
Durie and Salmon multiple myeloma
  clinical staging
Duroziez disease
durum
    papilloma d.
dusky erythema
dust
    blood d.
    d. cell
    chromatin d.
    d. corpuscle
    nuclear d.
Dutch classification
Dutcher body
DUTP
    deoxyuridine triphosphate
Dutton
    D. disease
    D. relapsing fever
    D. spirochete
Duttonella
duttonii
    Borrelia d.
Duverney gland
dux
    Sarcophaga d.
DVT
    deep vein thrombosis
D5W, D$_5$W
    5 percent dextrose in water
D/W
    dextrose in water (percent)
dwarf
    achondroplastic d.
    d. colony
    constitutional d.
    d. kidney
    pituitary d.
    primordial d.
    d. tapeworm
dwarfism
    achondroplastic d.
    acromelic d.
    chondrodystrophic d.
    Fröhlich d.

    Laron d.
    lethal d.
    Lorain d.
    mesomelic d.
    micromelic d.
    phocomelic d.
    pituitary d.
    polydystrophic d.
    senile d.
    Silver-Russell d.
    snub-nose d.
    thanatophoric d.
DxI 800 immunoassay system
D-xylose
    D-x. absorption
    D-x. absorption test
    D-x. tolerance test
dyad
Dyadobacter fermentans
dydrogesterone
dye
    acid d.
    acidic d.
    acidophilic d.
    acridine d.
    aminoanthraquinone d.
    aminoketone d.
    amphoteric d.
    aniline d.
    anionic d.
    anthraquinone d.
    arsenazo III d.
    azin d.
    azo d.
    azocarmine d.
    azoic d.
    basic d.
    cationic d.
    d. content
    DAPI d.
    diphenylmethane d.
    endolymphatic d.
    d. exclusion test
    d. excretion test
    fluorescent d.
    Hoechst d.
    hydroxyketone d.
    indamine d.
    indigoid d.
    indophenol d.
    ketonimine d.
    lactone d.

D

NOTES

dye (*continued*)
    metachromatic d.
    methine d.
    methylene blue d. (MBD)
    natural d.
    NBT d.
    nitro d.
    nitroblue tetrazolium d.
    nitroso d.
    oxazin d.
    patent blue V d.
    phthalocyanine d.
    polycationic d.
    polymethine d.
    quinoline d.
    quinolinium d.
    rosanilin d.
    salt d.
    stilbene d.
    sulfur d.
    synthetic d.
    thiazin d.
    thiazole d.
    triarylmethane d.
    triphenylmethane d.
    vital d.
    xanthene d.
dye-binding capacity (DBC)
dye-dilution curve
dyed starch method
Dyggve-Melchior-Clausen syndrome
Dyke-Davidoff-Masson syndrome
dyn
    dyne
DyNA block 1000 microtiter plate
dynamic
    d. equilibrium
    d. ileus
    d. isomerism
    d. pulmonary compliance
    d. real-time telepathology
    d. storage allocation
    d. viscosity
dynamite heart
dyne (dyn)
dynein arm
Dynex Immulon 1B microtiter plate
dyphylline
Dyrenium
dysautonomia
    familial d.
dysbarism
dysbetalipoproteinemia
    familial d.
dysbolism
dyscephalia mandibulooculofacialis
dyschondrogenesis
dyschondroplasia with hemangiomas
dyschondrosteosis

dyscohesion
    cellular d.
dyscrasia
    blood d.
    lymphatic d.
    plasma cell d.
dyscrasic, dyscratic
dysembryoma
dysembryoplastic neuroepithelial tumor
dysemia
dysencephalia splanchnocystica
dysenteriae
    Amoeba d.
    Bacillus d.
    Shigella d.
dysentery
    amebic d.
    d. antitoxin
    bacillary d.
    d. bacilli
    balantidial d.
    bilharzial d.
    catarrhal d.
    ciliary d.
    ciliate d.
    epidemic d.
    flagellate d.
    Flexner d.
    fulminant d.
    giardiasis d.
    malarial d.
    protozoal d.
    scorbutic d.
    Sonne d.
    spirillar d.
    sporadic d.
    viral d.
    winter d. of cattle
dyserythropoiesis
dyserythropoietic congenital anemia
dysfibrinogenemia
dysfunction
    autonomic d.
    bladder d.
    constitutional hepatic d.
    enterostomy d.
    infarctive placental d.
    minimal brain d. (MBD)
    multiorgan d.
    ovarian d.
    papillary muscle d.
    phagocyte d.
    pituitary d.
    placental d.
    ventricular d.
dysfunctional uterine bleeding
dysgammaglobulinemia
    type I, II d.

dysgenesis
    familial gonadal d.
    gonadal d.
    pure gonadal d. (PGD)
    renal tubular d. (RTD)
    reticular d. (RD)
    seminiferous tubule d.
    testicular d.
    XO gonadal d.
    XX gonadal d.
    XY gonadal d.
dysgenetic testes
dysgerminoma
dysglobulinemia
dysgonic
Dysgonomonas
    D. capnocytophagoides
    D. gadei
    D. mossii
dysgranulopoiesis
dyshematopoiesis
dyshematopoietic
dyshemopoiesis
dyshemopoietic anemia
dyshesion
dyshesive
dyshidrosis
dyshormonogenesis
dyshormonogenic goiter
dyskaryosis
dyskaryotic
dyskeratoma
    warty d.
dyskeratosis
    benign d.
    d. congenita
    hereditary benign intraepithelial d.
    intraepithelial d.
    malignant d.
dyskeratotic
dyskinesia
    tracheobronchial d.
dyslipoproteinemia
dysmaturity
    placental d.
dysmenorrhea
dysmetabolic iron overload
dysmorphia
dysmorphic erythrocyte
dysmorphism
    mandibulooculofacial d.
dysmorphogenesis

dysmorphologist
dysmorphology
dysmotility
    esophageal d.
dysmyelopoietic syndrome
dysosteogenesis
dysostosis
    acrofacial d.
    cleidocranial d.
    craniofacial d.
    Crouzon craniofacial d.
    mandibuloacral d.
    mandibulofacial d.
    metaphysial d.
    d. multiplex
    orodigitofacial d.
    otomandibular d.
    peripheral d.
dysoxidative carbonuria
dyspallia
dyspepsia
    nonulcer d.
dysphagia
    d. lusoria
    sideropenic d.
dysphagocytosis
    congenital d.
dysphasia
    cementoosseous d. (COD)
    local cementoosseous d. (LOCD)
dysphonia
    diplopia, dysphagia, dysarthria, d. (4Ds)
dyspigmentation
dysplasia
    acquired d.
    anhidrotic ectodermal d.
    anterofacial d.
    anteroposterior facial d.
    arrhythmogenic right ventricular d.
    asphyxiating thoracic d.
    atriodigital d.
    bronchopulmonary d. (BPD)
    cerebral d.
    cervical d.
    chondroectodermal d.
    cleidocranial d.
    congenital ectodermal d.
    congenital thymic d. (CTD)
    cortical d.
    craniocarpotarsal d.
    craniodiaphysial d.

NOTES

dysplasia *(continued)*
  craniometaphysial d.
  dentin d.
  diaphysial d.
  ectodermal hereditary d.
  endocervical glandular d. (EGD)
  d. epiphysialis hemimelia
  d. epiphysialis multiplex
  d. epiphysialis punctata
  epithelial d.
  faciodigitogenital d.
  fibromuscular d.
  fibrous familial d.
  fibrous monostotic d.
  florid cementoosseous d.
  florid local cementoosseous d.
    (FLCOD)
  glandular d.
  hereditary renal-retinal d.
  hidrotic ectodermal d.
  high grade d.
  hypohidrotic ectodermal d.
  intestinal neuronal d. (IND)
  low-grade d. (LGD)
  lymphopenic thymic d.
  mammary d.
  mandibulofacial d.
  metaphysial d.
  monostotic fibrous d.
  mucoepithelial d.
  multiple epiphysial d.
  neuronal intestinal d.
  nonsyndromal d.
  OAV d.
  oculoauriculovertebral d.
  oculodentodigital d.
  oculovertebral d.
  ODD d.
  OMM d.
  ophthalmomandibulomelic d.
  periapical cemental d.
  pigmentary d.
  polyostotic fibrous d.
  postradiation d. (PRDX)
  precancerous d.
  pseudoachondroplastic
    spondyloepiphysial d.
  renal-retinal d.
  right ventricular d.
  septooptic d.
  spondyloepiphyseal d. (SED)
  squamous d.
  syndromal d.
  thymic d.
  trilineage d.
  T-zone d.
  ventriculoradial d.
  vesical d.
  Zenker d.

dysplasia-associated
  d.-a. lesion
  d.-a. lesion or mass (DALM)
  d.-a. mass
dysplastic
  d. epithelium
  d. focus
  d. neuroepithelial tumor (DNET)
  d. nevus
  d. nevus syndrome
  d. nodule
dyspoiesis
dysprosium
dysproteinemia
  angioimmunoblastic
    lymphadenopathy with d. (AILD)
dysproteinemic neuropathy
dysprothrombinemia
dysraphic anomaly
dysregulation
  gene d.
dysrhythmia
dyssebacia
dysspondylism
dyssynchronous
dyssynergia
  biliary d.
  d. cerebellaris myoclonica
  d. cerebellaris progressive
  detrusor-external sphincter d.
  detrusor-sphincter d.
  progressive cerebellar d.
  vesico-sphincter d.
dystonia
dystonic
dystopia
dystopic
dystroglycan
  alpha d.
dystrophia
  d. brevicollis
  d. unguium
dystrophic
  d. calcification
  d. calcinosis
  d. neurite
dystrophica
  epidermolysis bullosa d.
dystrophin
  d. antibody
  d. gene
dystrophy
  adiposogenital d.
  asphyxiating thoracic d. (ATD)
  Becker muscular d. (BMD)
  Biber-Haab-Dimmer corneal
    lattice d.
  congenital muscular d.
  craniocarpotarsal d.

distal muscular d.
distal-type progressive muscular d.
Duchenne muscular d. (DMD)
facioscapulohumeral-type progressive
  muscular d.
infantile neuroaxonal d. (INAD)
Landouzy-Dejerine progressive
  muscular d.
limb-girdle muscular d.
lipoid d.
muscular d. (MD)
myotonic d. (DM)

ocular muscle d. (OMD)
ophthalmoplegic-type progressive
  muscular d.
progressive muscular d. (PMD)
reflex sympathetic d.
Reis-Bücklers corneal lattice d.
Thiel-Behnke corneal lattice d.
thoracic asphyxiant d. (TAD)
thoracic-pelvic-phalangeal d.
vulvar d.
dystrophy-dystocia syndrome (DDS)
dysuria-pyuria syndrome

NOTES

D

E
> erythrocyte
> extraction fraction
> glutamic acid
>> E antigen
>> chlorazol black E
>> E erythrocyte rosette assay
>> factor E
>> E rosette-forming cell
>> E test

E₁
> estrone

E₂
> estradiol

E₃
> estriol

E₄
> estetrol

EA
> early antigen
> erythrocyte antibody

EAA
> endotoxin activity assay
> extrinsic allergic alveolitis

EABA
> endogenous avidin-binding activity

EAC
> erythrocyte antibody complement
>> EAC rosette assay

Eadie-Hofstee equation

EAE
> experimental allergic encephalomyelitis

EAF
> eosinophilic angiocentric fibrosis

EAG
> experimental autoimmune glomerulonephritis

EaggEC
> enteroaggregative *Escherichia coli*

Eagle
>> E. basal medium
>> E. essential medium
>> E. minimum essential medium (EMEM)
>> E. syndrome

EAHF
> eczema, asthma, hay fever

EAHLG
> equine antihuman lymphoblast globulin

EAHLS
> equine antihuman lymphoblast serum

Eales disease

EAN
> experimental allergic neuritis

EAP
> epiallopregnanolone

ear
>> cauliflower e.
>> e. crystal
>> e. culture
>> e. lobule
>> scroll e.

eardrum

Earle
>> E. L fibrosarcoma
>> E. solution

early
>> E. Aberration Reporting System (EARS)
>> e. antigen (EA)
>> e. B cell
>> e. invasion
>> e. myeloid progenitor cell
>> e. neonatal death
>> e. reaction
>> e. stage of inflammation
>> E. Surveillance Project (ESP)

early-phase response

EARS
> Early Aberration Reporting System

earth
>> diatomaceous e.

earwax

eAST
> erythrocyte aspartate aminotransferase activity

East African (Rhodesian) trypanosomiasis

Eastern
>> E. equine encephalitis virus titer
>> E. equine encephalomyelitis (EEE)
>> E. equine encephalomyelitis virus
>> E. subtype Russian spring-summer encephalitis

eating cell

Eaton
>> E. agent
>> E. agent pneumonia

Eaton-Lambert syndrome

EB
> epidermolysis bullosa
> estradiol benzoate
>> EB virus

ebb phase

EBER
> Epstein-Barr encoded RNA
>> EBER ISH

EBER1 riboprobe

E

Eberth
    E. line
    E. perithelium
Eberthella typhi
EBL
    estimated blood loss
eBL
    endemic Burkitt lymphoma
EBNA
    Epstein-Barr nuclear antigen
Ebner
    E. gland
    imbrication line of von E.
    incremental line of von E.
    E. reticulum
Ebola
    E. hemorrhagic fever
    E. virus
    E. virus disease
"Ebola-like viruses"
Ebolavirus
Ebstein
    E. anomaly
    E. disease
    E. lesion
    E. malformation
ebur dentis
eburnation
eburnea
    substantia e.
eburneous
EBV
    Epstein-Barr virus
    EBV culture
EC
    electron capture
    enteric-coated
    enterochromaffin cell hyperplasia
    extracellular
    EC detector
ECA
    ethacrynic acid
E-cadherin
    epithelial cadherin
    E-c. calcium-dependent molecule
    E-c. gene
    E-c. immunohistochemistry
ecarin clotting time test card
ECBO
    enteric cytopathogenic bovine orphan
    ECBO virus
ECBV
    effective circulating blood volume
ECC
    endocervical curettage
eccentric
    e. hypertrophy
    e. nucleus

eccentrica
    hyperkeratosis e.
    keratoderma e.
eccentrochondroplasia
ecchondroma
ecchordosis physalifora
ecchymoma
ecchymosed
ecchymosis, pl. ecchymoses
    cadaveric ecchymoses
    Tardieu ecchymoses
ecchymotic
eccrine
    e. acrospiroma
    e. gland
    e. poroma
    e. spiradenoma
    e. sweat gland secretion
    e. tumor
eccrinology
eccyesis
ECD
    Erdheim-Chester disease
ECDO
    enterocytopathogenic dog orphan
    ECDO virus
ECE1
    endothelin-converting enzyme
ECF
    extracellular fluid
ECF-A
    eosinophil chemotactic factor of
    anaphylaxis
ECFV
    extracellular fluid volume
ecgonine
echidninus
    Laelaps e.
Echidnophaga gallinacea
echinata
    Memnoniella e.
echinate
Echinobotryum
Echinochasmus
echinocciasis
echinococcosis
    polyvisceral e.
    e. serological test
    unilocular e.
Echinococcus
    E. granulosus
    E. multilocularis
    E. vogeli
echinococcus
    E. cyst
    E. disease
echinocyte
echinocytosis
Echinoparyphium recurvatum

Echinorhynchus gadi
echinosis
Echinostoma
>   *E. ilocanum*
>   *E. lindoensis*
>   *E. malayanum*
>   *E. perfoliatum*
>   *E. revolutum*

echinostomiasis
echinulate
ECHO
>   enteric cytopathogenic human orphan
>   ECHO virus

echovirus
echt
>   cresyl e.

ECIS
>   endometrial carcinoma in situ

Ecker plug
ECL
>   electrogenerated chemiluminescence
>   extracapillary lesion

eclampsia
>   puerperal e.
>   uremic e.

ECLIA
>   electrochemiluminescence immunoassay

eclipse
>   e. period
>   e. phase

ECLT
>   euglobulin clot lysis time

ECM
>   erythema chronicum migrans
>   extracellular material
>   extracellular matrix

ECMO
>   enteric cytopathogenic monkey orphan
>   extracorporeal membrane oxygenation
>   ECMO virus

ecogenetics
ecoid
ecologic niche
ecology
Economo disease
economy class syndrome
Eco RI enzyme
ecospecies
ecosystem
ecotaxis
ecotropic virus

ECP
>   eosinophilic cationic protein
>   erythropoietic coproporphyria

ecphyma
ECSO
>   enteric cytopathogenic swine orphan
>   ECSO virus

EC-SOD
>   extracellular superoxide dismutase

ecstrophe
ECT
>   ectomesenchymal chondromyxoid tumor
>   euglobulin clot test

ECt$_{50}$
>   effective Ct$_{50}$

ectacolia
ectasia
>   congenital biliary e.
>   e. cordis
>   diffuse arterial e.
>   gastric antral vascular e. (GAVE)
>   hypostatic e.
>   mammary duct e.
>   mucinous ductal e.
>   papillary e.
>   senile e.
>   vascular e.
>   e. ventriculi paradoxa

ectasis
ectatic aneurysm
ecthyma
>   contagious e.
>   e. gangrenosum
>   e. infectiosum
>   e. infectiosum virus

ecthymatiform
ecthymiform
ectoantigen
ectoblastic cell
ectocervical smear
ectocornea
ectocyst
ectoderm
>   stomodeal e.

ectodermal
>   e. cell
>   e. defect
>   e. hereditary dysplasia

ectodermatosis
ectodermosis
>   e. erosiva pluriorificialis

ectogenous

E

NOTES

ectoglobular
ectomerogony
ectomesenchymal chondromyxoid tumor
  (ECT)
ectomesenchyme
ectomesenchymoma
ectonucleotide pyrophosphohydrolase
ectoparasite
ectoparasiticide
ectoparasitism
ectoperitonitis
ectophyte
ectopia
    e. cloacae
    e. renis
    e. testis
    e. vesicae
ectopic
    e. ACTH syndrome
    e. anus
    e. decidua
    e. focus (EF)
    e. gastric mucosa
    e. hormone
    e. hormone production
    e. pancreatic tissue
    e. pinealoma
    e. pregnancy (EP)
    e. testis
    e. thyroid tissue
ectoplasm
ectoplasmatic
ectopy
ectoretina
ectosarc
ectosteal
ectostosis
ectothrix infection
ectotoxin
Ectotrichophyton
ectozoic
ectozoon, pl. ectozoa
ectromelia virus
ectromelus
ectrometacarpia
ectropion
ECV
  effective circulating volume
  extracellular volume
ECW
  extracellular water
eczema
    allergic e.
    e., asthma, hay fever (EAHF)
    baker's e.
    chronic e.
    e. erythematosum
    facial e.
    e. herpeticum

    e. hypertrophicum
    lichenoid e.
    e. marginatum
    nummular e.
    e. vaccinatum
    e. verrucosum
    e. vesiculosum
eczematoid dermatitis
eczematous dermatitis
ED
  effective dose
  epileptiform discharge
ED$_{50}$
  median effective dose
EDC
  expected date of confinement
E-DCIS
  endocrine ductal carcinoma in situ
Eddowes syndrome
eddy
    e. current
    squamous e.
eddy-current loss
edema
    allergic pulmonary e.
    alveolar e.
    angioneurotic e.
    blue e.
    brain e.
    brown e.
    bullous e.
    cardiac e.
    cerebral e.
    circumscribed e.
    congestive e.
    cytotoxic e.
    dependent e.
    e. factor (EF)
    heat e.
    hereditary angioneurotic e. (HANE)
    inflammatory e.
    laryngeal e.
    lymphatic e.
    malignant e.
    e. neonatorum
    noncardiogenic pulmonary e.
    noninflammatory e.
    periodic e.
    periorbital e.
    peripheral e.
    pitting e.
    pulmonary e. (PE)
    Quincke e.
    solid e.
    stromal e.
edematization
edematous
edentate
    dicobalt e.

edentatus
>*Strongylus e.*

edetate
>calcium disodium e.
>sodium calcium e.

edetic acid

edge
>e. effect
>spiculated e.

Edinger-Westphal nucleus

Edlefsen reagent

Edman reaction

Edmondson-Steiner hepatocellular carcinoma grading classification

Edmondson tumor grading system

EDRF
>endothelium-derived relaxing factor

edrophonium
>e. chloride
>e. chloride test

EDS
>Ehlers-Danlos syndrome
>energy dispersed x-ray analysis
>energy dispersive spectrometer
>energy dispersive x-ray spectroscopy

Edsall disease

EDTA
>ethylenediaminetetraacetic acid
>>EDTA contamination of specimen
>>K3 EDTA
>>potassium EDTA (K3 EDTA)

EDTA-associated leukoagglutination

EDTA-dependent pseudothrombocytopenia

Edwardsiella tarda

Edwardsielleae

Edwards-Patau syndrome

Edwards syndrome

EEC
>endometrioid endometrial carcinoma
>enteropathogenic *Escherichia coli*

EEE
>Eastern equine encephalomyelitis
>>EEE virus

EEO
>electroendosmosis

E-EPE
>established extraprostatic extension

EF
>ectopic focus
>edema factor

encephalitogenic factor
>EF protein

EFA
>essential fatty acid

EFC
>endogenous fecal calcium

EFE
>endocardial fibroelastosis

effacement of lymph node architecture

Effapoxy resin

effect
>antimuscarinic e.
>Arias-Stella e.
>Auger e.
>biochemically mediated e.
>blast e.
>Bohr e.
>booster e.
>carry-over e.
>copper wire e.
>Crabtree e.
>crowding e.
>cytopathic e.
>defibrinogenating e.
>Doppler e.
>edge e.
>end-organ e.
>excitatory e.
>Faraday e.
>e. of fertilization
>founder e.
>Haldane e.
>intracellular signal transduction e.
>matrix e.
>monotypic e.
>muscarinic e.
>oxygen e.
>passenger leukocyte e.
>Pasteur e.
>photoelectric e.
>photographic e.
>piezoelectric e.
>polytopic e.
>radiation e.
>side e.
>Somogyi e.
>Soret e.
>Staub-Traugott e.
>Tyndall e.
>Whitten e.
>Wolff-Chaikoff e.
>zonation e.

E

NOTES

effective
e. circulating blood volume (ECBV)
e. circulating volume (ECV)
e. Ct_{50} (ECt_{50})
e. dose (ED)
e. half-life
e. oxygen transport (EOT)
e. refractory period (ERP)
e. renal blood flow (ERBF)
e. renal plasma flow
e. temperature (ET)
effectiveness
relative biological e. (RBE)
effector
allosteric e.
e. cell
frangible anchor-linker e. (FRALE)
effemination
efferens
vas e.
efferent
e. duct
e. ductule
gamma e.
e. lymphatic vessel
effervescent sodium phosphate
efficacy
efficiency
geometric e.
photopeak detection e.
efficiens
Corynebacterium e.
efflorescence
efflux
effusa
Hydrocarboniphaga e.
effuse colony
effusion
chylous e.
e. cytology
exudative e.
exudative pleural e.
joint e.
lymphoid-rich e.
malignant pleural e.
pericardial e.
pleural e.
pleurisy with e.
serofibrinous e.
serosanguineous e.
serous e.
transudative pleural e.
EFV
extracellular fluid volume
EGC
endocrine granule constituent
EGD
endocervical glandular dysplasia

EGE
eosinophilic gastroenteritis
EGF
epidermal growth factor
EGFP
enhanced green fluorescent protein
EGFR
epidermal growth factor receptor
egg
e. count
e. passage
Eggel tumor classification
Eggerthella lenta
egg-shell calcification
egg-white lysozyme (EWL)
egg-yolk agar
EGL
eosinophilic granuloma of lung
eglandulous
Eglis gland
EGOT
erythrocyte glutamic oxaloacetic transaminase
EGP-2
epithelial glycoprotein-2
EGTA
ethylene glycol tetraacetic acid
Egyptian splenomegaly
EH
epithelioid hemangioendothelioma
essential hypertension
EHBA
extrahepatic biliary atresia
EHBF
estimated hepatic blood flow
exercise hyperemia blood flow
EHE
epithelioid hemangioendothelioma
EHEC
enterohemorrhagic *Escherichia coli*
EHF
exophthalmos-hyperthyroid factor
ehimensis
Paenibacillus e.
EHL
endogenous hyperlipidemia
Ehlers-Danlos syndrome (EDS)
EHLL
epithelial hyperplastic laryngeal lesion
EHO
extrahepatic obstruction
EHP
excessive heat production
Ehrenreich and Churg membranous nephropathy staging system
Ehrlich
E. acid hematoxylin stain
E. anemia
E. aniline crystal violet stain

E. ascites carcinoma
E. benzaldehyde reaction
E. diazo reaction
E. diazo reagent
E. hematoxylin
E. inner body
E. phenomenon
E. postulate
E. side-chain theory
E. test
E. triacid stain
E. triple stain
E. tumor
E. unit (EU)
Ehrlichia
    E. canis
    E. chaffeensis
    E. equi
    E. phagocytophila
    E. risticii
    E. sennetsu
Ehrlichiaceae
Ehrlichieae
ehrlichiosis
    human granulocytic e. (HGE)
    human monocytic e. (HME)
EI
    enzyme inhibitor
    eosinophilic index
EIA
    enzyme-multiplied immunoassay
        EIA interface
EIC
    endometrial intraepithelial carcinoma
    enzyme immunochromatography
    epidermal inclusion cyst
    extensive intraductal component
Eichhorst corpuscle
eicosanoid
eicosapentaenoic acid (EPA)
EID
    electroimmunodiffusion
EIEC
    enteroinvasive *Escherichia coli*
eighth nerve tumor
Eijkman lactose broth
Eikenella corrodens
eiloid
Eimeria sardinae
Eimeriidae

Einarson
    E. gallocyanin-chrome alum
    E. gallocyanin-chrome alum stain
Einheit
    antitoxin E. (AE)
einsteinium
Einthoven law
Eisenlohr syndrome
Eisenmenger
    E. syndrome
    tetralogy of E.
eisodic
ejaculate
ejaculatorius
    ductus e.
ejaculatory duct
ejection murmur (EM)
EK
    erythrokinase
Ekbom syndrome
EKC
    epidemic keratoconjunctivitis
ekiri
Ektachem
EL
    electroluminescence
eLabNotebook
Eladia
Elaeophora schneideri
elaidic acid
E-LAM
    endothelial-leukocyte adhesion molecule
elastance
elastase
elastic
    e. cartilage
    e. fiber
    e. fiber stain
    e. lamellae
    e. laminae of artery
    e. layer of artery
    e. layer of cornea
    e. membrane
    e. scattering
    e. skin
    e. tissue
elastica
    cutis e.
    Helvella e.
    tela e.
    tunica e.

E

NOTES

elastica (continued)
  e. van Gieson (EVG)
  e. van Gieson stain
elasticity
  wound e.
elasticum
  pseudoxanthoma e. (PXE)
elastin
  e. stain
  Weigert stain for e.
elastin-binding protein
elastofibrolipoma
elastofibroma
  e. dorsi
  mediastinal e.
elastoid degeneration
elastoma
  juvenile e.
  Miescher e.
elastomer envelope
elastorrhexis
elastosis
  e. colloidalis conglomerata
  e. perforans serpiginosa
  senile e.
  solar e.
elastotic degeneration
ELAT
  enzyme-linked antiglobulin test
elaunin
Elavil
elbow
  pitcher's e.
  tennis e.
Elder malignant melanoma classification
Elecsys
  E. Anti-HBe assay
  E. free PSA immunoassay
  E. 2010 modular immunoassay
    analyzer
  E. PreciControl Anti-HBe control
  E. proBNP immunoassay
  E. RBC folate hemolyzing reagent
  E. total PSA immunoassay
  E. total PSA test
  E. troponin T immunoassay system
elective culture
Electra 1400C, 1800C coagulation system
electric
  e. chromatography
  e. field vector
  e. potential
  e. potential difference
  e. susceptibility
electrical artifact
electroblot analysis

electrochemical cell
electrochemiluminescence immunoassay (ECLIA)
electrochemistry
electrode
  active e.
  bipolar needle e.
  calomel e.
  carbon dioxide e.
  Clark oxygen e.
  e. of first kind
  glass e.
  hydrogen e.
  e. impedance
  indicator e.
  indifferent e.
  inert e.
  ion-selective e. (ISE)
  Orion e.
  pH e.
  Po_2e.
  e. potential
  quinhydrone e.
  recording e.
  reference e.
  e. response time
  e. of second kind
  e. sensitivity
  Severinghaus e.
  silver/silver chloride e.
  standard hydrogen e.
electroendosmosis (EEO)
electrogenerated chemiluminescence (ECL)
electroimmunoassay
electroimmunodiffusion (EID)
electroluminescence (EL)
electrolysis
  Faraday law of e.
electrolyte
  amphoteric e.
  e. balance and homeostasis
  colloidal e.
  fecal e.'s
  e. imbalance
  inorganic e.
  protein e.
  serum e.
  stool e.'s
electrolytic
  e. capacitor
  e. cell
  e. stripping
electromagnet
electromagnetic
  e. flowmeter (EMF)
  e. pulse (EMP)
  e. radiation
  e. unit (emu)

electrometer amplifier
electromotance
electromotive
    e. force (EMF)
    e. force cell
electron
    Auger e.
    e. beam
    e. capture (EC)
    e. capture detector
    conduction e.
    conversion e.
    free e.
    e. K-capture
    e. lens
    e. lucent granule
    e. micrograph
    e. microprobe
    e. microscope (EM)
    e. microscopy (EM)
    e. multiplier tube
    e. pair
    e. pair bond
    paramagnetic resonance of e.'s
    e. paramagnetic resonance
    e. spin resonance (ESR)
    e. transport chain
    e. transport chain complex I–IV
    e. transport inhibitor
    valence e.
    e. volt (eV)
electron-dense
    e.-d. droplet
    e.-d. hump
electronegative
electronegativity
electronic
    e. cell counter
    e. focal spot
    E. Surveillance System for the
      Early Notification of Community-
      based Epidemics (ESSENCE)
electron-lucent
    e.-l. fluff
    e.-l. vesicle
electronograph
electronystagmography
electroosmosis
electroosmotic flow
electroparacentesis
electropathology

electropherogram
    capillary electrophoresis e.
electrophile
electrophoresis (EP)
    acid e.
    acrylamide gel e.
    agar gel e.
    agarose gel e.
    alkaline phosphatase isoenzyme e.
    capillary e.
    capillary zone e. (CE)
    cerebrospinal fluid protein e.
    citrate agar gel e.
    creatine kinase isoenzyme e.
    denaturing density gradient e.
      (DDGE)
    denaturing gradient gel e. (DGGE)
    disc e.
    DNA gel e.
    gel e.
    globin-chain e.
    gradient gel e.
    hemoglobin e.
    high-resolution protein e. (HRE)
    high-voltage e. (HVE)
    IEF gel e.
    immunofixation e. (IFE)
    isoelectric focusing e.
    isoenzyme e.
    lipoprotein e. (LPE)
    moving-boundary e.
    polyacrylamide gel e. (PAGE)
    protein e.
    pulsed field gel e.
    pulsed field gradient gel e.
      (PFGE)
    SDS gel e.
    serum immunofixation e.
    serum protein e. (SPE, SPEP)
    sodium dodecyl sulfate-
      polyacrylamide gel e. (SDS-
      PAGE)
    temperature-gradient gel e. (TGGE)
    temporal temperature gradient
      gel e. (TTGE)
    e. test
    thin-layer e. (TLE)
    thyroxine-binding protein e.
    two-dimensional gel e.
    two-dimensional polyacrylamide
      gel e.
    urine protein e. (UPEP)

E

NOTES

electrophoresis *(continued)*
  zonal e.
  zone e.
ElectrophoresisTUTOR
electrophoretic
  e. mobility
  e. mobility shift assay
electrophysiology study
electropositive
electroscope
electrospray (ES)
electrostatic unit (ESU)
electrosynthesis
electrotonic
  e. junction
  e. synapse
electrotransfer test
elegans
  Apophysomyces e.
  Cunninghamella e.
  Granulicatella e.
  Phaeoannellomyces e.
  Prosthenorchis e.
eleidin
Elek test
element
  anatomical e.
  e. disorder
  extrachromosomal e.
  labile e.
  morphologic e.
  neoplastic e.
  putative peroxisome proliferator
    response e. (PPRE)
  rare earth e.
  sacculotubular e.
  secretory acinar e.
  symmetry e.
  trace e.
  transposable e.
  ultra-trace e.
elementary
  e. body
  e. charge
  e. granule
  e. particle
eleoma
elephantiac, elephantiasic
elephantiasis
  e. congenita angiomatosa
  congenital e.
  e. neuromatosa
  nevoid e.
  e. nostras
  e. scroti
  e. telangiectodes
  e. verrucosa nostrum
  e. vulva

elephantis
  Mycobacterium e.
elephant leg
Eleutherascus
elevate blood calcium level
elfin facies
elicitor
  bacterial lipochitooligosaccharide
    compound e.
elimination
  e. diet
  first-order e.
  immune e.
  e. reaction
  single breath nitrogen e.
elinin
ELISA
  enzyme-linked immunosorbent assay
    N-MID osteocalcin ELISA
    ELISA titer assay
ELISPOT enzymatic test assay
elite
  Hemoccult Sensa e.
elizabethae
  Bartonella e.
ellipse
ellipsoid
ellipsoidal
elliptical
elliptocyte
elliptocytic anemia
elliptocytosis
  hereditary e. (HE)
  spherocytic hereditary e.
  stomatocytic hereditary e.
Ellis
  E. type 1 glomerulonephritis
  E. types 1, 2 nephritis
Ellis-van Creveld syndrome
Ellsworth-Howard test
ELMS
  epithelioid leiomyosarcoma
elongata
  Tetrasphaera e.
elongated cell
elongation factor
elongatus
  Metastrongylus e.
elongin
elongisporus
  Lodderomyces e.
ELT
  euglobulin lysis time
El Tor vibrio
  Vibrio cholerae biotype El Tor
eluate
**Elucigene CF29 analyte-specific reagent
  kit**
eluent

elusive ulcer
elute
elution
    Kleihauer acid e.
    Kleihauer-Betke acid e.
elutriate
elutriation
    counterflow centrifugal e.
elyakovii
    Pseudoalteromonas e.
EM
    ejection murmur
    electron microscope
    electron microscopy
    erythema migrans
    erythrocyte mass
EMA
    epithelial membrane antigen
    EMA antibody
emaciation
emarginate
emargination
EMB
    eosin-methylene blue
    EMB Levine agar
Embadomonas
Embden-Meyerhof pathway
embed
embedding
    e. agent
    e. wax
Embellisia
EMBLT
    endocervical mucinous borderline tumor
embolemia
emboli (*pl. of* embolus)
embolic
    e. abscess
    e. aneurysm
    e. gangrene
    e. glomerulonephritis
    e. infarct
embolism
    air e.
    amniotic fluid e.
    arterial e.
    atheroma e.
    atheromatous e.
    bacillary e.
    bland e.
    bone marrow e.
    capillary e.

    cellular e.
    cerebral e.
    cholesterol e.
    chorionic villus e.
    coronary e.
    cotton-fiber e.
    fat e.
    gas e.
    infective e.
    lipid e.
    lymph e.
    lymphogenous e.
    miliary e.
    obturating e.
    oil e.
    pantaloon e.
    paradoxic e.
    paradoxical e.
    plasmodium e.
    pulmonary e. (PE)
    pyemic e.
    retinal e.
    retrograde e.
    riding e.
    saddle e.
    spinal e.
    straddling e.
    systemic air e.
    trichinous e.
    tumor e.
    venous e.
embolization
    trophoblastic e.
embolomycotic aneurysm
embolus, pl. **emboli**
    air e.
    amniotic fluid e.
    arrest of tumor emboli
    atheromatous e.
    bland e.
    bone marrow e.
    cholesterol emboli
    fat e.
    foreign body e.
    massive e.
    paradoxical e.
    parasitic e.
    recent e.
    septic e.
    tumor e.
    valvular tissue e.

NOTES

E

embryo
    e. biopsy
    cylindrical e.
    nodular e.
    stunted e.
embryocardia
embryogenesis
embryoid body
embryoma of the kidney
embryonal
    e. adenoma
    e. carcinosarcoma
    e. cell carcinoma
    e. duct cyst
    e. leukemia
    e. metaplasia
    e. nephroma
    e. rest
    e. rhabdomyosarcoma (ERMS)
    e. teratoma
    e. tumor
embryonate
embryonic
    e. competence
    e. germ cell
    e. hemoglobin
    e. neural crest
    e. sphere
    e. spot
    e. stem cell
    e. tumor
embryoniform
embryonization
embryonum
    smegma e.
embryophore
embryotoxicity
EMBT
    endocervical mucinous borderline tumor
EMC
    encephalomyocarditis
    extraskeletal myxoid chondrosarcoma
    EMC virus
EMEC
    epithelial-myoepithelial carcinoma
emeiocytosis (*var. of* emiocytosis)
EMEM
    Eagle minimum essential medium
emergency
    E. Medical Treatment and Labor
      Act (EMTALA)
    e. response planning guideline
      (ERPG)
    e. response to terrorism (ERT)
emerging virus
Emericella nidulans
Emericellopsis
emetica
    Russula e.

emetine
EMF
    electromagnetic flowmeter
    electromotive force
    endomyocardial fibrosis
    erythrocyte maturation factor
EMG
    exomphalos, macroglossia, and gigantism
      EMG syndrome
EMH
    extramedullary hematopoiesis
emigration
    e. theory
    e. of white cells
eminence
    Doyère e.
    median e.
    olivary e.
emiocytosis, emeiocytosis
emission
    e. line
    e. spectroscopy
    e. spectrum
    thermionic e.
EMIT
    enzyme-multiplied immunoassay
    technique
emitter
    beta e.
Emmens S/L test
EMMM
    epidermotropic metastatic malignant
    melanoma
Emmon modification of Sabouraud dextrose agar
Emmonsia
    E. parva var. *crescens*
    E. parva var. *parva*
Emmonsiella capsulata
emmprin
emotional leukocytosis
EMP
    electromagnetic pulse
    extramedullary solitary plasmacytoma
    EMP device
emperipolesis
    megakaryocytic e.
    thymic cell e.
emphraxis
emphysema
    bullous e.
    centriacinar e.
    centrilobular e.
    chronic pulmonary e. (CPE)
    compensatory e.
    congenital lobar e.
    cutaneous e.
    diffuse e.
    endolymphatic e.

familial e.
gangrenous e.
generalized e.
interstitial e.
intestinal e.
obstructive e.
panacinar e.
panlobular e.
paraseptal e.
pink puffer e.
pulmonary interstitial e. (PIE)
subcutaneous e.
surgical e.
vesicular e.

emphysematosa
colpohyperplasia e.
vaginitis e.

emphysematous
e. asthma
e. bleb
e. cholecystitis
e. gangrene
e. phlegmon
e. vaginitis

empirical
emprosthotonos, emprosthotonus
empty
e. marrow
e. sella
e. sella syndrome

empyema
e. articuli
e. benignum
latent e.
loculated e.
e. necessitatis
e. of pericardium
pulsating e.
subdural e.

empyemic
empyocele
EMS
eosinophilia-myalgia syndrome
EMTALA
Emergency Medical Treatment and Labor Act
emu
electromagnetic unit
emulsify fat
emulsion
bacillary e. (tuberculin) (BE)

EN
erythema nodosum
en
en bloc
en face section
en grappe
en thyrse
ENA
extractable nuclear antigen
extractable nuclear antigen antibody
ENaC
epithelial sodium channel
enamel
e. cell
e. crypt
e. epithelium
e. fiber
e. hypoplasia
interrod e.
e. layer
e. membrane
mottled e.
e. niche
e. organ
e. prism
e. rod
e. rod sheath
e. tuft
enamelin
enamelogenesis imperfecta
enameloid
enamelum
Enamovirus
enanthem
palatal e.
enantiobiosis
enantiomer
enantiomerism
enantiomorph
enantiomorphism
en-bloc stain
encainide
encapsulans
peritonitis e.
encapsulated
e. *Bacillus anthracis*
e. hemoglobin
encapsulation
encapsulatum
peritonitis fibroplastica e.
encapsuled
encarditis (*var. of* endocarditis)

NOTES

encelitis, enceliitis
encephalemia
encephalitis, pl. **encephalitides**
  acute hemorrhagic e.
  acute necrotizing e.
  allergic e.
  arthropod-borne virus e.
  Australian X e.
  bacterial e.
  California e. (CE)
  coxsackievirus e.
  Dawson e.
  Eastern subtype Russian spring-
    summer e.
  epidemic e.
  equine e.
  experimental allergic e.
  Far East Russian e.
  e. hemorrhagica
  herpes simplex virus e. (HSVE)
  hyperergic e.
  Ilhéus e.
  inclusion body e.
  Japanese B e. (JBE)
  e. japonica
  lead e.
  lethargic e.
  e. lethargica
  limbic e.
  Mengo e.
  Murray Valley e. (MVE)
  necrotizing e.
  e. neonatorum
  e. periaxialis concentrica
  postinfectious allergic e.
  postvaccinal e.
  postvaccination allergic e.
  Powassan e.
  purulent e.
  e. pyogenica
  Russian autumn e.
  Russian tick-borne e.
  secondary e.
  St. Louis e. (SLE)
  subacute inclusion body e.
  e. subcorticalis chronica
  suppurative e.
  tick-borne e. (Central European
    subtype)
  tick-borne e. (Eastern subtype)
  varicella e.
  Venezuelan equine e.
  vernal e.
  e. virus
  von Economo e.
  Western e. (WE)
  Western equine e.

  Western subtype Russian spring-
    summer e.
  woodcutter's e.
encephalitogen
encephalitogenic factor (EF)
Encephalitozoon
  E. cuniculi
  E. hellem
  E. intestinalis
encephalocele
encephaloclastic microcephaly
encephalocraniocutaneous lipomatosis
encephalocystocele
encephalodysplasia
encephaloid cancer
encephaloma
encephalomalacia
encephalomeningitis
encephalomeningocele
encephalomeningopathy
encephalomyelitis
  acute disseminated e. (ADEM)
  acute necrotizing hemorrhagic e.
  allergic e.
  autoimmune e.
  avian infectious e.
  benign myalgic e.
  Eastern equine e. (EEE)
  enzootic e.
  epidemic myalgic e.
  equine e.
  experimental allergic e. (EAE)
  granulomatous e.
  herpes B e.
  infectious porcine e.
  postinfectious e.
  postvaccination e. (PVEM)
  Venezuelan equine e. (VEE)
  viral e.
  Western e. (WE)
  Western equine e. (WEE)
  zoster e.
encephalomyelocele
encephalomyeloneuropathy
encephalomyelopathy
  carcinomatous e.
  epidemic myalgic e.
  infantile necrotizing e. (INE)
  necrotizing e.
  paracarcinomatous e.
  paraneoplastic e.
encephalomyeloradiculitis
encephalomyeloradiculopathy
encephalomyocarditis (EMC)
  e. virus
encephalopathia addisonia
encephalopathy
  anoxic e.
  bilirubin e.

Binswanger e.
bovine spongiform e.
demyelinating e.
hepatic e.
HIV e.
hypercapnic e.
hypernatremic e.
hypertensive e.
hypoglycemic e.
hypoxic e.
ischemic e.
lead e.
metabolic e.
palindromic e.
pancreatic e.
portal-systemic e. (PSE)
progressive subcortical e.
recurrent e.
saturnine e.
spongiform e.
subacute necrotizing e.
subacute spongiform e.
subcortical arteriosclerotic e.
thyrotoxic e.
transmissible mink e.
transmissible spongiform e. (TSE)
traumatic progressive e.
uremic e.
Wernicke e.
Wernicke-Korsakoff e.
encephalotrigeminal angiomatosis
enchondral
enchondroma
enchondromatosis
enchondromatosum
myxoma e.
enchondromatous
enchondrosarcoma
enclave
encode
encoder
encoding
encopresis
encrustation hypothesis
encysted
e. calculus
e. papillary lesion
e. pleurisy
encystment
end
e. artery
blunt e.

e. bulb
e. cell
e. organ
e. piece
e. piece of spermatozoon
e. plate
e. point
e. product
e. stage
e. of tape
endadelphos
Endamoeba
endangiitis, endangitis
e. obliterans
endaortitis
bacterial e.
endarterectomy
carotid e.
endarteritis
bacterial e.
e. deformans
e. obliterans
obliterating e.
obliterative e.
e. proliferans
proliferating e.
end-brush
end-bulb
endemia
endemic
e. Burkitt lymphoma (eBL)
e. colic
e. disease
e. fluorosis
e. funiculitis
e. goiter
e. hemoptysis
e. hypertrophy
e. index
e. murine typhus
e. nonbacterial infantile
gastroenteritis
e. syphilis
e. typhus
endemicum
granuloma e.
endemicus
Clonorchis e.
endemoepidemic
endergonic reaction
endermosis
end-feet

E

NOTES

ending
    annulospiral e.
    caliciform e.
    epilemmal e.
    flower-spray e.
    free nerve e.
    grape e.
    hederiform e.
    intraneural nerve e.
    nerve e.
    sole-plate e.
    synaptic e.
Endo agar
endoamylase
endoangiitis
endoaortitis
endoappendicitis
endoarteritis
Endobacteria
endobiotic
endobioticum
    Synchytrium e.
endobody
endobronchial
    e. tuberculosis
    e. tumor
endocardial
    e. cushion defect
    e. fibroelastosis (EFE)
    e. plaque
    e. sclerosis
endocarditic
endocarditis, encarditis
    abacterial thrombotic e.
    acute bacterial e.
    acute infective e.
    atypical verrucous e.
    bacteria-free stage of bacterial e.
    bacterial e. (BE)
    cachectic e.
    Candida e.
    e. chordalis
    constrictive e.
    infectious e.
    infective e.
    isolated parietal e.
    Libman-Sacks e.
    Löffler e.
    malignant e.
    marantic e.
    mural e.
    nonbacterial thrombotic e. (NBTE)
    nonbacterial verrucous e.
    polypous e.
    Q fever e.
    rheumatic e.
    septic e.
    Streptococcus e.
    subacute bacterial e. (SBE)
    subacute infective e.
    terminal e.
    thrombotic nonbacterial e.
    valvular e.
    vegetative e.
    verrucal atypical e.
    verrucal nonbacterial e.
    verrucous e.
endocardium
endocellular complement
endocervical
    e. cancer
    e. carcinoma
    e. cell
    e. curettage (ECC)
    e. glandular dysplasia (EGD)
    e. smear
endocervical/transformation zone data on Pap test
endocervicitis
endocervicosis
endocervix
    vagina, ectocervix, e. (VCE)
endochondral
    e. bone
    e. ossification
endochondromatosis
    multiple e.
endochondromatous myxoma
Endoconidiophora
endocrinae
    glandulae e.
endocrine
    e. adenomatosis
    e. cell
    e. disease
    e. ductal carcinoma in situ (E-DCIS)
    familial multiple e.
    e. gland
    e. granule
    e. granule constituent (EGC)
    e. marker
    e. myopathy
    e. phenotype
    e. polyglandular syndrome
endocrinoma
    multiple e.
endocrinopathy
    multiple e.
endocyst
endocystitis
endocytosis
    receptor-mediated e.
endocytotically active
endodeoxyribonuclease
endodermal
    e. cell

e. pharyngeal pouch
e. sinus tumor
Endodermophyton
endodyocyte
endodyogeny
endoenteritis
endoenzyme
endoesophagitis
endogamous
endogamy
endogastritis
endogenote
endogenous
e. aneurysm
e. antigen
e. antigen cell-bound antibody reaction
e. antigen-circulating antibody reaction
e. antigen-transferred cell-bound antibody reaction
e. antioxidant enzyme
e. avidin-binding activity (EABA)
e. bacterium
e. creatinine clearance
e. fecal calcium (EFC)
e. hemosiderosis
e. hyperglyceridemia
e. hyperlipidemia (EHL)
e. infection
e. peroxidase
e. pigments and deposits
e. pneumoconiosis
e. synthesis
e. variable
endoglobular, endoglobar
endointoxication
Endolimax nana
endolymph
endolympha
endolymphatic
e. duct
e. dye
e. emphysema
e. hydrops
e. stromal myosis
endolymphaticus
ductus e.
endolymphic
endomerogony
endometria (*pl. of* endometrium)

endometrial
e. adenocarcinoma
e. atrophy
e. biopsy
e. blood supply
e. brush
e. carcinoma
e. carcinoma in situ (ECIS)
e. cast
e. cavity
e. cell
e. curettage
e. cyst
e. cytology
c. functionalis
e. gestational alteration
e. hyperplasia
e. intraepithelial carcinoma (EIC)
e. polyp
e. smear
e. stromal sarcoma (ESS)
e. stromatosis
endometrioid
e. carcinoma
e. endometrial carcinoma (EEC)
e. tumor
endometrioma
endometriosis
micronodular stromal e.
stromal e.
uterine e.
vesical e.
endometritis
chronic specific e.
decidual e.
e. dissecans
granulomatous e.
syncytial e.
endometrium, pl. **endometria**
e. anaerobic culture
aspiration of e.
atrophic e.
cystic hyperplasia of e.
16-day e.
decidualized e.
disordered proliferative e.
FIGO adenocarcinoma of e.
proliferative e.
regenerative e.
secretory e.
Swiss cheese e.
endomitosis

E

NOTES

Endomyces
  E. albicans
  E. capsulatus
  E. epidermidis
  E. geotrichum
Endomycetales
Endomycopsis
endomyocardial
  e. biopsy
  e. fibroelastosis
  e. fibrosis (EMF)
  e. sclerosis
endomyocarditis
endomyometritis
endomysial
  e. antibody
  e. collagen
endomysium
  fibrocyte in e.
endoneurial fibroblast
endoneurium
endonuclease
  restriction e.
endonucleolus
endoparasite
endoparasitism
endopeptidase
  zinc-containing e.
endoperiarteritis
endopericarditis
endoperimyocarditis
endoperitonitis
endoperoxide
  cyclic e.
  prostaglandin e.
endophlebitis
endophthalmitis
  phacoanaphylactic e.
endophyte
endophytic
endophyticus
  Bacillus e.
endoplasm
endoplasmic reticulum (ER)
endoplast
endoplastic
endopolygeny
endopolyploidy
endoreduplication
  chromosomal e.
endoreplication
end-organ
  e.-o. damage
  e.-o. effect
endoribonuclease
endorphin
  e. assay
  beta e.

endosalpingiosis
endosalpingitis
endosalpinx
endosarc
endoscopic
  e. autopsy
  e. retrograde
    cholangiopancreatography
  e. ultrasonography
endosmosis
endosome
endosperm
endospore
endostatin
endosteal scalloping
endosteitis, endostitis
endosteoma
endosteum
endostitis (*var. of* endosteitis)
endostoma
endosulfan
endotendineum
endothelia (*pl. of* endothelium)
endothelial
  e. cell
  e. cyst
  e. differentiation
  high e.
  e. immunoglobin family adhesion
    protein
  e. leukocyte
  e. lining of vessel
  e. marker
  e. metaplasia
  e. myeloma
  e. phagocyte
  e. relaxing factor
  e. sarcoma
  e. thromboresistance
  e. tubuloreticular inclusion
endothelial-leukocyte adhesion molecule
  (E-LAM)
endothelin-1 receptor antagonist
endothelin-2
endothelin-3 (ET3)
endothelin-A, -B receptor
endothelin-converting enzyme (ECE1)
endothelin-receptor-B (ENDRB)
endotheliocyte
endothelioid habit
endotheliolytic serum
endothelioma
endotheliosis
endothelium, pl. endothelia
  e. of anterior chamber
  e. camerae anterioris
  continuous e.

discontinuous e.
fenestrated e.
endothelium-derived relaxing factor (EDRF)
endothermic
Endothia
endothrix
endotoxemia
gram-negative e.
endotoxicosis
endotoxic shock
endotoxin
e. activity assay (EAA)
e. shock
endotracheal
e. abnormality
e. insufflation
endotrachelitis
endovasculitis
hemorrhagic e. (HEV)
endovasculopathy
hemorrhagic e.
endovenitis
end-piece
endplate
motor e.
end-point measurement
end-product repression
ENDRB
endothelin-receptor-B
endrin
end-systolic pressure (ESP)
end-tidal CO$_2$ tension
endyma
eneae
Bosea e.
energetics
biochemical e.
energy
activation e.
binding e.
bond e.
e. dispersed x-ray analysis (EDS)
e. dispersive spectrometer (EDS)
e. dispersive x-ray microanalysis
e. dispersive x-ray spectroscopy (EDS)
free e.
kinetic e. (KE)
oxidative e.
potential e.
radiant e.

e. resolution
standard free e.
enflagellation
Engelmann disease
Engel-von Recklinghausen disease
engineering
biomedical e.
genetic e.
human e.
English disease
englobe
englobement
Engman disease
engraftment
cell e.
engulfment
cytologic e.
Engyodontium album
enhanced green fluorescent protein (EGFP)
enhancement
autometallographic silver e.
immunologic e.
immunological e.
enhancer
enhancing antibody
enhematospore
Enhygromyxa salina
enkephalin
ENL
erythema nodosum leprosum
enlargement
cardiac e. (CE)
diffuse e.
left atrial e. (LAE)
left ventricular e. (LVE)
right atrial e. (RAE)
right ventricular e. (RVE)
enoeca
Prevotella e.
enol
enolase
neuron-specific e. (NSA, NSE)
enostosis
enoyl-coenzyme A hydratase
enrichment
e. culture
e. medium
ENS
enteric nervous system
ensheathing callus

E

NOTES

345

Ensifer
> E. arboris
> E. fredii
> E. kostiensis
> E. kummerowiae
> E. medicae
> E. meliloti
> E. saheli
> E. terangae
> E. xinjiangensis

entactin
entamebiasis
Entamoeba
> E. buccalis
> E. buetschlii
> E. chattoni
> E. coli
> E. dispar
> E. gingivalis
> E. hartmanni
> E. histolytica
> E. histolytica serological test
> E. kartulisi
> E. moshkovskii
> E. nana
> E. nipponica
> E. polecki
> E. tetragena
> E. tropicalis
> E. undulans

entanii
> Gluconacetobacter e.

enteramine
enterectasis
enterelcosis
enteric
> e. bacillus
> e. cytopathogenic bovine orphan (ECBO)
> e. cytopathogenic human orphan (ECHO)
> e. cytopathogenic monkey orphan (ECMO)
> e. cytopathogenic swine orphan (ECSO)
> e. helminthic zoonosis
> e. nervous system (ENS)
> e. orphan virus
> e. tularemia

enteric-coated (EC)
enteric-type adenocarcinoma
entericus
> Streptococcus e.

enteritidis
> Bacillus e.
> Salmonella e.
> E. salmonella

enteritis
> e. anaphylactica
> bovine e. (BE)
> chronic cicatrizing e.
> diphtheritic e.
> eosinophilic e.
> feline infectious e.
> granulomatous e.
> e. of mink
> e. necroticans
> phlegmonous e.
> e. polyposa
> radiation e.
> regional e. (RE)
> staphylococcal e.
> transmissible e.
> typhoid e.

enteroaggregative *Escherichia coli* (EaggEC)
Enterobacter
> E. aerogenes
> E. agglomerans
> E. alvei
> E. cloacae
> E. cowanii
> E. gergoviae
> E. hafniae
> E. liquefaciens
> E. pneumonia
> E. sakazakii
> E. subgroup C.
> E. urinary tract infection

Enterobacteriaceae
enterobiasis
Enterobius vermicularis
enterobrosia
enterobrosis
enterocele
enterocholecystostomy
enterochromaffin
> e. cell
> e. cell hyperplasia (EC)
> e. staining

enterochromaffin-like cell hyperplasia
enteroclysis
Enterococcus
> E. canis
> E. faecalis
> E. faecium
> E. gilvus
> E. haemoperoxidus
> E. hermanniensis
> E. italicus
> E. moraviensis
> E. pallens
> E. phoeniculicola
> E. porcinus
> E. ratti
> E. urinary tract infection

vancomycin-resistant *E.* (VRE)
  E. villorum
enterococcus, pl. **enterococci**
enterocolitica
  Pasteurella e.
  Yersinia e.
enterocolitis, pl. **enterocolitides**
  acute necrotizing e.
  antibiotic e.
  cicatrizing e.
  diarrheogenic bacterial e.
  Hirschsprung-associated e. (HAEC)
  infectious enterocolitides
  lymphocytic e.
  necrotizing e.
  neonatal necrotizing e.
  pericrypt eosinophilic e.
  pseudomembranous e.
  radiation e.
  regional e.
  Yersinia-related e.
enterocutaneous fistula
enterocyst
enterocystoma
enterocyte
  rapid antigen uptake into the
    cytosol e.'s (RACE)
enterocytopathogenic dog orphan
  (ECDO)
Enterocytozoon bieneusi
enteroendocrine cell
enteroenteric fistula
enterogastritis
enterogastrone
enterogenous
  e. cyanosis
  e. cyst
  e. methemoglobinemia
enteroglucagon
enterohemorrhagic *Escherichia coli*
  (EHEC)
enterohepatitis
enteroinvasive *Escherichia coli* **(EIEC)**
enterokinase
enterolith
enterolithiasis
enteromegalia
enteromegaly
Enteromonas hominis
enteromycosis
enteronitis

enteropathica
  acrodermatitis e.
enteropathogen
enteropathogenic *Escherichia coli* **(EEC,**
  EPEC)
enteropathy
  acrodermatitis e.
  autoimmune e.
  familial e.
  gluten-induced e.
  gluten-sensitive e. (GSE)
  protein-losing e.
  tufting e.
enteropathy-associated T-cell lymphoma
enteropeptidase
enterophila
  Oerskovia e.
enteroptosia
enteroptosis
enteroptotic
enterosepsis
enterostenosis
enterostomy dysfunction
enterotoxic *Escherichia coli* **(ETEC)**
enterotoxigenic
  e. bacteria
  e. *Escherichia coli* (ETEC)
enterotoxin
  Clostridium perfringens e.
  Escherichia coli e.
  staphylococcal e.
  staphylococcal e. B (SEB)
enterovaginal fistula
enterovesical fistula
Enterovibrio norvegicus
enteroviral meningitis
Enterovirus
enterovirus
  e. culture
  e. type 71 (EV 71)
enterozoic
enterozoon, pl. **enterozoa**
enthalpy of reaction
enthesitis
enthesopathic
enthesopathy
enthetic
Entner-Doudoroff pathway
entochoroidea
entocornea
entodermal cell
Entoloma sinuatum

E

NOTES

Entomobirnavirus
entomology
Entomophthora coronata
Entomophthorales
entomophthoramycosis,
  entomophthoromycosis
    e. basidiobolae
    e. conidiobolae
Entomoplasmataceae
Entomoplasmatales
entomopox virus
Entomopoxvirus A, B, C
entopic
entoplasm
entoretina
entosarc
Entozoa
entozoal
entozoic
entozoon
entrance wound
entrapment
    e. neuropathy
    tendon e.
    ulnar nerve e.
entropion
entropy
entry
    e. wound
    e. zone
enucleate
enucleation
enumeration of hematopoietic stem cells
envelope
    cell e.
    cistern of nuclear e.
    corneocyte e.
    elastomer e.
    nuclear e.
    viral e.
envenomation
environment
    chemical e.
    a hypotonic e.
environmental
    e. illness
    E. Protection Agency (EPA)
    e. sample
    e. stress
    e. toxicology
EnVision non-avidin-biotin detection system
enz.
    enzymatic
Enzact
    Pro-PredictRx E.
enzanensis
    Actinokineospora e.
Enzinger tumor classification

enzootic
    e. bovine leukosis
    e. encephalomyelitis
    e. encephalomyelitis virus
    e. infection
enzymatic (enz.)
    e. adaptation
    e. antigen unmasking
    e. digestion
    e. digestion method
    e. fat necrosis
    e. liquidation
    e. poisoning
enzyme
    activating e.
    acyl e.
    adaptive e.
    allosteric e.
    alpha glucan-branching e.
    amino acid-activating e.
    amylolytic e.
    e. analyzer
    angiotensin-converting e.
    angiotensin I-converting e.
    e. antagonist
    antitumor e.
    e. assay
    autolytic e.
    bacterial e.
    e. balance
    BamH1 e.
    beta site APP cleaving e. (BACE)
    brancher e.
    branching e.
    brush border e.
    catabolic e.
    cathepsin D e.
    catheptic e.
    cholinesterase e.
    citrate condensing e.
    coagulating e.
    constitutive e.
    converting e.
    cryptic e.
    cyclooxygenase e.
    debranching e.
    e. deficiency anemia
    deficiency of pancreatic e.
    delta-5 desaturase e.
    e. demonstration method
    drug metabolizing e. (DME)
    Eco RI e.
    endogenous antioxidant e.
    endothelin-converting e. (ECE1)
    extracellular matrix-degrading e.
    FADD-like interleukin-1 beta
      converting e. (FLICE)
    fatty acid beta oxidation e.
    glucan-branching e.

glycogen branching e.
glycolytic e.
hydrolytic e.
immobilized e.
e. immunochromatography (EIC)
inducible e.
e. induction
e. inhibition
e. inhibitor (EI)
inhibitory e.
inverting e.
key e.
lipocortin e.
lipolytic e.
e. marker
microsomal e.
Nagao e.
poly-ADP-ribose-polymerase e.
proteolytic e.
receptor-destroying e. (RDE)
e. repression
restriction e.
serum e.
steatolytic e.
e. study
telomerase e.
terminal addition e.
topoisomerase II e.
e. unit (EU)
urease e.
enzyme-assisted immunoassay technique
enzyme-deficient anemia
enzyme-dependent colorimetric technique
enzyme-enhancement immunoassay
enzyme-labeled oligonucleotide
enzyme-linked
e.-l. antibody test
e.-l. antiglobulin test (ELAT)
e.-l. immunosorbent assay (ELISA)
enzyme-multiplied
e.-m. immunoassay (EIA)
e.-m. immunoassay technique (EMIT)
enzymes/isoenzymes
cardiac e./i.
enzymic fat necrosis
enzymolysis
eo
eosinophil
Eobacteria
E6-oncoprotein
E7-oncoprotein

eos
eosinophilic leukocyte
eosin
alcohol-soluble e.
e. B, Y
ethyl e.
hematoxylin and e. (H&E)
e. I bluish
e. Y derivative of fluorescein stain
e. yellowish
e. Ys
eosin-methylene
e.-m. blue (EMB)
eosinocyte
Eosinofix reagent
eosinopenia
eosinophil, eosinophile (eo)
e. adenoma
e. chemotactic factor
e. chemotactic factor of anaphylaxis (ECF-A)
e. count
e. granule
e. leukocytic infiltrate
polymorphonuclear e. (PME)
e. smear
e. stimulation promoter (ESP)
eosinophilia
angiolymphoid hyperplasia with e.
clonal e.
granulomatous angiitis with e.
nonallergic rhinitis with e. (NARES)
peripheral blood e.
pulmonary e.
pulmonary infiltration and e. (PIE)
sclerosing mucoepidermoid carcinoma with e. (SMECE)
simple pulmonary e.
tropical e.
eosinophilia-myalgia syndrome (EMS)
eosinophilic
e. abscess
e. angiocentric fibrosis (EAF)
e. cationic protein (ECP)
e. cell metaplasia
e. cellulitis
e. colitis
e. cystitis
e. cytoplasm
e. endomyocardial disease
e. enteritis

E

NOTES

eosinophilic *(continued)*
  e. esophagitis
  e. fasciitis
  e. gastritis
  e. gastroenteritis (EGE)
  e. granularity
  e. granule
  e. granuloma
  e. granuloma of lung (EGL)
  e. granulomatosis
  e. hyperplasia
  e. index (EI)
  e. leukemia
  e. leukocyte (eos)
  e. leukocytosis
  e. leukopenia
  e. lung
  e. macronucleus
  e. marrow
  e. meningoencephalitis
  e. metamyelocyte
  e. myelocyte
  e. pneumonia
  e. pneumonitis
  e. promyelocyte
  e. proteinaceous granular material
  e. pustular folliculitis
  e. viral inclusion body
eosinophilocytic leukemia
eosinophil protein X (EPX)
eosinophiluria
eosinotactic
eosin-stained microscopic section
EOT
  effective oxygen transport
EP
  ectopic pregnancy
  electrophoresis
    EP test
    EP toxicity
EPA
  eicosapentaenoic acid
  Environmental Protection Agency
EPC
  epilepsia partialis continua
EPD
  extramammary Paget disease
EPE
  extraprostatic extension
EPEC
  enteropathogenic *Escherichia coli*
ependyma
ependymal
  e. cell
  e. cyst
  e. layer
  e. zone
ependymitis
ependymoblastoma

ependymocyte
ependymoma
  epithelial e.
  grade I-IV e.
  malignant e.
  myxopapillary e.
  papillary e.
Eperythrozoon
EPF
  exophthalmos-producing factor
  exposed protruding form
ephapse
ephedrine
ephelis, pl. **ephelides**
ephemeral
  e. fever of cattle
  e. fever virus
Ephemerovirus
epiallopregnanolone (EAP)
epiblast
epiboly, epibole
epibulbar
epicanthal fold
epicardial
epicardium of atrium
epicatechin gallate
epichlorohydrin
Epicoccum purpurascens
epicondylitis
  lateral e.
  medial e.
Epics
  E. Altra cell sorting system
  E. C flow cytometer
  E. Profile flow cytometer
  E. XL, XLMCL flow cytometer
    system
epicutaneous testing
epicystitis
epicyte
epidemic
  e. benign dry pleurisy
  e. cerebrospinal meningitis
  e. curve
  e. diaphragmatic pleurisy
  e. disease
  e. dysentery
  Electronic Surveillance System for
    the Early Notification of
    Community-based E.'s (ESSENCE)
  e. encephalitis
  e. exanthema
  e. gastroenteritis virus
  e. hemoglobinuria
  hemorrhagic fever e.
  e. hemorrhagic fever
  e. hepatitis
  E. Information Exchange (Epi-X)
  e. keratoconjunctivitis (EKC)

e. keratoconjunctivitis virus
e. louse-borne typhus
e. myalgia
e. myalgia virus
e. myalgic encephalomyelitis
e. myalgic encephalomyelopathy
e. myositis
e. nausea
e. nonbacterial gastroenteritis
e. parotitides
parotitis virus e.
e. parotitis virus
e. pleurodynia
e. pleurodynia virus
e. polyarthritis
e. roseola
e. transient diaphragmatic spasm
e. tremor
typhus e.
e. vomiting
epidemica
nephropathia e.
epidemicity
epidemiography
epidemiology
hospital e.
molecular e.
E. Program Office (EPO)
epiderm
epidermal
e. dermal nevus
e. growth factor (EGF)
e. growth factor receptor (EGFR)
e. inclusion cyst (EIC)
e. ridge
epidermalization
epidermal-melanin unit
epidermic
e. cell
e. pearl
epidermica
cladosporiosis e.
Saccharomyces e.
epidermic-dermic nevus
epidermides (*pl. of* epidermis)
epidermidis
nonpenicillinase-producing
Staphylococcus e.
Staphylococcus e.
stratum basale e.
stratum corneum e.

stratum granulosum e.
stratum spinosum e.
epidermidization of cervix
epidermidosis
epidermis, pl. **epidermides**
clear layer of e.
corneal layer of e.
granular layer of e.
horny layer of e.
keratohyalin granule of e.
epidermitis
epidermodysplasia verruciformis
epidermoid
e. cancer
e. carcinoma
e. carcinoma in situ
e. inclusion cyst
e. metaplasia
epidermolysin
epidermolysis
e. bullosa (EB)
e. bullosa acquisita
e. bullosa dystrophica
e. bullosa lethalis
e. bullosa simplex
epidermolytic hyperkeratosis
epidermophytid
Epidermophyton
E. floccosum
E. inguinale
E. rubrum
epidermophytosis
epidermosis
epidermotropic metastatic malignant melanoma (EMMM)
epidermotropism
epididymal cyst
epididymidis
coni e.
ductus e.
lobuli e.
epididymis, pl. **epididymides**
duct of e.
lobule of e.
epididymitis
epididymoorchitis
epidural
e. abscess
e. hematoma
e. meningitis
epifluorescence microscopy
epigastric hernia

E

NOTES

epigastrius parasiticus
epigenesis
epigenetics
epigenetic silencing
epigenotype
epiglottiditis
epiglottis
epignathus
epihyal bone
epi-illumination
epilamellar
epilating dose
epilation
epilemma
epilemmal ending
epilepidoma
epilepsia partialis continua (EPC)
epilepsy
> familial myoclonic e.
> focal cortical e.
> grand mal e.
> jacksonian e.
> minor e.
> myoclonic e.
> petit mal e.
> posttraumatic e.
> psychomotor e.
> rolandic e.
> sudden unexplained death in e.
> (SUDEP)
> temporal lobe e.
> uncinate e.

epilepticus
> status e.

epileptiform discharge (ED)
epileptogenic
> e. focus
> e. zone

epiloia
epimastical fever
epimastigote
epimembranous glomerulonephritis
epimer
epimerase
epimerite
epimerization
epimicroscope
epimorphic regeneration
epimyoepithelial carcinoma
epimysium
epinephrine
> ferric chloride reaction of e.
> iodate reaction of e.
> iodine reaction of e.
> e. and norepinephrine assays
> urine e.

epinephros
epineurial
epineurium

epionychium
epiotic center
epiphenomenon
epiphenotype
epiphrenic diverticulum
epiphysial, epiphyseal
> e. arrest
> e. aseptic necrosis
> e. giant cell tumor
> e. plate

epiphysis, pl. epiphyses
> e. cerebri
> stippled e.

epiphysitis
epiphyte
epiploic
epiploica
episcleralis
> lamina e.

episcleral lamina
episcleritis
> rheumatoid e.

episialin
episode
> e. of care
> mitochondrial encephalopathy, lactic acidosis, and strokelike e.'s (MELAS)
> transient cerebral ischemic e. (TCIE)
> transient ischemic e. (TIE)

episomal
episome
> resistance transferring e.

epispadias
episplenitis
epistasis
epistasy
epistatic
epistaxis
Episthmium caninum
epitaxy
epitendineum
epitenon
epitestosterone
epithalaxia
epithelia (*pl. of* epithelium)
epithelial
> e. apoptosis
> e. attachment
> e. attachment of Gottlieb
> e. basement membrane
> e. cadherin (E-cadherin)
> e. cancer
> e. cell disease
> e. cell urinary cast
> e. choroid layer
> e. differentiation
> e. displacement

e. dysplasia
e. ependymoma
e. foot process
e. glycoprotein-2 (EGP-2)
human ovarian surface e. (HOSE)
e. hyperchromasia
e. hyperplasia
e. inclusion cyst
e. lamina
e. marker immunohistochemistry
e. membrane antigen (EMA)
e. neoplasm
e. nest
e. pearl
e. pigment
e. predominant blastoma
renal tubular e. (RTE)
e. rest
e. reticular cell
e. sodium channel (ENaC)
e. thymoma
e. tissue
e. tumor
epithelialis
lamina choroidea e.
epithelialization
epithelial-myoepithelial carcinoma (EMEC)
epithelial-stromal tumor
epitheliitis
epitheliocyte
thymic e.
tumor of thymic e.
epitheliofibril
epithelioglandular
epithelioid
e. cell
e. cell cluster
e. cell melanoma
e. cell nevus
e. hemangioendothelioma (EH, EHE)
e. histiocyte
e. leiomyoma
e. sarcoma (ES)
e. soft-tissue neoplasm (ESTN)
epitheliolysis
epitheliolytic
epithelioma
e. adenoides cysticum
basal cell e.
benign e.

Borst-Jadassohn type intraepidermal e.
calcifying e. of Malherbe
chorionic e.
e. contagiosum
e. cuniculatum
Malherbe calcifying e.
multiple self-healing squamous e.
sebaceous e.
epitheliomatous
epitheliopathy
epitheliosis
epitheliotropism
epithelium, pl. epithelia
adenomatous e.
androgen-normal e.
e. anterius corneae
Barrett e.
calicoblastic e.
carcinomatous e.
ciliated e.
classification of e.
columnar e.
crevicular e.
crypt e.
cuboidal e.
cylindrical e.
displacement of e.
distinctive e.
e. ductus semicircularis
dysplastic e.
enamel e.
external dental e.
foveolar e.
germinal e.
gingival e.
glandular e.
inner dental e.
junctional e.
laminated e.
e. of lens
e. lentis
mesenchymal e.
metaplastic columnar e.
muscle e.
neoplastic e.
nonkeratinized stratified squamous e.
nonneoplastic mucinous hyperplastic e.
odontogenic e.
olfactory e.

E

NOTES

epithelium *(continued)*
oncocytic e.
pavement e.
pigment e.
pseudostratified columnar e.
reduced enamel e.
respiratory e.
seminiferous e.
simple columnar e.
simple cuboidal e.
simple squamous e.
specialized e.
squamous e.
stratified ciliated columnar e.
stratified cuboidal e.
stratified squamous
nonkeratinized e.
sulcular e.
surface e.
transitional e.
vaginal e.
e. with mitotic figure
epithelium-lined ductal portion
epithelization
epitope
discontinuous e.
e. mapping
e. masking
phosphorylation-
dependent/independent
neurofilament e.
phosphorylation-independent NF-
H/M e.
e. retrieval
e. unmasking
epitoxoid
epitrichium
epituberculous infiltration
epitype
Epi-X
Epidemic Information Exchange
epizoic
epizoon
epizootic
anthrax e.
e. cellulitis
e. disease, category A, B
e. hemorrhagic disease of deer
e. lymphangitis
EPM
extraosseous plasmacytoma of the
mediastinum
EPO
Epidemiology Program Office
Epon-Araldite resin
Epon tissue-embedding medium
eponychium
epoophori
tubuli e.

epoophoron
transverse ductules of e.
e-positive RBCs
epoxide
heptachlor e.
e. leukotriene LTA4
e. reductase
epoxyeicosatrienoic acid
epoxy resin
EPP
erythropoietic protoporphyria
Eppendorf
E. 5702 centrifuge
E. filtertip
E. MicroChisel
E. MicroDissector
E. Repeater Pro pipette
E. tube
EPS
exophthalmos-producing substance
Epsilobacteria
epsilon
e. acid
e. antigen
e. clostridial toxin
e. component
e. isoform
e. staphylolysin
Epsilonretrovirus
Epstein
E. disease
E. syndrome
Epstein-Barr
E.-B. encoded RNA (EBER)
E.-B. nuclear antigen (EBNA)
E.-B. virus (EBV)
E.-B. virus antibody assay
E.-B. virus culture
E.-B. virus-encoded RNA in situ
hybridization
E.-B. virus serology
epulis, pl. **epulides**
e. cell
pigmented e.
EPX
eosinophil protein X
eq
equivalent
equal
bilateral, symmetrical, and e. (BSE)
equation
alveolar air e.
Arrhenius e.
Bohr e.
chemical e.
Cockcroft-Gault e.
Eadie-Hofstee e.
Friedewald e.
Hanes e.

Hasselbalch e.
Henderson-Hasselbalch e.
Hill e.
Hüfner e.
Lineweaver-Burk e.
Michaelis-Menten e.
Nernst e.
Scatchard e.
Svedberg e.
van der Waals e.
equational division
equi
    Corynebacterium e.
    Crossiella e.
    Ehrlichia e.
    Lactobacillus e.
    Papulaspora e.
    Rhodococcus e.
equilibration
equilibrium
chemical e.
e. constant
dynamic e.
physiologic e.
radioactive e.
secular e.
sedimentation e.
thermal e.
thermodynamic e.
transient e.
equina
    Setaria e.
    Taenia e.
equine
e. abortion virus
e. antihuman lymphoblast globulin (EAHLG)
e. antihuman lymphoblast serum (EAHLS)
e. arteritis virus
e. coital exanthema virus
e. encephalitis
e. encephalomyelitis
e. encephalomyelitis virus
e. gonadotropin unit
e. infectious anemia
e. infectious anemia virus
e. influenza
e. influenza virus
e. morbillivirus (Hendra virus)
e. rhinopneumonitis (ERP)
e. rhinopneumonitis virus

e. rhinovirus
e. serum hepatitis
e. viral arteritis
equinum
    Fusobacterium e.
    Trichophyton e.
    Trichophyton equinum var. *e.*
    Trypanosoma e.
equinus
    Rhizopus e.
    Strongylus e.
equiperdum
    Trypanosoma e.
equipment
eyewash e.
individual protective e. (IPE)
personal protective e. (PPE)
equipotential line
equivalence
e. point
e. relation
zone of e.
e. zone
equivalent (eq)
age e. (AEq)
lethal e.
metabolic e. (MET)
nitrogen e.
tissue e.
toxic e.
equorum
    Ascaris e.
    Parascaris e.
equuli
    Actinobacillus e.
ER
endoplasmic reticulum
estrogen receptor
Er
erbium
ERA
estrogen receptor assay
eradication therapy
Eranko fluorescence stain
Erb
E. disease
E. syndrome
erb
e. A oncogene
e. B, B-2 oncogene
e. B protooncogene
Erb-Charcot disease

NOTES

E

355

ERBF
  effective renal blood flow
Erb-Goldflam disease
erbium (Er)
ERC
  erythropoietin-responsive cell
Erdheim
  E. disease
  E. rest
  E. tumor
Erdheim-Chester disease (ECD)
erectile
  e. myxoma
  e. tissue
Eremascus
Eremomyces langeronii
Eremothecium
ergastoplasm
ERGIC-53 gene product
ergocalciferol
ergoloid mesylate
ergometer
ergonovine provocation test
ergoreceptor activation
ergosterol
ergot
  corn e.
ergothioneine
ergotism
ergotoxine
eriksonii
  Actinomyces e.
  Bifidobacterium e.
erinacei
  Trichophyton e.
  Trichophyton mentagrophytes var. *e.*
Erlanger and Gasser peripheral nerve assay
Erlenmeyer
  E. flask
  E. flask deformity
  E. flask-like
ERMS
  embryonal rhabdomyosarcoma
erode
E-rosette test
erosion
erosive
  e. adenomatosis of nipple
  e. aneurysm
  e. cystitis
  e. esophagitis
  e. gastritis
  e. inflammation
eroticum
  curiosum e.
ERP
  effective refractory period

  equine rhinopneumonitis
  estrogen receptor protein
ERPG
  emergency response planning guideline
Errantivirus
erraticus
  Ornithodoros e.
error
  coincidence e.
  e. detector
  machine e.
  preanalytic e.
  probable e.
  random e.
  e. rate
  standard e. (SE)
  systematic e.
  type I, II e.
ERRT
  extrarenal rhabdoid tumor
ERT
  emergency response to terrorism
ER-Tracker blue-white DPX
eruption
  bullous e.
  creeping e.
  Kaposi varicelliform e.
  macular e.
  maculopapular e.
  polymorphic light e.
  polymorphous e.
  varicelliform e.
eruptive fever
Erwinia
  E. amylovora
  E. herbicola
  E. papayae
Erwinieae
erysipelas
erysipeloid
Erysipelothrix
  E. inopinata
  E. insidiosa
  E. rhusiopathiae
Erysipelotrichaceae
Erysiphe graminis
erythema
  e. ab igne
  e. annulare centrifugum
  e. chronicum migrans (ECM)
  e. dose
  dusky e.
  e. dyschromicum perstans
  e. elevatum diutinum
  e. exfoliativa
  figurate e.
  e. figuratum
  gyrate e.
  e. gyratum repens

e. induratum
e. infectiosum
e. iris
e. keratodes
macular e.
e. marginatum
e. marginatum rheumaticum
e. migrans (EM)
mottled e.
e. multiforme
e. multiforme bullosum
e. multiforme exudativum
necrolytic migratory e.
e. neonatorum
e. nodosum (EN)
e. nodosum leprosum (ENL)
Osler e.
palmar e.
e. pernio
e. perstans
e. polymorphe
toxic e.
e. toxicum
erythematosum
anetoderma e.
eczema e.
erythematosus
acute disseminated lupus e.
discoid lupus e. (DLE)
disseminated acute lupus e.
lupus e. (LE)
pemphigus e.
systemic lupus e. (SLE)
erythrasma
erythremia
erythremic myelosis
erythrinae
Samsonia e.
erythritol
Erythrobacillus
Erythrobacter
E. citreus
E. flavus
E. longus
Erythrobasidium
erythroblast
basophilic e.
definitive e.
polychromatophilic e.
primitive e.
erythroblastemia

erythroblastic
e. anemia
e. island
erythroblastoma
erythroblastomatosis
erythroblastopenia
erythroblastosis
fetal e.
e. fetalis
e. neonatorum
erythroblastotic
erythrocatalysis
erythrochromia
erythroclasis
erythroclast
erythroclastic
erythrocuprein
erythrocytapheresis
erythrocyte (E)
e. adherence phenomenon
e. adherence test
e. antibody (EA)
e. antibody complement (EAC)
e. antibody complement rosette assay
e. antigen
e. aspartate aminotransferase activity (eAST)
e. in capillary
e. count
dichromatic e.
dysmorphic e.
e. fragility
e. fragility test
free e. protoporphyrin (FEP, FEPP)
e. glutamic oxaloacetic transaminase (EGOT)
hypochromic microcytic e.
e. indices
e. mass (EM)
e. maturation factor (EMF)
e. membrane
microcytic e.
normocytic e.
e. protoporphyrin test
reticulated e.
e. rosette
e. sedimentation
e. sedimentation rate (ESR)
sickled e.

E

NOTES

erythrocyte *(continued)*
    e. transketolase
    e. zinc protoporphyrin
erythrocyte-sensitizing substance (ESS)
erythrocythemia
erythrocytic
    e. blood cell
    e. marrow
    e. series
erythrocytoblast
erythrocytolysin
erythrocytolysis
erythrocytometer
erythrocytometry
erythrocytopenia
erythrocytophagy
erythrocytopoiesis
erythrocytorrhexis
erythrocytoschisis
erythrocytosis
    absolute e.
    leukemic e.
    e. megalosplenica
    relative e.
    stress e.
erythrocyturia
erythrodegenerative
erythroderma
    e. exfoliativa
    Sézary e.
erythrodextrin
erythrodysesthesia syndrome
erythrogenesis imperfecta
erythrogenic toxin
erythroglutinin
    Phaseolus vulgaris e. (PHA-E)
erythrogonium, pl. erythrogonia
erythrohepatic porphyria
erythroid
    e. aplasia
    e. colony assay
    e. hyperplasia
    e. hypoplasia
    e. leukemia
    e. precursor
    e. precursor cell
erythroidine
    beta e.
erythrokeratodermia variabilis
erythrokinase (EK)
erythrokinetics
erythrokinetic study
erythroleukemia
    acute e. (M6)
erythroleukosis
erythrolysin
erythrolysis
erythromelalgia
erythromelia

erythromyeloblastic leukemia
erythron
erythroneocytosis
erythropenia
erythrophage
erythrophagia
erythrophagocytosis
erythrophil
erythrophilic
erythrophobic
erythrophore
erythroplakia
erythroplasia of Queyrat
erythropoiesis
    extramedullary e.
    increased e.
    ineffective e.
    megaloblastic e.
erythropoietic
    e. coproporphyria (ECP)
    e. hormone
    e. porphyria
    e. porphyrin
    e. protoporphyria (EPP)
erythropoietic-stimulating factor (ESF)
erythropoietin
    inappropriate production of e.
    recombinant e.
    e. test
erythropoietin-responsive cell (ERC)
erythropyknosis
erythrorrhexis
erythrose
erythrosin B
Erythrovirus
Erythroxylon coca
erythruria
ES
    electrospray
    epithelioid sarcoma
    Ewing sarcoma
ES300-Cardiac T ELISA troponin T immunoassay system
Esbach reagent
escape
    e. mask
    e. mutant
eschar
    localized black e.
Escherich bacillus
Escherichia
    E. adecarboxylata
    E. albertii
    E. aurescens
    E. blattae
    E. coli
    E. coli enterotoxin
    E. coli 0157:h7
    E. coli pneumonia

E. *coli* urinary tract infection
enterohemorrhagic E. *coli* (EHEC)
enteroinvasive E. *coli* (EIEC)
E. fergusonii
E. *hermanii*
E. *vulneris*
Escherichieae
escomelis
Trypanosoma e.
esculenta
Gyromitra e.
Helvella e.
esculin hydrolysis test
ESF
erythropoietic-stimulating factor
ES-FISH
extra signal FISH
ESFT
Ewing sarcoma family of tumors
Eskimo traditional food
ESN
endometrial stromal nodule
esodic
esoethmoiditis
esogastritis
esophageae
glandulae e.
esophageal
e. achalasia
e. acid infusion test
e. acidity
e. aperistalsis
e. apudoma
e. atresia
e. carcinoma
e. dysmotility
e. gland
e. gland proper
e. hernia
e. hypomotility
e. motility study
e. perforation
e. reflux
e. ring
e. rupture
e. smear
e. spasm
e. stricture
e. tumor
e. varices
e. web
esophagectasia

esophagectasis
esophagi (*pl. of* esophagus)
esophagitis
Candida e.
corrosive e.
cytomegalovirus e.
eosinophilic e.
erosive e.
fungal e.
herpes e.
infectious e.
irradiation e.
monilial e.
peptic e.
pill e.
pill-induced e.
reflux e.
esophagogastric junction
esophagogastritis
esophagomalacia
esophagomycosis
esophagoptosia
esophagoptosis
esophagosalivary reflex
esophagostenosis
esophagostomiasis
esophagus, pl. **esophagi**
Barrett e.
cardiac gland of e.
e. communicate
tunica mucosa esophagi
tunica muscularis esophagi
esosphenoiditis
ESP
Early Surveillance Project
end-systolic pressure
eosinophil stimulation promoter
ESP II system
espundia
ESR
electron spin resonance
erythrocyte sedimentation rate
ESR assay
ESRA-10 erythrocyte sedimentation rate analyzer
ESR-Auto Plus sedimentation rate analyzer
ESR-Chex hematology control
ESS
endometrial stromal sarcoma
erythrocyte-sensitizing substance

NOTES

ESSENCE
    Electronic Surveillance System for the Early Notification of Community-based Epidemics
essential
    e. albuminuria
    e. asthma
    e. atrophy
    e. fatty acid (EFA)
    e. fever
    e. fructosuria
    e. hematuria
    e. hypercholesterolemia
    e. hyperlipemia
    e. hypertension (EH)
    e. macroglobulinemia
    e. monoclonal gammopathy
    e. oil
    e. pentosuria
    e. telangiectasia
    e. thrombocythemia (ET)
    e. thrombocytopenia
    e. thrombocytosis
established cell line
ester
    acridinium e.
    cholesterol e. (ChE)
    Cori e.
    fatty acid methyl e. (FAME)
    hexosephosphoric e.'s
    nonfluorescent acetoxymethyl e.
    tetra-methylrhodamine ethyl e. (TMRE)
esterase
    alpha-naphthyl acetate e. (ANAE)
    C1 e.
    chloracetate e.
    chloroacetate e. (CAE)
    cholesterol e.
    leukocyte e.
    naphthol-AS-D-chloracetate e. (NASDCE)
    neuron-specific e. (NSE)
    neuropathy target e. (NTE)
    nonspecific e. (NSE)
    e. staining method
    e. test
    urine leukocyte e.
esterification
estetrol (E$_4$)
esthesioneuroblastoma
    olfactory e.
esthesioneurocytoma
esthiomene
esthiomenous
estimate
    biased e.
    consistent e.
    dose e.

    interval e.
    median unbiased e.
    point e.
    pooled e.
    standard error of e. (SEE)
    unbiased e.
estimated
    e. blood loss (EBL)
    e. hepatic blood flow (EHBF)
Estlander flap
ESTN
    epithelioid soft-tissue neoplasm
estradiol (E$_2$)
    e. assay
    e. benzoate (EB)
    e. benzoate unit
    17 beta e.
    e. receptor
    e. test
Estren-Dameshek anemia
estriol (E$_3$)
    e. assay
    conjugated e.
    free e.
    maternal urine e.
    serum e.
    total e.
    unconjugated e.
    urinary e.
    urine placental e.
estrogen
    absence of e.
    plant e.
    e. receptor (ER)
    e. receptor alpha
    e. receptor assay (ERA)
    e. receptor beta
    e. receptor protein (ERP)
    e. stimulation test
    total urine e.
    urine total e.
    e. withdrawal bleeding (EWB)
estrogenic hormone
estrone (E$_1$)
    e. unit
estunensis
    Acetobacter e.
ESU
    electrostatic unit
ET
    effective temperature
    essential thrombocythemia
    etiology
    exchange transfusion
ET3
    endothelin-3
eta
    e. cell
    e. isoform

état mamelonné
ETEC
    enterotoxic *Escherichia coli*
    enterotoxigenic *Escherichia coli*
ethacrynic acid (ECA)
ethambutol
ethane
ethanedial
ethanedinitrile
ethanoic acid
ethanol
    e. assay
    e. gelation test
    e. level
ethanolamine
    arachidonic containing
      phosphatidyl e.
ethchlorvynol assay
ethene
ether
    bischloromethyl e.
    dimethyl e.
    ethyl e.
    petroleum e.
    e. storage
ethidium
    e. bromide
    e. bromide stain
ethiodized oil
ethion
ethionamide
ethionine
ethmoid
ethmoidal
    e. cell
    e. sinus
ethmoidales
    cellulae e.
    sinus e.
ethmoidalia
    antra e.
ethmoidalis
    fovea e.
    lamina cribrosa ossis e.
ethmoiditis
ethosuximide assay
ethoxazene hydrochloride
ethyl
    e. acetate
    e. alcohol (ETOH, EtOH)
    e. alcohol poisoning
    e. cyanide

    e. eosin
    e. ether
    e. green
    e. orange
    e. violet azide broth
ethylbromoacetate grenade
ethylcocaine
ethyldichloroarsine
ethylene
    e. chlorohydrin
    e. dibromide
    e. dichloride
    e. glycol
    e. glycol assay
    e. glycol dinitrate
    e. glycol intoxication
    e. glycol poisoning
    e. glycol tetraacetic acid (EGTA)
    e. oxide
    e. tetraacetic acid
ethylenediaminetetraacetate
ethylenediaminetetraacetic
    e. acid (EDTA)
    calcium e. (Ca-EDTA)
ethylidene dichloride
ethylphosphonofluoridate
    NATO code for nerve agent isopropyl e. (GE)
ethylphosphonothioate
    NATO code for nerve agent O-ethyl S-[2-(diethylamino)ethyl] e. (VE)
ethyne
etiocholanolone
etiol
    etiology
etiologic
    e. agent
    e. factor
etiology (ET, etiol)
    common viral e.
    genetic e.
    pyrexia of unknown e. (PUE)
    unknown e.
    villitis of unknown e. (VUE)
etiopathogenic factor
ETOH, EtOH
    ethyl alcohol
etorphine
EU
    Ehrlich unit
    enzyme unit

NOTES

eubacteria
Eubacteriales
Eubacterieae
Eubacteriineae
Eubacterium
 E. *aerofaciens*
 E. *aggregans*
 E. *alactolyticum*
 E. *combesi*
 E. *contortum*
 E. *crispatum*
 E. *endocarditis*
 E. *filamentosum*
 E. *lentum*
 E. *limosum*
 E. *minutum*
 E. *moniliforme*
 E. *parvum*
 E. *poeciloides*
 E. *pseudotortuosum*
 E. *pyruvativorans*
 E. *quartum*
 E. *quintum*
 E. *rectale*
 E. *tenue*
 E. *tortuosum*
 E. *ventriosum*
eucalyptus oil
eucapnia
eucaryote (*var. of* eukaryote)
eucaryotic (*var. of* eukaryotic)
Eucestoda
eucholia
euchromatic
euchromatin
 nucleus containing predominantly e.
Eucoleus
Euflagellata
Euglena
 E. *gracilis*
 E. *viridis*
Euglenidae
euglenoid movement
euglobin lysis time
euglobulin
 e. clot lysis
 e. clot lysis time (ECLT)
 e. clot test (ECT)
 e. lysis test
 e. lysis time (ELT)
euglycemia
euglycemic
eugnosia
eugonic
Eugregarinida
eukaryon
eukaryosis
Eukaryotae
eukaryote, eucaryote

eukaryotic, eucaryotic
 e. cell cycle
eukeratin
Eulenburg disease
eumelanin
eumelanosome
eumetria
eumorphism
eumycetes
Eumycetozoea
eumycotic mycetoma
eunuchoid
eunuchoidism
 hypogonadotropic e.
euosmia
euparal
Euparyphium
Eupenicillium
euplasia
euplastic lymph
euploid
euploid-polyploid pattern
euploidy
eupraxia
Euproctis chrysorrhoea
Eurasina
europaeiscabiei
 Streptomyces e.
europaeus
 Ulex e. (UE)
European
 E. blastomycosis
 E. hookworm
 E. rat flea
europium
Eurotium
Eurotium malignum
Euryarchaeota
eurystrepta
 Spirochaeta e.
eurytherma
 Amycolatopsis e.
eurythermal
Eurythermea
Eurytrema pancreaticum
euscope
Eusimulium
eustachian
 e. tonsil
 e. tube
eustachiana, eustachii
 tuba e.
Eustoma rotundatum parasitic worm
Eustrongylides
Eustrongylus
eutectic temperature
euthyroidism
euthyroid sick state
eutonic

Eutriatoma
Eutrombicula alfreddugesi
eutropha
>*Nitrosomonas e.*
>*Wautersia e.*
eutrophic
euvolemic
>e. hypotonic hyponatremia
>e. volume
EV
>extravascular
EV 71
>enterovirus type 71
eV
>electron volt
evagination
evaluation
>acute physiology and chronic health e. (APACHE)
>buccal smear for sex chromatin e.
>forensic e.
>hormonal e.
>pneumonectomy e.
>rapid on-site specimen cytologic e.
>tilt table e.
Evans
>E. blue
>E. syndrome
evansi
>*Trypanosoma e.*
evaporation
event
>agroterrorist e.
>late e.
>low probability, high consequence e. (LPHC)
>sentinel e.
eventration of diaphragm
eversion
EVG
>elastica van Gieson
evidence
>collection of forensic e.
>e. gathering process
>short-lived e.
evil
>king's e.
evisceration
evisceroneurotomy
evocative testing
evolutus
>*Peptostreptococcus e.*

EWB
>estrogen withdrawal bleeding
Ewing
>E. sarcoma (ES)
>E. sarcoma gene
>E. sarcoma/peripheral neuroectodermal tumor
Ewingella
EWL
>egg-white lysozyme
EWS/PNET
>Ewing sarcoma/primitive neuroectodermal tumor
EWS-WT1 chimeric transcript
ex
>exophthalmos
>ex vivo
>ex vivo platelet clumping
ExacTech blood glucose meter test
examination
>bile fluid e.
>cytologic e.
>dark-field e.
>digital rectal e. (DRE)
>direct wet mount e.
>double-contrast e.
>duodenal contents e.
>fecal e.
>full blood e. (FBE)
>gastric residue e.
>national e.
>ova and parasite e.
>Pap e.
>pericardial fluid e.
>peritoneal fluid e.
>permanent stained smear e.
>pleural fluid e.
>postmortem e.
>semen e.
>sputum e.
>stool e.
>synovial fluid e.
examiner
>Diplomate of the National Board of Medical E.'s
>medical e. (ME)
exanthema, exanthem, pl. **exanthemas, exanthemata**
>Boston e.
>epidemic e.
>e. subitum
>vesicular e.

NOTES

exanthematous
e. disease
e. fever
e. inflammation
exanthesis arthrosia
excavatio
e. disci
e. papillae
excavation
e. of optic disc
physiologic e.
excavatum
congenital pectus e.
pectus e.
excess (XS)
antibody e.
antigen e.
base e. (BE)
negative base e.
excessive
e. cornification
e. fatigue
e. heat production (EHP)
e. lacrimation
e. sweating
e. tearing
e. weakness
e. weight gain
e. weight loss
exchange
bidirectional information e.
Epidemic Information E. (Epi-X)
fetomaternal molecular e.
gas e.
lungs of gaseous e.
e. pairing
plasma e.
therapeutic plasma e.
e. transfusion (ET)
exchangeable
e. mass
e. sodium
exchanger
anion e. 1 (AE1)
excipient
excision
marginal e. (ME)
excisional biopsy
excitation spectrum
excitatory effect
excited
e. delirium
e. skin syndrome
e. state
exciter filter
excitomotor
excitotoxin protein

exclusion
allelic e.
confidential unit e. (CUE)
exconjugant
excoriation
excrescence
Lambl e.
mesothelial/monocytic incidental cardiac e. (MICE)
papillary e.
polypoid e.
excretion
phenolsulfonphthalein e.
pseudouridine e.
excretorius
ductus e.
excretory
e. duct
e. duct of seminal vesicle
e. duct of sweat
e. duct of sweat gland
e. duct of tracheal gland
e. ductules of lacrimal gland
e. portion
e. urogram (XU)
excurrent duct system
excystation
execute
execution time
exencephalia
exencephalic
exencephalocele
exencephalous
exencephaly
exenteration
exenteritis
exercise
e. hyperemia blood flow (EHBF)
e. intolerance
exercise-induced asthma
exergonic reaction
exflagellation
exfoliatin
exfoliation
exfoliativa
dermatitis e.
erythema e.
erythroderma e.
keratolysis e.
exfoliative
e. cytodiagnosis
e. cytologic alteration
e. cytology
e. dermatitis
e. gastritis
e. psoriasis
exhalans
Nocardiopsis e.

exhaust
    slot e.
exhaustion
    e. atrophy
    secretory e.
exhumation
Exidia
exigua
    Slackia e.
Exiguobacterium
    E. antarcticum
    E. undae
existence proof
exit
    e. access
    e. discharge
    e. dose
    e. wound
exiting projectile
exoantigen test
Exobasidium
exocellular
exocervix
exochorial pregnancy
exocrine
    e. cell
    e. gland
    e. pancreas
    e. phenotype
exocytosis
exodus
exoenzyme
exoerythrocytic plasmodium
Exoflagellata
exogamy
exogenetic
exogenote
exogenous
    e. aneurysm
    e. anticoagulant coagulation
    e. antigen
    e. antigen cell-bound antibody reaction
    e. antigen-circulating antibody reaction
    e. bacterium
    e. creatinine clearance
    e. creatinine clinoscope
    e. growth factor
    e. hemochromatosis
    e. hemosiderosis
    e. hyperglyceridemia

    e. infection
    e. lipid pneumonia
    e. obesity
    e. pigmentation
    e. variable
exomphalos, macroglossia, and gigantism (EMG)
exon
exonuclease
exopeptidase
Exophiala
    E. jeanselmei
    E. mycetoma
    E. pisciphila
    E. werneckii
exophthalmica
    cachexia e.
exophthalmic goiter
exophthalmos (ex)
exophthalmos-hyperthyroid factor (EHF)
exophthalmos-producing
    e.-p. factor (EPF)
    e.-p. substance (EPS)
exophyte
exophytic
    e. growth
    e. papilla
exoplasm
exoribonuclease
exoskeleton
exosmosis
exosome
exospore
Exosporina
exosporium
exostosis, pl. **exostoses**
    e. bursata
    e. cartilaginea
    chondromatous e.
    diaphysial juxtaepiphysial e.
    hereditary multiple exostoses
    ivory e.
    multiple e.
    osteocartilaginous e.
    solitary osteocartilaginous e.
exotaxin/CCL11 gene
exothermic
exotoxic
exotoxin product of bacteria
exotropia
expander
    plasma volume e.

E

NOTES

expansa
    Moniezia e.
expansion
    clonal e.
    volume e.
ExPEC
    extraintestinal pathogenic *Escherichia coli*
expected date of confinement (EDC)
expectoration
    prune juice e.
experiment
    control e.
    double-blind e.
    double-masked e.
experimental
    e. allergic encephalitis
    e. allergic encephalomyelitis (EAE)
    e. allergic neuritis (EAN)
    e. autoimmune glomerulonephritis (EAG)
    e. pathology
explant
explantation
explode
exploding crypt cell
explosion
    depleted uranium-containing e.
explosion-proof
explosive
    e. atmosphere
    chemical, biological, radiological, nuclear, e. (CBRNE)
    high e.
    e. limit
    low e.
    e. material
Expo 32 flow cytometry software
exponent
    hydrogen e.
exponential
    e. decay
    e. function
    e. phase
exposure
    neutron e.
expressed RNA
expression
    active protein e.
    calretinin e.
    CEACAM1 e.
    constitutive e.
    cytokeratin e.
    FMC7 e.
    gene e.
    hNIS gene e.
    inhibin e.
    latent membrane protein-1 e.
    myoid marker e.

    phosphorylated protein e.
    p57 KIP^2 e.
    podoplanin e.
    profile of gene e.
    reduced Fhit protein e.
    serial analysis of gene e. (SAGE)
    serological expression of cDNA e. (SEREX)
    surface e.
    total protein e.
    TRK-A gene e.
    underphosphorylated protein e.
    e. vector
expressivity
exsanguinate
exsanguination
exsanguine
Exserohilum longirostratum
exsiccant
exsiccate
exsiccated sodium sulfite
exsiccation
exsiccosis
exstrophy
    e. of the bladder
    e. of the cloaca
    cloacal e.
extended insulin zinc suspension
extension
    cytoplasmic e.
    established extraprostatic e. (E-EPE)
    extraprostatic e. (EPE)
    focal extraprostatic e. (F-EPE)
extensive
    e. accumulation
    e. regression
extensum
    hemangioma planum e.
externa
    hepatitis e.
    muscularis e.
    otitis e.
    pachymeningitis e.
    theca e.
    tunica e.
external
    e. decontamination
    e. dental epithelium
    e. elastic lamellae
    e. elastic lamina
    e. fistula
    e. hemorrhoid
    e. irradiation
    e. meningitis
    e. pillar cell
    e. pudendal vein
    e. pyocephalus
    e. pyramidal layer
    e. root sheath

e. salivary gland
e. spiral sulcus
e. storage
externum
perimysium e.
externus
sulcus spiralis e.
exteroceptor
extima
tunica e.
extinction coefficient
extinguishing
extra
e. electron density
e. signal FISH (ES-FISH)
extraabdominal
e. desmoid
e. fibromatosis
extracapillary lesion (ECL)
extracapsular
e. ankylosis
e. tumor
extracellular (EC)
e. aggregate alteration lipid
e. ATP
e. cholesterolosis
e. in distribution
e. fibril alteration
e. fluid (ECF)
e. fluid volume (ECFV, EFV)
e. granule
e. ground substance
e. lipid aggregate
e. macromolecule aggregate
e. material (ECM)
e. matrix (ECM)
e. matrix alteration
e. matrix-degrading enzyme
e. matrix glycoprotein
e. matrix protein
e. parasite
e. plasma
e. structural alteration
e. superoxide dismutase (EC-SOD)
e. tachyzoite
e. toxin
e. vacuole
e. volume (ECV)
e. water (ECW)
extrachorial placentation

extrachromosomal
e. element
e. inheritance
extracorporeal
e. photophoresis
e. photophoresis technique
extracorpuscular
extract
adipose tissue e.
adrenocortical e. (ACE)
allergenic e.
allergic e.
anterior pituitary e. (APE)
Büchner e.
ceanothus e.
lipopolysaccharide e.
parathyroid e. (PTE)
pollen e.
streptomycin assay agar with
yeast e.
whole ragweed e. (WRE)
extractable
e. nuclear antigen (ENA)
e. nuclear antigen antibody (ENA)
extraction
Baker pyridine e.
e. coefficient
countercurrent e.
differential e.
e. fraction (E)
Gibco-BRL TriZol DNA e.
guanidinium e.
solvent e.
testicular sperm e. (TESE)
Extract-N-Amp Blood PCR kit
extractor
RNAzol Reagent e.
extracystic
extradural hematorrhachis
extraembryonic mesoblast
extrafollicular colloid
extrafusal muscle fiber
extraglomerular mesangium
extragonadal germ cell tumor
extrahepatic
e. biliary atresia (EHBA)
e. obstruction (EHO)
extraintestinal
e. manifestation
e. pathogenic *Escherichia coli*
(ExPEC)

E

NOTES

extralobar sequestration
extramammary Paget disease (EPD)
extramedullary
    e. erythropoiesis
    e. hematopoiesis (EMH)
    e. myelogenous leukemia
    e. myelopoiesis
    e. solitary plasmacytoma (EMP)
extramembranous glomerulonephritis
extramural
extraneural
extranodal
    e. marginal zone
    e. marginal zone lymphoma
extranuchal nuchal fibroma
extranuclear
extraosseous
    e. ameloblastoma
    e. plasmacytoma
extraparenchymal
extrapineal pinealoma
extraplacental
extrapleural
extrapolation
extraprostatitis
extrapulmonary tuberculosis
extrapyramidal disease
extrarenal
    e. azotemia
    e. rhabdoid tumor (ERRT)
extraserous
extraskeletal
    e. chondroma
    e. myxoid chondrosarcoma (EMC)
    e. osteosarcoma
extratarsal
extrathymic tissue
extrauterine-extraovarian endometrioid
  stromal tumor
extrauterine pregnancy
extravasate
extravasation
    bile e.
    blood e.
    e. cyst
    e. feces
    e. gas
    mucus e.
extravascular (EV)
    e. hemolysis
    e. migratory metastasis mechanism
    e. site
    e. space
extreme
    e. capsule
    e. gastric hypersecretion
extremity
    broomstick e.

extremorientalis
    Pseudomonas e.
extrication
extrinsic
    e. allergic alveolitis (EAA)
    e. asthma
    e. compression
    e. factor
    e. hemolysis
    e. pathway
    e. semiconductor
    e. system
extructa
    Bulleidia e.
extrude
extrusion
exuberant
    e. infection
    e. tumor
exudate
    acute inflammatory e.
    bloody inflammatory e.
    fibrinonecrotic e.
    inflammatory e.
    mucopurulent e.
exudation
    e. cell
    e. corpuscle
    e. cyst
exudative
    e. arthritis
    e. bronchiolitis
    e. effusion
    e. glomerulonephritis
    e. granulomatous inflammation
    e. pleural effusion
exudativum
    erythema multiforme e.
exude
exulcerans
exuvia, pl. **exuviae**
eye
    fibrous tunic of e.
    owl e.
    raccoon's e.
    e. spot
    e. tumor
    e. tumor localization
    vascular layer of choroid coat
      of e.
    white of e.
eyelid
    conjunctival layer of e.
    heliotrope e.
eyepiece
    comparison e.
    compensated e.
    high eyepoint e.
    huygenian e.

Ramsden e.
widefield e.
eyepoint
eyespot

eyewash equipment
eyeworm
EZ-HP *Helicobacter pylori* **test**
ezrin

NOTES

E

F
Fahrenheit
farad
feces
female
force
gilbert (unit of magnetomotive force)
    F agent
    F antigen
    F body
    F distribution
    F donor
    F factor
    F genote
    F pili
    F plasmid
    F thalassemia
F_1
first filial generation
F_2
second filial generation
F^+ cell
FA
fluorescent antibody
    FA technique
FAA protein
FAB
French-American-British
    FAB leukemia classification
    FAB tumor staging
Fab
    F. fragment
    F. piece
Fabavirus
Faber
    F. anemia
    F. syndrome
fabism (*var. of* favism)
Fabry disease
face
    adenoid f.
    cleft f.
    hippocratic f.
    f. of polyhedron (P)
    f. shield
    trans f.
    f. velocity of laboratory hood
facet
    f. joint arthrography
    f. joint injection
    f. syndrome
facial
    f. diprosopus duplication
    f. eczema

    f. hemiatrophy
    f. myiasis
    f. palsy
    f. trophoneurosis
faciale
    granuloma f.
    tinea f.
facies, pl. **facies**
    adenoid f.
    cherubic f.
    cushingoid f.
    elfin f.
    f. hepatica
    hippocratic f.
    hound-dog f.
    hurloid f.
    Hutchinson f.
    leonine f.
    leprechaun f.
    Marshall Hall f.
    Parkinson f.
    Potter f.
    scaphoid f.
facilitated diffusion
facilitation of sympathetic activity
facility
    high-containment BSL4 f.
    medical treatment f. (MTF)
faciodigitogenital dysplasia
facioscapulohumeral-type progressive
    muscular dystrophy
Facklam classification scheme
Facklamia
    F. miroungae
    F. sourekii
    F. tabacinasalis
FAC protein
FACS
fluorescence-activated cell sorter
FACScalibur flow cytometer
FACScan flow cytometer
FACSort flow cytometer
FACStar Plus flow cytometer
FACSVantage flow cytometer
F-actin
    F-a. binding protein
    F-a. ring
factitia
    thyrotoxicosis f.
factitial panniculitis
factitious
    f. dermatitis
    f. melanin
    f. urticaria

F

factor

f. I, II, III, IV, V, VII, VIII,
VIII:C, VIII:R, IX, X, Xa, XI,
XII, XIII, XIIIa
f. A
ABO f.
accelerator f.
acquired genetic f.
activated clotting f.
adipocyte determination and
differentiation f. 1 (ADD1)
adrenocorticotropic hormone-
releasing f. (ACTH-RF)
AHG f.
f. alpha
amplification f.
anabolism-promoting f. (APF)
angiogenesis f.
animal protein f. (APF)
antialopecia f.
antianemic f.
anticomplementary f.
antigen-specific helper f.
antigen-specific suppressor f.
antihemophilic f. (AHF)
antihemophilic f. A, B
antiheparin f.
antinuclear f. (ANF)
antipernicious anemia f. (APA)
atrial natriuretic f.
autocrine growth f.
autocrine motility f. (AMF)
automated motility f.
f. B
bacteriocin f.
basic fibroblast growth f. (bFGF)
basic helix-loop-helix
transcription f. (bHLH)
basophil chemotactic f. (BCF)
B-cell activating f. (BAFF)
B-cell differentiating f.
B-cell differentiation/growth f.
B-cell growth f. I, II
B-cell stimulating f.
Bittner milk f.
blastogenetic f. (BF)
blood coagulation f.
B-lymphocyte stimulatory f. (BSF)
brain-derived neurotrophic f.
(BDNF)
f. V Cambridge
CAMP f.
cAMP response element binding
activation transcription f.
(CREB/ATF)
Castle f.
CDX1 intestine-specific
transcription f.

CDX2 intestine-specific
transcription f.
chemotactic f. (CF)
Christmas f. (CF)
citrovorum f. (CF)
clearing f.
clone-inhibiting f. (CIF)
cloning inhibitory f.
clotting f.
C3 Nef f.
coagulation f. I–XIII
cobra venom f.
colony-stimulating f. (CSF)
complement chemotactic f.
conglutinogen-activating f.
connective tissue growth f.
cord f.
coronary risk f.
correction f.
corticotropin-releasing f. (CRF)
f. VIII-crossed
immunoelectrophoresis
cryoprecipitated antihemophilic f.
crystal-induced chemotactic f.
f. D
decay accelerating f. (DAF)
decay antibody-accelerating f.
f. I, II, V, VII, VIII, IX, X, XI
deficiency
f. deficiency anemia
deficiency of plasma clotting f.
dose-reduction f. (DRF)
Duran-Reynals permeability f.
f. E
edema f. (EF)
elongation f.
encephalitogenic f. (EF)
endothelial relaxing f.
endothelium-derived relaxing f.
(EDRF)
eosinophil chemotactic f.
epidermal growth f. (EGF)
erythrocyte maturation f. (EMF)
erythropoietic-stimulating f. (ESF)
etiologic f.
etiopathogenic f.
exogenous growth f.
exophthalmos-hyperthyroid f. (EHF)
exophthalmos-producing f. (EPF)
extrinsic f.
F f.
Fc f.
fertility f.
fibrin stabilizing f. (FSF)
fibroblast growth f. (FGF)
Fitzgerald f.
Fitzgerald-Williams-Flaujeac f.
Flaujeac f.
Fletcher f.

G f.
f. II gene
glass f.
glial cell line-derived neurotropic f. (GDNF)
glucose tolerance f. (GTF)
gonadotropin-releasing f. (GRF)
granulocyte colony-stimulating f. (G-CSF)
granulocyte-macrophage colony-stimulating f. (GM-CSF)
growth hormone-releasing f. (GH-RF, GRF)
growth inhibitory f.
Hageman f. (HF)
hemophilic f. A
hepatocyte growth f. (HGF)
hepatocyte growth factor/scatter f. (HGF/SF)
histamine-releasing f. (HRF)
homeodomain transcription f.
human antihemophilic f.
humoral thymic f. (THF)
hydrazine-sensitive f.
hyperglycemic-glycogenolytic f. (HGF)
hypoxia inducible f. (HIF)
hypoxia inducible f. 1 (HIF-1)
immunoglobulin-binding f. (IBF)
immunoglobulin M-rheumatoid f. (IgM-RF)
inherited genetic f.
inhibiting f.
inhibition f.
f. inhibitor
initiation f.
insulinlike growth f.
insulinlike growth f.-1 (IGF-1)
intrinsic f. (IF)
labile f.
Lactobacillus bulgaricus f. (LBF)
Laki-Lorand f. (LLF)
LE f.
Leiden f.
f. V Leiden mutation test
lethal f. (LF)
leukemia inhibitory f. (LIF)
leukocyte inhibitory f.
leukocytosis-promoting f. (LPF)
leukopenic f.
ligand-activated transcription f.
L-L f.

load f.
luteinizing hormone-releasing f. (LH-RF)
lymph node permeability f. (LNPF)
lymphocyte-activating f.
lymphocyte blastogenic f.
lymphocyte mitogenic f.
lymphocyte-transforming f.
lymphocytosis-promoting f. (LPF)
macrophage activation f. (MAF)
macrophage agglutination f. (MAggF)
macrophage chemotactic f. (MCF)
macrophage chemotactic and activating f. (MCAF)
macrophage colony stimulating f. (M-CSF)
macrophage-derived growth f.
macrophage growth f.
macrophage inhibiting f. (MIF)
macrophage migration inhibition f.
megakaryocyte growth and development f. (MGDF)
melanocyte-stimulating hormone inhibiting f. (MIF)
melanocyte-stimulating hormone releasing f. (MRF)
microphthalmia-associated transcription f. (MITF)
migration inhibition f. (MIF)
migration-inhibitory f.
milk f.
mitogenic f.
monocyte-derived neutrophil chemotactic f. (MDNCF)
f. III multimer assay
myocardial depressant f. (MDF)
natural killer cell-stimulating f. (NKSF)
necrotizing f.
nephritic f.
nerve growth f. (NGF)
neurohumoral f.
neurotrophic f.
neutrophil activating f. (NAF)
neutrophil chemotactant f.
neutrophil chemotactic f. (NCF)
neutrophilic chemotactic f.
Nod f.
obligate osteogenic transcription f.
orexigenic f.
osteoclast activating f. (OAF)

F

NOTES

factor *(continued)*
  Ovenstone f. (OF)
  Passovoy f.
  peptide regulatory f. (PRF)
  pivotal transcription f.
  plasma atrial natriuretic f.
  plasma clotting f.
  plasma labile f.
  plasma thromboplastin f. (PTF)
  plasma thromboplastin f. B
  plasma f. X
  plasmin prothrombin conversion f.
    (PPCF)
  platelet f. 1–4
  platelet-activating f. (PAF)
  platelet-aggregating f. (PAF)
  platelet-derived growth f. (PDGF)
  platelet tissue f.
  polymorphonuclear neutrophil
    chemotactic f.
  postulated pathogenetic f.
  preadipocyte f. (Pref-1)
  predisposing f.
  prognostic f.
  prolactin-inhibiting f. (PIF)
  prolactin-releasing f. (PRF)
  proliferation inhibitory f. (PIF)
  properdin f. A, B, D, E
  prothrombokinase f.
  Prower f.
  Prower-Stuart f.
  quality f. (QF)
  R f.
  RB1 protein transcription f.
  recognition f.
  recombinant human insulin-like
    growth f. (rhIGF)
  recombinant platelet-derived
    growth f. (rPDGF)
  releasing f. (RF)
  renal erythropoietic f. (REF)
  resistance f.
  resistance inducing f. (RIF)
  resistance transfer f. (RTF)
  Rh f.
  rheumatoid f. (RF)
  rheumatoid arthritis f. (RAF)
  rho f.
  ripple f.
  risk f.
  rough f.
  secretor f.
  serum prothrombin conversion
    accelerator f.
  sex f.
  Simon septic f.
  skin-reactive f. (SRF)
  somatotroph release inhibiting f.
  somatotropin-releasing f. (SRF)

  SPCA f.
  specific macrophage-arming f.
    (SMAF)
  spreading f.
  stable f.
  stem cell f. (SCF)
  stem cell renewal f.
  Stuart f.
  Stuart-Prower f.
  sulfation f.
  T f.
  T-cell growth f. (TGF)
  T-cell replacing f. (TRF)
  termination f.
  testis-determining f. (TDF)
  thymic humoral f.
  thymic lymphopoietic f.
  thymic replacing f.
  thyroid-stimulating hormone-
    releasing f. (TSH-RF)
  thyrotoxic complement-fixation f.
  thyrotropin-releasing f. (TRF)
  tissue f.
  tissue-coding f. (TCF, TSF)
  tissue-damaging f. (TF)
  tissue plasminogen f.
  transcription f.
  transfer f. (TF)
  transforming growth f. X
  translocation f.
  trefoil family f. (TFF)
  tumor angiogenic f. (TAF)
  tumor-cell migration-inhibition f.
    (TMIF)
  tumor necrosis f. (TNF)
  tumor receptor-associated f. (TRAF)
  undegraded insulin f. (UIF)
  upstream binding f.
  uterine-relaxing f. (URF)
  vascular endothelial growth f.
    (VEGF)
  vascular permeability f.
  virulence f.
  von Willebrand f.
  W f.
  Williams f.
  wnt inhibitory f. (WIF)
  f. X for *Haemophilus*
factor-1
  T-cell growth f.-1
  thyroid transcription f.-1 (TTF-1)
factor-2
  T-cell growth f.-2
factorial
facultative
  f. anaerobe
  f. autotroph
  f. bacterium
  f. coccobacillus

f. heterochromatin
f. histiocyte
f. organism
f. parasite

FAD
flavin adenine dinucleotide

FADD
FAS-associated death domain protein

FADD-like interleukin-1 beta converting enzyme (FLICE)

FADF
fluorescent antibody dark-field

faecale
Trichosporon f.

Faecalibacterium prausnitzii

faecalis
Alcaligenes f.
Enterococcus f.
Psychrobacter f.
Rhodopseudomonas f.
Streptococcus f.
Zimmermannella f.

faecium
Enterococcus f.
Streptococcus f.

faeni
Frigoribacterium f.
Micropolyspora f.
Sphingomonas f.

faggot cell
Fahey and McKelvey method
Fahr disease
Fahrenheit (F)
F. thermometer

failure
acute renal f. (ARF)
acute respiratory f. (ARF)
adrenal f.
f. of all vital forces (FOAVF)
anemia associated with chronic renal f.
anemia of chronic renal f.
backward f.
bone marrow f.
cardiac f. (CF)
chronic renal f. (CRF)
chronic respiratory f.
circulatory f.
congestive cardiac f. (CCF)
congestive heart f. (CHF)
forward f.
fulminant hepatic f. (FHF)

heart f. (HF)
high-output cardiac f.
left ventricular f. (LVF)
liver f.
mean time between f.'s
multiple organ system f. (MOSF)
myonecrosis, myoglobinuria, renal f.
ovarian f.
peripheral circulatory f.
pituitary gonadotropic f.
f. rate
renal f.
respiratory f.
right ventricular f.
testicular f.
f. to thrive
ventilatory f.

Fajersztajn crossed sciatic sign
FAK
focal adhesion kinase

falcate
falcatus
Stellantchasmus f.

falciform
falciforme
Cephalosporium f.

falciparum
f. fever
f. malaria
Plasmodium f.

falcular
fallax
Clostridium f.

falling drop procedure
fallonii
Legionella f.

fallopian
f. tube cancer
f. tube tumor

Fallot
F. syndrome
tetralogy of F. (tet, TF)

false
f. abrasion collar
f. agglutination
f. albuminuria
f. anemia
f. aneurysm
f. cast
f. cyanosis
f. cyst
f. dextrocardia

NOTES

F

375

false *(continued)*
f. diphtheria
f. diverticulum
f. hematuria
f. hypertrophy
f. knot (umbilical cord)
f. labor
f. membrane
f. mole
f. negative
f. neuroma
f. positive
false-negative (FN)
f.-n. reaction
false-positive (FP)
biologic f.-p. (BFP)
chronic f.-p. (CFP)
f.-p. reaction
false-resistant
false-susceptible
falx cerebri
FAME
fatty acid methyl ester
familial
f. adenomatous polyposis (FAP)
f. adenomatous polyposis coli
f. benign pemphigus
f. cancer
f. cardiomyopathy
f. cerebellar ataxia
f. clival chordoma
f. cyclic neutropenia
f. cystinuria
f. dysautonomia
f. dysbetalipoproteinemia
f. emphysema
f. enteropathy
f. erythroblastic anemia
f. erythrophagocytic
lymphohistiocytosis (FEL)
f. fibrous dysplasia of jaw
f. gigantiform cementoma (FGC)
f. goiter
f. gonadal dysgenesis
f. hemolytic anemia
f. hemophagocytic
lymphohistiocytosis (FMLH)
f. hypercholesterolemia (FH)
f. hyperlipoproteinemia I, II, IIa,
IIb, III–V
f. hypertriglyceridemia
f. hypocalciuric hypercalcemia
f. hypoceruloplasminemia
f. hypoplastic anemia
f. intestinal polyposis
f. juvenile nephrophthisis (FJN)
f. juvenile polyp (FJP)
f. Mediterranean fever (FMF)
f. mental retardation (FMR)

f. microcytic anemia
f. multiple endocrine
f. multiple endocrine adenomatosis,
type 1, 2
f. myoclonic epilepsy
f. nephritis
f. nephronophthisis
f. nephrosis
f. nonhemolytic jaundice
f. paroxysmal polyserositis
f. paroxysmal rhabdomyolysis
f. periodic paralysis
f. polycythemia
f. polyposis
f. polyposis coli
f. primary systemic amyloidosis
f. pyridoxine-responsive anemia
f. recurrent polyserositis
f. splenic anemia
familial-type symptomatic porphyria
family
cancer f.
human ABC transporter f.
melanoma antigen-encoding gene f.
MyoD gene f.
14-3-3 protein f.
ras gene f.
septin gene f.
FAN
fuchsin, amido black, and naphthol
yellow
fan
macular f.
FANA
fluorescent antinuclear antibody
FANA test
Fañanás
cell of F.
Fanconi
F. anemia
F. pancytopenia
F. syndrome
Fanconi-Zinsser syndrome
fan-in
Fannia
F. canicularis
F. scalaris
fan-out
FAP
familial adenomatous polyposis
farad (F)
Faraday
F. constant
F. effect
F. law of electrolysis
faradic shock
Farber
F. disease
F. lipogranulomatosis

F. syndrome
F. test
Farber-Uzman syndrome
farciminosus
Histoplasma *f.*
farcinica
Nocardia *f.*
farcy
Far East Russian encephalitis
farmer's
f. lung disease
f. skin
Farr
F. law
F. test
farraginis
Bacillus *f.*
Farrant
F. medium
F. mounting fluid
FAS
fatty acid synthase
FAS-associated death domain protein (FADD)
fascia, pl. **fasciae, fascias**
f. adherens
deep f.
Denonvilliers f.
Gerota f.
Monakow f.
paraconal f.
perirenal f.
renal f.
f. renalis
fascial fibrosarcoma
fasciatus
Nosopsyllus *f.*
Pulex *f.*
fascicle
herringbone f.
muscle f.
nerve f.
fascicular
f. pattern
f. sarcoma
fasciculata
f. cell
zona f.
fasciculate bladder
fasciculation
fasciculus, pl. **fasciculi**
f. atrioventricularis

Bürdach cuneate f.
f. gracilis
fasciitis, fascitis
eosinophilic f.
infiltrative f.
necrotizing f.
nodular f.
parosteal f.
proliferative f.
pseudosarcomatous f.
fascin
Fasciola
F. gigantica
F. hepatica
fasciolaris
Cysticercus *f.*
fascioliasis
fasciolid
Fascioloides magna
fasciolopsiasis
Fasciolopsis
F. buski
F. rathouisi
fascitis (*var. of* fasciitis)
Fas-Fas ligand protein
Fas ligand
FAST
fluorescent allergosorbent test
fast
f. action potential
f. green
f. green FCF stain
f. hemoglobin
low-voltage f. (LVF)
f. smear
f. therapeutic turnaround time of results
f. turnaround time
f. x-scanning
f. yellow
fasted state
fastidiosa
Amycolatopsis *f.*
Desulfofaba *f.*
fastidious bacterium
fastigium
fasting
f. blood sugar (FBS)
f. plasma glucose (FPG)
fastness
fastosum
Platynosomum *f.*

F

NOTES

FastPack blood analyzer system
FAT
fluorescent antibody test
fat
f. absorption
f. absorption study
f. absorption test
f. assay
brown f.
f. cell
f. depot
f. droplet
f. embolism
f. embolism syndrome
f. embolus
emulsify f.
f. free
multilocular f.
f. necrosis
f. necrosis of pancreas
redistribution of body f.
f. staining
f. in stool
subcutaneous f.
f. tide
total body f. (TBF)
unilocular f.
white f.
yellow f.
fatal
f. dose (FD)
f. granulomatous disease (FGD)
fat-deficiency disease
fat-free
f.-f. dry weight (FFDW)
f.-f. mass (FFM)
f.-f. wet weight (FFWW)
fat-induced hyperlipidemia
fat-mobilizing
f.-m. hormone
f.-m. substance (FMS)
fat-pad
Imlach f.-p.
fat-storing cell
fatty
f. acid
f. acid assay
f. acid beta oxidation enzyme
f. acid methyl ester (FAME)
f. acid oxidation
f. acid oxidation disorder (FOD)
f. acid profile
f. acid synthase (FAS)
f. acid synthesis
f. ascites
f. atrophy
f. change
f. cirrhosis
f. degeneration

f. deposition
f. heart
f. infiltration
f. intraosseous tissue
f. kidney
f. liver
f. metamorphosis
f. oil
f. phanerosis
f. urinary cast
fauces
Fauchard disease
faucial tonsil
faucitis
faucium
Mycoplasma f.
faulty union
faun tail nevus
FAV
feline ataxia virus
faveolate
faveolus
favic chandelier
favid
favism, fabism
favisporus
Paenibacillus f.
favosa
porrigo f.
tinea f.
trichomycosis f.
Favre-Racouchot disease
favus
FB
foreign body
FBE
full blood examination
F-box protein
FBP
fibrinogen breakdown product
FBS
fasting blood sugar
fetal bovine serum
FC
flow cytometry
Fc
Fc fragment
Fc piece
Fc receptor
FCA
ferritin-conjugated antibody
FCC
follicular center cell
FCCP
carbonyl cyanide p-
(trifluoromethoxy)phenylhydrazone
trifluorocarbonylcyanide
phenylhydrazone
protonophore FCCP

FCF
  fast green FCF stain
FCL
  follicle center lymphoma
    FCL cell
FCM
  flow cytometry
FCS
  fluorescence correlation spectroscopy
FD
  fatal dose
FD$_{50}$
  median fatal dose
FDC
  follicular dendritic cell
FDNB
  fluoro-2,4-dinitrobenzene
FDP
  fibrin degradation product
  fibrin/fibrinogen degradation product
  fibrinogen degradation product
F-duction
Fe
  iron
feathery degeneration
feature
  chordoid f.'s
  clinical manifestations, etiologic
    factors, anatomic involvement,
    pathophysiologic f.'s (CEAP)
  fibroblastic-myofibroblastic f.
  general f.
  morphologic f.
  organotypic f.
febricitans
  pes f.
febrile
  f. agglutination
  f. agglutination test
  f. agglutinin
  f. albuminuria
  f. nonhemolytic transfusion reaction
    (FNHTR)
  f. urine
febrilis
  calor f.
  herpes f.
FEC
  free erythrocyte coproporphyrin
fecal
  f. abscess
  f. antigen

  f. carbohydrate
  f. chloride
  f. chymotrypsin
  f. color
  f. concentration
  f. consistency
  f. electrolytes
  f. examination
  f. fat
  f. fat stain
  f. fat test
  f. fistula
  f. impaction
  f. incontinence
  f. leukocyte
  f. leukocyte count
  f. lipids
  f. marker
  f. mucus
  f. muscle fiber
  f. nitrogen
  f. occult blood test (FOBT)
  f. osmolality
  f. pH
  f. porphyrin
  f. porphyrin analysis
  f. potassium
  f. reducing substances test
  f. sodium
  f. trypsin
  f. tumor
  f. urobilinogen (FU)
  f. vomitus
fecalith
fecaloma
fecal-oral transmission
feces (F)
  bloody f.
  chemical examination of f.
  extravasation f.
  impacted f.
  leukocytes in f.
Fechner tumor
Fechtner syndrome
FED
  forward fluorescence detector
Fede disease
feedback
  f. inhibition mutation
  f. loop
feed forward loop

F

NOTES

feeleii
> *Legionella f.*

Feer disease

feet (*pl. of* foot)

FEF
> forced expiratory flow

Fehleisen streptococcus

Fehling
> F. solution
> F. test

FEL
> familial erythrophagocytic
> lymphohistiocytosis

Felicola subrostratus

feline
> f. agranulocytosis
> f. ataxia virus (FAV)
> f. distemper
> f. infectious enteritis
> f. infectious peritonitis
> f. leukemia
> f. leukemia-sarcoma virus complex
> f. leukemia virus (FeLV)
> f. panleukopenia virus
> f. rhinotracheitis virus
> f. viral rhinotracheitis

felineum
> *Microsporum f.*

felineus
> *Opisthorchis f.*

felinum
> *Corynebacterium f.*

felis
> *Afipia f.*
> *Chlamydophila f.*
> *Haemophilus f.*
> *Isospora f.*
> *Rickettsia f.*

Felix-Weil reaction (FWR)

felleae
> tunica mucosa vesicae f.
> tunica muscularis vesicae f.
> tunica serosa vesicae f.

Fellomyces

Felton phenomenon

feltwork
> Kaes f.

Felty syndrome

FeLV
> feline leukemia virus

female (F)
> f. carrier
> f. castration
> f. genital tract (FGT)
> f. genital tract carcinosarcoma
> (FGTCS)
> f. hormone
> f. pseudohermaphrodite
> f. pseudohermaphroditism

> f. sex chromatin pattern
> XY f.

femininae
> glandulae urethrales f.
> tunica mucosa urethrae f.
> tunica muscularis urethrae f.

feminization
> f. syndrome, adrenal
> testicular f.

feminizing tumor

femoral
> f. hernia
> f. puncture

femorocele

femoropopliteal occlusive disease

femtoliter (fL)

femtometer (fm)

femtomole (fmol)

femur
> proximal f.

FENa
> fractional excretion of sodium

fenac

fenestra, pl. fenestrae
> alveolar f.
> f. cochleae
> hepatic f.
> f. ovalis
> f. rotunda
> f. of the vestibule
> f. vestibuli

fenestrata
> placenta f.

fenestrated
> f. capillary
> f. capillary showing
> f. endothelium
> f. membrane
> f. placenta

fenestration
> atrophic f.

Fennellia

fennelliae
> *Campylobacter f.*
> *Helicobacter f.*

Fennellomyces

fenofibrate

fentanyl

fenthion insecticide

Fenton reaction

Fenwick disease

Fenwick-Hunner ulcer

FEP, FEPP
> free erythrocyte protoporphyrin

F-EPE
> focal extraprostatic extension

fergusonii
> *Escherichia f.*

ferintoshensis
    Lactobacillus f.
ferment
fermentans
    Acidaminococcus f.
    Dyadobacter f.
    Geothrix f.
    Halanaerobium f.
    Mycoplasma f.
fermentation
    mannitol f.
    mixed acid f.
    salicin f.
    f. test
    f. tube
Fermentotrichon
fermentum
    Amphibacillus f.
    Lactobacillus f.
fermium (Fm)
Fernandez reaction
Fernbach flask
ferning
fern test
ferox
    Dinobdella f.
    prurigo f.
Ferrata cell
ferredoxin
Ferrein
    F. pyramid
    F. tube
    F. vasa aberrantia
ferreini
    processus f.
Ferribacterium limneticum
ferric
    f. ammonium sulfate stain
    f. chloride, perchloric acid, nitric acid (FPN)
    f. chloride reaction of epinephrine
    f. chloride test
    f. ferricyanide reduction test
    f. ferrocyanide
    f. iron
    f. oxide
ferricyanide
    ferrous f.
    potassium f.
ferrihemoglobin
ferrimagnetic
Ferrimonadaceae

ferriorganovorum
    Thermovenabulum f.
ferriphilum
    Leptospirillum f.
ferriprotoporphyrin (FPP)
ferrireducens
    Geovibrio f.
    Rhodoferax f.
ferrite
ferritin assay
ferritin-conjugated antibody (FCA)
ferritin-coupled antibody
Ferrobacteria
ferrocalcinosis
ferrochelatase deficiency
ferrocyanide
    ferric f.
ferroflocculation
ferrokinetics study
ferrooxidans
    Acidithiobacillus f.
    Leptospirillum f.
ferrophilus
    Palaeococcus f.
Ferroplasma acidiphilum
Ferroplasmaceae
ferrous
    f. citrate Fe 59
    f. ferricyanide
    f. iron
ferroxidase
ferrugination
ferruginea
    Asanoa f.
ferrugineum
    Microsporum f.
ferrugineus
    Pseudorhodobacter f.
ferruginosa
    Tubifera f.
ferruginous
    f. body
    f. micelles
fertile eunuch syndrome
fertility
    f. agent
    f. factor
    f. inhibition
fertilization
    effect of f.
fertilizer truck bomb

F

NOTES

FertilMARQ
    F. fertility screening test
    F. male fertility screening test kit
fervens
    calor f.
Fervidobacterium pennivorans
FES
    flame emission spectroscopy
    forced expiratory spirogram
fester
festoon
festooning
festucae
    Rathayibacter f.
FET
    forced expiratory time
fetal
    f. abnormality
    f. activity-acceleration determination
    f. adenocarcinoma
    f. adenoma
    f. adrenal cortex
    f. adrenal insufficiency
    f. alcohol syndrome
    f. antigen
    f. antigen test
    f. biophysical profile
    f. bovine serum (FBS)
    f. cotyledon
    f. death
    f. distress
    f. duplication
    f. erythroblastosis
    f. face syndrome
    f. fat cell lipoma
    f. fibronectin (FFN, fFN)
    f. hemoglobin (HbF)
    f. hemoglobin test
    f. hydantoin syndrome
    f. karyotyping in mid-trimester
      IUFD
    f. life
    f. lobulation
    f. lung maturity (FLM)
    f. neuron
    f. nuchal translucency
    f. oxygen saturation monitoring
    f. prematurity
    f. repertoire gradient
    f. reticularis
    f. stem artery thrombosis
    f. trimethadione syndrome
    f. vaccinia
    f. zone
fetalis
    Alishewanella f.
    chondromalacia f.
    erythroblastosis f.
    Hb Bart hydrops f.

    hydrops f.
    ichthyosis f.
    keratosis diffusa f.
    rachitis f.
fetalization
fetal-maternal erythrocyte distribution
FETI
    fluorescence excitation transfer
      immunoassay
fetid rhinitis
fetoglobulin
    alpha-1 f.
fetomaternal
    f. hemorrhage
    f. incompatibility
    f. molecular exchange
fetoplacental anasarca
fetoprotein
    alpha f. (AFP)
    alpha-1 f.
    beta fetoprotein
    gamma f.
    maternal serum alpha f. (MSAFP)
fetoscopic laser coagulation of vascular
    connection
fetoscopy
fetotoxicity
FETS
    forced expiratory time in seconds
fetus, pl. **fetuses**
    f. acardiacus
    f. amorphus
    Campylobacter fetus subsp. *f.*
    f. compressus
    f. in fetu
    harlequin f.
    hydropic f.
    macerated f.
    minimum dose causing death or
      malformation of 100% of fetuses
      (T/LD$_{100}$)
    f. papyraceus
    parasitic f.
    f. sanguinolentis
    stunted f.
Feuerstein-Mims syndrome
Feulgen
    F. cytometry
    F. reaction
    F. stain
    F. test
FEV-1
    forced expiratory volume at 1 second
fever
    abortus f.
    acute rheumatic f. (ARF)
    Aden f.
    aestivoautumnal f.
    African hemorrhagic f.

African swine f.
African tick-borne f.
aphthous f.
Argentinean hemorrhagic f.
blackwater f.
f. blister
Bolivian hemorrhagic f.
bouquet f.
boutonneuse f.
bovine ephemeral f.
breakbone f.
Bullis f.
Bunyamwera f.
Bwamba f.
camp f.
cat-bite f.
f. caused by infection (FI)
cave f.
Central European tick-borne f.
cerebrospinal f.
chikungunya hemorrhagic f.
childbed f.
classical swine f.
Colorado tick f.
continued f.
Crimean-Congo hemorrhagic f.
dandy f.
date f.
death f.
dengue hemorrhagic f.
desert f.
diphasic milk f.
Dumdum f.
Dutton relapsing f.
Ebola hemorrhagic f.
eczema, asthma, hay f. (EAHF)
ephemeral f. of cattle
epidemic hemorrhagic f.
epimastical f.
eruptive f.
essential f.
exanthematous f.
falciparum f.
familial Mediterranean f. (FMF)
Flinders Island spotted f.
flood f.
food f.
Fort Bragg f.
glandular f.
Haverhill f.
hay f.
hematuric bilious f.

hemoglobinuric f.
hemorrhagic f. (HF)
herpetic f.
hospital f.
Ilhéus f.
intermittent malarial f.
inundation f.
island f.
jail f.
Japanese river f.
jungle yellow f.
Katayama f.
kedani f.
Kenya tick f.
Korean hemorrhagic f.
Lassa hemorrhagic f.
laurel f.
louse-borne relapsing f.
malarial f.
malignant tertian f.
Malta f.
Manchurian hemorrhagic f.
Marseilles f.
marsh f.
Mediterranean f.
metal fume f.
miliary f.
miniature scarlet f.
monoleptic f.
mud f.
Omsk hemorrhagic f.
O'nyong-nyong f.
Oroya f.
paludal f.
pappataci f.
paratyphoid f., types A, B, C
parrot f.
Pel-Ebstein f.
pharyngoconjunctival f.
phlebotomus f.
polka f.
polyleptic f.
Pontiac f.
protein f.
puerperal f.
Pym f.
pyogenic f.
Q f.
quartan f.
Queensland tick f.
quotidian f.
rat-bite f.

NOTES

F

383

fever *(continued)*
    recrudescent typhus f.
    relapsing f.
    remittent malarial f.
    rheumatic f. (RF)
    Rift Valley f.
    Rocky Mountain spotted f. (RMSF)
    Ross River f.
    sandfly f.
    San Joaquin Valley f.
    scarlet f. (SF)
    septic f.
    sequela of rheumatic f.
    ship f.
    Siberian tick f.
    Sindbis f.
    slow f.
    solar f.
    spotted f.
    steroid f.
    swamp f.
    swine f.
    symptomatic f.
    syphilitic f.
    tertian f.
    three-day f.
    tick f.
    traumatic f.
    trench f.
    tsutsugamushi f.
    typhoid f.
    f. of undetermined origin (FUO)
    undifferentiated type f.
    undulant f.
    f. of unknown origin (FUO)
    uveoparotid f.
    valley f.
    viral hemorrhagic f. (VHF)
    vivax f.
    Wesselsbron f.
    West African f.
    West Nile f.
    Whitmore f.
    Wolhynia f.
    wound f.
    yellow f.
    Zika f.
feverish urine
FFA
    free fatty acid
FFDW
    fat-free dry weight
FFF
    Fuzzy Functional Form
      FFF technology
FFL
    floral variant of follicular lymphoma
FFM
    fat-free mass

FFN, fFN
    fetal fibronectin
      FFN test
FFP
    fresh frozen plasma
FFPE
    formalin-fixed paraffin-embedded
FFWW
    fat-free wet weight
FGC
    familial gigantiform cementoma
FGD
    fatal granulomatous disease
FGF
    fibroblast growth factor
FGT
    female genital tract
      FGT cytologic smear
FGTCS
    female genital tract carcinosarcoma
FH
    familial hypercholesterolemia
    follicular hyperplasia
FH$_4$
    N_5-formyl F.
FHF
    fulminant hepatic failure
FHIT
    fragile histidine triad
      FHIT gene
      FHIT protein
FI
    fever caused by infection
FIA
    fluorescent immunoassay
fiber
    A f.
    amianthoid collagen f.'s
    anastomosing f.
    argyrophilic f.
    astral f.
    Bergmann f.
    binucleate f.
    branching cardiac f.
    Burdach f.
    chromatic f.
    circular f.
    climbing f.
    collagen f.
    collagenous f.
    cone f.
    connective tissue f.
    delta f.
    f. density
    dentinal f.
    elastic f.
    enamel f.
    extrafusal muscle f.
    fecal muscle f.

f. FISH analysis
gamma f.
gray f.
intrafusal f.
Korff f.
f. of lens
Mahaim f.
meat f.
medullated nerve f.
mossy f.
Müller f.
myelinated nerve f.
nerve f.
nonmedullated f.
nuclear bag f.
nuclear chain f.
nucleus of muscle f.
osteocollagenous f.
osteogenetic f.
oxytalan f.
perforating f.
periodontal ligament f.
pilomotor f.
precollagenous f.
Prussak f.
Purkinje f.
red f.
Remak f.
reticular f.
reticulin f.
Retzius f.
rod f.
Rosenthal f.
Sharpey f.
skeinoid f.
skeletal muscle f.
sling f.
f. spectrum
spindle f.
stool muscle f.
stress f.
striatonigral f.
sudomotor f.
target f.
tautomeric f.
thin elastic f.
Tomes f.
transseptal f.
U f.
unmyelinated f.
white f.

yellow f.
zonular f.
fiber-FISH
    fiber fluorescence in situ
      hybridization
fiberoptic
fibra, pl. **fibrae**
    fibrae circulares
    fibrae lentis
    fibrae meridionales muscularis
     ciliaris
    fibrae obliquae tunicae muscularis
    fibrae zonulares
fibremia
Fibricola seoulensis
fibril
    Alzheimer f.
    amyloid f.
    anchoring f.
    beta-amyloid f.
    collagen f.
    fibronectin f.
    muscular f.
fibrilla, pl. **fibrillae**
fibrillar
    f. astrocyte
    f. basket
fibrillary
    f. astrocyte
    f. astrocytoma
    f. gliosis
    f. glomerulonephritis
    f. neuroma
fibrillate
fibrillated
Fibrillenstruktur
fibrillin gene
fibrillogenesis
fibrin
    f. body
    f. breakdown product
    f. calculus
    f. cap
    f. clot retraction assay
    f. degradation product (FDP)
    f. degradation product method
    f. deposition
    Fraser-Lendrum stain for f.
    f. glue
    f. histochemical stain
    intervillous f.
    lighter layer of f.

NOTES

F

fibrin *(continued)*
    f. matrix
    f. monomer
    Nitabuch f.
    perivillous f.
    f. plate lysis
    reptilase f.
    f. stabilizing factor (FSF)
    f. stabilizing factor test
    f. staining
    f., subchorionic
    subchorionic f.
    f. thrombus
    f. titer
    f. titer test
    Weigert stain for f.
fibrinase
fibrin/fibrinogen degradation product (FDP)
fibrin-like proteinaceous material
fibrinocellular
fibrinogen
    f. assay
    f. breakdown product (FBP)
    f. bridge
    cryoprecipitated f.
    f. deficiency
    f. degradation product (FDP)
    functional intact f. (FiF)
    f. I-125
    f. method
    f. split product (FSP)
    f. titer test
fibrinogenase
fibrinogenemia
fibrinogen-fibrin conversion syndrome
fibrinogenic
fibrinogenolysis
fibrinogenopenia
fibrinogenous
fibrinohemorrhagic peritonitis
fibrinoid
    f. degeneration
    f. necrosis
    f. necrotizing inflammation
fibrinokinase
fibrinolysin
    f. coagulation
    seminal f.
    streptococcal f.
fibrinolysis
    primary f.
fibrinolysokinase
fibrinolytic
    f. disorder
    f. protein
    f. purpura
    f. split product (FSP)

    f. system
    f. therapy
fibrinonecrotic exudate
fibrinopenia
fibrinopeptide
    fibrinopeptide A, B
    f. test
fibrinopurulent inflammation
fibrinous
    f. acute lobar pneumonia
    f. acute pleuritis
    f. adhesion
    f. bronchitis
    f. cast
    f. degeneration
    f. exudation
    f. inflammation
    f. lymph
    f. pericarditis
    f. peritonitis
    f. pleurisy
    f. polyp
    f. pseudomembrane
fibrin-split product
fibrinuria
fibrivorans
    Cellvibrio f.
fibroadenoma
    f. of breast
    giant f.
    intracanalicular f.
    juvenile f.
    pericanalicular f.
fibroadenosis
fibroadipose tissue
fibroameloblastic
    f. dentinoma
    f. odontoma
fibroareolar
fibroblast
    chick embryo f. (CEF)
    f. culture
    endoneurial f.
    f. and fibrocyte
    f. growth factor (FGF)
    f. interferon
    pericryptal f.
    proliferation of f.
    radiation f.
fibroblastic
    f. lesion
    f. meningioma
fibroblastic-myofibroblastic feature
fibroblastoma
    desmoplastic f.
    giant cell f. (GCF)
    perineural f.
fibrocalcific nodule
fibrocarcinoma

fibrocartilage
> degenerated intervertebral f.
> f. matrix alteration

fibrocartilaginous

fibrocartilago

fibrocaseous
> f. inflammation
> f. peritonitis

fibrocellular

fibrochondritis

fibrochondroma

fibrocollagenous stroma

fibrocongestive
> f. hypertrophy
> f. splenomegaly

fibrocontractive disease

fibrocyst

fibrocystic
> f. condition of breast
> f. disease
> f. disease of breast
> f. disease of pancreas
> f. mastitis
> f. mastopathy

fibrocystoma

fibrocyte
> f. in endomysium
> fibroblast and f.

fibrodysplasia ossificans progressiva

fibroelastic

fibroelastogenesis

fibroelastosis
> endocardial f. (EFE)
> endomyocardial f.
> intimal f.

fibroenchondroma

fibroepithelial
> f. papilloma
> f. polyp

fibroepithelioma

fibrofatty plaque

fibrofolliculoma

fibrogenesis imperfecta ossium

fibrogliosis

fibrohistiocytic lesion

fibrohistiocytoma

fibrohyaline tissue

fibrohyalinosis

fibroid
> f. adenoma
> f. inflammation

> f. tumor
> f. uterus

fibroin

fibroinflammatory lesion

fibrointimal thickening

fibrokeratoma
> acquired f.
> digital f.

fibrolamellar liver cell carcinoma

fibroleiomyoma

fibrolipoma

fibroliposarcoma

fibroma
> ameloblastic f.
> aponeurotic f.
> cementifying f.
> cementoossifying f. (COF)
> chondromyxoid f. (CMF)
> collagenous f.
> concentric f.
> desmoplastic f.
> extranuchal nuchal f.
> garlic-clove f.
> giant cell f.
> irritation f.
> juvenile ossifying f.
> localized f.
> f. molle
> f. molle gravidarum
> myxoid f.
> f. myxomatodes
> nonossifying f.
> nuchal f.
> odontogenic f.
> ossifying f.
> periosteal f.
> peripheral odontogenic f.
> periungual f.
> pleomorphic f.
> pleural f.
> rabbit f.
> senile f.
> Shope f.
> telangiectatic f.

fibromatoid

fibromatosis
> abdominal f.
> aggressive infantile f.
> f. colli
> congenital generalized f.
> desmoid f.
> desmoid-type f. (DTF)

F

NOTES

387

fibromatosis *(continued)*
    Dupuytren f.
    extraabdominal f.
    inclusion body f.
    infantile digital f.
    juvenile hyalin f.
    juvenile palmoplantar f.
    mesenteric f.
    musculoaponeurotic f.
    nodular palmar f.
    palmar f.
    penile f.
    plantar fascia f.
    retroperitoneal f.
fibromatous
fibromembranous
fibrometer
fibromuscular
    f. dysplasia
    f. hyperplasia
fibromyalgia
fibromyoma
fibromyositis
fibromyxoid sarcoma
fibromyxolipoma
fibromyxoma
fibromyxosarcoma
fibronectin
    cellular f.
    fetal f. (FFN, fFN)
    f. fibril
    plasma f.
    tissue f.
fibroneuroma
fibronexus junction
fibroodontoma
    ameloblastic f.
fibroosseous lesion
fibroosteoma
fibropapilloma
fibroplasia
    retrolental f. (RLF)
fibroplastic
fibroplastica
    gastritis f.
fibroplate
fibropolypus
fibroreticularis
    lamina f.
fibroreticulate
fibrosa
    localized osteitis f.
    multifocal osteitis f.
    myositis f.
    osteitis f.
    periosteitis f.
    tunica f.
fibrosarcoma (FS)
    ameloblastic f.

    congenital f. (CFS)
    congenital infantile f. (CIF)
    Earle L f.
    fascial f.
    infantile f.
    inflammatory f.
    medullary f.
    odontogenic f.
    periosteal f.
    sclerosing epithelioid f.
fibrosarcomatous variant of dermatofibrosarcoma protuberans (FS-DFSP)
fibrosclerosing lesion
fibrose
fibroserous
fibrosiderotic nodule
fibrosing
    f. adenomatosis
    f. adenosis
    f. alveolitis
fibrosis
    blood vessel f.
    bridging f.
    centrilobular f.
    condensation f.
    congenital hepatic f.
    cystic f. (CF)
    diffuse interstitial f.
    endomyocardial f. (EMF)
    eosinophilic angiocentric f. (EAF)
    focal f.
    hepatic f.
    honeycomb f.
    idiopathic endomyocardial f.
    idiopathic pulmonary f. (IPF)
    idiopathic retroperitoneal f. (IRF)
    inflammation with f.
    interstitial pulmonary f.
    islet cell focal f.
    leptomeningeal f.
    marrow f.
    mediastinal f.
    multifocal f.
    nodular subepidermal f.
    pancreatic f.
    pericellular f.
    pericentral f.
    perimuscular f.
    periportal f.
    pipestem f.
    pleural f.
    portal f.
    postinflammatory pulmonary f.
    progressive massive f. (PMF)
    pulmonary f.
    replacement f.
    retroperitoneal f.
    striped form of interstitial f.

subadventitial f.
subepidermal f.
subsinusoidal f.
Symmers clay pipestem f.
fibrositis
FIBROSpec test
fibrosum
adenoma f.
lipoma f.
molluscum f.
myxoma f.
pericardium f.
fibrosus
anulus f.
fibrothecoma
fibrothorax
fibrotic
fibrous
f. adhesion
f. ankylosis
f. articular capsule
f. astrocyte
f. astrocytoma
f. bacterial virus
f. body
f. cavernitis
f. cortical defect
f. degeneration
f. dysplasia of bone
f. dysplasia of jaw
f. dysplasia protuberans
f. familial dysplasia
f. goiter
f. hamartoma of infancy
f. histiocytoma
f. hypertrophic pachymeningitis
f. layer
f. long-spacing collagen (FLS)
f. membrane of joint capsule
f. mesothelioma
f. monostotic dysplasia
f. nodule
f. obliteration
f. osteoma
f. plug
f. polyp
f. protein
f. pseudotumor
f. repair
f. replacement
f. spindle cell lipoma
f. streak

f. tendon sheath
f. thyroiditis
f. tissue (FT)
f. tubercle
f. tunic of corpus spongiosum
f. tunic of eye
f. union
f. xanthoma
fibrovascular septum
fibroxanthoma
atypical f. (AFX)
ficin
Fick
F. bacillus
F. law
F. principle
Ficoll-Hypaque technique
Ficoll-Paque purified cell
ficulneum
Leuconostoc f.
FID
flame ionization detector
fidelis
Shewanella f.
Fiedler
F. disease
F. myocarditis
field
Cohnheim f.
depth of f.
f. effect transistor
high-power f. (HPF)
low-power f. (LPF)
magnetic f.
f. method
f. of microscope
microscopic f.
oil immersion f. (OIF)
F. rapid stain
red blood cells per high-power f. (RBC/hpf)
spiral visual f.
tubular visual f.
f. of view
f. vole
white blood cells per high-power f. (WBC/hpf)
fieldingi
Cooperia f.
Fielding membrane
Fiessinger-Leroy-Reiter syndrome

F

NOTES

FIF
> forced inspiratory flow

FiF
> functional intact fibrinogen
>> FiF assay
>> FiF test

fifth
> f. disease
> f. disease virus

FIGLU
> formiminoglutamic acid
>> FIGLU excretion test

FIGO
> International Federation of Gynecology
> and Obstetrics
>> FIGO adenocarcinoma of
>> endometrium
>> FIGO classification of tumor
>> staging

Figueira syndrome

figurata
> keratosis rubra f.

figurate erythema

figure
> f. description
> epithelium with mitotic f.
> flame f.
> mitotic f.
> myelin f. (MF)

fig wart

Fijivirus

filaceous

filaggrin

filaggrin-like immunoreactivity

filamen

filament
> actin f.
> algal f.
> Ammon f.
> axial f.
> cytokeratin f.
> cytoskeletal f.
> filopodia-like f.
> glial f.
> intermediate f. (IF)
> keratin f.
> myosin f.
> f. polymorphonuclear
> f. polymorphonuclear leukocyte
> spermatic f.
> thick f.
> thin f.
> Z f.

filamenta (*pl. of* filamentum)

filamented neutrophil

filament-nonfilament count

filamentosum
> *Eubacterium* f.

filamentous
> f. bacterial virus
> f. bacteriophage

filamentum, pl. filamenta
> *Prototheca filamenta*

filar
> f. mass
> f. micrometer
> f. substance

Filaria
> *F. bancrofti*
> *F. conjunctivae*
> *F. demarquayi*
> *F. hominis oris*
> *F. juncea*
> *F. labialis*
> *F. lentis*
> *F. loa*
> *F. lymphatica*
> *F. medinensis*
> *F. ozzardi*
> *F. palpebralis*
> *F. philippinensis*
> *F. sanguinis*
> *F. tucumana*
> *F. volvulus*

filaria, pl. filariae
> Ozzard f.
> persistent f.

filarial
> f. arthritis
> f. chylothorax
> f. funiculitis

filariasis
> Bancroft f.
> lymphatic f.
> Malayan f.
> onchocerciasis-type f.
> f. peripheral blood preparation
> f. serological test

filaricidal

filaricide

filariform

Filarioidea

Filaroides hirthi

Filatov, Filatow
> F. disease

file
> Indian f.
> master f.
> Rare Donor F.

filensin

Filifactor alocis

filiform
> f. growth pattern
> f. hyperkeratosis
> f. papillae
> f. process
> f. wart

filiformes
  papillae f.
filiformis
  verruca f.
filigree pattern
filipin fluorometry
filling defect
film
  blood f.
  f. density calibration
  fixed blood f.
  gelatin f.
  spot f.
  sulfa f.
  X-Omat AR f.
Filobacillus milosensis
Filobasidiella
  F. bacillisporus
  F. neoformans
Filobasidium
Filomicrobium fusiforme
filopodia-like filament
filopodium
filovaricosis
Filoviridae
Filovirus
filovirus
filter
  autoadhesive cellulose nitrate f.
  bacterial f.
  barrier f.
  Berkefeld f.
  Bird Nest f.
  f. bleeding time
  blocking f.
  blood f.
  f. capacitor
  Centriflo f.
  Chamberland f.
  collodion f.
  exciter f.
  gelatin f.
  Gelman f.
  glass fiber f.
  HEPA f.
  high-pass f.
  Hybond N f.
  f. hybridization
  inherent f.
  interference f.
  line f.
  low-pass f.

  membrane f.
  microaggregate f.
  Millex-GS plasma f.
  Millipore f.
  Nalgene capsule f.
  Nuclepore f.
  f. paper
  f. paper chromatography
  f. paper microscopic (FPM)
  f. paper microscopic test
  f. photometer
  polyether sulfone f.'s
  Seitz f.
  Selas f.
  Tetko nylon mesh f.
  Wratten f.
filterable, filtrable
  f. virus
filtering
filtertip
  Eppendorf f.
filtrable (*var. of* filterable)
FiltraCheck-UTI
  F.-U. colorimetric filtration system
  F.-U. disposable colorimetric
    bacteriuria detection system
  F.-U. test
filtrate
  bouillon f. (bf)
  glomerular f.
  tuberculin f. (TF)
filtration
  cascade f.
  gel f.
  glomerular f.
  lymph f.
  Millipore f.
  f. slit
  f. space
filum terminale
fimbria, pl. **fimbriae**
  fimbriae tubae uterinae
  fimbriae of uterine tube
fimbriate
fimbriated
finding
  pathologic f.
  in situ f.
FineFix
Finegoldia magna
finegoldii
  Alistipes f.

NOTES

F

finely stippled chromatin pattern
fine-needle
> f.-n. aspiration (FNA)
> f.-n. aspiration biopsy (FNAB)
> f.-n. aspiration cytology (FNAC)
> f.-n. cytopuncture

fine structure
finger
> clubbed f.
> dead f.
> drumstick f.
> hippocratic f.
> mallet f.
> promyelocytic leukemia zinc f. (PLZF)
> rudimentary f.
> sausage f.
> spade f.
> waxy f.
> webbed f.

fingerprint
> f. deposit
> DNA f.
> genetic f.
> high-resolution f. (HRF)
> f. pattern

fingerprinting
> DNA f.
> plasmid f.

finite element modeling
Fink-Heimer stain
Finn chamber patch test
FiO$_2$
> fractional concentration of inspired oxygen

fire
> range of f.
> Saint Anthony's f.

Firmicutes
firmware
first
> f. arch syndrome
> F. Check Ecstasy test kit
> F. Check home-screening test
> f. filial generation (F$_1$)
> f. morning urine specimen
> f. responder

first-degree
> f.-d. burn
> f.-d. frostbite
> f.-d. heart block
> f.-d. radiation injury

first-order
> f.-o. elimination
> f.-o. kinetics
> f.-o. reaction

first-pass metabolism
first-set graft rejection

Fischer
> F. burner
> F. exact test
> F. projection

fischeri
> *Neosartorya f.*
> *Trichophyton f.*

FISH
> fluorescence in situ hybridization
> double-fusion FISH (D-FISH)
> extra signal FISH (ES-FISH)
> multicolored FISH

fish
> f. gelatin
> f. skin
> f. tapeworm
> f. tapeworm anemia

Fishberg concentration test
Fisher
> F. exact test
> F. Scientific Histo-freeze 2000 freezing spray
> F. syndrome

fisherii
> *Aspergillus f.*

Fisher-Race nomenclature
Fishman-Lerner unit
fish-slime disease
fission
> binary f.
> f. fungus
> f. product
> uncontrolled f.

fissiparity
fissiparous
fissura, pl. **fissurae**
> fissurae cerebelli

fissural cyst
fissure
> Ammon f.
> anal f.
> f. in ano
> anterior median f.
> Bichat f.
> Bürdach f.
> cerebellar f.
> Henle f.
> Rolando f.
> Santorini f.

fissured nucleus
fist.
> fistula

fistula, pl. **fistulae**, **fistulas** (**fist.**)
> abdominal f.
> amphibolic f.
> amphibolous f.
> anal f.
> f. in ano
> arteriovenous f. (AVF)

biliary f.
f. bimucosa
blind f.
branchial f.
bronchoesophageal f.
bronchopleural f.
carotid cavernous f.
cervical f.
cholecystoduodenal f.
coccygeal f.
colocutaneous f.
coloileal f.
colonic f.
colovaginal f.
colovesical f.
complete f.
duodenal f.
enterocutaneous f.
enteroenteric f.
enterovaginal f.
enterovesical f.
external f.
fecal f.
gastric f.
gastrocolic f.
gastrocutaneous f.
gastroduodenal f.
gastrointestinal f.
genitourinary f.
hepatic f.
hepatopleural f.
horseshoe f.
incomplete f.
inflammatory f.
internal f.
intestinal f.
lacteal f.
mammary f.
metroperitoneal f.
mouth f.
nuisance f.
parietal f.
perineovaginal f.
pilonidal f.
pulmonary arteriovenous f. (PAF)
rectolabial f.
rectourethral f.
rectovaginal f.
rectovesical f.
rectovestibular f.
rectovulvar f.
salivary f.

sigmoidovesical f.
spermatic f.
stercoral f.
thoracic duct f. (TDF)
thyroglossal f.
tracheobiliary f.
tracheoesophageal f. (TEF)
umbilical f.
urachal f.
ureterocutaneous f.
ureterovaginal f.
urethrovaginal f.
urinary bladder f.
urogenital f.
uteroperitoneal f.
vesical f.
vesicocolic f.
vesicocutaneous f.
vesicointestinal f.
vesicouterine f.
vesicovaginal f.
vesicovaginorectal f.
fistulation
Fistulina
fistulization
fistulous
FITC
    fluorescein isothiocyanate
Fite
    F. method
    F. stain
Fite-Faraco stain
fitter cell theory
fitting
    curve f.
Fitzgerald factor
Fitzgerald-Williams-Flaujeac factor
Fitz-Hugh and Curtis syndrome
Fitz syndrome
fix
    B-plus F.
    F. and Perm Cell Permeabilization Kit
fixation
    alcohol f.
    AMeX f.
    f. artifact
    autotrophic f.
    carbon dioxide f.
    complement f. (CF)
    cytospray f.
    microwave f.

F

NOTES

fixation *(continued)*
   f. reaction
   secondary f.
   f. test
   Treponema pallidum complement f.
    (TPCF)
fixative
   acetone f.
   AFA f.
   alcohol-glycerin f.
   aldehyde f.
   Altmann f.
   B5 f.
   Bouin picroformol-acetic f.
   Brasil f.
   buffered formalin f.
   Carnoy f.
   Champy f.
   chromic acid f.
   coating f.
   CytoLyt f.
   CytoRich Red f.
   Flemming f.
   formaldehyde f.
   formalin f.
   formol-calcium f.
   formol-Müller f.
   formol-saline f.
   formol-Zenker f.
   Gendre f.
   glacial acetic acid f.
   glutaraldehyde f.
   Golgi osmiobichromate f.
   Helly f.
   Hermann f.
   Jores f.
   Kaiserling f.
   Karnovsky f.
   lead f.
   Luft potassium permanganate f.
   Marchi f.
   mercuric f.
   methanol f.
   Millonig phosphate-buffered
    formalin f.
   Müller f.
   neutral buffered formalin f.
   Newcomer f.
   Orth f.
   osmic acid f.
   Park-Williams f.
   periodate-lysing-paraformaldehyde f.
   Permount slide f.
   picric acid f.
   picroformol f.
   PreservCyt f.
   PVA f.
   Regaud f.
   Saccomanno f.

   SAF f.
   Schaudinn f.
   Shandon f.
   single vial f.
   Spray-Cyte slide f.
   Supermount slide f.
   Thoma f.
   Trump f.
   wick f.
   Zenker f.
fixative/solution
   Hollande f./s.
   isopentane f./s.
   methylbutane f./s.
fixed
   f. blood film
   f. cell
   f. macrophage
   f. oil
   f. sediment method
   f. virus
fixed-point variable
fixed-time method
FJN
   familial juvenile nephrophthisis
FJP
   familial juvenile polyp
FL
   follicular lymphoma
Fl
   fluorine
   follicle lysis
fL
   femtoliter
fl
   fluid
FL11 gene
flaccid
flaccidity
flagella (*pl. of* flagellum)
flagellar
   f. agglutination
   f. agglutinin
   f. antigen
Flagellata
flagellated
flagellate dysentery
flagellin
flagellosis
flagellum, pl. **flagella**
flail
   f. chest
   f. scallop
Flajani disease
flaky paint dermatitis
flame
   f. background
   capillary f.
   f. cell

f. emission spectrophotometry
f. emission spectroscopy (FES)
f. figure
f. intensity zone
f. ionization detector (FID)
manometric f.
f. nevus
f. photometer
f. photometry
flame-shaped retinal hemorrhage
flammability
flammable
flammeus
nevus f.
Flammulina
flank bruit
flap
Bakamjian deltopectoral f.
Estlander f.
Gillies f.
Karapandzic f.
Wookey skin f.
flash burn
flash-point temperature
flask
f. culture
Dewar f.
Erlenmeyer f.
Fernbach f.
Florence f.
hatching f.
vacuum f.
volumetric f.
flask-like
Erlenmeyer f.
flask-shaped heart
flat
f. bipolar cell
f. condyloma
f. smallpox
f. substrate method
f. urothelial hyperplasia
f. wart
Flatau-Schilder disease
flat-field objective
flattened
f. cell
f. shape
flatworm
Flaujeac factor
flava
macula f.

medulla ossium f.
Neisseria f.
Saccharopolyspora f.
flavescens
Aedes f.
Mycobacterium f.
Neisseria f.
Trichophyton f.
flavianic acid
flavida
Kribbella f.
flavin
f. adenine dinucleotide (FAD)
f. mononucleotide (FMN)
flavirostris
Anopheles f.
flaviscutellata
Lutzomyia f.
flaviscutellatus
Phlebotomus f.
flavithermus
Anoxybacillus f.
flaviverrucosa
Lentzea f.
Flaviviridae
Flavivirus
flavivirus
Flavobacteria
Flavobacteriaceae
Flavobacterium
F. aquatile
F. breve
F. degerlachei
F. frigidarium
F. frigoris
F. gelidilacus
F. gillisiae
F. limicola
F. meningosepticum
F. micromati
F. omnivorum
F. xanthum
F. xinjiangense
flavoenzyme
flavogenita
Stemonitis f.
flavoprotein
flavum
Oxalicibacterium f.
flavus
Arthrobacter f.
Aspergillus f.

NOTES

F

flavus (continued)
 Erythrobacter f.
 Plantibacter f.
flaxseed oil
FLCOD
 florid local cementoosseous dysplasia
flea
 American rat f.
 dog f.
 European rat f.
 human f.
 Indian rat f.
 plague-infected f.
flea-bitten kidney
Flegel disease
Fleischer ring
Fleischner syndrome
Fleitmann test
Flemming
 F. fixative
 germinal center of F.
 intermediate body of F.
 F. triple stain
flesh
 proud f.
fleshfly
fleshy
 f. mole
 f. polyp
Fletcher factor
fleurettii
 Staphylococcus f.
flexilis
 Thiothrix f.
Flexistipes sinusarabici
Flexner
 F. bacillus
 F. dysentery
 F. serum
flexneri
 Shigella f.
Flexner-Strong bacillus
Flexner-Wintersteiner rosette
FlexSure
 F. HP
 F. OBT
flexure
 splenic f.
FLICE
 FADD-like interleukin-1 beta converting
 enzyme
FLICE-like inhibitory protein (FLIP)
flight
 time of f.
Flinders Island spotted fever
flint
 F. arcade
 f. disease
 f. glass

FLIP
 FLICE-like inhibitory protein
flipped pattern of lactate dehydrogenase
FLM
 fetal lung maturity
 fluorescence lifetime imaging
 FLM imaging
 FLM microscopy
floater
floating
 f. beta disease
 f. organ
floating-point variable
floc
 flocculation
floccose
floccosum
 Acrothesium f.
 Epidermophyton f.
 Trichophyton f.
flocculable
flocculans
 Balneimonas f.
 Rubritepida f.
floccular degeneration
flocculate
flocculation (floc)
 cephalin f.
 cephalin-cholesterol f. (CCF)
 limes f. (Lf)
 limit of f. (LF)
 f. reaction (FR)
 f. test
 thymol f. (TF)
floccule
 toxoid-antitoxoid f. (TAF)
flocculence
flocculent
flocculus, pl. flocculi
flood
 f. fever
 f. plate
 f. source
floor cell
flora
 intestinal f.
 oral f.
floral
 f. variant
 f. variant of follicular lymphoma
 (FFL)
Florence
 F. crystal
 F. flask
Florey unit
florid
 f. cementoosseous dysplasia

f. local cementoosseous dysplasia (FLCOD)
f. oral papillomatosis

Florisil

flotation
f. bath
centrifugal f.
direct centrifugal f. (DCF)
f. rate
f. technique
f. test
f. unit

flow
abnormal f.
f. birefringence
cerebral blood f. (CBF)
f. chart
coronary blood f. (CBF)
f. cytometer
f. cytometric assay
f. cytometric crossmatch
f. cytometric immunophenotyping
f. cytometric platelet counting procedure
f. cytometric reticulocyte analysis
f. cytometry (FC, FCM)
f. cytophotometry
effective renal blood f. (ERBF)
effective renal plasma f.
electroosmotic f.
estimated hepatic blood f. (EHBF)
exercise hyperemia blood f. (EHBF)
forced expiratory f. (FEF)
forced inspiratory f. (FIF)
gene f.
hepatic blood f. (HBF)
high f. (HF)
inspiratory f.
maximal midexpiratory f. (MMEF)
maximum expiratory f. (MEF)
maximum inspiratory f. (MIF)
peak expiratory f. (PEF)
peak inspiratory f. (PIF)
penile blood f.
pseudopod f.
pulmonary blood f.
f. rate (FR)
reactive hyperemia blood f. (RHBF)
renal plasma f. (RPF)
splanchnic blood f. (SBF)

uterine blood f. (UBF)
f. volume loop

flower
collagen f.

flower-spray
f.-s. ending
f.-s. organ of Ruffini

flowing hyperostosis

flowmeter (FM)
electromagnetic f. (EMF)

flow-sorted aneuploid fraction

FLS
fibrous long-spacing collagen

FLSA
follicular lymphosarcoma

flu
influenza

fluctuation
IP3 dependent calcium f.

flucytosine

fludrocortisone

fluff
electron-lucent f.

fluid (fl)
Altmann f.
amniotic f.
anthrax-infected body f.
ascitic f.
f. balance
f. balance and homeostasis
Bensley osmic dichromate f.
body f.
Bouin f.
bronchoalveolar lavage f. (BALF)
Burnett disinfecting f.
Callison f.
cerebrospinal f. (CSF)
Ciaccio f.
Clarke f.
crevicular f.
f. culture
culture of vesicular f.
de Castro f.
Delafield f.
dentinal f.
extracellular f. (ECF)
Farrant mounting f.
gastric f. (GF)
Gendre f.
gingival f.
Helly f.
interstitial f.

F

NOTES

fluid *(continued)*
  intracellular f. (ICF)
  intraocular f.
  looped f.
  microscopic examination of cerebrospinal f.
  f. mosaic model
  Orth f.
  pleural f.
  prostatic f.
  proteinaceous f.
  Rees-Ecker f.
  respiratory tract f. (RTF)
  f. retention
  Saccomanno collection f.
  seminal f.
  serous f.
  f. shear stress
  spinal f.
  subretinal f. (SRF)
  sulcular f.
  synovial f.
  tissue f.
  transcellular f.
  tubular f. (TF)
  f. volume (FV)
  Zamboni f.
  Zenker f.
fluid-borne agent
fluke
  blood f.
  cat liver f.
  Chinese liver f.
  giant intestinal f.
  giant liver f.
  lancet f.
  liver f.
  lung f.
  Manson blood f.
  Oriental blood f.
  Oriental lung f.
  sheep liver f.
  vesical blood f.
  Yokogawa f.
fluminea
  Nocardia f.
FLU OIA A/B rapid test
fluor
fluorescein
  f. isothiocyanate (FITC)
  f. mercuric acetate
  f. sodium
fluorescein-labeled antibody
fluorescein-to-protein ratio (F:P)
fluorescence
  f. correlation spectroscopy (FCS)
  f. decay difference
  dual-color f.

  f. excitation transfer immunoassay (FETI)
  f. intensity of telomere spot
  laser-activated f.
  f. lifetime imaging (FLM)
  f. microscope
  f. microscopy
  perikaryal f.
  f. plus Giemsa stain
  f. polarization immunoassay (FPIA)
  f. quenching
  relative f. (RF)
  resonance f.
  f. resonance energy transfer (FRET)
  f. in situ hybridization (FISH)
  f. spectrum
  time-resolved f. (TRF)
fluorescence-activated cell sorter (FACS)
fluorescens
  Pseudomonas f.
fluorescent
  f. allergosorbent test (FAST)
  f. antibody (FA)
  f. antibody dark-field (FADF)
  f. antibody technique
  f. antibody test (FAT)
  f. antinuclear antibody (FANA)
  f. antinuclear antibody test
  f. cytoprint assay
  f. dye
  f. immunoassay (FIA)
  f. material
  f. microscope
  f. microscopy
  f. probe
  f. protection assay
  f. resonance energy transfer (FRET)
  f. in situ hybridization
  f. staining
  f. treponemal antibody (FTA)
  f. treponemal antibody-absorption (FTA-ABS, FTA-AB)
  f. treponemal antibody-absorption test
fluoride
  f. assay
  hydrogen f.
  f. number
  sodium f.
fluorine (Fl)
  f. 18
fluorite objective
fluoroacetamide
fluoroacetate
  f. assay
  sodium f.
fluorocarbon assay

fluorochrome
  molecule of equivalent soluble f. (MESF)
fluorochrome-avidin/streptavidin conjugate
fluorochrome-conjugated DNA
fluorochroming
fluorocyte
5-fluorocytosine
fluorodeoxyuridine (FUDR)
fluoro-2,4-dinitrobenzene (FDNB)
Fluorognost HIV-1 IFA assay kit
fluoroimmunoassay
  dissociation enhanced lanthanide f. (DELFIA)
  polarization f.
fluoro jade staining
fluorometry
  filipin f.
  time-resolved f. (TRF)
fluorophosphonate
  methylarachidonyl f. (MAFP)
fluoroscopic diaphragmatic paralysis sniff test
fluorosilicate
  sodium f.
fluorosis
  dental f.
  endemic f.
  skeletal f.
Fluorospheres
  Immuno-Brite F.
fluosol-DA
Flury
  F. strain rabies virus
  F. strain vaccine
fluvialis
  Vibrio f.
fluviatilis
  Anopheles f.
flux
  luminous f.
  magnetic f.
FLx/TDx immunoassay analyzer
fly
  f. agaric
  black f.
  dog f.
  fruit f.
  larva f.
  f. larva
  stable f.

  tsetse f.
  warble f.
flying spot microscope
Flynn-Aird syndrome
FM
  flowmeter
Fm
  fermium
fm
  femtometer
FMC7 expression
FMD
  foot-and-mouth disease
    FMD virus
fMet-Leu-Phe (*var. of* fMLP))
FMF
  familial Mediterranean fever
FMH
  familial hemiplegic migraine
FMLH
  familial hemophagocytic lymphohistiocytosis
fMLP, fMet-Leu-Phe
  formyl methionyl leucyl phenylalanine
    fMLP receptor
FMN
  flavin mononucleotide
fmol
  femtomole
FMR
  familial mental retardation
FMR-I gene
FMS
  fat-mobilizing substance
fms oncogene
FN
  false-negative
FNA
  fine-needle aspiration
FNAB
  fine-needle aspiration biopsy
FNAC
  fine-needle aspiration cytology
FNH
  focal nodular hyperplasia
FNHTR
  febrile nonhemolytic transfusion reaction
FN-MCD
  familial nephronophthisis-medullary cystic disease
    FN-MCD complex

F

NOTES

foam
  f. cell
  f. stability index (FSI)
  f. stability test
foam/shake test
foamy
  f. agent
  f. cytoplasm
  f. degeneration
  f. degeneration of hepatocytes
  f. gland prostate cancer
  f. histiocyte
  f. macrophage
  f. virus
FOAVF
  failure of all vital forces
FOBT
  fecal occult blood test
focal
  f. adhesion kinase (FAK)
  f. amyloidosis
  f. appendicitis
  f. atrophy
  f. axonal injury
  f. bone marrow defect
  f. bronchopneumonia
  f. calcification
  f. cortical epilepsy
  f. dermal hypoplasia
  f. dermal hypoplasia syndrome
  f. disease
  f. distance
  f. embolic glomerulonephritis
  f. epithelial hyperplasia
  f. fibrosis
  f. granulomatous inflammation
  f. hemorrhagic necrotizing
    pneumonic lesion
  f. hypertrophy
  f. infarct
  f. infection
  f. involvement
  f. length
  f. lymphocytic thyroiditis
  f. necrosis
  f. necrotizing glomerulonephritis
  f. plane
  f. plaque rupture
  f. pneumonia
  f. proliferative lupus nephritis
  f. reaction
  f. regression
  f. sclerosing glomerulopathy
  f. segmental distribution
  f. segmental glomerulosclerosis
  f. ulcer
  f. zone
FocalCheck microsphere
focus, pl. **foci**

  aberrant crypt f.
  conjugate f.
  depth of f.
  disseminated foci (DF)
  dysplastic f.
  ectopic f. (EF)
  epileptogenic f.
  fibrotic f.
  Ghon f.
  Ghon-Sachs f.
  low-voltage f. (LVF)
  metastatic f.
  natural f. of infection
  necrotic f.
  principal f.
  proliferating f.
focused grid
focusing
  isoelectric f. (IEF)
FOD
  fatty acid oxidation disorder
foenisicii
  Paneolus f.
foetidus
  Peptostreptococcus f.
foetus
  Trichomonas f.
fog oil (SGF2)
foil
  air f.
Foix-Alajouanine myelitis
Foix syndrome
folate
  f. deficiency
  f. deficiency anemia
  red cell f. (RCF)
  f. reductase
  sodium f.
  whole-blood f. (WBF)
fold
  ciliary f.
  epicanthal f.
  giant gastric f.
  Kerckring f.
  longitudinal f.
  mucobuccal f.
  numerous mucosal f.'s
folded
  f. cell
  f. nucleus
folded-cell index
folded-lung syndrome
folding
  sarcolemmal f.
foliacée
  lamé f.
foliaceous
  pemphigus f.
folia linguae

foliar
foliatae
    papillae f.
foliate papillae
folic
    f. acid
    f. acid assay
    f. acid deficiency
    f. acid deficiency anemia
    f. acid receptor
Folin
    F. test
    F. and Wu (FW)
    F. and Wu method
Folin-Ciocalteu
    F.-C. reagent
    F.-C. test
folinic acid
Folin-Looney test
foliose
folium
follicle
    anovular ovarian f.
    antral f.
    atretic ovarian f.
    f. center lymphoma (FCL)
    f. cyst
    cystic ovarian f.
    dental f.
    gastric f.
    graafian f.
    granular layer of a vesicular ovarian f.
    growing ovarian f.
    hair f.
    intestinal f.
    Lieberkühn f.'s
    lingual f.
    lymphatic f.
    lymphoid f.
    f. lysis (Fl)
    mature ovarian f.
    Montgomery f.
    multilaminar primary f.
    nabothian f.
    ovarian f.
    polyovular ovarian f.
    primary lymphoid f.
    primary ovarian f.
    primordial ovarian f.
    regressively transformed f.
    sebaceous f.

    secondary lymphoid f.
    secondary ovarian f.
    solitary f.
    splenic lymph f.
    thyroid f.
    f. of thyroid gland
    unilaminar primary f.
    vellus anagen f.
    vellus telogen f.
    vesicular ovarian f.
follicle-cell lymphoma
follicle-stimulating
    f.-s. hormone (FSH)
    f.-s. hormone assay
    f.-s. hormone releasing hormone (FSH-RH)
    f.-s. principle
follicular
    f. abscess
    f. adenoma
    f. ameloblastoma
    f. antrum
    f. atresia
    f. cell center
    f. cell lymphoma cell
    f. center cell (FCC)
    f. cholecystitis
    f. conjunctivitis
    f. cyst
    f. cystitis
    f. dendritic cell (FDC)
    f. dendritic cell sarcoma
    f. dermatitis
    f. epithelial cell
    f. gland
    f. goiter
    f. hyperplasia (FH)
    f. inflammation
    f. infundibula
    f. inverted keratosis
    f. lymphoma (FL)
    f. lymphosarcoma (FLSA)
    f. mucinosis
    f. ovarian cell
    f. and papillary adenocarcinoma
    f. pattern
    f. pharyngitis
    f. predominantly large cell lymphoma
    f. predominantly small cleaved cell lymphoma
    f. salpingitis

NOTES

follicular *(continued)*
    f. stigma
    f. urethritis
follicularis
    cystitis f.
    isolated dyskeratosis f.
    keratosis f.
    f. keratosis
folliculi *(pl. of* folliculus)
folliculitis
    f. abscedens et suffodiens
    f. barbae
    f. decalvans
    eosinophilic pustular f.
    f. keloidalis
    pseudolymphomatous f.
    f. ulerythematosa reticulata
folliculocentricity
folliculogenesis
folliculoma
folliculorum
    Acarus f.
    Demodex f.
    Simonea f.
folliculosis
folliculotropic mycosis fungoides
folliculus, pl. **folliculi**
    folliculi glandulae thyroideae
    folliculi linguales
    folliculi lymphatici aggregati
    folliculi lymphatici aggregati
      appendicis vermiformis
    folliculi lymphatici gastrici
    folliculi lymphatici laryngei
    folliculi lymphatici lienales
    folliculi lymphatici recti
    folliculi lymphatici solitarii
    f. lymphaticus
    f. ovaricus primarius
    f. ovaricus vesiculosus
    f. pili
    theca folliculi
    tunica externa thecae folliculi
    tunica interna thecae folliculi
Folling disease
followup
    lost to f. (LTF)
fomes, pl. **fomites**
Fomitopsis
Fonio solution
Fonsecaea
    F. compactum
    F. dermatitidis
    F. jeanselmei
    F. pedrosoi
Fontana
    F. methenamine silver stain
    F. space

Fontana-Masson
    F.-M. silver stain
    F.-M. staining method
fontislapidosi
    Idiomarina f.
food
    f. allergy
    f. ball
    f. deprivation
    Eskimo traditional f.
    f. fever
    f. intolerance
    Inuit traditional f.
    medical f.
    f. poisoning
food-based bioterrorism
foodborne
    f. botulism
    f. infection
    f. pathogen
foodSCAN food allergy test
foot, pl. **feet**
    athlete's f.
    basal feet
    Dupuytren disease of the f.
    fungous f.
    Hong Kong f.
    Madura f.
    Morand f.
    mossy f.
    perivascular end feet
    f. plate (*var. of* footplate)
    f. process
    F. reticulin impregnation stain
    F. reticulin method
    sandal f.
    trench f.
foot-and-mouth
    f.-a.-m. disease (FMD)
    f.-a.-m. disease virus
    f.-a.-m. disease virus vaccine
footplate, foot plate
foramen, pl. **foramina**
    Bichat f.
    f. of Luschka
    foramina nervosa
    f. nutricium
    nutrient f.
    obturator f.
    f. ovale
    foramina papillaria renis
Foraminifera
foraminiferous
foraminosus
    tractus spiralis f.
foraminulum
Forbes-Albright syndrome
Forbes disease

forbidden clone
force (F)
    centrifugal f.
    centripetal f.
    Chemical Biological Incident
      Response F. (of the U.S. Marine
      Corps) (CBIRF)
    electromotive f. (EMF)
    failure of all vital f.'s (FOAVF)
    London f.
    relative centrifugal f. (RCF)
    van der Waals f.'s
forced
    f. expiratory flow (FEF)
    f. expiratory spirogram (FES)
    f. expiratory time (FET)
    f. expiratory time in seconds
      (FETS)
    f. expiratory volume at 1 second
      (FEV-1)
    f. inspiratory flow (FIF)
    f. inspiratory oxygen
    f. vital capacity (FVC)
forceps
    air powered f.
    large-cup f.
    Spencer-Wells f.
Forcipomyia glauca
fordii
    Bacillus f.
Fordyce
    F. angiokeratoma
    F. disease
    F. granule
    F. spot
foregut
    f. carcinoid
    f. cyst
forehead
    olympian f.
foreign
    f. body (FB)
    f. body aspiration
    f. body embolus
    f. body giant cell
    f. body granuloma
    f. body odditis
    f. body reaction
    f. body salpingitis
    f. body tumorigenesis
    f. material deposition
    f. protein

    f. protein therapy
    f. serum
forensic
    f. anthropology
    f. anthropometry
    f. autopsy
    f. dentistry
    f. documentation
    f. evaluation
    f. evaluation of handgun wound
    f. medicine
    f. odontology
    f. photograph
    f. radiology
    f. toxicology
    f. urine drug testing (FUDT)
forespore
Forestier disease
forest yaws
fork
    replication f.
forkhead box J1 gene
form
    accolé f.
    appliqué f.
    attenuated viral f.
    band f.
    f. birefringence
    cell wall-deficient bacterial f.
      (CWDF)
    cornifying f.
    diffuse proliferative f.
    distinctive f.
    exposed protruding f. (EPF)
    Fuzzy Functional F. (FFF)
    ghost f.'s
    intramural protruding f. (IPF)
    involution f.
    myocardial infarction in
      dumbbell f.
    noncornifying f.
    replicative f.
    ring f.
    spore f.
    sunburst f.
    ulcerating f. (UF)
Formad kidney
formaldehyde
    aniline, sulfur, f. (ASF)
    f. dehydrogenase
    f. fixative
    f. solution

NOTES

F

formaldehyde-induced fluorescence method
formalin
    alcoholic f.
    f. ammonium bromide
    B5 sodium acetate-sublimate f.
    buffered neutral f.
    calcium acetate f.
    Carson f.
    f. fixative
    phosphate buffered f.
    f. pigment
    f. solution
    zinc f.
formalin-ether
    f.-e. sedimentation concentration
    f.-e. sedimentation method
formalin-ethyl acetate sedimentation concentration
formalin-fixed
    f.-f. paraffin-embedded sample
    f.-f. skin biopsy
    f.-f. tissue
    f.-f. tissue section
formalinize
formamide
    deionized f.
format
    low-volume air thermal cycle f.
formatexigens
    Bryantella f.
formatio, pl. **formationes**
    f. reticularis
formation
    coffin f.
    crescent f.
    cytokine f.
    de novo tissue f.
    formazan f.
    ketone body f.
    localized plaque f. (LPF)
    mesencephalic reticular f. (MRF)
    morule f.
    palisade f.
    peroxynitrite f.
    phagolysosome f.
    reticular f.
    Roman bridge f.
    rouleau f.
    standard enthalpy of f.
    tubule f.
formative cell
formazan
    blue f.
    f. formation
forme
    f. fruste
    f. tardive

formic
    f. acid
    f. aldehyde
formication
formicigenerans
    Dorea f.
formicigenes
    Tepidibacter f.
formicophilia
formiminoglutamic acid (FIGLU)
formin
formol-calcium fixative
formol-gel test
formol-Müller fixative
formol-saline fixative
formol-Zenker fixative
formonitrile
Formosa algae
formula, pl. **formulas, formulae**
    Arneth f.
    Arrhenius f.
    Bird f.
    Christison f.
    Häser f.
    Haworth f.
    Long f.
    Poisson-Pearson f.
    Ranke f.
    Reuss f.
    Runeberg f.
    Trapp f.
    Trapp-Häser f.
    Van Slyke f.
formulary
formyl methionyl leucyl phenylalanine (fMLP, fMet-Leu-Phe)
Forney syndrome
fornicalis
    Lactobacillus f.
fornix, pl. **fornices**
forskolin-stimulated intracellular cAMP accumulation
Forssman
    F. antibody
    F. antigen
    F. antigen-antibody reaction
    F. lipoid
    F. shock
Förster disease
forsythensis
    Tannerella f.
Fort Bragg fever
fortis
    Bacillus f.
    Vibrio f.
fortuitum
    Mycobacterium f.
fortuitum-chelonae
    Mycobacterium f.-c.

forward
> f. bias
> f. blood typing
> f. dot-blot
> f. failure
> f. fluorescence detector (FED)
> f. mutation
> f. scatter (FSC)

Foshay test
fosphenytoin
fossa, pl. **fossae**
> adipose f.
> infratemporal f.
> f. navicularis

fossula, pl. **fossulae**
Foster Kennedy syndrome
Fothergill disease
Fouchet
> F. reagent
> F. stain
> F. test

founder effect
four
> f. locus
> f. subunit

Fourier
> F. analysis
> F. transform infrared
> microspectroscopy (FTIR)

Fournier
> F. disease
> F. gangrene
> syphiloma of F.

fourth-degree
> f.-d. burn
> f.-d. frostbite
> f.-d. radiation injury

fourth venereal disease
fovea, pl. **foveae**
> f. centralis
> f. centralis maculae luteae
> f. ethmoidalis

foveate
foveated chest
Foveavirus
foveola, pl. **foveolae**
> f. gastrica
> f. papillaris

foveolar
> f. cell of stomach
> f. epithelium
> f. hyperplasia

foveolate
foveolin
Foville syndrome
fowl
> f. diphtheria
> f. erythroblastosis virus
> f. leukosis
> f. lymphomatosis
> f. lymphomatosis virus
> f. myeloblastosis virus
> f. neurolymphomatosis virus
> f. paralysis
> f. pest
> f. plague
> f. plague virus

fowleri
> *Naegleria f.*

Fowler solution
fowlpox virus
fox encephalitis virus
Fox-Fordyce disease
fozii
> *Psychrobacter f.*

FP
> false-positive
> freezing point
> frozen plasma

F:P
> fluorescein-to-protein ratio

FPG
> fasting plasma glucose

FPIA
> fluorescence polarization immunoassay

FPM
> filter paper microscopic

FPN
> ferric chloride, perchloric acid, nitric acid
> FPN reagent

FPP
> ferriprotoporphyrin

FR
> flocculation reaction
> flow rate

Fr
> francium

FRA
> fibrin-related antigen

fract
> fracture

fractal texture
fraction
> amorphous f. of adrenal cortex

F

NOTES

fraction *(continued)*
    blood plasma f.
    branching f.
    catecholamine f.
    cerebrospinal fluid lactate
      dehydrogenase f.'s
    extraction f. (E)
    flow-sorted aneuploid f.
    growth f.
    heparin-precipitable f. (HPF)
    f. of inspired oxygen
    mole f.
    O_2Hb f.
    plasma protein f. (PPF)
    saponifiable f.
    S-phase f.
    urine estradiol f.
    urine estriol f.
fractional
    f. allelic loss
    f. concentration of inspired oxygen
      (FiO_2)
    f. distillation
    f. excretion of sodium (FENa)
    f. sterilization
    f. uptake of carbon monoxide
    f. urinalysis
fractionated
    f. alkaline phosphatase
    f. erythrocyte porphyrin
fractionation
    Cohn f.
    lipoprotein-cholesterol f.
    nucleocytoplasmic f.
    protein f.
fracture (fract)
    avulsion f.
    f. callus
    cervical f.
    chip f.
    clay shoveler's f.
    closed f.
    comminuted f.
    compound comminuted f. (CCF)
    compound multiple f.'s
    compressed f.
    compression f.
    coronoid process f.
    craniofacial f.
    depressed f.
    f. dislocation
    Frykman hand f.
    greenstick f.
    healed f.
    Hunt and Hess hand f.
    impacted f.
    Judet epiphysial f.
    linear f.
    Neer shoulder f. I–III

    nonunion f.
    oblique f.
    orbital f.
    pathologic f.
    Pauwel femoral neck f.
    pelvic f.
    result of severe f.
    Salter-Harris 1–5 f.
    scaphoid f.
    simple f.
    spiral f.
    stellate f.
    stress f.
    transverse f.
    ununited f.
fractured transverse process
frag
    fragility
fragi
    Pseudomonas f.
fragile
    Desulfofrigus f.
    f. histidine triad gene
    f. X chromosome
    f. X syndrome
fragilis
    Bacteroides f.
    Dientamoeba f.
fragilitas
    f. ossium
    f. sanguinis
fragility (frag)
    f. of the blood
    capillary f.
    erythrocyte f.
    mechanical f.
    osmotic f.
    red cell f.
    f. test
fragilocyte
fragilocytosis
fragment
    antiuvomorulin Fab f.
    C-terminal f.
    Fab f.
    Fc f.
    Klenow f.
    f. length
    N-terminal f.
    N-terminal mid f. (NMID)
    P-radiolabeled DNA probe f.
    retained placental f.
    telomeric restriction f. (TRF)
    f. Y
fragmentation
    f. myocarditis
    f. of the myocardium
fragmenting projectile

fragmentography
mass f.
FRALE
frangible anchor-linker effector
Fraley syndrome
frambesia
frame
Deiters terminal f.
open reading f. (ORF)
reading f.
frame-scanning segment
frameshift mutation
framework
Franceschetti-Jadassohn syndrome
Franceschetti syndrome
Francis
F. disease
F. skin test
Francisella
F. philomiragia
F. tularensis
F. tularensis biovar Jellison type A, B
francium (Fr)
François syndrome
frangible anchor-linker effector (FRALE)
Frankiaceae
Frankineae
Frankl-Hochwart disease
Franklin disease
frank megaloblastic anemia
Frank-Starling mechanism
Fraser-Lendrum stain for fibrin
Fraser syndrome
frataxin gene
fraterna
Hymenolepis nana var. *f.*
fraternal twins
FRC
functional reserve capacity
functional residual capacity
freckle
Hutchinson melanotic f.
melanotic f.
frederiksbergense
Mycobacterium f.
frederiksbergensis
Pseudomonas f.
frederiksenii
Yersinia f.

fredii
Ensifer f.
Fredrickson dyslipoproteinemia classification
free
f. beta test
f. catecholamine fractionation
f. cell
f. electron
f. energy
f. erythrocyte coproporphyrin (FEC)
f. erythrocyte protoporphyrin (FEP, FEPP)
f. estriol
fat f.
f. fatty acid (FFA)
gluten f. (GF)
f. macrophage
f. nerve ending
f. protein S test
f. radical
f. ribosome
f. T_4
f. thyroxine index (FT_4I, FTI)
f. toxicology
f. T_4 ratio
f. triiodothyronine (FT_3)
f. triiodothyronine index (FT_3I)
f. (unbound) thyroxine (FT_4)
f. urinary cortisol test
f. water clearance
freeborni
Anopheles f.
freedom
degrees of f. (df)
Freeman-Sheldon syndrome
FreeStyle blood glucose monitoring system
free/total
f./t. PSA index
f./t. PSA ratio test
freeze-clamp
freeze-cleave method
freeze-drying
freeze-etch method
freeze-fracture
f.-f. replica
f.-f. technique
freeze-fracture-etch method
freezer
-86C ULT f.

F

NOTES

freezer *(continued)*
    CryoMed f.
    Gentle Jane Snap F.
freeze-substitution
freezing
    f. injury
    f. microtome
    f. point (FP)
    f. point depression osmometer
Frei
    F. antigen
    F. disease
    F. test
Freiberg disease
Frei-Hoffmann reaction
French-American-British (FAB)
French proof agar
freneyi
    Corynebacterium f.
Frenkel anterior ocular traumatic syndrome
frenulum linguae
frequence-time histogram
frequency
    angular f.
    f. counter
    crossover f.
    cutoff f.
    discharge f.
    f. distribution
    gene f.
    high f. (HF)
    mean dominant f. (MDF)
    medium f. (MF)
    f. polygon
    recombination f.
    urinary f.
    very-high f.
Frerichs theory
fresconis
    Brachybacterium f.
fresh frozen plasma (FFP)
Fresnel fringe
FRET
    fluorescence resonance energy transfer
    fluorescent resonance energy transfer
freudenreichii
    Propionibacterium f.
Freund
    F. anomaly
    F. complete adjuvant
    F. incomplete adjuvant
freundii
    Citrobacter f.
Frey syndrome
friable
Friderichsen-Waterhouse syndrome
fried egg colony
Friedewald equation

Friedländer
    F. bacillus
    F. bacillus pneumonia
    F. disease
    F. pneumobacillus
    F. stain for capsules
Friedmann
    F. disease
    F. vasomotor syndrome
Friedmanniella
    F. lacustris
    F. spumicola
Friedman test
Friedreich disease
Friend
    F. disease
    F. leukemia virus
frigidarium
    Flavobacterium f.
frigidity
frigoramans
    Subtercola f.
Frigoribacterium faeni
frigoris
    Clostridium f.
    Flavobacterium f.
frigorism
frill
    iris f.
fringe
    Fresnel f.
    synovial f.
frisingense
    Herbaspirillum f.
fritillariae
    Okibacterium f.
friuliensis
    Actinoplanes f.
frog test
Fröhlich
    F. dwarfism
    F. syndrome
Frohn reagent
Froin syndrome
Froment paper sign
Frommel-Chiari syndrome
Frommel disease
frond
    papillary f.
frondosum
    chorion f.
frontotemporal dementias with parkinsonism linked to chromosome 17 (FTDP-17)
Froriep induration
frostbite
    first-degree f.
    fourth-degree f.

second-degree f.
third-degree f.
frosted
f. heart
f. liver
frotteurism
frozen
f. blood
f. pelvis
f. plasma (FP)
f. red blood cells
f. section (FS, FZ)
f. section method
fructofuranose
fructokinase
fructopyranose
fructosamine
AccuMeter f.
fructose
f. assay
f. bisphosphate
f. 1,6-diphosphatase deficiency
f. diphosphate
f. intolerance
f. test
fructose-bisphosphate aldolase
fructosemia
fructosum
Leuconostoc f.
fructosuria
essential f.
fructosyl
fruit fly
fruiting body
frumenti
Lactobacillus f.
frustrated phagocytosis
frutescens
Capsicum f.
Frykman hand fracture
Fryn syndrome
fryxellensis
Loktanella f.
FS
fibrosarcoma
frozen section
FSC
forward scatter
FS-DFSP
fibrosarcomatous variant of
dermatofibrosarcoma protuberans

FSF
fibrin stabilizing factor
FSGS
focal segmental glomerular sclerosis
FSGSH
focal segmental glomerular sclerosis and
hyalinosis
FSH
follicle-stimulating hormone
FSH assay
FSH-RH
follicle-stimulating hormone releasing
hormone
FSH-RH assay
FSI
foam stability index
FSP
fibrinogen split product
fibrinolytic split product
FSR
fusiform skin revision
FT
fibrous tissue
FT₃
free triiodothyronine
FT₄
free (unbound) thyroxine
FTA
fluorescent treponemal antibody
FTA-ABS, FTA-AB
fluorescent treponemal antibody-
absorption
FTA-ABS test
FTDP-17
frontotemporal dementias with
parkinsonism linked to chromosome 17
FTI
free thyroxine index
FT₃I
free triiodothyronine index
FT₄I
free thyroxine index
FTIR
Fourier transform infrared
microspectroscopy
FU
fecal urobilinogen
FU-48 Zenker fixative solution
Fuchs
F. adenoma
F. syndrome
fuchsianus

NOTES

F

409

fuchsin
    acid f.
    aldehyde f. (AF)
    f., amido black, and naphthol
      yellow (FAN)
    aniline f.
    basic f.
    f. body
    diamond f.
    new f.
    f. stain
fuchsinophil
    f. cell
    f. granule
    f. reaction
fuchsinophilia
fuchsinophilic
fuchuensis
    Lactobacillus f.
fucicola
    Cellulophaga f.
fucosidosis
fucosyl moiety
FUDR
    fluorodeoxyuridine
FUDT
    forensic urine drug testing
fugacity
fugax
    amaurosis f.
fugitive swelling
Fuhrman
    F. grade tumor
    F. nuclear grade
    F. system
fujisawaense
    Methylobacterium f.
Fujiwara reaction
full
    f. blood examination (FBE)
    f. house pattern
    f. scale
full-body x-ray
fuller's earth pneumoconiosis
full-mutation allele
full-series biopsy
full-thickness burn
full-wave rectifier
full-width half-maximum
fulminans
    purpura f.
fulminant
    f. colitis
    f. dysentery
    f. hepatic failure (FHF)
    f. hepatitis
    f. myocarditis

fulminating
    f. anoxia
    f. smallpox
Fulvimarina pelagi
Fulvimonas soli
fulvum
    Microsporum f.
fulvus
    Cellvibrio f.
fumagillin
fumarase
fumarate hydratase
fumaric acid
fumarioli
    Bacillus f.
fume hood
fumigation
fumigatus
    Aspergillus f.
Funalia
functio laesa
function
    abnormal beta cell f.
    autocorrelation f.
    Boolean f.
    cardiopulmonary f.
    continuous f.
    delayed graft f.
    density f.
    detector transfer f. (DTF)
    discriminant f.
    distribution f.
    exponential f.
    line-spread f.
    liver f.
    Maddrey discriminant f.
    modulation transfer f.
    monocular f.
    neonatal biliary f.
    progressive impairment of renal f.
    quadratic f.
    respiratory f.
    secretin test for exocrine
      pancreatic f.
    split renal f. (SRF)
    step f.
    telomerase f.
    transfer f.
functional
    f. aerobic impairment
    f. affinity
    f. albuminuria
    f. bleeding
    f. constipation
    f. correlation
    f. death
    f. disease
    f. disorder
    f. group

f. group isomerism
f. hypertrophy
f. intact fibrinogen (FiF)
f. pathology
f. reserve capacity (FRC)
f. residual capacity (FRC)
f. terminal innervation ratio
f. tumor

functionale
stratum f.

functionalis
endometrial f.

functionally patent foramen ovale

fundamentalis
substantia f.

Fundibacter jadensis

fundic
f. gland
f. mucosa

funduliformis
Bacteroides f.

funestus
Anopheles f.

fungal
f. antibody screen
f. cast
f. esophagitis
f. hyphae
f. pericarditis
f. pneumonia
F. Prions
f. serology
f. skin testing
f. spore
f. stain

Fungalase-F stain
fungate
fungating
f. adenocarcinoma
f. sore

fungemia
fungi (*pl. of* fungus)
fungicidal
fungicide
fungiformes
papillae f.

fungiform papillae
fungilliform
fungiphilus
Azonexus f.

fungistatic
fungitoxic

fungitoxicity
fungivorans
Collimonas f.

Fungizone
fungoid
fungoides
folliculotropic mycosis f.
mycosis f. (MF)

fungoma
fungorum
Burkholderia f.

fungosity
fungous foot
fungus, pl. **fungi**
ascospore-forming f.
f. ball
f. cerebri
f. culture
cutaneous f.
dematiaceous f.
dimorphic pathogenic f.
fission f.
Fusarium f.
Gridley stain for fungi
imperfect f.
F. Imperfecti
mosaic f.
mycelial f.
Penicillium f.
perfect f.
f. smear
f. staining
thrush f.
yeast f.

funicular
f. myelitis
f. myelosis

funiculitis
endemic f.
filarial f.

funiculus
Bacillus f.

funis
funisitis
necrotizing f.

funkei
Actinomyces f.

funnel
f. breast
f. chest
separatory f.

NOTES

F

FUO
>fever of undetermined origin
>fever of unknown origin

furan

furanose

furanoside

furazolidone

furcal

furcate

furcosus
>*Bacteroides f.*

furens
>*Culicoides f.*

furfur
>*Malassezia f.*
>*Microsporum f.*
>*Pityrosporum f.*

furfural
>f. reaction
>f. reagent

furfurans
>porrigo f.

furnissii
>*Vibrio f.*

Furovirus

furrow
>Liebermeister f.

Furstner disease

Furst-Ostrum syndrome

furuncle

furunculoid

furunculosa
>*Leishmania f.*

furunculosis

fusariomycosis

Fusarium
>*F. fungus*
>*F. moniliforme*
>*F. oxysporum*
>*F. solanae*

fusca
>membrana f.
>*Mollisia f.*
>*Thermomonas f.*

fuscans
>*Trichosporon f.*

fuscicauda
>*Sarcophaga f.*

fuscidula
>*Aposphaeria f.*

fuseau

fused
>f. glandular pattern
>f. kidney
>f. novel gene

Fusellovirus

Fusibacter paucivorans

fusible calculus

Fusicoccum

fusidate
>sodium f.

Fusidium

fusiform
>f. aneurysm
>f. bacillus
>f. bronchiectasis
>f. cell
>f. cell of cerebral cortex
>f. layer
>f. skin revision (FSR)

fusiforme
>*Filomicrobium f.*

fusiformis
>*Bacteroides f.*
>*Sarcocystis f.*

Fusiformis necrophorus

fusimotor

fusion
>cell f.
>centric f.
>critical flicker f. (CFF)
>f. protein
>protoplast f.
>splenogonadal f.
>testicular-splenic f.
>whole-arm f.

fusispora
>*Acrophialophora f.*

Fusobacterium
>*F. aquatile*
>*F. equinum*
>*F. fusiforme*
>*F. glutinosum*
>*F. gonidiaformans*
>*F. mortiferum*
>*F. naviforme*
>*F. necrophorum*
>*F. nucleatum*
>*F. plauti-vincentii*
>*F. prausnitzii*
>*F. russii*
>*F. symbiosum*
>*F. varium*

fusocellular

fusospirillary

fusospirillosis

fusospirochetal

fusospirochetosis

fustic

futile cycle

fuzzy
>f. coat
>F. Functional Form (FFF)

FV
>fluid volume

FVC
>forced vital capacity

FVPTC
follicular variant of papillary thyroid
carcinoma
FW
Folin and Wu
FW method
FWR
Felix-Weil reaction
Fx
Icon Fx

Fya
Duffy antibody Fya
Fy antigen
Fyb
Duffy antibody Fyb
FZ
frozen section

NOTES

F

G

gauss
giga
gonidial (colony)
    G agent
    aggregated human immunoglobulin
      G (AHuG)
    G antigen
    G to A stage tumor transition
    azocarmine G
    G banding
    G cell
    G factor
    G protein
    G protein-linked receptor
    G syndrome
    G unit of streptomycin

g

gram

G_0 phase
G_1 phase
G_2 phase
GA

genetic algorithm
gestational age
NATO code for tabun

GAA repeat in the frataxin gene
GABA

gamma-aminobutyric acid

GAD

glutamic acid decarboxylase

Gadd153 gene
Gaddum and Schild test
gadei

    Dysgonomonas g.

gadfly
gadi

    Echinorhynchus g.

gadolinium
Gadus
gaetbuli

    Shewanella g.

Gaeumannomyces
Gaffky

    G. scale
    G. table

Gaffkya tetragena
GAG

glycosaminoglycan

gag reflex
Gail index of breast cancer risk
gain

    antigen g.
    current g.

gain-of-function abnormality

Gairdner disease
Gaisböck

    G. disease
    G. syndrome

galactan
galactanivorans

    Zobellia g.

galactic
galacticolus

    Saccharomyces g.

galactitol
galactoblast
galactocele
galactocerebroside beta galactosidase
galactography
galactokinase deficiency
galactolipid
galactolipin
galactometer
Galactomyces geotrichum
galactophore
galactophori

    tubuli g.

galactophoritis
galactophorous duct
galactopoietic hormone
galactorrhea
galactosamine
galactose

    g. assay
    g. breath test
    g. oxidase Schiff reaction
    g. phosphate uridyltransferase
    (GPUT)
    g. tolerance test

galactose-1-phosphate uridyltransferase (GALT)
galactosemia
galactosidase

    alpha g. A
    beta g.
    galactocerebroside beta g.
    o-nitrophenyl beta g.

galactoside
galactosidilyticus

    Bacillus g.

galactosuria
galactosylceramidase
galactosylhydrolase
galacturia
galacturonic acid
GA LAW

    glucose, age, lactate dehydrogenase,
    aspartate aminotransferase, white blood
    cells

G

Galeati gland
galectin
Galerina autumnalis
gall
    g. body
    g. duct
gallate
    epicatechin g.
gallbladder
    calcified g.
    g. carcinoma
    diffuse intramural calcification of
      the g.
    hourglass g.
    g. hydrops
    g. polyp
    porcelain g.
    sandpaper g.
    strawberry g.
Gallego differentiating solution
gallein
Gallibacterium anatis
Gallicola barnesae
gallicus
    Vibrio g.
gallinacea
    Echidnophaga g.
gallinaceus
    Streptococcus g.
gallinae
    Acarus g.
    Dermanyssus avium et g.
    Microsporum g.
gallinarum
    neurolymphomatosis g.
    osteopetrosis g.
    Trichomonas g.
gallinatum
    pectus g.
gallinifaecis
    Ochrobactrum g.
Gallionellaceae
gallisepticum
    Mycoplasma g.
gallium-67
gallium citrate
gallocyanin, gallocyanine
gallopava
    Dactylaria g.
gallstone ileus
gallus adenolike virus
Gallyas
    G. method
    G. silver staining technique
galoche chin
GALT
    galactose-1-phosphate uridyltransferase
    gastrointestinal associated lymphoid
      tissue

    gut-associated lymphoid tissue
      GALT deficiency
GaLV
    gibbon ape lymphosarcoma virus
galvanic
    g. cell
    g. skin response (GSR)
galvanism
galvanometer
GAL virus
gambiae
    Anopheles g.
Gambian trypanosomiasis
gambiense
    Trypanosoma brucei g.
gametangium
gamete
gametic
    g. chromosome
    g. disease
gametocide
gametocyst
gametocyte
gametocytemia
gametogonia
gametogony
gametoid theory
gametokinetic
gametophagia
gamma
    g. antigen
    g. camera
    g. cell
    g. cell of pancreas
    g. chain disease
    g. efferent
    g. fetoprotein
    g. fiber
    g. globulin (GG)
    g. heavy-chain disease
    g. hemolysis
    IFN g.
    interferon g.
    g. loop
    g. metachromasia
    g. motor neuron
    g. motor system
    g. phage lysis
    g. photo
    g. ray
    g. spectrometer
    g. spectrometry
    g. staphylolysin
    g. streptococcus
    g. thalassemia
    g. well counter
gamma-aminobutyrate
gamma-aminobutyric acid (GABA)
gamma-carboxyglutamate

gammaglobulinopathy
gamma-glutamyltransferase (GGT)
gamma-glutamyl transpeptidase (GGTP)
gamma-ray spectrum
Gammaretrovirus
gammatolerans
    Thermococcus g.
gammopathy
    benign monoclonal g. (BMG)
    biclonal g.
    essential monoclonal g.
    monoclonal g.
    polyclonal g.
Gamna disease
Gamna-Favre body
Gamna-Gandy
    G.-G. body
    G.-G. nodule
gamogony
gamont
gamophagia
Gamsia
Gamstorp syndrome
gandavensis
    Arthrobacter g.
    Cellvibrio g.
Gandy-Gamna
    G.-G. nodule
    G.-G. spleen
Gandy-Nanta disease
ganghwensis
    Nocardioides g.
    Thalassomonas g.
    Zooshikella g.
ganglia (*pl. of* ganglion)
gangliitis
ganglioblast
gangliocyte
gangliocytoma
    hypothalamic g.
ganglioglioma
    desmoplastic infantile g.
gangliolysis
    percutaneous radiofrequency g.
ganglioma
ganglion, pl. **ganglia, ganglions**
    aberrant g.
    Acrel g.
    Andersch g.
    Arnold g.
    Auerbach ganglia
    Bezold g.

g. cell
g. cell of dorsal spinal root
g. cell of retina
Corti g.
g. cyst
diffuse g.
Ganser g.
Lobstein g.
nerve g.
nodose g.
periosteal g.
Soemmerring g.
Troisier g.
unipolar neuron of dorsal root g.
ganglioneuroblastoma (GNB, GNBL)
ganglioneuroma
    central g.
    dumbbell g.
ganglioneuromatosis
ganglionic
    g. blocking agent (GBA)
    g. layer of cerebellar cortex
    g. layer of cerebral cortex
    g. layer of optic nerve
    g. motor neuron
ganglionitis
ganglionopathy
ganglions (*pl. of* ganglion)
ganglioside
    g. GD2 stain
    g. GM_1
    g. GM_2
gangliosidosis
    generalized g.
    GM_1 g.
    GM_2 g.
gangosa
gangrene
    arteriosclerotic g.
    cold g.
    diabetic g.
    dry g.
    embolic g.
    emphysematous g.
    Fournier g.
    gas g.
    hemorrhagic g.
    hot g.
    Meleney g.
    moist g.
    presenile spontaneous g.
    progressive bacterial synergistic g.

G

NOTES

gangrene *(continued)*
    static g.
    symmetrical g.
    thrombotic g.
    trophic g.
    venous g.
    wet g.
    white g.
gangrenescens
    granuloma g.
gangrenosa
    phagedena g.
    vaccinia g.
gangrenosum
    pyoderma g. (PG)
gangrenosus
gangrenous
    g. appendicitis
    g. emphysema
    g. granulomatous inflammation
    g. necrosis
    g. pharyngitis
    g. pneumonia
    g. stomatitis
ganmani
    Helicobacter g.
gannister's disease
Ganoderma
Ganser
    basal nucleus of G.
    G. commissure
    G. ganglion
    nucleus basalis of G.
    G. syndrome
GANT
    gastrointestinal autonomic nerve tumor
gap
    anion g.
    auscultatory g.
    chromatid g.
    isochromatid g.
    g. junction
    g. junction intercellular
      communication
    osmolal g.
    osmolar g.
gap$_0$ period
gap$_1$ period
gap$_2$ period
GAPDH
    glyceraldehyde phosphate dehydrogenase
gapes
gapeworm
gapped ligase chain reaction
Garciella nitratireducens
Gardner-Diamond syndrome
Gardnerella vaginalis
Gardner syndrome
gargantuan mastitis

gargoylism type of histiocyte
garinii
    Borrelia g.
garlic-clove fibroma
garnhami
    Leishmania mexicana g.
Garré
    G. disease
    G. sclerosing osteomyelitis
Gärtner bacillus
Gartner cyst
garvieae
    Streptococcus g.
gas
    g. abscess
    g. amplification
    arsine g.
    arterial blood g. (ABG)
    blood g.
    BTPS conditions of g.
    carrier g.
    g. chromatograph
    g. chromatography (GC)
    g. chromatography-mass
      spectrometry (GC-MS)
    combustible g.
    g. constant
    CS g.
    g. cyst
    D-Stoff (phosgene g.)
    g. embolism
    g. exchange
    extravasation g.
    g. gangrene
    g. gangrene antitoxin
    green cross (phosgene g.)
    HCN g.
    hemolytic g.
    hepatic portal venous g. (HPVG)
    ideal g.
    g. law
    mustard g.
    nettle g.
    oxidizing g.
    P-50 blood g.
    g. peritonitis
    g. phlegmon
    g. retention
    sneeze g.
    g. sterilizer
    g. storage limit
    STPD conditions of g.
    tear g.
    g. thermometer
    tritiated g.
    water g.
    Yperite (mustard g.)
gas-containing abdominal structure
GASDirect test

gaseous spectrum
gasicomitatum
    Leuconostoc g.
gasigenes
    Clostridium g.
Gaskell bridge
gas-liquid chromatography (GLC)
gasometry
gasping disease
Gasser syndrome
gas-solid chromatography (GSC)
Gasteromycetes
Gasterophilidae
Gasterophilus
gastradenitis, gastroadenitis
gastrectasia
gastrectasis
gastri
    Mycobacterium g.
gastric
  g. acid
  g. acid stimulation test
  g. algid malaria
  g. analysis
  g. argentaffin cell
  g. aspirate cell count
  g. atrophy
  g. calculus
  g. carcinoma
  g. carcinoma of the inner stomach
  g. chromoscopy
  g. culture
  g. emptying half time (GET1/2)
  g. emptying time (GET)
  g. fistula
  g. fluid (GF)
  g. follicle
  g. function test
  g. gland
  g. incisura
  g. inhibitory peptide (GIP)
  g. inhibitory polypeptide (GIP)
  g. lamina propria
  g. lavage
  g. lymphoid nodule
  g. mucosa
  g. myiasis
  g. parietal cell (GPC)
  g. parietography
  g. phenotype lesion
  g. pit
  g. polyp

  g. residua
  g. residue examination
  g. smear
  g. tubular adenoma
  g. tumor
  g. ulcer (GU)
  g. volvulus
  g. zymogenic cell
gastrica
  foveola g.
  tunica mucosa g.
gastricae
  glandulae g.
gastrici
  folliculi lymphatici g.
gastrin
  g. assay
  g. releasing peptide (GRP)
gastrin-calcium infusion stimulation test
gastrinoma triangle
gastrin-protein stimulation test
gastrin-secretin stimulation test
gastritis
  acute hemorrhagic erosive g.
  antral g.
  atrophic chronic g.
  autoimmune g.
  catarrhal g.
  chemical g.
  chemotherapy g.
  chronic atrophic g. (CAG)
  chronic hypertrophic g.
  g. cystica polyposa
  g. cystica profunda
  diffuse antral g. (DAG)
  eosinophilic g.
  erosive g.
  exfoliative g.
  g. fibroplastica
  giant hypertrophic g.
  granulomatous g.
  Helicobacter g.
  hemorrhagic g.
  hypertrophic g.
  interstitial g.
  lymphocytic g.
  multifocal atrophic g. (MAG)
  phlegmonous g.
  polypous g.
  pseudomembranous g.
  radiation g.
  reflux g.

G

NOTES

gastritis *(continued)*
    sclerotic g.
    Sydney classification for g.
    varioliform g.
gastroadenitis *(var. of* gastradenitis)
Gastroccult test
gastrocele
gastrocolic fistula
gastrocolitis
gastrocoloptosis
gastrocutaneous fistula
Gastrodiscoides hominis
Gastrodiscus hominis
gastroduodenal fistula
gastroduodenitis
gastroenteritis
    acute infectious nonbacterial g.
    endemic nonbacterial infantile g.
    eosinophilic g. (EGE)
    epidemic nonbacterial g.
    infantile g.
    porcine transmissible g.
    transmissible g.
    transmissible g. virus of swine
    viral g.
    g. virus type A, B
gastroenterocolitis
gastroenteroptosis
gastroesophageal
    g. reflux
    g. reflux disease (GERD)
gastroesophagitis
gastroileitis
gastrointestinal (GI)
    g. adsorbent
    g. anthrax
    g. anthrax infection
    g. associated lymphoid tissue
      (GALT)
    g. autonomic nerve tumor (GANT)
    g. blast injury
    g. bleeding
    g. bleed localization study
    g. blood loss test
    g. cancer
    g. contents
    g. disease
    g. fistula
    g. hemorrhage
    g. hormone
    g. ischemia
    g. mucosal cell
    g. pacemaker cell
    g. pacemaker cell tumor (GIPACT)
    g. protein loss test
    g. smooth muscle tumor
    g. stromal tumor (GIST)
    g. tract carcinoma

    g. tuberculosis
    upper g. (UGI)
gastrojejunal
gastrolienal
gastrolith
gastrolithiasis
gastromalacia
gastromegaly
gastropathy
    hypertrophic hypersecretory g.
gastropexy
Gastrophilidae
Gastrophilus
gastropod
Gastropoda
gastroptosia
gastroptosis
gastrorrhagia
gastrorrhexis
gastroschisis
gastrosia fungosa
Gastrospirillum hominis
gastrostaxis
gastrostenosis
gastrotoxin
gate
gathering
    mass g.
gating
Gaucher
    G. cell
    G. disease
    G. type of histiocyte
gauge
    vacuum g.
Gauma virus
gauss (G)
gaussian distribution
GAVE
    gastric antral vascular ectasia
gay
    G. gland
    g. lymph node syndrome
Gay-Lussac law
gay-related immunodeficiency disease
GB
    NATO code for sarin
GB-7 antibody
GBA
    ganglionic blocking agent
G-banding stain
GBIA
    Guthrie bacterial inhibition assay
GBM
    glioblastoma
    glomerular basement membrane
GC
    gas chromatography
    germinal center

gonococcus
gonorrhea culture
guanine cytosine
GC agar
GC OIA
GC OID
GC value
GCA
germinal cell aplasia
g-cal
gram-calorie
GCC
giant cell collagenoma
glassy cell carcinoma
GCC of the uterine cervix
GCDFP
gross cystic disease fluid protein
GCDFP-15 protein
G-cell tumor
GCF
giant cell fibroblastoma
GCH
giant cell hepatitis
GCIS
isolated gland carcinoma in situ
GCKD
glomerulocystic kidney disease
g-cm
gram-centimeter
GC-MS
gas chromatography-mass spectrometry
G-CSF
granulocyte colony-stimulating factor
GCTB
giant cell tumor of bone
GCT-LMP
giant cell tumor of low malignant
potential
GCTTS
giant cell tumor of tendon sheath
GD
NATO code for soman
gDNA
genomic deoxyribonucleic acid
GDNF
glial cell line-derived neurotropic factor
GDP
guanosine 5′-diphosphate
GDP-L-fucose
GDP-D-mannose

GE
NATO code for nerve agent isopropyl
ethylphosphonofluoridate
G:E
granulocyte/erythroid ratio
Ge antigen
Gedoelstia
gedoelstiosis
Gee disease
Gee-Herter disease
Gee-Herter-Heubner disease
Gee-Thaysen disease
Gegenbaur cell
Geiger-Müller (GM)
G.-M. counter
gel
aluminum hydroxide g.
Coomassie blue-stained g.
denaturing g.
g. diffusion
g. diffusion precipitin test
g. diffusion precipitin test in one
dimension
g. diffusion precipitin test in two
dimensions
g. diffusion reaction
g. electrophoresis
g. electrophoresis pattern
g. filtration
g. and flow cytometry
hydrophilic g.
hydrophobic g.
NuPAGE Bis-Tris g.
polyacrylamide g.
silica g.
Gelasinospora
gelatin
g. agar
g. film
g. filter
fish g.
g. hydrolysis
g. slide adhesive
g. sponge particle
g. zymography
gelatinase
gelatini
Bacillus g.
gelatinoid
gelatinolytic activity
gelatinosa
substantia g.

G

NOTES

gelatinous
    g. acute inflammation
    g. acute pneumonia
    g. adenocarcinoma
    g. ascites
    g. atrophy
    g. carcinoma
    g. infiltration
    g. polyp
    g. substance
    g. tissue
gelatinovorans
    Ruegeria g.
gelation
gel-embedded GA-fixed skeleton
gel-filtration chromatography
gelida
    Desulfofaba g.
Gelidibacter
    G. algens
    G. mesophilus
gelidilacus
    Flavobacterium g.
Gélineau syndrome
Gell
    G. and Coombs classification
    G. and Coombs reaction
Gelman filter
gelosis
gel-permeation chromatography
Gelria glutamica
gem-diol
Gemella
    G. cuniculi
    G. morbillorum
    G. palaticanis
    G. sanguinis
geminate
geminatus
    Anaeroglobus g.
geminin gene
gemistocyte
gemistocytic
    g. astrocyte
    g. astrocytoma
    g. cell
    g. tumor
gemistocytoma
GEMM
    granulocyte, erythrocyte, monocyte, and
    megakaryocyte
gemma
Gemmatimonadaceae
Gemmatimonadales
Gemmatimonadetes
Gemmatimonas aurantiaca
gemmation
gemmule
    Hoboken g.

genal gland
genavense
    Mycobacterium g.
GenBank database
gender reassignment
Gendre
    G. fixative
    G. fluid
gene
    adducin g.
    Aire g.
    allelic g.
    alpha globin g.
    amino acid transporter E16 g.
    g. amplification
    androgen receptor g.
    APC g.
    apoptosis g.
    g. arrangement study
    ataxin g.
    ATP7B g.
    atrophin g.
    autosomal g.
    g. bank
    Bax apoptosis g.
    bcl-1 g.
    beta-catenin g.
    beta globin g.
    bone morphogenetic protein 7 g.
    BRCA1 g.
    BRCA2 g.
    candidate tumor suppressor g.
    caretaker g.
    cationic trypsinogen g.
    CAV1 g.
    CAV2 g.
    CDH1 g.
    CDK4 g.
    cell death g.
    CFTR g.
    chimeric g.
    g. chip technology
    c-Ki-ras g.
    Clara cell secretory protein g.
    claudin 4 g.
    ClCN7 g.
    g. cloning
    c-myc g.
    g. code
    codominant g.
    COL4A5 g.
    collagen type IX alpha 2 g.
    competence g.
    complementary g.
    g. complex
    cyclin D1 g.
    cystic fibrosis transmembrane
      conductance regulator g.
    cytochrome b5 reductase g.

DEL1 g.
g. deletion
derepressed g.
DLK1 g.
dominant g.
g. dosage
DPC4 g.
g. dysregulation
dystrophin g.
E-cadherin g.
Ewing sarcoma g.
exotaxin/CCL11 g.
g. expression
g. expression pattern
g. expression profiling
g. expression signature
factor II g.
FHIT g.
fibrillin g.
FL11 g.
g. flow
FMR-I g.
forkhead box J1 g.
fragile histidine triad g.
frataxin g.
g. frequency
fused novel g.
GAA repeat in the frataxin g.
Gadd153 g.
geminin g.
glucocerebrosidase g.
G6PD g.
Grb7 g.
Grb14 g.
H g.
heme oxygenase-1 g.
HER-2 g.
HER-2/neu g.
hexon g.
hexosaminidase A g.
HFE g.
histocompatibility g.
HLA-DM g.
hMLH 1 g.
holandric g.
hologynic g.
homeobox g.
hPMS2 g.
H-ras g.
human androgen receptor g.
  (HUMARA)
huntingtin g.

IGH g.
immune response g.
Ir g.
Is g.
Jagged1 g.
jumping g.
g. knockout
lethal g.
g. library
LYP g.
major g.
g. mapping
marker g.
MCC g.
Melan-A (MART-1) g.
merlin g.
mismatch repair g.
MLH1 g.
MMR g.
mobile g.
modifying g.
Mrf4 g.
MSH-2 g.
MTND2 g.
MTND5 g.
MTTA g.
mutant g.
mutator g.
myf3 g.
myf4 g.
myf5 g.
MYH9 g.
MyoD family of g.'s
MyoD1 regulatory g.
myopodin g.
myotonin protein kinase g.
NEDD8 g.
neurofibromin g.
NF-1 g.
NOD2 g.
nonfunctional factor VIII-related g.
nonstructural g.
N-ras g.
NuMA g.
operator g.
p15 g.
p16 g.
p53 g.
PAX2 g.
PcG g.
PIG-A g.
p16INK4A g.

G

NOTES

gene *(continued)*
    PMP22 g.
    PMS-1, -2 g.
    pol g.
    g. pool
    p22phox g.
    PRAD1 g.
    procollagen alpha1(I) g.
    g. product
    programmed cell death 4 g.
      (PDCD4)
    prothrombin g.
    prothrombin g. 20210A
    PTEN tumor suppressor g.
    ras g.
    RB g.
    g. rearrangement
    recessive g.
    regulator g.
    regulatory g.
    repressor g.
    retinoblastoma g. (RB1)
    retinoic acid binding protein 1 g.
    14-3-3s g.
    S100A g.
    S100 calcium binding protein
      A1 g.
    secretor g.
    selenoprotein P g.
    SEPT9 g.
    sex-linked g.
    SHH g.
    g. silencing
    silent g.
    single copy g.
    SMN telomeric g.
    SMO g.
    specific g.
    g. splicing
    split g.
    steroid sulfatase g.
    structural g.
    STS g.
    suicide g.
    superoxide dismutase g.
    supplementary g.
    suppressor g.
    survival motor neuron telomeric g.
    synaptopodin g.
    tau g.
    g. therapy
    thioredoxin reductase g.
    g. transcription
    transfer g.
    transforming g.
    TSC1 g.
    TSC2 g.
    tumor suppressor g.
    type I collagen g.

    UPII g.
    UPIII g.
    UP1a uroplakin g.
    UP1b uroplakin g.
    VHL g.
    von Hippel-Lindau g.
    wild-type g.
    WRN g.
    wt1 g.
    XLA g.
    X-linked g.
    XLP g.
    Y-linked g.
    zinc finger g.
    ZYF g.

**GeneAmp PCR System 9600
  thermocycler**
GeneChip
GenePhor
    G. DNA fragment analyzer
    G. DNA silver staining kit
genera (*pl. of* genus)
general
    g. anatomy
    g. dissection technique
    g. feature
    g. gonadotropic activity (GGA)
    g. immunity
    g. paresis (GP)
    g. pathology
    g. peritonitis
    g. radiation
    g. transduction
    g. tuberculosis
generalisata
    hyperostosis corticalis g.
generalisatus
    herpes g.
generalized
    g. activation of thrombosis
    g. anaphylaxis
    g. chondromalacia
    g. cortical hyperostosis
    g. emphysema
    g. eruptive histiocytoma
    g. gangliosidosis
    g. linear mixed model (GLMM)
    g. panhypopituitarism
    g. pustular psoriasis of Zambusch
    g. Sanarelli-Shwartzman reaction
      (GSSR)
    g. Shwartzman phenomenon
    g. Shwartzman reaction (GSR)
    g. transduction
    g. transudation
    g. tuberculosis
    g. vaccinia
    g. xanthelasma

generation
    alternation of g.'s
    first filial g. (F_1)
    parental g. (P_1)
    second filial g. (F_2)
    site of action potential g.
    spontaneous g.
    g. time
generative cell
generator
    aerosol g.
    diazomethane g.
    random number g.
generic
    g. name
    g. substitution
genesistasis
genestatic
gene-targeting
genetic
    g. abnormality
    g. abnormality analysis
    g. adaptation
    g. anemia
    g. balance
    g. code
    g. counseling
    g. determinant
    g. drift
    g. engineering
    g. etiology
    g. fingerprint
    g. hits
    g. linkage analysis
    g. map
    g. mapping
    g. marker
    g. recombination
    g. regulation
    g. screening
    g. susceptibility
    G. Systems HIV-1 Western blot
        test
genetically
    g. abnormal cell
    g. significant dose (GSD)
genetics
    bacterial g.
    bacteriophage g.
    behavior g.
    biochemical g.
    clinical g.

    immunogenetic
    mathematical g.
    medical g.
    mendelian g.
    microbial g.
    molecular g.
    phage g.
    population g.
    reverse g.
    somatic cell g.
Gengou phenomenon
genic balance
genicula (*pl. of* geniculum)
geniculata
    Curvularia g.
geniculocalcarine tract
geniculotemporal tract
geniculum, pl. **genicula**
genioglossus muscle
geniohyoid
genital
    g. condyloma
    g. corpuscle
    g. culture
    g. disorder
    g. gland
    g. herpes
    g. mycoplasma
    g. tract actinomycosis
    g. tubercle
    g. wart
genitalia
    ambiguous external g.
    appearance of external g.
    corpuscula g.
genitalis
    herpes g.
    Treponema g.
genitalium
    Mycoplasma g.
genitourinary
    g. fistula
    g. malformation
    g. myiasis
genoblast
genocopy
genodermatosis
genome
    haploid g. (n)
    human g.
    g. sequencing

G

NOTES

genome *(continued)*
    g. stability
    viral g.
GenomeLab SNPstream genotyping system
genomic
    g. deoxyribonucleic acid (gDNA)
    g. DNA clone (chromosomal)
    g. imprinting
    g. integration
    g. probe
genophenotypic
genospecies
genote
    F g.
genotype
    PiMM g.
    PiMZ g.
genotypic blot hybridization
genotyping
    hereditary hemochromatosis g.
GenProbe
Gen-S
    G.-S automated cell counting instrument
    G.-S hematology analyzer
Gensoul disease
GenSpin gDNA purification kit
Genta
    G. slide
    G. stain
gentian
    g. aniline water
    g. orange stain
    g. violet (GV)
    g. violet stain
gentianophil, gentianophile
gentianophilous
gentianophobic
gentiobiase
Gentle Jane Snap Freezer
Gentra Systems Puregene DNA isolation kit
genu, pl. **genua**
    g. recurvatum
    g. valgum
    g. varum
genus, pl. **genera**
Geobacillus
    G. caldoxylosilyticus
    G. kaustophilus
    G. stearothermophilus
    G. subterraneus
    G. thermocatenulatus
    G. thermodenitrificans
    G. thermoglucosidasius
    G. thermoleovorans
    G. toebii
    G. uzenensis

Geobacter
    G. bremensis
    G. chapellei
    G. grbiciae
    G. hydrogenophilus
    G. pelophilus
    G. sulfurreducens
Geobacteraceae
Geobacteria
Geodermatophilaceae
Geodermatophilus
Geoglobus ahangari
geographic
    g. necrosis
    g. pathology
    g. tongue
geolei
    Thermosipho g.
geometric
    G. Data Miniprep slide maker
    g. efficiency
    g. isomerism
    g. optics
geometrical model
Geomyces pannorus
geophagia
geophilic
Geophilus
geophylla
    Inocybe g.
Georgenia muralis
Georgetown
    hemoglobin C G.
georgianum
    Oesophagostomum g.
Geothrix fermentans
Geotrichoides
geotrichosis
Geotrichum
    G. candidum
    G. immite
geotrichum
    Endomyces g.
    Galactomyces g.
geotropism
Geovibriales
Geovibrio
    G. ferrireducens
    G. thiophilus
Geraghty test
geranylgeranyl diphosphate
Gerbich blood group system
Gerbich-negative
    G.-n. phenotype
    G.-n. red cell
Gerbode defect
GERD
    gastroesophageal reflux disease

Gerhardt
- G. disease
- G. dullness
- G. ferric chloride test
- G. reaction
- G. syndrome
- G. test for acetoacetic acid
- G. test for urobilin in the urine

GERL
Golgi endoplasmic reticulum lysosome

Gerlach
- G. tonsil
- G. valvula

Gerlier disease

germ
- aberrant g.
- g. cell
- g. cell aplasia
- g. cell neoplasm
- g. cell tumor
- g. free (GF)
- g. layer
- g. line
- g. theory
- g. tube
- g. tube test

German
- G. measles
- G. measles virus

germanium
germicidal
germicide
germinal
- g. cell
- g. center (GC)
- g. center of Flemming
- g. center of lymphatic nodule
- g. center of lymph node
- g. epithelial inclusion cyst
- g. epithelium
- g. spot
- g. vesicle

germination tube test
germinativa
- macula g.

germinative
- g. layer
- g. layer of nail

germinativum
- stratum g.

germinoma
- hypophysial stalk g.
- pineal g.

Germiston virus
germline (GL)
- g. configuration
- g. mosaicism
- unrearranged g.
- g. variant

gerneri
- *Acinetobacter* g.

geroderma osteodysplastica
geromarasmus
gerontine
Gerota
- G. capsule
- G. fascia
- G. method

Gerronema
Gerstmann±Straussler±Scheinker disease (Indiana kindred), tau pathology class I
Gerstmann syndrome
gestagen
gestational
- g. age (GA)
- g. alteration
- g. choriocarcinoma
- g. proteinuria
- g. trophoblastic disease (GTD)
- g. trophoblastic neoplasia

gestationis
- herpes g.
- prurigo g.

gestosis
GET
- gastric emptying time

GET1/2
- gastric emptying half time

geV
- giga electron volt

GF
- gastric fluid
- germ free
- gluten free
- NATO code for cyclosarin
- NATO code for nerve agent cyclohexyl methylphosphonofluoridate

GFAP
- glial fibrillary acidic protein

GFP
- green fluorescence protein

NOTES

G

GFR
glomerular filtration rate
GG
gamma globulin
GGA
general gonadotropic activity
GGT
gamma-glutamyltransferase
GGT assay
GGTP
gamma-glutamyl transpeptidase
GH
growth hormone
GHD
growth hormone deficiency
Ghent
albumin G.
GH-IH
growth hormone-inhibiting hormone
Ghon
G. complex
G. focus
G. primary lesion
G. tubercle
Ghon-Sachs
G.-S. bacillus
G.-S. complex
G.-S. focus
G.-S. primary lesion
G.-S. tubercle
ghost
g. bands
blood g.
g. cell
g. corpuscle
g. forms
ghoul hand
GH-RF
growth hormone-releasing factor
GH-RH
growth hormone-releasing hormone
GH-RIH
growth hormone release inhibiting
hormone
GHz
gigahertz
GI
gastrointestinal
Gi
gilbert (unit of magnetomotive force)
Giannuzzi
G. crescent
G. demilune
Gianotti-Crosti syndrome
giant
g. anorectal condyloma acuminatum
g. baby
g. band
g. blue nevus

g. cell
g. cell aortitis
g. cell arteritis
g. cell carcinoma
g. cell carcinoma of thyroid gland
g. cell collagenoma (GCC)
g. cell fibroblastoma (GCF)
g. cell fibroma
g. cell glioblastoma
g. cell hepatitis (GCH)
g. cell interstitial pneumonia (GIP)
g. cell myeloma
g. cell myocarditis
g. cell reaction
g. cell reparative granuloma
g. cell thyroiditis
g. cell tumor
g. cell tumor of bone (GCTB)
g. cell tumor of lung
g. cell tumor of tendon sheath
(GCTTS)
g. colon
g. condyloma
g. condyloma of Buschke-
Löwenstein
g. fibroadenoma
g. follicle lymphoma
g. follicular lymphoblastoma
g. follicular lymphoma
g. gastric fold
g. hairy nevus
g. hamartoma
g. hives
g. hypertrophic gastritis
g. hypertrophy of gastric mucosa
g. intestinal fluke
g. intracanalicular fibroadenoma
g. liver fluke
g. melanosome
g. mitochondrion
g. neutrophil
g. neutrophilia
g. osteoid osteoma
g. pigmented nevus
g. platelet
g. platelet disease
g. platelet syndrome
g. rugal hypertrophy
g. urticaria
giantism
Giardia
G. intestinalis
G. lamblia
giardiasis dysentery
Giardiavirus
Gibberella
gibbon ape lymphosarcoma virus
(GaLV)
gibbus deformity

Gibco-BRL TriZol DNA extraction
Gibney disease
Gibson-Cooke sweat test
gibsoniae
> *Desulfotomaculum* g.

gibsonii
> *Streptomyces* g.

Giemsa
> G. chromosome banding stain
> G. method

Gierke
> G. cell
> G. corpuscle
> G. disease

Gieson
> elastica van G. (EVG)
> Verhoeff-van G. (VVG)

giga (G)
> g. electron volt (geV)

gigahertz (GHz)
gigantea
> *Calvatia* g.

giganteus
> *Aspergillus* g.

gigantica
> *Fasciola* g.

gigantism
> exomphalos, macroglossia, and g. (EMG)

gigantocellular glioma
gigantomastia
Gigantorhynchus
gigohm
GIK
> glucose, insulin, and potassium

gilardii
> *Roseomonas* g.
> *Wautersia* g.

gilbert
> G. disease
> gilbert (unit of magnetomotive force) (F, Gi)
> G. syndrome

Gilchrist
> G. disease
> G. mycosis

gill-arch skeleton
Gilles de la Tourette syndrome
Gill #2 hematoxylin blue stain
Gillies flap
gillisiae
> *Flavobacterium* g.

Gillisia limnaea
Gilmaniella
gilvus
> *Enterococcus* g.

GIM
> gonadotropin-inhibitory material

Gimenez stain
gingival
> g. cyst
> g. epithelium
> g. fluid
> g. hyperplasia
> g. tissue

gingivalis
> *Entamoeba* g.

gingivitis
> acute necrotizing ulcerative g.
> diphenylhydantoin g.
> hypertrophic g.
> necrotizing ulcerative g. (NUG)
> scorbutic g.

gingivodental ligament
gingivosis
gingivostomatitis
> herpetic g.
> necrotizing ulcerative g.

ginkgetin
ginkgolide
GIP
> gastric inhibitory peptide
> gastric inhibitory polypeptide
> giant cell interstitial pneumonia

GIPACT
> gastrointestinal pacemaker cell tumor

Girard
> G. method
> G. reagent

GISA
> glycopeptide-insensitive *Staphylococcus aureus*

GIST
> gastrointestinal stromal tumor

gitalin
gitaloxin
Gitelman syndrome
gitoxin
GITT
> glucose insulin tolerance test

gitter cell, gitterzelle
GKA
> glucokinase activator

G

NOTES

GL
  germline
  greatest length
glabellar
glabra
  verruca g.
glabrata
  Biomphalaria g.
  Candida g.
  Torulopsis g.
glabrosa
glabrous skin
glacial
  g. acetic acid
  g. acetic acid fixative
glaciale
  Brumimicrobium g.
Glaciecola
  G. mesophila
  G. pallidula
  G. polaris
  G. punicea
gland
  accessory lacrimal g.
  accessory parotid g.
  accessory suprarenal g.
  accessory thyroid g.
  acid g.
  acinic cell tumor of salivary g.
  acinotubular g.
  acinous g.
  admaxillary g.
  adrenal g.
  aggregate g.
  agminate g.
  albuminous g.
  alveolar g.
  anal g.
  anterior lingual g.
  apical g.
  apocrine sweat g.
  areolar g.
  arteriococcygeal g.
  arytenoid g.
  Avicenna g.
  axillary sweat g.
  Bauhin g.
  g. of biliary mucosa
  Blandin g.
  Bowman g.
  brachial g.
  bronchial g.
  Bruch g.
  Brunner g.
  buccal g.
  bulbourethral g.
  BUS g.'s
  cardiac g.
  ceruminous g.

cervical g.
chief cell of parathyroid g.
Ciaccio g.
ciliary g.
circumanal g.
clear cell carcinoma of salivary g.
clear cell hyperplasia of
  parathyroid g.
coccygeal g.
coil g.
compound exocrine g.
conjunctival g.
convoluted endometrial g.
Cowper g.
g. crowding
ductless g.
duct of Skene g.
duodenal g.
Duverney g.
Ebner g.
eccrine g.
Eglis g.
endocrine g.
esophageal g.
g. of eustachian tube
excretory duct of sweat g.
excretory duct of tracheal g.
excretory ductules of lacrimal g.
exocrine g.
external salivary g.
follicle of thyroid g.
follicular g.
fundic g.
Galeati g.
gastric g.
Gay g.
genal g.
genital g.
giant cell carcinoma of thyroid g.
Gley g.
greater vestibular g.
Guérin g.
hair-independent sebaceous g.
hemal g.
hematopoietic g.
hemolymph g.
hibernating g.
holocrine g.
hyperplastic g.
internal salivary g.
g. of internal secretion
interscapular g.
interstitial g.
intestinal g.
intraepithelial g.
jugular g.
Knoll g.
Krause g.
labial g.

labial salivary g. (LSG)
lacrimal g.
lactiferous g.
laryngeal g.
lesser vestibular g.
Lieberkühn g.'s
Littre g.
lobe of mammary g.
lobule of mammary g.
lobule of thyroid g.
Luschka cystic g.
lymph g.
major salivary g.
malpighian g.
mammary g.
marrow-lymph g.
master g.
maxillary g.
medulla of adrenal g.
meibomian g.
merocrine g.
mesenteric g.
milk g.
minor salivary g.
mixed tumor of salivary g.
Moll g.
g. of mouth
mucilaginous g.
muciparous g.
mucous acini of the posterior
  lingual g.
mucus secreting cervical g.
mucus secreting labial g.
nasal g.
nodular myofibroblastic stromal
  hyperplasia of the mammary g.
Nuhn g.
odoriferous g.
oil g.
olfactory g.
oxyntic g.
pacchionian g.
palatine g.
palpebral g.
parathyroid g.
paraurethral g.
parotid g.
pectoral g.
peptic g.
perspiratory g.
Peyer g.
pharyngeal g.

Philip g.
pileous g.
pineal g.
pituitary g.
Poirier g.
polymorphous low-grade carcinoma
  of salivary g.
prehyoid g.
preputial g.
prostate g.
pyloric g.
racemose g.
Rivinus g.
Rosenmüller g.
saccular g.
salivary g.
sebaceous g.
secretory g.
sentinel g.
seromucous g.
serous g.
Serres g.
sexual g.
Sigmund g.
simple branched g.
Skene g.
solitary g.
stroma of thyroid g.
sublingual g.
submandibular salivary g.
submaxillary g.
sudoriferous g.
suprahyoid g.
suprarenal g.
Suzanne g.
sweat g.
target g.
tarsal g.
Terson g.
Theile g.
thymus g.
thyroid g.
Tiedemann g.
tracheal g.
trachoma g.
tubular g.
tubuloacinar g.
tubuloalveolar mucous g.
tympanic g.
Tyson g.
unbranched simple tubular
  exocrine g.

NOTES

G

gland *(continued)*
    unicellular g.
    uterine g.
    vaginal g.
    vascular g.
    vesical g.
    vestibular g.
    vulvovaginal g.
    Waldeyer g.
    Wasmann g.
    Weber g.
    Wepfer g.
    Wölfler g.
    Wolfring g.
    Zeis g.
glanders
    g. bacillus
    g. pneumonia
glandes (*pl. of* glans)
gland-forming malignancy
glandilemma
glandula, pl. **glandulae**
    g. atrabiliaris
    g. basilaris
    g. bulbourethralis
    glandulae circumanales
    ductuli excretorii g.
    glandulae intestinales
    g. lacrimalis
    g. lingualis anterior
    g. mammaria
    g. mucosa
    g. parathyroidea
    g. parotidea
    g. parotidea accessoria
    g. parotis
    g. parotis accessoria
    g. pituitaria
    g. prostatica
    g. salivaria
    g. seromucosa
    g. serosa
    g. sublingualis
    g. submandibularis
    g. suprarenalis
    g. thyroidea
    g. thyroidea accessoria
    g. vestibularis major
glandulae
    g. areolares
    g. buccales
    g. ceruminosae
    g. cervicales uteri
    g. ciliares
    g. conjunctivales
    g. cutis
    g. duodenales
    g. endocrinae
    g. esophageae

    g. gastricae
    g. glomiformes
    g. labiales
    g. lacrimales accessoriae
    g. laryngeae
    g. mucosae biliosae
    g. nasales
    g. olfactoriae
    g. oris
    g. palatinae
    g. pharyngeales
    g. preputiales
    g. pyloricae
    g. sebaceae
    g. sine ductibus
    g. sudoriferae
    g. suprarenales accessoriae
    g. tarsales
    g. tracheales
    g. tubariae
    g. urethrales femininae
    g. urethrales masculinae
    g. uterinae
    g. vestibulares minores
glandular
    g. budding
    g. cancer
    g. carcinoma
    g. cell
    g. dysplasia
    g. epithelium
    g. fever
    g. hyperplasia
    g. mastitis
    g. metaplasia
    g. odontogenic cyst
    g. pharyngitis
    g. proliferation
    g. schwannoma
    g. structure
    g. substance of prostate
    g. system
glandularis
    cystitis g.
    g. proliferans cholecystitis
    pyelitis g.
    ureteritis g.
glandule
glandulous
glans, pl. **glandes**
Glanzmann
    G. disease
    G. thrombasthenia
Glanzmann-Naegeli thrombasthenia
Glanzmann-Riniker syndrome
GLA-protein
    bone GLA-p. (BGP)
glass
    g. body

cover g.
g. electrode
g. factor
g. fiber filter
flint g.
ground g.
heat-resistant g.
low-actinic g.
object g.
optical g.
Wood g.
glass-bead retention method
glass-blower's mouth
glass-ceramic
glasses
safety g.
glassy
g. cell carcinoma (GCC)
g. cytoplasm
g. membrane
glauca
Forcipomyia g.
glauciflava
Actinomadura g.
glaucoma
angle closure g.
congenital g.
infantile g.
open-angle g.
primary g.
secondary g.
glaucomatous
g. habit
g. pannus
glaucosuria
glaucum
Corynebacterium g.
glaucus
Aspergillus g.
GLC
gas-liquid chromatography
Gleason
G. pattern
G. prostate carcinoma score
G. tumor grade
Glénard disease
Glenner-Lillie stain for pituitary
glenohumeral joint instability
Glenospora graphii
Gley
G. cell
G. gland

glia
Bergmann g.
g. cell
gliacyte
gliadin
gliae
membrana limitans g.
glial
g. cell
g. cell line-derived neurotropic factor (GDNF)
g. fibrillary acidic protein (GFAP)
g. filament
glicentin
glioblast
glioblastoma (GBM)
g. cell line
giant cell g.
g. multiforme
gliocladium
Aspergillus g.
gliofibrillary acidic protein
glioma
brainstem g.
gigantocellular g.
lipidized g.
malignant g.
mixed g.
nasal g.
g. of optic chiasm
optic nerve g.
g. of the spinal cord
subependymal g.
telangiectatic g.
Gliomastix murorum
gliomatosis
g. cerebri
peritoneal g.
g. peritonei
gliomatous
gliomyxoma
glioneuroma
gliosarcoma
gliosis
g. of brain stem
fibrillary g.
isomorphous g.
pulvinar g.
g. uteri
gliotoxin

NOTES

G

433

Glisson
    G. cirrhosis
    G. disease
glissonian sheath
glissonitis
glitter cell
GLMM
    generalized linear mixed model
GLOB collection
globe cell anemia
globi (*pl. of* globus)
Globicatella sulfidifaciens
Globidium
globin-chain
    g.-c. electrophoresis
    g.-c. synthesis
globin insulin
globispora
    Sporosarcina g.
Globocephalus
globoid
    g. cell leukodystrophy
    g. encapsulated tumor
globose specialization
globoside
globular
    g. leukocyte
    g. monomer
    g. protein
    g. space of Czermak
    g. sputum
    g. thrombus
    g. value
globular-fibrous transformation
globule
    acidophilic yolk g.
    dentin g.
    hyaline g.
    polar g.
globuliferous phagocyte
globulin
    accelerator g. (AcG)
    alpha g.
    alpha-1 g.
    alpha-2 g.
    antidiphtheritic g.
    antihemophilic g. (AHG)
    antihemophilic g. A, B
    antihuman g. (AHG)
    antilymphocyte g. (ALG)
    antilymphocytic g.
    antimacrophage g. (AMG)
    antithoracic duct lymphocytic g.
    (ATDLG)
    antithymocyte g. (ATG)
    beta-1A g.
    beta-1C g.
    beta-1E g.
    beta-1F g.

    Bence Jones g.
    beta g.
    bovine gamma g. (BGG)
    chickenpox immune g. (human)
    corticosteroid-binding g. (CBG)
    cortisol-binding g. (CBG)
    equine antihuman lymphoblast g.
    (EAHLG)
    gamma g. (GG)
    hepatitis B immune g. (HBIG)
    horse antihuman thymus g.
    (HAHTG)
    human-derived botulism immune g.
    human gamma g. (hGG)
    human milk factor g.
    human rabies immune g. (HRIG)
    immune serum g. (ISG)
    liver-derived sex steroid-binding g.
    measles immune g. (human)
    pertussis immune g.
    plasma accelerator g.
    poliomyelitis immune g. (human)
    rabies immune g.
    $Rh_o(D)$ immune g.
    serum accelerator g.
    sex hormone-binding g.
    specific immune g. (human)
    steroid hormone binding g.
    (SHBG)
    g. test
    testosterone-estradiol binding g.
    (TeBG)
    tetanus immune g.
    thyroid-binding g. (TBG)
    thyroxine-binding g. (TBG)
    unbound thyroxine-binding g.
    (UTBG)
    vaccinia immune g. (VIG)
    g. X
    zoster immune g. (ZIG)
globulinemia
    IgA g.
globulinuria
globulomaxillary cyst
globulus
globus, pl. **globi**
Gloeobacterales
Gloeobacteria
Gloeocystidiellum
Gloeophyllum
Gloeosporium
glomangioma
glomangiomatous osseous malformation syndrome
glomangiopericytoma
glomangiosis
    pulmonary g.
glome
glomera (*pl. of* glomus)

glomerata
    Actinocorallia g.
Glomerella
glomerular
    g. barrier
    g. basal lamina
    g. basement membrane (GBM)
    g. basement membrane antibody
    g. basement membrane disease
    g. crescent
    g. cyst
    g. disorder
    g. filtrate
    g. filtration
    g. filtration rate (GFR)
    g. layer of olfactory bulb
    g. nephritis
    g. sclerosis
    g. tuft
glomerular-like cluster
glomerule
glomeruli (*pl. of* glomerulus)
glomerulitis
glomeruloid hemangioma
glomerulonephritis,
  pl. **glomerulonephritides (GN)**
    acute g. (AGN)
    acute crescentic g.
    acute exudative g.
    acute hemorrhagic g.
    acute poststreptococcal g.
    acute proliferative g.
    antibasement membrane g.
    Berger focal g.
    chronic g. (CGN)
    chronic membranous g. (CMGN)
    crescentic anti-GBM g.
    cryoglobulinemic g.
    diffuse extracapillary proliferative g.
    Ellis type 1 g.
    embolic g.
    epimembranous g.
    experimental autoimmune g. (EAG)
    extramembranous g.
    exudative g.
    fibrillary g.
    focal embolic g.
    focal necrotizing g.
    healed g.
    hemorrhagic g.
    hypocomplementemic g.

    idiopathic pauciimmune necrotizing crescentic g.
    immune complex g.
    immunotactoid g.
    induced g.
    lobular g.
    local g.
    membranoproliferative g. (MPGN)
    membranous g. (MGN)
    mesangial proliferative g.
    mesangiocapillary g.
    mesangioproliferative g.
    necrotizing g.
    pauciimmune g.
    pauciimmune crescentic and necrotizing g.
    postinfectious g.
    poststreptococcal g. (PSGN)
    proliferative g.
    rapidly progressive g. (RPGN)
    segmental g.
    subacute g.
    type II membranoproliferative g.
glomerulopathy
    focal sclerosing g.
    immune complex g.
    immunotactoid g.
    nonmyloidotic fibrillary g.
    proliferative g.
glomerulosa
    g. cell
    zona g.
glomerulosclerosis
    cirrhotic g.
    diabetic g.
    focal segmental g.
    intercapillary g.
    nodular g.
glomerulose
glomerulus, pl. **glomeruli**
    bloodless glomeruli
    capsula glomeruli
    malpighian g.
    g. of mesonephros
    obsolescent g.
    olfactory g.
    g. of pronephros
    Ruysch glomeruli
glomiformes
    glandulae g.
glomus, pl. **glomera**
    glomera aortica

G

NOTES

glomus (*continued*)
  g. body
  g. caroticum
  g. cell
  g. coccygeum
  g. jugulare tumor
  paraganglioma g.
  g. pulmonale
  g. vagale
gloriae
  Trichophyton g.
Glossina
  G. morsitans
  G. pallidipes
  G. palpalis
glossinidius
  Sodalis g.
glossitis
  atrophic g.
  Hunter g.
  median rhomboid g.
glottis, pl. **glottides**
glove juice technique
gloves
  chemical-resistant inner g.
  chemical-resistant outer g.
  Skinsense g.
glow modulator tube
Glu
  glutamic acid
glucagon
  gut g.
  g. hypersecretion
  immunoreactive g. (IRG)
  plasma g.
  g. response test
glucagonoma
glucaldrate
  potassium g.
glucan-branching
  g.-b. enzyme
  g.-b. glycosyltransferase
Glucatell beta-glucagan blood test kit
glucitol
glucocerebrosidase gene
glucocerebroside
glucocorticoid
  g. receptor (GR)
  g. suppressible aldosteronism
  g. therapy
glucocorticoid-glucocorticoid receptor complex
glucocorticoid-GR complex
glucocorticosteroid
glucofuranose
glucogenesis
glucogenic amino acid
glucohemia
glucokinase activator (GKA)

Gluconacetobacter
  G. entanii
  G. intermedius
  G. johannae
  G. oboediens
gluconate
  potassium g.
gluconeogenesis
gluconeogenetic
glucopenia
glucopyranose
glucosamine
glucose
  g., age, lactate dehydrogenase, aspartate aminotransferase, white blood cells (GA LAW)
  g. assay
  Benedict test for g.
  blood g. (BG)
  buffered desoxycholate g. (BDG)
  cerebral metabolic rate of g. (CMRG)
  cerebrospinal fluid g.
  conversion of g.
  dexamethasone, insulin, and g. (DIG)
  fasting plasma g. (FPG)
  g. fingerstick test
  g., insulin, and potassium (GIK)
  g. insulin tolerance test (GITT)
  maximal tubular reabsorption of g. (T_{mg})
  g. metabolism
  mole of g.
  g. oxidase
  g. oxidase method
  g. oxidase paper strip test
  g. oxidase test
  postprandial g.
  premeal g.
  renal threshold for g.
  g. suppression test
  g. tolerance (GT)
  g. tolerance factor (GTF)
  g. tolerance test (GTT)
  urine g.
glucose-format broth
glucose-nitrogen ratio (G:N)
glucose-6-phosphatase
  absence of g.-6-p.
  g.-6-p. hepatorenal deficiency glycogenosis
glucosephosphate
  g. isomerase
  g. isomerase assay
  g. isomerase deficiency
glucose-1-phosphate
glucose-6-phosphate
  g.-6-p. dehydrogenase (G6PD)

G

NOTES

glycerinated lymph
glycerin-potato broth
glycerol gelatin medium
glycerolization
glycerolize
glycerol-3-phosphate oxidase (GOI)
glycerophosphate
    potassium g.
glycerophosphatide
glyceryl triacetate
glycine (Gly)
    g. assay
    urine g.
glycine-arginine reaction
glycinemia
glycine-rich beta-glycoprotein
glycinuria
Glyciphagus
    G. buski
    G. domesticus
Glycobacteria
glycocalyx
glycochenodeoxycholate
glycochenodeoxycholic acid
glycocholate
glycocholic acid
glycoconjugate
    lipid-linked g.
glycodeoxycholic acid
glycogen
    g. acanthosis
    accumulation of g.
    g. branching enzyme
    cytoplasmic g.
    g. degradation
    g. digestion
    g. granule
    hepatic g.
    g. infiltration
    intracytoplasmic g.
    g. particle
    g. phosphorylase
    g. phosphorylase isoenzyme BB
    (GPBB)
    g. stain
    g. staining
    g. (starch) synthase
    g. storage
    g. storage disease (GSD)
    g. storage disorder (GSD)
    g. storage test
    g. synthesis
    tissue g.
glycogenesis
glycogenic acanthosis
glycogenolysis
glycogenolytic

glycogenosis
    glucose-6-phosphatase hepatorenal
     deficiency g.
    hepatophosphorylase deficiency g.
    hepatorenal g.
    idiopathic generalized g.
    myophosphorylase deficiency g.
    type V g.
glycogen-rich squamous cell carcinoma
glycoglycinuria
glycohistochemistry
glycol
    ethylene g.
    g. methacrylate
    polyethylene g.
    propylene g.
glycolate
    sodium g.
glycolic
    g. acid
    g. acid test
    g. aciduria
glycolipid
    g. layer
    g. lipidosis
    g. stain
    g. staining
glycolithocholic acid
glycolysis
    anaerobic g.
glycolytic enzyme
Glycomycetaceae
Glycomycineae
glycone
glyconeogenesis
glycopenia
glycopeptide
glycopeptide-insensitive *Staphylococcus aureus* (GISA)
Glycophagus
glycophorin A staining
glycoprotein (GP)
    acid g.
    alpha acid g.
    alpha-1 acid g.
    biliary g. (BGP)
    cell surface g.
    extracellular matrix g.
    gpIa g.
    gpIc g.
    gpIIa g.
    gpIIb g.
    gpIIIa g.
    g. hormone
    nonlineage specific
     transmembrane g.
    platelet membrane g.
    g. receptor
    g. stain

g. staining
submaxillary g.
thrombomodulin g. (TM)
tumor-associated g. (TAG)
glycoprotein-1
glycoprotein-2
epithelial g. (EGP-2)
glycoproteinase
glycoptyalism
glycopyrrolate
glycopyrronium bromide
glycorrhachia
glycorrhea
glycosaminoglycan (GAG)
glycosaminolipid
glycosialia
glycosidase
glycoside
cardiac g.
cyanophoric g.
digitalis g.
sterol g.
glycosphingolipid
glycosuria
alimentary g.
benign g.
digestive g.
normoglycemic g.
pathologic g.
phloridzin g.
renal g.
toxic g.
glycosuric melituria
glycosylase
uracil DNA g. (UDG)
glycosylated
g. hemoglobin
g. hemoglobin assay
g. hemoglobin test
glycosylation
N-linked g.
glycosyl ceramide
glycosylphosphatidylinositol (GPI)
g. specific phospholipase D (GPI-PLD)
glycosyltransferase
alpha glucan-branching g.
glucan-branching g.
glycuresis
glycuronuria
glycyl (Gly)
glycyl-glycine dipeptidase

glycyl-leucine dipeptidase
glycyltryptophan test
Glycyphagus domesticus
glyodin
glyoxylate reductase
glyoxylic acid test
GM
Geiger-Müller
GM instrument
g-m
gram-meter
GM-CSF
granulocyte-macrophage colony-stimulating factor
Gmelin test
GM$_1$ gangliosidosis
GM$_2$ gangliosidosis
GMP
guanosine monophosphate
cyclic GMP
3′:5′-GMP
GMS
Grocott methenamine silver
GMS stain
GMW
gram molecular weight
GN
glomerulonephritis
gram-negative
GN broth
G:N
glucose-nitrogen ratio
gnat
Gnathostoma
G. doloresi
G. hispidum
G. nipponicum
G. siamense
G. spinigerum
gnathostomiasis
GNB, GNBL
ganglioneuroblastoma
GNID
gram-negative intracellular diplococci
Gnomonia
Gnomoniopsis
gnotobiology
gnotobiota
gnotobiote
gnotobiotic
gnotophoresis

NOTES

G

GnRH
gonadotropin-releasing hormone
goatpox
goat's milk anemia
goblet
g. cell
g. cell adenocarcinoma
g. cell carcinoid
Godwin tumor
Gofman test
GOG
gynecologic oncology group
goggles
safety g.
GOI
glycerol-3-phosphate oxidase
goiter
aberrant g.
acute g.
adenomatous g.
colloid g.
congenital g.
cystic g.
diffuse nontoxic g.
diving g.
dyshormonogenic g.
endemic g.
exophthalmic g.
familial g.
fibrous g.
follicular g.
lingual g.
lymphadenoid g.
microfollicular g.
multinodular g.
multiple colloid adenomatous g.
  (MCAG)
nodular colloid g.
nodular hyperplastic g.
nontoxic g. (NTG)
parenchymatous g.
simple g.
sporadic diffuse g.
sporadic nodular g.
substernal g.
suffocative g.
thoracic g.
toxic g. (TG)
wandering g.
goitrous
gold
g. assay
g. chloride
g. chloride reagent
colloidal g. (CG)
7C g. urine protein test
g. cyanide (AuCN)
g. particle
protein A g. (PAG)

g. sol test
g. standard
g. therapy
g. toning
gold-198
Goldberg-Maxwell syndrome
Goldblatt
G. hypertension
G. kidney
Goldenhar syndrome
Goldflam disease
Goldflam-Erb disease
Goldscheider disease
Goldstein disease
Goldz-Gorlin syndrome
golf hole ureteral orifice
Golgi
G. apparatus
G. cavity alteration
G. cell
G. complex
G. endoplasmic reticulum lysosome
  (GERL)
G. internal reticulum
G. membrane alteration
G. osmiobichromate fixative
G. stain
G. tendon organ
G. vacuole alteration
G. vesicle alteration
G. zone
Golgi-Mazzoni corpuscle
golgiokinesis
Goltz syndrome
GOM
granular osmiophilic material
Gomori
G. aldehyde fuchsin stain
G. chrome alum hematoxylin-
  phloxine stain
G. methenamine silver stain
G. method for chromaffin
G. nonspecific acid phosphatase
  stain
G. nonspecific alkaline phosphatase
  stain
G. one-step trichrome stain
G. silver impregnation stain
**Gomori-Jones periodic acid-methenamine
silver stain**
Gomori-Takamatsu
G.-T. procedure
G.-T. stain
gonad
streak g.
gonadal
g. agenesis
g. aplasia
g. dysgenesis

g. endocrine disorder
g. ridge
g. shield
g. streak
g. stromal tumor
gonadoblastoma
gonadotrope adenoma
gonadotroph
gonadotropic hormone (GTH)
gonadotropin
chorionic g. (CG, CGT)
deficiency of g.
human chorionic g. (HCG, hCG)
human menopausal g. (HMG)
human pituitary g. (hPG)
menopausal g.
pituitary g.
pregnant mare serum g. (PMSG)
g. test
total urinary g. (TUG)
urinary chorionic g. (UCG)
gonadotropin-inhibitory material (GIM)
gonadotropin-producing adenoma
gonadotropin-releasing
g.-r. agent (GRA)
g.-r. factor (GRF)
g.-r. hormone (GnRH)
g.-r. hormone stimulation test
gonarthritis
gonatagra
gonatocele
gondii
Toxoplasma g.
gondwanensis
Psychroflexus g.
gonecystolith
gonensis
Anoxybacillus g.
Gongronella
Gongylonema pulchrum
gongylonemiasis
gonidial (colony) (G)
gonioma
gonitis
gonocele
gonococcal
g. arthritis
g. arthritis-dermatitis syndrome
g. conjunctivitis
g. ophthalmia
g. peritonitis

gonococcemia
gonococcus, pl. **gonococci (GC)**
gonocyte
gonohemia
gonophage
gonorrhea culture (GC)
gonorrheal
g. ophthalmia
g. rheumatism
g. salpingitis
gonorrhoeae
chromosomally mediated resistant
Neisseria g.
Neisseria g.
gonorrhoica
macula g.
gonotoxemia
gonotoxin
gonotyl
Gonyaulax catanella
Good
G. antigen
G. syndrome
goodfellowii
Leptotrichia g.
Goodpasture
G. stain
G. syndrome
Goormaghtigh cell
Gopalan syndrome
Gordius
G. *aquaticus*
G. *robustus*
Gordon
G. agent
G. body
G. and Sweets stain
G. syndrome
G. test
gordonae
Mycobacterium g.
Gordonia
G. *aichiensis*
G. *amarae*
G. *amicalis*
G. *bronchialis*
G. *desulfuricans*
G. *hirsuta*
G. *hydrophobica*
G. *namibiensis*
G. *nitida*
G. *paraffinivorans*

NOTES

G

Gordonia (continued)
    G. *polyisoprenivorans*
    G. *rubropertincta*
    G. *sihwensis*
    G. *sinesedis*
    G. *sputi*
    G. *terrae*
    G. *westfalica*
Gordoniaceae
gordoniae
    Rhodococcus g.
gordonii
    Streptococcus g.
Gordon-Sweet staining
Gorham disease
Goriaew rule
Gorlin-Chaudhry-Moss syndrome
Gorlin-Goltz syndrome
Gorlin-Psaume syndrome
Gorlin syndrome
gormanii
    Legionella g.
Gorman syndrome
gorondou
gossypol compound
GOT
    glutamic-oxaloacetic transaminase
Göthlin capillary fragility test
Gottlieb
    epithelial attachment of G.
Gottron papule
gottschalkii
    Anaerobranca g.
Gougerot-Blum
    G.-B. disease
    G.-B. syndrome
Gougerot-Carteaud syndrome
gougerotii
    Sporotrichum g.
Gougerot-Ruiter disease
Gougerot-Sjögren disease
goundou
gourvilii
    Trichophyton g.
gout
    abarticular g.
    articular g.
    calcium g.
    lead g.
    g. nephropathy
    saturnine g.
    tophaceous g.
gouty
    g. arthritis
    g. nephropathy
    g. tophus
    g. urine
Gower
    G. 1, 2 hemoglobin

Gowers
    G. solution
    G. syndrome
GP
    general paresis
    glycoprotein
    gram-positive
GPAIS
    guinea pig antiinsulin serum
GPBB
    glycogen phosphorylase isoenzyme BB
GPC
    gastric parietal cell
G6PD
    glucose-6-phosphate dehydrogenase
        A or B isozyme of G6PD
        G6PD gene
        G6PD Mediterranean variant
        mutation
        G6PD test
G6PH deficiency anemia
GPI
    glycosylphosphatidylinositol
    gram-positive identification
        Vitek GPI
gpIa glycoprotein
gpIc glycoprotein
gpIIa glycoprotein
gpIIb glycoprotein
GPIIb/IIIa
    platelet GPIIb/IIIa
gpIIIa glycoprotein
GPIPID
    guinea pig intraperitoneal infectious dose
GPI-PLD
    glycosylphosphatidylinositol specific
        phospholipase D
GPK
    guinea pig kidney
        GPK antigen
GPKA
    guinea pig kidney absorption (test)
GPO-DAOS method
GPS
    gray platelet syndrome
    guinea pig serum
GPT
    glutamic-pyruvic transaminase
GPT-binding protein
GPUT
    galactose phosphate uridyltransferase
GR
    glucocorticoid receptor
    glutathione reductase
GRA
    gonadotropin-releasing agent
graafian follicle
grab urine specimen

gracile
> *Trichosporon* g.

Gracilibacillus
> *G. dipsosauri*
> *G. halotolerans*

Gracilicutes

gracilis
> *Desulfovibrio* g.
> *Euglena* g.
> fasciculus g.
> *Hylemonella* g.
> *Nitrospina* g.
> g. syndrome

grade
> ACS g.
> analytical reagent g.
> AR g.
> g. I–IV astrocytoma
> g. I-IV ependymoma
> Fuhrman nuclear g.
> Gleason tumor g.
> high g. (HG)
> histological tumor g.
> g. 1, 2 neuroendocrine carcinoma
> Nottingham histologic g.
> prostatic intraepithelial neoplasia, mild dysplasia or low g. (PIN 1)
> prostatic intraepithelial neoplasia, moderate dysplasia or high g. (PIN 2)
> prostatic intraepithelial neoplasia, severe dysplasia or high g. (PIN 3)
> reagent g.
> weapon g.

Gradenigo syndrome

gradient
> average g.
> chemotactic g.
> colloidal silica g.
> fetal repertoire g.
> g. gel electrophoresis
> serum ascites albumin g. (SAAG)
> sucrose density g. (SDG)
> transmural g.

grading
> cytologic nuclear g.
> histologic g.
> Kernohan malignant astrocytoma g.
> Nottingham modification of Scarff-Bloom-Richardson g.
> tumor g.

graduated
> g. cylinder
> g. pipette

Graefe disease

Graffi virus

graft
> allogeneic g.
> autogeneic g.
> autologous g.
> autoplastic g.
> bone g. (BG)
> coronary artery bypass g. (CABG)
> heterologous g.
> heteroplastic g.
> heterospecific g.
> homologous g.
> homoplastic g.
> interspecific g.
> isogeneic g.
> isologous g.
> isoplastic g.
> material g.
> g. rejection
> serum chemistry g. (SCG)
> skin g. (SG)
> split-thickness skin g. (STSG)
> syngeneic g.
> g. versus host disease (GVHD)
> g. versus host reaction (GVHR)
> white g.
> xenogeneic g.

Graham
> G. law
> G. Little syndrome

Graham-Cole test

Grahamella

grain
> corps g.'s
> g. count halving time
> g. itch
> g. itch mite

gram (g)
> g. iodine
> g. ion
> g. method
> g. molecular weight (GMW)
> G. solution
> G. stain
> G. stain of stool

gram-calorie (g-cal)

gram-centimeter (g-cm)

Gram-chromotrope stain

NOTES

G

443

gramicidin
graminis
    Erysiphe g.
    Paenibacillus g.
    Puccinia g.
graminophila
    Heterodera g.
gram-meter (g-m)
gram-negative (GN)
    g.-n. bacillus
    g.-n. bacterium
    g.-n. broth
    g.-n. cocci
    g.-n. endotoxemia
    g.-n. intracellular diplococci (GNID)
grampicola
    Crassicauda g.
gram-positive (GP)
    g.-p. bacillus
    g.-p. bacterium
    g.-p. cocci
    g.-p. identification (GPI)
Gram-Sure reagent
Gram-Weigert stain
grana
granddaughter cyst
grandis
    Diplogonoporus g.
grand mal epilepsy
Grandry corpuscle
Granger method
Granit loop
granivorans
    Paenibacillus g.
Gr antigen
granular
    g. atrophy
    g. cell ameloblastoma
    g. cell myoblastoma
    g. cell schwannoma
    g. cell tumor
    g. conjunctivitis
    g. degeneration
    g. deposition
    g. endoplasmic reticulum
    g. golden appearance
    g. kidney
    g. layer of cerebellar cortex
    g. layer of cerebral cortex
    g. layer of epidermis
    g. layer of a vesicular ovarian
      follicle
    g. leukoblast
    g. leukocyte
    g. pharyngitis
    g. pneumocyte
    g. pneumonocyte
    g. urethritis

    g. urinary cast
    g. vaginitis
granulare
    Trichophyton g.
granularity
    eosinophilic g.
granularum
    Acholeplasma g.
    Mycoplasma g.
granulatio, pl. granulationes
    granulationes arachnoideae
granulation
    arachnoid g.
    Bayle g.
    cytoplasmic g.
    pacchionian g.
    g. tissue
    toxic g.
granule
    acidophil g.
    acrosomal g.
    acrosome g.
    alpha g.
    Altmann g.
    amphophil g.
    argentaffin g.
    autophagic g.
    azurophil g.
    azurophilic g.
    Babès-Ernst g.
    basal g.
    basophil g.
    basophilic g.
    Bensley specific g.
    beta g.
    Birbeck g.
    Bollinger g.
    bull's eye g.
    g. cell
    g. cell of connective tissue
    chromatic g.
    chromatophilic g.
    chromophil g.
    chromophobe g.
    cone g.
    Crooke g.
    delta g.
    dense-core neurosecretory g.
    dense secondary g.
    g.'s of developing neutrophils
    diazo stain for argentaffin g.'s
    electron lucent g.
    elementary g.
    endocrine g.
    eosinophil g.
    eosinophilic g.
    Fordyce g.
    fuchsinophil g.
    glycogen g.

Grawitz g.
haloed g.
Heinz g.
intranuclear perichromatin g.
iodophil g.
juxtaglomerular g.
kappa g.
keratohyalin g.
keratohyalin-like g.
lamellar g.
Langerhans g.
Langley g.
light-staining g.
lipofuscin g.
membrane-coating g.
metachromatic g.
mucigen g.
mucinogen g.
neurosecretory g.'s
Neusser g.
neutrophil g.
Nissl g.
oxyphil g.
paravacuolar g.
pentalaminar g.
pigment g.
primary g.
proacrosomal g.
prosecretion g.
rod g.
round secretory g.
sand g.
Schüffner g.
secondary g.
secretory g.
seminal g.
siderocytic g.
siderotic g.
smoker's g.
specific g.
sulfur g.
toxic g.
Zimmermann g.
zymogen g.
Granulicatella
  G. adiacens
  G. balaenopterae
  G. elegans
granuloblast
granulocyte
  band form g.
  coelomic g.

g. colony-stimulating factor (G-CSF)
g. concentrate
hypersegmented g.
hypogranular g.
hyposegmented g.
immature g.
g. pheresis
polymorphonuclear g.
g. recovery
segmented g.
g. transfusion
g. transfusion support
granulocyte, erythrocyte, monocyte, and megakaryocyte (GEMM)
granulocyte/erythroid ratio (G:E)
granulocyte-macrophage
  colony-forming unit g.-m. (CFU-GM)
  g.-m. colony-stimulating factor (GM-CSF)
granulocytic
  g. aplasia
  g. blood cell
  g. hyperplasia
  g. hypoplasia
  g. leukemia
  g. precursor cell
  g. sarcoma (GS)
  g. series
granulocytopenia
granulocytopoiesis
granulocytopoietic
granulocytosis
granulogenesis
granuloma
  amebic g.
  g. annulare
  apical g.
  barium g.
  beryllium g.
  bilharzial g.
  calcified g.
  caseating g.
  Churg-Strauss g.
  coccidioidal g.
  cutaneous extravascular necrotizing g.
  dental g.
  g. endemicum
  eosinophilic g.
  g. faciale

NOTES

G

445

granuloma *(continued)*
    foreign body g.
    g. gangrenescens
    giant cell reparative g.
    histiocytic g.
    Hodgkin g.
    infectious g.
    g. inguinale
    g. inguinale tropicum
    intramucosal loose g.
    Kaposi sarcoma-like g.
    laryngeal g.
    lethal midline g.
    lipoid g.
    lipophagic g.
    Majocchi g.
    malignant g.
    midline lethal g.
    midline malignant reticulosis g.
    mineral oil g.
    multifocal eosinophilic g.
    necrobiotic g.
    noncaseating g.
    nonnecrotizing g.
    oily g.
    palisading g.
    paracoccidioidal g.
    parasitic g.
    periapical g.
    pericryptal g.
    plasma cell g. (PCG)
    pulmonary hyalinizing g. (PHG)
    pyogenic g.
    g. pyogenicum
    reparative giant cell g.
    reticulohistiocytic g.
    ring g.
    sarcoid g.
    g. sarcoid
    sarcoidal g.
    schistosome g.
    sea urchin g.
    silica g.
    silicone g.
    spermatocytic g.
    spermatogenic g.
    suture g.
    swimming pool g.
    g. telangiectaticum
    tuberculoid g.
    tuberculoid-type g.
    unifocal eosinophilic g.
    uterine g.
    Windelmann g.
    zirconium g.

granulomatis
    Calymmatobacterium g.
    Cephalosporium g.
    Donovania g.

granulomatosis
    allergic g.
    angiitic g.
    benign lymphocytic angiitis and g.
    bronchocentric g. (BCG)
    g. disciformis chronica et progressiva
    eosinophilic g.
    Langerhans cell g. (LCG)
    lipophagia g.
    lipophagic intestinal g.
    lymphomatoid g. (LYG)
    Miescher g.
    necrotizing sarcoid g. (NSG)
    g. siderotica
    Wegener g.

granulomatous
    g. angiitis with eosinophilia
    g. colitis
    g. disease
    g. disease of childhood
    g. encephalomyelitis
    g. endometritis
    g. enteritis
    g. gastritis
    g. hepatitis
    g. inflammation
    g. lesion
    g. mastitis
    g. orchitis
    g. polyp
    g. process
    g. thyroiditis

granulomere
granulopenia
granuloplasm
granuloplastic
granulopoiesis
granulopoietic
granulopoietin
granulosa
    g. cell carcinoma
    g. cell tumor
    g. lutein cell
    membrana g.
    Oospora g.
    pars g.

granulosa-stromal cell tumor
granulosa-theca cell tumor
granulosis
    Noguchia g.
    g. rubra nasi

granulosity
granulosum
    Propionibacterium g.
    stratum g.
    Trichophyton g.
    Trichosporon g.

granulosus
> *Echinococcus* g.
> *Noguchia* g.
> *Oceanicola* g.

granulovacuolar degeneration
Granulovirus
granum
granzyme B
grape
> Carswell g.
> g. cell
> g. ending
> g. mole

graph
> Davenport g.
> g. tablet

graphesthesia, graphanesthesia
graphic
> g. analysis
> g. terminal

graphii
> *Glenospora* g.

graphite pneumoconiosis
Graphium
graphomotor
graphospasm
grappe
> en g.

grating
> diffraction g.
> replica g.

gravel
> coarse g.

Graves disease
grave wax
gravidarum
> fibroma molle g.
> hyperemesis g.
> molluscum fibrosum g.
> nephritis g.
> striae g.

gravimetric
Gravindex pregnancy test
gravis
> anemia g.
> colitis g.
> icterus g.
> myasthenia g.

gravitation abscess

gravity
> g. concentration
> specific g. (SG, sp gr)

gravity-settling culture (GSC)
Gravlee jet wash
Grawitz
> G. basophilia
> G. granule
> G. tumor

gray
> g. area
> g. commissure
> g. degeneration
> g. fiber
> g. hepatization
> g. induration
> g. infiltration
> g. patch
> g. platelet syndrome (GPS)
> g. scale
> g. zone lymphoma

grayi
> *Listeria* g.

grayish-white colony
gray-patch ringworm
Grb7 gene
Grb14 gene
grbiciae
> *Geobacter* g.

great
> g. alveolar cell
> g. pestilence
> G. Smokies Diagnostic Laboratories intestinal permeability test kit
> g. vessel

greater
> g. omentum
> g. vestibular gland

greatest length (GL)
green
> brilliant g.
> bromcresol g.
> g. cancer
> g. cross (phosgene gas)
> ethyl g.
> fast g.
> g. fluorescence protein (GFP)
> g. hemoglobin
> indocyanine g. (ICG)
> malachite g.
> methyl g.
> g. monkey virus

NOTES

G

green *(continued)*
    Paris g.
    g. pus
    g. sickness
    g. sputum
Greenfield disease
Greenhow disease
greenstick fracture
gregaloid
Gregarina
gregarine
Gregarinia
gregarinosis
Greig syndrome
**Greiner Vacuette coagulation plastic
    tube**
Gremmeniella
grenade
    ethylbromoacetate g.
grenz
    g. ray
    g. zone
gresilensis
    Legionella g.
Grey Turner sign
GRF
    gonadotropin-releasing factor
    growth hormone-releasing factor
grid
    aligned g.
    Bucky g.
    copper g.
    crossed g.
    focused g.
    g. index
    Kova Glasstic Slide #10 with g.'s
    g. line
    nickel g.
    ocular g.
    parallel g.
    Potter-Bucky g.
    g. ratio
    Westgard selection g.
Gridley
    G. stain
    G. stain for fungi
Griesinger disease
Griess reagent
griffe
    main en g.
griffin
    G. beaker
    g. claw
Griffith
    G. classification
    G. point
Grifola
grignonense
    Ochrobactrum g.

Grimelius
    G. argyrophil reaction
    G. argyrophil stain method
    G. stain
Grimontia hollisae
grimontii
    Acinetobacter g.
    Pseudomonas g.
grinder
    Potter-Elvehjem handheld tissue g.
grinder's asthma
grip
    devil's g.
Griphosphaeria corticola
grippe
    Balkan g.
Griscelli syndrome
grisea
    commissura anterior g.
    Madurella g.
griseofulvin
Grisonella ratellina
gristle
Grocott-Gomori
    G.-G. methenamine silver method
    G.-G. methenamine silver stain
groin ulcer
Grönblad-Strandberg syndrome
Groome assay
groove
    Blessig g.
    coffee-bean g.
    complementary g.
    Harrison g.
    Liebermeister g.
    g. of nail matrix
    nuclear g.
    peptide-binding g.
    g. sign
    skin g.
gross
    g. cystic disease fluid protein
    (GCDFP)
    g. deletion
    g. description
    G. disease
    g. hematuria
    g. lesion
    G. leukemia virus
    G. virus antigen (GSA)
ground
    g. glass
    g. glass appearance colony
    g. glass attenuation
    g. glass cell
    g. glass cytoplasm
    g. glass hepatocyte
    g. glass opacity
    g. itch anemia

g. lamella
g. state
g. substance

group
g. A beta hemolytic streptococci throat culture
ABO blood g.
acetyl g.
g. of activating substance
acyloxy g.
g. agglutination
g. agglutinin
g. A hapten
alkyl g.
g. antigens
arbovirus g. A, B, C
aryl g.
g. A *Streptococcus*
g. B arbor virus
blood g.
Bombay blood g.
g. B *Streptococcus*
g. 1 carcinogen
CH/RG blood g.
concentration-time product for 50% of exposed g. (Ct_{50})
connective tissue g.
control g.
coryneform g.
cross-reactive g. (CREG)
cytophil g.
determinant g.
g. D *Streptococcus*
functional g.
guanidinium g.
gynecologic oncology g. (GOG)
high mobility g. (HMG)
hydroxyl g.
I blood g.
g. I-IV mycobacteria
g. immunity
isogenous g.
Kell blood g. (K)
Kell-Cellano blood g.
keto g.
Kidd blood g.
Lewis blood g.
Lutheran blood g.
MNSs blood g.
National Bladder Cancer Collaborative G. (NBCCG)
g. N *Streptococcus*

P blood g.
PDC kinase molecule g.
Pediatric Oncology G. (POG)
peptide g.
platinum g.
polycomb g.
P-related blood g.
prenyl g.
prosthetic g.
proteus g.
psittacosis-lymphogranuloma venereum-trachoma g.
g. reaction
Rh blood g.
salmonella g.
g. specific amplification (GSA)
g. specific antigen
spotted fever g. (SFG)
sulfhydryl g.
symmetry g.
thiocarbonyl g.
g. transfer
ventral respiratory g.

grouping
antigenic structural g.
blood g.
haptenic g.
Lancefield g.
reverse g.

Grover disease
grower
rapid g.

growing
g. ovarian follicle
g. point

growth
g. acceleration
accretionary g.
g. alteration
appositional g.
g. arrest
autonomous g.
auxetic g.
g. disorder
disordered epithelial g.
exophytic g.
g. fraction
g. fraction with Ki-67
g. hormone (GH)
g. hormone deficiency (GHD)
g. hormone-inhibiting hormone (GH-IH)

NOTES

G

growth (*continued*)
  g. hormone-producing adenoma
  g. hormone release inhibiting hormone (GH-RIH)
  g. hormone-releasing factor (GH-RF, GRF)
  g. hormone-releasing hormone (GH-RH)
  g. hormone suppression test
  g. by hypertrophy
  g. inhibitory factor
  interstitial g.
  intussusceptive g.
  multiplicative g.
  new g.
  g. pattern
  g. plate
  Regaud pattern of g.
  g. retardation
  Schmincke pattern of g.
  turban g.
growth-stimulating hormone (GSH)
GRP
  gastrin releasing peptide
Gruber syndrome
Gruber-Widal reaction
Grubyella
grumous
gryochrome
GS
  granulocytic sarcoma
GSA
  Gross virus antigen
  group specific amplification
GSC
  gas-solid chromatography
  gravity-settling culture
GSD
  genetically significant dose
  glycogen storage disease
  glycogen storage disorder
GSE
  gluten-sensitive enteropathy
GSH
  glutathione
  growth-stimulating hormone
GSR
  galvanic skin response
  generalized Shwartzman reaction
  gunshot residue
    GSR test
GSSG
  glutathione disulfide
  oxidized glutathione
GSSR
  generalized Sanarelli-Shwartzman reaction

GT
  glucose tolerance
  glutamyl transpeptidase
GTD
  gestational trophoblastic disease
GTF
  glucose tolerance factor
GTH
  gonadotropic hormone
GTP
  guanosine triphosphate
GTPase-activating protein
GTT
  glucose tolerance test
GU
  gastric ulcer
guaiac
    stool g.
    g. test
guaiac-based fecal occult blood test
guaiacin
guaiacolsulfonate
    potassium g.
Guam
    amyotrophic lateral sclerosis/parkinsonism±dementia complex of G.
Guama virus
Guanarito virus
guanase
guanidine isothiocyanate method
guanidinemia
guanidinium
    g. extraction
    g. group
guanidino-aminovaleric acid
guanine
    g. cell
    g. cytosine (GC)
    cytosine phosphate g. (CpG)
    g. deaminase
    g. deaminase assay
guanosine
    g. 3′,5′-cyclic phosphate
    g. diphosphate
    g. 5′-diphosphate (GDP)
    g. monophosphate (GMP)
    g. 5′-phosphate
    g. triphosphate (GTP)
guanylic acid
guanyl-nucleotide-binding protein
guanylyl
guard cell
Guarnieri body
Guaroa virus
guaymasensis
    Persephonella g.
Gubler
    G. line

G. paralysis
G. syndrome
G. tumor
Gudden atrophy
Guérin gland
guideline
emergency response planning g.
(ERPG)
Guignardia
Guillain-Barré syndrome
Guilliermondella
guilliermondi
Candida g.
guinea
g. green B
g. pig antigen
g. pig antiinsulin serum (GPAIS)
g. pig intraperitoneal infectious
dose (GPIPID)
g. pig kidney (GPK)
g. pig kidney absorption (test)
(GPKA)
g. pig serum (GPS)
g. worm infection
Guinon disease
Gulf War syndrome
Gull disease
Gull-Sutton syndrome
Gulosibacter molinativorax
gumma, pl. **gummata, gummas**
syphilitic g.
tuberculous g.
gummatous
g. abscess
g. syphilid
g. ulcer
gummosa
periarteritis g.
scrofuloderma g.
gummy
Gumprecht shadow
gums
strawberry g.
Gun Hill hemoglobin
Gunning-Lieben test
Gunn syndrome
gunpowder
g. mark lesion
g. stippling
gunshot
g. residue (GSR)
g. wound

Günther disease
Günzberg
G. reagent
G. test
Gussenbauer artificial larynx
gustation
gustatorius
caliculus g.
porus g.
gustatory
g. bud
g. cell
g. organ
g. pore
g. sweating syndrome
gustus
organum g.
gut-associated lymphoid tissue (GALT)
gut glucagon
Guthrie
G. bacterial inhibition assay
(GBIA)
G. card
G. test
Gutman unit
guttata
morphea g.
parapsoriasis g.
Guttavirus
gutter
paracolic g.
guttiformis
Staleya g.
guttural duct
gutturotetany
Gutzeit test
guyanensis
Leishmania braziliensis g.
GV
gentian violet
GVHD
graft versus host disease
GVHR
graft versus host reaction
gyiorum
Kerstersia g.
Gymnamoebida
Gymnascella
Gymnoascaceae
Gymnoascus dankaliensis
Gymnodinium breve
Gymnophalloides seoi

G

NOTES

Gymnopilus
gymnothecium
gynandrism
gynandroblastoma
gynandromorphism
gynecogen
gynecoid
gynecologic oncology group (GOG)
gynecomastia, gynecomasty
gypseum
    Microsporum g.
gyrata
    cutis verticis g.

gyrate
    g. atrophy
    g. erythema
gyrectomy
gyrochrome cell
Gyrodactylus
Gyromitra esculenta
GyroTwister
Gyrovirus
gyrus
    cingulate g.

H
   Hauch
   Holzknecht unit
   Hounsfield unit
   NATO code for impure sulfur mustard
      H agglutination
      H agglutinin
      H antibody
      H antigen
      H band
      H chain
      H colony
      cytolipin H
      H disc
      H and E staining
      H gene
      H substance
H-2
      H-2 antigen
      H-2 complex
H3
   tritium
H+
      increased arterial H.
h
   Planck constant
h
   Planck
¹H
   protium
HA
   hyaluronic acid
HAA
   hepatitis-associated antigen
Ha-1A monoclonal antibody
Haagensen test
habenulae perforatae
Habermann disease
Haber syndrome
Haber-Weiss reaction
habit
      endothelioid h.
      glaucomatous h.
      leukocytoid h.
habitual abortion
habituation
Habronema
      H. majus
      H. megastoma
      H. microstoma
      H. muscae
habronemiasis
HACA
   human antichimeric antibody

HACEK
   Haemophilus, Actinobacillus,
      Cardiobacterium, Eikenella, Kingella
Haddad syndrome
Hadfield-Clarke syndrome
Hadobacteria
Hadrurus
HAEC
   Hirschsprung-associated enterocolitis
Haemadipsa ceylonica
Haemagogus
Haemamoeba
Haemaphysalis
      H. cinnabarina
      H. concinna
      H. leachi
      H. leporis-palustris
      H. spinigera
haematobium
      Schistosoma h.
Haematopinus
Haematopota
Haemobartonella
haemocanis
      Mycoplasma h.
Haemococcidium
Haemodipsus ventricosus
haemofelis
      Mycoplasma h.
haemoglobinophilus
      Haemophilus h.
Haemogregarina
haemolytica
      Pasteurella h.
      Thermomonas h.
haemolyticum
      Arcanobacterium h.
      Clostridium h.
haemolyticus
      Haemophilus h.
      Staphylococcus h.
haemomuris
      Mycoplasma h.
Haemonchus
      H. contortus
      H. placei
haemoperoxidus
      Enterococcus h.
Haemophileae
haemophilum
      Mycobacterium h.
Haemophilus
      H., Actinobacillus, Cardiobacterium,
         Eikenella, Kingella (HACEK)
      H. actinomycetemcomitans

H

Haemophilus *(continued)*
  H. aegyptius
  H. aphrophilus
  H. bovis
  H. bronchisepticus
  H. ducreyi
  H. duplex
  factor X for *H.*
  H. felis
  H. haemoglobinophilus
  H. haemolyticus
  H. influenzae
  H. influenzae pneumonia
  Koch-Weeks *H.*
  H. parahaemolyticus
  H. parainfluenzae
  H. parapertussis
  H. paraphrophilus
  H. paratropicalis
  H. pertussis vaccine (HPV)
  H. segnis
  H. suis
  H. vaginalis
Haemoproteus
haemorrhoidalis
  Sarcophaga h.
Haemosporida
Haemosporina
Haenszel test
haeundaensis
  Paracoccus h.
Haff disease
Haffkine vaccine
Hafnia alvei
hafnium
Hageman factor (HF)
hageni
  Otomyces h.
Haglund disease
Hagner disease
Hahella chejuensis
Hahn oxine reagent
HAHTG
  horse antihuman thymus globulin
HAI
  hemagglutinin inhibition
  histologic activity index
  HAI titer
Hailey-Hailey disease
hair
  h. analysis
  auditory h.
  h. ball
  beaded h.
  h. bulb
  h. cell (HC)
  club h.
  corkscrew h.
  h. cross

cuticle of h.
h. cycle
h. disc
h. follicle
ingrown h.
lanugo h.
h. papilla
h. root
Schridde cancer h.
taste h.
telogen h.
vellus h.
hair-independent sebaceous gland
hair-like filamentous projection
hairpin
  h. DNA
  h. loop
**hairpin-mediated polymerase slippage
  model**
HAIRscreen drug test
hairworm
hairy
  h. cell
  h. cell leukemia (HCL)
  h. heart
  h. mole
Hakim syndrome
Halanaerobacter salinarius
Halanaerobiaceae
Halanaerobiales
Halanaerobium
  H. fermentans
  H. kushneri
Halberstaedter-Prowazek body
Haldane
  H. effect
  H. hypothesis
Hale colloidal iron stain
half-bandwidth
half-cell
half-life
  biologic h.
  biological h.
  effective h.
  physical h.
  terminal h. (T$\frac{1}{2}$)
half-maximum
  full-width h.
half-moon
  red h.-m.
half-reaction
half time
half-value layer (HVL)
half-wave
  h.-w. potential
  h.-w. rectifier
Haliangium
  H. ochraceum
  H. tepidum

Halicephalobus
halichoeri
    Streptococcus h.
halide
halisteresis phenomenon
halisteretic
Hall
    H. disease
    H. method
Haller
    H. cone
    H. line
    H. tunica vasculosa
    H. vas aberrans
    H. vascular tissue
Hallermann-Streiff-François syndrome
Hallermann-Streiff syndrome
Hallervorden-Spatz
    H.-S. disease
    H.-S. disease, tau pathology class
    H.-S. syndrome
Hallervorden syndrome
Hallgren syndrome
hallmark
    h. of protein-secreting cell
    h. of steroid-secreting cell
Hallopeau disease
Hallopeau-Siemens syndrome
hallucination
    shared h.
hallucinogen
halo
    anemic h.
    h. melanoma
    h. nevus
    perinuclear h.
Haloarcula quadrata
Halobacillus
    H. karajensis
    H. locisalis
    H. salinus
Halobacteria
Halobacteriaceae
Halobacteriales
Halobacteroidaceae
Halobiforma
    H. haloterrestris
    H. nitratireducens
Halococcus dombrowskii
halocynthiae
    Halomonas h.

halodurans
    Alkalilimnicola h.
    Roseivivax h.
haloed granule
Haloferax
    H. alexandrinus
    H. lucentense
halogen
halogenated hydrocarbon assay
halogenation
halogenoderma
Halomebacteria
halometer
Halomicrobium mukohataei
Halomonadaceae
Halomonas
    H. alimentaria
    H. anticariensis
    H. axialensis
    H. boliviensis
    H. campisalis
    H. halocynthiae
    H. hydrothermalis
    H. magadiensis
    H. marisflavi
    H. maura
    H. muralis
    H. neptunia
    H. organivorans
    H. sulfidaeris
    H. ventosae
Halonatronum saccharophilum
Halon system
haloperidol assay
halophila
    Desulfocella h.
    Hongiella h.
    Nitrosomonas h.
    Prauserella h.
    Saccharomonospora h.
halophile
halophilus
    Aestuariibacter h.
    Algoriphagus h.
    Halothiobacillus h.
haloprogin
halorespirans
    Sulfurospirillum h.
Halorhabdus utahensis
Halorhodospira neutriphila
Halorubrum
    H. tebenquichense

NOTES

H

455

Halorubrum (continued)
   H. terrestre
   H. tibetense
   H. xinjiangense
Halosimplex carlsbadense
Halospirulina tapeticola
halosteresis
haloterrestris
   Halobiforma h.
Haloterrigena
   H. thermotolerans
   H. turkmenica
halothane
   h. assay
   h. hepatitis
Halothiobacillus
   H. halophilus
   H. hydrothermalis
   H. kellyi
   H. neapolitanus
halotolerans
   Corynebacterium h.
   Gracilibacillus h.
   Jeotgalicoccus h.
   Nesterenkonia h.
   Nocardiopsis h.
   Roseivivax h.
   Yania h.
Halsted
   H. law
   H. mastectomy
Halteridium
halzoun
HAM
   HTLV-1 associated myelopathy
   human alveolar macrophage
   HAM 56 antibody
Ham
   H. paroxysmal nocturnal
     hemoglobinuria test
   H. test for anemia
HAMA
   human antimouse antibody
   human antimurine antibody
Hamamatsu high-sensitivity
  photomultiplier tube
hamartia
hamartin protein
hamartoblastoma
hamartochondromatosis
hamartoma
   cystic h.
   giant h.
   leiomyomatous h.
   mesenchymal h.
   neurocristic h.
   neurovascular h.
   peribiliary gland h.
   pulmonary h.

   renal h.
   urothelial leiomyomatous h.
hamartomatous
   h. polyp
   h. tumor
hamburgensis
   Nitrobacter h.
Hamburger
   H. law
   H. phenomenon
hamelinense
   Roseibium h.
Hamel test
Hamigera
Hamilton
   H. pseudophlegmon
   H. Rating Scale (HRS)
Hamman
   H. disease
   H. syndrome
Hamman-Rich
   H.-R. disease
   H.-R. syndrome
Hammarsten
   H. reagent
   H. test
hammered copper colony
Hammerschlag method
Hammersmith hemoglobin
hammock ligament
Hammond disease
hamster
   h. egg penetration assay
   h. egg penetration test
hamulosa
   Cheilospirura h.
HAN
   Health Alert Network
hand
   crab h.
   H. disease
   ghoul h.
   mechanic's h.
   opera-glass h.
   skeleton h.
   spade h.
   trident h.
hand-foot-and-mouth
   h.-f.-a.-m. disease
   h.-f.-a.-m. disease virus
hand-foot syndrome
hand-foot-uterus syndrome
handgun
   semiautomatic h.
handling
   toxic chemical h.
Hand-Schüller-Christian
   H.-S.-C. disease
   H.-S.-C. type of histiocyte

HandyStep electronic repeating pipette
HANE
    hereditary angioneurotic edema
Hanes equation
Hanger test
hanging-block culture
hanging-drop culture
Hanhart syndrome
Hanker-Yates reagent
Hannebertia
Hanot
    H. cirrhosis
    H. disease
Hanot-Chauffard syndrome
Hansel stain
Hanseman cell
Hansemann macrophage
Hansen
    H. bacillus
    H. disease
Hanseniaspora
hansenii
    Debaryomyces h.
    Desulfofaba h.
    Desulfomusa h.
Hansenula
Hantaan virus
hantavirus pulmonary syndrome
HAP
    heredopathia atactia polyneuritiformis
HAP1
    huntingtin-associated protein 1
HAPA
    hemagglutinating antipenicillin antibody
hapalonychia
Haplographium
haploid
    h. cell
    h. genome (n)
    h. number
haploidy
haploinsufficiency
haploinsufficient
Haplorchis
Haplosporangium parvum
Haplosporidia
haplotype association study
happy puppet syndrome
Hapsburg
    disease of H.
hapten
    conjugated h.

    group A h.
    h. inhibition of precipitation
    h. X, Y antigen
haptenic grouping
haptoglobin (hp)
    h. assay
    h., Hp^1 and Hp^2
    h. test
Harada-Mori filter paper strip culture
Harada syndrome
Ha-ras mutation
hard
    h. chancre
    h. pad disease
    h. pad virus
    h. papilloma
    h. sore
    h. tissue
    h. tubercle
    h. ulcer
hardened pelvis
harderoporphyria
Harding-Passey melanoma
Hardy-Weinberg law
harei
    Peptoniphilus h.
Hare syndrome
Hargraves cell
haricot broth
Harleco synthetic resin
Harlem
    hemoglobin C H.
harlequin
    h. color change
    h. fetus
Harley disease
harmaline
harmine
harmonic
Harris
    H. alum hematoxylin
    H. and Ray test
    H. staining method
    H. syndrome
Harrison
    H. groove
    H. test
Hartmann
    H. pouch
    H. solution

NOTES

H

Hartmannella
>   *H. hyalina*
>   *H. veriformis*

hartmannellae
>   *Neochlamydia h.*

hartmanni
>   *Entamoeba h.*

Hartnup
>   H. disease
>   H. syndrome

Harvard criteria of irreversible coma

harvest
>   h. bug
>   h. mite

Harzia

Hasegawaea

Häser formula

HASH
>   human achaete-scute homolog

Hasharon hemoglobin

HASHD
>   hypertensive arteriosclerotic heart disease

Hashimoto
>   H. disease
>   H. struma
>   H. thyroiditis

Hassall
>   H. body
>   H. concentric corpuscle

Hassall-Henle wart

Hasselbalch equation

hassiacum
>   *Novosphingobium h.*

Hassin syndrome

HAT
>   heparin-associated thrombocytopenia
>   hypoxanthine-aminopterin-thymidine

hatchetti
>   *Acanthamoeba h.*

hatching
>   h. flask
>   h. test

hathewayi
>   *Clostridium h.*

Hauch (H)
>   ohne H.

Haute
>   hemoglobin Terre H.

HAV
>   hepatitis A virus

Haverhill fever

Haverhillia
>   *H. moniliformis*
>   *H. multiformis*

haversian
>   h. canal
>   h. lamella
>   h. space
>   h. system

Hawaii agent

hawaiiensis
>   *Bipolaris h.*

hawkinsin

hawkinsinuria

Hawkins sign

Haworth formula

hay
>   h. asthma
>   h. bacillus
>   h. fever

Hayem
>   H. hematoblast
>   H. solution

Hayem-Widal
>   H.-W. anemia
>   H.-W. syndrome

Hayflick limit

Haygarth node

hazard
>   h. identification
>   radiation h.
>   h. symbol

hazardous
>   h. concentration
>   h. material
>   h. materials labeling
>   H. Materials Response Unit (HMRU)
>   h. substance

HB
>   heart block

Hb
>   hemoglobin
>>   Hb Bart
>>   Hb Bart hydrops fetalis
>>   Hb Chesapeake
>>   Hb CS
>>   Hb D
>>   Hb Kansas
>>   Hb Köln

HBA71 antigen

HB$_c$Ab
>   antibody to hepatitis B core antigen
>   hepatitis B core antibody

HB$_c$Ag
>   hepatitis B core antigen

HBc antigen immunodetection

HbCO, HbCo
>   carboxyhemoglobin

HBD, HBDH
>   hydroxybutyrate dehydrogenase

HB$_e$Ab
>   hepatitis Be antibody

HB$_e$Ag
>   hepatitis Be antigen

HBF
>   hepatic blood flow

HbF
fetal hemoglobin
HBI
high serum-bound iron
HBIG
hepatitis B immune globulin
HBLV
human B lymphotropic virus
HBME 1
human mesothelial cell membrane
HBME 1 antibody
HbO$_2$
oxyhemoglobin
HbS
sickle cell hemoglobin
sulfhemoglobin
HB$_s$Ab
hepatitis B surface antibody
HB$_s$Ag
hepatitis B surface antigen
HbSS
homozygous hemoglobin S
HBV
hepatitis B virus
HBV DNA marker
HBW
high birth weight
HC
hair cell
Huntington chorea
hydroxycorticoid
NATO code for military obscurant smoke
(zinc oxide and hexachloroethane,
grained aluminum)
hc2
Hybrid Capture 2
hc2 CMV DNA test
hc2 HPV DNA test
HCA
hepatocellular adenoma
h-caldesmon (HCD)
HCC
hepatocellular carcinoma
hydroxycholecalciferol
metastatic hepatocellular carcinoma
HCCC
hyalinizing clear cell carcinoma
HCC-CC
clear cell hepatocellular carcinoma
HCD
h-caldesmon

HCG, hCG
human chorionic gonadotropin
HCG alpha subunit
beta HCG
HCG beta subunit
Icon II HCG
HCL
hairy cell leukemia
HCN
hydrogen cyanide
HCN gas
NATO code for HCN (AC)
HCO$_3$
bicarbonate
HCO$_3$ concentration
HCP
hereditary coproporphyria
HCR
hypocretin
hCSM
human chorionic somatomammotropin
HCT
homocytotrophic
hydrochlorothiazide
Hct
hematocrit
HCU
homocystinuria
HCV
hepatitis C virus
HCVD
hypertensive cardiovascular disease
HD
heart disease
high dosage
Hirschsprung disease
Hodgkin disease
Huntington disease
hydatid disease
NATO code for distilled (neat) sulfur
mustard
HD allele version
HDA
heteroduplex analysis
HDAC
histone deacetylase
HDAC inhibitor
HDC
histidine decarboxylase
hyperdiploid cell
HDCT
high-dose chemotherapy

NOTES

H

HDCV
  human diploid cell rabies vaccine
HDGC
  hereditary diffuse gastric cancer
HDH
  heart disease history
HDI
  histologically detectable iron
HDJ1 protein
HDL
  high-density lipoprotein
    AccuMeter HDL
    HDL cholesterol assay
    HDL direct test prefilled cartridge
HDL-C
  high-density lipoprotein-cholesterol
HDMEC
  human dermal microvascular endothelial
    cell
HDN
  hemolytic disease of newborn
    alloimmune HDN
    Kell HDN
HDRA
  histoculture drug response assay
HDS
  herniated disc syndrome
HDV
  hepatitis delta virus
  hepatitis D virus
HDW
  hemoglobin distribution width
HE
  hereditary elliptocytosis
  human enteric (virus)
H&E
  hematoxylin and eosin
    H&E stain
head
    angle h.
    bulldog h.
    h. cap
    deceleration of h.
    hydrophilic h.
    H. line
    h. louse
    Medusa h.
    h. and neck squamous cell
      carcinoma (HNSCC)
    h. space analysis
headache
    tension h.
healed
    h. appendicitis
    h. fracture
    h. Ghon complex
    h. glomerulonephritis
    h. infarct

    h. tuberculosis
    h. ulcer
healing
    h. appendicitis
    scarless h.
    wound h.
health
    H. Alert Network (HAN)
    immediately dangerous to life
      or h. (IDLH)
    H. Insurance Portability and
      Accountability Act (HIPAA)
    National Institute for Occupational
      Safety and H. (NIOSH)
    National Institutes of H. (NIH)
    h. physics
    H. Resources and Services
      Administration (HRSA)
HealthCheck
    H. HDL home-screening test
    H. One-Step One Minute
      pregnancy test
    H. total cholesterol home-screening
      test
healthy control
He antigen
heart
    h. antigen
    armored h.
    athletic h.
    beer h.
    beriberi h.
    h. block (HB)
    boat-shaped h.
    bony h.
    chaotic h.
    compensatory hypertrophy of the h.
    conducting system of h.
    dextroposition of the h.
    dextroversion of the h.
    h. disease (HD)
    h. disease history (HDH)
    disordered action of h. (DAH)
    drop h.
    dynamite h.
    h. failure (HF)
    h. failure cell
    fatty h.
    h. fatty acid binding protein (H-
      FABP)
    flask-shaped h.
    frosted h.
    hairy h.
    hypoplastic h.
    icing h.
    h. infusion agar
    luxus h.
    movable h.
    muscle of h.

myocytolysis of h.
myxedema h.
ox h.
parchment h.
pendulous h.
right and left fibrous rings of h.
sabot h.
senile amyloidosis of h.
stone h.
tabby cat h.
thrush breast h.
tiger h.
tiger lily h.
trilocular h.
h. tumor
valvular disease of h. (VDH)
heart-hand syndrome
heart-lung preparation
heartwater
heartworm
HEAT
  human erythrocyte agglutination test
heat
  h. antigen retrieval protocol
  h. capacity
  h. coagulation test
  h. of combustion
  h. content
  h. edema
  h. of formation
  h. of fusion
  h. instability test
  h. intolerance
  h. killed (HK)
  h. labile
  h. labile test
  latent h.
  h. precipitation test
  h. of reaction
  h. shock factor 1 (HSF1)
  h. shock protein (HSP)
  h. shock response
  h. sink
  h. of solution
  specific h.
  h. stability test
  h. of sublimation
  h. unit (HU)
  h. of vaporization
heater
  SlidePro slide h.

heat-extracted antigen
heat-induced epitope retrieval (HIER)
heat-killed *Listeria monocytogenes* (HKLM)
heat-labile
  h.-l. antibody
  h.-l. protein
heat-mediated antigen retrieval
heat-resistant glass
heat-stable (HS)
  h.-s. alkaline phosphatase
  h.-s. lactic dehydrogenase (HLDH)
heavy
  h. chain
  h. chain disease
  h. metal
  h. metal poisoning
  h. metal screen
  h. metal screening test
  h. water
hebeiensis
  Streptomyces h.
Hebeloma mesophaeum
Heberden
  H. disease
  H. node
Hebra
  H. disease
  prurigo of H.
hebraeum
  Amblyomma h.
hecateromeric
hecatomeral
Hecht pneumonia
Heckathorn disease
heckeshornense
  Mycobacterium h.
hectogram
hectometer
hederiform ending
hedgehog
  sonic h. (SHH)
heel
  cracked h.
Heerfordt
  H. disease
  H. syndrome
Hegglin
  H. anomaly
  H. syndrome
heidelberg
  Salmonella enteritidis serotype h.

NOTES

H

Heidenhain
- H. azan stain
- H. crescent
- H. demilune
- H. iron hematoxylin
- H. iron hematoxylin stain
- H. syndrome

height (ht)
- peak h.

heilmannii
- *Helicobacter h.*

Heine-Medin disease

Heinz
- H. body
- H. body hemolytic anemia
- H. body stain
- H. body test
- H. granule

Heinz-Ehrlich body

HEK
- human embryo kidney
- human embryonic kidney
- HEK cell

Hektoen
- H. enteric agar
- H. phenomenon

HEL
- human embryo lung
- HEL cell

HeLa cell

Helcococcus sueciensis

Heleidae

helenine

helgolandensis
- *Jannaschia h.*

helianthine

helical

helicase protein

helices (*pl. of* helix)

helicis
- chondrodermatitis nodularis chronica h.

Helicobacter
- H. aurati
- H. canadensis
- H. cinaedi
- H. fennelliae
- H. ganmani
- H. gastritis
- H. heilmannii
- H. hepaticus
- H. mesocricetorum
- H. pylori
- H. pylori breath test
- H. pylori gII test
- H. pylori serology
- H. pylori urease
- H. pylori urease test and culture
- H. typhlonius

Helicostylum

helicotrema

Helicotylenchus

Helie bundle

heliencephalitis

Heliobacterium
- H. sulfidophilum
- H. undosum

Heliorestis
- H. baculata
- H. daurensis

heliotrinireducens
- *Slackia h.*

heliotrope eyelid

Heliozoea

Helisal rapid blood test

helium equilibration time (HET)

helix, pl. **helices**
- alpha h.
- double h.
- right-handed alpha h.

helix-loop-helix protein

hellem
- *Encephalitozoon h.*

hellenicus
- *Staphylothermus h.*

Heller-Döhle disease

helle zellen (pale cells)

HELLP
- hemolysis, elevated liver enzymes, and low platelets
- HELLP syndrome

Helly
- H. fixative
- H. fluid

helmet cell

helminthagogue

helmintheca
- *Neorickettsia h.*

helminthemesis

helminthiasis

helminthic disease

helminth identification procedure

helminthism

helminthoid

helminthology

helminthoma

Helminthosporium oryzae

helmintic

Heloderma

Helophilus

Helotium

helper
- h. T cell
- h. T lymphocyte
- h. virus

helper/suppressor cell ratio

Helvella
    H. elastica
    H. esculenta
helvola
    Zimmermannella h.
helvolus
    Pseudoclavibacter h.
Helweg-Larssen syndrome
hemachromatosis (*var. of* hemochromatosis)
hemachrome
hemachrosis
hemacytometer
hemacytozoon
hemadsorption
    h. inhibition test
    mixed h. (MHA)
    h. virus test
    h. virus type 1, 2
hemafacient
hemagglutinating
    h. antipenicillin antibody (HAPA)
    h. cold autoantibody
    h. unit (HU)
hemagglutination
    indirect h. (IHA)
    h. inhibition (HI)
    h. inhibition assay
    h. inhibition titer
    passive h. (PHA)
    reverse passive h.
    h. test
    treponemal h. (TPH)
    h. treponemal test for syphilis
    Treponema pallidum h. (TPH)
    viral h.
hemagglutination-inhibition
    h.-i. antibody (HIA)
    h.-i. test (HIT)
hemagglutinin
    autologous h.
    cold h.
    heterologous h.
    homologous h.
    h. inhibition (HAI)
    warm h.
hemal
    h. gland
    h. node
hemalum
    Mayer h.
hemamebiasis

hemanalysis
hemangiectatic hypertrophy
hemangioblast
hemangioblastoma
hemangioendothelial sarcoma
hemangioendothelioblastoma
hemangioendothelioma
    epithelioid h. (EH, EHE)
    infantile hepatic h.
    retiform h.
    h. tuberosum multiplex
hemangiofibroma
    juvenile h.
hemangiolipoma
hemangioma
    ameloblastic h.
    arterial h.
    capillary h.
    cavernous h.
    choroidal h.
    circumscribed choroidal h. (CCH)
    h. congenitale
    dyschondroplasia with h.'s
    glomeruloid h.
    infantile h.
    microvenular h.
    nuchal h.
    placental h.
    h. planum extensum
    racemose h.
    renal h.
    sclerosing h.
    senile h.
    h. simplex
    targetoid hemosiderotic h.
hemangioma-thrombocytopenia syndrome
hemangiomatosis
    pulmonary capillary h. (PCH)
hemangioperic-like
hemangiopericytic
hemangiopericytoma (HPC)
    lipomatous h. (LHPC)
    orbital h.
hemangiopericytomatous growth pattern
hemangiosarcoma
    splenic h.
hemapheic
hemaphein
hemapheism
hemapheresis
hemarthrosis
Hemastainer

NOTES

H

hemastrontium
HemataCHEK hematology reference control
hematapostema
HemataSTAT Easy Read centrifuge
hematein
    Baker acid h.
    h. test
Hematek 2000 slide stainer
hematemesis
hematencephalon
Hematest reagent tablet test
hematherapy
hemathidrosis
hemathorax
hematic
hematid
hematidrosis
hematimeter
hematin
    acid formaldehyde h.
    h. albumin
    h. pigmentation
    reduced h.
hematinemia
hematinic principle
hematite pneumoconiosis
hematobilia
hematobium
    Schistosoma h.
hematoblast
    Hayem h.
hematocele
hematocelia
hematocephaly
hematochezia
hematochlorin
hematochyluria
hematocolpos
hematocrit (Hct)
    large vessel h. (LVH)
    mean circulatory h.
    total body h. (TBH)
    venous h. (VH)
    whole-blood h. (WBH)
hematocrystallin
hematocyst
hematocystis
hematocyte
hematocytoblast
hematocytolysis
hematocytometer
hematocytozoon
hematocyturia
hematodyscrasia
hematodystrophy
hematogen
hematogenesis
hematogenic

hematogenous
    h. abscess
    h. dissemination
    h. hyalin
    h. jaundice
    h. metastasis
    h. osteitis
    h. pigment
    h. theory of endometriosis
hematogone
hematohistioblast
hematohyaloid
hematoid
hematoidin
    h. crystal
    h. pigmentation
hematological anthropology
hematologic malignant neoplasm
hematologist
hematology
hematolymphangioma
hematolymphoid
    h. chimerism
    h. malignancy
hematolysis
hematolytic
hematoma
    chronic subdural h. (CSH)
    corpus luteum h.
    delayed traumatic intracerebral h. (DTICH)
    epidural h.
    intracranial h.
    intramural h.
    organized h.
    puerperal h.
    retroplacental h.
    subdural h.
hematometra
hematometry
hematomyelia
hematomyelopore
hematonic
hematopathology
hematopathy
hematopenia
hematophagia
hematophagous
hematophagus
hematophilia
hematoplastic
hematopneic index
hematopoiesis
    extramedullary h. (EMH)
    intrathoracic extramedullary h.
hematopoietic
    h. aplasia
    h. cell cytoplasmic alteration
    h. cell origin

h. cord blood cell
h. gland
h. hyperplasia
h. hypoplasia
h. malignancy
h. maturation
h. maturation alteration
h. maturation arrest
h. progenitor cell (HPC)
h. progenitor cell transplantation
h. stem cell (HSC)
h. system
h. tissue
hematopoietin
hematoporphyrinemia
hematoporphyrinuria
hematorrhachis
h. externa
extradural h.
h. interna
subdural h.
hematosalpinx, pl. **hematosalpinges**
hematosepsis
hematoside
hematosis
hematospectroscope
hematospectroscopy
hematospermatocele
hematospermia
hematostatic
hematostaxis
hematotoxic
hematotoxin
hematotropic
hematoxic
hematoxin
hematoxylin
alum h.
h. body
Boehmer h.
Carazzi h.
chrome h.
Clara h.
Cole h.
Delafield h.
Ehrlich h.
h. and eosin (H&E)
Harris alum h.
Heidenhain iron h.
iron h.
Lillie h.
Mayer h.

phosphotungstic acid h. (PTAH)
silver nitrate with h.
h. stain
Weigert iron h.
hematoxylin-malachite green-basic fuchsin stain
hematoxylin-phloxine B stain
hematoxylin-phloxine-saffron (HPS)
hematozoon
hematuria
benign familial h.
essential h.
false h.
gross h.
initial h.
microscopic h.
nonglomerular h.
renal h.
terminal h.
total h.
urethral h.
vesical h.
hematuric bilious fever
heme
h. moiety
h. oxygenase (HO)
h. oxygenase-1 (HO 1)
h. oxygenase/carbon monoxide (HO/CO)
h. oxygenase-1 gene
h. synthetase (HS)
h. test
hemendothelioma
heme-porphyrin fecal occult blood test
hemerythrin
HemeSelect
hemiacardius
hemiacetal
hemianopsia
binasal h.
bitemporal h.
hemiaplasia
hemiatrophy
facial h.
hemiballismus
hemiblock
hemic calculus
Hemichorda
Hemichordata
hemidesmosome
hemidrosis
hemiglobin

NOTES

H

hemiglobincyanide
hemiglobinemia
hemiglobinuria
hemihidrosis
hemihyperhidrosis
hemilesion
hemimelia
    dysplasia epiphysialis h.
hemimetabolous
hemin
Hemiptera
hemipterus
    Cimex h.
hemipyonephrosis
Hemispora stellata
hemisyndrome
hemithoracic duct
hemithoracicus
    ductus h.
Hemivirus
hemizygosity
hemizygous deletion
hemoagglutination
hemoagglutinin
hemoantitoxin
Hemobartonella
hemobilia
hemoblast
    Pappenheim h.
hemoblastosis
hemocatharsis
hemocatheresis
hemocatheretic
Hemoccult
    H. fecal occult blood test
    H. II Sensa fecal occult blood test
    H. Sensa
    H. Sensa elite
hemocele
hemocholecyst
hemocholecystitis
hemochromatosis, hemachromatosis
    autosomal dominant h.
    exogenous h.
    hereditary h. (HH, HHC)
    juvenile h.
    neonatal h.
    non-HFE-related h.
    secondary h.
hemochromogen
Hemochron
    H. Jr. Citrate PT assay
    H. P214 glass-activated ACT tube
hemoclasia
hemoclasis
hemoclastic
    h. reaction
    h. shock
hemoconcentration

hemoconia
hemoconiosis
hemocryoscopy
HemoCue
    H. B-Glucose analyzer
    H. hemoglobin test system
hemocyanin
    keyhole-limpet h. (KLH)
hemocystinuria
hemocyte
hemocytoblast
hemocytocatheresis
hemocytolysis
hemocytometer
    Neubauer h.
hemocytometry
hemocytotripsis
hemocytozoon
hemodiagnosis
hemodialyzer
    ultrafiltration h.
hemodilution
    acute normovolemic h. (ANH)
    h. test
hemodynamic collapse
hemodyscrasia
hemodystrophy
hemofiltration
hemoflagellate
    mitochondrion of h.
hemofuchsin
    Mallory stain for h.
hemofuscin pigmentation
hemogenesis
hemogenic
hemoglobin (Hb)
    h. A
    h. A_2
    aberrant h.
    h. A1c
    adult h.
    alkali-resistant h.
    h. Bart
    bile pigment h.
    h. carbamate
    carbon monoxide h.
    h. cast
    h. C disease
    h. C Georgetown
    h. C Harlem
    h. Chesapeake
    h. Constant Spring
    Constant Spring mutation of h.
    h. content of reticulocytes
    Cranston h.
    crossover h.
    h. D
    h. demonstration in tissue
    denatured h.

deoxygenated h.
h. distribution width (HDW)
h. D Punjab
h. E
h. electrophoresis
embryonic h.
encapsulated h.
h. E-thalassemia disease
h. E trait
h. F
fast h.
fetal h. (HbF)
h. F, H assay
glycosylated h.
Gower 1, 2 h.
h. G Philadelphia trait
green h.
Gun Hill h.
h. H
Hammersmith h.
Hasharon h.
h. H disease
hereditary persistence of fetal h.
  (HPFH)
homozygous h. S (HbSS)
h. I
h. Icaria
h. identification
h. Indianapolis
h. J
h. J Capetown
h. Kansas
Köln h.
h. Koya Dora
h. Lepore
h. Lepore trait
lipid vesicle-encapsulated h.
h. M
mean cell h. (MCH)
mean corpuscular h. (MCH)
h. M Hyde Park
h. M-Saskatoon
muscle h.
oxygenated h.
oxygen half-saturation pressure
  of h.
h. pigmentation
h. Portland
h. Rainier
reduced h. (HHb)
h. S
h. SC-alpha thalassemia

Seal Rock h.
sickle cell h. (HbS)
sickling h.
slow h.
h. SO Arab sickle cell disease
solubilized h.
h. S test
stroma-free h.
h. Terre Haute
total h.
total circulating h. (TCH)
unionized h. (HHb)
unstable h.
variant h.
h. Yakima
h. Zurich
hemoglobinated
hemoglobinemia
  paroxysmal nocturnal h.
hemoglobinocholia
hemoglobinolysis
hemoglobinometer
hemoglobinometry
hemoglobinopathy
  heterozygous h.
  homozygous h.
  mixed h.
hemoglobinopepsia
hemoglobinophilic
hemoglobin-polyoxyethylene
  pyridoxalated h.-p. (PHP)
hemoglobinuria
  bacillary h.
  cold h.
  epidemic h.
  intermittent h.
  malarial h.
  march h.
  paroxysmal cold h. (PCH)
  paroxysmal nocturnal h. (PNH)
  toxic h.
hemoglobinuric
  h. fever
  h. nephropathy
  h. nephrosis
hemogram
hemohistioblast
hemokinesis
hemolamella
hemoleukocyte
hemolith
hemology

NOTES

H

hemolymph
    h. gland
    h. heteroagglutinin
    h. node
hemolysate
hemolysin
    alpha h.
    bacterial h.
    beta h.
    cold h.
    DL h.
    Donath-Landsteiner biphasic h.
    heterophil h.
    immune h.
    natural h.
    h. saponin
    specific h.
    h. unit
    warm-cold h.
hemolysinogen
hemolysis
    absence of h.
    alpha h.
    beta h.
    bystander h.
    colloid osmotic h.
    DL biphasic h.
    h., elevated liver enzymes, and
      low platelets (HELLP)
    extravascular h.
    extrinsic h.
    gamma h.
    immune h.
    h. interference
    intramedullary h.
    intravascular h.
    macrovascular h.
    nonimmune h.
    osmotic h.
    passive h.
    pseudohyperkalemia in specimen h.
    traumatic h.
hemolytic
    h. amboceptor
    h. anemia
    h. anemia of newborn
    h. chain
    h. disease of newborn (HDN)
    h. disorder
    h. gas
    h. index
    h. jaundice
    h. malaria
    microangiopathic h.
    h. plaque assay
    h. reaction
    h. splenomegaly
    h. streptococcus
    h. substance

    h. transfusion reaction (HTR)
    h. tube assay
    h. unit
hemolytic-uremic syndrome (HUS)
hemolyticus
    Bacillus h.
hemolyzable
hemolyzation
hemolyze
hemometry
hemonchosis
hemonephrosis
hemopathology
hemopathy
hemoperfusion
hemopericardium
hemoperitoneum
hemopexin
hemophagia
hemophagocytic syndrome (HPS)
hemophagocytosis
hemophil
hemophilia
    h. A, B, C
    h. B Leyden
    h. Bm
    classic h.
    classical h.
    vascular h.
hemophiliac
hemophilic
    h. arthropathy
    h. factor A
hemophilus of Koch-Weeks
    (*Haemophilus aegypticus*)
hemophoresis
hemophthalmia
hemophthisis
hemoplastic
hemoplasty
hemopneumopericardium
hemopneumothorax
hemopoiesic diuretic
hemopoiesis
hemopoietic
hemopoietin
hemoprecipitin
hemoprotein
hemoptysis
    cardiac h.
    endemic h.
    Oriental h.
    parasitic h.
    vicarious h.
hemopyelectasia
hemopyelectasis
HemoQuant fecal blood test
hemorepellant

hemorrhage
    antepartum h. (APH)
    cerebral h.
    chorioamnionic h.
    Duret h.
    fetomaternal h.
    flame-shaped retinal h.
    gastrointestinal h.
    intracerebral h.
    intracranial h.
    intrapulmonary h.
    intraventricular h. (IVH)
    massive pulmonary h.
    maternal-fetal h.
    neonatal gastrointestinal h.
    perifollicular h.
    petechial h.
    pinpoint h.
    postpartum h. (PPH)
    punctate h.
    renal h.
    subarachnoid h. (SAH)
    transplacental h. (TPH)
    traumatic basal subarachnoid h.
      (TBSAH)
    traumatic subarachnoid h. (TSAH)

hemorrhagic
    acute h. ulceration
    h. anemia
    h. ascites
    h. bronchopneumonia
    h. chickenpox
    h. colitis
    h. colitis syndrome
    h. cyst
    h. cystitis
    h. dengue
    h. diathesis
    h. disease of deer
    h. disease of newborn
    h. disorder
    h. diverticulitis
    h. endovasculitis (HEV)
    h. fever (HF)
    h. fever epidemic
    h. fever with renal syndrome
    h. gangrene
    h. gastritis
    h. glomerulonephritis
    h. infarct
    h. inflammation
    h. lobar pneumonia

    h. malaria
    h. mediastinitis
    h. meningitis
    h. nephritis
    h. pachymeningitis
    h. pancreatitis
    h. pericarditis
    h. plague
    h. pleurisy
    h. rickets
    h. shock
    h. smallpox
    h. thoracic lymphadenitis
    h. thrombocythemia
    h. ulcer

hemorrhagica
    periorchitis h.
    purpura h.
    scarlatina h.
    variola h.

hemorrhagicum
    corpus h.
    cystic corpus h.

hemorrhagin unit

hemorrhoid
    cutaneous h.
    external h.
    internal h.
    thrombosed h.

hemorrhoidal
    h. artery
    h. nerve
    h. vein
    h. zone

hemosiderin
    h. deposition
    local deposition of h.
    h. stain
    stainable h.
    h. staining
    h. test

hemosiderin-laden macrophages
hemosiderinuria test
hemosiderosis
    basal h.
    endogenous h.
    exogenous h.
    idiopathic pulmonary h. (IPH)
    pulmonary h.
    secondary pulmonary h. (SPH)

HemoSite hemoglobin meter

NOTES

H

hemospermia
  h. spuria
  h. vera
Hemosporidium
hemosporines
hemostasis
hemostatic
hemosuccus pancreaticus
hemotherapy
hemothorax
hemotoxic anemia
hemotoxin
  cobra h.
hemotropic
hemozoic
hemozoin
hemozoon
HEMPAS
  hereditary erythrocytic multinuclearity
  with positive acidified serum
  HEMPAS cell
hemuresis
henchirensis
  Ramlibacter h.
Hench-Rosenberg syndrome
Henderson-Hasselbalch equation
Hendersonia
Henderson-Jones disease
Hendersonula toruloidea
Henipavirus
Henle
  H. ansa
  H. fenestrated elastic membrane
  H. fiber layer
  H. fissure
  loop of H.
  H. nervous layer
  H. plexus
  H. reaction
  H. sheath
  H. tubule
Henoch purpura
Henoch-Schönlein
  H.-S. purpura (HSP)
  H.-S. syndrome
henpuye
Henry
  H. fructose test
  H. law
henselae
  Bartonella h.
  Rochalimaea h.
Hensen
  H. canal
  H. cell
  H. disc
  H. duct
  H. line

  H. node
  H. stripe
HEP
  hepatoerythropoietic porphyria
HEPA
  high-efficiency particulate air
  HEPA filter
  HEPA filter mask
Hepacivirus
Hepadnaviridae
heparan
  h. sulfate
  h. sulfate proteoglycan
heparanese
  human h. II
heparan-*N*-sulfatase
heparin
  h. cofactor
  h. cofactor II deficiency
  h. unit
heparinase
heparin-associated thrombocytopenia (HAT)
heparinate
heparinemia
heparinic acid
heparin-induced
  h.-i. platelet activation assay (HIPA)
  h.-i. thrombocytopenia (HIT)
  h.-i. thrombocytopenia-thrombosis (HITT)
heparinize
heparinolytica
  Prevotella h.
heparin-precipitable fraction (HPF)
hepar lobatum
hepatarius
  Vibrio h.
hepatatrophia
hepatatrophy
hepatic
  h. abscess
  h. acinus
  h. adenoma
  h. arteriole
  h. blood flow (HBF)
  h. capsulitis
  h. coma
  h. cord
  h. cyst
  h. docimasia
  h. encephalopathy
  h. failure
  h. fenestra
  h. fibrosis
  h. fistula
  h. function test
  h. glycogen

h. hydrothorax
h. iron concentration (HIC)
h. iron index (HII)
h. laminae
h. lipase deficiency
h. lobule
h. porphyria
h. portal venous gas (HPVG)
h. progenitor cell
h. sinusoid
h. steatosis
h. stellate cell
h. transaminase
h. tumor
h. vein thrombosis
h. venoocclusive disease

hepatica
adiposis h.
Capillaria h.
Fasciola h.
Hepaticola
hepaticus
Helicobacter h.
hepatis
lobulus h.
peliosis h.
tunica fibrosa h.
tunica serosa h.
venae centrales h.
hepatitic
hepatitis, pl. **hepatitides**
h. A antibody
h. A, B, C, D, E
active chronic h.
acute focal h.
acute parenchymatous h.
acute viral h. (AVH)
alcoholic h.
anicteric virus h.
h. antibody
h. antigen
autoimmune h. (AIH)
A virus h.
h. A virus (HAV)
h. B core antibody (HBcAb)
h. B core antigen (HBcAg)
h. Be antibody (HBeAb)
h. Be antigen (HBeAg)
h. B immune globulin (HBIG)
h. B surface antibody (HBsAb)
h. B surface antigen (HBsAg)
h. B surface antigen test

h. B vaccine
h. B virus (HBV)
cholangiolitic h.
cholestatic h.
chronic active h. (CAH)
chronic interstitial h.
chronic lobular h. (CLH)
chronic persistent h. (CPH)
chronic viral h.
h. contagiosa canis
h. C serology
h. C virus (HCV)
delta h.
h. delta virus (HDV)
drug-induced h.
h. D serology
h. D virus (HDV)
epidemic h.
equine serum h.
"h. E-like viruses"
h. E virus (HEV)
h. externa
fulminant h.
h. GB virus (HGBV)
giant cell h. (GCH)
granulomatous h.
h. G virus (HGV)
halothane h.
icteric serum h. (ISH)
infectious h. (IH)
infectious canine h.
ischemic h.
La Brea h.
long incubation h.
lupoid h.
MS-1 h.
MS-2 h.
murine h.
NANB h.
neonatal h.
non-A h.
non-A, non-B h.
non-B h.
nonviral h.
peliosis h.
persistent chronic h.
plasma cell h.
posttransfusion h. (PTH)
sequela of chronic active h.
serum h. (SH)
short incubation h.
Simbu h.

NOTES

H

hepatitis *(continued)*
    subacute h.
    suppurative h.
    transfusion h.
    transfusion-mediated viral h.
    unresolved h.
    viral h., types A–E
    h. virus
    wilsonian fulminant h.
hepatitis-associated antigen (HAA)
hepatization
    gray h.
    red h.
    yellow h.
hepatobiliary cystadenoma
hepatoblastoma
hepatocarcinoma
hepatocavopathy
    obliterative h.
hepatocele
hepatocellular
    h. adenoma (HCA)
    h. bile duct carcinoma
    h. jaundice
    h. necrosis
hepatocholangitis
hepatocuprein
Hepatocystis
hepatocyte
    characteristics of h.
    foamy degeneration of h.'s
    ground glass h.
    h. growth factor (HGF)
    h. growth factor/scatter factor
    (HGF/SF)
    h. nuclear factor 1 alpha
hepatoerythropoietic porphyria (HEP)
hepatogenic
hepatogenous
    h. jaundice
    h. pigment
hepatohemia
hepatoid
hepatojugular reflux
hepatolenticular
    h. degeneration
    h. disease
hepatolienomegaly
hepatolith
hepatolithiasis
hepatolysin
hepatoma
    malignant h.
hepatomalacia
hepatomegaly, hepatomegalia
hepatomelanosis
hepatonecrosis
hepatonephromegaly

hepatoperitonitis
hepatophosphorylase deficiency
    glycogenosis
hepatophyma
hepatopleural fistula
hepatoptosis
hepatorenal
    h. glycogenosis
    h. glycogen storage disease
    h. syndrome
hepatorrhexis
hepatosplenitis
hepatosplenomegaly (HSM)
hepatotoxemia
hepatotoxic
hepatotoxicity type I, II
hepatotoxin
Hepatovirus
Hepatozoon
HepCheck whole blood control
HEPES buffer
HEPES-buffered KSOM
Hepevirus
HepPar1 antibody
heptabarbital
heptacarboxyporphyrin
    urine h.
heptachlor epoxide
heptafluorobutyric anhydride (HFBA)
heptane
Hepzyme
HER-2
    HER-2 gene
    HER-2 protein
herald patch
herbarius
    Alicyclobacillus h.
herbarum
    Curtobacterium h.
    Pleospora h.
Herbaspirillum
    H. chlorophenolicum
    H. frisingense
    H. lusitanum
    H. seropedicae
herbicide
    chlorophenoxy h.
herbicidovorans
    Sphingobium h.
Herbst corpuscle
HercepTest
    H. breast cancer
      immunohistochemical assay
    Dako H.
    H. IHC kit
    H. immunohistochemical test
Hercospora
herd immunity

hereditaria
    anemia hypochromica
      sideroachrestica h.
    porphyria cutanea tarda h.
    protocoproporphyria h.

hereditary
    h. acanthocytosis
    h. adynamia
    h. angioneurotic edema (HANE)
    h. benign intraepithelial dyskeratosis
    h. clubbing
    h. coproporphyria (HCP)
    h. deforming chondrodysplasia
    h. deforming chondrodystrophy
    h. diffuse gastric cancer (HDGC)
    h. disease
    h. elliptocytosis (HE)
    h. enzymatic-type
      methemoglobinemia
    h. erythroblastic multinuclearity
    h. erythrocytic multinuclearity with
      positive acidified serum
      (HEMPAS)
    h. fructose intolerance (HFI)
    h. hemochromatosis (HH, HHC)
    h. hemochromatosis genotyping
    h. hemolytic anemia (HHA)
    h. hemorrhagic telangiectasia (HHT)
    h. hemorrhagic thrombasthenia
    h. hypersegmentation
    h. hypersegmentation of neutrophils
    h. lymphedema
    h. methemoglobinemic cyanosis
    h. mixed polyposis syndrome
    h. multiple exostoses
    h. multiple trichoepithelioma
    h. nephritis (HN)
    h. nonhemolytic bilirubinemia
    h. nonpolyposis colon cancer
      (HNPCC)
    h. nonspherocytic hemolytic anemia
      (HNSHA)
    h. orotic aciduria
    h. osteoonychodysplasia (HOOD)
    h. persistence of fetal hemoglobin
      (HPFH)
    h. plasmathromboplastin component
      deficiency
    h. progressive arthroophthalmopathy
    h. pyropoikilocytosis (HPP)
    h. renal-retinal dysplasia
    h. sensory radicular neuropathy

    h. sideroblastic anemia
    h. spherocytosis (HS)
    h. stomatocytosis
    h. thrombophilia
    h. tyrosinemia

heredity
    autosomal h.
    sex-linked h.
    X-linked h.

heredodegenerative disease

heredopathia atactia polyneuritiformis
  (HAP)

HERF
    high-energy radiofrequency
      HERF device

Hericium

Hering
    canal of H.

Herlitz syndrome

hermanii
    Escherichia h.

Hermann fixative

hermanniensis
    Enterococcus h.

Hermansky-Pudlak syndrome

hermaphroditism

Hermetia illucens

hermetic seal

hermsi
    Ornithodoros h.

hermsii
    Borrelia h.

HER-2/neu
    HER-2/neu gene
    HER-2/neu oncogene
    HER-2/neu protein
    serum HER-2/neu
    HER-2/neu serum test

hernia
    cerebral h.
    diaphragmatic h.
    direct h.
    epigastric h.
    esophageal h.
    femoral h.
    hiatal h.
    hiatus h.
    incarcerated h.
    inguinal h.
    irreducible h.
    Larrey h.
    meningeal h.

NOTES

H

hernia *(continued)*
    Morgagni h.
    obturator h.
    peritoneal h.
    retrocolic h.
    retrosternal h.
    Richter h.
    rolling h.
    strangulated h.
    umbilical h.
    urinary bladder h.
    h. uteri inguinale
hernial aneurysm
herniated
    h. disc syndrome (HDS)
    h. nucleus pulposus (HNP)
herniation
    cerebral h.
    uncal h.
heroin-associated nephropathy
herophili
    torcular h.
herpangina virus
herpes
    h. B encephalomyelitis
    h. catarrhalis
    h. corneae
    h. cytology
    h. desquamans
    h. digitalis
    h. esophagitis
    h. facialis
    h. febrilis
    h. generalisatus
    genital h.
    h. genitalis
    h. gestationis
    h. gladiatorum
    h. iris
    h. labialis
    neonatal h.
    h. pneumonitis
    h. progenitalis
    h. simplex (HS)
    h. simplex antibody
    h. simplex lymphadenitis
    h. simplex virus (HSV)
    h. simplex virus culture
    h. simplex virus encephalitis (HSVE)
    h. simplex virus I (HSV I)
    h. simplex virus II (HSV II)
    h. simplex virus infection
    h. simplex virus isolation
    traumatic h.
    h. virus
    h. whitlow
    h. zoster
    h. zoster ophthalmicus
    h. zoster varicellosus
    h. zoster virus
HerpeSelect type specific IgG antibody detection kit
herpeslike virus (HLV)
herpes-type virus (HTV)
Herpesviridae
herpesvirus (HV)
    h. antigen
    canine h.
    caprine h.
    h. hominis (HVH)
    human h. 1–8 (HHV)
    h. papio 2
    H. simiae
    suid h.
herpetic
    h. fever
    h. gingivostomatitis
    h. keratitis
    h. keratoconjunctivitis
    h. meningoencephalitis
    h. paronychia
    h. stomatitis
    h. ulcer
    h. viral disease
    h. whitlow
herpetica
    pharyngitis h.
herpeticum
    eczema h.
herpetiformis
    dermatitis h.
    morphea h.
Herpetomonas
    H. donovani
    H. furunculosa
    H. tropica
Herpetoviridae
herpetovirus
    canine h.
    caprine h.
Herpotrichia
Herring body
herringbone
    h. fascicle
    h. pattern
herring-worm disease
Herrmann syndrome
Hers disease
Herter
    H. disease
    H. test
Herter-Heubner disease
hertz (Hz)
Herxheimer
    H. reaction
    H. spiral
hesitation wound

Hespellia
> *H. porcina*
> *H. stercorisuis*

hesperidum
> *Alicyclobacillus h.*

HET
> helium equilibration time

hetastarch
heterakid
Heterakis
heterauxesis
heteraxial
heterecious
heterecism
heteroagglutination
heteroagglutinin
> hemolymph h.

heteroallele
heteroantibody
heteroantigen
heteroantiserum
heteroatom
Heterobasidion
Heterobilharzia
heteroblastic
heterobrachial inversion
heterocellular
heterocentric
heterochromatic
heterochromatin
> constitutive h.
> facultative h.
> nuclear h.
> satellite-rich h.

heterochromatinization
heterochromia
heterochromic iridocyclitis
heterochromous
heterochthonous
heteroclitic antibody
heterocycle
heterocyclic compound
heterocytotropic antibody
Heterodera
> *H. graminophila*
> *H. marioni*
> *H. radicicola*

heterodermic
heterodimer
> TAP1/TAP2 h.

Heterodoxus spiniger
heteroduplex analysis (HDA)

heterodyne
heterofermentation
heterogametic sex
heterogamy
heterogeneic antigen
heterogeneity
heterogeneous
> h. assay
> h. nuclear RNA (hnRNA)
> h. nucleation
> h. pattern

heterogenetic
> h. antibody
> h. antigen

heterogenic enterobacterial antigen
heterogenote
heterogenous vaccine
heterogony
heterograft
heterokaryon
heterokaryotic twins
heterokeratoplasty
heterolactic
heteroligating antibody
heterologous
> h. antiserum
> h. bone
> h. chimera
> h. desensitization
> h. graft
> h. hemagglutinin
> h. protein
> h. serotype
> h. serum
> h. tumor

heterology
heterolysin
heterolysis
heterolysosome
heterolytic cleavage
heteromastigote
heteromeric cell
heterometabolous
heterometaplasia
heteromorphic
> h. bivalent
> h. chromosome

heteroosteoplasty
heteropathy
heterophagic vacuole
heterophagosome
heterophagy

NOTES

H

heterophil, heterophile
- h. agglutinin
- h. antibody
- h. antibody test
- h. antigen
- h. antigen reaction
- h. hemolysin

heterophilic leukocyte

Heterophyes
- *H. brevicaeca*
- *H. katsuradai*

heterophyiasis
heterophyid
Heterophyidae
Heterophyopsis continua
heteroplasia
heteroplasmy
heteroplastic graft
heteroplastid
heteroplasty
heteroploid
heteroploidy
heteropolymer
heteropolysaccharide
heteropyknotic chromatin
heteroscedasticity
heterosis
heterosomal aberration
heterosome
heterospecific graft
heterotaxia
- cardiac h.

heterotaxic
heterothallic
heterothallism
heterotopia
- intestinal h.
- neuronal nodular h.
- occult nodular h.

heterotopic transplantation
heterotopous
heterotransplantation
heterotremus
- *Paragonimus h.*

heterotroph
heterotrophic bacterium
heterovaccine therapy
heteroxenous
heterozygosity
- loss of h. (LOH)

heterozygote
- compound h.
- manifesting h.

heterozygous
- h. alpha thalassemia 1
- h. hemoglobinopathy
- h. point mutation
- h. thalassemia
- h. type of hemoglobin disorder

Heublein method
Heubner disease
heuristic method
HEV
- hemorrhagic endovasculitis
- hepatitis E virus
- high-endothelial venule

hexacanth
hexacarboxyporphyrin
- urine h.

hexachloride
- benzene h. (BHC)

hexachlorobenzene
1,2,3,4,5,6-hexachlorocyclohexane
hexachlorophene assay
hexadecimal
Hexadnovirus
hexafluorosilicate
- sodium h.

hexamer
hexamethonium bromide
hexamethylenetetramine
hexamethylpararosaniline
hexamethyl violet
Hexamita
hexamitiasis
hexane
hexanoic acid
hexaphosphate
- inositol h.

Hexaplex assay
Hexapoda
hexavalent
hexazonium salt
hexokinase method
hexon
- h. antigen
- h. gene

hexopyranose
hexosamine
hexosaminidase
- h. A, B
- h. A deficiency
- h. A gene
- total h.

hexose
- h. diphosphate
- h. monophosphate (HMP)
- h. monophosphate pathway
- h. monophosphate shunt (HMPS)

hexose-1-phosphate uridyltransferase
hexosephosphate
- h. dehydrogenase
- h. isomerase

hexosephosphoric esters
hexuronate
hexuronic acid
HF
- Hageman factor

heart failure
hemorrhagic fever
high flow
high frequency
H-FABP
heart fatty acid binding protein
HFAS
hereditary flat adenoma syndrome
HFBA
heptafluorobutyric anhydride
HFE gene
HFI
hereditary fructose intolerance
HFLL
hemosiderotic fibrohistiocytic lipomatous
lesion
HFR
HFR mutant
HFR strain
Hfr
high-frequency recombination
hFSH
human-derived follicle-stimulating
hormone
HG
high grade
Hg
mercury
Hg2+
inorganic mercury
HGA
homogentisic acid
HGBV
hepatitis GB virus
HgCN
mercury cyanide
HGE
human granulocytic ehrlichiosis
HGF
hepatocyte growth factor
hyperglycemic-glycogenolytic factor
HGF/SF
hepatocyte growth factor/scatter factor
hGG
human gamma globulin
hGH
human growth hormone
HGPRT
hypoxanthine guanine
phosphoribosyltransferase
HGPRT-deficient cell

HGSIL
high-grade squamous intraepithelial
lesion
HGV
hepatitis G virus
HH
hereditary hemochromatosis
HHA
hereditary hemolytic anemia
HHb
hypohemoglobin
reduced hemoglobin
unionized hemoglobin
HHC
hereditary hemochromatosis
HHD
hypertensive heart disease
HHF 35
HHF 35 antibody
HHF 35 stain
HHLL
histocytoid hemangioma-like lesion
HHT
hereditary hemorrhagic telangiectasia
HHV
human herpesvirus 1–8
HHV 8 antigen
HHV 8 DNA in sarcoidosis
HI
hemagglutination inhibition
HIA
hemagglutination-inhibition antibody
hians
Diphyllobothrium h.
hiatal hernia
hiatus hernia
hibernating
h. gland
h. myocardium
hibernica
Phoma h.
hibernoma
interscapular h.
HIC
hepatic iron concentration
Hickey-Hare test
**Hicks-Pitney thromboplastin generation
test**
HID
high iron diamine
hidden radiation source
hidebound disease

NOTES

H

477

hidradenitis
    h. axillaris of Verneuil
    neutrophilic eccrine h.
    h. suppurativa
hidradenocarcinoma
hidradenoma
    clear cell h.
    nodular h.
    papillary h.
hidroa
hidrocystoma
    apocrine h.
hidrosadenitis
hidrotic ectodermal dysplasia
HIER
    heat-induced epitope retrieval
hierarchical
    h. clustering
    h. clustering analysis
HIF
    hypoxia inducible factor
HIF-1
    hypoxia inducible factor 1
    HIF-1 alpha
high
    h. amplitude swelling
    h. anion gap acidosis
    h. birth weight (HBW)
    h. degree of unsaturation of fatty acid tail
    h. dosage (HD)
    h. egg-passage Flury strain rabies vaccine
    h. electrophoretic mobility
    h. endothelial
    h. endothelial postcapillary
    h. explosive
    h. eyepoint eyepiece
    h. flow (HF)
    h. frequency (HF)
    h. grade dysplasia
    h. iron diamine (HID)
    h. level
    h. magnification
    h. molecular weight (HMW)
    h. molecular weight cytokeratin (HMW-CK)
    h. molecular weight kininogen (HMWK)
    h. protein (HP)
    H. Pure PCR product purification kit
    h. serum-bound iron (HBI)
    h. trough concentration
    h. vacuum
    h. voltage
    h. yield histology
high-containment BSL4 facility

high-density
    h.-d. lipoprotein (HDL)
    h.-d. lipoprotein-cholesterol (HDL-C)
high-dose tolerance
high-efficiency particulate air (HEPA)
high-energy
    h.-e. bond
    h.-e. phosphate
    h.-e. radiofrequency (HERF)
higher bacteria
high-frequency
    h.-f. recombination (Hfr)
    h.-f. recombination mutant
    h.-f. transduction
high-grade
    h.-g. B-cell lymphoma
    h.-g. squamous intraepithelial lesion (HGSIL, HSIL)
    h.-g. TCC
highly
    h. complex series of reaction
    h. pathogenic avian influenza
Highman
    H. Congo red technique
    H. method
    H. method for amyloid
high-output cardiac failure
high-pass filter
high-performance
    h.-p. chromatofocusing (HPCF)
    h.-p. ion exchange chromatography (HPIEC)
    h.-p. liquid
    h.-p. liquid chromatography (HPLC)
    h.-p. size exclusion chromatography (HPSEC)
high-power field (HPF)
high-pressure liquid chromatography (HPLC)
high-resolution
    h.-r. banding
    h.-r. CT
    h.-r. protein electrophoresis (HRE)
high-velocity
    h.-v. missile (HVM)
    h.-v. steel-core round
high-voltage
    h.-v. electrophoresis (HVE)
    h.-v. transformer
Higoumenakia sign
HII
    hepatic iron index
Hikojima antigen
hila (*pl. of* hilum)
hilar
    h. cell
    h. cell tumor of ovary
    h. dance
    h. node (HN)

hilar-based fluffy infiltrate
Hildenbrand disease
hilitis
Hill equation
hillock
    axon h.
hilum, pl. **hila**
    h. of kidney
    h. lienis
    h. of lung
    h. of lymph node
    h. nodi lymphatici
    h. ovarii
    h. of ovary
    h. pulmonis
    h. renalis
    h. of spleen
    h. splenicum
hilus
    h. cell
    h. dance
Himasthla
hindrance
    steric h.
Hine-Duley phantom
Hines-Bannick syndrome
Hinfl solution
hinge region
hinshawii
    Arizona h.
Hinton test
hinzii
    Bordetella h.
HIP1
    huntingtin-interacting protein 1
hip
    congenital dislocation of h. (CDH)
HIPA
    heparin-induced platelet activation assay
HIPAA
    Health Insurance Portability and
    Accountability Act
Hippea maritima
hippei
    Propionispora h.
Hippelates
Hippel disease
Hippel-Lindau
    H.-L. disease
    von H.-L. (VHL)
Hippeutis
Hippobosca

Hippoboscidae
hippocampal sclerosis (HS)
hippocampi
    alveus h.
hippocampus
    alveus of h.
hippocoleae
    Arcanobacterium h.
hippocratic
    h. face
    h. facies
    h. finger
hippocratici
    digiti h.
hippurate
    h. broth
    methenamine h.
hippuratus
    Agromyces h.
hippuria
hippuric
    h. acid
    h. acid crystal
    h. acid excretion test
Hirano body
hiranonis
    Clostridium h.
hircus, pl. **hirci**
Hirneola
Hirschfeld disease
hirschfeldii
    Salmonella enteritidis serotype *h.*
hirschii
    Hydrogenophilus h.
Hirschowitz syndrome
Hirsch-Peiffer stain
Hirschsprung-associated enterocolitis
  (HAEC)
Hirschsprung disease (HD)
hirsuta
    Gordonia h.
hirsutism
    amenorrhea and h.
hirtellous
hirthi
    Filaroides h.
hirudin
hirudinaceus
    Macracanthorhynchus h.
Hirudinea
hirudiniasis
hirudinization

NOTES

H

479

Hirudo
  H. aegyptiaca
  H. japonica
  H. medicinalis
His
  H. bundle
  H. disease
  H. isthmus
  H. perivascular space
hispanica
  Arthropsis h.
  Borrelia h.
hispanicus
  Vibrio h.
hispidum
  Gnathostoma h.
Hiss capsule stain
Histalog test
histaminase
histamine
  h. flare test
  h. liberator
  h. receptor blocker
  h. shock
  h. stimulation test
histaminemia
histamine-releasing factor (HRF)
histaminergic
histaminiformans
  Allisonella h.
histaminuria
histangic
His-Tawara system
histidase
histidinase
histidine
  h. alpha deaminase
  analog of h. (AHH)
  h. decarboxylase (HDC)
  h. loading test
  urine h.
histidinemia
histidine-rich matrix protein
histidinuria
histidyl
histioblast
histiocyte
  cardiac h.
  crescentic h.
  epithelioid h.
  facultative h.
  foamy h.
  gargoylism type of h.
  Gaucher type of h.
  Hand-Schüller-Christian type of h.
  malignant lymphoma with a high
    content of epithelioid h.'s
  Niemann-Pick type of h.
  phagocytic h.

  sea-blue h.
  von Hansemann h.
histiocyte-rich B-cell lymphoma
  (HRBCL)
histiocytic
  h. granuloma
  h. leukemia
  h. lymphoma (HL)
  h. medullary reticulosis
histiocytoid carcinoma
histiocytoma
  ankle-type fibrous h.
  atypical fibrous h.
  cellular cutaneous fibrous h.
    (CCFH)
  fibrous h.
  generalized eruptive h.
  malignant fibrous h. (MFH)
  superficial malignant fibrous h.
histiocytosis
  kerasin h.
  Langerhans cell h. (LCH)
  lipid h.
  localized h.
  malignant h.
  nodular non-X h.
  nonlipid h.
  phosphatid h.
  phosphatid-type h.
  regressing atypical h. (RAH)
  sinus h. (SH)
  systemic h.
  h. X
histiogenic
histioid
histioma
histionic
histoangic
histoblast
histo-blood group antigen
histochemical stain
histochemistry
Histochoice
Histoclad
Histoclear slide processing solution
histocompatibility
  h. antigen
  h. assay
  h. assessment
  h. complex
  h. gene
  h. locus (HL)
  h. testing
histoculture drug response assay
  (HDRA)
histocyte
histocytoid hemangioma-like lesion
  (HHLL)
histocytologic research

histocytosis
  sea-blue h.
histodiagnosis
histodiagnostic marker
histodifferentiation
Histo-Dx
  histologic diagnosis
Histofine
  H. SAB-PO immunohistochemical staining kit
  H. staining method
histofluorescence
histogenesis
histogenetic
histogenous
histogeny
histogram
  cumulative-frequency h.
  frequence-time h.
  h. mode
  two-parameter h.
histography
histoid
  h. leprosy
  h. neoplasm
  h. tumor
histoincompatibility
histologic
  h. accommodation
  h. activity index (HAI)
  h. appearance
  h. grading
  h. lesion
  h. staining
  h. technician (HT)
histological
  h. chemistry
  h. pattern
  h. tumor grade
histologically detectable iron (HDI)
histologist
histology
  high yield h.
  pathologic h.
  tumor h.
histolysis
histolytic
histolytica
  Amoeba h.
  Entamoeba h.
histolyticum
  Clostridium h.

histolyticus
  Bacillus h.
histoma
histometaplastic
Histomonas meleagridis
histomoniasis
histomorphology
histomorphometry
histone deacetylase (HDAC)
histoneurology
histonomy
histonuria
Histopaque-1077
histopathogenesis
histopathology
  acid-fast staining h.
Histophilus somni
histophysiology
Histoplasma
  H. antibody assay
  H. capsulatum var. capsulatum
  H. capsulatum var. duboisii
  H. farciminosus
histoplasmin
histoplasmin-latex test
histoplasmoma
histoplasmosis
  African h.
  bronchopulmonary h.
  h. serology
histoprognostic
historadiography
historrhexis
history
  case h.
  heart disease h. (HDH)
histospectroscopy
histotechnologist
histotechnology
histotome
histotomy
histotope
histotoxic
  h. anoxia
  h. hypoxia
histotrophic
histotropic
histozoic
His-Werner disease
HIT
  hemagglutination-inhibition test

NOTES

H

481

HIT *(continued)*
  heparin-induced thrombocytopenia
  hypertrophic infiltrative tendinitis
Hitachi
    H. 704, 736, 911 analyzer
    H. 747-100 cholesterol analyzer
    H. 747 CK/MB analyzer
hitchhiker thumb
hits
    genetic h.
HITT
  heparin-induced thrombocytopenia-
    thrombosis
HIV
  human immunodeficiency virus
    HIV antibody test
    HIV culture
    HIV encephalopathy
    HIV quantitation
    HIV sialadenitis
    SI variant of HIV
HIV 2
HIV-1 serology
Hivagen test
HIVAN
  human immunodeficiency virus-
    associated nephropathy
hives
    giant h.
HJ
  Howell-Jolly
    HJ body
Hjärre disease
HK
  heat killed
hK2
  human kallikrein 2
hK3
  human kallikrein 3
HKLM
  heat-killed *Listeria monocytogenes*
HL
  histiocytic lymphoma
  histocompatibility locus
  hyperreactio luteinalis
HLA
  human leukocyte antigen
    HLA allele
    HLA BW 54 antigen
    HLA class I deficiency
    HLA complex
    HLA haplotype segregation
    HLA sequence in NK repertoire
    soluble HLA
    HLA typing
HLA-A antigen
HLA-B27
HLA-B antigen

HLA-B8 phenotype
HLA-C locus specificity
HLA-D antigen
HLA-DM gene
HLA-DR antigen
HLA-DR3 phenotype
HLDH
  heat-stable lactic dehydrogenase
hL-FABP
  human liver-type fatty acid-binding
    protein
HLH
  hemophagocytic lymphohistiocytosis
hLH
  human luteinizing hormone
hLT
  human lymphocyte transformation
HLV
  herpeslike virus
hMAM
  human mammaglobin
    hMAM RNA
HMB
  homatropine methylbromide
    HMB 45 antibody
    HMB 45 antigen
    HMB 45 marker
HMD
  hyaline membrane disease
HME
  human monocytic ehrlichiosis
HMFG-2 antibody
HMG
  high mobility group
  human menopausal gonadotropin
  hydroxymethylglutaryl
HML
  human milk lysozyme
hMLH 1 gene
HMO
  hypothetical mean organism
HMP
  hexose monophosphate
HMPS
  hexose monophosphate shunt
HMRU
  Hazardous Materials Response Unit
HMS
  hypothetical mean strain
HMSAS
  hypertrophic muscular subaortic stenosis
HMW
  high molecular weight
    HMW kininogen
HMW-CK
  high molecular weight cytokeratin
HMWK
  high molecular weight kininogen

HmX
    HmX hematology analyzer
    HmX H20 hematology system
HN
    hereditary nephritis
    hilar node
    NATO code for nitrogen mustard
HN1
    NATO code for nitrogen mustard 1
HN2
    NATO code for nitrogen mustard 2
HN3
    NATO code for nitrogen mustard 3
HN$_2$
    mechlorethamine
hNIS
    human sodium/iodide symporter
      hNIS gene expression
HNL
    histiocytic necrotizing lymphadenitis
    human neutrophil lipocalin
HNP
    herniated nucleus pulposus
HNPCC
    hereditary nonpolyposis colon cancer
    hereditary nonpolyposis colorectal cancer
hnRNA
    heterogeneous nuclear RNA
HNSCC
    head and neck squamous cell carcinoma
HNSHA
    hereditary nonspherocytic hemolytic
      anemia
h nucleus
HO
    heme oxygenase
HO 1
    heme oxygenase-1
hoagii
      Corynebacterium h.
Ho antigen
hobnail
    h. cell
    h. cell metaplasia
    h. liver
    h. nucleus
Hoboken
    H. gemmule
    H. nodule
HOC
    hydroxycorticoid

hock disease
HOCM
    hypertrophic obstructive cardiomyopathy
HO/CO
    heme oxygenase/carbon monoxide
Hodara disease
Hodgkin
    H. disease (HD)
    H. granuloma
    lymphocyte-rich classic H.
    H. lymphoma
    H. and Reed-Sternberg cell
    H. sarcoma
Hodgson disease
Hoechst dye
Hoesch test
hof
    perinuclear h.
    prominent nuclear h.
Hofbauer cell
Hoffa disease
Hoffman
    H. test
    H. violet
Hoffmann duct
Hoffmann-Werdnig syndrome
Hofmann bacillus
hofmannii
Hofmeister test
hofstadii
    Leptotrichia h.
hog
    h. cholera
    h. cholera serum
    h. cholera vaccine
    h. cholera virus
Hogben test
Hohenbuehelia
Höhn
    Physosporella H.
holandric
    h. gene
    h. inheritance
holarthritic
holarthritis
Hollande
    H. fixative/solution
    H. solution
Hollander test
Hollenhorst plaques
Hollerith code

NOTES

H

hollisae
>   *Grimontia h.*
>   *Vibrio h.*

hollow cathode lamp

Holmes
>   H. alkaline buffer
>   H. method
>   H. stain

Holmes-Adie syndrome
holmesii
>   *Bordetella h.*

Holmgren-Golgi canal
holmium
holoacardius
>   h. acephalus
>   h. acormus
>   h. amorphus

holocord
holocrine gland
holoendemic disease
holoenzyme
hologynic
>   h. gene
>   h. inheritance

holomastigote
holometabolous
Holophyra coli
holophytic
holoprosencephaly
holorachischisis
holotelencephaly
holothuriorum
>   *Salegentibacter h.*

holotrichous
holotype
holozoic
holsaticum
>   *Mycobacterium h.*

Holt-Oram syndrome
Holzer method
Holzknecht unit (H)
Homalomyia
homatropine methylbromide (HMB)
homaxial
home
>   H. Access hepatitis C Check test
>   h. canning

Homén syndrome
homeobox gene
homeodomain
>   h. protein
>   h. transcription factor

homeomorphous
homeoplasia
homeoplastic
homeostasis
>   electrolyte balance and h.
>   fluid balance and h.
>   immunologic h.

homeostatic
homeotherapy
Homer-Wright rosette
homing
hominis
>   *Blastocystis h.*
>   *Campylobacter h.*
>   *Cardiobacterium h.*
>   *Coccidium h.*
>   *Debaryomyces h.*
>   *Dermatobia h.*
>   *Enteromonas h.*
>   *Gastrodiscoides h.*
>   *Gastrodiscus h.*
>   *Gastrospirillum h.*
>   herpesvirus h. (HVH)
>   *Isospora h.*
>   *Mycoplasma h.*
>   *Oestrus h.*
>   *Pentatrichomonas h.*
>   poliovirus h.
>   *Polycytella h.*
>   *Psilorchis h.*
>   *Rhabditis h.*
>   *Saccharomyces h.*
>   *Sarcocystis h.*
>   *Staphylococcus h.*
>   *Taenia h.*
>   *Tetratrichomonas h.*
>   *Trichomonas h.*
>   *Trypanosoma h.*

hominivorax
>   *Cochliomyia h.*

homme rouge
homoallele
homobiotin
homocarnosine
homocentric
homochronous inheritance
homocyclic
homocysteine
>   h. desulfhydrase
>   h. testing

homocystine
>   h. testing
>   urine h.

homocystinemia
homocystinuria (HCU)
>   h. test

homocytotrophic (HCT)
homocytotropic antibody
homodimer
homofermentation
homogametic sex
homogenate
homogeneity
homogeneous
>   h. immersion

h. ligand assay
h. staining region (HSR)
homogenization
amphophilic h.
homogenize
homogenote
homogentisate
h. dioxygenase
h. 1,2-dioxygenase
h. oxidase
h. oxygenase
homogentisic
h. acid (HGA)
h. acid test
homogentisuria
homograft rejection
homoioplasia
homolactic
homolog, homologue
deltalike 1 h. (DLK1)
human achaete-scute h. (HASH)
human mismatch-repair protein
MutL h. (MLH1)
human MutS h.
phosphatase and tensin h.
smoothened h. (SMOH)
homologous
h. antigen
h. antiserum
h. artificial insemination (AIH)
h. chimera
h. chromosome
h. desensitization
h. graft
h. hemagglutinin
h. recombination
h. series
h. serotype
h. serum
h. serum jaundice
h. single-pass membrane
sialoglycoprotein
h. structure
h. tumor
homology
h. of chains
DNA h.
h. region
h. of strands
homolysin
homolysis
homolytic cleavage

homomorphic bivalent
homophil
homoplastic graft
homopolymer
homoscedasticity
homotetrameric complex
homothallic
homothallism
homotopic transplantation
homotransplantation
homovanillic
h. acid (HVA)
h. acid test
homozygosity
homozygote
homozygous
h. achondroplasia
h. alpha thalassemia 1, 2
h. hemoglobinopathy
h. hemoglobin S (HbSS)
h. point mutation
h. thalassemia
h. typing cell
homozygous-type hemoglobin disorder
hone
automatic h.
honei
Rickettsia h.
honeycomb
h. fibrosis
h. lung
h. macula
h. ringworm
h. tetter
honeycombing
cell h.
radiologic h.
honeycomb-like space
honey urine
Hong
H. Kong foot
H. Kong influenza
H. Kong toe
Hongia koreensis
Hongiella
H. halophila
H. mannitolivorans
H. marincola
H. ornithinivorans
hongkongensis
Actinomyces h.
Laribacter h.

NOTES

H

honing
HOOD
    hereditary osteoonychodysplasia
hood
    fume h.
    laboratory h.
    laminar flow h.
hooded chemical-resistant clothing
hoof-and-mouth disease
Hooke law
Hooker-Forbes test
hooklet
hookworm
    American h.
    h. anemia
    h. disease
    dog h.
    European h.
    New World h.
    Old World h.
Hopkins-Cole test
Hoplopsyllus anomalus
Hoppe-Goldflam disease
Hoppe-Seyler test
hordei
    Acarus h.
Hordeivirus
hordeolum
Horie tumor classification
horizontal
    h. cell of Cajal
    h. cell of retina
    h. transmission
Horm collagen reagent
horminium
    Salvia h.
Hormoconis
Hormodendrum
    H. carrionii
    H. cladosporioides
    H. compactum
    H. pedrosoi
Hormogoneae
Hormographiella
hormonal
    h. evaluation
    h. imbalance
    h. receptor
    h. therapy
hormone
    adaptive h.
    adenohypophysial h.
    adipokinetic h.
    adrenocortical h. (ACH)
    adrenocorticotropic h. (ACTH)
    adrenomedullary h.
    alpha melanocytic-stimulating h.
    androgenic h.
    anterior pituitary h. (APH)

antidiuretic h. (ADH)
antimüllerian h. (AMH)
Aschheim-Zondek h.
bovine growth h. (BGH)
chondrotrophic h.
chromaffin h.
chromatophorotropic h.
corpus luteum h.
cortical h.
corticotropin-releasing h. (CRH)
h. demonstration in tissue
diabetogenic h.
ectopic h.
erythropoietic h.
estrogenic h.
fat-mobilizing h.
female h.
follicle-stimulating h. (FSH)
follicle-stimulating hormone
  releasing h. (FSH-RH)
galactopoietic h.
gastrointestinal h.
glycoprotein h.
gonadotropic h. (GTH)
gonadotropin-releasing h. (GnRH)
growth h. (GH)
growth hormone-inhibiting h. (GH-
  IH)
growth hormone release
  inhibiting h. (GH-RIH)
growth hormone-releasing hormone
  (GH-RH)
growth-stimulating h. (GSH)
human-derived follicle-stimulating h.
  (hFSH)
human growth h. (hGH)
human luteinizing h. (hLH)
human pituitary follicle-
  stimulating h. (hPFSH)
hypersecretion of growth h.
hypophysiotropic h.
immunoreactive human growth h.
  (IRhGH)
inappropriate antidiuretic h. (IADH)
inhibiting h.
inhibitory h.
interstitial cell-stimulating h. (ICSH)
juvenile h.
ketogenic h.
lactogenic h.
langerhansian h.
lipolytic h.
luteal h.
luteinizing h. (LH)
luteinizing hormone-releasing h.
  (LH-RH)
lutein-stimulating h. (LSH)
luteotropic h. (LTH)
lymphocyte-stimulating h.

male h.
mammotropic h.
melanocyte-inhibiting h.
melanocyte-stimulating hormone release-inhibiting h.
melanocyte-stimulating hormone releasing h.
melanophore-stimulating h. (MSH)
neonatal thyroid-stimulating h.
neurohypophysial h.
orchidic h.
ovarian h.
ovine lactogenic h. (OLH)
pancreatic gut h.
parathyroid h. (PTH)
peptide h.
pituitary glycoprotein h.
pituitary growth h. (PGH)
placental h.
plasma luteinizing h.
posterior pituitary h.
progestational h.
prolactin release-inhibiting h.
prolactin-releasing h. (PRH)
proparathyroid h.
protein h.
prothoracicotropic h.
h. receptor
h. receptor status
regulatory h.
releasing h. (RH)
sex h. (SH)
somatotropic h. (STH)
somatotropin-releasing h. (SRH)
steroid h.
steroidogenic h.
syndrome of inappropriate secretion of antidiuretic h. (SIADH)
testicular h.
thyroid-stimulating h. (TSH)
thyrotropic h. (TTH)
thyrotropin-releasing h. (TRH)
TSH releasing h.
Hormonema dematioides
hormone-releasing
horn
Ammon h.
cicatricial h.
cutaneous h.
iliac h.
lateral gray h.
nail h.

sebaceous h.
warty h.
Horner syndrome
hornification
horny
h. cell
h. layer of epidermis
h. layer of nail
horror autotoxicus
horse
h. antihuman thymus globulin (HAHTG)
h. red blood cell (HRBC)
h. serum (HS)
h. serum block
horsefly
horsepox virus
horseradish
h. peroxidase (HRP)
h. peroxidase conjugated streptavidin-biotin complex
horseshoe
h. fistula
h. kidney
horseshoe-shaped nucleus
hortae
Piedraia h.
Hortaea werneckii
Hortega
H. cell
H. neuroglia stain
Horton
H. disease
H. syndrome
HOSE
human ovarian surface epithelial
HOSE cell
hose
drench h.
Hospidex microtiter plate
hospita
Burkholderia h.
hospital
h. epidemiology
h. fever
hospital-acquired
h.-a. gram-negative pneumonia
h.-a. penetration contact
host
accidental h.
alternate h.
amplifier h.

NOTES

H

487

host *(continued)*
    dead-end h.
    h. defenses
    definitive h.
    intermediate h.
    natural h.
    paratenic h.
    h. of predilection
    reservoir h.
    h. response
    h. stroma
    transfer h.
host-parasite relationship
host-range mutation
Hostuviroid
hot
    h. abscess
    h. antigen suicide
    h. cell
    h. gangrene
    h. lesion
    h. looping
    h. nodule
    h. spot
    h. zone
Hotchkiss-McManus PAS technique
Hottentot apron
houghtoni
    Diphyllobothrium h.
hound-dog facies
Hounsfield unit (H)
hour
    milligram per h. (mg/h)
2-hour
    2-h. postprandial blood sugar test
    2-h. postprandial plasma glucose
       test
hourglass
    h. gallbladder
    h. stomach
housefly
Houssay
    H. animal
    H. phenomenon
    H. syndrome
houstonense
    Mycobacterium h.
Howard test
Howell
    H. prothrombin test
    H. unit
Howell-Jolly (HJ)
Howship lacuna
Hoyer canal
HP
    high protein
    FlexSure HP
hp
    haptoglobin

HPA
    hybridization protection assay
HPC
    hemangiopericytoma
    hematopoietic progenitor cell
    hyperplastic-like mucosal change
HPCF
    high-performance chromatofocusing
HPF
    heparin-precipitable fraction
    high-power field
HPFH
    hereditary persistence of fetal
       hemoglobin
hPFSH
    human pituitary follicle-stimulating
       hormone
hPG
    human pituitary gonadotropin
HPIEC
    high-performance ion exchange
       chromatography
hPL
    human placental lactogen
HPLC
    high-performance liquid chromatography
    high-pressure liquid chromatography
       32 Karat software for HPLC
       System Gold HPLC
       HPLC water
hPMS2 gene
HPP
    hereditary pyropoikilocytosis
HPPA
    hydroxyphenylpyruvic acid
HPRC
    hereditary papillary renal cell carcinoma
hPrL
    human prolactin
HPRT
    hypoxanthine phosphoribosyltransferase
HPRT-deficient cell
HPS
    hematoxylin-phloxine-saffron
    hemophagocytic syndrome
    hypertrophic pyloric stenosis
HPSEC
    high-performance size exclusion
       chromatography
HPT
    hyperparathyroidism
HPV
    Haemophilus pertussis vaccine
    human papillomavirus
       HPV triage
HPVD
    hypertensive pulmonary vascular disease
HPVG
    hepatic portal venous gas

H.P. Wright method
HR
　hazard ratio
H-ras gene
HRBC
　horse red blood cell
HRBCL
　histiocyte-rich B-cell lymphoma
HRE
　high-resolution protein electrophoresis
HRF
　high-resolution fingerprint
　histamine-releasing factor
HRIG
　human rabies immune globulin
HRP
　horseradish peroxidase
HRS
　Hamilton Rating Scale
　Hodgkin and Reed-Sternberg
　　HRS cell
HRSA
　Health Resources and Services
　　Administration
HS
　heat-stable
　heme synthetase
　hereditary spherocytosis
　herpes simplex
　hippocampal sclerosis
　horse serum
　Hurler syndrome
HSA
　human serum albumin
HSC
　hematopoietic stem cell
　　totipotent HSC
HSF1
　heat shock factor 1
HSIL
　high-grade squamous intraepithelial
　　lesion
H-SLAP
　human stromelysin aggregated
　　proteoglycan
HSM
　hepatosplenomegaly
HSP
　heat shock protein
　Henoch-Schönlein purpura
　　HSP 40, 70, 90

HSR
　homogeneous staining region
HSU method
HSV
　herpes simplex virus
　　HSV culture
　　HSV isolation
HSVE
　herpes simplex virus encephalitis
HSV I
　herpes simplex virus I
HSV II
　herpes simplex virus II
HT
　histologic technician
　hypertension
5-HT
　5-hydroxytryptamine
ht
　height
H-tetanase
HTHD
　hypertensive heart disease
HTLV
　human T-cell leukemia-lymphoma virus
HTLV-I
　human T-cell lymphotropic virus type I
　　HTLV-I antibody
　　HTLV-1 associated myelopathy
　　(HAM)
HTLV-II
　human T-cell lymphotropic virus type II
HTLV-III
　human T-cell lymphotropic virus type III
HTN
　hypertension
HTP
　hydroxytryptophan
HTR
　hemolytic transfusion reaction
HTV
　herpes-type virus
HU
　heat unit
　hemagglutinating unit
　hydroxyurea
　hyperemia unit
Hu antigen
Huchard disease
Hucker-Conn
　H.-C. crystal violet solution
　H.-C. stain

NOTES

H

Huddleston agglutination test
Huebener-Thomsen-Friedenreich
  phenomenon
Hueck ligament
Huët-Pelger nuclear anomaly
Hüfner equation
Huhner test
hulunbeirensis
  Natrialba h.
human
  h. ABC transporter family
  h. achaete-scute homolog (HASH)
  h. alpha-1 proteinase inhibitor
  h. alveolar macrophage (HAM)
  h. androgen receptor gene
    (HUMARA)
  h. antichimeric antibody (HACA)
  h. antihemophilic factor
  antihemophilic plasma h.
  h. antimicrobial peptide
  h. antimouse antibody (HAMA)
  h. antimurine antibody (HAMA)
  h. B lymphotropic virus (HBLV)
  h. botulinum neurotoxin type A,
    B, E, F
  botulism immune globulin
    intravenous (h.) (BIG-IV)
  h. chorionic gonadotropin (HCG,
    hCG)
  h. chorionic gonadotropin injection
    test
  h. chorionic somatomammotropin
    (hCSM)
  h. dermal microvascular endothelial
    cell (HDMEC)
  h. diploid cell rabies vaccine
    (HDCV)
  h. embryo kidney (HEK)
  h. embryo lung (HEL)
  h. embryonic kidney (HEK)
  h. engineering
  h. enteric (virus) (HE)
  h. epidermal growth receptor 2
  h. erythrocyte agglutination test
    (HEAT)
  h. flea
  h. gamma globulin (hGG)
  h. genetic identity testing
  h. genome
  h. glandular kallikrein 3
  h. granulocytic ehrlichiosis (HGE)
  h. growth hormone (hGH)
  h. growth hormone deficiency
  h. growth hormone stimulation test
  h. heparanese II
  h. herpesvirus 1–8 (HHV)
  h. immunodeficiency virus (HIV)
  h. immunodeficiency virus culture
  h. kallikrein 2 (hK2)

  h. kallikrein 3 (hK3)
  h. leukemia-associated antigen
  h. leukocyte antigen (HLA)
  h. liver-type fatty acid-binding
    protein (hL-FABP)
  h. luteinizing hormone (hLH)
  h. lymphocyte antigen
  h. lymphocyte transformation (hLT)
  h. lymphoproliferative disease
  h. mammaglobin (hMAM)
  h. measles immune serum
  h. menopausal gonadotropin (HMG)
  h. mesothelial cell membrane
    (HBME 1)
  h. milk factor globulin
  h. milk lysozyme (HML)
  h. mismatch-repair protein MutL
    homolog (MLH1)
  h. monocytic ehrlichiosis (HME)
  h. MutS homolog
  h. neutrophil lipocalin (HNL)
  h. normal immunoglobulin
  h. ovarian surface epithelial
    (HOSE)
  h. papillomavirus (HPV)
  h. papillomavirus DNA probe test
  h. parvovirus B19
  h. pertussis immune serum
  h. pituitary follicle-stimulating
    hormone (hPFSH)
  h. pituitary gonadotropin (hPG)
  h. placental lactogen (hPL)
  h. progenitor cell antigen
  h. prolactin (hPrL)
  h. rabies immune globulin (HRIG)
  h. remains
  h. scarlet fever immune serum
  h. serum albumin (HSA)
  h. sodium/iodide symporter (hNIS)
  h. stromelysin aggregated
    proteoglycan (H-SLAP)
  h. T-cell leukemia-lymphoma virus
    (HTLV)
  h. T-cell lymphotropic virus type I
    (HTLV-I)
  h. T-cell lymphotropic virus type
    II (HTLV-II)
  h. T-cell lymphotropic virus type
    III (HTLV-III)
  h. telomerase reverse transcriptase
  h. thymus antiserum (HUTHAS)
  h. tubercle bacillus
  h. umbilical vein endothelial cell
    (HUVEC)
human-derived
  h.-d. botulism immune globulin
  h.-d. follicle-stimulating hormone
    (hFSH)

humanus
Pediculus humanus h.
HUMARA
human androgen receptor gene
humectant
Humicola
humidifier lung
humilata
Cellulomonas h.
humiphilum
Ornithinimicrobium h.
humor
aqueous h.
h. aquosus
Morgagni h.
ocular h.
plasmoid h.
production of aqueous h.
vitreous h.
h. vitreus
humoral
h. antibody
h. hypercalcemia of malignancy
h. immune response
h. immunity
h. pathology
h. regulator
h. thymic factor (THF)
hump
h. deposit
electron-dense h.
Hünermann syndrome
hungatei
Butyrivibrio h.
Clostridium h.
hungry bone syndrome
Hunner
H. cystitis
H. stricture
H. ulcer
Hunt
H. disease
H. and Hess hand fracture
H. syndrome
Hunter
H. glossitis
H. membrane
H. syndrome
Hunter-Hurler syndrome
Hunter-Schreger
H.-S. band
H.-S. line

huntingtin
h. gene
h. protein
huntingtin-associated protein 1 (HAP1)
huntingtin-interacting protein 1 (HIP1)
Huntington
H. chorea (HC)
H. disease (HD)
Hurler
H. disease
H. syndrome (HS)
hurloid facies
Hürthle
H. cell
H. cell adenocarcinoma
H. cell adenoma
H. cell carcinoma
H. cell metaplasia
H. cell tumor
HUS
hemolytic-uremic syndrome
hyaluronidase unit for semen
Huschke auditory teeth
HUT
hyperplasia of usual type
Hutchinson
H. crescentic notch
H. disease
H. facies
H. incisor
H. mask
H. melanotic freckle
H. patch
H. pupil
summer prurigo of H.
H. syndrome
H. teeth
H. triad
Hutchinson-Boeck disease
Hutchinson-Gilford
H.-G. disease
H.-G. syndrome
Hutchison syndrome
HUTHAS
human thymus antiserum
Hutinel disease
HUVEC
human umbilical vein endothelial cell
Huvos grading system
Huxley
H. layer

NOTES

H

491

Huxley *(continued)*
>   H. membrane
>   H. sheath

huygenian eyepiece

Huygens ocular

HV
>   herpesvirus

HVA
>   homovanillic acid
>> HVA test

HVE
>   high-voltage electrophoresis

hveragerdense
>> *Thermodesulfobacterium h.*

HVH
>   herpesvirus hominis

HVL
>   half-value layer

HVM
>   high-velocity missile

HVSD
>   hydrogen-detected ventricular septal defect

hwajinpoensis
>> *Bacillus h.*

hyacinthi
>> *Acarus rhizoglypticus h.*

hyalin
>   alcoholic h.
>   hematogenous h.
>   Laquer stain for alcoholic h.

hyalina
>> *Hartmannella h.*

hyaline
>   alcoholic h.
>   h. arteriolosclerosis
>   h. body of pituitary
>   h. capsule
>   h. cartilage
>   h. cartilage matrix
>   h. cell
>   h. Civatte body
>   h. core
>   h. degeneration
>   h. globule
>   h. leukocyte
>   Mallory h.
>   h. material
>   h. membrane
>   h. membrane disease (HMD)
>   h. membrane disease of newborn
>   h. necrosis
>   h. nephrosclerosis
>   h. perisplenitis
>   h. plaque
>   h. sclerosis
>   h. thickening
>   h. thrombus
>   h. tubercle

>   h. urinary cast
>   h. vascular angiofollicular lymph node hyperplasia

hyalinization

hyalinized
>   h. core
>   h. stroma

hyalinizing
>   h. clear cell carcinoma (HCCC)
>   h. spindle cell tumor with giant rosettes
>   h. trabecular tumor

hyalinosis
>   focal segmental glomerular sclerosis and h. (FSGSH)
>   systemic h.

hyalinuria

hyalocyte

Hyalodendron lignicola

hyalohyphomycosis

hyaloid
>   h. body
>   h. canal
>   h. membrane

hyaloidea
>   membrana h.
>   stella lentis h.

hyaloideus
>   canalis h.

hyalomere

Hyalomma
>> *H. anatolicum*
>> *H. marginatum*
>> *H. variegatum*

hyaloplasm
>   nuclear h.

hyaloplasmic

hyaloserositis

hyalosome

hyaluronate

hyaluronic acid (HA)

hyaluronidase
>   h. collagen
>   h. digestion
>   h. unit for semen (HUS)

hyaluronoglucosaminidase

hyaluronoglucuronidase

Hyams esthesioneuroblastoma classification

H-Y antigen

Hybond
>   H. N filter
>   H. N+ nylon membrane

hybrid
>   h. antibody
>   H. Capture 2 (hc2)
>   H. Capture 2 (cervical cancer screening) device
>   H. Capture 2 Chlamydia test

H. Capture 2 HPV DNA test
H. Capture system
h. cell
h. orbital
SV40-adenovirus h.

hybridization
array-based comparative genomic h. (aCGH)
cell h.
cellular h.
comparative genome h.
comparative genomic h. (CGH)
competition h.
cross h.
DNA h.
DNA-DNA h.
DNA-RNA h.
Epstein-Barr virus-encoded RNA in situ h.
fiber fluorescence in situ h. (fiber-FISH)
filter h.
fluorescence in situ h. (FISH)
fluorescent in situ h.
genotypic blot h.
in-solution h.
liquid-phase h.
liquid (solution) h.
molecular h.
nonisotopic in situ h. (NISH)
nucleic acid h.
h. protection assay (HPA)
quantitative fluorescence in situ h. (Q-FISH)
RNA-driven h.
RNA-RNA h.
sandwich h.
saturation h.
sequencing by h. (SBH)
in situ h. (ISH)
solid-phase h.
solution h.
suppression subtractive h.

hybridize
hybridized probe
hybridoma
h. antibody
h. supernatant
h. technique

Hybritech
H. free PSA test
H. Ostase bone metabolism marker

H. PSA blood test
H. PSA determination system

hydantoin
hydatid
alveolar h.
alveolar h. disease
h. cyst
h. degeneration
h. disease (HD)
h. mole
h. of Morgagni
osseous h.
h. polyp
h. pregnancy
h. rash
sessile h.
Virchow h.

hydatidiform mole
hydatidocele
hydatidoma
hydatidosis
hydatiduria
hydatigena
Taenia h.
Hydatigera
H. infantis
H. taeniaeformis
Hyde disease
Hydnopolyporus
hydradenitis
hydradenoma
hydralazine lupus
hydranencephaly
hydrargyromania
hydrarthrosis
hydratase
aconitate h.
fumarate h.
hydrate
chloral h.
sodium h.
hydrated alumina
hydration
water of h.
hydrazide
isonicotinic acid h.
thiophen-2-carboxylic acid h. (TCH)
hydrazine
alpha h.
h. yellow
hydrazine-sensitive factor
hydremia

NOTES

H

hydrencephalocele
hydrencephalomeningocele
hydrencephalus
hydride
  antimony h.
  arsenic h.
  arsenious h.
  phenyl h.
hydroa
  h. aestivale
  h. febrile
  h. vesiculosum
hydroappendix
hydrocalycosis
hydrocarbon
  alicyclic h.
  aliphatic saturated h.
  aliphatic unsaturated h.
  aromatic h.
  carcinogenic h.
  cyclic h.
  polycyclic aromatic h.
  saturated h.
  unsaturated h.
Hydrocarboniphaga effusa
hydrocele
  h. sac
  h. spinalis
hydrocephalic
hydrocephalocele
hydrocephaloid disease
hydrocephalus
  communicating h.
  noncommunicating h.
  normal pressure h. (NPH)
hydrochloric
  h. acid
  secreting h.
hydrochloride
  acridine h.
  adiphenine h.
  aminoacridine h.
  arginine h.
  atabrine h.
  chloroguanide h.
  cocaine h.
  colestipol h.
  cyproheptadine h.
  diphenhydramine h.
  doxepin h.
  ethoxazene h.
  hydromorphone h.
  meperidine h.
  methadone h.
  methamphetamine h.
  phenazopyridine h.
  prazosin h.
  procaine h.

  quinacrine h.
  semicarbazide h.
hydrochlorothiazide (HCT)
hydrocholecystis
hydrocholeresis
hydrocholeretic
hydrocirsocele
hydrocortisone (compound F)
hydrocyanic acid
hydrocyst
hydrocystoma
hydrocytosis
hydroencephalocele
hydrofluoric acid
hydrogel coated slide
hydrogen
  h. acceptor
  h. arsenide
  arseniuretted h.
  h. bacterium
  h. bond
  h. chloride
  h. cyanide (HCN)
  h. electrode
  h. exponent
  h. fluoride
  h. ion
  h. ion concentration (pH)
  h. peroxide
  h. peroxide solution
  h. sulfide
hydrogenalis
  Anaerococcus h.
hydrogenase
hydrogenate
hydrogenation
hydrogen-detected ventricular septal defect (HVSD)
Hydrogenimonas thermophila
hydrogeniphila
  Persephonella h.
hydrogeniphilum
  Thermodesulfobacterium h.
hydrogeniphilus
  Caminibacter h.
Hydrogenobacter
  H. hydrogenophilus
  H. subterraneus
Hydrogenobaculum acidophilum
hydrogenolysis
Hydrogenophaga intermedia
hydrogenophilus
  Geobacter h.
  Hydrogenobacter h.
Hydrogenophilus hirschii
Hydrogenothermaceae
Hydrogenothermus marinus
hydrolability

hydrolase
    acetyl-CoA h.
    acid h.
    aminoacyl-tRNA h.
    aryl-ester h.
    diadenosine oligophosphate h.
    phosphoric monoester h.
    ubiquitin C-terminal h.
hydrolysate
    casein h.
    lactalbumin h. (LAH)
    protein h.
hydrolysis
    gelatin h.
hydrolytic enzyme
hydrolyze
hydroma
hydromeningocele
hydrometer scale
hydrometrocolpos
hydromicrocephaly
hydromorphone hydrochloride
hydromphalus
hydromyelia
hydromyelocele
hydromyoma
hydronephrosis
hydronephrotic
hydronium ion
hydropericardium
hydroperitoneum
hydroperitonia
hydroperoxide
hydrophila
    Aeromonas h.
hydrophilia
hydrophilic
    h. gel
    h. head
hydrophobia
hydrophobica
    Gordonia h.
hydrophobic gel
hydrophobicity
hydrophthalmos
hydropic
    h. abortus
    h. degeneration
    h. fetus
    h. swelling
hydropneumatosis
hydropneumopericardium

hydropneumoperitoneum
hydropneumothorax
hydrops
    h. abdominis
    h. amnii
    h. articuli
    cochlear h.
    endolymphatic h.
    h. fetalis
    h. folliculi
    gallbladder h.
    immune fetal h.
    labyrinthine h.
    nonimmune fetal h.
    h. tubae profluens
Hydropus
hydropyonephrosis
hydroquinone
hydrorchis
hydrosalpinx
hydrosarca
hydrosarcocele
hydrostatic
    h. pressure
    h. test
hydrosyringomyelia
Hydrotaea
hydrotaxis
hydrothermale
    Desulfacinum h.
hydrothermalis
    Desulfovibrio h.
    Halomonas h.
    Halothiobacillus h.
    Thermomonas h.
hydrothionemia
hydrothionuria
hydrothorax
    chylous h.
    hepatic h.
hydrotomy
hydrotropism
hydrotympanum
hydroureter
hydroxide
    aluminum h.
    h. ion
    potassium h. (KOH)
hydroxy-3-methylglutaric acidemia
hydroxyapatite
    h. assay
    h. exchange procedure

NOTES

H

hydroxybenzene
hydroxybenzoicus
>   *Sedimentibacter h.*

hydroxybutyrate
>   beta h. (BHBA)
>   h. dehydrogenase (HBD, HBDH)

hydroxybutyric
>   h. dehydrogenase
>   h. test

hydroxychloroquine cardiotoxicity
hydroxycholecalciferol (HCC)
hydroxycobalamin
hydroxycorticoid (HC, HOC)
17-hydroxycorticosteroid
>   17-h. assay
>   17-h. test

17-hydroxycorticosterone
18-hydroxycorticosterone
hydroxyethyl starch
5-hydroxyindoleacetic
>   5-h. acid
>   5-h. acid assay
>   5-h. test

hydroxyketone dye
hydroxyl
>   h. concentration (pOH)
>   h. group
>   h. radical

hydroxylase
>   dopamine h.
>   phenylalanine h.
>   proline h.
>   pyroglutamate h.
>   tyrosine h. (TH)

4-hydroxylase
>   prolyl 4-h.

21-hydroxylase
hydroxylation
>   h. kidney
>   h. liver

hydroxylysylpyridinoline
hydroxymethylglutaryl (HMG)
hydroxyphenylpyruvic acid (HPPA)
hydroxyphenyluria
hydroxyprogesterone
>   alpha h.

17-hydroxyprogesterone test
hydroxyproline
>   h. assay
>   h. index
>   h. oxidase
>   urinary h.
>   urine h.

hydroxyprolinemia
hydroxyprolinuria

hydroxystilbamidine isethionate
5-hydroxytryptamine (5-HT)
hydroxytryptophan (HTP)
>   hydroxytryptophan decarboxylase

hydroxyurea (HU)
25-hydroxyvitamin D assay
Hydrozoa
hygienic laboratory coefficient
hygroma, pl. **hygromata**
>   h. axillare
>   cervical h.
>   h. colli cysticum
>   cystic h.
>   subdural h.

hygrometer
hygrophilous
Hygrophoropsis
hygroscopic
hylemonae
>   *Clostridium h.*

Hylemonella gracilis
Hylemya
>   *H. antiqua*
>   *H. brassicae*

hylic tumor
hyloma
>   mesenchymal h.
>   mesothelial h.

hymen
>   imperforate h.

hymenal tag
Hymenobacter
>   *H. actinosclerus*
>   *H. aerophilus*
>   *H. roseosalivarius*

Hymenochaete
hymenoid
hymenolepiasis
hymenolepidid
Hymenolepididae
Hymenolepis
>   *H. diminuta*
>   *H. lanceolata*
>   *H. murina*
>   *H. nana*
>   *H. nana* var. *fraterna*

hymenology
Hymenomycetes
Hymenoptera
hymenoptera venom
Hymenoscyphus
Hymorphan
hyodysenteriae
>   *Treponema h.*

hyointestinalis
>   *Campylobacter h.*

Hyostrongylus rubidus
hypalbuminemia
Hypaque

hypazoturia
hyperacanthosis
hyperacidity
hyperactive glutamate receptor
hyperacute rejection
hyperadenosis
hyperadiposis
hyperadiposity
hyperadrenalism
hyperadrenocorticism
hyperaggregability
hyperalbuminemia
hyperalbuminosa
    polyemia h.
hyperaldosteronemia
hyperaldosteronism
    primary h.
    secondary h.
hyperalimentation
    intravenous h. (IVH)
hyperallantoinuria
hyperalphaglobulinemia
hyperaminoacidemia
hyperaminoaciduria
hyperammonemia I, II
hyperamylasemia
hyperamylasuria
hyperbaric chamber
hyperbetaalaninemia
hyperbetaglobulinemia
hyperbetalipoproteinemia
hyperbilirubinemia
    congenital h.
    conjugated h. I–III
    constitutional h.
    h. I, II
    unconjugated h.
hyperbilirubinuria
    obstructive h.
hyperbola
hyperbradykinism
hypercalcemia
    familial hypocalciuric h.
    idiopathic infantile h.
hypercalcemic
    h. crisis
    h. sarcoidosis
    h. uremia
hypercalcinuria
hypercalcitoninemia
hypercalcitoninism

hypercalciuria
    idiopathic h. (IHC)
hypercapnia
    permissive h.
hypercapnic
    h. acidosis
    h. encephalopathy
hypercarbia
hypercardia
hypercellular bone marrow
hypercellularity
    diffuse mesangial h. (DMH)
hyperchloremia
hyperchloremic metabolic acidosis
hyperchlorhydria
hyperchloruria
hypercholesteremia
hypercholesterolemia
    essential h.
    familial h. (FH)
hypercholesterolia
hypercholia
hyperchromasia
    epithelial h.
    nuclear h.
hyperchromatic
    h. anemia
    h. cell
    h. macrocythemia
    h. nucleus
hyperchromatin
hyperchromatism
hyperchromatosis
hyperchromemia
hyperchromia
    macrocytic h.
hyperchromic
    h. anemia
    h. shift
hyperchylomicronemia
hypercitraturia
hypercoagulability
hypercoagulable
    h. state
    h. state coagulation screen
hypercorticism
hypercortisolism
hypercupremia
hypercupruria
hypercyanotic
hypercythemia
hypercytochromia

NOTES

H

hypercytosis
hyperdiploid
hyperdistention
hyperdiuresis
hyperechoic
hyperelastica
    cutis h.
hyperelastosis cutis
hyperemesis gravidarum
hyperemia
    acute h.
    peristaltic h.
    reactive h. (RH)
    h. unit (HU)
hyperemic
hyperendemic disease
hypereosinophilia
hypereosinophilic syndrome
hyperergia
hyperergic encephalitis
hypererythrocythemia
hyperesthetic zone
hyperestrogenism
hyperextensible skin
hyperferremia
hyperfibrinogenemia
hyperfibrinolysis
hyperflexion
hyperfunction
    anterior pituitary h.
hypergammaglobulinemia
    monoclonal h.
    polyclonal h.
hyperganglionosis
hypergastrinemia
hypergenesis
hypergenetic
hypergenitalism
hypergia
hypergic
hyperglobulia
hyperglobulinemia
hyperglobulinemic purpura
hyperglobulism
hyperglycemia
    nonketotic h.
hyperglycemic
hyperglycemic-glycogenolytic factor
    (HGF)
hyperglyceridemia
    endogenous h.
    exogenous h.
hyperglycinemia
    ketotic h.
    nonketotic h. (NKHG)
hyperglycinuria
hyperglycosemia
hyperglycosuria
hyperglyoxylemia

hypergonadism
hypergonadotropic
hypergranulosis
hyperguanidinemia
hyperhemoglobinemia
hyperheparinemia
hyperhidrosis
hyperhomocystinemia
hyperhydropexis
hyperhydropexy
hyper-IgE syndrome
hyper-IgM syndrome
hyperimmune serum
hyperimmunity
hyperimmunization
hyperimmunoglobulinemia D, E, G, M
hyperindicanemia
hyperinfection
hyperinnervation
    nitrergic h.
hyperinosemia
hyperinosis
hyperinsulinemia
hyperinsulinism
hyperirritability
hyperisotonic
hyperkalemia
hyperkaluresis
hyperkaluria
hyperkeratinization
hyperkeratomycosis
hyperkeratosis
    h. congenita
    h. eccentrica
    epidermolytic h.
    h. figurata centrifuga atrophica
    h. filiform
    h. follicularis et parafollicularis
    h. lenticularis perstans
    h. penetrans
hyperkeratotic papilloma
hyperketonemia
hyperketonuria
hyperkinesis
hyperleukocytosis
hyperlipidemia
    carbohydrate-induced h.
    endogenous h. (EHL)
    fat-induced h.
hyperlipoproteinemia
    familial h. I, II, IIa, IIb, III–V
hyperliposis
hyperlithuria
hyperlucency of bone
hyperlucent lung
hyperlysinemia type I, II
hyperlysinuria
hypermagnesemia
hypermature

hypermelanosis
hypermenorrhea
hypermetaplasia
hypermethylation
hypermetropia
latent h.
hypermobility
apomorphine-induced h.
hypermutation
hypermyotrophy
hypernatremia
hypernatremic encephalopathy
hyperneocytosis
hypernephroid
hypernephroma
hyperoncotic
hyperonychia
hyperopia
manifest h.
hyperorchidism
hyperornithinemia
hyperorthocytosis
hyperorthokeratosis
hyperosmolality
hyperosmolar diabetic coma
hyperosmolarity
hyperosmotic
nonketotic h. (NKH)
hyperostosis
h. corticalis deformans
h. corticalis deformans juvenilis
h. corticalis generalisata
diffuse idiopathic skeletal h.
flowing h.
h. frontalis interna
generalized cortical h.
infantile cortical h.
streak h.
hyperostotic spondylosis
hyperoxaluria
hyperparakeratosis
hyperparasite
hyperparasitism
hyperparathyroidism (HPT)
primary h.
secondary h.
tertiary h.
hyperperfusion/hyperfiltration injury
hyperperistalsis
ureteral h.
hyperphenylalaninemia
hyperphosphatasemia

hyperphosphatasia
hyperphosphatemia
hyperphosphaturia
hyperphosphorylation of occludin
hyperpigmentation
hyperpituitarism
postpubertal h.
prepubertal h.
hyperplasia
adenoid h.
adenomatous h.
adrenal cortical h.
adrenocortical h.
alveolar pneumocyte h.
angiofollicular mediastinal lymph
node h.
antral G-cell h.
apocrine h. (ApoHyp)
atypical adenomatous h. (AAH)
atypical apocrine h.
atypical ductal h. (ADH)
atypical endometrial h.
atypical lobular h. (ALH)
atypical melanocytic h.
basal cell h.
basaloid h.
basophilic h.
benign florid lymphoid h.
benign giant lymph node h.
benign mediastinal lymph node h.
benign prostatic h.
bilateral micronodular adrenal h.
capsular synovial-like h. (CSH)
C-cell h.
clear cell cribriforming h.
columnar cell h.
complex endometrial h.
congenital adrenal h. (CAH)
congenital sebaceous h.
cortical stromal h. (CSH)
corticotroph cell h.
cutaneous lymphoid h. (CLH)
cystic endometrial h.
cystic hypersecretory h.
cystic prostatic h.
diffuse h.
ductal h.
endometrial h.
enterochromaffin cell h. (EC)
enterochromaffin-like cell h.
eosinophilic h.
epithelial h.

NOTES

H

499

hyperplasia *(continued)*
    erythroid h.
    fibromuscular h.
    flat urothelial h.
    focal epithelial h.
    focal nodular h. (FNH)
    follicular h. (FH)
    foveolar h.
    gingival h.
    glandular h.
    granulocytic h.
    hematopoietic h.
    hyaline vascular angiofollicular
      lymph node h.
    hypersecretory h.
    intracystic h.
    intraductal h.
    intravascular papillary endothelial h.
    lentiginous melanocytic h.
    Leydig cell h.
    lipomelanotic reticuloendothelial
      cell h.
    lobular epithelial h.
    lymph node h.
    lymphoid h.
    mast cell h.
    megakaryocytic h.
    megaloblastic h.
    mesonephric remnant h.
    microglandular h. (MGH)
    micronodular pneumocyte h. (MPH)
    myeloid h.
    myointimal h.
    neuronal h.
    neutrophilic h.
    nodular lymphoid h. (NLH)
    nodular mesothelial h.
    nodular regenerative h. (NRH)
    papillar villous h.
    papillary h.
    papillary endothelial h. (PEH)
    plasma cell angiofollicular lymph
      node h.
    polypoid h.
    postatrophic h.
    postsclerotic h.
    primary h.
    prostate h.
    pseudoangiomatous h.
    pseudoangiomatous stromal h.
      (PASH)
    pseudocarcinomatous h.
    pseudoepitheliomatous h.
    pulmonary lymphoid h. (PLH)
    reactive follicular h.
    reserve cell h.
    reticuloendothelial cell h.
    reticulum cell h.
    secondary h.

    senile sebaceous h.
    simple endometrial h.
    stromal h.
    stromovascular h.
    Swiss cheese h.
    thyrotroph h.
    transmural lymphoid h.
    h. of usual type (HUT)
    verrucous h.
    verumontanum mucosal gland h.
    vulvar squamous h.
    wasserhelle h.
    water-clear cell h.
hyperplasia/metaplasia
    complex atypical h. (CAHM)
hyperplastic
    h. arteriosclerosis
    h. bone marrow
    h. cholecystosis
    h. gland
    h. inflammation
    h. nephrosclerosis
    h. nodular goiter
    h. osteoarthritis
    h. polyp
hyperploid pattern
hyperploidy
hyperpolarization
hyperpotassemia
hyperprebetalipoproteinemia
hyperproduction of pituitary
    corticotropin
hyperproinsulinemia
hyperprolactinemia
hyperproliferation
hyperprolinemia
hyperproteinemia
hyperreactio luteinalis (HL)
hyperreactivity
    bronchial h.
hyperreninemia
hyperreninism
hypersalemia
hypersarcosinemia
hypersecretion
    extreme gastric h.
    glucagon h.
    h. of growth hormone
hypersecretory hyperplasia
hypersegmentation
    h. of granulocyte nuclei
    hereditary h.
    leukocytic h.
hypersegmented
    h. granulocyte
    h. neutrophil
hypersensitive
hypersensitivity
    h. angiitis

contact h.
delayed h.
delayed-type h. (DTH)
immediate h.
h. myocarditis
h. pneumonitis
h. pneumonitis serology
pulmonary h.
h. reaction, type I–IV
tuberculin-type h.
h. vasculitis
hypersensitization
hyperserotonemia
hyperskeocytosis
hypersomia
hypersplenism
hypersplenosis
hypersthenuria
hypersusceptibility
hypertelorism
ocular h.
hypertension (HT, HTN)
arterial h.
benign intracranial h. (BIH)
diastolic h.
essential h. (EH)
Goldblatt h.
idiopathic h.
intracranial h.
malignant h.
mineralocorticoid h.
orthostatic h.
paroxysmal h.
portal h.
primary plexogenic h. (PPHT)
primary pulmonary h. (PPH)
pulmonary artery h.
renal h.
renovascular h.
systolic h.
thrombotic pulmonary h.
hypertensive
h. arteriopathy
h. arteriosclerosis
h. arteriosclerotic heart disease
(HASHD)
h. cardiovascular disease (HCVD)
h. encephalopathy
h. heart disease (HHD, HTHD)
h. pulmonary vascular disease
(HPVD)

hyperthecosis
stromal h.
testoid h.
hyperthelia
hyperthermia
malignant h.
hyperthrombinemia
hyperthymic
hyperthymism
hyperthymization
hyperthyroidism
hyperthyroiditis
hyperthyroxinemia
hypertonia polycythemica
hypertonica
polycythemia h.
hypertonic hyponatremia
hypertonicity
hypertrichosis
h. lanuginosa acquisita
nevoid h.
hypertriglyceridemia
familial h.
hypertrophia
hypertrophic
h. amphophil cell
h. anal papilla
h. arthritis
h. cervical pachymeningitis
h. chronic vulvitis
h. fibrous pachymeningitis
h. gastritis
h. gingivitis
h. hypersecretory gastropathy
h. infiltrative tendinitis (HIT)
h. interstitial neuropathy
h. lichen planus
h. muscular subaortic stenosis
(HMSAS)
h. obstructive cardiomyopathy
(HOCM)
h. polyneuritic-type muscular
atrophy
h. pulmonary osteoarthropathy
h. pyloric stenosis (HPS)
h. scar
hypertrophicum
eczema h.
hypertrophied chondrocyte
hypertrophy
adaptive h.
adenoid h.

NOTES

H

hypertrophy *(continued)*
    asymmetric septal h. (ASH)
    benign prostatic h. (BPH)
    h. of chamber wall
    combined ventricular h. (CVH)
    compensatory h.
    complementary h.
    concentric h.
    diffuse h.
    eccentric h.
    endemic h.
    false h.
    fibrocongestive h.
    focal h.
    functional h.
    giant rugal h.
    growth by h.
    hemangiectatic h.
    idiopathic myocardial h. (IMH)
    Kupffer cell h.
    left atrial h. (LAH)
    left ventricular h. (LVH)
    lipomatous h.
    myofibrillary h.
    numerical h.
    physiologic h.
    prostatic h. (PH)
    quantitative h.
    right atrial h. (RAH)
    right ventricular h. (RVH)
    simple h.
    simulated h.
    true h.
    ventricular h.
    vicarious h.
    virginal h.
hypertyrosinemia, Oregon type
hyperuremia
hyperuresis
hyperuricemia
hyperuricemic nephropathy
hyperuricosuria
hyperuricuria
hyperurobilinogenemia
hypervaccination
hypervalinemia
hypervariable region
hypervascular
    h. hepatocellular carcinoma
    h. nodule
hypervascularity
    villous capillary h.
hyperventilation syndrome
hyperviscosity syndrome
hypervitaminosis A, D
hypervolemia
hypervolemic hypotonic hyponatremia
hypha, pl. **hyphae**
    fungal hyphae

    racquet h.
    spiral h.
hyphal
hyphemia
Hypholoma
Hyphomicrobiaceae
Hyphomicrobiales
Hyphomicrobium
    H. chloromethanicum
    H. sulfonivorans
Hyphomonas
    H. adhaerens
    H. johnsonii
    H. rosenbergii
Hyphomyces destruens
Hyphomycetes
hyphomycosis
Hyphopichia
Hyphozyma
hypnocyst
hypnotic
hypnotoxin
hypnozoite
hypoacidity
hypoadrenalism
hypoadrenocorticism
    primary h.
    secondary h.
hypoalbuminemia
hypoaldosteronism
hypoaldosteronuria
hypoalphaglobulinemia
hypoazoturia
hypobaric
hypobetalipoproteinemia
hypobromous acid
hypocalcemia
hypocalcification
hypocalciuria
hypocapnia
hypocapnic
hypocarbia
hypocellularity of bone marrow
hypocellular stroma
hypoceruloplasminemia
    familial h.
hypochloremia
    dilutional h.
hypochloremic
    h. azotemia
    h. metabolic acidosis
hypochlorhydria
hypochlorite
    sodium h.
hypochlorous acid
hypochloruria
Hypochnicium
Hypochnus
hypocholesterolemia, hypocholesteremia

hypochondriac region
hypochondriasis
hypochondroplasia
hypochromasia
hypochromatic
hypochromatism
hypochromemia
    idiopathic h.
hypochromia
hypochromic
    h. microcytic anemia
    h. microcytic erythrocyte
    h. shift
hypochrosis
hypocitraturia
hypocomplementemia
hypocomplementemic glomerulonephritis
hypocorticoidism
Hypocrea
hypocretin (HCR)
    h. 1, 2
hypocupremia
hypocythemia
    progressive h.
hypocytosis
Hypoderaeum conoideum
hypoderm
Hypoderma bovis
hypodermatosis
hypodermic
    h. implantation
    h. microscope
hypodermis
hypodermolithiasis
hypodiploid
hypodipsia
    primary h.
hypoeosinophilia
hypoestrogenism
hypoferremia
hypoferric anemia
hypofibrinogenemia
hypofunction
    adrenal h.
hypogaea
    Arachis h.
hypogammaglobulinemia
    acquired h.
    common variable h. (CVH)
    congenital X-linked infantile h.
    physiologic h.
    primary h.

    secondary h.
    Swiss-type h.
    transient h.
    X-linked infantile h.
hypoganglionosis
hypogenesis
hypoglobulia
hypoglobulinemia
hypoglycemia
    alimentary h.
    leucine h.
    neonatal h.
    postabsorptive h.
    postprandial h.
    profound h.
hypoglycemic
    h. encephalopathy
    h. shock
hypoglycorrhachia
hypogonadism
hypogonadotropic eunuchoidism
hypogranular granulocyte
hypogranulocytosis
hypohemoglobin (HHb)
hypohidrotic ectodermal dysplasia
hypohydremia
hypohydrochloria
hypohyloma
hypoinsulinism
hypoisotonic
hypokalemia
hypokalemic
    h. alkalosis
    h. diarrhea
    h. nephropathy
    h. nephrosis
    h. periodic paralysis
hypokaluria
hypoleukemia
hypoleydigism
hypolipoproteinemia
hypoliposis
hypolymphemia
hypomagnesemia
hypomelanosis of Ito
hypomethylation
hypomineralization
hypomotility
    esophageal h.
Hypomyces
hyponatremia
    dead-space h.

NOTES

hyponatremia *(continued)*
>   drip-arm h.
>   euvolemic hypotonic h.
>   hypertonic h.
>   hypervolemic hypotonic h.
>   hypotonic h.
>   hypovolemic hypotonic h.
>   isotonic h.

hyponatruria
hyponeocytosis
hypooncotic
hypoorthocytosis
hypoparathyroidism
hypoperfusion
>   tissue h.

hypopharyngeal diverticulum
hypophosphatasia
>   congenital h.

hypophosphatemia
>   X-linked familial h.

hypophosphatemic rickets
hypophosphaturia
hypophyseal *(var. of* hypophysial)
hypophysectomy
hypophyseoportal system
hypophyseos
>   lobus anterior h.
>   lobus glandularis h.
>   lobus posterior h.
>   pars nervosa h.
>   pars pharyngea h.

hypophysial, hypophyseal
>   h. stalk germinoma
>   h. syndrome

hypophysiotropic hormone
hypophysis
>   alpha cell of anterior lobe of h.
>   anterior lobe of h.
>   basophil cell of anterior lobe
>   of h.
>   basophilic cell of anterior lobe
>   of h.
>   beta cell of anterior lobe of h.
>   h. cerebri
>   chromophobe cell of anterior lobe
>   of h.
>   delta cell of anterior lobe of h.
>   diagram of the h.
>   pharyngeal h.
>   posterior lobe of h.
>   h. staining procedure

hypophysitis
>   lymphocytic h.
>   lymphoid h.
>   purulent h.

hypopigmentation
hypopigmentation-immunodeficiency
disease
hypopituitarism

hypoplasia
>   cartilage-hair h. (CHH)
>   crypt h.
>   erythroid h.
>   focal dermal h.
>   granulocytic h.
>   hematopoietic h.
>   lymphoid h.
>   megakaryocytic h.
>   oligonephronic h.
>   renal h.
>   right ventricular h.
>   thymic h.

hypoplasminogenemia
hypoplastic
>   h. anemia
>   h. bone marrow
>   h. heart

hypoploid
hypoploidy
hypopotassemia
hypoproaccelerinemia
hypoproconvertinemia
hypoproteinemia
>   prehepatic h.

hypoprothrombinemia
hypopyon
hyporegenerative anemia
hyporeninemia
hyporeninemic
hyposalemia
hyposarca
hyposecretion
hyposegmentation
>   leukocytic nuclear h.

hyposegmented granulocyte
hyposensitivity
hyposensitization
hyposialadenitis
hyposkeocytosis
hyposmotic
hypospadias
hyposplenism
hypostasis
>   postmortem h.
>   pulmonary h.

hypostatic
>   h. abscess
>   h. congestion
>   h. ectasia
>   h. pneumonia

hyposthenuria
hypostome
hyposulfite
>   sodium h.

hypotension
>   orthostatic h.

hypotensive
hypotetraploid cell

hypothalamic gangliocytoma
hypothalamic-pituitary-testicular axis
hypothalamohypophysial
    h. portal system
    h. tract
hypothalamoneurohypophysial system
hypothalamus
    lateral h.
hypothermia
hypothesis, pl. **hypotheses**
    alternative h.
    autocrine h.
    Benditt h.
    biogenic amine h.
    cardionector h.
    chemiosmotic h.
    encrustation h.
    Haldane h.
    lattice h.
    Lyon h.
    metabolic h.
    monoclonal h.
    omnibus h.
    proton-motive h.
    h. testing
    thrombogenic h.
    unitarian h.
    wobble h.
hypothetical
    h. mean organism (HMO)
    h. mean strain (HMS)
hypothrombinemia
hypothromboplastinemia
hypothyroid
hypothyroidism
hypothyroxinemia
hypotonia
    vasomotor h.
hypotonic hyponatremia
hypotonicity
hypotonus
hypotransferrinemia
hypotriploid
hypouricemia
hypouricuria
hypoventilation
Hypovirus

hypovitaminosis
hypovolemia
hypovolemic
    h. hypotonic hyponatremia
    h. shock
hypoxanthine
    h. guanine phosphoribosyltransferase (HGPRT)
    h. phosphoribosyltransferase (HPRT)
hypoxanthine-aminopterin-thymidine (HAT)
hypoxemia
hypoxia
    anemic h.
    histotoxic h.
    hypoxic h.
    h. inducible factor (HIF)
    h. inducible factor 1 (HIF-1)
    ischemic h.
    oxygen affinity h.
    stagnant h.
    tissue h.
hypoxic
    h. anoxia
    h. cell
    h. cell injury
    h. encephalopathy
    h. hypoxia
    h. nephrosis
    h. vasoconstriction
Hypoxylon
hypsiloid cartilage
Hypsizygus
hypsochrome
hypsochromic shift
hysteratresia
hysteresis loop
hysterical blindness
Hysterolecitha
hysterolith
hysteromyoma
hysterotonin
hystrix
    ichthyosis h.
Hz
    hertz

NOTES

H

I

I
iodine
I antigen
I band
I blood group
I cell
I disc
I region
^{123}**I**
^{125}**I**
^{127}**I**
^{131}**I**
^{131}I uptake test
^{132}**I**
iodine-132
Ia antigen
IADH
inappropriate antidiuretic hormone
IAHA
immune adherence hemagglutination assay
IAHS
infection-associated hemophagocytic syndrome
IASD
interatrial septal defect
IAT
invasive activity test
iodine-azide test
iatrogenic
i. agent
i. anemia
i. artifact
i. disease
i. immunosuppression
IB
immune body
inclusion body
Ibaraki virus
IBC
iron-binding capacity
IBD
inflammatory bowel disease
IBD First Step test
IBF
immunoglobulin-binding factor
IBL
immunoblastic lymphadenopathy
IBM
inclusion body myositis
IBR
infectious bovine rhinotracheitis
IBR virus
IBU
International benzoate unit

IBV
infectious bronchitis virus
IBW
ideal body weight
IC
infection control
intermittent claudication
interstitial cystitis
irritable colon
isovolumic contraction
ICA
immunocytochemical assay
intracranial aneurysm
islet cell antibody
ICAM-1
intercellular adhesion molecule-1
ICAO
internal carotid artery occlusion
Icaria
hemoglobin I.
ICC
immunocompetent cell
Indian childhood cirrhosis
ICD
International Classification of Diseases
ICE
iridocorneal endothelial syndrome
ice
i. point
i. water calorics test
iceberg phenomenon
I-cell disease
ICF
intracellular fluid
ICG
indocyanine green
ICG excretion test
Ichnovirus
ichorous pus
ichorrhea
ichthyoacanthotoxism
ichthyohemotoxism
Ichthyophthirius multifiliis
ichthyosarcotoxism
ichthyosis
acquired i.
i. congenita
i. congenita neonatorum
i. fetalis
i. hystrix
i. intrauterina
lamellar i.
i. linguae
nacreous i.
i. palmaris et plantaris

507

ichthyosis *(continued)*
  i. sauroderma
  i. scutulata
  i. sebacea
  i. sebacea cornea
  i. simplex
  i. spinosa
  i. uteri
  i. vulgaris
  X-linked i.
ichthyotic
ichthyotoxin
icing
  i. heart
  i. liver
ICM
  interference-contrast microscopy
ICOD
  infectious cause of death
Icon
  I. Fx
  I. 25 hCG test
  I. II HCG
  I. MicroALB
icosahedral symmetry
ICSH
  International Committee for
    Standardization in Hematology
  interstitial cell-stimulating hormone
ICSI
  intracytoplasmic sperm injection
ICT
  inflammation of connective tissue
  insulin coma therapy
ICt_{50}
  incapacitating Ct_{50}
"Ictalurid herpes-like viruses"
icteric serum hepatitis (ISH)
icteroanemia
icterogenic spirochetosis
icterohematuric
icterohemoglobinuria
icterohemolytic anemia
icterohepatitis
icteroid
icterus
  acquired hemolytic i.
  benign familial i.
  chronic familial i.
  congenital familial i.
  congenital hemolytic i.
  cythemolytic i.
  i. gravis
  i. gravis of newborn
  i. index (ict ind)
  i. index test
  i. interference
  i. melas

  i. neonatorum
  i. praecox
ict ind
  icterus index
Ictotest reagent tablet
ICW
  intracellular water
ID
  identification
  immunodiffusion
  infecting dose
  infective dose
ID_{50}
  median infectious dose
IDA
  image display and analysis
  iminodiacetic acid
  iron deficiency anemia
Idaeovirus
IDC
  infiltrating ductal carcinoma
  interdigitating dendritic cell
IDCS
  interdigitating dendritic cell sarcoma
IDDM
  insulin-dependent diabetes mellitus
IDDRT
  Infectious Disease Death Review Team
ideal
  i. body weight (IBW)
  i. gas
  i. gas law
  i. solution
identical twins
identification (ID)
  antibody i.
  arthropod i.
  definitive organism i.
  gram-positive i. (GPI)
  hazard i.
  hemoglobin i.
  victim i.
identifier
  biometric i.
identity pattern
Ide test
idioagglutinin
idiocy
  amaurotic familial i.
  late infantile amaurotic familial i.
idiogram
idioheteroagglutinin
idioheterolysin
idioisoagglutinin
idioisolysin
idiolysin
Idiomarina
  I. abyssalis
  I. baltica

I. fontislapidosi
I. loihiensis
I. ramblicola
I. zobellii
Idiomarinaceae
idiopathic
    i. Bamberger-Marie disease
    i. bone cavity
    i. brachial plexopathy
    i. cardiomyopathy
    i. endomyocardial fibrosis
    i. etiology
    i. fibrous mediastinitis
    i. fibrous retroperitonitis
    i. generalized glycogenosis
    i. hemosiderosis
    i. hypercalcemia of infants
    i. hypercalcemic sclerosis of infants
    i. hypercalciuria (IHC)
    i. hypertension
    i. hypertrophic osteoarthropathy (IHO)
    i. hypertrophic subaortic stenosis (IHSS)
    i. hypochromemia
    i. infantile hypercalcemia
    i. megacolon
    i. mesenteric phlebosclerosis
    i. myelofibrosis
    i. myocardial hypertrophy (IMH)
    i. myocarditis
    myometrial hypertrophy (IMH)
    i. myxedema
    i. nephrotic syndrome (INS)
    i. Parkinson disease
    i. paroxysmal rhabdomyolysis
    i. pauciimmune necrotizing crescentic glomerulonephritis
    i. pentosuria
    i. pericarditis
    i. polyneuritis
    i. proctitis
    i. pulmonary fibrosis (IPF)
    i. pulmonary hemosiderosis (IPH)
    i. refractory sideroblastic anemia (IRSA)
    i. respiratory distress syndrome (IRDS)
    i. thrombocytopenia
    i. thrombocytopenic purpura (ITP)
    i. warm autoimmune hemolytic anemia

idiopathica
    dermatitis chronica atrophicans i.
idiopathy
    toxic i.
idiosyncrasy
idiosyncratic
    i. reaction
    i. sensitivity
idiotope
idiotype
    i. antibody
    i. autoantibody
    set of i.'s
idiotypic
    i. antigen
    i. antigenic determinant
IDI-Strep B test
iditol
    i. dehydrogenase
    i. dehydrogenase assay
IDL
    intermediate-density lipoprotein
IDLH
    immediately dangerous to life or health
ID-Micro typing system
idoxuridine (IDU)
IDR
    intradermal reaction
IDS
    immunity deficiency state
IDU
    idoxuridine
    iododeoxyuridine
iduronic
    i. acid
    i. sulfatase
iduronidase
IE
    immunoelectrophoresis
I/E
    inspiratory:expiratory
IED
    improvised explosive device
      incendiary IED
IEF
    isoelectric focusing
      IEF gel electrophoresis
IEM
    immune electron microscopy
IEOP
    immunoelectroosmophoresis

NOTES

IEP
  immunoelectrophoresis
IF
  immunofluorescence
  interfollicular
  intermediate filament
  intrinsic factor
IFA
  immunofluorescence assay
  indirect fluorescent antibody
IFC
  intrinsic factor concentrate
IFCC
  International Federation of Clinical
    Chemistry
IFE
  immunofixation electrophoresis
Iflavirus
IFN
  interferon
    IFN alpha
    IFN beta
    IFN gamma
IFR
  inspiratory flow rate
IFRA
  indirect fluorescent rabies antibody (test)
IFV
  intracellular fluid volume
Ig
  immunoglobulin
IgA
  immunoglobulin A
    IgA endomysial antibody
    IgA globulinemia
    IgA II-HA assay test kit
    IgA immunodeficiency
    IgA myeloma
    IgA nephropathy
    secretory IgA
IgA-antigliadin antibody
IGCN
  intratubular germ cell neoplasia
IGCNU
  intratubular germ cell neoplasia,
    unclassified type
IgD
  immunoglobulin D
    IgD myeloma
IgE
  immunoglobulin E
    IgE antibody
    latex-specific IgE
    IgE myeloma
    specific IgE
    total serum IgE
IgE-mediated disease
IGF-1
  insulinlike growth factor-1

IgG
  immunoglobulin G
    IgG desmoplakin antibody
    IgG index
    IgG index method
    IgG myeloma
    IgG ratio
IgG:albumin ratio
IGH gene
IgM
  immunoglobulin M
    IgM antibody
    IgM anti-hepatitis A virus
    IgM II-HA assay test kit
    IgM nephropathy
    VCA IgM
IgM-RF
  immunoglobulin M-rheumatoid factor
    IgM-RF antibody
**Ig-mutated chronic lymphocytic
  leukemia**
ignava
    Cryomorpha i.
    Johnsonella i.
    Tepidimonas i.
Ignavigranum ruoffiae
Ignicoccus
    I. islandicus
    I. pacificus
ignitability
igniterrae
    Thermus i.
ignition
    i. point
    i. source control
    i. temperature
ignorata
    Nocardia i.
IGPD
  inherited giant platelet disorder
IGSS
  immunogold-silver staining
**Ig-unmutated chronic lymphocytic
  leukemia**
IGV
  intrathoracic gas volume
IH
  infectious hepatitis
IHA
  indirect hemagglutination
IHBTD
  incompatible hemolytic blood transfusion
    disease
IHC
  idiopathic hypercalciuria
  immunohistochemical
  immunohistochemistry
IHD
  ischemic heart disease

iheyensis
> *Oceanobacillus i.*

IHO
> idiopathic hypertrophic osteoarthropathy

IHSA
> iodinated human serum albumin

IHSS
> idiopathic hypertrophic subaortic stenosis

I/i antigen

IIF
> indirect immunofluorescent

I-125 iodinated human serum albumin

I-131 iodinated human serum albumin

Ikegami video camera

IL
> interleukin
> > IL test liquid antithrombin

IL-1–IL-18
> interleukin 1–18

IL-2 receptor alpha-chain deficiency

ILA
> insulinlike activity

Ilarvirus

ILC
> infiltrating lobular carcinoma

ILD
> ischemic leg disease
> ischemic limb disease

ileal intussusception

ileitis
> backwash i.
> Crohn i.
> distal i.
> postcolectomy i.
> prestomal i.
> regional i. (RI)
> terminal i.

ileocecal intussusception

ileocolic intussusception

ileocolitis ulcerosa chronica

ileojejunitis

ileostomy
> Koch i.

ileum
> i. duplex
> duplex i.
> terminal i.

ileus
> adynamic i.
> dynamic i.
> gallstone i.
> mechanical i.

meconium i.
paralytic i.
spastic i.
i. subparta
ureteral i.

Ilhéus
> I. encephalitis
> I. fever
> I. virus

iliac
> i. horn
> i. roll

ill
> louping i.

ill-defined

illinoisensis
> *Alkanindiges i.*

illness
> environmental i.
> neuroparalytic i.
> respiratory i. (RI)
> severity of i.

illudens
> *Omphalotus i.*

illuminance

illumination
> critical i.
> diffuse i.
> Köhler i.

illustris
> *Lucilia i.*

ILNR
> intralobar nephrogenic rest

ilocanum
> *Echinostoma i.*

Ilosvay reagent

ILVEN
> inflammatory linear verrucous epidermal
> nevus

Ilyobacter insuetus

IM
> infectious mononucleosis
> intestinal metaplasia
> intracellular macroadenoma

IMA
> immunometric assay

IMAA
> iodinated macroaggregated albumin

I(Ma) antigen

image
> confocal i.
> i. cytology

NOTES

image *(continued)*
    i. cytometry
    i. display and analysis (IDA)
    I. Titer
image-guided
    i.-g. breast biopsy
    i.-g. core biopsy
imaging
    FLM i.
    fluorescence lifetime i. (FLM)
    postmortem i.
    in vivo tissue i.
Imago broth
imbalance
    allelic i.
    calcium i.
    chloride i.
    electrolyte i.
    hormonal i.
    magnesium i.
    phosphate i.
    potassium i.
    sodium i.
    sympathetic i.
imbed
imbibition
imbricata
imbricate
imbrication line of von Ebner
IMBT
    intestinal mucinous borderline tumor
IMC
    immunohistochemical
Imerslund-Grasbeck syndrome
IMH
    idiopathic myocardial hypertrophy
    myometrial hypertrophy
imidazole
imidazolepyruvic acid
imide
imine
imino acid
iminodiacetic acid (IDA)
iminoglycinuria
imipramine and desipramine assays
Imlach fat-pad
Immage
    I. Anti-DNaseB
    I. immunochemistry system
immature
    i. granulocyte
    i. neutrophil
    i. teratoma
immediate
    i. allergy
    i. contagion
    i. hypersensitivity
    i. hypersensitivity reaction
    i. principle

    i. radiation toxicity
    triage i.
immediately dangerous to life or health (IDLH)
immediate-phase skin response
immediate-spin crossmatch
immersion
    i. foot
    homogeneous i.
    i. microscopy
    i. objective
    oil i.
    i. syndrome
    water i.
immersion-submersion
imminent abortion
immiscible
immite
    Geotrichum i.
immitis
    Coccidioides i.
    Dirofilaria i.
immobilization
    Treponema pallidum i. (TPI)
immobilized
    i. enzyme
    i. postoperative patient
immobilizing antibody
immortalization
immotile cilia syndrome
immotility
ImmuKnow immune cell function assay
Immulite
    I. 2000 chemiluminescent analyzer
    I. Dynamic Duo analyzer
    I. 2000 free PSA
    I. free PSA assay
    I. 1000, 2000, 2500 immunoassay system
    I. 2000 PSA assay
    I. 2500 SMS immunoassay system
    I. 2000 third-generation PSA
    I. third-generation PSA assay
Immu-Mark immunostaining kit
immune
    i. adherence
    i. adherence hemagglutination assay (IAHA)
    i. adherence phenomenon
    i. adhesion test
    i. adsorption
    i. agglutination
    i. agglutinin
    i. barrier
    i. body (IB)
    i. clearance
    i. complex
    i. complex assay
    i. complex disease

i. complex disorder
i. complex glomerulonephritis
i. complex glomerulopathy
i. complex-mediated hypersensitivity reaction
i. complex-mediated inflammatory lesion
i. complex nephritis
i. complex nephropathy
i. cytolysis
i. deficiency
i. deviation
i. dysfunction syndrome
i. electron microscopy (IEM)
i. elimination
i. fetal hydrops
i. hemolysin
i. hemolysis
i. inflammation
i. inflammatory reaction
i. interferon
i. lactoglobulin
i. opsonin
i. paralysis
i. precipitation
i. protein
i. rejection of seminoma
i. response (Ir)
i. response gene
i. serum
i. serum globulin (ISG)
i. surveillance
i. system
i. thrombocytopenia
i. thrombocytopenic purpura
i. tolerance
immune-deposit disease
immune-mediated
　　i.-m. destruction
　　i.-m. mechanism
　　i.-m. process
immune-privileged
immune-stimulating complex (ISCOM)
immunifacient
immunity
　　acquired i.
　　active i.
　　adoptive i.
　　antibody-dependent i.
　　antiviral i.
　　artificial active i.
　　artificial passive i.

bacteriophage i.
cell-mediated i. (CMI)
cellular i.
combinatorial i.
concomitant i.
cross-protective i.
i. deficiency
i. deficiency state (IDS)
general i.
group i.
herd i.
humoral i.
infection i.
innate i.
local i.
maternal i.
natural i.
nonspecific i.
passive i.
relative i.
specific active i.
specific passive i.
i. substance
immunization
　　active i.
　　paratyphoid i.
　　passive i.
　　postexposure i.
　　preexposure i.
　　i. reaction poliomyelitis
　　Rh i.
　　smallpox i.
immunize
immunizing unit (IU)
immunoadjuvant
immunoadsorbent
immunoadsorption
immunoaffinity
　　i. chromatography
　　i. purification
immunoagglutination
immunoalkaline phosphatase stain
immunoamyloidosis
immunoarchitectural appearance
ImmunoAssay
　　Optical I. (OIA)
immunoassay
　　agglutination i.
　　Asserachrom APA i.
　　chemiluminescent i.
　　cloned enzyme donor i. (CEDIA)
　　Cobas Integra Cyclosporine I.

NOTES

513

immunoassay *(continued)*
    coenzyme-labeled i.
    competitive heterogeneous
      enzyme i.
    direct quenching fluorescent i.
    DNA-enzyme i. (DEIA)
    double antibody i.
    Elecsys free PSA i.
    Elecsys proBNP i.
    Elecsys total PSA i.
    electrochemiluminescence i.
      (ECLIA)
    enzyme-enhancement i.
    enzyme-multiplied i. (EIA)
    fluorescence excitation transfer i.
      (FETI)
    fluorescence polarization i. (FPIA)
    fluorescent i. (FIA)
    ImmunoCard STAT! rotavirus i.
    ImmunoCard STAT! strep A i.
    ligand i.
    light-scattering i.
    lymphocyte transformation i.
    MAb-based enzyme i.
    microparticle capture enzyme i.
      (MEIA)
    microparticle enzyme i. (MEIA)
    nephelometric i.
    noncompetitive heterogeneous
      enzyme i.
    nonradioisotopic i.
    OncoChek i.
    particle concentration fluorescence i.
      (PCFIA)
    particle-enhanced turbidimetric
      inhibition i. (PETINIA)
    passive immunodiffusion i.
    radioisotopic i.
    i. reagent
    solid phase i.
    solid phase fluorescence i. (SPFIA)
    sperm-ubiquitin tag i. (SUTI)
    substrate-labeled fluorescence i.
      (SLFIA)
    substrate-labeled fluorescent i.
      (SLFIA)
    thin-layer i.
    time-resolved fluorescence i.
    turbidimetric i.
immunobiology
immunoblast
immunoblastic
    i. lymphadenopathy (IBL)
    i. lymphoma
    i. sarcoma
immunoblot test
immunoblotting
Immuno-Brite Fluorospheres

ImmunoCard
    I. STAT! rotavirus immunoassay
    I. STAT! rotavirus test
    I. STAT! strep A immunoassay
immunocatalysis
immunochemical
    i. assay
    i. fecal occult blood test
immunochemistry
    i. reagent
    ultrastructural i.
immunochromatography
    enzyme i. (EIC)
immunocompetence
immunocompetent cell (ICC)
immunocomplex
immunocompromised
immunoconcentration assay
immunoconglutinin
ImmunoCyt cytopathology recurrent
  bladder cancer test
immunocyte
immunocytoadherence
immunocytochemical
    i. assay (ICA)
    i. localization
immunocytochemical assay (ICA)
immunocytochemically
immunocytochemistry
immunocytoma
immunocytopenia
immunodeficiency
    B-cell i.
    combined i.
    common variable i. (CVID)
    i. disease
    IgA i.
    immunoglobulin A i.
    phagocytic dysfunction disorder i.
    secondary i.
    severe combined i. (SCID)
    i. syndrome
    T-cell i.
    i. with hypoparathyroidism
immunodeficient
immunodepressant
immunodepression
immunodepressor
immunodetection
    HBc antigen i.
immunodiagnosis
immunodiffusion (ID)
    double i.
    Ouchterlony i.
    Oudin i.
    radial i. (RID)
    single i.
    single-diffusion radial i.
ImmunoDip urinary albumin test

immunodominance
ImmunoDOT Mono G, M test kit
Immuno 1 DPD assay
immunoelectroosmophoresis (IEOP)
immunoelectrophoresis (IE, IEP)
    countercurrent i. (CIE, CIEP)
    crossed i.
    double-crossed i.
    factor VIII-crossed i.
    Laurell rocket i.
    reverse i.
    rocket i.
    two-dimensional i.
immunoenhancement
immunoenhancer
immunoenzymometric
    i. assay
    i. staining
immunoferritin
immunofiltration
    analytical i.
    preparative i.
immunofixation
    i. electrophoresis (IFE)
    i. by subtraction
immunofixation electrophoresis (IFE)
immunofluorescence (IF)
    adenovirus i.
    i. assay (IFA)
    direct i.
    lumpy-bumpy i.
    i. method
    i. microscopy
    mixed i. (MIF)
    i. technique
    i. test
immunofluorescent
    i. assay
    i. assay kit
    indirect i. (IIF)
    i. stain
    i. staining
immunogen
immunogenetic
immunogenic determinant
immunogenicity
immunogenotyping
immunogenum
    Mycobacterium i.
immunoglobulin (Ig)
    i. A (IgA)
    i. A, D, G, M test

i. A immunodeficiency
    antibody deficiency with near-
    normal i.'s
anti-D i.
cerebrospinal fluid i.
chickenpox i.
i. class
i. D (IgD)
i. disorder
i. domain
i. E (IgE)
i. family adhesion protein
i. G (IgG)
i. gene rearrangement
human normal i.
i. M (IgM)
measles i.
monoclonal i.
i. M-rheumatoid factor (IgM-RF)
pertussis i.
poliomyelitis i.
quantitative i.
rabies i.
$Rh_o(D)$ i.
secretory i.
i. subclass
i. supergene
surface i. (sIg)
tetanus i.
thyroid-stimulating i. (TSI)
TSH binding inhibitory i. (TBII)
immunoglobulin-binding factor (IBF)
immunoglobulinopathy
immunogold
    i. electron microscopy
    i. labeling
    i. probe
immunogold-silver staining (IGSS)
immunohematology
immunohemolytic anemia
immunohistochemical (IHC, IMC)
    i. analysis
    i. marker
    i. parameter
    i. pattern
    i. stain
    i. staining
    i. stain for T cell
    i. technique
immunohistochemistry (IHC)
    anticytokeratin i.
    E-cadherin i.

NOTES

immunohistochemistry (*continued*)
    epithelial marker i.
    i. reagent
immunohistofluorescence
immunohistology
    qualitative i.
    quantitative i.
immunoincompetent
immunoinhibition
immunolabeling
    double i.
immunologic
    i. competence
    i. enhancement
    i. high-dose tolerance
    i. homeostasis
    i. memory
    i. paralysis
    i. pregnancy test
    i. unresponsiveness
immunological
    i. competence
    i. deficiency
    i. enhancement
    i. mechanism
    i. paralysis
    i. surveillance
    i. tolerance
immunologically
    i. activated cell
    i. competent cell
    i. privileged site
immunologist
immunology
    armchair i.
    transplantation i.
immunoluminometric assay
immunomagnetic cell separation
immunomarker
immunometric assay (IMA)
immunomodulation
immunomodulator
immunomodulatory
    i. agent
    i. treatment
immunomorphology
immunoparalysis
immunopathogenesis
immunopathology
immunoperoxidase
    PAP i.
    paraffin i. (PIP)
    i. stain
    i. staining method
    i. technique
    i. test
immunophenotype
    myofibroblastic i.

immunophenotypic
    i. signature
    i. study
immunophenotypical
immunophenotyping
    cell surface i.
    flow cytometric i.
    leukemia i.
    lymphoma i.
    quantitative flow cytometric i.
immunophilin
immunopositivity
    S-100 protein i.
immunopotency
immunopotentiation
immunopotentiator
immunoprecipitation
    automated i. (AIP)
ImmunoPrep reagent system
immunoprofile
immunoproliferative
    i. disorder
    i. small intestinal disease (IPSID)
immunoprophylaxis
immunoradioassayable human chorionic somatomammotropin (IRHCS)
immunoradiometric assay (IRMA)
immunoradiometry
immunoreaction
immunoreactive (IR)
    i. glucagon (IRG)
    i. human growth hormone (IRhGH)
    i. insulin (IRI)
immunoreactivity
    caspase i.
    cytokeratin i.
    cytoplasmic i.
    filaggrin-like i.
    somatostatin-like i. (SLI)
immunoreceptor
    i. tyrosine activation motif (ITAM)
    i. tyrosine inhibitory motif (ITIM)
immunoregulation
    disordered i.
immunoselection
immunosenescence
immunosilent
immunosorbent antibody
immunostain
    BG8 i.
    CD99 i.
    Dako hepatocyte i.
    MIB1 nuclear i.
    pancytokeratin i.
    S-100 i.
    TDT i.
    tryptase i.
immunostainer
    Shandon Cadenza i.

TechMate 1000 i.
Ventana automated i.
Ventana NexES i.
Ventana TechMate 100 i.
immunostaining
clusterin i.
keratin i.
MyoD1 i.
immunostimulant
immunostimulation
immunosubtraction (ISUB)
immunosuppressant
immunosuppression
iatrogenic i.
immunosuppressive
immunosurveillance
immunotactoid
i. glomerulonephritis
i. glomerulopathy
Immunotech
I. immunoassay component
I. immunoassay kit
immunotherapy
adoptive i.
biological i.
immunotolerance
immunotransfusion
Immuno-trol cell
immunotyping
ImmuSTRIP HAMA test kit
impact
i. loading
I. on-site drug and alcohol test
system
planar i.
projectile i.
i. splatter
impacted
i. feces
i. fracture
i. tooth
impaction
fecal i.
i. lesion
impaired clot retraction
impaired utilization of iron
impairment
functional aerobic i.
impalpable
impatiens
Saccharospirillum i.

impedance
electrode i.
output i.
imperfect
i. fungus
i. stage
i. state
i. yeast
imperfecta
amelogenesis i.
dentinogenesis i.
enamelogenesis i.
erythrogenesis i.
osteogenesis i.
Imperfecti
Fungi I.
imperforate
i. anus
i. hymen
imperforation
impermeable junction
impetiginized
impetigo
bullous i.
i. contagiosa
i. neonatorum
i. vulgaris
impingement syndrome
implant
buffered i.
carcinomatous i.
invasive i.
noninvasive i.
silicone breast i. (SBI)
synchronous peritoneal i.
Zyplast i.
implantation
i. bleeding
circumferential i.
i. cone
i. cyst
i. dermoid
hypodermic i.
interstitial i.
periosteal i.
i. site
superficial i.
i. test (IT)
implosion
impotence
imprecision

NOTES

impregnation
    silver i.
    Watanabe silver i.
impression
    i. cytology
    i. preparation
    rifling i.
imprint
    maternal i.
    paternal i.
    touch i.
    Wright-Giemsa stained touch i.
imprinting
    genomic i.
improvement
    quality i. (QI)
improvised explosive device (IED)
impulse sealing
impulsive loading
impurity
IMR
    infant mortality rate
IMT
    inflammatory myofibroblastic tumor
IMViC
    indole, methyl red, Voges-Proskauer, and citrate
        IMViC test
IMx analyzer
In
    indium
^{111}In
    indium 111
in
    In Charge diabetes control system
    in situ
    in situ DNA nick end labeling
    in situ finding
    in situ hybridization (ISH)
    in situ nick end labeling
    in tela
    in utero
    in vacuo
    in vitro
    in vitro invasion assay
    in vitro transcription/translation (IVTT)
    in vivo
    in vivo adhesive platelet (IVAP)
    in vivo compatibility test
    in vivo tissue imaging
Inaba antigen
inactivate
inactivated
    i. leukocytolytic serum
    i. poliovirus vaccine (IPV)
    i. ricin toxoid vaccination

inactivation
    complement i.
    i. mechanism
inactivator
    anaphylatoxin i.
inactive tuberculosis
INAD
    infantile neuroaxonal dystrophy
inadvertent
    i. inoculation
    i. inoculation of vaccinia virus
inanition
inapparent infection
inappropriate
    i. antidiuretic hormone (IADH)
    i. antidiuretic hormone syndrome
    i. production of erythropoietin
INB
    internuclear bridging
inborn
    i. error of vitamin D metabolism
    i. lysosomal disease
inbreeding
    coefficient of i.
    i. coefficient
incapacitate
incapacitating
    i. chemical agent
    i. Ct_{50} (ICt_{50})
    i. dose
incaprettamento (ritual ligature strangulation)
incarcerated hernia
incendiary IED
inch
    pounds per square i. (psi)
inchonensis
    Tsukamurella i.
incidence
    angle of i.
    i. of hepatocellular carcinoma
    i. increase
    peak i.
    i. rate
incident
    criticality i.
    i. light
    mass casualty i. (MCI)
    mass fatality i.
incineration
incised wound
incisional biopsy
incisor
    Hutchinson i.
incisura
    i. angularis
    Anthomyia i.
    gastric i.

incisure
> Lanterman i.
> Schmidt-Lanterman i.

inclusion
> i. blennorrhea
> blennorrhea i.
> i. body (IB)
> i. body disease
> i. body encephalitis
> i. body fibromatosis
> i. body myositis (IBM)
> cell i.
> i. cell
> i. cell disease
> i. conjunctivitis
> i. conjunctivitis virus
> i. cyst
> cytoplasmic i.
> i. dermoid
> Döhle i.
> endothelial tubuloreticular i.
> intranuclear i.
> leukocyte i.
> neural i. (NI)
> neuronal intranuclear i.
> ubiquitinated i.
> viral i.

incognita
> *Oxyuris i.*

incohesive

incompatibility
> ABO i.
> blood i.
> chemical i.
> fetomaternal i.
> physiologic i.
> Rh i.

incompatible
> i. blood transfusion
> i. blood transfusion reaction
> i. chemical
> i. hemolytic blood transfusion
> disease (IHBTD)

incompetence
> aortic i. (AI)
> mitral i.
> pulmonary i. (PI)
> tricuspid i. (TI)
> valvular i.

incompetent
> i. aortic valve
> i. cervix

> i. foramen ovale valve
> i. mitral valve
> i. pulmonic valve
> i. tricuspid valve
> i. valve foramen ovale

incomplete
> i. abortion
> i. agglutinin
> i. amnion
> i. amputation
> i. antibody
> i. antigen
> i. compound fracture
> i. conjoined twins
> i. differentiation (cardiac valve)
> i. dislocation
> i. dominance
> i. fistula
> i. hernia
> i. muzzle contusion
> i. neurofibromatosis
> i. penetrance
> i. regeneration
> i. right bundle branch block
> i. transposition

inconstans
> *Proteus i.*

incontinence
> fecal i.
> i. of pigment
> urinary i.

incontinentia
> i. pigmenti
> i. pigmenti achromians

incorporation of irradiation

increase
> absolute cell i.
> incidence i.

increased
> i. arterial H+
> i. basal metabolism
> i. capillary fragility
> i. erythropoiesis
> i. flow
> i. metabolism
> i. pressure
> i. sodium retention
> i. specific gravity
> i. temperature
> i. turbidity
> i. urine urobilinogen

NOTES

increased *(continued)*
    i. viscosity
    i. volume
increment
incremental
    i. line
    i. line of von Ebner
increta
    placenta i.
incrustation
incubate
incubation period (IP)
incubative stage
incubator
    Sagian 180 CO2 i.
incubatory carrier
incurable
IND
    intestinal neuronal dysplasia
    IND A, B
indamine dye
indenization
indentation
independence
    anchorage i.
independent
    i. assortment
    i. practice association
    i. variable
indeterminate
    i. calcification
    i. cell adenocarcinoma
    i. colitis
    i. leprosy
    i. pattern
    i. range entrance wound
index, pl. **indices, indexes**
    absorbency i.
    acidophilic i.
    activity i.
    amniotic fluid foam stability i.
    antitryptic i.
    apoptotic i.
    Arneth i.
    bacteriological i. (BI)
    blood indices
    body mass i. (BMI)
    Breslow tumor i.
    Broders tumor i.
    burn i. (BI)
    carbohydrate metabolism i. (CMI)
    cardiac i.
    i. case
    cephalic i.
    cerebrospinal fluid albumin i.
    cerebrospinal fluid IgG i.
    cerebrospinal fluid-to-serum
     albumin i.
    chemotherapeutic i. (CI)

chronicity i.
Colour I. (C.I.)
coronary prognostic i. (CPI)
creatinine height i. (CHI)
crowded cell i.
degenerative i.
development-at-birth i. (DBI)
DNA i. (DI)
endemic i.
eosinophilic i. (EI)
erythrocyte indices
foam stability i. (FSI)
folded-cell i.
free thyroxine i. (FT_4I, FTI)
free/total PSA i.
free triiodothyronine i. (FT_3I)
grid i.
hematopneic i.
hemolytic i.
hepatic iron i. (HII)
histologic activity i. (HAI)
hydroxyproline i.
icterus i. (ict ind)
IgG i.
international prognostic i.
International Sensitivity I. (ISI)
iron i.
juxtaglomerular granulation i. (JGI)
karyopyknotic i. (KI)
Ki-67 i.
Knodell histology activity i.
Kovats i.
Krebs leukocyte i.
labeling i.
leukopenic i.
lymphocyte proliferation/regression i.
  (LPI/LRI)
mass i.
maturation i.
Mentzer MCV i.
metacarpal i.
mitosis-karyorrhexis i. (MKI)
mitotic i.
mitotic activity i. (MAI)
myelofibrosis
  proliferation/regression i.
  (MPI/MRI)
Nottingham Prognostic I. (NPI)
nucleoplasmic i. (NP)
O'Grady prognostic indices
opsonic i.
peripheral blood labeling i.
phagocytic i.
phenylalanine tolerance i.
phosphate excretion i. (PEI)
plasma-cell labeling i.
proliferative i. (PI)
PSA i.
pyknotic i.

red cell indices
i. of refraction
refractive i. (RI)
i. register
Reid i.
relative value i. (RVI)
retention i.
reticulocytic production i. (RPI)
saturation i. (SI)
Schilling i.
sedimentation i.
Sertoli cell i. (SCI)
short increment sensitivity i. (SISI)
splenic i.
squamous cell i.
staphyloopsonic i.
steroid protein activity i. (SPAI)
stratification i.
thoracic i. (TI)
thyroxine-binding i. (TBI)
time-tension i. (TTI)
topo-II-alpha i.
tuberculoopsonic i.
tubular-fertility i. (TFI)
uricolytic i.
volume i.

India
I. ink capsule stain
I. ink method
I. ink mount
I. ink preparation
I. rubber man syndrome

Indian
I. childhood cirrhosis (ICC)
I. file
I. rat flea

Indianapolis
hemoglobin I.

Indian-file pattern

indica
Pseudomonas i.

indican
metabolic i.
plant i.
i. test

indicanidrosis
indicanuria
indicated
method of collection not i. (MOCNI)

indicator
acid-base i.

alizarin i.
Andrade i.
clinical i.
i. culture medium
i. electrode
i. organism
oxidation-reduction i.
i. paper
pH i.
redox i.
i. system
i. tube

indicator-dilution curve
indices (*pl. of* index)
indicus
Bacillus i.
Deinococcus i.
Thermodesulfatator i.

Indiella
indifferent
i. cell
i. electrode
i. neutrotaxis

indigenous bacterium
indigo
i. blue
i. calculus
i. carmine

indigo-carmine
i.-c. stain
i.-c. test

indigoferae
Rhizobium i.

indigoid dye
indigotin
indiguria
indirect
i. addressing
i. agglutination
i. antiglobulin test
i. assay
i. bilirubin test
i. Coombs test
i. fluorescent antibody (IFA)
i. fluorescent antibody test
i. fluorescent rabies antibody (test) (IFRA)
i. hemagglutination (IHA)
i. hemagglutination test
i. hernia
i. immunofluorescence test
i. immunofluorescent (IIF)

NOTES

indirect *(continued)*
    i. maternal death
    i. reacting bilirubin
    i. suffocation
    i. transport
indiscriminate lesion
indium (In)
    i. leukocyte scan
indium 111 (^{111}In)
    i. 111 chloride
    i. 111 trichloride
individual protective equipment (IPE)
indocyanine
    i. green (ICG)
    i. green test
indolacetic acid
indolaceturia
indolaceturic acid
indolelactic acid
indole, methyl red, Voges-Proskauer, and citrate (IMViC)
indole-nitrate broth
indolent ulcer
indolicus
    Peptoniphilus i.
indolifex
    Oceanibulbus i.
indologenes
    Kingella i.
    Suttonella i.
indoluria
indonesiensis
    Acetobacter i.
    Desulfovibrio i.
    Streptomyces i.
indophenol
    i. dye
    i. method
    i. test
indoxyl sulfate
indoxyluria
induced
    i. abortion
    i. allergic encephalomyelitis
    i. allergic neuritis
    i. aspermatogenesis
    i. glomerulonephritis
    i. phagocytosis
    i. sensitivity
    i. thyroiditis
    i. uveitis
inducer cell
inducible
    i. enzyme
    i. nitric oxide synthetase (iNOS)
inducing
    syncytium i. (SI)
inductance

induction
    enzyme i.
    lysogenic i.
    magnetic i.
    negative control enzyme i.
    i. period
    positive control enzyme i.
    sputum i.
    i. therapy
inductive
    i. phase
    i. reactance
inductor
indulin
indulinophil, indulinophile
indurated
induration
    collapse i.
    cyanotic i.
    Froriep i.
    gray i.
    plastic i.
    red i.
indurative myocarditis
induratum
    erythema i.
indusium
industrial
    i. poison
    i. toxicology
INE
    infantile necrotizing encephalomyelopathy
ineffective erythropoiesis
inelastic scattering
Inermicapsifer madagascariensis
inert electrode
inertia
inevitable abortion
inexpectatum
    Albidovulum i.
inf
    infusion
infancy
    chronic pneumonitis of i. (CPI)
    fibrous hamartoma of i.
    melanotic neuroectodermal tumor of i.
    spongy degeneration of i.
    sudden unexpected death in i. (SUDI)
    transient hypogammaglobulinemia of i.
infant
    i. botulism
    i. death
    idiopathic hypercalcemia of i.'s
    idiopathic hypercalcemic sclerosis of i.'s

low birth weight i. (LBWI)
i. mortality rate (IMR)
premature i.
splenic anemia of i.'s

infantarius
   Streptococcus i.
   Streptococcus i. subsp. *infantarius*

infantile
   i. amaurotic familial idiocy
   i. celiac disease
   i. cortical hyperostosis
   i. digital fibromatosis
   i. fibrosarcoma
   i. gastroenteritis
   i. gastroenteritis virus
   i. glaucoma
   i. hemangioma
   i. hepatic hemangioendothelioma
   i. muscular atrophy
   i. myofibromatosis
   i. myxedema
   i. necrotizing encephalomyelopathy
    (INE)
   i. neuroaxonal dystrophy (INAD)
   i. paralysis
   i. polycystic kidney disease
   i. progressive spinal muscular
    dystrophy
   i. purulent conjunctivitis
   i. respiratory distress syndrome
   i. SMA
   i. spasm
   i. type coarctation
   i. uterus

infantilis
   poliodystrophia cerebri
    progressiva i.
   roseola i.

infantilism
   tubal i.

infantis
   Bifidobacterium i.
   Hydatigera i.
   Salmonella enteritidis serotype *i.*

infantum
   dermatitis exfoliativa infantum
   dermatitis gangrenosa i.
   Leishmania donovani i.

infarct
   acute i.
   anemic i.

anterior lateral myocardial i.
  (ALMI)
anteroseptal myocardial i. (ASMI)
bile i.
bland i.
bone i.
Brewer i.
cerebral i.
digital i.
embolic i.
focal i.
healed i.
hemorrhagic i.
microscopic i.
old i.
pale i.
posterior wall i. (PWI)
pulmonary i.
recent i.
red i.
reddish-brown i.
ruptured myocardial i.
septic i.
thrombotic i.
uric acid i.
white i.
Zahn i.

infarction
   acute myocardial i. (AMI)
   anterior wall i. (AWI)
   anterior wall myocardial i.
    (AWMI)
   atrial i.
   bowel i.
   cardiac remodeling after acute
    myocardial i.
   cerebral i. (CI)
   inferior wall myocardial i. (IWMI)
   intestinal i.
   lymph node i.
   maternal floor i.
   mesenteric i.
   myocardial i. (MI)
   myocardial infarction in H-form
   nontransmural myocardial i.
   old myocardial i. (OMI)
   postmyocardial i.
   pulmonary i. (PI)
   renal i.
   silent myocardial i.
   subendocardial myocardial i.

NOTES

infarction *(continued)*
>> through-and-through myocardial i.
>> transmural myocardial i.

infarctive placental dysfunction
infected abortion
infecting dose (ID)
infection
>> abortive i.
>> airborne i.
>> atypical mycobacteria i.
>> bacterial i.
>> biliary tract i.
>> *Chlamydia* i.
>> colonization i.
>> concurrent i.
>> i. control (IC)
>> cross i.
>> cryptogenic i.
>> cutaneous anthrax i.
>> cytomegalovirus i.
>> dragon worm i.
>> droplet i.
>> ectothrix i.
>> endogenous i.
>> *Enterobacter* urinary tract i.
>> *Enterococcus* urinary tract i.
>> enzootic i.
>> *Escherichia coli* urinary tract i.
>> exogenous i.
>> exuberant i.
>> fever caused by i. (FI)
>> focal i.
>> foodborne i.
>> gastrointestinal anthrax i.
>> guinea worm i.
>> herpes simplex virus i.
>> i. immunity
>> inapparent i.
>> inhalational anthrax i.
>> intestinal parasitic i.
>> *Klebsiella* urinary tract i.
>> latent i.
>> lower urinary tract i.
>> mass i.
>> medina worm i.
>> meningococcal i.
>> meningococcus i.
>> mixed i.
>> mycobacteria i.
>> *Mycobacterium avium* i.
>> *Mycoplasma* i.
>> nosocomial i.
>> opportunistic i.
>> oral i.
>> orf i.
>> parainfluenza virus i.
>> parvovirus B19 i.
>> pelvic i.
>> persistent i.

>> persistent tolerant i. (PTI)
>> postoperative i.
>> *Proteus* urinary tract i.
>> *Providencia* urinary tract i.
>> *Pseudomonas* urinary tract i.
>> puerperal i.
>> pulmonary i.
>> pyogenic i.
>> recurrent bacterial i.
>> recurrent hepatitis C virus i.
>> recurrent sinus and pulmonary i.
>> recurrent upper respiratory tract i. (RURTI)
>> reservoir of i.
>> respiratory syncytial virus i.
>> rickettsial i.
>> secondary i.
>> second-strain i.
>> serpent i.
>> *Serratia* urinary tract i.
>> spinal cord i.
>> *Staphylococcus aureus* urinary tract i.
>> streptococcal i.
>> suppurative i.
>> i. surveillance and control program (ISCP)
>> upper respiratory i. (URI)
>> upper respiratory tract i. (URTI)
>> urea-splitting bacterial i.
>> urinary tract i. (UTI)
>> viral respiratory i. (VRI)
>> whipworm i.
>> zoonotic i.
infection-associated hemophagocytic syndrome (IAHS)
infection-immunity
infectiosity
infectiosum
>> erythema i.
infectious
>> i. agent
>> i. anemia
>> i. arteritis
>> i. arteritis virus of horses
>> i. arthritis
>> i. avian bronchitis
>> i. bovine rhinotracheitis (IBR)
>> i. bovine rhinotracheitis virus
>> i. bronchitis virus (IBV)
>> i. bulbar paralysis
>> i. canine hepatitis
>> i. cause of death (ICOD)
>> i. colitis
>> i. disease
>> I. Disease Death Review Team (IDDRT)
>> I. Disease Surveillance Information System (ISIS)

i. disorder
i. ectromelia virus
i. eczematoid dermatitis
i. endocarditis
i. enterocolitides
i. esophagitis
i. granuloma
i. hepatitis (IH)
i. hepatitis virus
i. mononucleosis (IM)
i. mononucleosis screening test
i. myocarditis
i. myositis
i. myxoma
i. nucleic acid
i. papilloma of cattle
i. papilloma virus
i. parotitis
i. plasmid
i. polyneuritis
i. porcine encephalomyelitis
i. porcine encephalomyelitis virus
i. wart
i. waste
"infectious laryngo-tracheitis-like viruses"
infectiousness
infectiva
  polioencephalitis i.
infective
  i. dose (ID)
  i. embolism
  i. endocarditis
  i. thrombus
infectivity
infectoria
  Lewia i.
inferior
  i. complete closed dislocation
  i. complete compound dislocation
  i. dislocation
  i. displacement
  ductulus aberrans i.
  i. lipodystrophy
  i. petrosal sinus sampling
  i. petrosal vein sampling
  tarsus i.
  tela choroidea i.
  i. wall myocardial infarction
    (IWMI)
infernum
  Desulfacinum i.
infertility screen

infestans
  Phytophthora i.
infestation
  parasitic i.
  saprophytic i.
  Trichomonas i.
infidelity
  lineage i.
infiltrate
  acute inflammatory i.
  Assmann tuberculous i.
  brisk i.
  central-patch i.
  eosinophil leukocytic i.
  hilar-based fluffy i.
  inflammatory i.
  infraclavicular i.
  Jessner lymphocytic i.
  leukocytic i.
  lymphocytic inflammatory i.
  lymphoplasmacytic i.
  microscopic inflammatory i.
  monocytic inflammatory i.
  neutrophilic i.
  nonbrisk i.
  plasma cell i.
  plasmacytic i.
  polymorphonuclear leukocytic i.
  polymorphous lymphoid i.
  pulmonary i.
infiltrating
  i. comedocarcinoma
  i. cribriform carcinoma
  i. duct adenocarcinoma
  i. ductal carcinoma (IDC)
  i. lipoma
  i. lobular carcinoma (ILC)
  i. papillary carcinoma
infiltration
  adipose i.
  calcareous i.
  cellular i.
  epituberculous i.
  fatty i.
  gelatinous i.
  glycogen i.
  gray i.
  intratumoral i.
  i. of leukemic cell
  lipomatous i.
  lymphocytic i.
  lymphoplasmacytic i.

NOTES

infiltration (*continued*)
    muconodular i.
    pulmonary interstitial lymphocytic i.
    sanguineous i.
    tuberculous i.
    tubular i.
infiltrative
    i. disease
    i. fasciitis
    i. margin
    i. ophthalmopathy
infinite
infinitely miscible
infinitesimal
infinity
inflamed ulcer
inflammable
inflammation
    active chronic i.
    acute and chronic i.
    acute hemorrhagic i.
    adhesive i.
    allergic i.
    alterative i.
    atrophic i.
    blennorrhagic i.
    bullous granulomatous i.
    calcified granulomatous i.
    caseating granulomatous i.
    caseous i.
    catarrhal i.
    cavitating i.
    chronic active i.
    chronic nonspecific i.
    circumscribed i.
    confluent i.
    i. of connective tissue (ICT)
    croupous i.
    cystic acute i.
    cystic chronic i.
    cystic granulomatous i.
    degenerative i.
    diffuse acute i.
    diffuse chronic i.
    disseminated i.
    early stage of i.
    erosive i.
    exanthematous i.
    exudative granulomatous i.
    fibrinoid necrotizing i.
    fibrinopurulent i.
    fibrinous i.
    fibrocaseous i.
    fibroid i.
    focal granulomatous i.
    follicular i.
    gangrenous granulomatous i.
    gelatinous acute i.
    granulomatous i.

    hemorrhagic i.
    hyperplastic i.
    immune i.
    interstitial i.
    localized i.
    lymphoplasmacytic i.
    membranous acute i.
    miliary granulomatous i.
    multifocal i.
    necrotic i.
    necrotizing granulomatous i.
    neutrophilic i.
    nonnecrotizing granulomatous i.
    obliterative i.
    organizing i.
    ossifying i.
    i. of the ovary
    productive i.
    proliferative i.
    pseudomembranous acute i.
    purulent i.
    pustular i.
    recurrent i.
    respiratory i.
    sclerosing i.
    serofibrinous i.
    serous acute i.
    sinusoidal i.
    spinal cord i.
    subacute i.
    suppurative acute i.
    suppurative chronic i.
    suppurative granulomatous i.
    testis i.
    transudative i.
    ulcerative i.
    uremic i.
    vesicular acute i.
    vesicular granulomatous i.
    i. with fibrosis
inflammatoria
    crusta i.
inflammatory
    i. adenocarcinoma
    i. arthritis
    i. bowel disease (IBD)
    i. carcinoma
    i. cavity
    i. cell
    i. cell debris
    i. corpuscle
    i. dermatosis
    i. disorder
    i. edema
    i. exudate
    i. fibromyxoid tumor
    i. fibrosarcoma
    i. fistula
    i. infiltrate

i. lymph
i. macrophage
i. mediator
i. membrane
i. myofibroblastic lesion
i. myofibroblastic tumor (IMT)
i. myofibrohistiocytic proliferation
i. myopathy
i. necrosis
i. odontogenic cyst
i. pelvic disease (IPD)
i. perforation
i. polyp
i. pseudomembrane
i. pseudotumor
i. reaction
i. rheumatism
i. rupture
i. sinus tract
i. transudate
inflation
inflatum
   Scedosporium i.
inflatus
   Wardomyces i.
inflection
   point of i.
influenza (flu)
   i. A, B, C
   i. A, B titer
   avian i.
   equine i.
   highly pathogenic avian i.
   Hong Kong i.
   Spanish i.
   swine i.
   i. test
   i. virus
   i. virus culture
   i. virus vaccine
influenzae
   Bacillus i.
   Haemophilus i.
Influenzavirus A, B, C
infolding
   papillary i.
   VSMC i.
information
   i. retrieval
   i. theory
informed consent

infra
   vide i.
infraclavicular infiltrate
infradian rhythm
infragranular layer
infrared
   i. CO_2 analyzer
   i. microscope
   i. spectrophotometry (IRS)
   i. spectroscopy
infrasubspecific
infratemporal fossa
infraumbilical
infundibula
   follicular i.
infundibular
   i. part
   i. stalk
   i. stem
   i. stenosis
infundibularis
   pars i.
infundibuloma
infundibulum
   Choanotaenia i.
infusion (inf)
   brain-heart i. (BHI)
   peripheral blood stem cell i.
   total-dose i. (TDI)
Infusoria
infusorian
ingestion challenge test
ingestive
ingluviei
   Lactobacillus i.
ingrown
   i. hair
   i. toenail
inguinale
   granuloma i.
   hernia uteri i.
   lymphogranuloma i.
   Trichophyton i.
inguinal hernia
inhae
   Leuconostoc i.
inhalant
   i. antigen
   i. corticosteroid
inhalation
   i. injury

NOTES

527

inhalation *(continued)*
    i. pneumonia
    volatile substance i.
inhalational
    i. anthrax
    i. anthrax infection
    i. botulism
inherent filter
inheritance
    alternative i.
    amphigenous i.
    autosomal dominant i.
    autosomal recessive i.
    biparental i.
    codominant i.
    complemental i.
    cytoplasmic i.
    dominant i.
    extrachromosomal i.
    holandric i.
    hologynic i.
    homochronous i.
    intermediate i.
    maternal i.
    mendelian i.
    mitochondrial i.
    multifactorial i.
    i. pattern
    polygenic i.
    quantitative i.
    quasicontinuous i.
    quasidominant i.
    recessive i.
    sex-linked i.
    supplemental i.
    unit i.
    X-linked dominant i.
    X-linked recessive i.
inherited
    i. albumin variant
    i. cancer
    i. disease
    i. genetic factor
    i. giant platelet disorder (IGPD)
inhibens
    Carnobacterium i.
inhibin
    i. A
    i. expression
inhibiting
    i. antibody
    i. factor
    i. hormone
inhibition
    allogeneic i.
    allosteric i.
    competitive i.
    contact i.

    enzyme i.
    i. factor
    fertility i.
    hemagglutination i. (HI)
    hemagglutinin i. (HAI)
    neurogenic i.
    RAST i.
    i. test
    tetrazolium reduction i. (TRI)
    tissue thromboplastin i. (TTI)
inhibitor
    alloantibody i.
    alpha-2 macroglobulin i.
    alpha-1 protease inhibitor
    alpha-1 trypsin i.
    i. assay
    carbonic anhydrase i.
    cell-cycle i.
    C1 esterase i. (C1EInh)
    cholinesterase i.
    coagulation factor i.
    cyclin-dependent kinase i. (CDKI)
    electron transport i.
    enzyme i. (EI)
    factor i.
    HDAC i.
    human alpha-1 proteinase i.
    inter-alpha-trypsin i. (ITI)
    lupus erythematosus i.
    malonate i.
    monoamine oxidase i.
    noggin protein i.
    noncompetitive i.
    oxidative phosphorylation i.
    plasminogen activator i. (PAI)
    plasminogen activator i. I, II
    protease i. (PI)
    proteinase i.
    soybean trypsin i. (SBTI)
    tissue factor pathway i. (TFPI)
    i. of transcription
    Trojan horse i.
    trypsin i.
    Z-dependent protease i. (ZPI)
inhibitory
    i. enzyme
    i. hormone
    i. mold agar
in-house consultation
iniencephaly
initial
    i. hematuria
    i. oliguric phase
    i. prognostic score (IPS)
    i. segment
    i. syphilitic lesion
initialization
initiating agent

initiation
>   i. codon
>   i. factor

initio
>   ab i.

initis

injection
>   facet joint i.
>   intracytoplasmic sperm i. (ICSI)
>   lactated Ringer i.
>   i. mass
>   peritumoral i.
>   Ringer i.
>   sensitizing i.

injurious agent

injury
>   auditory blast i.
>   avulsion i.
>   birth i.
>   blast i.
>   blunt head i.
>   cell i.
>   cold i.
>   compression i.
>   crush i.
>   decompensation i.
>   decompression i.
>   diffuse axonal i.
>   first-degree radiation i.
>   focal axonal i.
>   fourth-degree radiation i.
>   freezing i.
>   gastrointestinal blast i.
>   hyperperfusion/hyperfiltration i.
>   hypoxic cell i.
>   inhalation i.
>   markers of myocardial i.
>   miscellaneous blast i.
>   posterior dislocation i.
>   primary blast i.
>   pulmonary blast i.
>   quaternary blast i.
>   radiation i.
>   red blood cell i.
>   reperfusion i.
>   reversible i.
>   rotator cuff i.
>   secondary blast i.
>   second-degree radiation i.
>   severity of fibrosis after lung i.
>   spinal cord i.
>   tendon i.

>   tertiary blast i.
>   third-degree radiation i.
>   torsion i.
>   transfusion-related acute lung i.
>   (TRALI)
>   traumatic brain i. (TBI)

inkin
>   *Sarcinosporon i.*
>   *Trichosporon i.*

In-Line Strep A test

innate immunity

innatus
>   calor i.

inner
>   i. circular muscle layer
>   i. circumferential lamella
>   i. dental epithelium
>   i. hair cell
>   i. neural layer
>   i. phalangeal cell

innervation
>   motor i.

innidiation

innocens
>   diabetes i.

innocent
>   i. bystander cell
>   i. tumor

innocuous

innominate

innoxious

inochondritis

inoculability

inoculable

inoculate

inoculating loop

inoculation
>   inadvertent i.
>   i. smallpox

inoculum

Inocybe geophylla

inohanensis
>   *Nocardia i.*

Inonotus

inopectic

inopexia

inopinata
>   *Erysipelothrix i.*
>   *Scardovia i.*

inorganic
>   i. acid
>   i. chemistry

NOTES

inorganic *(continued)*
    i. component
    i. electrolyte
    i. mercury (Hg2+)
    i. phosphate
    i. pyrophosphatase
    i. pyrophosphate
inornata
    Culiseta i.
iNOS
    inducible nitric oxide synthetase
inoscopy
inosemia
inosinate
inosine
    i. cyclohydrolase
    i. dehydrogenase
    i. diphosphate
    i. monophosphate
    i. phosphate
    i. phosphorylase
    i. pyrophosphorylase
    i. triphosphate
inosine-5′-phosphate
inosinic acid
inosita
    melituria i.
inosite-free broth
inosithin neutralization test
inositol
    i. dehydrogenase
    i. hexanitrate
    i. hexaphosphate
    i. niacinate
myo-**inositol**
inosituria
inosuria
inotropic
Inoviridae
Inovirus
inquiline
Inquilinus limosus
inquiry
INR
    International Normalized Ratio
INS
    idiopathic nephrotic syndrome
inscription
    tendinous i.
inscriptio tendinea
insect
    i. bite
    i. virus
Insecta
insectarium
insecticide
    chlorfenthion i.
    fenthion i.

    organochlorine i.
    organophosphate i.
insemination
    homologous artificial i. (AIH)
insensible water loss
insertion
    battledore i.
    i. mutation
    promoter i.
    i. sequence
    velamentous i.
insertional
    i. activity
    i. mutagenesis
    i. translocation
insheathed
insidiosa
    Erysipelothrix i.
    Ralstonia i.
insidiosum
    Pythium i.
Insight digital camera
insipidus
    central diabetes i.
    diabetes i.
    nephrogenic diabetes i. (NDI)
insol
    insoluble
insolitus
    Achromobacter i.
insoluble (insol)
    i. complement-bound aggregate
    i. Prussian blue
    i. salt
in-solution hybridization
insolutum
    Polypaecilum i.
inspiratory
    i. flow
    i. flow rate (IFR)
    i. reserve capacity (IRC)
    i. reserve volume (IRV)
inspiratory:expiratory (I/E)
    i.:e. phase ratio
inspissate
inspissated
inspissation
inspissator
INSS
    International Neuroblastoma Staging
    System
instability
    chromosomal i. (CIN)
    glenohumeral joint i.
    microsatellite i. (MIN)
    nuclear excision repair i. (NIN)
    vasomotor i.
InstaCheck Med+ immunoassay for drugs of abuse

instantaneous rigor mortis
instant thin-layer chromatography
(ITLC)
Instant-View fecal occult blood test
instar
instillation
institute
> American National Standards I.
> (ANSI)
> National Cancer I. (NCI)
> I. of Virus Preparations
instructive theory
instrument
> Advia 60, 120 automated cell
> counting i.
> Cell-Dyn 1200, 3200, 4000
> automated cell counting i.
> Gen-S automated cell counting i.
> GM i.
> ionizing chamber i.
> MLA-100 coagulation i.
> STKS automated cell counting i.
> Sysmex CA-6000 coagulation i.
instrumentation
> advanced breast biopsy i. (ABBI)
insudate
insudation
> plasmatic i.
insuetus
> *Ilyobacter i.*
insufficiency
> adrenal i.
> adrenocortical i.
> aortic valvular i.
> arterial i.
> circulatory i.
> coronary i. (CI)
> fetal adrenal i.
> metabolic i.
> mitral i.
> ovarian i.
> pancreatic exocrine function i.
> primary adrenal i.
> pulmonary i.
> renal i.
> respiratory i.
> tricuspid i. (TI)
> uteroplacental i. (UPI)
> velopharyngeal i.
> venous i.
insufficient signal (IS)

insufflation
> cranial i.
> endotracheal i.
> perirenal i.
> presacral i.
> retroperitoneal gas i.
insula, pl. insulae
insular
> i. carcinoma
> i. sclerosis
insulated gate field effect transistor
insulator
insulin
> i. antagonist
> i. antibody
> atypical i.
> i. clearance (C_{in})
> i. clearance test
> i. coma therapy (ICT)
> crystalline i. (CI)
> crystalline zinc i.
> globin i.
> i. hypoglycemia test
> immunoreactive i. (IRI)
> i. lipoatrophy
> i. lipodystrophy
> potassium, glucose, and i. (PGI)
> prompt zinc i.
> protamine zinc i.
> i. receptor and signal transduction
> i. resistance
> i. sensitivity test (IST)
> i. shock
> i. shock therapy (IST)
> soluble i. (SI)
> i. tolerance test (ITT)
> i. unit
insulinase
insulin-dependent diabetes mellitus
(IDDM)
insulinemia
insulin-glucose tolerance test
insulinlike
> i.-l. activity (ILA)
> i.-l. growth factor
> i.-l. growth factor-1 (IGF-1)
insulinoma
insulinopenic
insulinotropic
insulitis
Insul-Tote
insusceptibility

NOTES

intake
  prolonged alcohol i.
intake and output (I/O)
integer oocyte
integral
  i. dose
  i. protein
Integrated Core system
integrating microscope
integration
  genomic i.
  large-scale i.
  medium-scale i.
  plasmid i.
  very large scale i. (VLSI)
integrator
integrin alpha1beta1
integrity
  sarcolemmal i.
integument
integumentary system
integumentum commune
intense inflammatory reaction
intensely basophilic cytoplasm
intensity
  luminous i.
interacinar
interacinous
interaction
  bacterial-fungal i.
  cell i. (CI)
  cell-cell i.
  CTLA-4 i.
  drug i.
  i. of radiation with matter
  sample i.
interactive processing
inter-alpha-globulin
inter-alpha-trypsin inhibitor (ITI)
interalveolar
  i. pore
  i. septum
interalveolare
  septum i.
interannular segment
interatrial septal defect (IASD)
interband
intercalary
  i. cell
  i. deletion
  i. neuron
intercalate
intercalated
  i. cell of the renal cortex
  i. disc
  i. duct
intercalatum
  Schistosoma i.

intercapillary
  i. cell
  i. glomerulosclerosis
  i. nephrosclerosis
intercarotid body
intercellular
  i. adhesion molecule-1 (ICAM-1)
  i. bridge
  i. canaliculus of parietal cell
  i. cement
  i. junction
  i. lymph
  i. prickle
Intercept
  I. oral fluid drug testing
  I. platelet system
interchange
interchromosomal aberration
intercommunicating network
intercristal space
intercurrent disease
interdigitale
  Trichophyton i.
  Trichophyton mentagrophytes var. *i.*
interdigitating
  i. cell sarcoma
  i. dendritic cell (IDC)
  i. dendritic cell sarcoma (IDCS)
  i. dendritic cell tumor
  i. papillary neoplasm
  i. reticulum cell
interdigitation
  cell membrane i.
interelectrode distance
interface
  air-liquid i.
  alveolar-capillary i.
  dermoepidermal i.
  EIA i.
interfacial canal
interfascicular connective tissue
interference
  anion i.
  background i.
  bacterial i.
  cation i.
  centromere i.
  chemical i.
  chromatid i.
  constructive i.
  destructive i.
  drug i.
  i. filter
  hemolysis i.
  icterus i.
  ionization i.
  i. microscope

spectral i.
i. test
interference-contrast microscopy (ICM)
interfering
defective i. (DI)
interferon (IFN)
i. alpha
antigen i.
i. beta
fibroblast i.
i. gamma
immune i.
leukocyte i.
i. regulatory factor 1 (IRF1)
interfibrillar
interfibrous
interfilamentous
interfollicular (IF)
interganglionic
intergemmal
interglobular
i. space
i. space of Owen
interglobulare
spatium i.
interieur
milieu i.
interindividual CNV
interjectum
Mycobacterium i.
interkinesis
interlamellar
interleukin (IL)
interleukin 1–18 (IL-1–IL-18)
interlobar duct
interlobitis
interlobular
i. connective tissue septum
i. duct
i. ductule
i. pleurisy
interlobulares
ductuli i.
interlobularis
pneumonia i.
intermedia
alpha thalassemia i.
Brevundimonas i.
Hydrogenophaga i.
pars i.
Prevotella i.

thalassemia i.
Yersinia i.
intermediary
i. metabolism
i. system
intermediate
i. body of Flemming
i. carcinoma
i. cell
i. coliform bacteria
i. disc
i. filament protein
i. host
i. inheritance
i. junction
i. lamella
malignant teratoma, i. (MTI)
i. normoblast
i. part
i. range entrance wound
reaction i.
intermediate-density lipoprotein (IDL)
intermedin
unit of i.
intermedium
Paracolobactrum i.
intermedius
Gluconacetobacter i.
Lutzomyia i.
Peptostreptococcus i.
Phlebotomus i.
Streptococcus i.
intermittent
i. albuminuria
i. claudication (IC)
i. hemoglobinuria
i. malaria
i. malarial fever
i. parasite
i. sterilization
interna
hyperostosis frontalis i.
lamina elastica i.
lamina rara i.
pachymeningitis i.
theca i.
internal
i. adhesive pericarditis
i. carotid artery occlusion (ICAO)
i. carotid stenosis
i. cavity
i. conversion

NOTES

internal *(continued)*
    i. decontamination
    i. elastic lamellae
    i. elastic lamina
    i. elastic membrane
    i. fistula
    i. hemorrhoid
    i. meningitis
    i. pathology
    i. pillar cell
    i. pyocephalus
    i. resistance (IR)
    i. root sheath
    i. salivary gland
    i. standard
    i. storage
internalized vesicle
international
    I. benzoate unit (IBU)
    I. Classification of Diseases (ICD)
    I. Committee for Standardization in Hematology (ICSH)
    I. Federation of Clinical Chemistry (IFCC)
    I. Federation of Gynecology and Obstetrics (FIGO)
    I. Neuroblastoma Staging System (INSS)
    I. Normalized Ratio (INR)
    I. prognostic index
    I. Prostate Symptom Score (IPPS)
    I. Sensitivity Index (ISI)
    I. Society for Urological Pathology (ISUP)
    I. Standards Organization (ISO)
    I. System of Units (SI)
    I. Union of Pure and Applied Chemistry (IUPAC)
    I. unit (IU)
interneuron
internexin
    alpha i.
internodal
    i. pathway
    i. segment
internodale
    segmentum i.
internode
internuclear bridging (INB)
internum
    perimysium i.
internuncial
    i. cell
    i. neuron
interobserver variability
interocclusal clearance
interoceptive
interoceptor
interosseous cartilage

interpapillary ridge
interphalangeal
    proximal i. (PIP)
interphase
interphyletic
interplant
interplanting
interpolation
interrod enamel
interrogans
    Leptospira i.
interscapular
    i. gland
    i. hibernoma
intersection
    tendinous i.
intersectio tendinea
intersex syndrome
intersheath space of optic nerve
interspace
interspecific graft
interspersed repeats
interspongioplastic substance
interstice
interstitial
    i. cell of Leydig
    i. cell-stimulating hormone (ICSH)
    i. cell tumor of testis
    i. cystitis (IC)
    i. deletion
    i. emphysema
    i. fluid
    i. gastritis
    i. giant cell pneumonia
    i. gland
    i. growth
    i. implantation
    i. inflammation
    i. keratitis
    i. lamella
    i. lung disease
    i. mastitis
    i. myositis
    i. nephritis
    i. plasma cell pneumonia
    i. pneumonitis
    i. pulmonary fibrosis
    i. tissue
    i. water (ISW)
interstitium
intertriginis
    Trichophyton i.
intertriginous
intertrigo
intertropical anemia
interval
    asymptomatic i.
    calibration i.
    confidence i. (CI)

i. estimate
postmortem i. (PMI)
reference i. (RI)
rupture-delivery i. (RDI)
i. scale
systolic time i. (STI)
time i. (TI)
tolerance i.
intervening sequence
interventricular septal defect (IVSD)
intervertebralis
anulus fibrosus disci i.
calcinosis i.
intervillositis
chronic i.
intervillous
i. fibrin
i. microabscess
i. perfusion
i. space
intestinal
i. absorption
i. amebiasis
i. atresia
i. botulism
i. calculus
i. ceroid deposition
i. chronic graft-versus-host disease
i. colic
i. crypt cell
i. emphysema
i. fistula
i. flora
i. flow disorder
i. follicle
i. gland
i. heterotopia
i. infarction
i. lipodystrophy
i. lymphangiectasis
i. malrotation
i. metaplasia (IM)
i. mucosa
i. myiasis
i. necrosis
i. neuronal dysplasia (IND)
i. obstruction (IO)
i. parasite
i. parasitic infection
i. phenotype lesion
i. sand
i. sepsis

i. tract carcinoid
i. villus
intestinales
villi i.
intestinalis
Collinsella i.
Encephalitozoon i.
Giardia i.
Lamblia i.
Ligula i.
mycosis i.
pneumatosis cystoides i. (PCI)
Retortamonas i.
Roseburia i.
Septata i.
tonsilla i.
intestinal-type mucin
intestine
absorptive cell of i.
aggregated lymphatic follicle of small i.
circular fold of small i.
nonrotation of i.
papillary adenoma of large i.
solitary nodule of i.
intestinotoxin
intima
aortic tunica i.
tunica i.
intimal
i. cell
i. fibroelastosis
i. surface
intimitis
proliferative i.
intolerance
cold i.
exercise i.
fructose i.
heat i.
hereditary fructose i. (HFI)
lactose i.
lysine i.
lysinuric protein i. (LPI)
sucrose i.
intoxication
acid i.
alcohol i.
alkaline i.
anaphylactic i.
botulism i.
citrate i.

NOTES

intoxication *(continued)*
    ethylene glycol i.
    methanol i.
    neuronal cell i.
    salicylate i.
    septic i.
    serum i.
    TCDD i.
    vitamin A, D i.
    water i.
intraabdominal adhesion
intraacinous
intraarterial
intraauricular
intrabuccal
intracanalicular fibroadenoma
intracapsular ankylosis
intracartilaginous
intracavernous
    i. aneurysm
    i. injection test
intracavitary
intracellular
    i. accumulation
    i. canaliculus
    i. coccobacillus
    i. fluid (ICF)
    i. fluid volume (IFV)
    i. free cholesterol
    i. myofibril
    i. NADPH
    i. parasite
    i. receptor analysis
    i. signal transduction effect
    i. thrombosis
    i. toxin
    i. water (ICW)
intracellulare
    Mycobacterium i.
intracerebral hemorrhage
intrachain disulphide bond
intrachange
intrachromosomal aberration
intracisternal
    i. microtubule
    i. space
intracorporeal
intracorpuscular
intracranial
    i. aneurysm (ICA)
    i. hematoma
    i. hemorrhage
    i. hypertension
    i. tumor
intracrine
intracristal space
intracutaneous
    i. allergy testing

    i. reaction
    i. tuberculin skin testing
intracystic
    i. hyperplasia
    i. papillary carcinoma
    i. papillary lesion of the breast
    i. papillary nodule
    i. papilloma
intracytoplasmic
    i. crystal
    i. glycogen
    i. inclusion cell
    i. microfilament
    i. mucin
    i. vacuole
intradepartmental consultation
intradermal
    i. allergy testing
    i. nevus
    i. reaction (IDR)
    i. test (IT)
intraductal
    i. hyperplasia
    i. papillary carcinoma (IPC)
    i. papillary mucinous neoplasm (IPMN)
    i. papillary mucinous tumor (IPMT)
    i. papillary projection
    i. papilloma
    i. papillomatosis
intraepidermal
    i. basal cell epithelioma, Borst-Jadassohn type
    i. squamous cell carcinoma
intraepidermic bulla
intraepiphysial
intraepithelial
    i. carcinoma
    i. dyskeratosis
    i. gland
    i. lymphocyte
    i. lymphocytosis
    i. neoplasia
intraesophageal pH test
intrafascicular
intrafilar
intrafusal fiber
intragemmal
intraglandular
intraglobular
intraglomerular crystallization
intrahepatic vascular obstruction
intrahyoid
intralesional
intralobar
    i. reticulation
    i. sequestration

intralobular
  i. duct
  i. ductule
  i. lesion
intramedullary hemolysis
intramembranous
  i. ossification
  i. space
intramucosal loose granuloma
intramural hematoma
intraneural nerve ending
intranuclear
  i. inclusion
  i. perichromatin granule
  i. spot
intraobserver variability
intraocular
  i. fluid
  i. foreign body (IOFB)
intraoperative
  i. cytology
  i. touch preparation
intraoperative cell salvage
intraosseous
intraosteal
intraperitoneal air
IntraPrep permeabilization reagent
intraprotoplasmic
intrapulmonary
  i. hemorrhage
  i. spindle cell thymoma
intrarenal
intrasinusoidal cytokeratin-positive
  mesothelial cell
Intrasporangiaceae
intrastromal
intratesticular tumor
intrathoracic
  i. extramedullary hematopoiesis
  i. gas volume (IGV)
intratubular germ cell neoplasia (IGCN)
intratumoral (IT)
  i. infiltration
  i. lymph vessel density
intratumor microvessel density
intrauterina
  ichthyosis i.
  rachitis i.
intrauterine
  i. asphyxia
  i. contraceptive device (IUD)
  i. fetal death (IUFD)

  i. fetal transfusion (IVT)
  i. foreign body (IUFB)
  i. growth rate (IUGR)
  i. malnutrition (IUM)
intravasation
intravascular
  i. agglutination
  i. coagulation of blood
  i. coagulation screen
  i. consumption coagulopathy
    (IVCC)
  i. coronary ultrasound
  i. hemolysis
  i. lymph
  i. mass (IVM)
  i. papillary endothelial hyperplasia
  i. space
intravenous
  I. glucose tolerance test (IVGTT)
  I. hyperalimentation (IVH)
  I. leiomyomatosis (IVL)
  I. tolbutamide tolerance test
    (IVTTT)
intraventricular
  i. conduction defect (IVCD)
  i. hemorrhage (IVH)
intravital
  i. microscopy
  i. stain
intra vitam necrosis
intrinsic
  i. asthma
  i. factor (IF)
  i. factor antibody
  i. factor concentrate (IFC)
  i. pathway
  i. semiconductor
  i. system
  i. tyrosine kinase
introduction of air into circulation
intron
intron-exon distribution
introversion
intumesce
intumescence
intumescent
intussusception
  colic i.
  double i.
  ileal i.
  ileocecal i.
  ileocolic i.

NOTES

intussusception (*continued*)
    jejunogastric i.
    retrograde i.
intussusceptive growth
intussusceptum
intussuscipiens
Inuit traditional food
inulin clearance
inundation fever
InV
    I. allotype
    I. group antigen
invaccination
invadens
    Trichomaris i.
invagination
    plasmalemmal i.
invariant chain
invasin
invasion
    angiolymphatic i.
    benign pheochromocytoma with histological i. (BPCHI)
    early i.
    lymphatic vessel i. (LVI)
    lymphovascular i.
    lymphovascular space i. (LVSI)
    melanomatous follicular i.
    perineural i. (PNI)
    regulator of i.
    Rosen criteria for lymphovascular i.
    stromal i.
    vascular i. (VI)
invasive
    i. activity test (IAT)
    i. aspergillosis
    i. ductal carcinoma
    i. fibrous thyroiditis
    i. implant
    i. lobular carcinoma
    i. mole
    i. papillary carcinoma
    i. squamous cell carcinoma (ISCC)
invasiveness
inventory
    vendor managed i.
invermination
inverse anaphylaxis
inverse-square law
inversion
    carbohydrate i.
    chromosomal i.
    heterobrachial i.
    overlapping i.
    pericentric i.
    i. of uterus
    visceral i.

inversus
    dextrocardia with situs i.
    situs i.
invertase
inverted
    i. follicular keratosis
    i. papilloma
    i. repeat
    i. testis
inverter
inverting enzyme
invert sugar
investigation
    crime scene i.
    CSF morphologic i.
investing tissue
invisible differentiation
invisus
    Dialister i.
Invitrogen TA cloning kit
invocatus
    Brevibacillus i.
involucra (*pl. of* involucrum)
involucre
involucrin
involucrum, pl. **involucra**
involuntary muscle
involution
    i. cyst
    i. form
    senile i.
involutus
    Paxillus i.
involvement
    bladder neck margin i.
    central nervous system i.
    focal i.
    lymph node i.
    nodal i.
    NSLN i.
    systemic sclerosis with lung i.
IO
    intestinal obstruction
I/O
    intake and output
    I/O device
io
    Automeris io
IOBeads magnetic beads
Iodamoeba
    I. bütschlii
    I. williamsi
iodate
    potassium i.
    i. reaction of epinephrine
iodemia
iodic acid
iodide
    i. assay

bismuth i.
potassium mercuric i.
propidium i.
radioactive i. (RAI)
saturated solution of potassium i.
  (SSKI)
sodium i.
i. transport defect
iodimetry
iodinated
i. human serum albumin (IHSA)
i. macroaggregated albumin (IMAA)
i. thyroglobulin
iodine (I)
butanol-extractable i. (BEI)
i. cyst
i. deficiency
i. escape peak
gram i.
Lugol i.
i. mumps
i. number
i. overload
plasma inorganic i. (PII)
propidium i. (PI)
protein-bound i. (PBI)
radioactive i. (RAI)
i. reaction of epinephrine
serum precipitable i. (SPI)
serum protein-bound i. (SPBI)
i. solution
i. stain
i. staining
i. test
tincture of i.
i. value
iodine-123
iodine-125
iodine-127
iodine-131
i. thyroid metastatic survey
i. uptake test
iodine-132 (^{132}I)
iodine-azide test (IAT)
iodine-131-6 beta iodomethyl-19-
  norcholesterol
iodinism
iodinophil, iodinophile
iodinophilous
iodobismuthate
iodochlorhydroxyquin

iodocholesterol
iododeoxyuridine (IDU, IUDR)
5-iododeoxyuridine
iododerma
iodometric
iodometry
iodophil granule
iodophilia
iodophor
iodoplatinate
iodotyrosine deiodinase defect
ioduria
IOFB
intraocular foreign body
iometer
ion
alkoxide i.
bicarbonate i.
calcium i. (Ca2+)
carbonium i.
carboxylate i.
i. channel
i. concentration
i. counter
cytosolic concentration of
  calcium i.'s
dipolar i.
i. disorder
gram i.
hydrogen i.
hydronium i.
hydroxide i.
magnesium i. (Mg2+)
i. microscope
oxonium i.
i. pair
ion-exchange
i.-e. chromatography
i.-e. column
i.-e. resin
ionic
i. bond
i. charge
i. concentration
i. strength
ionization
avalanche i.
i. chamber
i. constant
i. interference
specific i.
ionize

NOTES

ionized
    i. calcium
    i. calcium assay
ionizing
    i. chamber instrument
    i. radiation
ionogram
ionopherogram
ionophore
ion-selective electrode (ISE)
iontophoresis
    pilocarpine nitrate i.
IOPath immunohistochemistry reagent
iota
    Clostridium perfringens
    enterotoxin i. (CPI)
IOTest monoclonal antibody
IP
    incubation period
IP3 dependent calcium fluctuation
IPA
    isopropyl alcohol
IPC
    intraductal papillary carcinoma
IPD
    inflammatory pelvic disease
IPE
    individual protective equipment
IPF
    idiopathic pulmonary fibrosis
    intramural protruding form
IPH
    idiopathic pulmonary hemosiderosis
IPHP
    inflammatory papillary hyperplasia of the palate
i(12p) marker chromosome
IPMN
    intraductal papillary mucinous neoplasm
IPMT
    intraductal papillary mucinous tumor
Ipomoea
Ipomovirus
IPPS
    International Prostate Symptom Score
iproniazid
IPS
    initial prognostic score
ipsefact
IPSID
    immunoproliferative small intestinal disease
ipsilateral intraductal carcinoma
IPV
    inactivated poliovirus vaccine
IR
    immunoreactive
    internal resistance

Ir
    immune response
    Ir gene
iranensis
    Cellulomonas i.
IRC
    inspiratory reserve capacity
IRDS
    idiopathic respiratory distress syndrome
IRF
    idiopathic retroperitoneal fibrosis
IRF1
    interferon regulatory factor 1
IRG
    immunoreactive glucagon
IRHCS
    immunoradioassayable human chorionic somatomammotropin
IRhGH
    immunoreactive human growth hormone
IRI
    immunoreactive insulin
irides (*pl. of* iris)
iridescent virus
iridica
    stella lentis i.
iridis (*gen. of* iris)
iridium
iridocapsulitis
iridochoroiditis
iridocorneal endothelial syndrome (ICE)
iridocornealis
    spatia anguli i.
iridocyclitis
    heterochromic i.
    i. septica
iridokeratitis
Iridoviridae
Iridovirus
iris, gen. **iridis**, pl. **irides**
    crypt of i.
    i. frill
    herpes i.
    ligamentum pectinatum iridis
    pectinate ligaments of i.
    pigment cell of i.
    pigmented layer of i.
    pillar of i.
    stratum pigmenti iridis
    stroma iridis
    stroma of i.
iritis
IRM
    idiopathic retractile mesenteritis
IRMA
    immunoradiometric assay
iron (Fe)
    i. absorption
    i. assay

bound serum i. (BSI)
i. broth
decreased serum i.
i. deficiency anemia (IDA)
i. deposit
ferric i.
ferrous i.
i. hematoxylin
i. hematoxylin stain
high serum-bound i. (HBI)
histologically detectable i. (HDI)
impaired utilization of i.
i. index
low serum-bound i. (LBI)
i. overload
i. plasma clearance
i. protein
serum i. (SI)
i. stain
stainable i.
iron-binding
i.-b. capacity (IBC)
i.-b. capacity test
total i.-b. capacity (TIBC)
unsaturated i.-b. capacity (UIBC)
iron-positive pigment demonstration
iron-storage disease
iron-sulfide protein
Irpex
irradiated
i. casualty
i. CPD blood
irradiation
contamination i.
i. CVS/CNS syndrome
i. damage
i. esophagitis
external i.
i. hematopoietic syndrome
incorporation of i.
time of vomiting following i.
ultraviolet i.
ultraviolet blood i. (UBI)
irreducible hernia
irregular
i. border colony
i. fried egg morphology
i. margin
irregularis
Cephaliophora i.
irregularly round colony

irreversible
i. coma
i. damage
i. reaction
irreversibly sickled cell (ISC)
irrigation
Ringer i.
irritability
irritable
i. bowel syndrome
i. colon (IC)
irritans
Pulex i.
Siphona i.
irritant
primary i.
irritation
i. cell
i. fibroma
irritative lesion
irruption
irruptive
IRS
infrared spectrophotometry
IRSA
idiopathic refractory sideroblastic anemia
IRV
inspiratory reserve volume
Irvine syndrome
IS
insufficient signal
Isaacson classification
Isambert disease
Isamine blue
Isaria
Isavirus
ISC
irreversibly sickled cell
ISCC
invasive squamous cell carcinoma
ischemia
basilar artery i.
gastrointestinal i.
mesenteric i.
mucosal i.
myocardial i.
i. retinae
small bowel i.
transient cerebral i. (TCI)
ischemic
i. bowel disease
i. colitis

NOTES

ischemic *(continued)*
    i. contracture
    i. encephalopathy
    i. heart disease (IHD)
    i. hepatitis
    i. hypoxia
    i. leg disease (ILD)
    i. limb disease (ILD)
    i. muscular atrophy
    i. necrosis
ischial tuberosity
ischiopagus
ischiorectal abscess
ISCOM
    immune-stimulating complex
ISCP
    infection surveillance and control
      program
ISE
    ion-selective electrode
isethionate
    hydroxystilbamidine i.
ISG
    immune serum globulin
Is gene
ISH
    icteric serum hepatitis
    in situ hybridization
      EBER ISH
ishikariensis
    Asanoa i.
Ishikawa cell line
ISI
    International Sensitivity Index
ISIS
    Infectious Disease Surveillance
    Information System
island
    blood i.
    bony i.
    i.'s of Calleja
    CpG i.
    i. disease
    erythroblastic i.
    i. fever
    Langerhans i.'s
    i.'s of Langerhans
    i.'s of pancreas
    pancreatic i.'s
    pathogenicity i.
islandicus
    Ignicoccus i.
    Thermodesulfovibrio i.
islands
island-sparing plaques
islet
    i. alpha cell
    i. beta cell
    i.'s of Calleja

    i. cell adenoma
    i. cell antibody (ICA)
    i. cell antibody screening test
    i. cell carcinoma
    i. cell focal fibrosis
    i. cell hyperinsulinism
    i. cell hyperplasia
    i. cell tumor
    i. delta cell
    delta cell i.
    i. hormone
    i.'s of Langerhans
    pancreatic i.
    i. tissue
ISO
    International Standards Organization
isoagglutination
isoagglutinin
isoagglutinogen
isoallele
isoallelism
isoallotypic determinant
isoalloxazine
isoanaphylaxis
isoantibody
    platelet i.
isoantigen
    Rh i.
Isobaculum melis
isobar
isobaric
isobuteine
isobutyl alcohol
isobutyric acid
isocellular
isochromatic
isochromatid
    i. break
    i. gap
isochromatophil, isochromatophile
isochromic anemia
isochromosome
isochronal rhythm
isochronous
isochrous
isocitrate
    i. dehydrogenase
    i. dehydrogenase assay
    i. dehydrogenase test
isocitric
    i. acid
    i. dehydrogenase
IsoCode Stix device
isocortex
isocyanate
isocytolysin
isodactylism
isodesmosine
isodisomy

isoelectric
    i. focusing (IEF)
    i. focusing electrophoresis
    i. level
    i. point
isoenzyme
    i. A
    alkaline phosphatase i.
    cerebrospinal fluid lactate
      dehydrogenase i.'s
    creatine kinase i.
    i. electrophoresis
    lactate dehydrogenase i.
    PKC i.
    protein kinase C i.
    Regan i.
    skeletal muscle component of
      cardiac i.'s (MM)
isoerythrolysis
    neonatal i.
isoferritin
    acidic i.
isoflow
    volume of i.
isoform
    beta i.
    Cbfal/Runx2 i.
    epsilon i.
    eta i.
    sigma i.
    zeta i.
isogamy
isogeneic, isogenic
    i. graft
isogenous
    i. chondrocyte
    i. chondrocyte in lacuna
    i. group
    i. nest
isograft
isohemagglutination
isohemagglutinin
isohemolysin
isohemolysis
isohydric shift
isohydruria
isohypercytosis
isohypocytosis
isoimmune
    i. antibody
    i. hemolytic anemia
    i. neonatal

    i. neonatal purpura
    i. neonatal thrombocytopenia
isolate
    Towne CMV low passage
      clinical i.
isolated
    i. cleft palate
    i. conotruncal heart defect
    i. dextrocardia
    i. dyskeratosis follicularis
    i. gland carcinoma in situ (GCIS)
    i. levocardia
    i. parietal endocarditis
    i. proteinuria
    i. sinistrocardia
isolation
    body substance i. (BSI)
    CMV i.
    cytomegalovirus i.
    herpes simplex virus i.
    HSV i.
    i. of nucleic acid
    postexposure i.
Isolator
    I. blood culture system
    I. lysis-centrifugation tube
isolectin B4
isoleucine
    urine i.
isoleucyl
isoleucyl-RNA synthetase
isoleukoagglutinin
Isolex 300i magnetic cell selection
  system
isologous
    i. chimera
    i. graft
isolysin
isolysis
isolytic
isomaltase
isomastigote
isomer
    optical i.
isomerase
    glucosephosphate i.
    hexosephosphate i.
    triosephosphate i.
isomeric transition (IT)
isomerism
    chain i.
    dynamic i.

NOTES

isomerism *(continued)*
    functional group i.
    geometric i.
    nuclear i.
    optical i.
    position i.
    spatial i.
    stereochemical i.
    structural i.
isomerization
isometric
isomicrogamete
isomorphic response
isomorphous gliosis
isomuscarine
isoniazid
    i. assay
    i. phenotype test
isonicotinic acid hydrazide
isonormocytosis
isoolomoucine
isoosmolar
isoosmotic
Isopaque
Isoparorchis trisimilitubis
isopathy
isopentane-dry ice bath
isopentane fixative/solution
isophagy
isophil antibody
isophile antigen
isoplastic graft
isopleth
isoprecipitin
isoprene
isoprenoid
isopropanol
    i. assay
    i. precipitation test
isopropyl alcohol (IPA)
Isoptericola variabilis
isopyknic
isopyknotic
isosbestic point
isosensitize
isoserum treatment
isosexual pseudoprecocity
isosmotic
Isospora
    I. belli
    I. bigemina
    I. canis
    I. felis
    I. hominis
    I. rivolta
    I. suis
isosporiasis
isosthenuria
isosulfan blue

isothermal
isothiocyanate
    fluorescein i. (FITC)
    tetramethylrhodamine i. (XRITC)
isotone
isotonic
    i. coefficient
    i. hyponatremia
    i. sodium chloride solution
isotope dilution-mass spectrometry
isotopic dilution
isotransplantation
isotropic disc
isotype switching
isotypic
isovaleric acid
isovalericacidemia
isovaleryl-CoA dehydrogenase
isovolumic contraction (IC)
isozyme
israelensis
    Chromohalobacter i.
israelii
    Actinomyces i.
issachenkonii
    Pseudoalteromonas i.
Issatchenkia orientalis
IST
    insulin sensitivity test
    insulin shock therapy
isthmus, pl. **isthmi, isthmuses**
    His i.
ISUB
    immunosubtraction
ISUP
    International Society for Urological
    Pathology
ISW
    interstitial water
IT
    implantation test
    intradermal test
    intratumoral
    isomeric transition
itai-itai disease
italicus
    Enterococcus i.
ITAM
    immunoreceptor tyrosine activation motif
Itaqui virus
ITAS
    internal telomerase standard
itch
    barber's i.
    Cuban i.
    dhobie i.
    grain i.
    jock i.
    mad i.

Malabar i.
prairie i.
swimmer's i.
winter i.

iteration
iterative process
Iteravirus
ITI
inter-alpha-trypsin inhibitor
ITIM
immunoreceptor tyrosine inhibitory motif
ITLC
instant thin-layer chromatography
Ito
I. cell
hypomelanosis of I.
I. nevus
Ito-Reenstierna test
ITP
idiopathic thrombocytopenic purpura
I-TRAC Plus transfusion system
ITT
insulin tolerance test
IU
immunizing unit
international unit
IUD
intrauterine contraceptive device
IUDR
iododeoxyuridine
IUFB
intrauterine foreign body
IUFD
intrauterine fetal death
fetal karyotyping in mid-trimester
IUFD
IUGR
intrauterine growth rate
IUM
intrauterine malnutrition
IUPAC
International Union of Pure and Applied
Chemistry
IVAP
in vivo adhesive platelet
IVBAT
intravascular sclerosing
bronchioloalveolar tumor
IVCC
intravascular consumption coagulopathy

IVCD
intraventricular conduction defect
Ivemark syndrome
IVGTT
intravenous glucose tolerance test
IVH
intravenous hyperalimentation
intraventricular hemorrhage
IVL
intravenous leiomyomatosis
IVM
intravascular mass
ivorii
Peptoniphilus i.
ivory exostosis
IVSD
interventricular septal defect
IVT
intrauterine fetal transfusion
IVTT
in vitro transcription/translation
IVTT assay
IVTTT
intravenous tolbutamide tolerance test
Ivy
I. bleeding time test
I. method
I. method of bleeding time
I. template bleeding time
IWMI
inferior wall myocardial infarction
Ixodes
I. bicornis
I. cavipalpus
I. cookei
I. dammini
I. frequens
I. holocyclus
I. pacificus
I. persulcatus
I. rasus
I. ricinus
I. scapularis
I. spinipalpis
ixodiasis
ixodic
ixodid
Ixodidae
Ixodoidea

NOTES

J
joule
J chain
hemoglobin J
J receptor
J_{Capetown}
J6-HC, J6-MC, J6-MI high capacity centrifuge
Jaa antigen
jaagsiekte sheep retrovirus
Ja antigen
Jab1
Jun activation domain binding protein 1
Jaccoud
J. arthritis
J. arthropathy
J. syndrome
jacketed high-velocity round
jacksonian epilepsy
Jackson syndrome
Jacobsson method
Jacod syndrome
Jacquemin test
Jadassohn
cyst of J.
J. nevus
Jadassohn-Lewandowski syndrome
Jadassohn-Tièche nevus
jadensis
Alcanivorax j.
Fundibacter j.
Jaffe
J. assay
J. reaction
J. test
Jaffe-Campanacci syndrome
Jaffe-Lichtenstein disease
Jagged1 gene
Jahnke syndrome
jail fever
JAK kinase
Jakob-Creutzfeldt
J.-C. disease
J.-C. pseudosclerosis
Jakob disease
Jaksch disease
jalaludinii
Mitsuokella j.
Jamaican vomiting sickness
Jamestown Canyon virus
jamilae
Paenibacillus j.
Jamshidi needle
Janet disease
Janeway lesion

Janibacter
J. brevis
J. terrae
janiceps
Jannaschia
J. cystaugens
J. helgolandensis
jannaschii
Thialkalivibrio j.
Jansen disease
Jansky-Bielschowsky disease
Jansky human blood group classification
Janus green B
Japanese
J. B encephalitis (JBE)
J. B encephalitis virus
J. river fever
japonica
Amycolatopsis j.
Hirudo j.
Rickettsia j.
Shewanella j.
Tetrasphaera j.
japonicum
Pseudospirillum j.
Rhizobium j.
Schistosoma j.
japonicus
Cellvibrio j.
Debaromyces j.
Thermosipho j.
jar
anaerobic j.
Coplin j.
Jarisch-Herxheimer reaction
Jass staging system
Jatlow-Nadim procedure
Jatropha kurcas
jaundice
acholuric j.
acute febrile j.
black j.
catarrhal j.
cholestatic j.
chronic acholuric j.
chronic familial j.
chronic idiopathic j.
congenital familial nonhemolytic j.
congenital hemolytic j.
familial nonhemolytic j.
hematogenous j.
hemolytic j.
hepatocellular j.
hepatogenous j.

jaundice *(continued)*
    homologous serum j.
    leptospiral j.
    malignant j.
    mechanical j.
    nonhemolytic j.
    nonobstructive j.
    obstructive j.
    painless j.
    regurgitation j.
    retention j.
    spherocytic j.
    toxemic j.
javensis
    Streptomyces j.
jaw
    familial fibrous dysplasia of j.
    fibrous dysplasia of j.
    lumpy j.
    progonoma of j.
Jaworski
    J. body
    J. corpuscle
    J. test
JBE
    Japanese B encephalitis
JCAHO
    Joint Commission on Accreditation of
    Healthcare Organizations
JCML
    juvenile chronic myelogenous leukemia
JC virus
jeanselmei
    Exophiala j.
    Fonsecaea j.
Jeanselme nodule
Jeghers-Peutz syndrome
jeikeium
    Corynebacterium j.
jejuense
    Clostridium j.
jejuensis
    Kribbella j.
jejuni
    Campylobacter j.
jejunitis cystica profunda
jejunogastric intussusception
jejunoileitis
jejunostomy
Jellison
    Francisella tularensis biovar J.
    type A, B
jelly
    Wharton j.
JEM-100CX electron microscope
Jendrassik-Grof method
jenensis
    Oerskovia j.

Jenner
    J. method
    J. stain
Jenner-Giemsa stain
Jenner-Kay unit
Jensen
    J. classification
    J. disease
    J. sarcoma
jensenii
    Lactobacillus j.
    Propionibacterium j.
Jeol
    J. 100 S transmission electron
    microscope
    J. 1200 transmission electron
    microscope
jeotgali
    Bacillus j.
    Psychrobacter j.
Jeotgalibacillus alimentarius
Jeotgalicoccus
    J. halotolerans
    J. pinnipedialis
    J. psychrophilus
Jerne
    J. plaque assay
    J. technique
Jervell and Lange-Nielsen syndrome
Jessner lymphocytic infiltrate
jet lesion
Jeune syndrome
Jewett
    J. bladder carcinoma
    J. bladder carcinoma classification
    J. and Strong staging
jeyporiensis
    Anopheles j.
JGCT
    juvenile granulosa cell tumor
    juxtaglomerular cell tumor
JGI
    juxtaglomerular granulation index
JH virus
jigger
Jimson weed
jinjuensis
    Pseudomonas j.
Jk antigen
JM
    juxtamembrane
JMML
    juvenile myelomonocytic leukemia
Jobbins antigen
Job syndrome
jock itch
Jod-Basedow phenomenon
Joest body

johannae
>   *Gluconacetobacter j.*

Johne
>   J. bacillus
>   J. disease

johnin

Johns Hopkins Center for Civilian Biodefense Studies

Johnson-Dubin syndrome

Johnsonella ignava

johnsonii
>   *Hyphomonas j.*

Johnson-Steven disease

joint
>   j. abnormality
>   j. adhesion
>   j. calculus
>   j. capsule
>   Clutton j.
>   J. Commission on Accreditation of Healthcare Organizations (JCAHO)
>   j. disease
>   j. effusion
>   j. oil
>   J. Task Force for Civil Support (of the Defense Department) (JTF-CS)

jointed bamboo-rod cellular appearance

Joklik buffer

Jolles test

Jolly body

Jones
>   Bence J. (BJ)
>   J. methenamine silver stain
>   J. method

Jones-Cantarow test

Jonesiaceae

Jonesia dentrificans

Jones-Mote reaction

joostei
>   *Chryseobacterium j.*

Jordan anomaly

Jores fixative

Joseph syndrome

jostii
>   *Rhodococcus j.*

joule (J)
>   J. law

Jourdain disease

journal
>   telehealth j.

JRA
>   juvenile rheumatoid arthritis

Js antigen

J-sella deformity

J-series prostaglandin

JTF-CS
>   Joint Task Force for Civil Support (of the Defense Department)

juccuya

Judet epiphysial fracture

jugular gland

juice
>   cancer j.
>   pancreatic j.

jumbo biopsy

jump
>   conditional j.
>   unconditional j.

jumping
>   j. disease
>   j. gene

Jun activation domain binding protein 1 (Jab1)

junction
>   adhering j.
>   j. capacitor
>   cell j.
>   cervical-vaginal j.
>   choledochoduodenal j.
>   communicating j.
>   corneoscleral j.
>   corticomedullary j.
>   dermal epidermal j.
>   electrotonic j.
>   esophagogastric j.
>   fibronexus j.
>   j. field effect transistor
>   gap j.
>   impermeable j.
>   intercellular j.
>   intermediate j.
>   mucocutaneous j.
>   muscle-tendon j.
>   myoneural j.
>   neuromuscular j.
>   j. nevus
>   occipitoatlantoaxial j.
>   j. potential
>   sclerocorneal j.
>   squamocolumnar j. (SCJ)
>   tight j. (TJ)
>   ureteropelvic j.

J

NOTES

junctional
  j. complex
  j. cyst
  j. epidermolysis bullosa
  j. epithelium
  j. expansion nodule
  j. nevus
Jung
  J. Autostainer XL
  J. CV 5000 Robotic Coverslipper
  J. muscle
jungle yellow fever
Jüngling disease
Junin virus
justifiable abortion
justify
juvenile
  j. angiofibroma
  j. carcinoma
  j. cell
  j. cerebellar astrocytoma
  j. chronic myelogenous leukemia (JCML)
  j. cirrhosis
  j. diabetes mellitus
  j. elastoma
  j. fibroadenoma
  j. granulosa cell tumor (JGCT)
  j. hemangiofibroma
  j. hemochromatosis
  j. hormone
  j. hyalin fibromatosis
  j. kyphosis
  j. melanoma
  j. myelomonocytic leukemia (JMML)
  j. neutrophil
  j. ossifying fibroma
  j. osteoporosis
  j. Paget disease
  j. palmoplantar fibromatosis
  j. papillomatosis
  j. pernicious anemia
  j. pilocytic astrocytoma
  j. polyp
  j. polyposis coli
  j. polyposis syndrome
  j. rheumatoid arthritis (JRA)
  j. SMA
  j. xanthogranuloma (JXG)
  j. xanthoma
juvenile-onset diabetes
juvenilis
  osteochondritis deformans j.
  verruca plana j.
juxtaarticular nodule
juxtacortical
  j. chondroma
  j. osteogenic sarcoma
juxtaglomerular
  j. apparatus
  j. body
  j. cell
  j. cell tumor (JGCT)
  j. complex
  j. granulation index (JGI)
  j. granule
juxtamedullary
juxtamembrane (JM)
juxtanuclear Golgi reactivity
juxtaoral organ of Chievitz
juxtapapillaris
  retinochoroiditis j.
juxtapulmonary-capillary receptor
juxtatumoral stroma
JXG
  juvenile xanthogranuloma

K
Kell blood group
kelvin
lysine
potassium
K antigen
K cell
K and k antigen
K virus

k
constant
kelvin temperature scale

KA
ketoacidosis

Kabatiella
Kabatina
kabure
Kaes
K. feltwork
K. line
Kaes-Bekhterev
K.-B. band
K.-B. layer
K.-B. stripe
Kaffir pox
Kahlbaum disease
Kahler
K. disease
K. law
Kahn test
kaikoae
Psychromonas k.
kainate receptor
Kaiserling
K. fixative
K. method
K. solution
kala azar
kalemia
kaliopenia
kaliopenic
Kalischer disease
kalium
kaliuresis
kaliuretic
kallidin
kallikrein
human k. 2 (hK2)
human k. 3 (hK3)
plasma k.
k. system
kallikrein-inhibiting unit (KIU)
Kallmann syndrome
kaluresis
kaluretic

Kamino body
Kanagawa phenomenon
kanaloae
Vibrio k.
kanamycin
Kandinskii-Clerambault syndrome
kanei
Trichophyton k.
Kangiella
K. aquimarina
K. koreensis
kangri
k. burn carcinoma
k. cancer
Kanner syndrome
Kansas
hemoglobin K.
kansasii
Mycobacterium k.
kaodzera
kaolin
k. partial thromboplastin time (KPTT)
k. pneumoconiosis
kaolin-clotting time
kaolinosis
Kapetanakis purpura
Kaplan-Meier staining method
Kaposi
K. sarcoma
K. sarcoma-like granuloma
K. varicelliform eruption
kaposiform
kappa
k. chain specificity
k. granule
k. light chain
k. opioid receptor (KOR)
karajensis
Halobacillus k.
Karapandzic flap
32 Karat software for HPLC
Karmen unit (KU)
Karnofsky status
Karnovsky
K. fixative
K. II solution
Kartagener syndrome
kartulisi
Entamoeba k.
karwari
Anopheles k.
karyochrome cell
karyoclasis
karyocyte

K

karyogamy
karyogonad
karyokinesis
karyology
karyolymph
karyolysis
karyolytic
karyomere
karyomicrosome
karyomitome
karyomorphism
karyon
karyophage
karyoplasm
karyoplasmolysis
karyoplast
karyoplastin
karyopyknosis
karyopyknotic index (KI)
karyorrhectic nuclear debris
karyorrhexis
karyostasis
karyotheca
karyotype
    k. aberration
    numerical k.
    spectral k.
    X k.
    XO k.
    XX k.
    XXX k.
    XXY k.
    XY k.
    XYY k.
karyotyping
    digital k.
    spectral k.
karyozoic
Kasabach-Merritt syndrome
Kashin-Bek disease
Kasten
    K. fluorescent Feulgen stain
    K. fluorescent PAS stain
    K. fluorescent Schiff reagent
Kast syndrome
kat
    katal
katal (kat)
Katayama
    K. fever
    K. test
katharometer
Kato thick smear technique
katsuradai
    Heterophyes k.
Katzenstein and Peiper criteria
KAU
    King-Armstrong unit
Kauffman-White classification

kaustophilus
    Geobacillus k.
Kawasaki disease
kayaii
    Photorhabdus luminescens subsp. *k.*
Kayser disease
Kayser-Fleischer ring
KB
    ketone body
kbp
    kilobase pair
kc
    kilocycle
KC1 Delta coagulation analyzer
kcal
    kilocalorie
K-capture
    electron K-c.
KCl
    potassium chloride
KCN
    potassium cyanide
kcps
    kilocycles per second
kDa
    kilodalton
KD antigen
KE
    kinetic energy
Kearns-Sayre syndrome
Kearns syndrome
kedani
    k. disease
    k. fever
    k. mite
K3 EDTA
    potassium EDTA
kefirgranum
    Lactobacillus kefiranofaciens subsp. *k.*
Keissleriella
Keith bundle
Keith-Wagener (KW)
    K.-W. classification
Keith-Wagener-Barker (KWB)
    K.-W.-B. classification
Kelev strain rabies virus
Kell
    K. antigen
    K. blood group (K)
    K. blood group system
    K. body antibody type
    K. HDN
Kell-Cellano blood group
kellicotti
    Paragonimus k.
kellyi
    Halothiobacillus k.

keloid
    Addison k.
keloidosis
kelosomia
kelvin (K)
    k. temperature scale (k)
    k. thermometer
Kendall Company Telfa pad
Kennedy syndrome
Kent bundle
Kent-His bundle
kentuckyensis
    Amycolatopsis k.
Kenya tick fever
kerasin histiocytosis
keratan sulfate
keratiasis
keratic
keratin
    k. cocktail
    k. filament
    k. immunostaining
    k. pearl
    k. polypeptide
    k. stain
    k. staining
    k. whorl
    wide-spectrum k.
keratiniphila
    Amycolatopsis k.
    Amycolatopsis k. subsp. *keratiniphila*
keratinization
    metaplastic k.
keratinize
keratinized cell
keratinizing
    k. invasive squamous cell
      carcinoma (KISCC)
    k. squamous cell carcinoma
      (KSCC)
keratinocyte
    apoptotic k.
keratinocyte growth factor 2 (KGF2)
keratinophilic
keratinosome
keratinous cyst
keratitic precipitate (KP)
keratitis
    Acanthamoeba k.
    acne rosacea k.
    k. bullosa
    k. disciformis

    herpetic k.
    interstitial k.
    mycotic k.
    parenchymatous k.
    reticular k.
    sclerosing k.
    serpiginous k.
    suppurative k.
    vascular k.
    vesicular k.
    zonular k.
keratoacanthoma
keratoacanthosis
keratoangioma
keratoatrophoderma
keratoconjunctivitis
    chronic follicular k.
    epidemic k. (EKC)
    herpetic k.
    phlyctenular k.
    k. sicca
    superior limbic k. (SLKC)
    virus k.
keratoconus posticus circumscriptus
keratocyst
    odontogenic k. (OKC)
keratocyte
keratoderma
    k. acquisitum
    k. blennorrhagica
    k. climactericum
    k. eccentrica
    lymphedematous k.
    mutilating k.
    k. palmaris et plantaris
    palmoplantar k.
    k. plantare sulcatum
    punctate k.
    senile k.
    k. symmetrica
keratodermatitis
keratodes
    erythema k.
keratohyalin
    k. granule
    k. granule of epidermis
keratohyaline alteration
keratohyalin-like granule
keratoid
keratolysis exfoliativa
keratolytic

K

NOTES

keratoma
    k. disseminatum
    k. hereditarium mutilans
    k. plantare sulcatum
    senile k.
keratomalacia
keratomycosis
keratonosis
keratopathy
    band k.
keratoplasia
keratose
keratosis, pl. **keratoses**
    actinic k.
    arsenic k.
    arsenical k.
    k. blennorrhagica
    clonal seborrheic k.
    k. diffusa fetalis
    follicularis k.
    k. follicularis
    inverted follicular k.
    lichenoid k.
    nevus follicularis k.
    k. nigricans
    k. palmaris et plantaris
    pilaris k.
    preexisting actinic k.
    k. punctata
    k. rubra figurata
    seborrheic k.
    k. seborrheica
    senile k.
    k. senilis
    solar k.
    tar k.
    k. vegetans
keratotic
    k. micaceous balanitis
    k. papilloma
Kerckring
    K. fold
    K. valve
kerion
    Celsus k.
Kerley A, B lines
Kernia
kernicterus
Kernig meningeal sign
Kernohan
    K. malignant astrocytoma grading
    K. notch
kern-plasma relation theory
keroid
Kerstersia gyiorum
kerstersii
    Comamonas k.
Keshan disease

kestanbolensis
    Anoxybacillus k.
ketal
ketimine
    aminoethylcysteine k.
keto
    k. acid
    k. group
ketoacidosis (KA)
    alcoholic k.
    diabetic k. (DKA)
    starvation k.
ketoaciduria
    branched-chain k.
ketoconazole
Keto-Diastix urine ketone and glucose test
keto-enol tautomer
ketogenesis
ketogenic
    k. amino acid
    k. corticoid test
    k. hormone
    k. steroid (KGS)
17-ketogenic
    17-k. steroid
    17-k. steroids assay
ketogenic/antiketogenic ratio
ketoglutarate
    alpha k.
Ketogulonicigenium
    K. robustum
    K. vulgare
ketohexokinase
ketohexose
ketone
    k. body (KB)
    k. body formation
    k. body test
    k. body utilization
    dimethyl k.
    methyl butyl k.
    methyl ethyl k. (MEK)
    methyl isobutyl k.
ketonemia
ketonimine dye
ketonuria
    branched-chain k.
ketopentose
ketose
ketosis
ketosteroid (KS)
17-ketosteroid
    17-k. assay
    17-k. fractionation
Ketostix
ketosuria
ketotic hyperglycinemia
ketotransferase

ketotriose
Ketron-Goodman pagetoid reticulosis
Kety-Schmidt method
keV
 kiloelectron volt
key
  k. enzyme
  k. vein
keyhole-limpet hemocyanin (KLH)
KFAb
 kidney-fixing antibody
KFD
 Kikuchi-Fujimoto disease
KFS
 Klippel-Feil syndrome
kg
 kilogram
kg-cal
 kilogram-calorie
KGF2
 keratinocyte growth factor 2
KGS
 ketogenic steroid
Khuskia
kHz
 kilohertz
KI
 karyopyknotic index
Ki-1
  Ki-1 antibody
  Ki-1 antigen
Ki-67
  Ki-67 antibody
  Ki-67 antigen
  growth fraction with Ki-67
  Ki-67 immunohistochemical well-
   differentiated gastric carcinoma
   analysis
  Ki-67 immunophenotypic marker
  Ki-67 index
  Ki-67 oncogene
  Ki-67 positive cell
  Ki-67 protein
Ki-1+ lymphoma
KIA
 Kliger iron agar
Kidd
  K. antigen
  K. blood antibody type
  K. blood group
  K. blood group system

kidney
 amyloid k.
 Armanni-Ebstein k.
 arteriolosclerotic k.
 arteriosclerotic k.
 artificial k.
 Ask-Upmark k.
 atrophic k.
 k. biopsy
 cake k.
 k. cancer
 k. carbuncle
 clear cell sarcoma of the k.
  (CCSK)
 contracted k.
 convoluted tubule of k.
 k. cortex
 cow k.
 crush k.
 cystic k.
 disc k.
 doll's k.
 duplex k.
 dwarf k.
 embryoma of the k.
 fatty k.
 flea-bitten k.
 Formad k.
 fused k.
 Goldblatt k.
 granular k.
 guinea pig k. (GPK)
 hilum of k.
 horseshoe k.
 human embryo k. (HEK)
 human embryonic k. (HEK)
 hydroxylation k.
 malignant rhabdoid tumor of k.
  (MRTK)
 malpighian body of k.
 maximal tubular excretory capacity
  of k.'s (T_m)
 medullary sponge k.
 monkey k. (MK)
 mortar k.
 multicystic dysplasia of k.
  (MCDK)
 multicystic dysplastic k. (MCDK)
 multilocular cystic k.
 nonrotation of k.
 pancake k.
 papillary foramina of k.

K

NOTES

kidney *(continued)*
    pelvic k.
    polycystic disease of k.'s
    primary African green monkey k. (PAGMK)
    k. profile
    putty k.
    pyelonephritic k.
    rabbit k.
    rhabdoid tumor of the k. (RTK)
    rhesus monkey k. (RMK)
    Rose-Bradford k.
    sclerotic k.
    k. stone analysis
    straight venule of k.
    supernumerary k.
    k. transplant rejection
    waxy k.
kidney-fixing antibody (KFAb)
KidneyScreen
    K. At·Home mail-in test
    K. At·Home testing kit
kielensis
    Ahrensia k.
Kiel non-Hodgkin lymphoma classification
Kienböck
    K. atrophy
    K. disease
Kiernan space
kieselguhr
Ki-FDC1p antibody
Kikuchi
    K. disease
    K. lymphadenitis
Kikuchi-Fujimoto
    K.-F. disease (KFD)
    K.-F. lymphadenitis
Kilham rat virus
killed
    heat k. (HK)
    k. measles virus vaccine (KMV)
    k. vaccine (KV)
killer
    k. cell
    k. immunoglobulin-like receptor (KIR)
    k. lymphocyte
    T-natural k. (TNK)
kilobase pair (kbp)
kilocalorie (kcal)
kilocycle (kc)
    k.'s per second (kcps)
kilodalton (kDa)
kiloelectron volt (keV)
kilogram (kg)
kilogram-calorie (kg-cal)
kilohertz (kHz)
kilohm

Kiloh-Nevin syndrome
kilojoule (kJ)
kilometer (km)
kilonensis
    Pseudomonas k.
kilopascal (kPa)
kiloton (kT)
kilovolt (kV)
    k. ampere (kVA)
    k. peak (kVp)
kilovoltage
    peak k.
kilowatt (kW)
kilowatt-hour (kWh)
Ki-M1p antibody
Ki-M4p antibody
kimchii
    Lactobacillus k.
    Leuconostoc k.
    Weissella k.
Kimex
Kimmelstiel-Wilson
    K.-W. disease
    K.-W. lesion
    K.-W. nodule
    K.-W. syndrome
Kimura disease
kinase
    adenosine k.
    adenylate k.
    anaplastic lymphoma k. (ALK)
    aspartate k.
    Bruton tyrosine k. (BTK)
    cAMP-dependent protein k.
    conserved helix-loop-helix ubiquitous k. (CHUK)
    creatine k. (CK)
    cyclin-dependent k. (CDK)
    cyclin-dependent k. 5 (CDK5)
    cyclin-dependent protein k. 1 (Cdk1)
    focal adhesion k. (FAK)
    intrinsic tyrosine k.
    JAK k.
    macrocreatine k.
    mitochondrial creatine k. (mtCK)
    phosphoglycerate k.
    phosphorylase k.
    pyruvate k. (PK)
    receptor tyrosine k.
    Ser-Thr k.
    serum creatine k. (SCK)
    thymidine k.
kind
    electrode of first k.
    electrode of second k.
kindred
kinematic viscosity
Kineococcus radiotolerans

Kineosphaera limosa
kinetic
>k. analyzer
>k. energy (KE)
>k. measurement

kinetics
>cell k.
>cellular k.
>first-order k.
>simulation k. (simkin)
>tumor cell k.
>zero-order k.

kinetochore
kinetocyte
kinetoplasm
kinetoplast
kinetosome
Kinevac
kingae
>*Kingella* k.
>*Moraxella* k.

King-Armstrong unit (KAU)
Kingella
>*K. denitrificans*
>*Haemophilus, Actinobacillus, Cardiobacterium, Eikenella, K.* (HACEK)
>*K. indologenes*
>*K. kingae*

king's evil
King unit
kinin
>plasma k.
>k. system

kininogen
>high molecular weight k. (HMWK)
>HMW k.
>low molecular weight k.

kinky hair disease
Kinnier Wilson disease
kinocentrum
kinocilium
kinoplasm
kinoplasmic
Kinsbourne syndrome
Kinyoun carbolfuchsin stain
KIP
>kinase inhibitory protein

KIR
>killer immunoglobulin-like receptor
>>KIR sequence in NK repertoire

Ki-ras mutation

Kirby-Bauer
>K.-B. method
>K.-B. test

Kirchoff law
Kiricephalus
Kirkland disease
Ki-S5 antibody
KISCC
>keratinizing invasive squamous cell carcinoma

Kisenyi sheep disease virus
kissing disease
KIT
>kinase tyrosine

kit (*See also* assay, test)
>A1c At·Home testing k.
>active total PSA ELISA k.
>adenovirus test k.
>Amersham Life Science PCR product presequencing k.
>Amersham Life Science Thermo Sequenase sequencing k.
>Ana-Sal HIV home test k.
>ApopTag Plus k.
>Asserachrom D-Dimer k.
>Babystart fertility test k.
>BD-CHEK intestinal inflammation k.
>Bindazyme ANA Screening ELISA k.
>Bioshaf automated one-step fertility k.
>Boehringer Mannheim DIG-Nucleic Detection k.
>Boehringer Mannheim DIG-Oligonucleotide Tailing k.
>Boehringer in vitro transcription k.
>CAS DNA staining k.
>Cellquant K.
>CEP 12 SpectrumOrange DNA probe k.
>CEP X, Y SpectrumOrange DNA probe k.
>Coulter Manual CD4 K.
>cyanide antidote k.
>DakoCytomation EGFR pharmDx colorectal cancer diagnostic k.
>Dako large volume LSAB2 alkaline phosphatase k.
>Diatest diabetes breath test k.
>Directigen Flu A + B test k.

NOTES

K

kit *(continued)*

Elucigene CF29 analyte-specific reagent k.
Extract-N-Amp Blood PCR k.
FertilMARQ male fertility screening test k.
First Check Ecstasy test k.
Fix and Perm Cell Permeabilization K.
Fluorognost HIV-1 IFA assay k.
GenePhor DNA silver staining k.
GenSpin gDNA purification k.
Gentra Systems Puregene DNA isolation k.
Glucatell beta-glucagan blood test k.
Great Smokies Diagnostic Laboratories intestinal permeability test k.
HercepTest IHC k.
HerpeSelect type specific IgG antibody detection k.
High Pure PCR product purification k.
Histofine SAB-PO immunohistochemical staining k.
IgA II-HA assay test k.
IgM II-HA assay test k.
Immu-Mark immunostaining k.
ImmunoDOT Mono G, M test k.
immunofluorescent assay k.
Immunotech immunoassay k.
ImmuSTRIP HAMA test k.
Invitrogen TA cloning k.
KidneyScreen At·Home testing k.
Legionella urinary antigen ELISA test k.
LUA ELISA test k.
manual CD4 k.
Melastatin test k.
MERmaid-Spin k.
MOM basic k.
MOM fluorescein k.
MOM peroxidase k.
nerve agent antidote k. (NAAK)
PathVysion HER-2 DNA probe k.
pH-stat titration application k.
Pierce Micro BCA Assay k.
PowerPlex 1.2 genetic identification k.
protein S-free k.
k. protooncogene
PSA IRMA k.
Puregene DNA isolation k.
QIAamp DNA blood biorobot k.
Qiagen QIAquick gel extraction k.
QIAquick PCR 96 purification k.
Quanta Lite ANA ELISA test k.
Quanta Lite CCP ELISA k.

Quanta Lite ELISA autoimmune k.
rapid drug screen multiple drug screen standard k.
Redquant k.
RLP-Cholesterol Immunoseparation Assay k.
spill control k.
Staclot Protein S test k.
STA Liatest D-DI coagulation/inflammation test k.
Staller k.
Takara Biomedicals One-Step RNA PCR k.
Taq DyeDeoxy Terminator Cycle Sequencing k.
Taq Master Mix k.
True test k.
TruGene HIV-1 genotyping k.
Universal ISH detection k.
UroVision bladder cancer recurrence k.
Vectastain ABC Elit k.
Vectastain Universal Elite ABC k.
Vectastain Universal Quick k.
Vector MOM k.
Ventana alkaline phosphatase blue detection k.
Vidas total PSA assay k.
Vielle menopause home test k.
Vitros HBsAg confirmatory k.
Wako NEFA test k.
ZstatFlu test k.

Kitasato broth
kitasatonis
Lactobacillus k.
Kitasatospora
K. niigatensis
K. putterlickiae
Kittrich stain
KIU
kallikrein-inhibiting unit
kJ
kilojoule
Kjeldahl
K. method
K. procedure
Klatskin tumor classification
Klauder syndrome
Klebanoff reaction
Klebs disease
Klebsiella
K. mobilis
K. oxytoca
K. pneumonia
K. pneumoniae
K. pneumoniae subsp. *ozaenae*
K. pneumonia rhinoscleromatis
K. urinary tract infection
K. variicola

Klebsielleae
Klebs-Löffler bacillus
Kleihauer
    K. acid elution
    K. stain
    K. test
Kleihauer-Betke
    K.-B. acid elution
    K.-B. stain
    K.-B. test
Klein bacillus
Kleine-Levin syndrome
Klein-Gumprecht shadow nuclei
Klemperer disease
Klenow fragment
KLH
    keyhole-limpet hemocyanin
Kliger iron agar (KIA)
Klinefelter syndrome (KS)
Klinger-Ludwig acid-thionin stain for sex chromatin
Klippel disease
Klippel-Feil
    K.-F. deformity
    K.-F. syndrome (KFS)
Klippel-Trenaunay syndrome
Klippel-Trenaunay-Weber syndrome
Kloeckera
Klump and Bieth method
Klumpke-Dejerine syndrome
Klumpke paralysis
Klüver-Barrera Luxol fast blue stain
Klüver-Bucy syndrome
Kluyvera
kluyveri
    Clostridium k.
Kluyveromyces
Km
    Km allotype
    Km antigen
km
    kilometer
KMV
    killed measles virus vaccine
knee
    Brodie k.
    dashboard k.
    septic k.
    k. synoviocyte
Knemidokoptes
Kniest syndrome

knife
    microtome k.
    souvenir k.
knife-rest crystal
knight disease
knizocyte
knob
    aortic k.
    malarial k.
knockout
    gene k.
Knodell histology activity index
Knoellia
    K. sinensis
    K. subterranea
Knoll gland
knot
    syncytial k.
knotting
    syncytial k.
Knott technique
knowlesi
    Plasmodium k.
KO89-kit antibody
Kobelt cyst
Kober test
Köbner phenomenon
Koch
    K. bacillus
    K. ileostomy
    K. law
    K. old tuberculin
    K. phenomenon
    K. postulate
Kocher-Debré-Semelaigne syndrome
Kocher dilatation ulcer
kochi
    Plasmodium k.
kochii
    Borrelia k.
Koch-Weeks
    K.-W. bacillus
    K.-W. *Haemophilus*
Kocuria
    K. marina
    K. polaris
    K. rhizophila
Kodak
    K. Ektachem DT-60 cholesterol analyzer
    K. Ektachem Vitros 250, 750, 950 cholesterol analyzer

K

NOTES

Koebner phenomenon
koehlerae
    Bartonella k.
Koenen tumor
Koenig syndrome
Koerber-Salus-Elschnig syndrome
Kogoj
    K. abscess
    pustules of K.
    spongiform pustule of K.
KOH
    potassium hydroxide
    KOH preparation
    KOH test
Köhler
    K. disease
    K. illumination
Köhlmeier-Degos disease
Kohn
    K. one-step staining technique
    K. pore
koilocyte
koilocytosis
koilocytotic
    k. atypia
    k. cell
koilonychia
kokoi venom
Kokoskin stain
koleovorans
    Paenibacillus k.
Kölliker
    K. layer
    K. reticulum
Kolmer
    K. test
    K. test with Reiter protein (KRP)
Köln
    Hb K.
    K. hemoglobin
kongjuensis
    Pseudonocardia k.
koningi
    Scopulariopsis k.
koniocortex
Konzo
Koongol virus
Koplik spot
KOR
    kappa opioid receptor
    KOR agonist
Kordia algicida
Korean
    K. hemorrhagic fever
    K. hemorrhagic fever virus
koreense
    Planomicrobium k.
koreensis
    Arthrobacter k.

    Catellatospora k.
    Comamonas k.
    Hongia k.
    Kangiella k.
    Kribbella k.
    Paenibacillus k.
    Pseudomonas k.
    Rhodococcus k.
    Sphingomonas k.
    Weissella k.
Korff fiber
Korsakoff syndrome
Koser citrate broth
koseri
    Citrobacter k.
Koshevnikoff disease
Kossa stain
kostiensis
    Ensifer k.
Kostmann
    K. agranulocytosis
    K. syndrome
Kova Glasstic Slide #10 with Grids
Kovalevsky canal
Kovats index
Kowarsky test
Kozakia baliensis
KP
    keratitic precipitate
KP1
    K. antibody
    K. immunohistochemical reagent
KP1/CD68 monoclonal antibody
kPa
    kilopascal
KPTT
    kaolin partial thromboplastin time
Kr
    krypton
Kr85
    krypton 85
Krabbe
    K. disease
    K. leukodystrophy
    K. syndrome
Krafft point
krajdenii
    Trichophyton k.
kra-kra
K-ras
    K-r. mutation
    K-r. oncogene
kraurosis vulvae
Krause
    K. end bulb
    K. gland
    K. syndrome
Krauss and Neubecker morphologic
    criteria

KRB
    Krebs-Ringer bicarbonate buffer
Krebs
    K. cycle
    K. leukocyte index
Krebs-Henseleit cycle
Krebs-Ringer
    K.-R. bicarbonate buffer (KRB)
    K.-R. phosphate (KRP)
    K.-R. solution
Kribbella
    K. antibiotica
    K. flavida
    K. jejuensis
    K. koreensis
    Lachnobacterium K.
    K. sandramycini
    K. solani
kribbensis
    Paenibacillus k.
kriegii
    Oceanobacter k.
kringle
Krishaber disease
Krisovski sign
kristensenii
    Yersinia k.
Krokiewicz test
Krompecher carcinoma
Kronecker stain
KRP
    Kolmer test with Reiter protein
    Krebs-Ringer phosphate
Krukenberg
    K. spindle
    K. tumor
    K. vein
krulwichiae
    Bacillus k.
Krumwiede triple sugar agar
krungthepensis
    Asaia k.
krusei
    Candida k.
Kruskal-Wallis test
krypton (Kr)
    k. 85 (Kr85)
KS
    ketosteroid
    Klinefelter syndrome
KSCC
    keratinizing squamous cell carcinoma

KSOM
    potassium simplex optimized medium
    HEPES-buffered KSOM
kT
    kiloton
KU
    Karmen unit
kubicae
    Mycobacterium k.
Kuehneromyces
Kufs disease
Kugelberg-Welander disease
Kühne
    K. methylene blue
    K. spindle
    K. terminal plate
Kuhnt-Junius disease
Kulchitsky cell
kullae
    Pigmentiphaga k.
Külz cylinder
Kumba virus
Kümmell disease
Kümmell-Verneuil disease
kummerowiae
    Ensifer k.
    Sinorhizobium k.
Kunin antigen
Kunitz domain-containing protein
Kunkel
    K. syndrome
    K. test
kunsanensis
    Nocardiopsis k.
Kupffer
    K. cell
    K. cell hypertrophy
    K. cell iron deposition
    K. cell sarcoma
kurcas
    Jatropha k.
Kurthia
kurtosis
kuru plaque
kururiensis
    Burkholderia k.
Kurzrok-Ratner test
kushneri
    Halanaerobium k.
Kuskokwim syndrome
Kussmaul
    K. disease

K

NOTES

Kussmaul *(continued)*
K. paralysis
K. respiration
Kussmaul-Kien respiration
Kussmaul-Landry paralysis
Kussmaul-Maier disease
Kuwabara paper
kuzendorf
Salmonella cholerae suis var. *k.*
KV
killed vaccine
kV
kilovolt
kVA
kilovolt ampere
Kveim
K. antigen
K. test
Kveim-Stilzbach
K.-S. antigen
K.-S. test
kVp
kilovolt peak
KW
Keith-Wagener

kW
kilowatt
kwashiorkor
marasmic k.
kwashiorkor-marasmus syndrome
KWB
Keith-Wagener-Barker
kweiyangensis
Anopheles k.
kWh
kilowatt-hour
Kyasanur
K. Forest disease
K. Forest disease virus
kyphos
kyphoscoliosis
kyphoscoliotic pelvis
kyphosis
juvenile k.
kyphotic pelvis
Kyrle disease
Kytococcus schroeteri

L
　lethal
　leucine
　lewisite
　light
　liter
　NATO code for lewisite
　　L chain
　　L dose
　　L layer
　　L layer
　　L unit of streptomycin
L1
　lewisite 1
L2
　lewisite 2
L3
　lewisite 3
L_0, Lo
　limes zero
　　L_0 dose
l-
　levorotatory
L-
　sterically related to L-glyceraldehyde
l1307K gene mutation
L26 antibody
LA
　latex agglutination
　lupus anticoagulant
　　Staclot LA
La
　　La Brea hepatitis
　　La Crosse virus
LAA
　leukocyte ascorbic acid
lab
　laboratory
Laband syndrome
Labbé neurocirculatory syndrome
label
　affinity l.
　ligand-conjugate l.
　radioactive l.
　l. variable
labeled
　l. antigen
　l. streptavidin biotin (LSAB)
labeling
　cohort l.
　double fluorescence l.
　hazardous materials l.
　l. of hazardous materials
　immunogold l.
　l. index

　ligand-conjugate l.
　ruthenium red l.
　in situ DNA nick end l.
　in situ nick end l.
　T-cell antibody l.
　TdT-mediated dUTP nick-end l.
　　(TUNEL)
labia (*pl. of* labium)
labial
　l. gland
　l. salivary gland (LSG)
　l. salivary gland biopsy
labiales
　glandulae l.
labii (*gen. of* labium)
labile
　l. cell
　l. element
　l. factor
　heat l.
labiomycosis
labium, gen. **labii**, pl. **labia**
　l. limbi tympanicum laminae
　　spiralis ossei
　l. limbi vestibulare laminae
　labia majus
Labophot-2 microscope
labor
　false l.
laboratorian
laboratory (lab)
　bacteriology l.
　clinical l.
　controlled access l.
　l. diagnosis
　face velocity of l. hood
　l. hood
　LRN BioWatch l.
　l. manifestation
　national l.
　public health l.
　QuestDirect direct to consumer l.
　reference l.
　l. reference (LR)
　L. Response Network (LRN)
　restricted access l.
　sentinel l.
　Venereal Disease Research L.
　　(VDRL)
　virology l.
Labpette FX pipette
labranchiae
　Anopheles l.
labrocyte

L

labstation
T/T Mega advanced multifunction microwave l.
labyrinth
Ludwig l.
renal l.
labyrinthica
otitis l.
labyrinthine
l. defect (LD)
l. hydrops
l. space
labyrinthus
Lacazia loboi
Laccaria
lacerated wound
laceration
laceyi
Streptomyces l.
Lachesis
Lachnellula
Lachnobacterium
L. *bovis*
L. *Kribbella*
LaChrom HPLC system
laciniae tubae
lacis cell
lack of collagen
lac operon
lacrimal
l. calculus
l. gland
l. gland tumor
l. sac tumor
lacrimalis
glandula l.
Peptoniphilus l.
lacrimator
lactacidemia
lactacidosis
lactaciduria
lactalbumin hydrolysate (LAH)
lactamica
Neisseria l.
Lactarius
lactase deficiency
lactate
accumulation of l.
cerebrospinal fluid l.
l. dehydrogenase (LD)
l. dehydrogenase, aspartate aminotransferase, white blood cells (LAW)
l. dehydrogenase assay
l. dehydrogenase isoenzyme
l. dehydrogenase isoenzyme determination
l. dehydrogenase test

l. dehydrogenase virus
sodium l.
lactated
l. Ringer injection
l. Ringer solution (LRS)
lactate-pyruvate ratio (L:P)
lactatifermentans
Clostridium l.
lactating adenoma
lactational mastitis
lactea
macula l.
lacteal
central l.
l. cyst
l. fistula
l. vessel
lactenin
lactescence
lacteus
Mycetocola l.
lactic
l. acid
l. acid assay
l. acid bacteria
l. acidemia
l. acidosis
l. dehydrogenase (LD)
l. dehydrogenase test
l. dehydrogenase virus (LDV)
lacticacidemia
lactiferi
ductus l.
tubuli l.
lactiferous
l. duct
l. gland
l. sinus
lactis
Paenibacillus l.
Lactobacillaceae
lactobacillary milk
Lactobacilleae
Lactobacillus
L. *acidipiscis*
L. *acidophilus*
L. *algidus*
L. *amylolyticus*
L. *arizonensis*
L. *bifidus*
L. *brevis*
L. *buchneri*
L. *bulgaricus*
L. *bulgaricus* factor (LBF)
L. *casei*
L. *catenaformis*
L. *coleohominis*
L. *crispatus*
L. *curvatus*

L. cypricasei
L. delbrueckii
L. diolivorans
L. durianis
L. equi
L. ferintoshensis
L. fermentum
L. fornicalis
L. frumenti
L. fuchuensis
L. ingluviei
L. jensenii
L. kefiranofaciens subsp. *kefirgranum*
L. kimchii
L. kitasatonis
L. leichmannii
L. mindensis
L. minor
L. mucosae
L. nagelii
L. pantheris
L. paracollinoides
L. paralimentarius
L. perolens
L. plantarum
L. psittaci
L. saerimneri
L. salivarius
L. spicheri
L. thermotolerans
L. trichodes
L. versmoldensis

lactobacillus, pl. **lactobacilli**
    Boas-Oppler l.
lactobezoar
lactocele
lactoferrin
lactogen
    human placental l. (hPL)
    placental l. (PL)
lactogenic hormone
lactoglobulin
    beta l. (BLG)
    immune l.
lactolyticus
    Anaerococcus l.
lactone dye
lactoperoxidase radioiodination
lactophenol cotton blue stain

lactose
    l. intolerance
    l. tolerance test
lactose-litmus broth
lactoside
    ceramide l.
lactosidosis
lactosuria
lactosyl ceramide
lactotrope adenoma
lactotroph
    pituitary l.
lactotrophic
lacuna, pl. **lacunae**
    cartilage l.
    chondrocyte l.
    Howship l.
    isogenous chondrocyte in l.
    osseous l.
    resorption lacunae
lacunar
    l. abscess
    l. cell
    l. resorption
lacunata
    Moraxella l.
lacune
    vascular l.
lacunule
lacus
    Mycobacterium l.
lacuscaerulensis
    Silicibacter l.
lacusekhoensis
    Nesterenkonia l.
lacusfryxellense
    Clostridium l.
lacustris
    Friedmanniella l.
lacZ-tagged cell
LAD
    leukocyte adhesion deficiency
Ladd
    L. band
    L. syndrome
ladder
    180-bp l.
    sequence l.
Ladendorff test
LAE
    left atrial enlargement
Laelaps echidninus

L

NOTES

Laënnec
    L. cirrhosis
    L. disease
    L. pearl
laesa
    functio l.
Laetiporus sulphureus
Laetrile
laeve
    chorion l.
Lafora
    L. body
    L. disease
lag
    anaphase l.
    nitrogen l.
    phase l.
    l. phase
    l. time
lagena
    Torulomyces l.
Lagochilascaris minor
Lagovirus
lagunensis
    Caldisphaera l.
LAH
    lactalbumin hydrolysate
    left atrial hypertrophy
lahorensis
    Ornithodoros l.
laidlawii
    Acholeplasma l.
LAIT
    latex agglutination-inhibition test
laiteuse
    tache l.
LAK
    lymphokine-activated killer cell
lake
    acellular mucus l.
    bile l.
    red cell l.
    subchorial l.
    vascular l.
    venous l.
laked blood agar
Laki-Lorand factor (LLF)
laky blood
LAL
    Limulus amoebocyte lysate
    LAL gram-negative bacteria test
Lallemand body
LAM
    lymphangioleiomyomatosis
    lymphangiomyomatosis
    pulmonary LAM

LAMB
    lentigines, atrial myxoma, mucocutaneous
    myxomas, and blue nevi
    LAMB syndrome
lambda
    l. carrageenin
    l. chain specificity
    l. light chain
Lambert
    L. canal
    L. law
Lambert-Eaton
    L.-E. myasthenic syndrome (LEMS)
    L.-E. syndrome
Lambl excrescence
lamblia
    Giardia l.
    L. intestinalis
lambliasis
lambo lambo
lamé foliacée
lamella, pl. **lamellae**
    annulate lamellae
    articular l.
    l. of bone
    circumferential l.
    concentric l.
    cornoid l.
    elastic lamellae
    external elastic lamellae
    ground l.
    haversian l.
    inner circumferential l.
    intermediate l.
    internal elastic lamellae
    interstitial l.
    outer circumferential l.
    ovigerous l.
    triangular l.
    vitreous l.
lamellar
    l. body
    l. bone
    l. collagen
    l. granule
    l. ichthyosis
    l. necrosis
lamellate
lamellated
    l. collection of inspissated
      inflammatory debris
    l. corpuscle
lamellipodium
lamellosa
    corpuscula l.
lamina, pl. **laminae**
    basal l.
    l. basalis choroideae
    basement l.

basilar l.
l. basilaris cochleae
boundary l.
l. choriocapillaris
l. choroidea epithelialis
l. choroidocapillaris
l. cribrosa ossis ethmoidalis
l. cribrosa sclerae
l. densa
dense fibrous l. (DFL)
l. dentata
l. elastica anterior
l. elastica interna
l. elastica posterior
episcleral l.
l. episcleralis
epithelial l.
external elastic l.
l. fibroreticularis
l. fusca sclerae
glomerular basal l.
hepatic l.
internal elastic l.
labium limbi vestibulare l.
l. lateralis cartilaginis tubae auditivae
l. lateralis cartilaginis tubae auditoriae
l. of lens
l. limitans anterior corneae
l. limitans posterior corneae
l. lucida
l. medialis cartilaginis tubae auditivae
l. medialis cartilaginis tubae auditoriae
l. membranacea cartilaginis tubae auditivae
l. muscularis mucosae
osseous spiral l.
l. propria
l. propria mucosae
l. rara
l. rara interna
reticular l.
l. of Rexed
spiral l.
laminae spiralis ossei
successional l.
tympanic lip of limbus of spiral l.
l. vasculosa choroideae

vestibular lip of limbus of spiral l.
l. vitrea
laminar
l. cortical necrosis
l. cortical sclerosis
l. flow burner
l. flow hood
laminariae
Zobellia l.
laminated
l. epithelium
l. thrombus
lamination
laminin
l. antigen
l. chain
l. marker
l. receptor
laminitis
L-**amino acid oxidase**
lamins
lamotrigine
LAMP
lysosomal-associated membrane protein
LAMP-1
lysosomal-associated membrane protein-1
LAMP-2
lysosomal-associated membrane protein-2
lamp
hollow cathode l.
portable magnifier lab l.
slit l.
spirit l.
tungsten arc l.
tungsten halogen l.
VisionSaver lab l.
Wood l.
Lamprocystis purpurea
Lan antigen
Lancefield
L. classification
L. grouping
L. precipitation test
lanceolata
Drepanidotaenia l.
Hymenolepis l.
lanceolate myxoma
lanceolatus
Peptostreptococcus l.
lance-ovate spot
Lancereaux-Mathieu disease

L

NOTES

lancet
    l. fluke
    Laser l.
    Safe-T Lance Plus l.
Landouzy-Dejerine progressive muscular dystrophy
Landouzy disease
Landry
    L. disease
    L. syndrome
Landry-Guillain-Barré (LGB)
    L.-G.-B. syndrome
Landschutz tumor
land scurvy
Landsteiner classification
Landsteiner-Donath test
Landström muscle
Lane disease
Langdon-Down disease
Lange
    L. colloidal gold test
    L. solution
Langendorff apparatus
Langerhans
    L. cell granulomatosis (LCG)
    L. cell histiocytosis (LCH)
    L. granule
    islands of L.
    L. islands
    islets of L.
langerhansian hormone
Langer line
langeroni
    Arthrographis l.
langeronii
    Eremomyces l.
    Pithoascus l.
Langhans
    L. giant cell
    L. layer
    L. stria
    L. type of giant cell reaction
Langley granule
Lang test
lanienae
    Campylobacter l.
Lanosa nivalis
Lansing virus
Lanterman
    L. incisure
    L. segment
lanthanide
lanthanoid
lanthanum nitrate
lanuginosus
    Thermomyces l.
lanugo hair
LAP
    leucine aminopeptidase

    leukocyte alkaline phosphatase
    lymphangiomatous polyp
    lyophilized anterior pituitary
    LAP score
    LAP stain
    LAP test
laparomyositis
laparoscopic renal resection
lapinization
lapinized
Laplace law
Laquer stain for alcoholic hyalin
L-arabinose dehydrogenase
L-arabitol dehydrogenase
laramiense
    Clostridium estertheticum subsp. *l.*
larbish
lardaceous
    l. liver
    l. spleen
large
    l. calorie (C, Cal)
    l. deletion
    l. external transformation-sensitive (LETS)
    l. glandular pattern
    l. granular lymphocyte (LGL)
    l. granular lymphocyte leukemia
    l. particle sorting module (LPS)
    l. unstained cell (LUC)
    l. vein
    l. vessel hematocrit (LVH)
large-cell
    l.-c. acanthoma
    l.-c. immunoblastic lymphoma
    l.-c. neuroendocrine carcinoma (LCNEC)
large-cup forceps
large-needle aspiration biopsy (LNB)
large-scale integration
lari
    Campylobacter l.
Laribacter hongkongensis
Laricifomes
Laron dwarfism
Larrey
    L. cleft
    L. hernia
Larrey-Weil disease
larrymoorei
    Agrobacterium l.
    Rhizobium l.
Larsen
    L. disease
    L. syndrome
Larsen-Johansson disease
larva, pl. **larvae**
    Bacillus larvae
    l. currens

l. fly
fly l.
larva migrans
Lepidoptera l.
larval
larvicidal
larvicide
larviparous
larviphagic
laryngeae
glandulae l.
laryngeal
l. cancer
l. carcinoma
l. edema
l. gland
l. granuloma
l. intubation trauma
l. lupus
l. nodule
l. papillomatosis
l. polyp
l. tonsil
l. tuberculosis
l. web
laryngei
folliculi lymphatici l.
larynges (*pl. of* larynx)
laryngeus
Mammomonogamus l.
laryngis
pachyderma l.
tunica mucosa l.
laryngitis
laryngocele
laryngogram
laryngomalacia
laryngopharyngitis
laryngotracheitis
avian infectious l.
laryngotracheobronchitis (LTB)
larynx, pl. **larynges**
chondromalacia of l.
Gussenbauer artificial l.
lymphatic follicle of l.
Lasègue disease
laser
l. capture microdissection
l. confocal microscopy
l. diffraction particle size
L. lancet
l. microprobe

l. microscope
Tsunami l.
laser-activated fluorescence
laser-scanning confocal microscopy
LaserTweezer
Lasette
Lash casein hydrolysate-serum medium
Lasiodiplodia
Lasiohelea
L-asparaginase therapy
Lassa
L. hemorrhagic fever
L. virus
late
l. cortical T cell
l. effect poliomyelitis
l. event
l. infantile amaurotic familial idiocy
l. neonatal death
l. positive component (LPC)
l. reaction
l. replicating X chromosome
l. systolic murmur (LSM)
latency
distal l.
l. period (LP)
terminal l.
latent
l. allergy
l. coccidioidomycosis
l. empyema
l. heat
l. hypermetropia
l. infection
l. iron-binding capacity (LIBC)
l. membrane protein (LMP)
l. membrane protein 1 (LMP-1)
l. membrane protein-1 expression
l. microbism
l. period
l. porphyria
l. rat virus
l. stage
latentiation
late-phase response
lateral
l. aberrant thyroid carcinoma
l. cartilaginous plate
l. cell membrane
l. collateral ligament degeneration
l. epicondylitis

L

NOTES

lateral *(continued)*
    l. geniculate body
    l. gray horn
    l. hypothalamus
    l. plate of cartilaginous auditory tube
    l. semicircular canal
    l. vaginal wall smear
lateralis
    pharyngitis hypertrophica l.
latericius
    Arenibacter l.
lateris
    nevus unius l.
lateritium
    sedimentum l.
latex
    l. agglutination (LA)
    l. agglutination-inhibition test (LAIT)
    l. agglutination test
    l. agglutinin
    l. allergy
    l. fixation test
    l. flocculation test (LFT)
    l. particle agglutination test
    l. screen
    l. slide agglutination test
latex-specific IgE
lathyrism
lathyrus protein
latina
    Actinomadura l.
lato
    Borrelia burgdorferi sensu l.
Latrodectus
    L. bishopi
    L. geometricus
    L. mactans
LATS
    long-acting thyroid stimulator
    LATS assay
    LATS protector
    LATS test
lattice hypothesis
latum
    condyloma l.
    Diphyllobothrium l.
latus
    Bothriocephalus l.
    Dibothriocephalus l.
latyschewii
    Borrelia l.
Lauber disease
laudable pus
Launois-Bensaude syndrome
Launois-Cléret syndrome
Launois syndrome
laurel fever

Laurell
    L. rocket immunoelectrophoresis
    L. technique
Laurence-Biedl syndrome
Laurence-Moon-Bardet-Biedl syndrome
Laurence-Moon-Biedl syndrome
Laurence-Moon syndrome
Lauren classification
Laurén criteria
lauric acid
lauryl sulfate broth
Lauth violet
LAV
    lymphadenopathy-associated virus
lavage
    bronchoalveolar l. (BAL)
    bronchopulmonary l.
    cervicovaginal l.
    ductal l.
    gastric l.
    peritoneal l.
lavamentivorans
    Parvibaculum l.
Lavdovsky nucleoid
lavender cytoplasm
Laverania
LAW
    lactate dehydrogenase, aspartate aminotransferase, white blood cells
law
    Ambard l.'s
    Ångström l.
    Avogadro l.
    Baumé l.
    Beer l.
    Beer-Boguer l.
    Behring l.
    Bell-Magendie l.
    Bernoulli l.
    Bouguer l.
    Boyle l.
    Charles l.
    Coulomb l.
    Courvoisier l.
    Dalton l.
    Einthoven l.
    Farr l.
    Fick l.
    gas l.
    Gay-Lussac l.
    Graham l.
    Halsted l.
    Hamburger l.
    Hardy-Weinberg l.
    Henry l.
    Hooke l.
    ideal gas l.
    inverse-square l.
    Joule l.

Kahler l.
Kirchoff l.
Koch l.
Lambert l.
Laplace l.
Marfan l.
mass action l.
l. of mass action
Mendel l.
Ohm l.
Pascal l.
Planck radiation l.
Poiseuille l.
l. of priority
Profeta l.
Raoult l.
right-to-know l.
Snell l.
Starling l.
Stefan-Boltzmann l.
Stokes l.
Virchow l.

Lawford syndrome
Lawless stain
lawn plate
Lawrence-Seip syndrome
laxa

cutis l.

Laxitextum
layer

ameloblastic l.
anterior elastic l.
bacillary l.
basal cell l.
Bowman l.
brown l.
cambium l.
l. of cerebellar cortex
l. of cerebral cortex
Chievitz l.
choriocapillary l.
columnar l.
depletion l.
enamel l.
ependymal l.
epithelial choroid l.
external pyramidal l.
fibrous l.
fusiform l.
germ l.
germinative l.
glycolipid l.

half-value l. (HVL)
Henle fiber l.
Henle nervous l.
Huxley l.
infragranular l.
inner circular muscle l.
inner neural l.
Kaes-Bekhterev l.
Kölliker l.
L l.
Langhans l.
longitudinal l.
malpighian l.
membranous l.
Meynert l.
molecular cell l.
Nitabuch l.
odontoblastic l.
osteogenetic l.
outer longitudinal muscle l.
palisade l.
papillary l.
parabasal cell l.
photoreceptor l.
plasma l.
plexiform l.
polymorphous l.
posterior elastic l.
prickle cell l.
Purkinje cell l.
pyramidal cell l.
l. of retina
l. of rods and cones
Sattler elastic l.
l. of skin
sluggish l.
spindle-celled l.
spinous l.
still l.
subendocardial l.
subendothelial l.
subpapillary l.
suprabasal cell l.
Tomes granular l.
uteroplacental fibrinoid l.
vascular l.
ventricular l.
Weil basal l.

lazarine leprosy
Lazaro

mal de San L.

lazy leukocyte syndrome

NOTES

L

LBCL
large B-cell lymphoma
LBF
Lactobacillus bulgaricus factor
LBI
low serum-bound iron
LBM
lean body mass
LBW
low birth weight
LBWI
low birth weight infant
LC
large cell
lethal concentration
lymphocytic colitis
LCA
leukocyte common antigen
LCA antibody
LCAT
lecithin-cholesterol acyltransferase
LCAT deficiency
LCCSCT
large-cell calcifying Sertoli cell tumor
LCD
lipochondral degeneration
LCFA
long-chain fatty acid
LCG
Langerhans cell granulomatosis
LCH
Langerhans cell histiocytosis
L-chain
L-c. disease
L-c. myeloma
LCIS
lobular carcinoma in situ
LCL
Levinthal-Coles-Lillie
lymphocytic leukemia
lymphocytic lymphosarcoma
LCL bodies
LCM
left costal margin
lymphatic choriomeningitis
lymphocytic choriomeningitis
LCM virus
LCNEC
large-cell neuroendocrine carcinoma
LCNHL
large-cell non-Hodgkin lymphoma
LCPUFA
long-chain polyunsaturated fatty acid
LCR
ligase chain reaction
LCT
long-chain triglyceride
LCt
lethal concentration

LCt$_{50}$
lethal Ct$_{50}$
LD
labyrinthine defect
lactate dehydrogenase
lactic dehydrogenase
Legionnaires disease
lethal dose
living donor
lymphocyte-defined
LD 400 luminescence detector
LD$_{50}$
median lethal dose
LDHD
lymphocyte-depleted Hodgkin disease
LDL
low-density lipoprotein
LDL cholesterol assay
LDL direct test prefilled cartridge
LDL-C
low-density lipoprotein-cholesterol
L$^+$ dose
LDV
lactic dehydrogenase virus
LE
lupus erythematosus
LE body
LE cell
LE cell test
LE factor
LE phenomenon
Le
Le antigen
Le Veen shunt
leachi
Haemaphysalis l.
leaching
lead
l. anemia
l. assay
black l.
l. broth
l. chromate
chromate stain for l.
l. citrate
l. citrate stain
l. colic
l. core high-velocity round
l. demonstration in tissue
l. encephalitis
l. encephalopathy
l. fixative
l. gout
l. hydroxide stain
l. level
l. nephropathy
l. pigmentation
l. poisoning

l. snowstorm
l. stomatitis
leading strand
lead-pipe
l.-p. colon
l.-p. rigidity
leaflet
mitral valve cleft l.
outer l.
tricuspid valve cleft l.
leak
spinal fluid l.
leakage
vascular l.
lean body mass (LBM)
learning
distance l.
least
l. splanchnic nerve
l. squares regression
leather-bottle stomach
leave-one-out cross-validation analysis
Leber
L. disease
L. hereditary optic neuropathy (LHON)
L. optic atrophy
Lechtheimia corymbifera
lecithin
amniotic fluid unsaturated l.
lecithinase A
lecithin-cholesterol
l.-c. acyltransferase (LCAT)
lecithin/sphingomyelin ratio (L:S)
LECL
lymphoepithelioid cell lymphoma
Leclanché cell
Leclercia
lectin
mannose binding l. (MBL)
peanut l.
Ulex l.
lectotype
lectularia
Acanthia l.
lectularius
Cimex l.
lectus
Algibacter l.
Lecythophora
LED
lupus erythematosus disseminatus

Ledderhose disease
Leder
L. reaction
L. stain
Lederer anemia
leech
American l.
artificial l.
medicinal l.
leeching
Leeuwenhoek canal
Lee-White (LW)
L.-W. clotting test
L.-W. clotting time method
left
l. atrial enlargement (LAE)
l. atrial hypertrophy (LAH)
l. bundle branch block
l. costal margin (LCM)
deviation to the l.
shield to the l.
shift to the l.
l. shift
l. shift (increased band forms on WBC differential)
l. ventricular enlargement (LVE)
l. ventricular failure (LVF)
l. ventricular hypertrophy (LVH)
left-sided lesion
left-sidedness
bilateral l.
left-to-right ratio (L:R)
leg
Barbados l.
elephant l.
milk l.
white l.
Legal
L. disease
L. test
Legg-Calvé-Perthes disease
Legg disease
Legg-Perthes disease
Legionella
L. beliardensis
L. bozemanii
L. busanensis
L. drancourtii
L. drozanskii
L. dumoffii
L. fallonii
L. feeleii

NOTES

Legionella (continued)
- L. *gormanii*
- L. *gresilensis*
- L. *jordanis*
- L. *longbeachae*
- L. *micdadei*
- L. *pittsburgensis*
- L. *pneumophila*
- L. *pneumophila* culture
- L. *pneumophila* direct fA smear
- L. *rowbothamii*
- L. *taurinensis*
- L. urinary antigen (LUA)
- L. urinary antigen ELISA test kit
- L. *wadsworthii*

Legionellaceae
legionellosis
Legionnaires
- L. disease (LD)
- L. disease antibody

Leica
- L. VT1000 E fully automatic microtome
- L. VT1000 M semi-automatic microtome

Leiden
- L. factor
- L. mutation

Leifsonia
- L. *aquatica*
- L. *aurea*
- L. *cynodontis*
- L. *naganoensis*
- L. *poae*
- L. *rubra*
- L. *shinshuensis*
- L. *xyli*
- L. *xyli* subsp. *cynodontis*
- L. *xyli* subsp. *xyli*

Leigh disease
Leiner disease
leiodermia
leiomyoblastoma
leiomyofibroma
leiomyoma
- benign metastasizing l. (BML)
- bizarre l.
- clear cell l.
- l. cutis
- epithelioid l.
- parasitic l.
- uterine l.
- vascular l.

leiomyomatosis
- intravenous l. (IVL)
- l. peritonealis disseminata

leiomyomatous hamartoma
leiomyosarcoma (LMS)
- epithelioid l. (ELMS)

pleomorphic l.
uterine l. (ULMS)
Leipzig yellow
Leishman
- L. chrome cell
- L. stain

Leishman-Donovan body
Leishmania
- L. *aethiopica*
- L. *braziliensis braziliensis*
- L. *braziliensis guyanensis*
- L. *braziliensis panamensis*
- L. *caninum*
- L. *donovani archibaldi*
- L. *donovani chagasi*
- L. *donovani donovani*
- L. *donovani infantum*
- L. *furunculosa*
- L. *infantum*
- L. *mexicana amazonensis*
- L. *mexicana garnhami*
- L. *mexicana mexicana*
- L. *mexicana pifanoi*
- L. *mexicana venezuelensis*
- L. *nilotica*
- L. *peruviana*
- L. *tropica*
- L. *tropica major*
- L. *tropica mexicana*

leishmaniasis
- American l.
- l. americana
- anergic l.
- cutaneous l.
- lupoid l.
- mucocutaneous l.
- nasooral l.
- nasopharyngeal l.
- pseudolepromatous l.
- l. recidivans
- l. serological test
- l. tegumentaria diffusa
- visceral l.

Leishmaniavirus
leishmanicidal
leishmaniosis
leishmanoid
Leisingera methylohalidivorans
Leitz image analysis system
LEL
- lymphoepithelial lesion

LELC
- lymphoepithelioma-like carcinoma

Leloir disease
Leminorella
lemmocyte
lemniscus, pl. **lemnisci**
lemoignei
- *Paucimonas* l.

lemonnieri
> *Saccharomyces l.*

lemon sign

LEMS
> Lambert-Eaton myasthenic syndrome
> LEMS antibody

Lendrum
> L. inclusion body stain
> L. phloxine-tartrazine stain

Lenègre disease

length
> focal l.
> fragment l.
> greatest l. (GL)

Lenhossek process

Lennert
> L. classification
> L. lesion
> L. lymphoma

Lennox syndrome

lens
> achromatic l.
> l. antigen
> aplanatic l.
> cortex of l.
> l. dislocation
> electron l.
> epithelium of l.
> fiber of l.
> lamina of l.
> oil immersion l.
> opacification of l.
> l. star
> suspensory ligament of l.

lens-induced uveitis

lenta
> *Eggerthella l.*
> sepsis l.

Lentibacillus salicampi

lenticula

lenticular
> l. opacity
> l. papilla
> l. progressive degeneration
> l. protein

lenticularis
> dermatofibrosis l.

lenticulopapular

lentigines (*pl. of* lentigo)

lentiginosis
> periorificial l.

lentiginous
> l. melanocytic hyperplasia
> l. melanocytic structure

lentigo, pl. **lentigines**
> lentigines, atrial myxoma, mucocutaneous myxomas, and blue nevi (LAMB)
> l. maligna
> l. maligna melanoma
> malignant l.
> lentigines (multiple), electrocardiographic abnormalities, ocular hypertelorism, pulmonary stenosis, abnormalities of genitalia, retardation of growth, and deafness (sensorineural) (LEOPARD)
> PUVA l.
> solar l.

lentigomelanosis

Lentinula

Lentinus

lentis
> apparatus suspensorius l.
> cortex l.
> epithelium l.
> fibrae l.
> radii l.
> substantia l.
> tunica vasculosa l.

Lentisphaera araneosa

Lentisphaerae

Lentisphaerales

Lentivirinae

Lentivirus

lentivirus

Lentodium

lentogenic

lentum
> *Eubacterium l.*

lentus
> *Vibrio l.*

Lentzea
> *L. albida*
> *L. albidocapillata*
> *L. californiensis*
> *L. flaviverrucosa*
> *L. violacea*
> *L. waywayandensis*

Lenzites betulina

Lenz syndrome

L

NOTES

leonina
 Toxascaris l.
leonine facies
leontiasis ossea
Leon virus
LEOPARD
 lentigines (multiple), electrocardiographic abnormalities, ocular hypertelorism, pulmonary stenosis, abnormalities of genitalia, retardation of growth, and deafness (sensorineural)
 LEOPARD syndrome
Lepehne-Pickworth stain
leper
lepidic
Lepidoptera **larva**
lepidosis
Lepiota
Lepista
Lepore
 hemoglobin L.
 L. thalassemia
leporinum
 Arnium l.
Leporipoxvirus
leporis-palustris
 Haemaphysalis l.
lepra
 l. cell
 l. cell organism
 l. manchada
leprae
 Bacillus l.
 Mycobacterium l.
lepraemurium
 Mycobacterium l.
leprechaun facies
leprologist
leprology
leproma
lepromatous leprosy
lepromin
 l. reaction
 l. skin test
leprosarium, leprosery
leprose
leprostatic
leprosum
 erythema nodosum l. (ENL)
leprosus
 pemphigus l.
leprosy
 anesthetic l.
 articular l.
 l. bacillus
 borderline l.
 cutaneous l.
 dimorphous l.
 dry l.

histoid l.
indeterminate l.
lazarine l.
lepromatous l.
Lucio l.
macular l.
Malabar l.
murine l.
mutilating l.
nodular l.
smooth l.
trophoneurotic l.
tuberculoid l.
leprotic
leprous
leptin protein
leptochromatic
Leptoconops
leptocyte
leptocytosis
Leptodontium camptobactrum
Leptographium
leptokurtic
leptomeningeal
 l. carcinoma
 l. carcinomatosis
 l. cyst
 l. fibrosis
leptomeninges
leptomeningitis
 basilar l.
leptomonad
Leptomonas
leptonema
Leptoporus
Leptopsylla segnis
leptoscope
Leptosphaeria
Leptosphaerulina
Leptospira
 L. australis
 L. autumnalis
 L. biflexa
 L. canicola
 L. culture
 L. grippotyphosa
 L. hebdomidis
 L. hyos
 L. icterohaemorrhagiae
 L. interrogans
 L. pomona
 L. serodiagnosis
Leptospiraceae
leptospiral jaundice
leptospire
Leptospirillum
 L. ferriphilum
 L. ferrooxidans
 L. thermoferrooxidans

leptospirosis icterohemorrhagica
leptospiruria
leptotene
Leptothrix
Leptotrichia
    L. buccalis
    L. goodfellowii
    L. hofstadii
    L. shahii
    L. trevisanii
    L. wadei
Leptotrombidium
    L. akamushi
    L. deliense
Leptus
Leriche syndrome
Leri pleonosteosis
Leri-Weill
    L.-W. disease
    L.-W. syndrome
Lermoyez syndrome
Leroy disease
Lesch-Nyhan syndrome
lesion
    angiocentric immunoproliferative l. (AIL)
    angiocentric lymphoproliferative l.
    angioimmunoproliferative l. (AIL)
    Antopol-Goldman l.
    Armanni-Ebstein l.
    Baehr-Lohlein l.
    benign lymphoepithelial l.
    benign proliferative l.
    bird's nest l.
    bone marrow l.
    brain l.
    bull's eye l.
    Cameron l.
    cavitary l.
    central l.
    coin l.
    cold l.
    collar button l.
    complex sclerosing l.
    Councilman l.
    cryptolytic l.
    diffuse l.
    discrete l.
    dysplasia-associated l.
    Ebstein l.
    encysted papillary l.

epithelial hyperplastic laryngeal l. (EHLL)
extracapillary l. (ECL)
fibroblastic l.
fibrohistiocytic l.
fibroinflammatory l.
fibroosseous l.
fibrosclerosing l.
focal hemorrhagic necrotizing pneumonic l.
gastric phenotype l.
Ghon primary l.
Ghon-Sachs primary l.
granulomatous l.
gross l.
gunpowder mark l.
hemosiderotic fibrohistiocytic lipomatous l. (HFLL)
high-grade squamous intraepithelial l. (HGSIL, HSIL)
histocytoid hemangioma-like l. (HHLL)
histologic l.
hot l.
immune complex-mediated inflammatory l.
impaction l.
indiscriminate l.
inflammatory myofibroblastic l.
initial syphilitic l.
intestinal phenotype l.
intralobular l.
irritative l.
Janeway l.
jet l.
Kimmelstiel-Wilson l.
left-sided l.
Lennert l.
lobular proliferative l.
local l.
Lohlein-Baehr l.
low-grade squamous intraepithelial l. (LGSIL, LSIL)
lymphoepithelial l. (LEL)
lymphoplasmacytic l.
lytic l.
macroscopic l.
Mallory-Weiss l.
mass l.
melanocytic l.
mixed gastric and intestinal phenotype l.

L

NOTES

lesion *(continued)*
    molecular l.
    mucinous breast l.
    myofibroblastic l.
    nil l.
    nonexophytic l.
    noninvasive lobular l.
    nonodontogenic l.
    Nora l.
    null phenotype l.
    odontogenic l.
    onion scale l.
    onionskin l.
    organic l.
    papular l.
    papulonodular l.
    parenchymal l.
    partial l.
    periluminal l.
    peripheral l.
    pigmented skin l. (PSL)
    plexiform l.
    polar l.
    portal tract l.
    precancerous l.
    precursor l.
    premalignant epidermal l.
    prenecrotizing phagocytic l.
    primary l.
    pseudo-Kaposi l.
    punched out lytic bone l.
    punched out osteolytic l.
    Quilty l.
    radial sclerosing l.
    right-sided l.
    ring-wall l.
    satellite vesicular l.
    shagreen l.
    skip l.
    space-occupying l. (SOL)
    spitzoid melanocytic l.
    spontaneous l. (SPL)
    squamous intraepithelial l. (SIL)
    structural l.
    synchronous airway l. (SAL)
    synchronous mass l.
    systemic l.
    target l.
    total l.
    trophic l.
    tubulointerstitial l.
    tumefactive fibroinflammatory l. (TFL)
    tumor-like l.
    l. of vasculature
    verrucopapillary external genital l.
    wire-loop l.
lesser
    l. omentum

    l. splanchnic nerve
    l. vestibular gland
lesteri
    Anopheles l.
LET
    leukocyte esterase test
    linear energy transfer
LETC
    lymphoepithelioma-like thymic carcinoma
lethal (L)
    l. anthrax aerosol
    l. coefficient
    l. concentration (LC, LCt)
    l. Ct_{50} (LCt_{50})
    l. dose (LD)
    l. dwarfism
    l. equivalent
    l. factor (LF)
    l. gene
    l. midline granuloma
    l. mutation
    synthetic l.
lethalis
    epidermolysis bullosa l.
lethargic encephalitis
LETS
    large external transformation-sensitive
letter bomb
Letterer-Siwe disease
lettingae
    Thermotoga l.
Leu
    leucine
    Leu 1–22 antibody
    Leu 1 antigen
leucin
leucine (L, Leu)
    l. aminopeptidase (LAP)
    l. aminopeptidase test
    l. hypoglycemia
    l. tolerance test
    urine l.
leucinosis
leucinuria
Leucoagaricus
Leucobacter albus
leucocelaenus
    Aedes l.
Leucocoprinus
Leucocytozoon
leucocytozoonosis
leucofuchsin
leucomethylene blue
Leuconostoc
    L. ficulneum
    L. fructosum
    L. gasicomitatum
    L. inhae

L. *kimchii*
L. *mesenteroides*
leuco patent blue
leucosphyrus
   Anopheles l.
Leucosporidium
Leucostoma
Leucotrichaceae
leucovorin calcium
leucyl
leucyl-RNA synthetase
leukanemia
leukapheresis
leukasmus
leukemia
   acute biphenotypic l.
   acute granulocytic l. (AGL)
   acute lymphoblastic l. (ALL)
   acute lymphocytic l. (ALL)
   acute megakaryoblastic l.
   acute megakaryocytic l. (M7)
   acute monoblastic l. (AMoL)
   acute monocytic l. (AMoL, M5)
   acute monocytic l. with
     differentiation (M5b)
   acute monocytic l. without
     differentiation (M5a)
   acute myeloblastic l. with
     maturation (M2)
   acute myeloblastic l. without
     localized differentiation (M0)
   acute myeloblastic l. without
     maturation (M1)
   acute myelocytic l.
   acute myelogenous l.
   acute myeloid l. (AML)
   acute myelomonocytic l. (AMML,
     M4)
   acute nonlymphocytic l. (ANLL)
   acute promyelocytic l. (APL, M3)
   acute undifferentiated l. (AUL)
   adult T-cell l. (ATL)
   aleukemic granulocytic l.
   aleukemic lymphocytic l.
   aleukemic monocytic l.
   atypical chronic myeloid l. (aCML)
   basophilic l.
   basophilocytic l.
   B-cell acute lymphoblastic l. (B-
     ALL)
   B-cell chronic lymphocytic l.
     (BCLL)

B-cell precursor lymphoblastic l.
   (BCP-LBL)
B-cell prolymphocytic l. (B-PLL)
blast cell l.
chronic cell l.
chronic eosinophilic l. (CEL)
chronic granulocytic l. (CGL)
chronic lymphatic l. (CLL)
chronic lymphocytic l. (CLL)
chronic lymphosarcoma l. (CLSL)
chronic monoblastic leukemia
   (CMoL)
chronic monocytic l. (CMoL)
chronic myelocytic l. (CML)
chronic myelogenous l. (CML)
chronic myeloid l.
chronic myelomonocytic l. (CMML)
chronic neutrophilic l.
chronic prolymphocytic l.
compound l.
congenital l.
l. cutis
embryonal l.
eosinophilic l.
eosinophilocytic l.
erythroid l.
erythroleukemia
erythromyeloblastic l.
extramedullary myelogenous l.
feline l.
l. of fowls
granulocytic l.
hairy cell l. (HCL)
histiocytic l.
Ig-mutated chronic lymphocytic l.
Ig-unmutated chronic lymphocytic l.
l. immunophenotyping
l. inhibitory factor (LIF)
juvenile chronic myelogenous l.
   (JCML)
juvenile myelomonocytic l. (JMML)
large granular lymphocyte l.
leukemic l.
leukopenic l.
lymphatic l.
lymphoblastic l.
lymphocytic l. (LCL)
lymphoid l.
lymphosarcoma cell l.
mast cell l.
mature cell l.
megakaryocytic l.

L

NOTES

leukemia *(continued)*
    meningeal l.
    micromyeloblastic l.
    mixed cell l.
    mixed lineage l. (MLL)
    monoblastic l.
    monocytic l.
    monomyelocytic l.
    murine l.
    myeloblastic l.
    myelocytic l.
    myelogenic l.
    myelogenous l.
    myeloid l.
    myelomonocytic l.
    Nägeli type of monocytic l.
    natural killer cell l.
    neutrophilic l.
    nonlymphocytic l.
    null cell lymphoblastic l.
    Philadelphia chromosome-positive chronic myelogenous l. (Ph1$^+$ CML)
    plasma cell l.
    plasmacytic l.
    polymorphocytic l.
    progranulocytic l.
    prolymphocytic l. (PLL)
    promyelocytic l.
    putative l.
    Rai classification of chronic lymphocytic l.
    Rieder cell l.
    Schilling type of monocytic l.
    smoldering l.
    splenic l.
    stem cell l.
    subacute myelomonocytic l.
    subleukemic granulocytic l.
    subleukemic lymphocytic l.
    subleukemic monocytic l.
    T-cell acute lymphoblastic l. (T-ALL)
    T-cell chronic lymphocytic l.
    T-cell prolymphocytic l. (T-PLL)
    thrombocytic l.
    thymic l.
    thymus l. (TL)
leukemia-associated inhibitory activity (LIA)
leukemia/lymphoma
    adult T-cell l. (ATLL)
leukemic
    l. erythrocytosis
    l. leukemia
    l. meningitis
    l. myelosis
    l. phase of lymphoma

    l. reticuloendotheliosis
    l. reticulosis
leukemid
leukemogenesis
leukemogenic
leukemoid reaction
leukin
leukoagglutination
    EDTA-associated l.
leukoagglutinin test
leukobilin
leukoblast
    granular l.
leukoblastosis
leukochloroma
leukocidin
leukocoria
leukocytactic
leukocytal
leukocytaxia
leukocyte
    acidophilic l.
    l. acid phosphatase stain
    l. adherence assay test
    l. adhesion deficiency (LAD)
    l. adhesion molecule
    l. agglutinin
    agranular l.
    l. alkaline phosphatase (LAP)
    l. alkaline phosphatase method
    l. alkaline phosphatase score
    l. alloantibodies
    l. alloimmunization
    l. ascorbic acid (LAA)
    l. bactericidal assay test
    basophilic l. (baso)
    l. common antigen (LCA)
    l. count
    l. cream
    cystinotic l.
    l. cytochemistry
    l. differential count
    endothelial l.
    eosinophilic l. (eos)
    l. esterase
    l. esterase test (LET)
    fecal l.
    l. in feces
    filament polymorphonuclear l.
    globular l.
    granular l.
    heterophilic l.
    l. histamine release test
    hyaline l.
    l. inclusion
    l. inhibitory factor
    l. interferon
    lymphoid l.
    mast l.

mononuclear l. (mono)
motile l.
multinuclear l.
neutrophilic l.
nonfilament polymorphonuclear l.
nongranular l.
nonmotile l.
oxyphilic l.
polymorphonuclear l. (poly)
polynuclear l.
l. recruitment
segmented l. (segs)
stool l.
l. transfusion
transitional l.
l. transmigration
Türk irritation l.
vaginal l.

leukocyte-poor packed red blood cells
leukocyte-reduced
    l.-r. platelets
    l.-r. red blood cells
leukocythemia
leukocytic
    l. crystal
    l. hypersegmentation
    l. infiltrate
    l. margination
    l. marrow
    l. maturation alteration
    l. nuclear hyposegmentation
    l. sarcoma
leukocytoblast
leukocytoclasia
leukocytoclasis
leukocytoclastic
    l. angiitis
    l. vasculitis
leukocytogenesis
leukocytoid habit
leukocytolysin
leukocytolysis
leukocytolytic
leukocytoma
leukocytometer
leukocytopenia
leukocytoplania
leukocytopoiesis
leukocytosis
    absolute l.
    agonal l.
    basophilic l.

digestive l.
distribution l.
emotional l.
eosinophilic l.
lymphocytic l.
monocytic l.
neutrophilic l.
l. of the newborn
pathologic l.
physiologic l.
pure l.
relative l.
terminal l.

leukocytosis-promoting factor (LPF)
leukocytotactic
leukocytotaxia
leukocytotoxin
Leukocytozoon
leukocytozoonosis
leukocyturia
leukoderma
    acquired l.
    l. acquisitum centrifugum
leukodystrophy
    Alexander l.
    globoid cell l.
    Krabbe l.
    metachromatic l. (MLD)
    metachromatic-type l.
    spongy degenerative-type l.
    sudanophilic l.
leukoencephalitis
    acute epidemic l.
    acute hemorrhagic l. (AHLE)
    subacute sclerosing l.
leukoencephalopathy
    cerebral autosomal dominant
      arteriopathy with subcortical
      infarcts and l. (CADASIL)
    megaloencephalic l.
    multifocal progressive l.
    progressive multifocal l. (PML)
    subcortical arteriosclerotic l.
leukoerythroblastic
    l. anemia
    l. reaction
leukoerythroblastosis
leukogram
leukokeratosis
leukokinetic
leukokinetics
leukokinin

NOTES

L

leukokraurosis
leukolymphosarcoma
leukolysin
leukolysis
leukolytic
leukoma
leukomyelopathy
leukon
leukonecrosis
leukonychia
leukoparakeratosis
leukopathia
    acquired l.
leukopathy
leukopedesis
leukopenia
    autoimmune l.
    basophilic l.
    eosinophilic l.
    lymphocytic l.
    monocytic l.
    neutrophilic l.
leukopenic
    l. factor
    l. index
    l. leukemia
    l. myelosis
leukophagocytosis
leukophlegmasia dolens
leukophoresis
leukoplakia
    oral hairy l. (OHL)
    proliferative verrucous l. (PVL)
    l. vulva
leukoplakic vulvitis
leukopoiesis
leukopoietic
leukopoietin
leukoreduction
    poststorage l.
    prestorage l.
    universal l.
leukorrhea
leukosarcoma
leukosarcomatosis
leukosis
    avian l.
    enzootic bovine l.
    fowl l.
Leukosporidium
leukostasis
Leukostat stain
leukotactic assay
leukotaxia
leukotaxine
leukotaxis
leukotic
leukotome
leukotoxin

leukotriene A, B, C, D
leukotriene-dependent erythroid
   differentiation
Leukovirus
LeuM1
    LeuM1 antibody
    LeuM1 antigen
    LeuM1 immunoperoxidase stain
LeuM3 antibody
LeuM5 antibody
Leung stain
Levaditi
    L. method
    L. stain
levan
Levay antigen
Lev disease
level
    l. of agreement
    antibiotic l.
    barbiturate l.
    biosafety l. (BSL)
    biosafety l. 1 (BSL1)
    biosafety l. 2 (BSL2)
    biosafety l. 3 (BSL3)
    biosafety l. 4 (BSL4)
    blood calcium l.
    blood cholesterol l.
    ceruloplasmin l.
    cidal l.
    Clark l.
    confidence l.
    critical staining l.
    DNA adduct l.
    elevate blood calcium l.
    ethanol l.
    high l.
    isoelectric l.
    lead l.
    low l.
    minimal bactercidal l. (MBL)
    panic l.
    peak-and-trough l.
    plasma-acetaminophen l.
    salicylate l.
    serum drug l.
    signal l.
    significance l.
    sweat chloride l.
    therapeutic drug l.
    whole-blood mercury l.
Levey-Jennings chart
Lévi disease
Levine
    L. alkaline Congo red stain
    L. EMB agar
Levinea
    L. amalonatica

L. diversus
L. malonatica
Levine-Rosai tumor classification
Levinson test
Levinstein (*var. of* Löwenstein)
Levinthal-Coles-Lillie (LCL)
Leviviridae
Levivirus
levocardia
isolated l.
levodopa
levorotatory (*l-*)
levothyroxine (T4)
levulosemia
levulose tolerance test
levulosuria
Lévy-Roussy syndrome
Lewandowski
nevus elasticus of L.
Lewandowski-Lutz disease
Lewia infectoria
Lewinstein (*var. of* Löwenstein)
Lewis
L. acid
L. antibody
L. antigen
L. base
L. blood group
L. lung tumor
L. phenomenon
lewisi
Trypanosoma l.
lewisite (L)
NATO code for l. (L)
lewisite 1 (L1)
lewisite 2 (L2)
lewisite 3 (L3)
Lewis-X blood group antigen
Lewy body
lexingtonensis
Amycolatopsis l.
Leyden
L. crystal
L. disease
Leyden-Möbius syndrome
Leydig
L. cell adenoma
L. cell hyperplasia
L. cell tumor
interstitial cell of L.
L. interstitial cell
Leydig-Sertoli cell tumor

LF
lethal factor
limit of flocculation
LF protein
Lf
limes flocculation
Lf dose
L-form
LFT
latex flocculation test
liver function tests
localized fibrous tumor
L-fucose
LGB
Landry-Guillain-Barré
LGD
low-grade dysplasia
LGESS
low-grade endometrial stromal sarcoma
LGL
large granular lymphocyte
L-glyceric aciduria
LGSIL
low-grade squamous intraepithelial lesion
LGV
lymphogranuloma venereum
LGV-TRIC
lymphogranuloma venereum-trachoma
inclusion conjunctivitis
L-H
lymphocytic-histiocytic
L-H cell
LH
luteinizing hormone
LH 755 hematology Workcell
LH 500, 750, 1500 series
hematology analyzer
Lhermitte-McAlpine syndrome
L-histidine ammonia-lyase
LHM
lymphohistiocytoid mesothelioma
LHMT
low-range heparin management
LHMT test
LHON
Leber hereditary optic neuropathy
LHPC
lipomatous hemangiopericytoma
LH-RF
luteinizing hormone-releasing factor
LH-RH
luteinizing hormone-releasing hormone

L

NOTES

583

L-hydroxyacyl coenzyme A
LIA
    leukemia-associated inhibitory activity
Liacopoulos phenomenon
libanotica
    Actinocorallia l.
LIBC
    latent iron-binding capacity
liberae
liberator
    histamine l.
    L. universal locking stylet
Libertella
Libman-Sacks
    L.-S. disease
    L.-S. endocarditis
    L.-S. syndrome
library
    cDNA l.
    gene l.
LIBS
    ligand-induced binding site
LIC
    limiting isorrheic concentration
lice (*pl. of* louse)
lichen
    l. amyloidosis
    l. annularis
    atrophic l. planus
    l. aureus
    l. myxedematosus
    l. nitidus
    l. planopilaris
    l. planus
    l. sclerosus et atrophicus
    l. sclerosus of vulva
    l. scrofulosorum
    l. simplex chronicus
    l. striatus
lichenification
licheniformis
    Bacillus l.
lichenization
lichenoid
    l. eczema
    l. interface dermatitis
    l. keratosis
lichenoides
    parapsoriasis l.
Lichtheim
    L. disease
    L. syndrome
LID
    low-iron diamine
Liddle syndrome
lidocaine
    l. assay
    l. hydrochloride
L-iduronidase

Lieberkühn
    crypts of L.
    L. follicles
    L. glands
Liebermann-Burchard
    L.-B. reaction
    L.-B. test
Liebermeister
    L. furrow
    L. groove
lien
    l. accessorius
    l. mobilis
    l. succentorius
lienales
    folliculi lymphatici l.
lienalis
    Onchocerca l.
    peliosis l.
lienis
    hilum l.
    porta l.
    pulpa l.
    sinus l.
    tunica fibrosa l.
    tunica propria l.
lienomedullary
lienomyelogenous
Liesegang
    L. phenomenon
    L. ring
LIF
    leukemia inhibitory factor
life, pl. **lives**
    average l.
    fetal l.
    mean effective l.
    quality of l.
    l. table
    technologic l.
    L. Technologies TRIzol reagent
    useful l.
Li-Fraumeni cancer syndrome
ligament
    Arantius l.
    gingivodental l.
    hammock l.
    Hueck l.
    peridental l.
ligamentum, pl. **ligamenta**
    l. anulare bulbi
    l. pectinatum
    l. pectinatum anguli
    l. pectinatum iridis
    l. spirale cochleae
ligand
    addressing l.
    l. assay
    Fas l.

l. immunoassay
receptor activator of nuclear factor kappa B l. (RANKL)
ligand-activated transcription factor
ligand-conjugate
l.-c. label
l.-c. labeling
ligand-dependent dimerization
ligand-gated channel
ligandin
ligand-induced binding site (LIBS)
ligase
l. chain reaction (LCR)
DNA l.
polynucleotide l.
ubiquitin l.
ligation-dependent amplification
light (L)
l. band
black l.
l. cell of thyroid
l. chain
l. chain class-restricted B cell
l. chain deposition disease
l. chain Fanconi syndrome
l. green SF yellowish
incident l.
l. micrograph
l. microscope
l. microscopy (LM)
l. pipe
polarized l.
l. reaction (LR)
stray l.
strobe l.
ultraviolet l.
visible l.
l. water
Wood l.
LightCycler system
lighter layer of fibrin
light-scattering immunoassay
light-staining
l.-s. apical cytoplasm
l.-s. granule
Lightwood syndrome
Lignac
L. disease
L. syndrome
Lignac-Fanconi syndrome

ligneous
l. struma
l. thyroiditis
lignicola
Hyalodendron l.
lignieresii
Actinobacillus l.
lignoceric acid
ligroin
Ligula intestinalis
"λ-like viruses"
lilacinus
Paecilomyces l.
Lillie
L. allochrome connective tissue stain
L. allochrome method
L. azure-eosin stain
L. ferrous iron stain
L. hematoxylin
L. sulfuric acid Nile blue stain
limb-girdle muscular dystrophy
limbic encephalitis
limb lipodystrophy
limbus
l. corneae
l. penicillatus
l. striatus
limen, pl. **limina**
difference l. (DL)
limes
l. flocculation (Lf)
l. reacting (Lr)
l. zero (L_0, Lo)
limicola
Flavobacterium l.
Propionivibrio l.
limimaris
Desulfomonile l.
limina (*pl. of* limen)
limit
assimilation l.
l. check
critical l.
l. dextrin
l. dextrinosis
explosive l.
l. of flocculation (LF)
gas storage l.
Hayflick l.
permissible exposure l. (PEL)
quantum l.

L

NOTES

limit *(continued)*
    l. of resolution
    saturation l.
    storage l.
    tolerance l.
    within normal l.'s (WNL)
limitans
    membrana l.
limitation
    container size l.
limited scleroderma
limiting
    l. isorrheic concentration (LIC)
    l. layer of cornea
    l. membrane of retina
    l. reactant
limnaea
    Gillisia l.
limnaeum
    Chlorobaculum l.
limnaeus
    Thialkalicoccus l.
Limnatis nilotica
limnemia
limnemic
limneticum
    Ferribacterium l.
Limnobacter thiooxidans
limnology
Limnoperdon
limnophilus
    Brevibacillus l.
limosa
    Kineosphaera l.
limosum
    Eubacterium l.
limosus
    Inquilinus l.
limulus
    l. amebocyte lysate assay
    L. amoebocyte lysate (LAL)
    l. lysate test
    L. polyphemus
LIN
    laryngeal intraepithelial neoplasia
lincomycin
Linda
    Mycobacterium paratuberculosis L.
lindane
lindaniclasticus
    Rhodanobacter l.
Lindau
    L. disease
    L. tumor
Lindau-von Hippel disease
lindemanni
    Sarcocystis l.
Lindner body

lindoensis
    Echinostoma l.
line
    accretion l.
    Amici l.
    Baillarger l.
    Beau l.
    BeWo choriocarcinoma cell l.
    Blaschko l.
    cell l.
    cement l.
    cleavage l.
    D l.
    delay l.
    l. of demarcation
    dentate l.
    Eberth l.
    emission l.
    equipotential l.
    l. filter
    germ l.
    glioblastoma cell l.
    grid l.
    Gubler l.
    Haller l.
    Head l.
    Hensen l.
    Hunter-Schreger l.
    incremental l.
    Ishikawa cell l.
    Kaes l.
    Kerley A, B l.'s
    Langer l.
    LoVo human colorectal cancer cell l.
    M l.
    Muehrcke l.
    l. number
    Ohngren l.
    Owen l.
    Paris l.
    pectinate l.
    Raji cell l.
    Reid base l. (RBL)
    resonance l.
    Retzius l.
    l. of Retzius
    Schreger l.
    l. spectrum
    tender l.
    l. test
    Ullmann l.
    Wegner l.
    WiDr human colorectal cancer cell l.
    Z l.
    Zahn l.
    l.'s of Zahn
linea, pl. **lineae**

lineae albicantes
lineae atrophicae
l. pectinata canalis analis
l. splendens
lineage
l. infidelity
l. marker
ulcer associated cell l. (UACL)
linear
l. acceleration
l. amplifier
l. attenuation coefficient
l. deposition
l. discriminant algorithm
l. energy transfer (LET)
l. fracture
l. IgA bullous disease in children
l. regression
l. sebaceous nevus syndrome
l. ulcer
linearis
morphea l.
linearity
l. check
photometric l.
linens
Staphylococcus equorum subsp.
linens
line-spread function
Lineweaver-Burk equation
Lingelsheimia anitrata
lingua, pl. **linguae**
anthracosis linguae
folia linguae
frenulum linguae
tunica mucosa linguae
lingual
l. crypt
l. follicle
l. goiter
l. mandibular salivary gland defect
l. papilla
l. tonsil
linguales
folliculi l.
lingualis
papilla l.
tonsilla l.
Linguatula
L. rhinaria
L. serrata
linguatuliasis

Linguatulidae
linguloides
Diphyllobothrium l.
lini
Pseudomonas l.
lining cell
linin network
linitis plastica
linkage
l. analysis
chromosomal l.
l. disequilibrium
l. group
l. map
phosphatidylinositol glycan l. (PIG)
linnaean system of nomenclature
Linognathus
linoleate
linoleic acid
linolenic acid
linolic acid
Linstowiidae
liotrix
LIP
lymphocytic interstitial pneumonia
lymphocytic interstitial pneumonitis
lymphoid interstitial pneumonia
lip
cleft l.
pseudocolloid of l.'s
rhombic l.
liparocele
lipase
l. assay
clearing factor l.
lipoprotein l. (LPL)
pancreatic l.
l. 105 stain
l. test
triacylglycerol l.
lipedema
lipemia, lipohemia, lipoidemia
absorptive l.
alimentary l.
diabetic l.
postprandial l.
l. retinalis
lipemic
lipid
l. A
accumulation of complex l.'s
anisotropic l.

L

NOTES

lipid *(continued)*
    l. assay
    Ciaccio-positive l.
    l. degeneration
    l. depletion
    l. embolism
    extracellular aggregate alteration l.
    fecal l.'s
    l. histiocytosis
    l. metabolism
    l. nephrosis
    Niemann-Pick l.
    nuclear aggregate l.
    l. peroxidation
    l. peroxidation of intracellular
      membrane
    l. pigment
    l. pneumonia
    l. profile
    l. proteinosis
    l. stain
    stool l.'s
    l. storage disease
    l. synthesis
    l. test
    l. transport disorder
    l. vesicle-encapsulated hemoglobin
lipidemia
lipidized glioma
lipid-linked glycoconjugate
lipidosis, pl. **lipidoses**
    cerebroside l.
    glycolipid l.
    sphingomyelin l.
    stellate-cell l.
    sulfatide l.
lipid-rich neoplastic cell
lipiduria
Lipi+Plus
    L. direct HDL assay
    L. direct LDL assay
lipoarthritis
lipoatrophia
    l. annularis
    l. circumscripta
lipoatrophic diabetes
lipoatrophy
    insulin l.
    partial l.
lipoblastic lipoma
lipoblastoma
lipoblastomatosis
lipocalidus
    Syntrophothermus l.
lipocalin
    human neutrophil l. (HNL)
lipocele
lipochitooligosaccharide
lipochondral degeneration (LCD)

lipochondrodystrophy
lipochoristoma
lipochrome
    l. pigment
    l. pigmentation
LipoClear
    L. Plus lipemia clearing reagent
    L. reagent tube
lipocortin enzyme
lipocrit
lipocyte
lipodystrophia
    l. intestinalis
    l. progessiva superior
lipodystrophy
    congenital total l.
    inferior l.
    insulin l.
    intestinal l.
    limb l.
    mesenteric l.
    progressive l.
lipoedema
lipofibroma
lipofuscin
    l. accumulation
    ceroid l.
    l. granule
    l. pigment
lipofuscinosis
lipogenesis
lipogenic
lipogranuloma
lipogranulomatosis
    disseminated l.
    Farber l.
lipohemia *(var. of* lipemia*)*
lipoic acid
lipoid
    l. degeneration
    l. dermatoarthritis
    l. dystrophy
    Forssman l.
    l. granuloma
    l. nephrosis (LN)
    l. pneumonia
    l. proteinosis
    l. thesaurismosis
lipoidemia *(var. of* lipemia*)*
lipoidica
    necrobiosis l.
lipoidosis
lipolysis regulation
lipolysosome
lipolytic
    l. enzyme
    l. hormone
lipolytica
    Aequorivita l.

lipoma
l. annulare colli
l. arborescens
atypical l.
l. capsulare
l. cavernosum
chondroid l.
fetal fat cell l.
l. fibrosum
fibrous spindle cell l.
infiltrating l.
lipoblastic l.
l. myxomatodes
l. ossificans
l. petrificans
pleomorphic l.
l. sarcomatodes
l. sarcomatosum
soft tissue l.
spindle cell l.
telangiectatic l.
lipomatodes
nevus l.
lipomatoid
lipomatosa
macrodystrophia l.
lipomatosis, pl. **lipomatoses**
encephalocraniocutaneous l.
mediastinal l.
multiple symmetric l.
l. of nerve
l. neurotica
lipomatosum
myxoma l.
lipomatosus
nevus l.
lipomatous
l. hemangiopericytoma (LHPC)
l. hypertrophy
l. infiltration
l. myxoma
l. polyp
lipomelanic reticulosis
lipomelanin
lipomelanotic
l. reticuloendothelial cell hyperplasia
l. reticulosis
lipomeningocele
lipomucopolysaccharidosis
Lipomyces
lipomyelomeningocele

Liponyssoides
Liponyssus
lipopeliosis
lipopenia
lipopenic
lipophage
lipophagia granulomatosis
lipophagic
l. granuloma
l. intestinal granulomatosis
lipophagy
lipophanerosis
lipophilic
lipophilum
Mycoplasma l.
lipophyllodes tumor
lipopolysaccharide (LPS, OXK)
l. extract
OX2 l.
OX19 l.
Lipoprint
L. cholesterol subfraction test system
L. LDL subfraction test
lipoprotein (LP)
l. a (LpA)
acetylated low-density l. (AcLDL)
alpha l.
l. assay
beta l.
l. chylomicron
l. electrophoresis (LPE)
l. electrophoresis test
high-density l. (HDL)
intermediate-density l. (IDL)
l. lipase (LPL)
l. lipase deficiency
low-density l. (LDL)
oxidized low density l. (oxLDL)
l. phenotyping
l. polymorphism
pre-beta-l.
very-high-density l. (VHDL)
very-low-density l. (VLDL)
l. X (LpX)
lipoprotein-associated phospholipase A2
lipoprotein-cholesterol
l.-c. fractionation
high-density l.-c. (HDL-C)
low-density l.-c. (LDL-C)
lipoproteinemia

NOTES

liposarcoma
    dedifferentiated l.
    myxoid l.
liposis
liposome
Lipotena cervi
Lipothrixvirus
lipotrophic
lipotropic
lipotropin (LPH)
lipotropy
lipovaccine
lipoxenous
lipoxeny
lipoxin
lipoxygenase-induced apoptosis
lipoxygenase pathway
lipping
Lipschütz
    L. body
    L. cell
    L. disease
    L. ulcer
lipuria
lipuric
liquefaciens
    Aerobacter l.
    Aeromonas l.
    Enterobacter l.
    Moraxella l.
    Serratia l.
liquefacient
liquefaction
    l. degeneration
    l. necrosis
liquefactive
    l. degeneration
    l. necrosis
liquefy
Liquichek
    L. hematology-16 control
    L. hematology control (A)
    L. hematology control (C)
    L. immunology control
    L. qualitative urine toxicology
      control
    L. reticulocyte control and stain
    L. sedimentation rate control
    L. ToRCH Plus control
    L. urine toxicology control C2,
      C3, S1, S2 low opiate
liquid
    Altmann l.
    l. chromatography
    combustible l.
    Cotunnius l.
    l. crystal
    high-performance l.
    l. human serum

    l. junction potential
    l. scintillation counter
    l. scintillation counting
    l. scintillator
    l. (solution) hybridization
liquidation
    enzymatic l.
liquid-in-glass thermometer
liquid-liquid
    l.-l. chromatography
    l.-l. junction potential
liquid-phase
    l.-p. hybridization
    l.-p. hybridization protection assay
liquid-solid chromatography
liquiform
liquor
    l. cerebrospinalis
    l. cotunnii
    meconium-stained l.
    Morgagni l.
    l. puris
Lisch nodule
Lison-Dunn
    L.-D. method
    L.-D. stain
lissamine rhodamine B 200
Lissauer paralysis
lissencephalia, lissencephaly
lissencephalic
list
    l. mode
    l. structure
Listerella parodoxa
Listeria
    L. denitrificans
    L. grayi
    L. monocytogenes
listeriosis, listerosis
liter (L)
    milligram per l. (mg/L)
    millimole per l. (mmol/L)
    l. per minute (Lpm)
literal
lithiasis
    l. conjunctivae
    pancreatic l.
lithic acid
lithium
    l. assay
    l. carbonate
    l. carmine
    l. tungstate
lithium-drifted detector
Lithobius
lithocholate
lithocholic acid
lithogenesis
lithogenic

lithogenous
lithogeny
lithoid
lithonephritis
lithopedion
lithotripsy
lithotroph
lithotrophica
    Nautilia l.
lithotrophicum
    Balnearium l.
    Sulfurovum l.
lithuresis
lithureteria
lithuria
litmus
    l. paper
    l. whey
litoralis
    Bacteriovorax l.
    Oceanisphaera l.
    Thiocapsa l.
    Ulvibacter l.
litorea
    Alteromonas l.
Little disease
littoral
    l. cell
    l. cell angioma
Littre gland
littritis
livedo
    lupus l.
    postmortem l.
    l. racemosa
    l. reticularis
    l. reticularis idiopathica
    l. reticularis symptomatica
    l. telangiectatica
    l. vasculitis
livedoid
live oral poliovirus vaccine
liver
    l. abscess
    l. acinus
    acute yellow atrophy of l.
    amebic abscess of l.
    l. battery
    l. cancer
    capsular cirrhosis of l.
    cardiac fibrosis of the l.
    l. cell adenoma

    l. cell carcinoma
    l. cell necrosis
    centrilobular necrosis of the l.
    cyanotic atrophy of l.
    l. cyst
    l. failure
    fatty l.
    l. flocculation test
    l. fluke
    frosted l.
    l. function
    l. function tests (LFT)
    l. grooves
    hobnail l.
    hydroxylation l.
    icing l.
    lardaceous l.
    nodular transformation of the l.
    nutmeg l.
    l. palm
    polycystic l.
    portal lobule of l.
    l. profile
    l. rot
    septal fibrosis of l.
    stellate cell of l.
    sugar-icing l.
    venoocclusive disease of the l.
    wandering l.
    waxy l.
    yellow atrophy of l.
liver-derived sex steroid-binding globulin
liver-pancreas (LP)
lives (*pl. of* life)
lividity
    postmortem l.
living donor (LD)
livingstonensis
    Shewanella l.
livor mortis
lixiviation
LJM
    Lowenstein-Jensen medium
Ljubljana classification
LKM
    liver kidney microsomal
    LKM antibody
LLF
    Laki-Lorand factor
L-L factor
LLL
    localized leishmania lymphadenitis

L

NOTES

LLM
localized leukocyte mobilization
Lloyd reagent
L-lysine:NAD⁺ oxidoreductase
LM
light microscopy
LMC
lymphocyte-mediated cytotoxicity
LMC assay
LMD
low molecular weight dextran
LMP
latent membrane protein
low malignant potential
LMP-1
latent membrane protein 1
LMS
leiomyosarcoma
LMW
low molecular weight
LMWD
low molecular weight dextran
LN
lipoid nephrosis
lupus nephritis
lymph node
LN1 antibody
LN2 antibody
LN3 monoclonal antibody
LNB
large-needle aspiration biopsy
LNC
large noncleaved
LNGFR
low-affinity nerve growth factor receptor
LN-met
lymph node metastasis
LNPF
lymph node permeability factor
Lo (*var. of* L₀)
loa
Filaria l.
load
l. factor
magnum l.
viral l.
loading
l. buffer
l. dose
impact l.
impulsive l.
salt l.
lobar
l. cerebral atrophy
l. pneumonia
l. pulmonary atrophy
l. sclerosis
lobatum
hepar l.

lobe
l. of mammary gland
succenturiate l.
lobectomy
sleeve l.
lobi (*pl. of* lobus)
lobitis
Loboa loboi
Lobo disease
loboi
Lacazia l.
Loboa l.
Trichosporon l.
Lobomyces
lobomycosis
lobopodium
Lobstein
L. disease
L. ganglion
L. syndrome
lobster-claw deformity
lobular
l. adenocarcinoma
l. cancerization
l. carcinoma
l. carcinoma in situ (LCIS)
l. disarray
l. epithelial hyperplasia
l. glomerulonephritis
l. neoplasia
l. panniculitis
l. pattern
l. phenotype
l. pneumonia
l. proliferation
l. proliferative lesion
lobulation
fetal l.
lobule
classic liver l.
convoluted part of kidney l.
ear l.
l. of epididymis
hepatic l.
l. of mammary gland
peripheral l.
primary pulmonary l.
renal cortical l.
respiratory l.
secondary pulmonary l.
l. of testis
l. of thymus
thyroid l.
l. of thyroid gland
lobulet
lobuli (*pl. of* lobulus)
lobulitis
lymphocytic l.
lobulocentricity

lobulocentric pattern
lobulus, pl. **lobuli**
    l. corticalis renalis
    lobuli epididymidis
    lobuli glandulae mammariae
    lobuli glandulae thyroideae
    l. hepatis
    lobuli testis
    lobuli thymi
lobus, pl. **lobi**
    l. anterior hypophyseos
    lobi glandulae mammariae
    l. glandularis hypophyseos
    l. nervosus
    l. posterior hypophyseos
local
    l. anaphylaxis
    l. anemia
    l. cementosseous dysphasia
    (LOCD)
    l. death
    l. deposition of hemosiderin
    l. exhaust ventilation
    l. glomerulonephritis
    l. immunity
    l. lesion
    l. reaction
    l. recurrence
    l. replication
    l. skin memory
localization
    eye tumor l.
    immunocytochemical l.
    l. needle
    l. suture
localized
    l. arteriolar dilation
    l. black eschar
    l. fibroma
    l. histiocytosis
    l. inflammation
    l. leishmania lymphadenitis (LLL)
    l. leukocyte mobilization (LLM)
    l. mucinosis
    l. nodular tenosynovitis
    l. osteitis fibrosa
    l. peritonitis
    l. plaque formation (LPF)
    l. Schwartzman reaction
    l. scleroderma
locant

location
    storage l.
LOCD
    local cementosseous dysphasia
loci (*pl. of* locus)
locisalis
    Halobacillus l.
Locke-Ringer solution
Locke solution
lock-in amplifier
lockout
    criticality l.
locomotive cell
locoregional
loculated
    l. architecture
    l. empyema
loculation
loculus, pl. **loculi**
locus, pl. **loci**
    l. ceruleus
    cis-acting l.
    four l.
    histocompatibility l. (HL)
    major histocompatibility l.
    microsatellite l.
    l. niger
LOD
    logarithm of odds
    LOD score
Lodderomyces elongisporus
Loeb deciduoma
Loeffler (*var. of* Löffler)
loessense
    Rhizobium l.
Loevit cell
Loewenthal reaction
Löffler, Loeffler
    L. blood culture medium
    L. blood serum
    L. caustic stain
    L. coagulated serum medium
    L. disease
    L. endocarditis
    L. methylene blue
    L. myocarditis
    L. serum agar
    L. syndrome I, II
logarithm
    common l.
    napierian l.
    l. of odds (LOD)

L

NOTES

logarithmic
    l. amplifier
    l. curve
    l. phase
log dilution
logic
logical record
logit transformation
lognormal distribution
LOH
    loss of heterozygosity
    LOH assay
Lohlein-Baehr lesion
loiasis
loihiensis
    Idiomarina l.
Loktanella
    L. fryxellensis
    L. salsilacus
    L. vestfoldensis
Lomentospora
London force
long
    l. arm of chromosome
    L. coefficient
    L. formula
    l. incubation hepatitis
    l. terminal repeat sequence (LTR)
    l. tract
    l. tract sign
long-acting thyroid stimulator (LATS)
longbeachae
    Legionella l.
long-chain
    l.-c. fatty acid (LCFA)
    l.-c. polyunsaturated fatty acid (LCPUFA)
    l.-c. triglyceride (LCT)
longicatena
    Actinocorallia l.
    Dorea l.
longifusum
    Trichophyton l.
longior
    Tyroglyphus l.
longipalpis
    Lutzomyia l.
    Phlebotomus l.
longirostratum
    Exserohilum l.
longispicularis
    Trichostrongylus l.
longispiculata
    Nematodirella l.
Longispora albida
longissimespiculata
    Nematodirella l.
longitudinal
    l. fold

    l. layer
    l. layer of muscular tunic
    l. section
long-range wound
long-segment Hirschsprung disease
long-spacing
    segment l.-s. (SLS)
long-term
    l.-t. potentiation (LTP)
    l.-t. treatment with aspirin
longus
    Erythrobacter l.
lookback process
loop
    capillary l.
    l. diuretic
    l. electrosurgical excisional procedure
    feedback l.
    feed forward l.
    flow volume l.
    gamma l.
    Granit l.
    hairpin l.
    l. of Henle
    hysteresis l.
    inoculating l.
    nephronic l.
looped fluid
looping
    hot l.
loop-o-gram
loose
    l. contact wound
    l. irregular connective tissue
    l. skin
Looser-Milkman syndrome
Lophodermium
Lophophora
lophotrichous
Lorain
    L. disease
    L. dwarfism
Lorain-Lévi syndrome
lordoscoliosis
lordosis
lordotic
    l. albuminuria
    l. pelvis
lorgnette
    main en l.
loricrin
Losch nodule
loss
    allele-specific l.
    allelic l.
    blood l. (BL)
    body fluid l.
    conductive hearing l.

eddy-current l.
estimated blood l. (EBL)
l. of expression and prognosis
fractional allelic l.
l. of heterozygosity (LOH)
insensible water l.
occult blood l.
recurrent fetal l. (RFL)
third-space fluid l.
transepidermal water l. (TWL)

Lou Gehrig disease

Louis-Bar syndrome

Louisiana pneumonia

louping
l. ill
l. ill virus

louse, pl. **lice**
body l.
chicken l.
crab l.
dog l.
head l.
pubic l.
sucking l.

louse-borne
l.-b. relapsing fever
l.-b. typhus

lousiness

lousy

lova
Dracunculus l.

lovaniensis
Acetobacter l.

LoVo human colorectal cancer cell line

low
l. birth weight (LBW)
l. birth weight infant (LBWI)
l. density lipoprotein receptor
l. egg-passage vaccine
l. explosive
l. grade astrocytoma
l. level
l. magnification
l. malignant potential (LMP)
l. molecular weight (LMW)
l. molecular weight dextran (LMD, LMWD)
l. molecular weight kininogen
l. order
l. protein (LP)
l. serum-bound iron (LBI)

low-actinic glass

low-affinity nerve growth factor receptor (LNGFR)

low-compliance bladder

low-density
l.-d. lipoprotein (LDL)
l.-d. lipoprotein-cholesterol (LDL-C)

Lowe
L. disease
L. syndrome

Löwenberg
L. canal
L. scala

Löwenstein, Levinstein, Lewinstein
L. process

Lowenstein-Jensen
L.-J. agar
L.-J. medium (LJM)
L.-J. plate

Lowenthal test

lower
l. anal canal
l. motor neuron
l. nephron nephrosis
l. respiratory tract smear
l. ring
l. urinary tract infection

Lowe-Terrey-MacLachlan syndrome

low-fiber diet

low-frequency transduction

low-grade
l.-g. angiosarcoma
l.-g. endometrial stromal sarcoma (LGESS)
l.-g. fibromyxoid sarcoma
l.-g. squamous intraepithelial lesion (LGSIL, LSIL)
l.-g. TCC

low-iron diamine (LID)

Lown-Ganong-Levine syndrome

low-pass filter

low-power field (LPF)

low-range heparin management (LHMT)

low-temperature antigen retrieval (LTAR)

low-temperature, heat-mediated antigen retrieval (LTHMAR)

low-voltage
l.-v. fast (LVF)
l.-v. focus (LVF)
l.-v. high-resolution scanning electron microscopy (LV-HRSEM)

low-volume air thermal cycle format

L

NOTES

Loxosceles
    L. laeta
    L. reclusa
Loxotrema ovatum
LP
    latency period
    lipoprotein
    liver-pancreas
    low protein
    lymphocyte predominant
    lymphoid plasma
        LP antigen
L:P
    lactate-pyruvate ratio
LPA
    lysophosphatidic acid
LpA
    lipoprotein a
LPC
    late positive component
LPD
    lymphoproliferative disease
LPE
    lipoprotein electrophoresis
LPF
    leukocytosis-promoting factor
    localized plaque formation
    low-power field
    lymphocytosis-promoting factor
LPH
    lipotropin
L-phase variant
LPHC
    low probability, high consequence event
LPHD
    lymphocyte-predominant Hodgkin
        disease
LPI
    lysinuric protein intolerance
LPI/LRI
    lymphocyte proliferation/regression index
LPL
    lipoprotein lipase
    lymphoplasmacytoid lymphoma
Lpm
    liter per minute
LPS
    large particle sorting module
    lipopolysaccharide
LPT
    lymphocyte-predominant thymoma
LPV
    lymphotropic papovavirus
LpX
    lipoprotein X
LQTS Finnish founder mutation
LR
    laboratory reference
    light reaction

L:R
    left-to-right ratio
Lr
    limes reacting
        Lr dose
LRN
    Laboratory Response Network
        LRN BioWatch laboratory
LRP
    luciferase reporter mycobacteriophage
        LRP assay
LRS
    lactated Ringer solution
LRT
    low-risk tumor
L:S
    lecithin/sphingomyelin ratio
LSA
    lymphosarcoma
        LS 6500 liquid scintillation
            counting system
        LS 100Q/200/230 series laser
            diffraction particle size analyzer
        LS 13 320 series laser diffraction
            particle size analyzer
LSAB
    labeled streptavidin biotin
LSAB2 multistep detection system
L-saccharopine
LSA/RCS
    lymphosarcoma-reticulum cell sarcoma
LSD
    lysergic acid diethylamide
LSG
    labial salivary gland
        LSG biopsy
LSH
    lutein-stimulating hormone
LSIL
    low-grade squamous intraepithelial lesion
LSM
    late systolic murmur
LST
    lysis, storage, and transportation
        LST buffer
L-sulfoiduronate sulfatase
LT
    lymphotoxin
LTA4
    epoxide leukotriene LTA4
LTAR
    low-temperature antigen retrieval
LTB
    laryngotracheobronchitis
LTF
    lost to followup
LTH
    luteotropic hormone

LTHMAR
low-temperature, heat-mediated antigen retrieval
LTP
long-term potentiation
LTR
long terminal repeat sequence
LUA
Legionella urinary antigen
LUA ELISA test kit
Lu antigen
Lubarsch
crystal of L.
L. crystal
LUC
large unstained cell
Lucas-Championnière disease
lucent
lucentense
Haloferax l.
lucentensis
Thalassospira l.
Lucetina
Lucey-Driscoll syndrome
lucida
lamina l.
lucidum
stratum l.
luciferase reporter mycobacteriophage (LRP)
luciferensis
Bacillus l.
Lucilia
L. *caesar*
L. *illustris*
L. *sericata*
Lucio
L. leprosy
L. leprosy phenomenon
Lucké
L. adenocarcinoma
L. carcinoma
L. virus
lückenschädel
Lücke test
ludipueritiae
Teichococcus l.
Ludwig
L. angina
L. labyrinth
Luebering-Rapaport pathway
Luer lock glass syringe

lues
luetic
l. aneurysm
l. aortitis
Luft
L. disease
L. potassium permanganate fixative
Lugol
L. iodine
L. iodine solution
L. stain
Lukes-Butler
L.-B. histologic subclassification
L.-B. Hodgkin disease classification
L.-B. non-Hodgkin lymphoma classification
Lukes-Collins
L.-C. non-Hodgkin lymphoma classification
Luki aspirating tube
lumbago
lumbar
l. appendicitis
l. canal stenosis
l. puncture
l. spondylosis
lumbosacral
l. myelopathy
l. radiculopathy
l. spine ankylosis
lumbrical
lumbricidal
lumbricide
lumbricoid
lumbricoides
Ascaris l.
lumbricosis
lumbricus
lumen, pl. **lumina, lumens**
residual l.
steinstrasse (cobbled street ureteric l.)
lumican
luminal pattern
luminescence
luminescent
luminometer
luminometry
luminophore
luminous
l. flux

L

NOTES

luminous *(continued)*
    l. flux density
    l. intensity
Lumi-Phos solution
lumpy
    l. jaw
    l. skin disease
lumpy-bumpy
    l.-b. deposit
    l.-b. immunofluorescence
Luna-Ishak stain
lunar
lunata
    Curvularia l.
lunate
lung
    l. abscess
    acinic cell tumor of l.
    l. aspiration
    bilobed right l.
    l. biopsy
    bird-breeder's l.
    bird-fancier's l.
    black l.
    blast l.
    brown induration of the l.
    busulfan l.
    butterfly l.
    l. cancer
    l. carcinoid
    l. carcinoma
    cheese worker's l.
    collier's l.
    cystic disease of l.
    diffusing capacity of l.
    eosinophilic l.
    eosinophilic granuloma of l. (EGL)
    l. fluke
    l.'s of gaseous exchange
    giant cell tumor of l.
    hilum of l.
    honeycomb l.
    human embryo l. (HEL)
    humidifier l.
    hyperlucent l.
    malt-worker's l.
    maple bark stripper's l.
    mason's l.
    miner's l.
    mushroom-worker's l.
    pigment induration of the l.
    pizza l.
    rheumatoid l.
    rudimentary l.
    secondary malignant neoplasm, l.
    l. section
    shock l.
    silo-filler's l.
    thresher's l.

    l. tumor
    l. unit
    uremic l.
    welder's l.
    woodworker's l.
lunger disease
lungworm
lunotriquetral
Lunyo virus
lupi
    Spirocerca l.
lupiform
lupinine
lupinosa
    porrigo l.
lupoid
    l. hepatitis
    l. leishmaniasis
    l. ulcer
luposa
    tuberculosis cutis l.
lupous
lupus
    l. anticoagulant (LA)
    l. anticoagulant positive control
    l. band test
    cerebral l.
    chilblain l.
    chronic discoid l.
    chronic discoid l. erythematosus
    discoid l. erythematosus (DLE)
    l. erythematosus (LE)
    l. erythematosus cell
    l. erythematosus disseminatus
      (LED)
    l. erythematosus inhibitor
    l. erythematosus profundus
    hydralazine l.
    l. hypertrophicus
    laryngeal l.
    l. livedo
    l. lymphaticus
    l. mutilans
    neonatal l.
    l. nephritis (LN)
    l. panniculitis
    l. papillomatosus
    l. pernio
    l. pleuritis
    l. psoriasis
    l. sclerosus
    l. sebaceus
    l. serpiginosus
    subacute cutaneous l.
    l. superficialis
    l. tuberculosus
    l. tumidus
    l. verrucosus
    l. vulgaris

lurida
    Amycolatopsis l.
    Amycolatopsis orientalis subsp. *l.*
luridiscabiei
    Streptomyces l.
lusatiensis
    Defluvibacter l.
Luschka
    L. cystic gland
    L. duct
    foramen of L.
    L. tonsil
Luse body
lusitana
    Aquicella l.
lusitaniae
    Clavispora l.
lusitanum
    Herbaspirillum l.
lusoria
    dysphagia l.
lutea
    macula l.
    Pseudomonas l.
luteae
    fovea centralis maculae l.
luteal
    l. cell
    l. cyst
    l. hormone
Luteimonas mephitis
luteinalis
    hyperreactio l. (HL)
lutein cell
luteinization
luteinize
luteinized follicular cyst
luteinizing
    l. hormone (LH)
    l. hormone assay
    l. hormone-releasing factor (LH-RF)
    l. hormone-releasing hormone (LH-RH)
    l. hormone secretion
    l. principle
    l. tumor
luteinoma
lutein-stimulating hormone (LSH)
luteireticuli
    Streptomyces l.
Lutembacher syndrome

Luteococcus
    L. peritonei
    L. sanguinis
luteogenic
luteola
    Auchmeromyia l.
luteolum
    Brevibacterium l.
    Chlorobium l.
luteolus
    Agromyces l.
    Arthrobacter l.
luteolysis
luteolytic
luteoma
    pregnancy l.
    stromal l.
luteotropic hormone (LTH)
luteotropin
Luteovirus
lutetiensis
    Streptococcus l.
lutetium
luteum
    atretic corpus l.
    l. cell
    corpus l.
    cystic corpus l.
    punctum l.
luteus
    Micrococcus l.
Lutheran
    L. blood antibody type
    L. blood group
    L. blood group system
luti
    Psychrobacter l.
    Ruminococcus l.
lututrin
Lutzomyia
    L. flaviscutellata
    L. intermedius
    L. longipalpis
    L. peruensis
Lutz-Splendore-Almeida disease
luxation
Luxol fast blue stain
luxury perfusion
luxus heart
Luys
    L. body syndrome
    L. segregator

L

NOTES

LVE
left ventricular enlargement
LVF
left ventricular failure
low-voltage fast
low-voltage focus
LVH
large vessel hematocrit
left ventricular hypertrophy
LV-HRSEM
low-voltage high-resolution scanning
electron microscopy
LVI
lymphatic vessel invasion
LVSI
lymphovascular space invasion
LW
Lee-White
Lw antigen
lwoffi
Achromobacter l.
Acinetobacter calcoaceticus l.
LX4201 clinical system
LXi 725 clinical system
**LX20, LX200, LX2000 PRO clinical
system**
L-xylulose
L-x. dehydrogenase
L-x. reductase
L-xylulosuria
Ly antigen
lyase
adenylosuccinate l.
argininosuccinate l.
Lyb antigen
lycopenemia
lycoperdonosis
Lycoperdon perlatum
lycophora
lye
Lyell
L. disease
L. syndrome
LYG
lymphomatoid granulomatosis
LYM
lymphoma
Lymantria
Lyme
L. borreliosis
L. disease
L. disease serology
L. neuroborreliosis
Lymnaea
lymph
aplastic l.
blood l.
l. capillary
l. cell

l. cord
l. corpuscle
corpuscular l.
croupous l.
dental l.
l. embolism
euplastic l.
fibrinous l.
l. filtration
l. gland
glycerinated l.
inflammatory l.
intercellular l.
intravascular l.
l. node (LN)
l. node biopsy
l. node cancer
l. node hyperplasia
l. node infarction
l. node involvement
l. node permeability factor (LNPF)
l. node puncture
l. node sectioning
l. nodule
plastic l.
l. scrotum
l. sinus
l. space
tissue l.
vaccine l.
l. varix
lymphaden
lymphadenitis
acute suppurative l.
cytomegalovirus l.
dermatopathic l.
hemorrhagic thoracic l.
herpes simplex l.
histiocytic necrotizing l. (HNL)
Kikuchi l.
Kikuchi-Fujimoto l.
localized leishmania l. (LLL)
mediastinal l.
mesenteric l.
paratuberculous l.
postvaccinial l.
regional granulomatous l.
tuberculosis l.
tuberculous l.
lymphadenoid goiter
lymphadenoma
lymphadenomatosis
lymphadenopathy
angioimmunoblastic l.
dermatopathic l.
immunoblastic l. (IBL)
silicone l.
sinus histiocytosis with massive l.
(SHML)

l. syndrome
syphilitic l.
lymphadenopathy-associated virus (LAV)
lymphadenosis
benign l.
malignant l.
lymphadenovarix
lymphangeitis
lymphangiectasia
lymphangiectasis
cavernous l.
congenital pulmonary l. (CPL)
cystic l.
intestinal l.
simple l.
lymphangiectatic
lymphangiectatica
pachyderma l.
lymphangiectodes
lymphangiitis
lymphangioendothelial sarcoma
lymphangioendothelioma
lymphangiogram
lymphangioleiomyomatosis (LAM)
pulmonary l.
lymphangiology
lymphangioma
l. capillare varicosum
l. cavernosum
l. circumscriptum
l. cysticum
l. superficium simplex
l. tuberosum multiplex
l. xanthelasmoideum
lymphangiomatosis
pulmonary l.
lymphangiomatous
lymphangiomyomatosis (LAM)
lymphangiophlebitis
lymphangiosarcoma
lymphangitis
l. carcinomatosa
epizootic l.
l. epizootica
lymphapheresis
lymphatic
l. angina
l. cancer
l. choriomeningitis (LCM)
l. corpuscle
l. dissemination theory of
endometriosis

l. duct
l. dyscrasia
l. edema
l. endothelial hyaluronan receptor
(LYVE1)
l. filariasis
l. follicle
l. follicle of larynx
l. follicle of rectum
l. leukemia
l. mapping
l. nevus
l. sarcoma
l. sinus
l. stroma
l. tissue
l. tracking
lymphatica
anemia l.
Filaria l.
telangiectasia l.
lymphatici
cortex nodi l.
hilum nodi l.
lymphaticus
folliculus l.
lupus l.
nevus l.
nodulus l.
nodus l.
status l.
varix l.
lymphatitis
lymphatolysis
lymphatolytic
lymphectasia
lymphedema
congenital l.
hereditary l.
l. praecox
primary l.
lymphedematous keratoderma
lymphemia
lymphoadenoma
lymphoblast
lymphoblastic
l. leukemia
l. lymphoma
l. lymphosarcoma
l. plasma cell
lymphoblastoid

L

NOTES

lymphoblastoma
  giant follicular l.
lymphoblastosis
lymphocele
lymphocerastism
Lymphocryptovirus
lymphocutaneous sporotrichosis
lymphocyst
Lymphocystivirus
lymphocytapheresis
lymphocyte
  activated l.
  l. activation
  atypical l.
  B l.
  binucleated l.
  l. blastogenic factor
  bronchial l.
  bronchiolar l.
  circulating atypical l.
  cytologic T l. (CTL)
  Downey-type l.
  l. function associated antigen
  helper T l.
  l. homing receptor
  intraepithelial l.
  killer l.
  large granular l. (LGL)
  majority of peripheral blood l.
  mantle-zone l.
  l. marker assay
  massive infiltrate of l.'s
  l. microcytotoxicity assay
  l. mitogenic factor
  monocytoid l. (ML)
  neoplastic l.
  nodular poorly differentiated l.
    (NPDL)
  null l.
  peripheral blood l. (PBL)
  plasmacytoid l.
  reactive l.'s
  Rieder l.
  small l. (SL)
  splenic lymphoma with villous l.
    (SLVL)
  l. subset
  l. subset enumeration
  l. subset panel
  suppressor T l.
  T l.
  l. transfer test
  l. transformation
  l. transformation immunoassay
  l. transformation test
  transformed l.
  tumor-infiltrating l. (TIL)
  vacuolated l.
  Willemze type A l.

lymphocyte-activating factor
lymphocyte-defined (LD)
lymphocyte-mediated cytotoxicity (LMC)
lymphocyte-predominant Hodgkin disease
  (LPHD)
lymphocyte-stimulating hormone
lymphocyte transformation test
lymphocyte-transforming factor
lymphocythemia
lymphocytic
  l. adenohypophysitis
  l. blood cell
  l. choriomeningitis (LCM)
  l. choriomeningitis virus
  l. colitis (LC)
  l. cuffing
  l. enterocolitis
  l. gastritis
  l. hypophysitis
  l. infiltration
  l. infiltration of skin
  l. inflammatory infiltrate
  l. interstitial pneumonia (LIP)
  l. interstitial pneumonitis (LIP)
  l. leukemia (LCL)
  l. leukemia marker panel
  l. leukemoid reaction
  l. leukocytosis
  l. leukopenia
  l. lobulitis
  l. lymphoma
  l. lymphosarcoma (LCL)
  l. marrow
  l. series
  l. thymoma
  l. thyroiditis
  l. transformation
  l. vasculitis
lymphocytic-histiocytic (L-H)
lymphocytoblast
lymphocytolysis
lymphocytoma
lymphocytopenia
lymphocytopoiesis
lymphocytorrhexis
lymphocytosis
  intraepithelial l.
  neutrophilic l.
  peripheral blood l.
  persistent polyclonal B-cell l.
lymphocytosis-promoting factor (LPF)
lymphocytotoxic antibody
lymphocytotoxicity
lymphocytotoxin
lymphoderma perniciosa
lymphoepithelial lesion (LEL)
lymphoepithelioid cell lymphoma
  (LECL)

lymphoepithelioma
lymphoepithelioma-like carcinoma
 (LELC)
lymphogenesis
lymphogenic
lymphogenous
    l. embolism
    l. metastasis
lymphoglandula
lymphogranuloma
    l. benignum
    l. inguinale
    l. malignum
    Schaumann l.
    venereal l.
    l. venereum (LGV)
    l. venereum antigen
    l. venereum titer
    l. venereum-trachoma inclusion
     conjunctivitis (LGV-TRIC)
    l. venereum virus
lymphogranulomatosis
    Miyagawanella l.
lymphohematopoiesis
lymphohematopoietic
lymphohistiocytic vasculitis
lymphohistiocytoid mesothelioma (LHM)
lymphohistiocytosis
    familial erythrophagocytic l. (FEL)
    familial hemophagocytic l. (FMLH)
    hemophagocytic l. (HLH)
lymphoid
    l. aggregate
    l. aplasia
    l. corpuscle
    l. cuffing
    l. follicle
    l. follicles of the spleen
    l. hemoblast of Pappenheim
    l. hyperplasia
    l. hypophysitis
    l. hypoplasia
    l. interstitial pneumonia (LIP)
    l. leukemia
    l. leukocyte
    l. monoclonal antibody
    l. neoplasm
    l. nodule
    l. organ
    l. plasma (LP)
    l. polyp
    l. progenitor cell

    l. series
    l. stem cell
lymphoidei
    medulla nodi l.
lymphoidocyte
lymphoid-rich effusion
lymphokine
lymphokine-activated killer cell (LAK)
lympholeukocyte
lymphology
lymphoma (LYM)
    acute lymphoblastic leukemia
     secondary to Burkitt l.
    adult T-cell l. (ATL)
    anaplastic large cell l. (ALCL)
    anaplastic large cell malignant l.
    angiocentric T-cell l.
    angioimmunoblastic l. (AIL)
    angioimmunoblastic T-cell l. (AIL)
    angiotrophic l.
    B-cell l. (BCL)
    B-cell chronic lymphocytic
     leukemia/small lymphocytic l.
    B-cell non-Hodgkin l. (B-NHL)
    benign l.
    biphenotypic l.
    blastoid variant of mantel cell l.
     (BMCL)
    blastoma mantel cell l. (BMCL)
    Burkitt l. (BL)
    Burkitt-like l.
    centroblastic l.
    centrocytic l.
    centrocytic/mantle-cell l. (CC/MCL)
    classic Hodgkin l. (CHL)
    composite l.
    cutaneous l.
    cutaneous B-cell l. (CBCL)
    cutaneous T-cell l. (CTCL)
    diffuse histocytic l. (DHL)
    diffuse large B-cell l. (DLBCL)
    diffuse large cell l. (DLCL)
    diffuse poorly differentiated l.
     (DPDL)
    diffuse small cleaved cell l.
    discordant l.
    endemic Burkitt l. (eBL)
    enteropathy-associated T-cell l.
    extranodal marginal zone l.
    floral variant of follicular l. (FFL)
    follicle-cell l.
    follicle center l. (FCL)

NOTES

lymphoma *(continued)*
    follicular l. (FL)
    follicular predominantly large cell l.
    follicular predominantly small cleaved cell l.
    giant follicular l.
    gray zone l.
    high-grade B-cell l.
    histiocyte-rich B-cell l. (HRBCL)
    histiocytic l. (HL)
    Hodgkin l.
    immunoblastic l.
    l. immunophenotyping
    Ki-1+ l.
    large B-cell l. (LBCL)
    large-cell immunoblastic l.
    large-cell non-Hodgkin l. (LCNHL)
    Lennert l.
    leukemic phase of l.
    lymphoblastic l.
    lymphocytic l.
    lymphoepithelioid cell l. (LECL)
    lymphoplasmacytic l.
    lymphoplasmacytoid l. (LPL)
    lymphosarcoma-type malignant l.
    macrofollicular l.
    malignant l. (ML)
    MALT l.
    mantle cell l. (MCL)
    mantle cell lymphocytic l.
    mantle zone l. (MZL)
    marginal zone l.
    marginal zone B-cell l. (MZBCL)
    marginal zone cell l. (MZL)
    Mediterranean l.
    microvillus l.
    mixed large- and small-cell non-Hodgkin l. (MNHL)
    monocytoid B-cell l.
    mucosa-associated lymphoid tissue l. (MALToma)
    nasal angiocentric T-cell l. (NATL)
    nasal T/NK-cell l.
    natural killer cell l.
    NK l.
    nodal marginal zone B-cell l.
    nodular histiocytic l.
    nonepidermotropic primary cutaneous T-cell l.
    non-Hodgkin l. (NHL)
    non-MALT l.
    null cell l.
    null-type non-Hodgkin l.
    parafollicular B-cell l. (PBCL)
    paraimmunoblastic l.
    peripheral T-cell l. (PTCL, PTL)
    plaque-stage cutaneous T-cell l.
    plasmacytoid l.
    polymorphic B-cell l.
    poorly differentiated lymphocytic l. (PDLL)
    postthymic T-cell l. (PTCL)
    prethymic lymphoblastic l.
    primary bone l. (PBL)
    primary central nervous system l. (PCNSL)
    primary cutaneous anaplastic large cell l.
    primary cutaneous CD30+ large T-cell l.
    primary effusion l. (PEL)
    primary gastric l.
    pulmonary MALT l.
    pyothorax-associated l.
    respiratory angiocentric l.
    Revised European-American L. (REAL)
    small cell malignant l. (SCML)
    small lymphocytic l. (SLL)
    small noncleaved cell, non-Burkitt l.
    SNCC l.
    SNCC Burkitt l.
    SNCC non-Burkitt l.
    splenic marginal zone l. (SMZL)
    stem cell l.
    T-cell l.
    T-cell rich B-cell l. (TCRBCL)
    T-natural killer cell l.
    U-cell l.
    undifferentiated l. (UL)
    Waldeyer ring l.
    well-differentiated lymphocytic l. (WDLL)
    Western-type intestinal l.
lymphomagenesis
lymphoma/leukemia
    adult T-cell l. (ATLL)
lymphomatoid
    l. granulomatosis (LYG)
    l. papulosis (LyP)
    l. polyposis
lymphomatosa
    angina l.
    struma l.
lymphomatosis
    avian l.
    fowl l.
    ocular l.
    visceral l.
lymphomatosum
    adenocystoma l.
    cystadenoma l.
    papillary cystadenoma l.
lymphomatous
lymphomyeloma
lymphomyxoma

lymphopathia venereum
lymphopenia
 CD4 l.
 CD4/CD8 count
 CD44v6-specific probe
lymphopenic thymic dysplasia
lymphophagocytosis
lymphophilum
 Propionibacterium l.
 Propionimicrobium l.
lymphoplasmacytic
 l. infiltrate
 l. infiltration
 l. inflammation
 l. lesion
 l. lymphoma
 l. response
 l. synovitis
lymphoplasmacytoid
 l. cell
 l. lymphoma (LPL)
lymphoplasmapheresis
lymphopoiesis
 B cell l.
lymphopoietic
lymphoproliferative
 l. disease (LPD)
 l. disorder
 l. syndrome
 X-linked l. (XLP)
lymphoreticular
 l. aggregate
 l. cancer
 l. disease
 l. disorder
 l. malignancy
 l. neoplasia
 l. system
lymphoreticulosis
 benign inoculation l.
lymphorrhea
lymphorrhoid
lymphosarcoma (LSA)
 l. cell leukemia
 follicular l. (FLSA)
 lymphoblastic l.
 lymphocytic l. (LCL)
 reticulum cell l.
lymphosarcoma-reticulum cell sarcoma (LSA/RCS)
lymphosarcomatosis

lymphosarcoma-type malignant lymphoma
lymphoscintigraphy
lymphosis
lymphostatic verrucosis
lymphotoxicity
lymphotoxin (LT)
lymphotropic papovavirus (LPV)
lymphovascular
 l. invasion
 l. space invasion (LVSI)
lymphuria
Lynch syndrome tumor
Lyon hypothesis
lyonization
lyonize
lyophilization
lyophilize
lyophilized anterior pituitary (LAP)
Lyophyllum
LyP
 lymphomatoid papulosis
LYP gene
Lyphochek
 L. anemia control
 L. fertility control
 L. hypertension markers control
 L. maternal serum control
 L. tumor marker control
 L. whole blood control
Lyponyssus
Lys
 lysine
lysate
 Limulus amoebocyte l. (LAL)
lyse
lysemia
lysergic
 l. acid
 l. acid diethylamide (LSD)
 l. acid diethylamide assay
lysin
 beta l.
lysine (K, Lys)
 l. dehydrogenase
 l. intolerance
 l. ketoglutarate reductase
lysine-2-oxoglutaryl reductase
lysine-iron agar
lysinemia

L

NOTES

lysing
- l. agent
- l. reagent

lysinogen
lysinogenic
lysinuria
lysinuric protein intolerance (LPI)
lysis
- l. buffer
- bystander l.
- clot l.
- colloid-osmotic l.
- differential cell l.
- dilute blood clot l. (DBCL)
- diluted whole blood clot l.
- fibrin plate l.
- follicle l. (Fl)
- gamma phage l.
- preferential l.
- l., storage, and transportation (LST)

Lysobacteraceae
Lysobacterales
lysochrome
lysogen
lysogenesis
lysogenic
- l. bacterium
- l. induction
- l. strain

lysogenicity
lysogenization
lysogeny
lysokinase
lysolecithin
lysophosphatidate
lysophosphatide
lysophosphatidyl choline
lysophosphatidylethanolamine
lysophospholipase
lysosomal
- l. protease

- l. storage disease
- l. trafficking regulator protein (LYST)

lysosomal-associated
- l.-a. membrane protein (LAMP)
- l.-a. membrane protein-1 (LAMP-1)
- l.-a. membrane protein-2 (LAMP-2)

lysosome
- angulated l.
- definitive l.
- Golgi endoplasmic reticulum l. (GERL)
- primary l.
- secondary l.

lysostaphin
lysotype
lysozyme
- l. assay
- egg-white l. (EWL)
- human milk l. (HML)
- l. test
- urine l.

lysozymuria
lyssa
Lyssavirus
LYST
- lysosomal trafficking regulator protein

lysyl
lysyl-bradykinin
lysylpyridinoline
Lyt antigen
Lythoglyphopsis
lytica
- *Cellulophaga l.*

lytic lesion
Lytta
LYVE1
- lymphatic endothelial hyaluronan receptor

μ (*var. of* mu)
   micron
μω
   microhm
μbar
   microbar
μCi
   microcurie
μCi/hr
   microcurie-hour
μF
   microfarad
μH
   microhenry
μL
   microliter
μm
   micrometer
μmm
   micromillimeter
μs
   microsecond
μV
   microvolt
μW
   microwatt
M
   molar
     M antigen
     M band
     M cell
     M colony
     M component
     M concentration
     M line
     M phase
     M phase
     M protein
     M spike
M0
   acute myeloblastic leukemia without
     localized differentiation
   no cancer spread to other organs
   no evidence of distant metastases
M1
   acute myeloblastic leukemia without
     maturation
M2
   acute myeloblastic leukemia with
     maturation
M3
   acute promyelocytic leukemia
     M3 muscarinic acetylcholine
     receptor

M4
   acute myelomonocytic leukemia
M5
   acute monocytic leukemia
M6
   acute erythroleukemia
M7
   acute megakaryocytic leukemia
MΩ
   megohm
m
   meter
mμ
   millimicron
mμc
   millimicrocurie
mμg
   millimicrogram
MA
   metastatic adenocarcinoma
   monomorphic adenoma
   muscle actin
M5a
   acute monocytic leukemia without
     differentiation
mA
   milliampere
MAA
   macroaggregated albumin
maanshanensis
     Rhodococcus m.
MAb, mAB
   monoclonal antibody
MAb-based enzyme immunoassay
MAb 12C3
MAC
   membrane attack complex
   Mycobacterium avium-intracellulare
   complex
Mac387 antibody
Macaca
MacCallum patch
Macchiavello stain
MacConkey
     M. agar
     M. broth
macedonicum
     Phlebotomus m.
macedonicus
     Streptococcus gallolyticus subsp. *m.*
macerated
     m. fetus
     m. stillbirth
maceration

M

macestii
Desulfomicrobium m.
MacFarlane serum method
Machado-Guerreiro test
Mache unit (MU)
machine
m. error
Rosys Plato Gene M.
Sakura Seiki Autosmear automatic smear m.
Select-a-Fuge microcentrifuge m.
suicide m.
Ventana ES slide processor m.
Machlomovirus
Machupo virus
MacKenzie syndrome
Macleod
M. rheumatism
M. syndrome
Macluravirus
maclurin
macmurdoensis
Sporosarcina m.
MacNeal tetrachrome blood stain
Macracanthorhynchus hirudinaceus
macrencephaly
macroadenoma
intracellular m. (IM)
macroaggregate
macroaggregated albumin (MAA)
macroamylase
macroamylasemia
macroanatomic
macroangiopathic
macroarray
Macrobdella decora
macrobiote
macroblast
macrocephala
Acrocarpospora m.
macrocephalic
macrocephaly
macrochemistry
macrochilia
macrochylomicron
macrocolon
macroconidium, pl. **macroconidia**
macrocranium
macrocreatine kinase
macrocryoglobulin
macrocryoglobulinemia
macrocyst
macrocytase
macrocyte
oval m.
macrocythemia
hyperchromatic m.
macrocytic
m. achylic anemia

m. anemia of pregnancy
m. hyperchromia
macrocytosis
Macroduct
M. coil
M. collecting system
M. system for sweat stimulation and collection
macrodystrophia lipomatosa
macroencephalon
macroerythroblast
macroerythrocyte
macrofollicular
m. adenoma
m. lymphoma
m. variant
macrogamete
macrogametocyte
macrogamont
macrogamy
macrogastria
macrogenitosomia
m. praecox
m. praecox suprarenalis
macroglia, macroglial
m. cell
macroglobulin
alpha m.
alpha-2 m.
m. assay
macroglobulinemia
essential m.
Waldenström m. (WM)
macroglossia
macrogoltabida
Sphingopyxis m.
macrogyria
macrohomology
Macrohyporia
macro-Kjeldahl method
macrolabia
Macrolepiota
macroleukoblast
macrolide antibiotic
macromastia
macromelanosome
macromerozoite
macrometastasis
macromethod of Wintrobe
macromolecular
macromolecule
Macromonas
M. bipunctata
M. mobilis
macromonocyte
macromyeloblast
macronodular
macronormoblast

macronormochromoblast
macronucleolus, pl. **macronucleoli**
macronucleus, pl. **macronuclei**
    eosinophilic m.
macroorchidism
macroovalocyte
macroparasite
macropathology
macrophage
    activated m.
    m. activation factor (MAF)
    m. agglutination factor (MAggF)
    alveolar m.
    armed m.
    associated m.
    bone marrow m.
    m. chemotactic and activating factor (MCAF)
    m. chemotactic factor (MCF)
    m. colony stimulating factor (M-CSF)
    m. density
    fixed m.
    foamy m.
    free m.
    m. growth factor
    Hansemann m.
    hemosiderin-laden m.'s
    human alveolar m. (HAM)
    inflammatory m.
    m. inflammatory protein (MIP)
    m. inhibiting factor (MIF)
    m. migration inhibition factor
    m. migration inhibition test
    modified m.
    monocyte m.
    phagocytic m.
    m. phagocytosis
    m. presented antigen result
    pulmonary alveolar m. (PAM)
    starry-sky m.
    system of m.'s
    tingible body m.
    transmigration m.
    von Hansemann m.
macrophage-derived growth factor
macrophagocyte
Macrophoma
Macrophomina
macrophotography
    digital m.
macropolycyte

macroprolactinoma
macropromyelocyte
macrorchis
    Prosthogonimus m.
macroreticulocyte
macroscopic
    m. agglutination
    m. lesion
macroscopy
macrosigmoid
macrosis
macrosomia
macrospore
Macrosporium tomato
macrosporoidium
    Stemphylium m.
macrostomia
macrothrombocyte
macrotrabeculae
macrovascular hemolysis
macrovesicular
    m. fat droplet
    m. steatosis
mactans
    Latrodectus m.
macula, pl. **maculae**
    m. adherens
    m. albida
    m. atrophica
    m. cerulea
    m. communicans
    m. communis
    m. cribrosa
    m. densa
    m. flava
    m. germinativa
    m. gonorrhoica
    honeycomb m.
    m. lactea
    m. lutea
    mongolian m.
    neuroepithelium of m.
    m. pellucida
    m. retinae
    m. sacculi
    Saenger m.
    m. tendinea
    m. utriculi
macular
    m. amyloidosis
    m. atrophy
    m. eruption

M

NOTES

macular *(continued)*
    m. erythema
    m. fan
    m. leprosy
    m. star
maculatum
    Amblyomma m.
    atrophoderma m.
maculatus
    Anopheles m.
Maculavirus
macule
maculipennis
    Anopheles m.
maculoerythematous
maculopapular eruption
maculosa
    dermatitis atrophicans m.
madagascariensis
    Inermicapsifer m.
    Taenia m.
madarosis
madder
Maddrey discriminant function
Madelung
    M. disease
    M. neck
mad itch
Madura
    M. boil
    M. foot
madurae
    Actinomadura m.
Madurella
    M. grisea
    M. mycetomi
maduromycetoma
maduromycosis
maduromycotic mycetoma
maedi virus
MAF
    macrophage activation factor
    metanephric adenofibroma
Maffucci
    M. disease
    M. syndrome
MAFP
    methylarachidonyl fluorophosphonate
MAG
    multifocal atrophic gastritis
magadiensis
    Halomonas m.
    Tindallia m.
magaldrate
magenta
    m. I–III
    acid m.
    basic m.
    m. O

MAggF
    macrophage agglutination factor
maggot
    Congo floor m.
    rat-tail m.
Magitot disease
magna
    coxa m.
    Fascioloides m.
    Finegoldia m.
magnesium (Mg)
    m. ammonium phosphate
    m. assay
    m. imbalance
    m. ion (Mg2+)
    m. oxide (MgO)
    m. test
    urine m.
magnesium-activated ATPase
magnetic
    m. core
    m. core memory
    m. field
    m. field strength
    m. flux
    m. induction
    m. moment
    m. susceptibility
    m. tape
magneticus
    Desulfovibrio m.
magnetization
magnification (X)
    high m.
    low m.
    medium m.
magnifier
    Omnivue illuminated m.
magnitude
    signed m.
magnivelare
    Tricholoma m.
magnocellular hypothalamic neuron
magnum load
magnus
    Diplococcus m.
    Peptococcus m.
    Peptostreptococcus m.
Magnus and de Kleijn neck reflex
MAHA
    microangiopathic hemolytic anemia
Mahaim fiber
Maher disease
MAI
    mitotic activity index
    Mycobacterium avium-intracellulare
mail-in microalbumin test
main
    m. en griffe

m. en lorgnette
m. site of airway resistance
maintenance
minichromosome m.
MAIPA
monoclonal antibody-specific
immobilization of platelet antigen
maitriensis
Planococcus m.
Majocchi
M. disease
M. granuloma
M. purpura
major
m. agglutinin
m. basic protein (MBP)
beta thalassemia m.
ductus sublingualis m.
m. duodenal papilla
m. gene
glandula vestibularis m.
m. histocompatibility antigen
(MHA)
m. histocompatibility complex
(MHC)
m. histocompatibility locus
Leishmania tropica m.
m. outer membrane protein
(MOMP)
papilla duodeni m.
Phlebotomus m.
m. salivary gland
m. sublingual duct
thalassemia m.
m. tranquilizer
variola m.
majority of peripheral blood
lymphocyte
majus
Habronema m.
labia m.
MAK6 immunohistochemical reagent
maker
Geometric Data Miniprep slide m.
mal
m. de Cayenne
m. de San Lazaro
Malabar
M. itch
M. leprosy
malabarica
phlegmasia m.

malabsorption
m. disease
m. disorder
m. syndrome
malachite
m. green
m. green broth
m. green stain
malacia
malacic
malacoplakia, malakoplakia
m. vesicae
malacosis
malacotic
maladie de Roger
malakoplakia (*var. of* malacoplakia)
malaria
algid m.
benign tertian m.
bilious remittent m.
bovine m.
double tertian m.
falciparum m.
m. film test
gastric algid m.
hemolytic m.
hemorrhagic m.
intermittent m.
malariae m.
malignant tertian m.
ovale m.
pernicious m.
quartan m.
quotidian m.
remittent m.
m. smear
tertian m.
therapeutic m.
vivax m.
malariacidal
malariae
m. malaria
Plasmodium m.
malarial
m. cachexia
m. deposition pigment
m. dysentery
m. fever
m. hemoglobinuria
m. knob
m. parasite
m. pigment deposition

M

NOTES

malarial *(continued)*
    m. pigment stain
    m. rosette
malariology
malarious
malar rash
Malassez disease
Malassezia
    M. furfur
    M. ovalis
    M. pachydermatis
malate dehydrogenase
malathion
malaya
    microfilaria m.
Malayan
    M. filariasis
    M. pit viper venom
malayanum
    Echinostoma m.
malayensis
    Schistosoma m.
malayi
    Brugia m.
    Wuchereria m.
malaysiensis
    Angiostrongylus m.
Malbranchea
maldigestive disease
MALDIMS
    matrix-assisted laser desorption and
    ionization mass spectrometry
MALDI-TOF
    matrix-assisted laser desorption ionization
    time-of-flight
    MALDI-TOF mass spectrometry
Maldonado-San Jose stain
male
    m. castration
    m. frog test
    m. hormone
    m. pseudohermaphrodite
    m. reproductive system
    m. rudimentary uterus
    m. sex chromatin pattern
    m. toad test
    m. Turner syndrome
    47,XYY m.
malformation
    Arnold-Chiari m.
    arteriovenous m. (AVM)
    cardiac valvular m.
    cardiovascular m.
    cavernous m. (CM)
    cerebrovascular m. (CVM)
    chromosome dicentric m.
    congenital cardiovascular m.
    cutaneous m.
    cystic adenomatoid m.

    Dandy-Walker m.
    dicentric m.
    Dieulafoy m.
    Ebstein m.
    genitourinary m.
    spinal cord vascular m.
    m. syndrome
    vascular m.
malfunction
Malherbe
    M. calcifying epithelioma
    M. disease
Malibu disease
malic
    m. acid
    m. dehydrogenase (MDH)
maligna
    cynanche m.
    lentigo m.
    struma m.
    variola m.
malignancy
    B-cell m.
    borderline m.
    gland-forming m.
    hematolymphoid m.
    hematopoietic m.
    humoral hypercalcemia of m.
    lymphoreticular m.
    postthymic m.
malignancy-related ascites
malignant
    m. adenoma
    m. ameloblastoma
    m. anemia
    m. atrophic papulosis
    m. breast tumor
    m. bubo
    m. carbuncle
    m. carcinoid syndrome
    m. cartilaginous tumor
    m. dyskeratosis
    m. edema
    m. endocarditis
    m. endovascular papillary
    angioendothelioma
    m. ependymoma
    m. fibrous histiocytoma (MFH)
    m. giant cell tumor of bone
    m. giant cell tumor of soft parts
    m. glioma
    m. granuloma
    m. hepatoma
    m. histiocytosis
    m. Hodgkin and Reed-Sternberg
    cell
    m. hypertension
    m. hyperthermia
    m. jaundice

m. lentigo
m. lentigo melanoma
m. lymphadenosis
m. lymphoma (ML)
m. lymphoma with a high content of epithelioid histiocytes
m. melanoma in situ
m. melanoma staging
m. meningioma
m. mesenchymoma
m. mesothelioma
m. mixed mesodermal tumor (MMMT)
m. mixed müllerian tumor (MMMT)
m. mixed tumor (MMT)
m. myoepithelioma
m. neoplasm
m. nephrosclerosis
m. neurilemmoma
m. peripheral nerve sheath tumor (MPNST)
m. plasma cell tumor
m. pleural effusion
m. pustule
m. rhabdoid tumor of kidney (MRTK)
m. rhabdoid tumor of soft tissue (MRTS)
m. schwannoma
m. smallpox
m. synovioma
m. tertian fever
m. tertian malaria
m. thymoma
m. transformation
m. triton tumor (MTT)
m. trophoblastic teratoma (MTT)
m. tumors of the stomach
m. vascular tumor

maligni
    Bacillus oedematis m.

malignum
    lymphogranuloma m.

Malin syndrome

Mali syndrome

Mall
    periportal space of M.

mallei
    Actinobacillus m.
    Bacillus m.

    Burkholderia m.
    Malleomyces m.

malleinization

mallein test

Malleomyces
    M. mallei
    M. pseudomallei
    M. whitmori

malleosa
    pneumonia m.

mallet finger

Mallophaga

Mallory
    M. aniline blue stain
    M. body
    M. collagen stain
    M. hyaline
    M. iodine stain
    M. phloxine stain
    M. phosphotungstic acid
    M. phosphotungstic acid hematoxylin stain
    M. stain for *Actinomyces*
    M. stain for hemofuchsin
    M. trichrome stain
    M. triple stain

Mallory-Weiss
    M.-W. lesion
    M.-W. syndrome
    M.-W. tear

Malmejde test

malmoense
    Mycobacterium m.

Malmö protocol

malnutrition
    intrauterine m. (IUM)
    protein-calorie m. (PCM)

malocclusion

malonate inhibitor

malonatica
    Levinea m.

malondialdehyde concentrate

Maloney leukemia virus

malonic acid

malonitrile
    chlorobenzylidene m.

malononitrile
    NATO code for o-chlorobenzylidene m. (CS)

malonyl coenzyme A

malorum
    Acetobacter m.

M

NOTES

malperfusion
    placental m.
malpighian
    m. body
    m. body of kidney
    m. body of spleen
    m. capsule
    m. cell
    m. corpuscle
    m. gland
    m. glomerulus
    m. layer
    m. nodule
    m. rete
    m. stratum
    m. tuft
malpighii
    stratum m.
malposition
malrotation
    intestinal m.
MALT
    mucosa-associated lymphoid tissue
    MALT lymphoma
malt
    m. agar
    m. extract broth
Malta fever
maltaromaticum
    Carnobacterium m.
Maltese cross
MALToma
    mucosa-associated lymphoid tissue
    lymphoma
maltoma
maltophilia
    Pseudomonas m.
    Stenotrophomonas m.
    Xanthomonas m.
maltose
maltosuria
malt-worker's lung
malum
    m. articulorum senilis
    m. coxae senile
Mamastrovirus
mamelonated
mamelonation
mamelonné
    état m.
mamillary duct
mammaglobin
    human m. (hMAM)
Mammalian Prions
mammaria, gen. and pl. **mammariae**
    glandula m.
    lobi glandulae mammariae
    lobuli glandulae mammariae

mammary
    m. aspiration specimen (MAS)
    m. aspiration specimen cytology
      test (MASCT)
    m. calculus
    m. duct
    m. duct ectasia
    m. dysplasia
    m. fistula
    m. gland
    m. intraepithelial neoplasia
    m. Paget disease
    m. tumor virus (MTV)
    m. tumor virus of mice
mammilla, pl. **mammillae**
mammillitis
    bovine herpes m.
    bovine ulcerative m.
    bovine vaccinia m.
mammitis
mammographic microcalcification
Mammomonogamus laryngeus
mammosomatotroph cell
mammosomatotropic adenoma
Mammotome biopsy system
mammotroph
mammotropic hormone
mammotropin
management
    automation initiative in
      laboratory m.
    case m.
    component m.
    critical incident stress m. (CISM)
    low-range heparin m. (LHMT)
manager
    Cholesterol M.
Manan needle
manchette
Manchurian hemorrhagic fever
Mancini
    M. iodine stain
    M. method
mandelate
    methenamine m.
mandelii
    Pseudomonas m.
Mandelin reagent
mandibuloacral dysostosis
mandibulofacial
    m. dysostosis
    m. dysotosis syndrome
    m. dysplasia
mandibulooculofacial
    m. dysmorphia
    m. dysmorphism
    m. syndrome
mandibulooculofacialis
    dyscephalia m.

mandrake root
mandrillaris
    Balamuthia m.
maneuver
    Valsalva m.
manganese
    m. assay
    m. poisoning
    m. toxicity
manganic
manganism
manganous
manganoxidans
    Caldimonas m.
mange
    sarcoptic m.
mangiferae
    Dothiorella m.
    Nattrassia m.
manifest
    m. hyperopia
    phenotypically m.
manifesta
    spina bifida m.
manifestation
    abnormal clinical m.
    extraintestinal m.
    laboratory m.
manifesting heterozygote
manifold
    Visiprep solid-phase extraction
    vacuum m.
mannan
manner
    bimodal m.
    m. of death
mannitol fermentation
mannitolilytica
    Ralstonia m.
mannitolivorans
    Hongiella m.
Mann methyl blue-eosin stain
mannoheptulosuria
mannoprotein
mannose binding lectin (MBL)
mannose-6-phosphate (Man6P)
mannosidase
    alpha m.
mannosidosis
Mann-Whitney rank sum statistic
manometric flame

MANOVA
    multivariate analysis of variance
man-o'-war
    Portuguese m.-o.-w.
Man6P
    mannose-6-phosphate
    Man6P recognition marker
Manson
    M. blood fluke
    M. disease
Mansonella
    M. demarquayi
    M. ozzardi
    M. perstans
    M. streptocerca
    M. tucumana
mansonelliasis
mansoni
    Bothriocephalus m.
    Diphyllobothrium m.
    Oxyspirura m.
    Schistosoma m.
    Spirometra m.
Mansonia
mansonii
    Cladosporium m.
    Zygosporium m.
mansonoides
    Bothriocephalus m.
    Diphyllobothrium m.
    Spirometra m.
Mantel-Cox
    M.-C. method
    M.-C. procedure
M_1 antigen
mantle
    m. cell lymphocytic lymphoma
    m. sclerosis
    m. zone
mantle-zone lymphocyte
Mantoux
    M. conversion
    M. diameter (MD)
    M. pit
    M. skin test
manual
    m. CD4 kit
    m. optic planimeter
manuum
MAP
    megaloblastic anemia of pregnancy

M

NOTES

MAP *(continued)*
    microtubule-associated protein
    mitogen-activated protein
map
    chromosome m.
    cytogenetic m.
    genetic m.
    linkage m.
    memory m.
    restriction m.
    tumor m.
    m. unit
maple
    m. bark stripper's disease
    m. bark stripper's lung
    m. syrup urine disease (MSUD)
maplike skull
mapping
    epitope m.
    genetic m.
    lymphatic m.
    site-specific biopsy m.
maprotiline
MAPSS
    multiangle polarized scatter separation
maquilingensis
    Caldivirga m.
Marafivirus
Maragiliano body
Marañón syndrome
marantic
    m. atrophy
    m. endocarditis
    m. thrombosis
    m. thrombus
marasmic
    m. kwashiorkor
    m. thrombosis
    m. thrombus
Marasmius
marasmus
marble
    m. bone
    m. bone disease
Marboran
Marburg
    M. agent
    M. virus
    M. virus disease
"Marburg-like viruses"
Marburgvirus
marcescens
    Serratia m.
march
    m. albuminuria
    m. anemia
    M. disease
    m. hemoglobinuria

Marchand
    M. adrenal
    M. rest
    M. wandering cell
Marchesani syndrome
Marchi
    M. fixative
    M. reaction
    M. stain
Marchiafava-Bignami disease
Marchiafava-Micheli
    M.-M. anemia
    M.-M. syndrome
marcid
Marcus Gunn syndrome
Marcy agent
Marek
    M. disease
    M. disease virus
    M. herpesvirus disease (MDHV)
"Marek's disease-like viruses"
Marfan
    M. disease
    M. law
    M. syndrome
Margarinomyces
margaritifer
    Tepidiphilus m.
Margaritispora
Margaropus winthemi
margin
    corneal m.
    infiltrative m.
    irregular m.
    left costal m. (LCM)
    outer m.
    placental disc m.
    sclerotic m.
    seared wound m.
    slitlike m.
    true mucosal m.
marginal
    m. granulocyte pool (MGP)
    m. insertion of umbilical cord
    m. ulcer
    m. zone (MZ)
    m. zone lymphoma
marginated chromatin
margination
    leukocytic m.
marginatum
    Clinostomum m.
    eczema m.
    erythema m.
    Hyalomma m.
Margolis syndrome
maricaloris
    Pseudoalteromonas m.

Marie
    M. disease
    M. syndrome
Marie-Bamberger
    M.-B. disease
    M.-B. syndrome
Marie-Robinson syndrome
Marie-Strümpell disease
Marie-Tooth disease
marijuana, marihuana
marimammalium
    Actinomyces m.
marina
    Alteromonas m.
    Anisakis m.
    Blastopirellula m.
    Cobetia m.
    Kocuria m.
    Nitrosomonas m.
    Persephonella m.
    Pseudomonas m.
    Psychromonas m.
    Roseospira m.
    Thiocapsa m.
marincola
    Hongiella m.
    Psychrobacter m.
marine protein concentrate (MPC)
Marinesco-Garland syndrome
Marinesco-Sjögren syndrome
mariniglutinosa
    Pseudoalteromonas m.
marinintestina
    Shewanella m.
marinisedimentorum
    Reinekea m.
Marino and Muller-Hermelink (MMH)
marinum
    Aeromicrobium m.
    Mycobacterium m.
    plasma m.
marinus
    Bacteriovorax m.
    Dethiosulfovibrio m.
    Hydrogenothermus m.
    Prochlorococcus m. subsp. *marinus*
    Serinicoccus m.
Marion disease
marioni
    Heterodera m.
maris
    Williamsia m.

marisflavi
    Bacillus m.
    Halomonas m.
marismortui
    Chromohalobacter m.
    Salibacillus m.
    Virgibacillus m.
maritima
    Hippea m.
    Woodsholea m.
maritimum
    Tenacibaculum m.
maritimus
    Planococcus m.
    Psychrobacter m.
    Thermodiscus m.
Marituba virus
Marjolin ulcer
mark
    port-wine m.
    m. sense reader
    strawberry m.
    tape m.
    tide m.
    Unna m.
marked splenomegaly
marker
    allotypic m.
    B-cell m.
    biliary progenitor m.
    candidate tumor m.
    CDX2 immunohistochemical m.
    cell surface m.
    chromosomal m.
    m. chromosome
    chromosome 14q tumor m.
    clusterin m.
    collagen m.
    DNA m.
    endocrine m.
    endothelial m.
    enzyme m.
    fecal m.
    m. gene
    genetic m.
    HBV DNA m.
    histodiagnostic m.
    HMB 45 m.
    Hybritech Ostase bone
      metabolism m.
    immunohistochemical m.
    Ki-67 immunophenotypic m.

M

NOTES

marker *(continued)*
    laminin m.
    lineage m.
    Man6P recognition m.
    mesothelioma m.
    MIB1 cell proliferation m.
    microsatellite m.
    molecular m.
    m.'s of myocardial injury
    myogen m.
    myoid m.
    N-cadherin m.
    neuroendocrine m.
    nonlineage m.
    oncofetal m.
    Ostase biochemical m.
    Ostase bone metabolism m.
    panmacrophage m.
    pan-T m.
    phosphomannosyl recognition m.
    polymorphic genetic m.
    progenitor m.
    proliferation m.
    rapid intraoperative quantitative RT-PCR assessment of tumor m.
    m. rescue
    rhabdomyosarcoma m.
    S-100 m.
    single copy gene m.
    smooth muscle m.
    supernumerary m.
    surface m.
    tau molecular m.
    T-cell m.
    T-helper/inducer subset m.
    T-suppressor/cytotoxic subset m.
    tumor m.
    tumor progression m.
    utrophin m.
    VEGFR3 m.
marking
    coarse m.
markovian texture
Marme reagent
marmoratus
    status m.
marmoset virus
marmot
Maroteaux-Lamy syndrome
Marquis reagent
marrow
    aplastic bone m.
    basophilic m.
    bone m. (BM)
    m. cavity
    m. cell
    empty m.
    eosinophilic m.
    erythrocytic m.

    m. fibrosis
    hypercellular bone m.
    hypocellularity of bone m.
    leukocytic m.
    lymphocytic m.
    Maximow stain for bone m.
    mesodermal bone m.
    monocytic m.
    neutrophilic m.
    particle of bone m.
    red bone m.
    m. reticulin
    reticulocytic m.
    yellow bone m.
marrow-lymph gland
MARSA
    methicillin and aminoglycoside-resistant *Staphylococcus aureus*
Marseilles fever
marsh
    M. disease
    m. fever
Marshall
    M. Hall facies
    M. method
    M. syndrome
Marshallagia marshalli
marshalli
    Alcaligenes m.
    Marshallagia m.
Marshall-Marchetti (MM)
Marsonnina
Martin
    M. broth
    M. disease
Martininia
Martin-Lester agar
Martinotti cell
martius
    m. scarlet blue (MSB)
    m. yellow
Martorell syndrome
MAS
    mammary aspiration specimen
    McCune-Albright syndrome
mA-s
    milliampere-second
Masaoka
    M. classification
    M. staging criteria
    M. thymic cancer staging system
maschaladenitis
maschaloncus
MASCT
    mammary aspiration specimen cytology test
masculinae
    glandulae urethrales m.

masculinization
    ovarian m.
masculinovoblastoma
mask
    BLB m.
    escape m.
    HEPA filter m.
    Hutchinson m.
    m. of pregnancy
    tropical m.
masked
    m. message
    m. virus
masking
    epitope m.
Mason-Pfizer monkey virus
mason's lung
MASP
    MBL-associated serine protease
maspin nuclear staining
mass
    m. action law
    atomic m.
    m. attenuation coefficient
    body m. (BM)
    carbon gelatin m.
    m. casualty incident (MCI)
    circumscribed m.
    m. concentration
    critical m.
    cul-de-sac m.
    decrease in bone m.
    dysplasia-associated m.
    dysplasia-associated lesion or m.
      (DALM)
    erythrocyte m. (EM)
    exchangeable m.
    m. fatality incident
    fat-free m. (FFM)
    filar m.
    m. fragmentography
    m. gathering
    m. index
    m. infection
    injection m.
    intravascular m. (IVM)
    lean body m. (LBM)
    m. lesion
    mediastinal m.
    m. memory
    m. miniature radiography (MMR)
    molecular m.

    m. number
    parathyroid m.
    m. pinocytosis
    red blood cell m. (RBCM)
    m. spectrograph
    m. spectrometer
    m. spectrometry (MS)
    m. spectroscopy
    m. storage
    unit of m.
    whorled m.
massa, gen. and pl. **massae**
mass-casualty weapon (MCW)
massiliae
    Rickettsia m.
massiliensis
    Afipia m.
    Bosea m.
    Paenibacillus m.
massive
    m. collapse
    m. embolus
    m. hepatic necrosis (MHN)
    m. infiltrate of lymphocytes
    m. pulmonary hemorrhage
    m. transfusion
    m. vitreous retraction (MVR)
Masson
    M. argentaffin stain
    M. body
    M. humid meningioma
    M. pseudoangiosarcoma
    M. trichrome method
    M. trichrome stain
    M. tumor
Masson-Fontana
    M.-F. ammoniacal silver stain
    M.-F. ammoniac silver stain
    M.-F. method
MAST
    multiple antigen stimulation test
    multithread allergosorbent test
mast
    m. cell
    m. cell degranulation test
    m. cell disease
    m. cell hyperplasia
    m. cell leukemia
    m. cell sarcoma
    m. cell staining
    m. cell tryptase

M

NOTES

mast (*continued*)
    m. cell tumor
    m. leukocyte
mastadenitis
mastadenoma
Mastadenovirus
mastatrophy, mastatrophia
mastauxe
mastectomy
    Halsted m.
master
    m. file
    m. gland
    M. 2-step test
mastic test
Mastigomyces
Mastigophora
mastigophorous
mastigote
mastitis
    acute m.
    bovine m.
    chronic cystic m.
    cystic m.
    fibrocystic m.
    gargantuan m.
    glandular m.
    granulomatous m.
    interstitial m.
    lactational m.
    m. neonatorum
    parenchymatous m.
    periductal m.
    perilobular m.
    phlegmonous m.
    plasma cell m.
    puerperal m.
    retromammary m.
    submammary m.
    suppurative m.
mastocyte
mastocytogenesis
mastocytoma
mastocytosis
mastoid abscess
mastoidea
    otitis m.
mastoiditis
Mastomys natalensis
mastoncus
mastopathy
    cystic m.
    diabetic m.
    fibrocystic m.
Mastophora
mastoplasia
mastoscirrhus
Mastrevirus

matching
    CREG m.
mater
    dura m.
    pia m.
material
    Advia Centaur HBc IgM
     control m.
    biological matrix reference m.'ss
    biuret-reactive m. (BRM)
    calibration m.
    certified reference m.
    chromatin m.
    coarse m.
    control m.
    Cotasil silicone slide coating m.
    cross-reacting m. (CRM)
    diastase-resistant m.
    eosinophilic proteinaceous
     granular m.
    explosive m.
    extracellular m. (ECM)
    fibrin-like proteinaceous m.
    fluorescent m.
    gonadotropin-inhibitory m. (GIM)
    m. graft
    granular osmiophilic m. (GOM)
    hazardous m.
    hyaline m.
    labeling of hazardous m.'s
    matrix reference m.'s
    neurosecretory m. (NSM)
    particulate crystalline m.
    primary reference m.
    reactive m.
    reference m.
    m. safety data sheet (MSDS)
    secondary reference m.'s
    simulated matrix reference m.'s
    vasodepressor m. (VDM)
    vasoexcitor m. (VEM)
    weapons-grade nuclear m.
maternal
    m. age
    m. antibody
    m. cotyledon
    m. death
    m. floor infarction
    m. immunity
    m. imprint
    m. inheritance
    m. meiotic nondisjunction
    m. polyhydramnios
    m. serum alpha fetoprotein
    (MSAFP)
    m. urine estriol
maternal-fetal hemorrhage
mathematical genetics
Mathieu disease

mating
- assortative m.
- consanguineous m.
- negative assortative m.
- positive assortative m.
- random m.

matrass

matrical, matricial

matrices (*pl. of* matrix)

matrilineal

matrilysin

matritensis
- *Citeromyces m.*

matrix, pl. **matrices**
- bone m.
- m. calculus
- cartilage m.
- cell m.
- cytoplasmic m.
- m. effect
- extracellular m. (ECM)
- fibrin m.
- groove of nail m.
- hyaline cartilage m.
- m. metalloproteinase (MMP)
- m. metalloproteinase 1 (MMP 1)
- m. metalloproteinase 2 (MMP 2)
- mitochondrial m.
- m. mitochondrialis
- myxochondroid m.
- myxocollagenous m.
- myxoid m.
- osteoid m.
- m. reference materials
- territorial m.
- m. vesicle

matrix-assisted
- m.-a. laser desorption and ionization mass spectrometry (MALDIMS)
- m.-a. laser desorption ionization time-of-flight (MALDI-TOF)

matrix-producing carcinoma

matruchotii
- *Corynebacterium m.*

matter
- interaction of radiation with m.
- sclerosis of white m.
- white m.

mattheei
- *Schistosoma m.*

maturate

maturation
- accelerated villous m.
- acute myeloblastic leukemia with m. (M2)
- acute myeloblastic leukemia without m. (M1)
- m. arrest
- m. B cell
- m. division
- m. of gonadal structure
- m. index
- trilinear m.

mature
- m. abnormal chorion
- m. abnormal chorionic villus
- m. abnormal placenta
- m. adipocyte
- m. bacteriophage
- m. B cell
- m. cell leukemia
- m. neutrophil
- m. ovarian follicle
- m. spermatozoon
- m. teratoma

maturity
- fetal lung m. (FLM)
- m. onset diabetes of the young (MODY)

maturity-onset diabetes

Maunier-Kuhn disease

maura
- *Halomonas m.*

Maurer
- M. cleft
- M. dot

Mauriac syndrome

Mauthner sheath

MAV
- multinucleated atypia of the vulva

Max
- Strep A OIA M.

Maxcy disease

maxillary gland

maxillectomy cavity

maxillitis

maximal
- m. acid output
- m. growth temperature
- m. Histalog test
- m. inspiratory flow rate (MIFR)
- m. midexpiratory flow (MMEF)

M

NOTES

maximal *(continued)*
>m. midexpiratory flow rate (MMEFR)
>m. midflow rate (MMFR)
>m. permissible dose (MPD)
>m. sustained ventilatory capacity (MSVC)
>m. tubular excretory capacity of kidneys (T_m)
>m. tubular reabsorption of glucose (T_{mg})

Maximow stain for bone marrow

maximum
>m. expiratory flow (MEF)
>m. expiratory flow rate (MEFR)
>m. expiratory flow volume (MEFV)
>m. impurities reagent
>m. inhibiting dilution (MID)
>m. inspiratory flow (MIF)
>m. inspiratory pressure (MIP)
>m. permissible concentration (MPC)
>m. temperature
>m. thermometer
>m. urea clearance
>m. urinary concentration (MUC)
>m. voluntary ventilation (MVV)

Maxisorp microtiter plate
Max-Joseph space
MAXM hematology flow cytometer
maxwell (Mx)
Mayaro virus
maydis
>*Ustilago m.*

Mayer
>M. acid alum hematoxylin stain
>M. hemalum
>M. hemalum stain
>M. hematoxylin
>M. hematoxylin stain
>M. mucicarmine stain
>M. mucihematein stain

Mayer-Rokitansky-Küster syndrome
mayfly
May-Grünwald-Giemsa stain
May-Grünwald stain
May-Hegglin
>M.-H. anomaly
>M.-H. body

mazamorra
mazoplasia
Mazzoni corpuscle
mazzottii
>*Borrelia m.*

Mazzotti test
MB
>methylene blue
>microbiological assay
>MB band

MB1
>monoclonal antibody M.

Mb
>myoglobin

M5b
>acute monocytic leukemia with differentiation

mbar
>millibar

MBAS
>methylene blue active substance

MBC
>minimal bactericidal concentration

MbCO
>carbon dioxide myoglobin

MBD
>methylene blue dye
>minimal brain damage
>minimal brain dysfunction

MBL
>mannose binding lectin
>minimal bactercidal level

MBL-associated serine protease (MASP)
MbO_2
>deoxyhemoglobin

MBP
>major basic protein
>myelin basic protein
>>MBP assay

MBR
>major breakpoint region

MB-Redox system
MBT
>mucinous borderline tumor

MC
>medullary carcinoma
>mesenchymal chondrosarcoma
>mixed cellularity

mC
>millicoulomb

MCA
>microcarcinoma
>multichannel analyzer

MCAF
>macrophage chemotactic and activating factor

MCAG
>multiple colloid adenomatous goiter

McArdle disease
McArdle-Schmid-Pearson disease
MCB
>membranous cytoplasmic body

MCBR
>minimum concentration of bilirubin

MCC
>minimum complete-killing concentration
>mutated in colon cancer

Mycobacterium phlei cell wall DNA
  complex
    MCC gene
McCarey-Kaufman (M-K)
    M.-K. medium
McCune-Albright syndrome (MAS)
MCD
    mean cell diameter
    mean of consecutive differences
    mean corpuscular diameter
    medullary cystic disease
    multiple carboxylase deficiency
MCDK
    multicystic dysplasia of kidney
    multicystic dysplastic kidney
McEwen point
MCF
    macrophage chemotactic factor
MCFA
    medium-chain fatty acid
mcg
    microgram
MCH
    mean cell hemoglobin
    mean corpuscular hemoglobin
MCHC
    mean cell hemoglobin concentration
    mean corpuscular hemoglobin
      concentration
MCHD
    mixed-cellularity Hodgkin disease
MCI
    mass casualty incident
      trauma MCI
mCi
    millicurie
mCi-hr
    millicurie-hour
McKrae herpes simplex virus strain
MCL
    mantle cell lymphoma
McLean-Maxwell disease
McLeod blood phenotype
McMaster technique
mcmeekinii
    Planomicrobium m.
McNeer classification
McNemar test
MCP
    mitotic control protein
    monocyte chemoattractant protein

MCP 1
    monocyte chemoattractant protein 1
    monocyte chemotactic protein 1
McPhail test
MCR
    metabolic clearance rate
    minor cluster region
    mutation cluster region
M-CSF
    macrophage colony stimulating factor
MCT
    mast cell tryptase positive chymase
      negative
    mean circulation time
    mean corpuscular thickness
    medium-chain triglyceride
    mucinous cystic tumor
MCTC
    mast cell positive tryptase and chymase
MCTD
    mixed connective tissue disease
MCV
    mean cell volume
    mean corpuscular volume
    molluscum contagiosum virus
MCVr
    reticulocyte mean corpuscular volume
MCW
    mass-casualty weapon
MD
    Mantoux diameter
    moderately differentiated
    muscular dystrophy
Md
    mendelevium
MDA
    methylenedioxyamphetamine
    multiple displacement amplification
      MDA in WGA
MDC
    minimum detectable concentration
MDF
    mean dominant frequency
    myocardial depressant factor
MDH
    malic dehydrogenase
MDHV
    Marek herpesvirus disease
MDMA
    methylenedioxymethamphetamine

NOTES

MDNCF
monocyte-derived neutrophil chemotactic factor

MDR
multidrug resistance
multiple drug resistance

MDR1
multidrug resistance 1
MDR1 transporter

MDS
myelodysplastic syndrome
MDS system

MDT
median detection threshold

MDTR
mean diameter-thickness ratio

MDUO
myocardial disease of unknown origin

ME
marginal excision
medical examiner

M:E
myeloid-erythroid ratio

MEA
multiple endocrine adenomatosis

meal
test m.

mean
m. cell diameter (MCD)
m. cell hemoglobin (MCH)
m. cell hemoglobin concentration (MCHC)
m. cell threshold
m. cell volume (MCV)
m. circulation time (MCT)
m. circulatory hematocrit
m. of consecutive differences (MCD)
m. corpuscular diameter (MCD)
m. corpuscular hemoglobin (MCH)
m. corpuscular hemoglobin concentration (MCHC)
m. corpuscular thickness (MCT)
m. corpuscular volume (MCV)
m. diameter-thickness ratio (MDTR)
m. dominant frequency (MDF)
m. dose per unit cumulated activity
m. effective life
m. follicle size
m. generation time
m. hemolytic dose (MHD)
m. nuclear area (MNA)
m. platelet volume (MVP)
m. square deviation
m. time between failures

measles
m. antibody
atypical m.

m. convalescent serum
German m.
m. immune globulin (human)
m. immunoglobulin
m., mumps, and rubella (MMR)
m., mumps, and rubella vaccine
m. pneumonitis
three-day m.
tropical m.
m. virus
m. virus pneumonia
m. virus vaccine

measly

measurable
not m. (NM)

measurement
blood volume m.
carbon dioxide combining power m.
end-point m.
kinetic m.
oxygen saturation m.
right anterior m. (RAM)
total exchangeable potassium m.

measuring pipette

meat fiber

MEBMM
mixed epithelial papillary cystadenoma of borderline malignancy of müllerian type

MEC
mucoepidermoid carcinoma

5-MeC
5-methylcytosine

mechanical
m. agent
m. asphyxia
m. displacement
m. diuretic
m. fragility
m. ileus
m. jaundice
m. styptic
m. vector
m. ventilation

mechanic's hand

mechanism
autoimmune m.
compensatory m.
countercurrent m.
defense m.
extravascular migratory metastasis m.
Frank-Starling m.
immune-mediated m.
immunological m.
inactivation m.
perforin-dependent m.
ping-pong m.

mechanocyte

mechanoreceptor
mechlorethamine (HN$_2$)
mecillinam
Mecistocirrus
Meckel
    M. cave
    M. diverticulum
    M. plane
    M. syndrome
Meckel-Gruber syndrome
Mecke reagent
meconium
    m. aspiration
    m. ileus
    m. periorchitis
    m. peritonitis
    m. stain
meconium-stained liquor
MED
    minimal erythema dose
media (*pl. of* medium)
mediae
    cellulae ethmoidales m.
medial
    m. arteriosclerosis
    m. calcification
    m. cartilaginous plate
    m. collateral ligament degeneration
    m. collateral ligament tearing
    m. cystic necrosis
    m. epicondylitis
    m. necrosis of aorta
    m. plate of cartilaginous auditory tube
    m. preoptic nucleus
median
    m. bar of Mercier
    m. curative dose (CD$_{50}$)
    m. detection threshold (MDT)
    m. effective dose (ED$_{50}$)
    m. eminence
    m. fatal dose (FD$_{50}$)
    m. infectious dose (ID$_{50}$)
    m. lethal dose (LD$_{50}$)
    m. rhomboid glossitis
    m. tissue culture dose (TCD$_{50}$)
    m. tissue culture infective dose (TCID$_{50}$)
    m. unbiased estimate
mediastinal
    m. elastofibroma
    m. fibrosis
    m. lipomatosis
    m. lymphadenitis
    m. mass
    m. pericarditis
    m. shadow
mediastinitis
    hemorrhagic m.
    idiopathic fibrous m.
    sclerosing m.
mediastinopericarditis
mediastinum
    extraosseous plasmacytoma of the m. (EPM)
mediate
    m. agglutination
    m. contagion
mediated conversion
mediation
mediator
    m. cell
    chemical m.
    inflammatory m.
    vasoactive m.
medicae
    Ensifer m.
medical
    m. bacteriology
    m. equipment set (MES)
    m. examiner (ME)
    m. food
    m. genetics
    m. internal radiation dose (MIRD)
    m. laboratory technician
    m. mycology
    m. pathology
    m. radiology
    m. record
    m. review officer (MRO)
    m. technologist (MT)
    m. treatment facility (MTF)
medicamentosa
    dermatitis m.
    struma m.
medication-related diarrhea
medicinal
    m. leech
    m. scarlet red
medicine
    clinical m.
    forensic m.
    occupational m.
    preventive m.

M

NOTES

medicine *(continued)*
   systematized nomenclature of m.
      (SNOMED)
medicolegal autopsy
medina worm infection
Medin disease
medinensis
   Dracunculus m.
mediocanellata
   Taenia m.
medionecrosis
   m. of the aorta
   m. aortae idiopathica cystica
   cystic m.
mediterranea
   Pseudomonas m.
Mediterranean
   M. anemia
   familial M. fever (FMF)
   M. fever
   M. hemoglobin E disease
   M. lymphoma
mediterranei
   Amycolatopsis m.
   Nocardia m.
mediterraneus
   Desulfobulbus m.
   Sulfitobacter m.
medium, pl. **media**
   Acanthamoeba m.
   active m.
   aerotitis media
   aortic tunica media
   aqueous mounting m.
   m. artery
   Balamuth aqueous egg yolk
      infusion m.
   Balamuth culture m.
   bilateral otitis media (BOM)
   Boeck-Drbohlav-Locke egg-
      serum m.
   Bordet-Gengou culture m.
   brain-heart infusion broth m.
   Bruns glucose m.
   m. chocolatization
   chocolatization of blood culture m.
   cholesterol-free m.
   chopped meat m.
   clearing m.
   Columbia m.
   contrast m.
   Cryo-Gel embedding m.
   culture m.
   Czapek-Dox m.
   defined culture m.
   dermatophyte test m. (DTM)
   Diamond TYM m.
   dispersion m.
   dispersive m.

Eagle basal m.
Eagle essential m.
Eagle minimum essential m.
   (EMEM)
enrichment m.
Epon tissue-embedding m.
Farrant m.
m. frequency (MF)
Glycergel mounting m.
glycerol gelatin m.
m. incisural space
indicator culture m.
Lash casein hydrolysate-serum m.
Löffler blood culture m.
Löffler coagulated serum m.
Lowenstein-Jensen m. (LJM)
m. magnification
McCarey-Kaufman m.
minimum essential m. (MEM)
M-K m.
motility test m.
mounting m.
Nickerson m.
NNN culture m.
nonpermissive culture m.
nutrient m.
OF m.
otitis media (OM)
oxidation-fermentation m.
Paraplast Plus tissue embedding m.
passive m.
permissive culture m.
Petragnani m.
potassium simplex optimized m.
   (KSOM)
PVA lacto-phenol m.
radiopaque m.
Rees culture m.
refracting m.
RPMI 1640 m.
Sabouraud m.
scala media
secretory otitis media
selective m.
separating m.
serous otitis media
m. sized pyramidal cell
sodium chloride culture m.
sorbitol-MacConkey m.
support m.
suppurative chronic otitis media
tellurite m.
Thayer-Martin m.
thioglycolate m.
tissue culture m. (TCM)
Tobie, von Brand, and Mehlman
   diphasic m.
transport m.
tunica media

TY1-S-33 m.
TYSGM-9 m.
m. vein
von Apathy gum syrup m.
Weinman m.
Wickersheimer m.
xylene-soluble mounting m.
medium-chain
m.-c. fatty acid (MCFA)
m.-c. triglyceride (MCT)
medium-scale integration
Medlar body
medorrhea
medulla, pl. **medullae**
adrenal m.
m. of adrenal gland
cystic disease of renal m.
m. glandulae suprarenalis
m. of hair shaft
m. of lymph node
microcystic disease of renal m.
m. nodi lymphoidei
m. ossium
m. ossium flava
m. ossium rubra
medullar
medullare
osteoma m.
medullaris
substantia m.
medullary
m. adenocarcinoma
m. carcinoma of breast
m. carcinoma cell
m. carcinoma of thyroid
m. chemoreceptor
m. chromaffinoma
m. cord
m. cystic disease (MCD)
m. ducts of Bellini
m. fibrosarcoma
m. histiocytic reticulosis
m. interstitial cell
m. membrane
m. necrosis
m. ray
m. sarcoma
m. serotonergic network deficiency
m. sheath
m. sinus
m. sponge kidney
m. substance

m. T cell
m. thymoma
m. thyroid carcinoma (MTC)
medullated nerve fiber
medullation
medullization
medulloarthritis
medulloblast
medulloblastoma
desmoplastic m.
melanotic m.
medulloepithelial cell
medulloepithelioma
adult m.
medullomyoblastoma
medusa, pl. **medusae**
M. head
medusae
caput m.
MEF
maximum expiratory flow
MEFR
maximum expiratory flow rate
MEFV
maximum expiratory flow volume
MEG
megakaryocyte
megabladder
megacaryoblast (*var. of* megakaryoblast)
megacaryocyte (*var. of* megakaryocyte)
megacephaly
megacin
Megacollybia
megacolon
aganglionic m.
chronic idiopathic m.
congenital m.
m. congenitum
idiopathic m.
toxic m.
megacycle
megacystic syndrome
megacystis
megadolichocolon
megaelectron volt (MeV)
megaesophagus
megagamete
megahertz (MHz)
megakaryoblast, megacaryoblast
megakaryocyte, megacaryocyte (MEG)
basophilic m.
bizarre m.

M

NOTES

627

megakaryocyte *(continued)*
> colony-forming unit granulocyte, erythrocyte, monocyte, and m. (CFU-GEMM)
> granulocyte, erythrocyte, monocyte, and m. (GEMM)
> m. growth and development factor (MGDF)

megakaryocytic
> m. aplasia
> m. blood cell
> m. emperipolesis
> m. hyperplasia
> m. hypoplasia
> m. leukemia
> m. myelosis
> m. precursor

megakaryocytopoiesis
megakaryopoiesis
megalencephaly, megaloencephaly
megaloblast
> basophilic m.
> orthochromatic m.
> polychromatophilic m.

megaloblastic
> m. anemia
> m. anemia of pregnancy (MAP)
> m. erythropoiesis
> m. hyperplasia

megaloblastoid
megaloblastosis
megalocephaly
megalocystis
megalocyte
megalocythemia
megalocytic anemia
megalocytosis
megaloencephalic leukoencephalopathy
megaloencephalon
megaloencephaly *(var. of* megalencephaly)
megaloenteron
megalogastria
megalohepatia
megalokaryocyte
Megalopyge
megalosplenia
megalospore
megaloureter
megalourethra
megamerozoite
megamitochondria
meganucleus
megapoietin
megarectum
Megaselia
megasigmoid
Megasphaera
megaspore

megastoma
> *Habronema m.*

megaterium
> *Bacillus m.*

megathrombocyte
Megatrichophyton
megaureter
megaurethra
megavolt (MV)
megavoltage
meglumine
megninii
> *Trichophyton m.*

megohm (MΩ)
megoxycyte
megoxyphil, megoxyphile
MEIA
> microparticle capture enzyme immunoassay
> microparticle enzyme immunoassay

meibomian
> m. cyst
> m. gland
> m. stye

meibomitis, meibomianitis
Meige disease
Meigs syndrome
Meinicke
> M. test
> M. turbidity reaction (MTR)

meiocyte
meiosis
meiotic
> m. nondisjunction
> m. phase
> m. recombination

Meissel stain
Meissner
> M. corpuscle
> M. plexus

meissnerian differentiation
MEK
> methyl ethyl ketone

mekongi
> *Schistosoma m.*

Melan-A (MART-1) gene
melanemia
melaniferous phagocyte
melanimon
> *Aedes m.*

melanin
> artificial m.
> m. bleaching method
> factitious m.
> m. pigmentation
> smoky m.
> m. staining method
> m. test

melaninogenica
    Prevotella m.
melaninogenicus
    Bacteroides m.
melanism
melanoacanthoma
melanoameloblastoma
melanoblast
melanoblastoma
melanocarcinoma of anus
melanocortin
melanocyte
    cultured autologous m.
    m. specific MITF (MITF-M)
melanocyte-inhibiting hormone
melanocyte-stimulating
    m.-s. hormone inhibiting factor
    (MIF)
    m.-s. hormone release-inhibiting
    hormone
    m.-s. hormone releasing factor
    (MRF)
    m.-s. hormone releasing hormone
melanocytic
    m. lesion
    m. nevus
melanocytosis
    pagetoid m. (PM)
melanodendrocyte
melanodermatitis
melanodermic
melanogenemia
melanogenesis
melanogen test
melanoglossia
melanoid
Melanoides
melanokeratosis
Melanolestes picipes
melanoleukoderma
melanoma
    acral lentiginous m.
    amelanotic mucosal m.
    anorectal m.
    m. antigen-encoding gene family
    benign juvenile m.
    clinical variant of malignant m.
    Cloudman m.
    cutaneous malignant m. (CMM)
    desmoplastic m.
    epidermotropic metastatic
      malignant m. (EMMM)

    epithelioid cell m.
    halo m.
    Harding-Passey m.
    juvenile m.
    lentigo maligna m.
    malignant lentigo m.
    minimal deviation m.
    mucosal lentiginous m.
    multifocal choroidal m.
    nodular m.
    ocular m.
    oral-sinonasal m.
    m. in situ
    spindle cell m.
    Spitz-like m.
    subungual m.
    superficial spreading m.
    uveal m.
    verrucous m.
melanomatosis
    meningeal m.
melanomatous follicular invasion
Melanomma
melanonychia
melanopathy
melanophage
melanophagocyte
melanophore
melanophore-stimulating hormone (MSH)
melanoplakia
Melanoporia
melanosarcoma
melanosis
    m. circumscripta precancerosa
    m. coli
    m. corii degenerativa
    mucosal m.
    neurocutaneous m.
    oculodermal m.
    peritoneal m.
    precancerous m. of Dubreuilh
    primary acquired m.
    Riehl m.
    vagabond's m.
melanosome
    giant m.
melanotic
    m. ameloblastoma
    m. carcinoma
    m. freckle
    m. medulloblastoma
    m. neuroectodermal tumor

M

NOTES

melanotic *(continued)*
    m. neuroectodermal tumor of infancy
    m. pigment
    m. progonoma
    m. prurigo
    m. schwannoma
    m. stool
    m. whitlow
melanotroph
melanotropic cell
melanura
    Culiseta m.
melanuria
melanuric
MELAS
    mitochondrial encephalopathy, lactic acidosis, and strokelike episodes
    MELAS syndrome
melas
    icterus m.
melasma universale
Melastatin test kit
melatonin
Melchior syndrome
meleagridis
    Amoeba m.
    Histomonas m.
Meleda disease
melena
Meleney
    M. gangrene
    M. ulcer
melicera
meliceris
meliloti
    Ensifer m.
melioidosis
    Whitmore m.
melis
    Isobaculum m.
melitensis
    Brucella m.
melitis
melitose
melituria
    glycosuric m.
    m. inosita
    nondiabetic glycosuric m.
Melkersson-Rosenthal syndrome
Melkersson syndrome
mellis
    Saccharomyces m.
mellitus
    diabetes m.
    insulin-dependent diabetes m. (IDDM)
    noninsulin-dependent diabetes m. (NIDDM)

Melnick-Needles syndrome
Meloidae
Meloidogyne
melonis
    Sphingomonas m.
melon seed body
melophagium
    Trypanosoma m.
Melophagus
melorheostosis
melting
    m. point (MP)
    m. temperature (Tm)
MEM
    minimum essential medium
membrana, pl. **membranae**
    m. adventitia
    m. basalis ductus semicircularis
    m. basilaris
    m. carnosa
    m. choriocapillaris
    m. cordis
    m. decidua
    m. fibrosa capsulae articularis
    m. fusca
    m. granulosa
    m. hyaloidea
    m. limitans
    m. limitans gliae
    m. mucosa
    m. pituitosa
    m. preformativa
    m. propria ductus semicircularis
    m. pupillaris
    m. reticularis organi spiralis
    m. serosa
    m. statoconiorum
    m. synovialis
    m. tectoria ductus cochlearis
    m. tympani
    m. versicolor
    m. vestibularis ductus cochlearis
    m. vitellina
    m. vitrea
membranacea
    placenta m.
membranaceous
membranae (*pl. of* membrana)
membranaefaciens
    Pichia m.
membranate
membrane
    acellular basement m.
    acute inflammatory m.
    acute pyogenic m.
    air bleb m.
    alveolodental m.
    antiglomerular basement m. (anti-GBM)

artificial rupture of m.'s (ARM)
asymmetric unit m.
m. attack complex (MAC)
basement m.
basilar m.
basolateral m.
Bichat m.
m. bone
Bowman m.
Bruch m.
Brunn m.
canalicular m.
m. capacitance
cell m.
circular layer of tympanic m.
Corti m.
croupous m.
cutaneous layer of tympanic m.
cytoplasmic m.
Debove m.
decidual m.
deciduous m.
Descemet m.
diphtheritic m.
drum m.
Duddell m.
elastic m.
enamel m.
epithelial basement m.
erythrocyte m.
false m.
fenestrated m.
Fielding m.
m. filter
m. filter technique
glassy m.
glomerular basement m. (GBM)
Henle fenestrated elastic m.
human mesothelial cell m. (HBME 1)
Hunter m.
Huxley m.
hyaline m.
hyaloid m.
Hybond N+ nylon m.
inflammatory m.
internal elastic m.
lateral cell m.
lipid peroxidation of intracellular m.
medullary m.
mitochondrial m.

mucous m.
Nitabuch m.
nitrocellulose m.
nuclear m.
olfactory m.
osmiophilic cell surface m.
otolithic m.
outer mitochondrial m.
peridental m.
periodontal m.
photoreceptor m. (PRM)
pial-glial m.
pituitary m.
placental m.
plasma m.
postsynaptic m.
m. potential
premature rupture of (fetal) m.'s (PROM)
presynaptic m.
proligerous m.
prolonged rupture of fetal m.'s (PRFM)
prophylactic m.
m. protein
Puchtler-Sweat stain for basement m.'s
pyknotic nucleus with irregular m.
pyogenic m.
radiate layer of tympanic m.
Reissner m.
rupture of m.'s (ROM)
Ruysch m.
schneiderian m.
Schultze m.
semipermeable m.
serous m.
m. sidedness
m. skeleton
spiral m.
statoconial m.
subsurface basement m.
Sure Blot m.
synovial m.
torocyte m.
m. trafficking
m. transport
trophoblastic cell m.
tubular basement m. (TBM)
tympanic m.
m. of tympanum
m. type 1–6

M

NOTES

membrane *(continued)*
    undulating m.
    unit m.
    vaginal synovial m.
    vasculosyncytial m.
    vestibular m.
    vitreous m.
    Volkmann m.
    yolk m.
membrane-bound receptor analysis
membrane-coating granule
membranelle
membraniform
membranocartilaginous
membranoid
membranoproliferative glomerulonephritis (MPGN)
membranous
    m. acute inflammation
    m. cisternae
    m. cochlea
    m. cytoplasmic body (MCB)
    m. deciduitis
    m. glomerulonephritis (MGN)
    m. layer
    m. lupus nephritis
    m. nephropathy
    m. ossification
    m. pattern
    m. pharyngitis
    m. pregnancy
Memnoniella echinata
memory
    m. B, T cell
    cache m.
    core m.
    local skin m.
    magnetic core m.
    m. map
    mass m.
    scratch-pad m.
MEN
    multiple endocrine neoplasia
    MEN syndrome, type 1, 2, 2a, 2b, 3
menadione
menaquinone
Mendel-Bekhterev sign
mendelevium (Md)
mendelian
    m. character
    m. genetics
    m. inheritance
Mendel law
Mendosicutes
Ménétrier
    M. disease
    M. syndrome
Mengert shock syndrome

Menghini needle
Mengo
    M. encephalitis
    M. virus
Ménière
    M. disease
    M. syndrome
menin
meningeal
    m. carcinoma
    m. carcinomatosis
    m. hernia
    m. leukemia
    m. melanomatosis
    m. sarcoma
    m. sarcomatosis
meninges (*pl. of* meninx)
meningioangiomatosis
meningioma
    anaplastic m.
    angiomatous m.
    clear cell m.
    cutaneous m.
    fibroblastic m.
    malignant m.
    Masson humid m.
    meningothelial m.
    mucinous m.
    nonanaplastic invasive m.
    orbital m.
    psammomatous m.
    spinal m.
    suprasellar m.
meningiomatosis
    diffuse m.
meningismus
meningitic streak
meningitidis
    Neisseria m.
meningitis, pl. meningitides
    amebic m.
    anthrax m.
    aseptic m.
    bacterial m.
    basilar m.
    Candida m.
    cerebrospinal m. (CSM)
    cryptococcal m.
    enteroviral m.
    epidemic cerebrospinal m.
    epidural m.
    external m.
    hemorrhagic m.
    internal m.
    leukemic m.
    meningococcal m.
    Mollaret m.
    mycotic m.
    neoplastic m.

occlusive m.
otitic m.
plague m.
pyogenic m.
serous m.
subacute m.
syphilitic m.
torular m.
tuberculous m. (TBM)
viral m.
meningocele
meningocerebral cicatrix
meningocerebritis
meningococcal
m. infection
m. meningitis
meningococcemia
meningococcin
meningococcus, pl. **meningococci**
m. conjunctivitis
m. infection
meningocyte
meningoencephalitis
acute fulminating primary
amebic m.
acute primary hemorrhagic m.
amebic m.
biundulant m.
eosinophilic m.
herpetic m.
mumps m.
primary amebic m.
syphilitic m.
meningoencephalocele
meningoencephalomyelitis
meningoencephalopathy
carcinomatous m.
meningomyelitis
meningomyelocele
meningomyeloradiculitis
Meningonema peruzzii
meningoosteophlebitis
meningoradiculitis
meningosepticum
Chryseobacterium m.
Flavobacterium m.
meningothelial meningioma
meninguria
meninx, pl. **meninges**
meniscal
m. degeneration
m. tear

menisci (*pl. of* meniscus)
meniscitis
meniscocyte
meniscocytosis
meniscus, pl. **menisci**
degenerated m.
tactile m.
m. tactus
Menkes syndrome
menometrorrhagia
menopausal
m. gonadotropin
m. syndrome
menopause
delayed m.
m. home test
Menopon
menorrhagia
menostasis
menstrual
m. colic
m. cycle
m. sclerosis
m. stage
mentagrophytes
Trichophyton m.
Trichophyton m. var. *mentagrophytes*
Mentha
Mentzer MCV index
Menzies method
meperidine hydrochloride
mephenytoin
mephitis
Luteimonas m.
meprobamate assay
mEq
milliequivalent
MER
methanol-extruded residue
merbromin
mercaptan
mercaptoacetic acid
mercaptomerin sodium
mercaptopurine
mercaptopyrazidopyrimidine (MPP)
Mercier
median bar of M.
Merck new fuchsin stain
mercocresol
mercurialism
mercurial thermometer

M

NOTES

mercuric
> m. conjugate
> m. cyanide
> m. fixative

mercurous

mercury (Hg)
> m. assay
> m. cyanide (HgCN)
> inorganic m. (Hg2+)
> methyl m.
> millimeter of m. (mmHg)
> m. poisoning

mercury-wetted relay

Merfiluor DFA *Cryptosporidium/Giardia* detection procedure

meridiana
> *Pseudomonas* m.

meridiei
> *Desulfosporosinus* m.

meridional fiber of ciliary muscle

Meripilus

Merismodes

merispore

meristematic

meristic variation

Merkel
> M. cell tumor
> M. corpuscle
> M. tactile cell
> M. tactile disc

Merkel-Ranvier cell

merlin gene

MERmaid-Spin kit

Mermis nigrescens

mermithid

Mermithidae

Mermithoidea

merocrine gland

merogenesis

merogenetic

merogony
> diploid m.
> parthenogenetic m.

meromelia

meromicrosomia

meront

merorachischisis

merosporangium

merotomy

merozoite antigen

merozygote

mersalyl
> m. exchange assay
> m. exchange method

Merulius

Merzbacher-Pelizaeus disease

MES
> medical equipment set

MESA
> microsurgical epididymal sperm aspiration
> myoepithelial sialadenitis

mesameboid

mesangial
> m. cell
> m. deposit
> m. IgA nephropathy
> m. lupus nephritis
> m. proliferative glomerulonephritis
> m. ring

mesangiocapillary glomerulonephritis

mesangiolysis

mesangioproliferative glomerulonephritis

mesangium
> extraglomerular m.

mesaortitis

mesarteritis

mesaxon

mescal

mescaline

mesectic

mesencephalic reticular formation (MRF)

mesencephalitis

mesenchyma

mesenchymal
> m. cell
> m. chondrosarcoma (MC)
> m. differentiation
> m. epithelium
> m. hamartoma
> m. hyloma
> m. neoplasia
> m. stroma
> m. tissue
> m. tumor

mesenchyme
> myxoid m.
> splanchnic m.

mesenchymoma
> benign m.
> malignant m.

mesenteric
> m. adenitis
> m. fibromatosis
> m. gland
> m. infarction
> m. ischemia
> m. lipodystrophy
> m. lymphadenitis
> m. panniculitis
> m. phlebosclerosis
> m. thrombosis
> m. vascular obstruction

mesenteritis
> idiopathic retractile m. (IRM)

mesenteroides
  Leuconostoc m.
mesenteron
mesentery
MESF
  molecule of equivalent soluble
    fluorochrome
meshwork
  trabecular m.
mesnili
  Chilomastix m.
mesoappendiceal
mesoappendix
mesobacterium
mesoblast
  primitive m.
mesoblastic nephroma
mesocardia
Mesocestoides
  M. corti
  M. variabilis
Mesocestoididae
mesocolic
meso compound
mesocricetorum
  Helicobacter m.
mesodermal bone marrow
mesoderm cell
Mesogastropoda
mesogenic
mesoglia
mesoglial cell
mesolepidoma
mesolimbic dopaminergic system
mesolymphocyte
mesomelia
mesomelic dwarfism
mesometanephric carcinoma
mesometritis
meson
mesonephric
  m. adenocarcinoma
  m. cyst
  m. remnant
  m. remnant hyperplasia
  m. rest
  m. tissue
  m. tubule
mesonephroid tumor
mesonephroma
mesonephros
  glomerulus of m.

mesoneuritis
  nodular m.
mesophaeum
  Hebeloma m.
mesophil, mesophile
mesophila
  Glaciecola m.
mesophilica
  Pseudomonas m.
mesophilic bacterium
mesophilicum
  Methylobacterium m.
mesophilum
  Tenacibaculum m.
mesophilus
  Gelidibacter m.
mesophlebitis
mesophragma
mesosigmoiditis
mesosome
mesothelia (*pl. of* mesothelium)
mesothelial
  m. cell
  m. cyst
  m. hyloma
  m. sarcoma
**mesothelial/monocytic incidental cardiac
  excrescence (MICE)**
mesothelin
mesothelioma
  benign m.
  fibrous m.
  lymphohistiocytoid m. (LHM)
  malignant m.
  m. marker
  pleural m.
  sarcomatoid m.
mesothelium, pl. **mesothelia**
  peritoneal m.
Mesozoa
message
  masked m.
messeae
  Anopheles m.
messenger ribonucleic acid (mRNA)
messinensis
  Oleiphilus m.
mesylate
  deferoxamine m.
  ergoloid m.
MET
  metabolic equivalent

M

NOTES

metabiosis
metabisulfite test
metabolic
    m. acidosis
    m. alkalosis
    m. antagonism
    m. antagonist
    m. bone disease
    m. clearance rate (MCR)
    m. coma
    m. craniopathy
    m. detoxification
    m. disorder
    m. encephalopathy
    m. equivalent (MET)
    m. hypothesis
    m. indican
    m. insufficiency
    m. mucinosis
    m. pathway
    m. pool
    m. stone disease
    m. storage disease
    m. syndrome
metabolism
    aerobic m.
    anaerobic m.
    basal m.
    copper m.
    divalent ion m. (DIM)
    drug m.
    first-pass m.
    glucose m.
    inborn error of vitamin D m.
    intermediary m.
    lipid m.
    propionate m.
metabolite
    cyanohydrin m.
    PredictRx m.'s
    Pro-PredictRx m.
    reactive oxygen m. (ROM)
metabolizable
metacarpal index
metacarpophalangeal (MP)
metacentric
metacercaria
metacestode
metachromasia, metachromasy
    alpha m.
    beta m.
    gamma m.
metachromatic
    m. body
    m. dye
    m. granule
    m. leukodystrophy (MLD)
    m. stain
    m. stain test

metachromatic-type leukodystrophy
metachromatism
metachroming
metachromophil, metachromophile
metachronal rhythm
metachronous
    m. collagenous colitis
    m. seeding
metachrosis
metacryptozoite
metagenesis
metagglutinin
metaglobulin
metagonimiasis
Metagonimus
    M. ovatus
    M. yokogawai
metal
    alkali m.
    alkaline earth m.
    m. fume fever
    heavy m.
    m. oxide semiconductor field effect
      transistor
    m. sol
metal-catalyzed pseudoperoxidation
metaldehyde
metallic
    m. bond
    m. foreign body (MFB)
    m. thermometer
metallicus
    Nocardiopsis m.
metallidurans
    Ralstonia m.
    Wautersia m.
metallireducens
    Desulfitobacterium m.
metalloenzyme
metalloflavoprotein
metallophil cell
metallophilia
metalloprotease
    a disintegrin and m. (ADAM)
metalloprotein
metalloproteinase
    m. 1
    matrix m. (MMP)
    matrix m. 1 (MMP 1)
    matrix m. 2 (MMP 2)
    tissue inhibitor of m. (TIMP)
metalloscopy
metallothionein concentrate
metal-to-metal contact
metamere
metameric
metamerism
metamorphosis, pl. metamorphoses
    fatty m.

retrograde m.
syringomatous m.
metamyelocyte
  basophilic m.
  eosinophilic m.
  neutrophilic m.
metanephric
  m. adenoma
  m. adenosarcoma
  m. stromal tumor
  m. tubule
metanephrine
  m. assay
  m. test
  urine m.
metanephrogenic tissue
metaneutrophil, metaneutrophile
metaniline, metanil
  metaniline yellow
metaphase
  m. cell
  m. chromosome
  m. plate
metaphosphate
  potassium m.
metaphosphoric acid
metaphysial, metaphyseal
  m. dysostosis
  m. dysplasia
metaphysis, pl. metaphyses
metaphysitis
metaplasia
  agnogenic myeloid m.
  apocrine m.
  atypical squamous m. (ASM)
  autoparenchymatous m.
  Barrett m.
  bronchiolar m.
  cardia intestinal m. (CIM)
  cartilaginous m.
  celomic m.
  chondroid m.
  ciliated m.
  columnar m.
  decidual m.
  embryonal m.
  endothelial m.
  eosinophilic cell m.
  epidermoid m.
  glandular m.
  hobnail cell m.
  Hürthle cell m.

intestinal m. (IM)
myelofibrosis with myeloid m.
  (MMM)
myeloid m. (MM)
myelosclerosis with myeloid m.
oncocytic m.
osseous m.
pancreatic acinar m.
Paneth cell m.
primary myeloid m.
pseudopyloric m.
pyloric gland m.
secondary myeloid m.
smooth muscle m.
squamous m.
squamous m. of amnion
symptomatic myeloid m.
tuboendometrioid m.
metaplasis
metaplasm
metaplastic
  m. anemia
  m. carcinoma
  m. cell
  m. columnar epithelium
  m. keratinization
  m. ossification
  m. polyp
Metapneumovirus
metapyrone
Metarhizium
metarubricyte
  pernicious anemia-type m.
metastable state
metastasis, pl. metastases (mets)
  biochemical m.
  calcareous m.
  contralateral axillary m.
  distal m.
  distant organ m.
  hematogenous m.
  lymph node m. (LN-met)
  lymphogenous m.
  no evidence of distant metastases
  (M0)
  occult m.
  pathologic tumor-node m. (pTNM)
  pulsating m.
  satellite m.
  skip m.
metastasis-free survival
metastasize

M

NOTES

metastatic
- m. abscess
- m. bone survey
- m. calcification
- m. carcinoid syndrome
- m. carcinoma
- m. cascade
- m. cluster
- m. focus
- m. hepatocellular carcinoma (HCC)
- m. mumps
- m. neoplasm
- m. pain
- m. panniculitis
- m. pneumonia
- m. thermometer
- m. tumor

metastrongyle
Metastrongylus
- M. apri
- M. elongatus

metatroph
metatrophic
metatropic
metatypical carcinoma
metavinculin
Metavirus
metaxeny (*var. of* metoxeny)
Metazoa
metazoan parasite
metazoonosis
Metchnikoff theory
met-enkephalin
meteori
- *Agrobacterium m.*

meteorism
meter (m)
- φ 340, 350, 360, 390 benchtop pH/ISE m.
- count rate m.
- d'Arsonval m.
- φ 240, 250, 260 handheld pH/ISE m.
- φ 255, 265, 295 handheld waterproof pH/ISE m.
- HemoSite hemoglobin m.
- φ 660, 690 high-performance pH/ISE m.
- neutron m.
- oxygen saturation m. (OSM)
- pH m.
- rate m.
- survey m.

meter-kilogram-second (MKS)
- m.-k.-s. system
- m.-k.-s. unit

MeterPlus
- Triage M.

methacrylate
- butyl m.
- glycol m.
- m. resin

methacycline
methadone
- m. assay
- m. hydrochloride

methallenestril
methamphetamine hydrochloride
methanal
methandrostenolone
methane
Methanobacteria
Methanobacteriaceae
Methanobacteriales
Methanobacterium
Methanocaldococcaceae
Methanococcaceae
Methanococcales
Methanococci
Methanococcus
Methanocorpusculaceae
methanol
- m. assay
- m. fixative
- m. intoxication
- m. poisoning
- m. test

methanol-extruded residue (MER)
methanolica
- *Pseudomonas m.*

Methanomicrobiaceae
Methanomicrobiales
Methanoplanaceae
Methanopyraceae
Methanopyrales
Methanopyri
Methanosaetaceae
Methanosarcinaceae
Methanosarcinales
Methanospirillaceae
Methanothermaceae
Methanothermea
methaqualone assay
metHb
- methemoglobin

methemalbumin (MHA)
- m. assay

methemalbuminemia
methemalbuminuria
methemoglobin (metHb)
- m. reductase
- stroma-free m.

methemoglobinemia
- acquired m.
- congenital m.
- enterogenous m.
- hereditary enzymatic-type m.

primary m.
secondary m.
toxic m.
methemoglobinuria
methenamine
   m. hippurate
   m. mandelate
   periodic acid-silver m. (PAM, PASM)
   m. silver
   m. silver stain
methicillin and aminoglycoside-resistant *Staphylococcus aureus* (MARSA)
methicillin-resistant
   m.-r. coagulase-negative *Staphylococcus* (MRCNS)
   m.-r. *Staphylococcus aureus* (MRSA)
methicillin-susceptible
   m.-s. coagulase-negative *Staphylococcus* (MSCNS)
   m.-s. *Staphylococcus aureus* (MSSA)
methimazole
methine dye
methionine
   m. malabsorption syndrome
   N-formyl m.
   m. synthase
   m. test
methionyl
methionyl-RNA synthetase
methisazone
methocycline
method
   ABC staining m.
   Abell-Kendall m.
   AccuProbe m.
   acid anhydride m.
   acid-fast staining m.
   acridine orange m.
   aequorin recombinant m.
   agar diffusion m.
   AgNOR m.
   alkaline phosphatase m.
   Altmann-Gersh m.
   AMeX processing and embedding m.
   amidohydrolase m.
   analytic m.
   antialkaline phosphatase m.
   Ashby differential agglutination m.

Astrup m.
axon staining m.
Ayoub-Shklar m.
bacterial agar m.
bacterial antigen detection m.
Baker Sudan black m.
Bang m.
Barnett-Bourne acetic alcohol-silver nitrate method
Barrnett-Seligman dihydroxydinaphthyl disulfide m.
Barrnett-Seligman indoxyl esterase m.
Barroso-Moguel and Costero silver m.
Baumgartner m.
Beaver direct smear m.
Bence Jones protein m.
bench m.
Benedict m.
Bengston m.
Bennett sulfhydryl m.
Bennhold Congo red m.
Bensley aniline-acid fuchsin-methyl green m.
benzo sky blue m.
Berg chelate removal m.
bicinchoninic acid m. (BCA)
Bielschowsky m.
Billheimer m.
bioluminescent m.
biotin-streptavidin-alkaline phosphatase m.
biotin-streptavidin detection m.
biotin-streptavidin-peroxidase m.
black periodic acid m.
Bloch m.
Bodian m.
Borchgrevink m.
Born m.
bread-loaf m.
Brecher-Cronkite m.
Breen and Tullis m.
Cajal gold sublimate m.
Cajal uranium silver m.
Caldwell-Moloy m.
Camp-Gianturco m.
Caraway m.
carbolfuchsin-methylene blue staining m.
cellophane tape m.
cell separation m.

M

NOTES

method *(continued)*

Chang aniline-acid fuchsin m.
Chiffelle and Putt m.
chloranilate m.
chloride m.
cholesterol staining m.
chromate m.
chrome alum hematoxylin-
  phloxine m.
chromolytic m.
Ciaccio m.
Clark-Collip m.
clean-catch collection m.
m. of Cleary
cobaltinitrite m.
Coblentz test m.
Colcher-Sussman m.
collagen staining m.
m. of collection not indicated
  (MOCNI)
constitutive heterochromatin m.
cooled-knife m.
copper sulfate m.
Craigie tube m.
Credé m.
Crippa lead tetraacetate m.
cysteic acid m.
Dacie m.
Dale-Laidlaw clotting time m.
Dane m.
definitive m.
diazo staining m.
Dick m.
Dieterle m.
diffusion m.
digitonin m.
dilute blood clot lysis m.
disc sensitivity m.
double antibody m.
Duke m.
dyed starch method
enzymatic digestion m.
enzyme demonstration m.
esterase staining m.
Fahey and McKelvey m.
fibrin degradation product m.
fibrinogen m.
field m.
Fite m.
fixed sediment m.
fixed-time m.
flat substrate m.
Folin and Wu m.
Fontana-Masson staining m.
Foot reticulin m.
formaldehyde-induced
  fluorescence m.
formalin-ether sedimentation m.
freeze-cleave m.

freeze-etch m.
freeze-fracture-etch m.
frozen section m.
FW m.
Gallyas m.
Gerota m.
Giemsa m.
Girard m.
glass-bead retention m.
glucose oxidase m.
glycerin m.
GPO-DAOS m.
gram m.
Granger m.
Grimelius argyrophil stain m.
Grocott-Gomori methenamine
  silver m.
guanidine isothiocyanate m.
Hall m.
Hammerschlag m.
Harris staining m.
Heublein m.
heuristic m.
hexokinase m.
Highman m.
Histofine staining m.
Holmes m.
Holzer m.
H.P. Wright m.
HSU m.
IgG index m.
immunofluorescence m.
immunoperoxidase staining m.
India ink m.
indophenol m.
Ivy m.
Jacobsson m.
Jendrassik-Grof m.
Jenner m.
Jones m.
Kaiserling m.
Kaplan-Meier staining m.
Kety-Schmidt m.
Kirby-Bauer m.
Kjeldahl m.
Klump and Bieth m.
Lee-White clotting time m.
leukocyte alkaline phosphatase m.
Levaditi m.
Lillie allochrome m.
Lison-Dunn m.
MacFarlane serum m.
macro-Kjeldahl m.
Mancini m.
Mantel-Cox m.
Marshall m.
Masson-Fontana m.
Masson trichrome m.
melanin bleaching m.

melanin staining m.
Menzies m.
mersalyl exchange m.
micro-Astrup m.
micro-Kjeldahl m.
Miles-Misra m.
Millipore m.
ModAMeX section m.
Monte Carlo m.
Movat pentachrome m.
myelin staining m.
myoglobin identification m.
Nichols m.
Nikiforoff m.
Nuclepore m.
Ouchterlony m.
PAM m.
Pap m.
Pembrey m.
Penfield m.
periodic acid-Schiff m.
peroxidase staining m.
Pfeiffer-Comberg m.
Pisano m.
Pizzolato peroxide-silver m.
plasma thrombin clot m.
Ploton staining m.
point counting m.
polyvinyl alcohol fixative m.
protein separation m.
Puchtler alkaline Congo red m.
Puchtler Sirius red m.
push-wedge m.
PVA fixative m.
Quicgel m.
Quick m.
Rees-Ecker m.
reference m.
Rideal-Walker m.
RNAzol B RNA extraction m.
Sahli m.
Salzman m.
Sanger DNA sequencing m.
Schick m.
Scotch tape m.
SEM freeze-fracture m.
SEREX m.
Shaffer-Hartmann m.
Sheather sugar flotation m.
m. of Shiiki
solochrome azurine staining m.

Somogyi m.
special reference m.
Stovall-Black m.
streptavidin-biotin peroxidase m.
suction m.
Sweet m.
template bleeding time m.
thermodilution m.
Thoms m.
Tietz-Fiereck m.
two-slide m.
ultropaque m.
Van Slyke and Cullen m.
von Clauss m.
von Kossa m.
Warthin-Starry m.
Welker m.
Whipple m.
Wilson m.
Wintrobe and Landsberg m.
Wintrobe sedimentation rate m.
Ziehl-Neelsen m.
zinc sulfate flotation m.
ZSR m.
methodology
suicide m.
methotrexate
m. poisoning
methoxy-4-hydroxymandelic acid test
methoxychlor
methoxyhydroxymandelic acid (MOMA)
methyl
m. acetate
m. alcohol poisoning
m. aldehyde
m. blue
m. bromide
m. butyl ketone
m. chloroform
m. demeton
m. ethyl ketone (MEK)
m. green
m. green-pyronin stain
m. isobutyl ketone
m. mercury
m. orange
m. parathion
m. red (MR)
m. red test
m. red, Voges-Proskauer (MR-VP)
m. red, Voges-Proskauer broth

NOTES

methyl *(continued)*
    m. violet
    m. yellow
methylarachidonyl fluorophosphonate (MAFP)
methylation pattern diversity
methylbenzene
methylbromide
    homatropine m. (HMB)
methylbutane fixative/solution
3-methylcrotonylglycinuria
methylcytosine
5-methylcytosine (5-MeC)
methyldichloroarsine
methyldopa
    alpha m.
methylene
    m. azure
    m. blue (MB)
    m. blue active substance (MBAS)
    m. blue dye (MBD)
    m. blue test
    m. chloride
    m. dichloride
    m. violet
    m. white
methylenedioxyamphetamine (MDA)
3,4-methylenedioxyamphetamine assay
methylenedioxymethamphetamine (MDMA)
methylenetetrahydrofolate reductase (MTHFR)
methylenophil, methylenophile
methylenophilic
methylenophilous
methylisobutylketone
methylmalonic
    m. acid
    m. acidemia
    m. aciduria
methylmalonyl-CoA decarboxylase
methylmercaptan
methylmorphine
methylnitrosourea
Methylobacterium
    M. fujisawaense
    M. mesophilicum
    M. organophilum
    M. radiotolerans
    M. rhodesianum
    M. rhodinum
    M. zatmanii
Methylococcaceae
methylohalidivorans
    Leisingera m.
methylotrophus
    Arthrobacter m.
methylovorans
    Albibacter m.

methylparaben
methylphenylethylhydantoin (MPEH)
1-methyl-4-phenyl-1,2,3,6-tetrahydropyridine (MPTP)
methylphosphonofluoridate
    NATO code for nerve agent cyclohexyl m. (GF)
methylphosphonothioate
    NATO code for nerve agent O-ethyl S-[2-(diethylamino)ethyl] m. (VM)
5-methylresorcinol
methylrosaniline chloride
methyltetrahydrofolate
methylthymol blue
methyltransferase
    tetrahydropteroylglutamate m.
4-methylumbelliferyl phosphate (MUP)
methyprylon assay
metMb
    metmyoglobin
metmyoglobin (metMb)
Metopirone test
Metopium
Metorchis
metoxenous
metoxeny, metaxeny
metraterm
metratrophia
metratrophy
metria
metric
    m. data
    m. system
metritis
metrocyte
metrofibroma
metrolymphangitis
metromalacia
metromalacoma
metromalacosis
metronidazole assay
metroperitoneal fistula
metroperitonitis
metropolitan medical response system (MMRS)
metrorrhagia
metrosalpingitis
metrotrophic test
mets
    metastasis
metschnikovii
    Vibrio m.
Metschnikowia
Mett, Mette
    M. test tube
    M. unit
metyrapone stimulation test

MeV
  megaelectron volt
  million electron volts
mevalonate
mevinphos
Mexican
  M. hat cell
  M. hat corpuscle
mexicana
  Actinomadura m.
  Leishmania mexicana m.
  Leishmania tropica m.
  Petrotoga m.
mexicanus
  Desulfovibrio m.
  Paragonimus m.
  Streptomyces m.
Mexico
  albumin M.
mexiletine
Meyenburg
  M. complex
  M. disease
Meyenburg-Altherr-Uehlinger syndrome
meyerae
  Actinomadura m.
Meyer-Betz syndrome
Meyer disease
Meyer-Schwickerath and Weyers syndrome
Meynert
  M. cell
  M. layer
Meynet node
MF
  medium frequency
  mycosis fungoides
  myelin figure
mF
  millifarad
M'Fadyean stain
MFB
  metallic foreign body
MFH
  malignant fibrous histiocytoma
MFO system
MF/SS
  mycosis fungoides/Sézary syndrome
Mg
  magnesium
  Mg agglutinin

Mg2+
  magnesium ion
mg
  milligram
MGAB
  mucous gland adenoma of bronchus
MGC
  multinucleated giant cell
MGCT
  malignant giant cell tumor
  mixed germ cell tumor
MGDF
  megakaryocyte growth and development factor
mg/dL
  milligram per deciliter
MGH
  microglandular hyperplasia
mg/h
  milligram per hour
MG-intermedius
MGIT
  mycobacteria growth indicator tube
    Bactec MGIT 960
mg/L
  milligram per liter
MGN
  membranous glomerulonephritis
MgO
  magnesium oxide
    MgO nanoparticle
MGP
  marginal granulocyte pool
MGUS
  monoclonal gammopathy of undetermined significance
  monoclonal gammopathy of unknown significance
mH
  millihenry
MHA
  major histocompatibility antigen
  methemalbumin
  microangiopathic hemolytic anemia
  microhemagglutination assay
  mixed hemadsorption
MHA-TP
  microhemagglutination assay-*Treponema pallidum*
    MHA-TP test
MHC
  major histocompatibility complex

M

NOTES

MHC *(continued)*
    MHC I/calreticulin complex
    MHC restriction
MHD
    mean hemolytic dose
    minimum hemolytic dose
MHN
    massive hepatic necrosis
MHz
    megahertz
MI
    myocardial infarction
Mi-2 antigen
MIB1
    MIB1 antibody
    MIB1 antigen
    MIB1 cell proliferation marker
    MIB1 nuclear immunostain
MIBB
    minimally invasive breast biopsy
Mibelli
    M. angiokeratoma
    M. disease
    M. porokeratosis
MIC
    minimal inhibitory concentration
    minimal isorrheic concentration
    minimum inhibitory concentration
MIC2
    MIC2 antibody
    MIC2 oncogene
MICA
    mirror-image complementary antibody
micaceous
mica pneumoconiosis
micdadei
    Legionella m.
MICE
    mesothelial/monocytic incidental cardiac excrescence
mice (*pl. of* mouse)
micelle
    ferruginous m.
Michaelis-Gutmann body
Michaelis-Menten equation
Michel deformity
Micral
    M. chemstrip
    M. urine dipstick test
micranatomy
micrencephalous
micrencephaly, micrencephalia
microabscess
    intervillous m.
    Munro m.
    Pautrier m.
microabsorption spectroscopy
microacinar architectural pattern
microadenoma

microaerophila
    Thioalkalispira m.
microaerophile
microaerophilic streptococcus
microaerophilum
    Propionibacterium m.
microaggregate filter
MicroALB
    Icon M.
microalbinuria
microalbumin
    m. immunoturbidimetric assay
    m. test
microalbuminuria
microaleuriospore
microammeter
microampere
microanalysis
    energy dispersive x-ray m.
microanalytical EDS analysis
microanatomic
microanatomist
microanatomy
microaneurysm
    retinal m.
microangiopathic
    m. hemolytic
    m. hemolytic anemia (MAHA, MHA)
microangiopathy
    diabetic m.
    thrombotic m. (TMA)
microangioscopy
Microanthomyces alpinus
microarray
    Affymetrix U133A oligonucleotide m.
    DNA m.
    m. expression profiling assay
Microascus trigonosporus
micro-Astrup method
Microbacteriaceae
Microbacterium
Microbank cryopreservative
microbar (μbar)
microbe
microbeam
    P.A.L.M. ultraviolet laser m.
microbial
    m. antagonism
    m. associate
    m. genetics
    m. persistence
    m. variation
    m. vitamin
microbic dissociation
microbicidal
microbicide
microbid

Microbilharzia variglandis
microbioassay
microbiological assay (MB)
microbiologic assay
microbiologist
    National Registry of M.'s
microbiology
    m. automation
    m. identification system
microbiotic
microbism
    latent m.
microblast
microbody
microbore test
Microbotryum
microbroth
microburet
microcalcification
    mammographic m.
microcapillary bed
microcarcinoma (MCA)
microcell
microcentrifuge
    Microfuge 18 m.
    Microfuge 22R refrigerated m.
    MicroPrep 2 m.
microcentrum
microcephaly
    encephaloclastic m.
    schizencephalic m.
microchemical balance
microchemistry
microchimerism
MicroChisel
    Eppendorf M.
microchromosome
Micrococcaceae
Micrococcales
Micrococceae
micrococci (*pl. of* micrococcus)
Micrococcineae
Micrococcus
    M. conglomeratus
    M. luteus
    M. varians
micrococcus, pl. micrococci
microcolitis
microcolony

microcolumn chromatography
micro(computerized)tomography
  (microCT)
microconidium, pl. microconidia
microcoulomb
microcrypt
    atrophic m.
microcrystalline
microCT
    micro(computerized)tomography
microcurie (μCi)
microcurie-hour (μCi/hr)
microcyst
microcystic disease of renal medulla
Microcystis aeruginosa
microcyte
microcythemia
microcytic
    m. erythrocyte
    m. hypochromic anemia
microcytosis
microdeletion syndrome
microdensitometer
microdeposit
microdiffusion analysis
microdissected chief cell
microdissection
    laser capture m.
MicroDissector
    Eppendorf M.
microdochectomy
Microdochium
microdrepanocytic
    m. anemia
    m. disease
microdrepanocytosis
microdysgenesia
microelectrophoresis
microenvironment
microerythrocyte
microevolution
microfarad (μF)
microfibril
microfilament
    intracytoplasmic m.
    subplasmalemmal m.
microfilaremia
microfilaria, pl. microfilariae
    Brugia microfilariae
    m. diurna
    m. malaya
    sheathed m.

M

NOTES

microfilariasis
microflora
Microflow test
microfluorodensitometry
microfold cell
microfollicular
    m. adenoma
    m. goiter
    m. pattern
Microfuge
    M. 18 microcentrifuge
    M. 22R refrigerated microcentrifuge
microfuge tube
microgamete
microgametocyte
microgamont
microgamy
microglandular
    m. adenosis
    m. hyperplasia (MGH)
    m. pattern
microglia
    activated m.
    m. cell
microgliacyte
microglial
    m. cell
    m. nodule
microglioma
microgliomatosis
microgliosis
microglobulin
    beta-2 m.
    serum beta-2 m.
microglossia
micrognathia with peromelia
microgram (mcg)
micrograph
    acoustic m.
    electron m.
    light m.
    scanning electron m. (SEM)
micrography
microgyria
microhemagglutination
    m. assay (MHA)
    m. assay-*Treponema pallidum*
    (MHA-TP)
microhemagglutination-*Treponema*
    m.-*T.* pallidum **test**
microhematocrit
    m. centrifugation
    m. concentration
microhenry (μH)
microhistology
microhm (μω)
microhomology
microimmunofluorescence test
microincineration

microincinerator
microinfarct
microinjection
    piezo-actuated m.
microinjector
microinvasion
microinvasive carcinoma
microiontophoretically applied
micro-Kjeldahl method
microlesion
microleukoblast
microliter (μL)
microlith
microlithiasis
    pulmonary alveolar m. (PAM)
micrology
microlymphocytotoxicity
    m. assay
    double-fluorescence m.
    m. test
micromanipulation
micromanipulator
micromati
    Flavobacterium m.
micromelia
micromelica
    rachitis fetalis m.
micromelic dwarfism
micromerozoite
micrometastasis
    carcinomatous m.
micrometastatic
    m. disease
    m. vascular deposit
micrometer (μm)
    caliper m.
    filar m.
    ocular m.
    slide m.
micromethod
    buffy coat m.
micrometry
micromillimeter (μmm)
micromolar concentration
micromole
Micromonosporaceae
Micromonospora purpurea
Micromonosporineae
micromyeloblast
micromyeloblastic leukemia
micron (μ)
microneedle
Micronema
microneme
micronodularity
    regenerative m.
micronodular stromal endometriosis
micronucleus

microorganism
micropapillary component (MPC)
micropapilloma
microparasite
microparticle
    m. capture enzyme immunoassay
     (MEIA)
    m. enzyme immunoassay (MEIA)
    procoagulant platelet-derived m.
microparticulate
micropathology
microphage
microphagocyte
microphotograph
microphthalmia-associated transcription
  factor (MITF)
micropinocytosis
micropinocytotic vesicle
micropipette, micropipet
microplania
microplasia
microplethysmography
micropolygyria
Micropolyspora faeni
micropore filter technique
microprecipitation test
micropredation
micropredator
MicroPrep 2 microcentrifuge
microprobe
    electron m.
    laser m.
    Raman m.
microprocessor
microprogram
microprolactinoma
    pituitary m.
micropromyelocyte
microprotein
micropyle
microrefractometer
microRNA molecule
microroentgen
micros
    Peptostreptococcus m.
microsatellite
    m. analysis
    m. instability (MIN)
    m. locus
    m. marker
    m. polymorphism

microscope
    acoustic m.
    analytical electron m. (AEM)
    beta ray m.
    BHTU m.
    binocular m.
    capillary m.
    cellular debris centrifuge
     polarizing m.
    centrifuge m.
    color-contrast m.
    comparator m.
    comparison m.
    compound m.
    dark-field m.
    dark-ground m.
    dissecting m.
    electron m. (EM)
    fluorescence m.
    fluorescent m.
    flying spot m.
    hypodermic m.
    infrared m.
    integrating m.
    interference m.
    ion m.
    JEM-100CX electron m.
    Jeol 100 S transmission
     electron m.
    Jeol 1200 transmission electron m.
    Labophot-2 m.
    laser m.
    light m.
    Nomarski m.
    Olympus BH2 m.
    opaque m.
    phase m.
    phase-contrast m.
    Philips 301 electron m.
    polarizing m.
    projection x-ray m.
    reflecting m.
    Rheinberg m.
    scanning electron m. (SEM)
    schlieren m.
    simple m.
    stereoscopic m.
    stroboscopic m.
    television m.
    transmission electron m. (TEM)
    trinocular m.
    ultrasonic m.

NOTES

M

microscope *(continued)*
    ultraviolet m.
    x-ray m.
    Zeiss Axiophot fluorescent m.
    Zeiss Axioplan m.
    Zeiss Axioskop m.
    Zeiss LSM-10 laser m.
    Zeiss transmission electron m.

microscopic
    m. agglutination
    m. anatomy
    m. appearance
    m. colitis
    m. examination of cerebrospinal fluid
    m. examination of stool
    m. field
    filter paper m. (FPM)
    m. hematuria
    m. infarct
    m. inflammatory infiltrate
    m. polyangiitis
    m. section
    m. thymoma

microscopy
    atomic force m. (AFM)
    bright-field m.
    clinical m.
    confocal m.
    confocal laser scan m. (CLSM)
    cryoelectron m.
    dark-field m.
    deconvolution fluorescence m.
    electron m. (EM)
    epifluorescence m.
    FLM m.
    fluorescence m.
    fluorescent m.
    immersion m.
    immune electron m. (IEM)
    immunofluorescence m.
    immunogold electron m.
    interference-contrast m. (ICM)
    intravital m.
    laser confocal m.
    laser-scanning confocal m.
    light m. (LM)
    low-voltage high-resolution scanning electron m. (LV-HRSEM)
    phase-contrast m.
    polarized m.
    scanning electron m. (SEM)
    scanning probe m. (SPM)
    scanning transmission electron m.
    scanning tunneling m. (STM)
    transmission electron m. (TEM)
    urine m.
    video time-lapse m.
    widefield capillary m.

microsecond (μs)
microsection
microslide
microsomal
    m. enzyme
    m. enzyme system
    liver kidney m. (LKM)
    m. thyroid antibody
    m. thyroid antibody test

microsome
microspectrophotometry
microspectroscope
microspectroscopy
    Fourier transform infrared m. (FTIR)

Microsphaeraceae
Microsphaeropsis
microsphere
    aggregated m.
    FocalCheck m.
    trisacryl gelatin m.

microspherocyte
microspherocytosis
microsplanchnic
microsplenia
Microspora
Microsporasida
microspore
Microsporida
microsporidian
microsporidiasis
microsporidiosis
Microsporidium
microsporon
    Audouin m.

microsporosis
Microsporum
    M. audouinii
    M. canis
    M. canis var. *distortum*
    M. felineum
    M. ferrugineum
    M. fulvum
    M. furfur
    M. gallinae
    M. gypseum
    M. lanosum
    M. nanum
    M. persicolor
    M. vanbreuseghemi

microsteatosis
microstoma
    Habronema m.

microstomia
microsyringe
Microtatobiotes
microtear

microthrombocytopenia
   X-linked m.
microthrombus, pl. **microthrombi**
microti
   Babesia m.
   Mycobacterium m.
   Mycoplasma m.
microtiter plate
microtome
   cold m.
   freezing m.
   m. knife
   Leica VT1000 E fully
      automatic m.
   Leica VT1000 M semi-
      automatic m.
   rocker m.
   rocking m.
   rotary m.
   sliding m.
   Stadie-Riggs m.
microtomization
microtomy
microtonometer
microtoxicity assay
Microtrombidium
microtubule
   axon containing m.
   m. in cilia
   intracisternal m.
microtubule-associated protein (MAP)
Microtus
microunit
microvascular
microvenular hemangioma
microvesicle
microvesicular
microvessel
   decidual m.
   m. density (MVD)
microvillus, pl. **microvilli**
   brush-border m.
   m. inclusion disease
   m. lymphoma
   stubby m.
Microviridae
Microvirus
microvivisection
microvolt (μV)
microwatt (μW)
microwave fixation
microxyphil

microzoon
micrurgical
Micrurus
MID
   maximum inhibiting dilution
   minimal infecting dose
   minimum infective dose
Midas II automated stainer
midbody
midbrain
   red nucleus of m.
midcarpal
midcervical region
middle
   m. cell
   m. ear adenoma
   m. lobe syndrome
   m. molecule
   m. piece
   m. piece of spermatozoon
Middlebrook
   M. agar
   M. broth
Middlebrook-Dubos hemagglutination test
midge
midget bipolar cell
midkine protein
midline
   m. lethal granuloma
   m. malignant reticulosis granuloma
   m. shift
midstream urinalysis
midterminal spore
midthoracic region
midzonal necrosis
Mielke bleeding time
Miescher
   M. elastoma
   M. granulomatosis
   M. syndrome
miescheriana
   Sarcocystis m.
MIF
   macrophage inhibiting factor
   maximum inspiratory flow
   melanocyte-stimulating hormone
      inhibiting factor
   migration inhibition factor
   mixed immunofluorescence
   MIF test

M

NOTES

MIFC
  minimally invasive follicular carcinoma
MIFR
  maximal inspiratory flow rate
migraine
  familial hemiplegic m. (FMH)
migrans
  Agamonematodum m.
  cutaneous larva m.
  erythema m. (EM)
  larva m.
  ocular larva m.
  spiruroid larva m.
  thrombophlebitis m.
  visceral larva m.
migrating
  m. abscess
  m. bullet
  m. thrombophlebitis
migration
  m. inhibition factor (MIF)
  m. inhibition test
migration-inhibitory
  m.-i. factor
  m.-i. factor test
migratory
  m. cell
  m. pneumonia
  m. polyarthritis
Mikulicz
  M. cell
  M. disease
  M. syndrome
mild silver protein
Miles-Misra method
milia (*pl. of* milium)
miliaria
  apocrine m.
  m. profunda
  m. rubra
  sebaceous m.
miliary
  m. abscess
  m. aneurysm
  m. embolism
  m. fever
  m. granulomatous inflammation
  m. tuberculosis
milieu interieur
military
  m. nerve agent
  m. operation
milium, pl. **milia**
  colloid m.
  m. cyst
milk
  acidophilus m.
  m. anemia

m. cyst
m. duct
m. factor
m. gland
lactobacillary m.
m. leg
m. spot
milk-alkali syndrome
milker's
  m. nodes
  m. nodule
  m. nodule virus
Milkman syndrome
milkpox
milky
  m. ascites
  m. spot
  m. urine
mill
  Retsch MM200 mixer m.
Millard-Gubler
  M.-G. paralysis
  M.-G. syndrome
Miller-Dieker syndrome
Miller ocular disc
miller's asthma
Millex-GS plasma filter
milliamperage
milliampere (mA)
milliampere-second (mA-s)
millibar (mbar)
millicoulomb (mC)
millicurie (mCi)
millicurie-hour (mCi-hr)
milliequivalent (mEq)
millifarad (mF)
Milligan trichrome stain
milligram (mg)
  m. hour
  m. percent
  m. per deciliter (mg/dL)
  m. per hour (mg/h)
  m. per liter (mg/L)
millihenry (mH)
millijoule (mJ)
millikatal (mkat)
millilambert
milliliter (mL)
millimeter
  cubic m. (cmm, cu mm, mm^3)
  m. of mercury (mmHg)
millimicrocurie (mμc)
millimicrogram (mμg)
millimicron (mμ)
millimolar
millimole (mmol)
  m. per liter (mmol/L)
millinormal (mN)

million
    m. electron volts (MeV)
    parts per m. (ppm)
milliosmole (mOsm)
millipede
Millipore
    M. filter
    M. filtration
    M. method
millirad (mrad)
millirem (mrem)
milliroentgen (mR)
millisecond (ms, msec)
milliunit (mU)
millivolt (mV)
milliwatt (mW)
Millonig
    M. phosphate buffer
    M. phosphate-buffered formalin
    fixative
Millon-Nasse test
Millon reagent
Mills disease
Mills-Reincke phenomenon
milnei
    Culicoides m.
milosensis
    Filobacillus m.
Milroy disease
Miltenberger antigen
Milton disease
Mima polymorpha
mimicus
    Vibrio m.
MIN
    microsatellite instability
Minamata disease
minatitlanensis
    Bosea m.
mindensis
    Lactobacillus m.
mineral
    m. crystal
    m. nutrient
    m. oil aspiration
    m. oil foreign body
    m. oil granuloma
    ultrastructural morphology of
    bone m.
mineralization
mineralocorticoid
    m. deficiency

    m. hypertension
    m. receptor
miner's
    m. asthma
    m. lung
mini
    m. Hype-Wipe bleach towelette
    m. scissors
miniature scarlet fever
miniblock
    paraffin m.
minicell
minichromosome
    m. maintenance
    m. maintenance protein
minima
    Taenia m.
minimal
    m. bactercidal level (MBL)
    m. bactericidal concentration (MBC)
    m. brain damage (MBD)
    m. brain dysfunction (MBD)
    m. deviation melanoma
    m. erythema dose (MED)
    m. growth temperature
    m. hemolytic unit
    m. infecting dose (MID)
    m. inhibitory concentration (MIC)
    m. isorrheic concentration (MIC)
    m. lethal concentration
    m. lethal dose
    m. morbidostatic dose (MMD)
    m. reacting dose (MRD)
    m. residual disease (MRD)
    triage m.
minimal-change
    m.-c. disease
    m.-c. nephrotic syndrome
minimally
minimum
    m. bactericidal concentration
    m. bactericidal concentration test
    m. complete-killing concentration
    (MCC)
    m. concentration of bilirubin
    (MCBR)
    m. detectable concentration (MDC)
    m. dose causing death or
    malformation of 100% of fetuses
    (T/LD_{100})
    m. essential medium (MEM)
    m. hemolytic dose (MHD)

M

NOTES

minimum *(continued)*
    m. infective dose (MID)
    m. inhibitory concentration (MIC)
    m. lethal concentration (MLC)
    m. lethal dose (MLD)
    m. mission-oriented protective posture (MOPP)
    m. mycoplasmacidal concentration (MPC)
    Penicillium m.
    m. temperature
    m. thermometer
minimus
    Anopheles m.
    Scopulariopsis m.
minipool (MP)
    m. NAT
    m. nucleic acid testing
mink enteritis virus
Minkowski-Chauffard syndrome
minocycline
minor
    m. agglutinin
    beta thalassemia m.
    M. disease
    m. duodenal papilla
    m. epilepsy
    m. histocompatibility antigen
    m. histocompatibility complex
    Lactobacillus m.
    papilla duodeni m.
    m. salivary gland
    m. salivary gland biopsy
    Streptococcus m.
    m. sublingual duct
    thalassemia m.
    m. tranquilizer
    variola m.
    Weissella m.
minores
    ductus sublinguales m.
    glandulae vestibulares m.
Minot-von Willebrand syndrome
minus
    Spirillum m.
    m. strand
minuta
    Plasmodium vivax m.
minute
    count per m. (cpm)
    cycle per m. (c/min)
    liter per m. (Lpm)
    revolutions per m. (rpm)
    m. volume (MV)
minutisporangium
    Cryptosporangium m.
minutissima
    Phomatospora m.

minutissimum
    Corynebacterium m.
    Nocardia m.
minutum
    Eubacterium m.
mionectic
miostagmin reaction
MIP
    macrophage inflammatory protein
    maximum inspiratory pressure
mirabilis
    Proteus m.
miracidium, pl. miracidia
Mirchamp sign
MIRD
    medical internal radiation dose
Mirex
miricola
    Chryseobacterium m.
Mirizzi syndrome
miroungae
    Facklamia m.
mirror-image cell
miscarriage
miscellaneous blast injury
miscibility
miscible
    infinitely m.
    partially m.
mismatch
    m. repair (MMR)
    m. repair gene
    V/Q m.
missed abortion
missense mutation
missile
    high-velocity m. (HVM)
    m. wound
missplicing
mistranslation
mitchellae
    Aedes m.
Mitchell disease
mite
    grain itch m.
    harvest m.
    kedani m.
    parasitoid m.
    predaceous m.
    red m.
    trombiculid m.
    m. typhus
MITF
    microphthalmia-associated transcription factor
    melanocyte specific MITF (MITF-M)
MITF-M
    melanocyte specific MITF

MITGCN
   malignant intratubular germ-cell
      neoplasia
miticidal
miticide
mitis
   prurigo m.
   Streptococcus m.
mitochondria (*pl. of* mitochondrion)
mitochondrial
   m. aggregation
   m. antibody
   m. complex II
   m. creatine kinase (mtCK)
   m. crista alteration
   m. encephalopathy, lactic acidosis,
      and strokelike episodes (MELAS)
   m. enzyme desmolase
   m. inheritance
   m. matrix
   m. matrix alteration
   m. membrane
   m. membrane alteration
   m. myopathy
   m. pyruvate dehydrogenase
   m. sheath
   m. toxin
mitochondrialis
   matrix m.
mitochondrially inherited disorder
mitochondrion, pl. **mitochondria**
   crista of m.
   giant m.
   m. of hemoflagellate
mitogen
   m. assay
   pokeweed m. (PWM)
mitogen-activated protein (MAP)
mitogenesis
mitogenetic
mitogenic factor
mitokinetic
mitoplasm
mitosis, pl. **mitoses**
   abnormal m.
   m. of normoblast
   three-part m.
mitosis-karyorrhexis index (MKI)
mitotic
   m. activity index (MAI)
   m. arrest
   m. chromosome

   m. count
   m. cycle
   m. figure
   m. index
   m. period
   m. poison
   m. rate
   m. spindle
   m. spindle assembly checkpoint
   m. spindle defect
mitotic control protein (MCP)
MitoTracker Red CMXRos
Mitovirus
mitoxantrone
mitral
   m. atresia
   m. cell
   m. incompetence
   m. incompetency and stenosis
   m. insufficiency
   m. regurgitation
   m. valve
   m. valve calcification
   m. valve cleft leaflet
   m. valve prolapse (MVP)
Mitrophora
Mitsuda
   M. antigen
   M. reaction
mitsuokai
   Catenibacterium m.
Mitsuokella jalaludinii
Mittendorf dot
mixed
   m. acid fermentation
   m. agglutination
   m. agglutination reaction
   m. agglutination test
   m. anemia
   m. calculus
   m. cell leukemia
   m. chancre
   m. connective tissue disease
      (MCTD)
   m. cryoglobulinemia
   m. cryoglobulin syndrome
   m. dust pneumoconiosis
   m. epithelial-mesenchymal tumor
   m. epithelial papillary cystadenoma
      of borderline malignancy of
      müllerian type (MEBMM)
   m. epithelial tumor

M

NOTES

mixed *(continued)*
m. function oxidase system
m. gastric and intestinal phenotype lesion
m. glioma
m. hemadsorption (MHA)
m. hemoglobinopathy
m. hepatocellular carcinoma
m. immunofluorescence (MIF)
m. infection
m. leukocyte culture (MLC)
m. lineage leukemia (MLL)
m. lymphocyte culture (MLC)
m. lymphocyte culture assay
m. lymphocyte culture reaction
m. lymphocyte culture test
m. lymphocyte reaction (MLR)
m. lymphocyte-tumor culture (MLTC)
m. mesodermal tumor
m. multilocular thymic cyst
m. squamous cell carcinoma and adenocarcinoma
m. thalassemia
m. thrombus
m. tumor of salivary gland
m. tumor of skin
m. venous
m. venous blood
mixing
phenotypic m.
mixoploid
developmental m.
proliferative m.
mixoploidy
mixotrophic
mixture
dextrose solution m. (DSM)
dichloropropene-dichloropropane m.
racemic m.
Ringer m.
toxoid-antitoxoid m. (TAM)
mixtus
Cellvibrio m.
Miyagawa body
Miyagawanella
M. lymphogranulomatosis
M. ornithosis
M. pneumoniae
M. psittaci
Miyasato disease
mJ
millijoule
MK
monkey kidney
MK protein
M-K
McCarey-Kaufman
M-K medium

mkat
millikatal
MKI
mitosis-karyorrhexis index
MKS
meter-kilogram-second
MKS system
MKS unit
ML
malignant lymphoma
monocytoid lymphocyte
M:L
monocyte-lymphocyte ratio
mL
milliliter
MLA-100 coagulation instrument
MLC
minimum lethal concentration
mixed leukocyte culture
mixed lymphocyte culture
MLC assay
MLC test
MLD
metachromatic leukodystrophy
minimum lethal dose
MLH1
human mismatch-repair protein MutL homolog
MLH1 gene
MLL
mixed lineage leukemia
MLR
mixed lymphocyte reaction
MLTC
mixed lymphocyte-tumor culture
MLV
Moloney leukemogenic virus
mouse leukemia virus
MLVA
multilocus variable number (tandem repeat) analysis
MM
Marshall-Marchetti
multiple myeloma
myeloid metaplasia
skeletal muscle component of cardiac isoenzymes
MM band
MM virus
mm³
cubic millimeter
MMA
monomethylarsonic acid
MMD
minimal morbidostatic dose
MMEF
maximal midexpiratory flow
MMEFR
maximal midexpiratory flow rate

MMFR
    maximal midflow rate
MMH
    Marino and Muller-Hermelink
        MMH osteogenic classification
mmHg
    millimeter of mercury
MMM
    myelofibrosis with myeloid metaplasia
    myeloid metaplasia with myelofibrosis
MMMT
    malignant mixed mesodermal tumor
    malignant mixed müllerian tumor
mmol
    millimole
mmol/L
    millimole per liter
MMP
    matrix metalloproteinase
MMP 1
    matrix metalloproteinase 1
MMP 2
    matrix metalloproteinase 2
MMPC
    metastatic malignant pheochromocytoma
MMR
    mass miniature radiography
    measles, mumps, and rubella
    mismatch repair
        MMR gene
MMRS
    metropolitan medical response system
MMT
    malignant mixed tumor
MMTV
    mouse mammary tumor virus
mN
    millinormal
MNA
    mean nuclear area
mnemonic code
MNHL
    mixed large- and small-cell non-Hodgkin
        lymphoma
MNSs blood group
MO
    myositis ossificans
mobile
    Alkalispirillum m.
    Aminobacterium m.
    Anaerobaculum m.

    m. chilling unit
    cor m.
    m. gene
    m. phase
mobilis
    Klebsiella m.
    lien m.
    Macromonas m.
    Petrotoga m.
    Tistrella m.
mobility
    electrophoretic m.
    high electrophoretic m.
mobilization
    localized leukocyte m. (LLM)
    m. test
mobilizing agent
Mobiluncus
Möbius
    M. disease
    M. syndrome
MOC31 monoclonal antibody
MOCNI
    method of collection not indicated
modal centromere copy number
ModAMeX
    modified acetone methylbenzoate xylene
        ModAMeX section method
mode
    conversational m.
    decay m.
    histogram m.
    list m.
model
    Cox proportional hazards
        regression m.
    fluid mosaic m.
    generalized linear mixed m.
        (GLMM)
    geometrical m.
    hairpin-mediated polymerase
        slippage m.
    polymerase slippage m.
    unequal crossing over m.
modeling
    finite element m.
moderator band
Modestobacter multiseptatus
modification
    racemic m.
    Rye m.

M

NOTES

655

modified
- m. acetone methylbenzoate xylene (ModAMeX)
- m. acid-fast stain
- m. amino acid
- m. macrophage
- m. Masaoka thymic cancer staging system
- m. red blood cell
- m. smallpox
- m. Steiner stain
- m. TM agar
- m. type smallpox
- m. zinc sulfate centrifugal flotation technique

modifier

modifying gene

modular

modulate

modulation
- antigenic m.
- m. transfer function

module
- large particle sorting m. (LPS)

modulus

MODY
- maturity onset diabetes of the young

moesin

Mogibacterium
- *M. diversum*
- *M. neglectum*
- *M. pumilum*
- *M. timidum*

Mohr pipette

moiety
- ceramide m.
- fucosyl m.
- heme m.
- sialyl m.

moist
- m. desquamation
- m. gangrene
- m. necrosis
- m. papule
- m. wart

Mokola virus

mol
- mole

molal

molality

molar (M)
- m. absorptivity
- m. concentration
- m. heat capacity
- m. pregnancy
- m. villi
- m. weight

molarity

mold
- Cryo rubber m.
- pink bread m.

mole (mol)
- blood m.
- Breus m.
- carneous m.
- complete m.
- cystic m.
- false m.
- fleshy m.
- m. fraction
- m. of glucose
- grape m.
- hairy m.
- hydatid m.
- hydatidiform m.
- invasive m.
- spider m.
- vesicular m.

molecular
- m. allelotyping
- m. anemia
- m. assay
- m. biology
- m. cell layer
- m. chaperone
- m. characterization
- m. cloning
- m. cytogenetic analysis
- m. disease
- m. dispersion
- m. distillation
- m. epidemiology
- m. exclusion chromatography
- m. genetics
- m. hybridization
- m. layer of cerebellum
- m. layer of cerebral cortex
- m. layer of olfactory bulb
- m. layer of retina
- m. lesion
- m. marker
- m. mass
- m. pathology
- m. resistance testing
- m. sieve
- m. sieve chromatography
- m. staging
- m. typing
- m. weight (MW)

moleculare
- stratum m.

molecularly targeted therapy

molecule
- accessory m.
- adhesion m.
- carcinoembryonic antigen-related cell adhesion m. 1 (CEACAM1)

CD m.
cell adhesion m. (CAM)
cell-cell adhesion m.
cell-substrate adhesion m.
CI m.
costimulatory m.
E-cadherin calcium-dependent m.
endothelial-leukocyte adhesion m.
  (E-LAM)
m. of equivalent soluble
  fluorochrome (MESF)
intercellular adhesion m.-1 (ICAM-
  1)
leukocyte adhesion m.
microRNA m.
middle m.
neuron cell adhesion m.
phospholipid m.
vascular cell adhesion m.-1
  (VCAM-1)
molenkampi
  Prosthodendrium m.
molinativorax
  Gulosibacter m.
Molisch test
Moll
  adenocarcinoma of M.
  M. gland
Mollaret meningitis
molle
  fibroma m.
  papilloma m.
Möller-Barlow disease
Mollicutes
Mollisia fusca
mollities
mollusc (*var. of* mollusk)
Mollusca
mollusca (*pl. of* molluscum)
mollusciformis
  verruca m.
Molluscipoxvirus
molluscous animal
molluscum, pl. **mollusca**
  m. body
  m. contagiosum
  m. contagiosum virus (MCV)
  m. corpuscle
  m. fibrosum
  m. fibrosum gravidarum
  m. sebaceum virus
  m. verrucosum

mollusk, mollusc
Moloney
  M. leukemogenic virus (MLV)
  M. sarcoma virus (MSV)
  M. test
Molotov cocktail
Molten disease
molybdate
  ammonium m.
molybdenum
molybdic
molybdites
  Chlorophyllum m.
MOM
  mouse-on-mouse
  MOM basic kit
  MOM fluorescein kit
  MOM peroxidase kit
MOMA
  methoxyhydroxymandelic acid
moment
  dipole m.
  magnetic m.
momentum
MOMP
  major outer membrane protein
Monacrosporium
monad
Monakow
  M. bundle
  M. fascia
  M. stria
  M. syndrome
monamide
monaminergic
monaminuria
monarthritis
Monascus
monaxonic
Mönckeberg
  M. arteriosclerosis
  M. degeneration
  M. medial calcification
  M. medial calcific sclerosis
Mondor disease
Monera
moneran
Monge disease
mongol
mongolian
  m. macula
  m. spot

M

NOTES

mongolism
mongoloid
Moniezia
    M. benedeni
    M. expansa
Moniezia expansa
monilated
monilethrix
Monilia albicans
Moniliaceae
monilial esophagitis
moniliasis pneumonia
Moniliella
moniliform
moniliforme
    Eubacterium m.
moniliformis
    Armillifer m.
    Haverhillia m.
    Moniliformis m.
    Streptobacillus m.
Moniliformis moniliformis
Monilinia
monitor
    air m.
    Amplicor CMV M.
    chemical agent m. (CAM)
    Crit-Line fluid m.
    Sof-Tact glucose m.
monitoring
    atmospheric m.
    fetal oxygen saturation m.
    therapeutic drug m. (TDM)
monitorization
monkey
    m. B virus
    m. kidney (MK)
monkeypox virus
mono
    monocyte
    mononuclear leukocyte
    mononucleosis
    Acceava Mono
monoallelic
monoamine oxidase inhibitor
monoaminodicarboxylic acid
monoaminomonocarboxylic acid
monoaminuria
monoamniotic placenta twins
monoassociated
monobactam
monobasic
    m. acid
    m. potassium phosphate
    m. sodium phosphate
monoblast
monoblastic leukemia
Monocelis
monocentric

monocephalus
    m. tetrapus dibrachius
    m. tripus dibrachius
monochorionic
    m. diamniotic placenta
    m. diamniotic placenta twins
    m. monoamniotic placenta
monochroic
monochromatic
monochromatism
monochromatophil, monochromatophile
monochromator
monochromic
monochromophil, monochromophile
Monocillium
monoclonal
    m. antibody (MAb, mAB)
    m. antibody MB1
    m. antibody-specific immobilization
      of platelet antigen (MAIPA)
    m. antiepithelial membrane antigen
    m. band
    m. B-cell pattern
    m. free light chain
    m. gammopathy
    m. gammopathy of undetermined
      significance (MGUS)
    m. gammopathy of unknown
      significance (MGUS)
    m. hypergammaglobulinemia
    m. hypothesis
    m. immunoglobulin
    m. M spike
    m. paraprotein
    m. peak
    m. protein
    m. tumor
monoclonality
monocular function
monocyte (mono)
    m. chemoattractant protein (MCP)
    m. chemoattractant protein 1 (MCP
      1)
    m. function test
    m. macrophage
    plasmacytoid m.
monocyte-derived neutrophil chemotactic
    factor (MDNCF)
monocyte-lymphocyte ratio (M:L)
monocyte-macrophage system
monocytic
    m. angina
    m. blood cell
    m. inflammatory infiltrate
    m. leukemia
    m. leukemoid reaction
    m. leukocytosis
    m. leukopenia

m. marrow
m. precursor cell
monocytogenes
m. bacterium
Listeria m.
monocytoid
m. B-cell lymphoma
m. cell
m. lymphocyte (ML)
monocytopenia
monocytopoiesis
monocytosis
avian m.
monodermal teratoma
monodermoma
Monodictys nigrosperma
Mono-Diff test
monoenoic fatty acid
monoethylglycinexylidide
monofluorophosphate
sodium m.
monogenesis
monogenetic
monogenic character
monogenous
monoglyceride
monoglycosylated
monohistiocytic series
monohydric alcohol
monohydrochloride
arginine m.
monohydrolase
orthophosphoric ester m.
monoinfection
monoiodotyrosine
monokine
monolayer
cell m.
monoleptic fever
monolocular
monomastigote
monomelica
osteosis eburnisans m.
monomer
fibrin m.
globular m.
monomeric actin
monomethylarsonic acid (MMA)
monomicrobic
monomorphic adenoma (MA)
monomorphism
monomorphous

monomyelocytic leukemia
monomyositis
Mononchus
mononeme
mononeural
mononeuritis multiplex
mononeuropathy multiplex
mononuclear
m. cell
m. leukocyte (mono)
m. phagocyte
m. phagocyte system (MPS)
mononucleate
mononucleosis (mono)
differential test for infectious m.
infectious m. (IM)
posttransfusion m. (PTM)
spot test for infectious m.
mononucleotide
flavin m. (FMN)
m. repeat
monooxygenase
beta m.
dopamine m.
monopenia
monophasic
m. choriocarcinoma
m. synovial sarcoma (MSS)
m. wave
monophosphate
3′,5′-m.
adenosine m. (AMP)
adenosine 3′,5′-cyclic m. (cAMP)
concentration of adenosine m.
cyclic adenosine m. (cAMP)
cyclic guanosine m.
cytidine m. (CMP)
deoxyadenosine m. (dAMP)
deoxycytidine m.
deoxyguanosine m. (dGMP)
deoxyuridine m. (dUMP)
guanosine m. (GMP)
hexose m. (HMP)
inosine m.
thymidine m.
uridine m.
xanthosine m.
monophyletic theory
monophyletism
monoplasmatic
monoplast
monoplastic

M

NOTES

monoploid
monopolar
monoptychial
monorecidive chancre
monosaccharide
Monoscreen test
monosodium
    m. glutamate (MSG)
    m. urate (MSU)
    m. urate crystal
monosome
monosomic cell
monosomy
    mosaic autosomal m.
    m. X
monospecific direct Coombs test
Monosporium apiospermum
Monospot test
Monostichella
Monosticon Dri-Dot test
Monostoma
monostome
monostotic fibrous dysplasia
monostratal
monosynaptic bipolar cell
monotherapy
Monotospora
monotreme
Monotricha
monotrichate
monotrichous
monotypic effect
monounsaturated
Mono-Vacc test
monovalent antiserum
monoxenic culture
monoxenous
monoxide
    carbon m. (CO)
    diffusing capacity for carbon m.
      (D_{CO}, DCO)
    diffusing capacity of lung for
      carbon m. (DLCO)
    fractional uptake of carbon m.
    heme oxygenase/carbon m.
      (HO/CO)
monoxime
    diacetyl m.
monozoic
monozygosity
monozygotic twins
Monsel solution
monstrocellular sarcoma of Zülch
montana
    Rickettsia m.
montanus
    Diamanus m.
Monte Carlo method

montefiorense
    Mycobacterium m.
Montenegro skin test
montevideo
    Salmonella enteritidis serotype *m.*
Montevideo unit (MU)
Montgomery
    M. follicle
    M. tubercle
montoyai
    Penicillium m.
montpellierensis
    Veillonella m.
Montreal platelet syndrome (MPS)
moorei
    Solobacterium m.
mooreparkense
    Corynebacterium m.
Moore syndrome
mop bipolar cell
MOPP
    minimum mission-oriented protective
    posture
Morand foot
moraviensis
    Enterococcus m.
Morax-Axenfeld
    M.-A. bacillus
    diplococcus of M.-A.
    M.-A. diplococcus
Moraxella
    M. anatipestifer
    M. bovis
    M. catarrhalis
    M. conjunctivitis
    M. kingae
    M. lacunata
    M. liquefaciens
    M. nonliquefaciens
    M. osloensis
    M. phenylpyruvica
Moraxellaceae
morbidity rate
morbility
morbilli
morbilliform rash
Morbillivirus
morbillivirus
    equine m. (Hendra virus)
morbillorum
    Diplococcus m.
    Gemella m.
    Peptostreptococcus m.
    Streptococcus m.
morbus
Morchella
mordant solution
mordens
    Physaloptera m.

mordicans
morelense
  Sinorhizobium m.
Morel-Kraepelin disease
Morel syndrome
Morerastrongylus costaricensis
Morgagni
  M. column
  M. cyst
  M. disease
  M. hernia
  M. humor
  M. liquor
  M. nodule
  M. prolapse
  M. sphere
  M. syndrome
Morgagni-Adams-Stokes syndrome
Morgagni-Stewart-Morel syndrome
Morgan bacillus
Morganella morganii
morgani
  Chordodes m.
morganii
  Morganella m.
  Proteus m.
morgue
  m. capability
  m. operations
  m. service
moriens
  ultimum m.
morin
Moritella
  M. abyssi
  M. profunda
  M. viscosa
Moritellaceae
Mörner test
Morococcus cerebrosus
morphallactic regeneration
morphea
  m. acroterica
  m. alba
  m. guttata
  m. herpetiformis
  m. linearis
  m. pigmentosa
  m. profundus
morphine assay
morphodifferentiation

morphogenesis
morphologic
  m. abnormality
  m. criteria
  m. element
  m. feature
morphological analysis
morphology
  blood smear m.
  clear cell m.
  colony m.
  irregular fried egg m.
  red blood cell m.
  syncytial m.
  vascular m.
morphometric analysis
morphometry
morphon
Morquio
  M. disease
  M. syndrome
Morquio-Brailsford syndrome
Morquio-Ullrich
  M.-U. disease
  M.-U. syndrome
morrhuate
  sodium m.
Morris syndrome
Morrow Brown needle
morselize
morsitans
  Glossina m.
mors thymica
mortality rate (MR)
mortar kidney
Mortierella wolfii
mortiferum
  Fusobacterium m.
mortification
mortified
mortis
  instantaneous rigor m.
  livor m.
  rigor m.
Morton
  M. disease
  M. neuroma
  M. syndrome
mortuary science
morula
morular

M

NOTES

morule
  m. formation
  squamous m.
Morvan
  M. disease
  M. syndrome
mosaic
  m. autosomal monosomy
  m. fungus
  m. pattern
  ring m.
  Schmorl m.
  m. wart
mosaicism
  confined placental m. (CPM)
  diploid m.
  germline m.
  triploid m.
  trisomy 8 m.
  45,X/46,XY m.
Moschcowitz disease
moscoviensis
  Nitrospira m.
Mosenthal test
MOSF
  multiple organ system failure
Mosher
  air cell of M.
  M. air cell
moshkovskii
  Entamoeba m.
Mosler diabetes
mOsm
  milliosmole
mosquitocidal
mosquitocide
Moss classification
mosselii
  Pseudomonas m.
Mosse syndrome
mossii
  Dysgonomonas m.
mossy
  m. cell
  m. fiber
  m. foot
mote
  blood m.
moth-eaten pattern
mother
  m. cell
  m. cyst
moth patch
motif
  antigen receptor activation m.
    (ARAM)
  immunoreceptor tyrosine
    activation m. (ITAM)

  immunoreceptor tyrosine
    inhibitory m. (ITIM)
motile
  m. cell
  m. cilia
  m. leukocyte
  m. rod
  m. serum
motilin
motility
  m. test
  m. test medium
  tumor cell m.
motion
  brownian m.
  range of m. (ROM)
motor
  m. axon
  m. axon twig
  m. cell
  m. end plate
  m. endplate
  m. innervation
  m. neuron
  m. neuron disease
MOTT
  mycobacteria other than tubercle
Mott
  M. bacilli
  M. cell
mottled
  m. enamel
  m. erythema
mottling
  reddish-blue m.
Motulsky dye reduction test
moulage
Mounier-Kuhn syndrome
mount
  India ink m.
  wet m.
mountant
mounting medium
mouse, pl. **mice**
  cancer free white m. (CFWM)
  m. encephalomyelitis virus
  m. hepatitis virus
  m. leukemia virus (MLV)
  m. mammary tumor virus (MMTV)
  New Zealand m.
  m. parotid tumor virus
  pneumonia virus of mice (PVM)
  m. poliomyelitis virus
  m. thymic virus
  transgenic mice
  m. unit (MU)
  m. uterine unit (MUU)
mouse-on-mouse (MOM)

mousepox virus
mouse-specific lymphocyte antigen (MSLA)
mouth
    m. fistula
    gland of m.
    glass-blower's m.
    scabby m.
    sore m.
    tapir m.
    trench m.
mouthwash method collection of genomic DNA
movable
    m. heart
    m. testis
Movat
    M. pentachrome method
    M. pentachrome stain
movement
    ameboid m.
    m. artifact
    brownian m.
    doll's eye m.
    euglenoid m.
    nonrapid eye m. (NREM)
    streaming m.
moving-boundary electrophoresis
moving phase
Mowry colloidal iron stain
moyamoya disease
MP
    melting point
    metacarpophalangeal
    minipool
        MP NAT
MPC
    marine protein concentrate
    maximum permissible concentration
    micropapillary component
    minimum mycoplasmacidal concentration
MPD
    maximal permissible dose
MPEH
    methylphenylethylhydantoin
MPG
    malignant paraganglioma
MPGN
    membranoproliferative glomerulonephritis
MPH
    micronodular pneumocyte hyperplasia

MPIF1
    myeloid progenitor inhibitory factor 1
MPI/MRI
    myelofibrosis proliferation/regression index
MPNST
    malignant peripheral nerve sheath tumor
MPO
    myeloperoxidase
MPP
    mercaptopyrazidopyrimidine
MPPC
    malignant primary pheochromocytoma
MPS
    mononuclear phagocyte system
    Montreal platelet syndrome
    mucopolysaccharide
MPSC
    micropapillary serous carcinoma
MPTP
    1-methyl-4-phenyl-1,2,3,6-tetrahydropyridine
MR
    methyl red
    mortality rate
mR
    milliroentgen
mrad
    millirad
Mrakia
MRC
    medullary renal carcinoma
MRC-5 human diploid fibroblast cell
MRCNS
    methicillin-resistant coagulase-negative *Staphylococcus*
MRD
    minimal reacting dose
    minimal residual disease
mrem
    millirem
MRF
    melanocyte-stimulating hormone releasing factor
    mesencephalic reticular formation
Mrf4 gene
mRNA
    messenger ribonucleic acid
MRO
    medical review officer
MRP
    multidrug resistance protein

M

NOTES

MRSA
methicillin-resistant *Staphylococcus aureus*
MRT
malignant rhabdoid tumor
MRTK
malignant rhabdoid tumor of kidney
MRTS
malignant rhabdoid tumor of soft tissue
MRV
mononuclear Reed-variant
MR-VP
methyl red, Voges-Proskauer
MR-VP broth
MS
mass spectrometry
mucosubstance
multiple sclerosis
myeloid sarcoma
MS-1
MS-1 agent
MS-1 hepatitis
MS-2
MS-2 agent
MS-2 hepatitis
ms, msec
millisecond
MSA
muscle-specific actin
MSA antibody
MSAFP
maternal serum alpha fetoprotein
M-Saskatoon
hemoglobin M-S.
MSB
martius scarlet blue
MSB trichrome stain
MSCNS
methicillin-susceptible coagulase-negative *Staphylococcus*
MSDS
material safety data sheet
msec (*var. of* ms)
MSG
monosodium glutamate
MSH
melanophore-stimulating hormone
MSH-2 gene
MSLA
mouse-specific lymphocyte antigen
MSS
monophasic synovial sarcoma
MSSA
methicillin-susceptible *Staphylococcus aureus*
MSTS
Musculoskeletal Tumor Society
MSTS score
MSTS staging system

MSU
monosodium urate
MSU crystal
MSUD
maple syrup urine disease
MSV
Moloney sarcoma virus
murine sarcoma virus
MSVC
maximal sustained ventilatory capacity
MT
antimetallothionein antibody
medical technologist
MTB
Mycobacterium tuberculosis
MTC
medullary thyroid carcinoma
mtCK
mitochondrial creatine kinase
MTD
mean tubular diameter
MTF
medical treatment facility
MTHFR
methylenetetrahydrofolate reductase
MTI
malignant teratoma, intermediate
MTI antibody
MTND2 gene
MTND5 gene
MTR
Meinicke turbidity reaction
MTT
malignant teratoma, trophoblastic
malignant triton tumor
malignant trophoblastic teratoma
MTTA gene
MTU
malignant teratoma, undifferentiated
MTV
mammary tumor virus
MU
Mache unit
Montevideo unit
mouse unit
mU
milliunit
mu, μ
mu antigen
mu heavy chain disease
MUC
maximum urinary concentration
MUC1 gene derived glycoprotein assay
mucase
mucescens
Salipiger m.
Mucha disease

Mucha-Habermann
    M.-H. disease
    M.-H. syndrome
mucicarmine stain
mucid
muciferous
muciform
mucigen granule
mucigenous
mucihematein
mucilaginosa
    Rhodotorula m.
    Rothia m.
mucilaginosus
    Stomatococcus m.
mucilaginous gland
mucilloid
    psyllium hydrophilic m.
mucin
    allergic m.
    m. clot test
    m. depletion
    intestinal-type m.
    intracytoplasmic m.
    polymorphic epithelial m. (PEM)
    wispy intraluminal basophilic m.
mucin-depleted mucoepidermoid
  carcinoma
mucinemia
muciniphila
    Akkermansia m.
mucinogen granule
mucinoid degeneration
mucinosa
    alopecia m.
mucinosis
    cutaneous dermal m.
    cutaneous focal m.
    follicular m.
    localized m.
    metabolic m.
    papular m.
    reticular erythematous m. (REM)
    secondary m.
mucinous
    m. adenocarcinoma
    m. atrophy
    m. breast lesion
    m. bronchioloalveolar carcinoma
    m. cyst
    m. cystadenocarcinoma
    m. cystadenoma

    m. degeneration
    m. ductal ectasia
    m. meningioma
    m. stroma
mucinuria
muciparous gland
muciphage
mucitis
Muckle-Wells syndrome
mucoalbuminous cell
mucobuccal fold
mucocele
    orbital m.
    sinus m.
mucociliary
mucoclasis
mucocutaneous
    m. junction
    m. leishmaniasis
    m. lymph node syndrome
mucoenteritis
mucoepidermoid
    m. carcinoma (MEC)
    m. tumor
mucoepithelial dysplasia
mucohyaline stroma
mucoid
    m. adenocarcinoma
    m. colony
    m. medial degeneration
mucoides
    Trichosporon m.
Mucolexx
mucolipidosis, pl. **mucolipidoses**
    m. type I–IV
muconodular infiltration
mucopeptide
mucopolysaccharidase
mucopolysaccharide (MPS)
    acid m. (AMP)
    m. stain
    m. staining
    m. storage disease
    stromal m.
    sulfated acid m. (SAM)
    m. test
mucopolysaccharidosis,
  pl. **mucopolysaccharidoses**
    m. subgroup
    m. type IS
    m. type IVA, B
    m. type I–VIII

M

NOTES

mucopolysacchariduria
mucoprotein
   m. assay
   Tamm-Horsfall m. (THM)
   m. test
mucopurulent exudate
mucopus
Mucoraceae
mucormycosis
   pulmonary m.
mucoroides
   Aspergillus m.
Mucor racemosus
mucosa
   ectopic gastric m.
   fundic m.
   gastric m.
   giant hypertrophy of gastric m.
   gland of biliary m.
   glandula m.
   intestinal m.
   membrana m.
   muscular layer of m.
   Neisseria m.
   olfactory m.
   oxyntocardiac m.
   respiratory m.
   Roseomonas m.
   tunica m.
mucosa-associated
   m.-a. lymphoid tissue (MALT)
   m.-a. lymphoid tissue lymphoma
     (MALToma)
mucosae
   Lactobacillus m.
   lamina muscularis m.
   lamina propria m.
   muscularis m.
   m. nasi
   regio respiratoria tunicae m.
mucosal
   m. disease
   m. disease virus
   m. ischemia
   m. lentiginous melanoma
   m. melanosis
   m. neuroma
   m. neuroma syndrome
   m. prolapse syndrome
   m. ridge
   m. tunic
mucosanguineous
mucosanguinolent
mucoserous cell
mucositis
   plasma cell m.
mucosubstance (MS)
mucosulfatidosis

mucosum
   Treponema m.
mucosus
   Diplococcus m.
mucous
   m. acini of the posterior lingual
     gland
   m. acinus
   m. carcinoid
   m. cast
   m. colitis
   m. connective tissue
   m. cyst
   m. gland adenoma of bronchus
     (MGAB)
   m. gland of auditory tube
   m. membrane
   m. neck cell
   m. papule
   m. patch
   m. plaque
   m. plug
   m. polyp
   m. sheath of tendon
   m. thread
mucoviscidosis
mucro, pl. mucrones
   m. cordis
   m. sterni
mucron
Mucuna
mucus
   m. extravasation
   fecal m.
   m. retention
   m. secreting cervical gland
   m. secreting labial gland
   stool m.
muddy brown urinary cast
mud fever
Muehrcke line
Mueller-Hinton
   M.-H. agar
   M.-H. broth
Muellerius capillaris
Muir-Torre syndrome
mukohataei
   Halomicrobium m.
mulberry calculus
Mulder test
mule-spinner's cancer
muliebris
   corpus spongiosum urethrae m.
   dartos m.
"mu-like viruses"
Müller
   M. capsule
   M. fiber
   M. fixative

M. muscle
M. radial cell
Muller-Hermelink histological criteria
müllerian
m. adenosarcoma
m. rest
m. tumor
multiangle polarized scatter separation (MAPSS)
multiblock
m. technique
tissue m.
multicapsular
multicellular
multicentric
m. occurrence
m. reticulohistiocytosis
Multiceps
M. multiceps (Taenia multiceps)
M. serialis
multiceps
Multiceps m. (Taenia multiceps)
Taenia m.
multichannel analyzer (MCA)
multiclonal
multicolored FISH
multicolor FISH analysis
multicore disease
multicystic
m. ameloblastoma
m. dysplasia of kidney (MCDK)
m. dysplastic kidney (MCDK)
multidot pattern
multidrug
m. resistance (MDR)
m. resistance 1 (MDR1)
m. resistance protein (MRP)
multifactorial
m. inheritance
m. inherited disease
multifiliis
Ichthyophthirius m.
multifocal
m. choroidal melanoma
m. eosinophilic granuloma
m. fibrosis
m. inflammation
m. osteitis fibrosa
m. progressive leukoencephalopathy
multiformatter

multiforme
erythema m.
glioblastoma m.
multiformis
Haverhillia m.
prurigo chronica m.
multiform layer of cerebral cortex
multiglandular
multiinfarct dementia
multiinfection
multilamellar body
multilaminar primary follicle
multilobar
multilobated
multilobate placenta
multilobed
multilobular
multilocular
m. adipose tissue
m. cystic kidney
m. fat
m. hydatid cyst
multilocularis
Echinococcus m.
multiloculate hydatid cyst
multilocus variable number (tandem repeat) analysis (MLVA)
Multimek 96/384
multimeter
multimodal peak
multinodal
multinodular goiter
multinuclearity
hereditary erythroblastic m.
multinuclear leukocyte
multinucleated
m. atypia of the vulva (MAV)
m. cell
m. giant cell (MGC)
m. osteoclast
multinucleosis
multiorgan dysfunction
multipapillosa
Parafilaria m.
multiparameter flow cytometry
multipartial
multipartita
Nakamurella m.
placenta m.
multiphasic screening
multipixel spectral analysis

M

NOTES

multiple
m. access
m. adenoma
m. adenomatous polyps
m. allele
m. antigen stimulation test (MAST)
m. biotin-avidin amplification
m. carboxylase deficiency (MCD)
m. chemical sensitivity
m. colloid adenomatous goiter (MCAG)
m. displacement amplification (MDA)
m. drug resistance (MDR)
m. endochondromatosis
m. endocrine adenomatosis (MEA)
m. endocrine neoplasia (MEN)
m. endocrinoma
m. endocrinopathy
m. epiphysial dysplasia
m. event curve
m. exostosis
m. hamartoma syndrome
m. idiopathic hemorrhagic sarcoma
m. intestinal polyposis
m. lentigines syndrome
m. level sectioning
m. lymphomatous polyposis
m. marker screen
m. mucosal neuroma syndrome
m. myeloma (MM)
m. myelomatosis
m. myositis
m. organ dysfunction syndrome
m. organ system failure (MOSF)
m. osteochondromas
m. puncture tuberculin skin testing
m. puncture tuberculin test
m. red-to-purple skin plaque
m. sclerosis (MS)
m. self-healing squamous epithelioma
m. serositis
m. stage random sample
m. stain
m. symmetric lipomatosis
m. system atrophy
m. tumor
multiplex
dysostosis m.
hemangioendothelioma tuberosum m.
lymphangioma tuberosum m.
mononeuritis m.
mononeuropathy m.
myeloma m.
m. reverse transcription PCR enzyme hybridization assay
steatocystoma m.

multiplexed fluorescent microsphere immunoassay for TH1, TH2 cytokines
multiplication
vegetative m.
multiplicative growth
multiplier
multiploid adenoma
multiploidy
DNA m.
multipolar
m. cell
m. motor neuron
m. spindle
multipotent
multipuncture tuberculin skin test
multiresinivorans
Pseudomonas m.
multirule Shewhart procedure
multiseptatus
Modestobacter m.
Multisizer 3 Coulter counter
Multistix
multisynaptic
multithread allergosorbent test (MAST)
multitrichous
multivalent vaccine
multivariate
m. analysis
m. analysis of variance (MANOVA)
m. logistic regression
multivesicular body
multivorans
Dehalospirillum m.
Salana m.
Sulfurospirillum m.
multiwire proportional chamber
multocida
Pasteurella m.
mummification necrosis
mummified cell
mumps
m. antibody titer
iodine m.
m. meningoencephalitis
metastatic m.
m. sensitivity test
m. serology
m. skin test antigen
m. virus
m. virus culture
m. virus vaccine
Munchmeyer disease
Munich tumor classification system
munition
smoke-producing m.

Munro
  M. abscess
  M. microabscess
MUP
  4-methylumbelliferyl phosphate
mural
  m. aneurysm
  m. cell
  m. endocarditis
  m. nodule
  m. thrombus
muralis
  Citricoccus m.
  Georgenia m.
  Halomonas m.
muramic acid
muramidase
Murchison-Sanderson syndrome
murein
Murex *Candida albicans* **CA50 test**
murexide
muriatic acid
Muricauda ruestringensis
Muricoccus roseus
muriform
murina
  Hymenolepis m.
murine
  m. hepatitis
  m. leprosy
  m. leukemia
  m. sarcoma virus (MSV)
  m. typhus
muris
  Actinomyces m.
  Brachybacterium m.
muris-ratti
  Actinomyces m.-r.
murliniae
  Citrobacter m.
murmur
  ejection m. (EM)
  late systolic m. (LSM)
Muromegalovirus
murorum
  Gliomastix m.
Murphy-Pattee test
Murray
  M. Valley encephalitis (MVE)
  M. Valley rash
Murutucu virus
Musca domestica

muscae
  Habronema m.
muscaria
  Amanita m.
muscarine
muscarinic
  m. effect
  m. receptor
muscarinism
Muscidae
muscle
  m. action potential
  arrector pili m.
  m. biopsy
  m. bundle
  cardiac m.
  m. contractile protein
  cytoplasm of smooth m.
  dartos m.
  dilator pupillae m.
  m. epithelium
  m. fascicle
  m. of heart
  m. hemoglobin
  involuntary m.
  Jung m.
  Landström m.
  meridional fiber of ciliary m.
  Müller m.
  red m.
  Reisseisen m.
  Rouget m.
  ruptured papillary m.
  satellite cell of skeletal m.
  m. serum
  single unit smooth m.
  skeletal m.
  smooth m.
  m. spindle
  striated m.
  transverse perineal m.
  unstriated m.
  white m.
muscle-specific actin (MSA)
muscle-tendon
  m.-t. attachment
  m.-t. junction
musculamine
muscular
  m. artery
  m. atrophy
  m. cushion

M

NOTES

muscular *(continued)*
    m. dystrophy (MD)
    m. fibril
    m. layer of mucosa
    m. rheumatism
    m. rigidity
    m. subaortic stenosis
    m. substance of prostate
    m. tissue
    m. tunic
muscularis
    m. externa
    fibrae obliquae tunicae m.
    m. mucosae
    tunica m.
musculoaponeurotic fibromatosis
musculoskeletal
    M. Tumor Society (MSTS)
musculotropic
musculus skeleti
mushroom
    angel of death m.
    m. poisoning
mushroom-worker's lung
mustard
    m. gas
    NATO code for distilled (neat) sulfur m. (HD)
    NATO code for impure sulfur m. (H)
    NATO code for nitrogen m. (HN)
    NATO code for nitrogen m. 1 (HN1)
    NATO code for nitrogen m. 2 (HN2)
    NATO code for nitrogen m. 3 (HN3)
mustard-induced burn
mustargen
Musto stain
mutabilis
    Pholioata m.
mutagen
    chromosomal m.
mutagenesis
    insertional m.
mutagenic
mutagenicity test
mutans
    Streptococcus m.
mutant
    conditional-lethal m.
    conditionally lethal m.
    core promoter m.
    escape m.
    m. gene
    HFR m.
    high-frequency recombination m.
    precore m.

    suppressor-sensitive m.
    temperature-sensitive m.
mutarotation
mutase
    diphosphoglycerate m.
    S-methylmalonyl-CoA m.
mutated
    m. in colon cancer (MCC)
    m. crypt
mutation
    addition-deletion m.
    amber m.
    auxotrophic m.
    m. burden
    clear plaque m.
    cold-sensitive m.
    conditional lethal m.
    constitutive m.
    deletion m.
    dominant negative m.
    feedback inhibition m.
    forward m.
    frameshift m.
    G6PD Mediterranean variant m.
    Ha-ras m.
    heterozygous point m.
    homozygous point m.
    host-range m.
    insertion m.
    Ki-ras m.
    K-ras m.
    Leiden m.
    lethal m.
    l1307K gene m.
    LQTS Finnish founder m.
    missense m.
    NOD2/CARD15 m.
    nonsense m.
    ochre m.
    p53 m.
    phage-resistant m.
    pleiotropic m.
    point m.
    prothrombin G20210A m.
    prothrombin II m.
    rapid-lysis m.
    m. rate
    reading frame shift m.
    reverse m.
    semilethal m.
    sex-reversed m.
    silent m.
    somatic point m.
    spontaneous m.
    subvital m.
    suppressor m.
    temperature-sensitive m.
    transition m.
    transversion m.

t-s m.
ultraviolet light-induced m.
mutational analysis
mutator gene
mutilans
arthritis m.
keratoma hereditarium m.
lupus m.
rhinopharyngitis m.
mutilating
m. keratoderma
m. leprosy
m. wound
Mutinus
muton
mutualism
mutualist
MUU
mouse uterine unit
muzzle
m. abrasion
m. contusion
muzzled sperm
MV
megavolt
minute volume
mV
millivolt
MVC
microvessel count
MVD
microvessel density
MVE
Murray Valley encephalitis
MVE virus
MVP
mean platelet volume
mitral valve prolapse
MVR
massive vitreous retraction
MVV
maximum voluntary ventilation
MW
molecular weight
mW
milliwatt
Mx
maxwell
MY-10 clone stain
Myá disease

myalgia
cervical m.
epidemic m.
myasis
myasthenia gravis
myasthenic crisis
myatrophy
mycelia (*pl. of* mycelium)
mycelial
m. fungus
m. pathogen
mycelian
Myceligenerans xiligouense
mycelioid
Myceliophthora
mycelium, pl. **mycelia**
aerial m.
nonseptate m.
septate m.
Myceloblastanon
Mycena
mycete
mycetism
m. cerebralis
m. choliformis
m. nervosa
Mycetocola
M. lacteus
M. saprophilus
M. tolaasinivorans
mycetogenetic
mycetogenic
mycetogenous
mycetoides
Corynebacterium m.
mycetoma
actinomycotic m.
Bouffardi black m.
Bouffardi white m.
Brumpt white m.
Carter black m.
eumycotic m.
maduromycotic m.
Nicolle white m.
Vincent white m.
mycetomi
Madurella m.
MycoAKT latex bead agglutination test
mycobacteria (*pl. of* mycobacterium)
Mycobacteriaceae

M

NOTES

mycobacterial
    m. adjuvant
    m. DNA in sarcoidosis
Mycobacteriales
mycobacteriophage
    luciferase reporter m. (LRP)
mycobacteriosis
Mycobacterium
    M. africanum
    M. avium
    M. avium infection
    M. avium-intracellulare (MAI)
    M. avium-intracellulare complex
      (MAC)
    M. avium serovar 1–29
    M. balnei
    M. boenickei
    M. botniense
    M. bovis
    M. bovis BCG strain
    M. bovis subsp. *caprae*
    M. butyricum
    M. canariasense
    M. caprae
    M. chelonae subsp. *abscessus*
    M. chimaera
    M. doricum
    M. elephantis
    M. flavescens
    M. fortuitum
    M. fortuitum-chelonae
    M. frederiksbergense
    M. gastri
    M. genavense
    M. gordonae
    M. haemophilum
    M. heckeshornense
    M. holsaticum
    M. houstonense
    M. immunogenum
    M. interjectum
    M. intracellulare
    M. kansasii
    M. kubicae
    M. lacus
    M. leprae
    M. lepraemurium
    M. malmoense
    M. marinum
    M. microti
    M. montefiorense
    M. neworleansense
    M. nonchromogenicum
    M. palustre
    M. parascrofulaceum
    M. paratuberculosis
    M. paratuberculosis Linda
    M. parmense
    M. phlei

    M. phlei cell wall DNA complex
      (MCC)
    M. pinnipedii
    M. psychrotolerans
    M. saskatchewanense
    M. scrofulaceum
    M. septicum
    M. shottsii
    M. simiae
    M. smegmatis
    M. szulgai
    M. terrae
    M. triviale
    M. tuberculosis (MTB)
    M. ulcerans
    M. vanbaalenii
    M. xenopi
mycobacterium, pl. **mycobacteria**
    atypical mycobacteria
    Battey-type m.
    mycobacteria culture
    group I-IV mycobacteria
    m. growth indicator tube (MGIT)
    mycobacteria infection
    nonphotochromogenic mycobacteria
    nontuberculous mycobacteria (NTM)
    mycobacteria other than tubercle
      (MOTT)
    photochromogenic mycobacteria
    Runyon mycobacteria (group I–IV)
    scotochromogenic mycobacteria
mycobactin
mycobiotic agar
Mycocandida
Mycocentrospora acerina
mycocide
Mycococcus
mycoderma
    Saccharomyces m.
mycodermatitis
mycogastritis
Mycogone
Mycokluyveria
mycolic acid
mycologist
mycology
    medical m.
mycomyringitis
myc oncogene
mycophage
Mycoplana
    M. bullata
    M. dimorpha
Mycoplasma
    M. agar
    M. agassizii
    M. alligatoris
    M. buccale
    M. faucium

M. fermentans
M. gallisepticum
M. genitalium
M. granularum
M. haemocanis
M. haemofelis
M. haemomuris
M. hominis
M. infection
M. lipophilum
M. microti
M. orale
M. pneumoniae
M. primatum
M. pulmonis
M. salivarium
M. serology
M. suis
M. testudineum
M. wenyonii
mycoplasma
    genital m.
    T-strain m.
mycoplasmal pneumonia
Mycoplasmataceae
Mycoplasmatales
mycopus
mycoside
mycosis, pl. **mycoses**
    allergic bronchopulmonary m.
    (ABPM)
    m. cutis chronica
    m. fungoides (MF)
    m. fungoides d'emblée
    Gilchrist m.
    m. intestinalis
    opportunistic m.
    superficial m.
    systemic m.
Mycosphaerella
mycostatic
mycotic
    m. abscess
    m. aneurysm
    m. keratitis
    m. meningitis
    m. prostatitis
mycotica
    otitis m.
Mycotoruloides
mycotoxicosis

mycotoxin
    T2 m.
    trichothecene m.
    weaponized T2 m.
Mycotypha
mycovirus
myc **protooncogene**
mydriasis
myelapoplexy
myelatelia
myelauxe
myelemia
myelin
    m. basic protein (MBP)
    m. body
    m. degeneration
    m. figure (MF)
    neurokeratin network of
      dissolved m.
    m. sheath
    m. staining method
    Weigert stain for m.
myelinated
    m. nerve
    m. nerve fiber
myelination
myelinic degeneration
myelinization
myelinogenesis
myelinolysis
    central pontine m.
myelinosis
    central pontine m.
myelitis
    acute necrotizing m.
    acute transverse m.
    ascending m.
    bulbar m.
    concussion m.
    demyelinated m.
    Foix-Alajouanine m.
    funicular m.
    postinfectious m.
    postvaccinal m.
    subacute necrotizing m.
    systemic m.
    transverse m.
myeloablative therapy
myeloarchitectonics
myeloblast
myeloblastemia

M

NOTES

myeloblastic
    m. leukemia
    m. protein
myeloblastoma
myeloblastosis
    avian m.
myelocele
myelocyst
myelocystic
myelocystocele
myelocystomeningocele
myelocyte
    m. A, B, C
    basophilic m.
    eosinophilic m.
    neutrophilic m.
myelocythemia
myelocytic
    m. crisis
    m. leukemia
    m. leukemoid reaction
myelocytoma
myelocytomatosis
myelocytosis
myelodiastasis
myelodysplasia
myelodysplastic syndrome (MDS)
myelofibrosis
    m. anemia
    chronic idiopathic m. (CIMF)
    idiopathic m.
    myeloid metaplasia with m. (MMM)
    primary m.
    m. with myeloid metaplasia (MMM)
myelogenesis
myelogenetic
myelogenic
    m. leukemia
    m. osteopathy
    m. sarcoma
myelogenous
    m. callus
    m. leukemia
myelogone
myelogonium
myeloic
myeloid
    m. depression
    m. hyperplasia
    m. leukemia
    m. metaplasia (MM)
    m. metaplasia with myelofibrosis (MMM)
    m. metaplasia with polycythemia vera (PCV-M)
    m. reticulosis
    m. sarcoma (MS)

    m. series
    m. stem cell
    m. tissue
myeloid-erythroid ratio (M:E)
myeloidosis
myeloid progenitor inhibitory factor 1 (MPIF1)
myeloleukemia
myelolipoma
myelolymphocyte
myelolysis
myeloma
    amyloidosis of multiple m.
    Bence Jones m.
    m. cast nephropathy
    m. cell
    endothelial m.
    giant cell m.
    IgA m.
    IgD m.
    IgE m.
    IgG m.
    L-chain m.
    multiple m. (MM)
    m. multiplex
    nonsecretory m.
    plasma-cell m.
    plasmacytic m.
    m. protein
myelomalacia
    angiodysgenetic m.
myelomatosis
    multiple m.
    m. multiplex
myelomeningitis
myelomeningocele
myelomonocyte
myelomonocytic leukemia
myelonencephalitis
myelopathic
    m. anemia
    m. polycythemia
myelopathy
    carcinomatous m.
    cervical m.
    compressive m.
    diabetic m.
    HTLV-1 associated m. (HAM)
    lumbosacral m.
    paracarcinomatous m.
    transverse m.
    vascular m.
myeloperoxidase (MPO)
    m. deficiency
    m. H_2O_2 halide system
    m. stain
    m. system
myelopetal
myelophthisic anemia

myelophthisis
myeloplast
myelopoiesis
    extramedullary m.
myelopoietic
myeloproliferative
    m. disease
    m. disorder
    m. syndrome
myeloradiculitis
myeloradiculodysplasia
myeloradiculopolyneuronitis
myelorrhagia
myelorrhaphy
myelosarcoma
myelosarcomatosis
myeloschisis
myelosclerosis with myeloid metaplasia
myelosis
    aleukemic m.
    chronic nonleukemic m.
    erythremic m.
    funicular m.
    leukemic m.
    leukopenic m.
    megakaryocytic m.
    nonleukemic m.
    subleukemic m.
myelostimulatory theory
myelosuppression
myelosyringosis
myelotoxic
myenteric
    m. nerve
    m. plexus
myenteron
myf3 gene
myf4 gene
myf5 gene
MYH9
    myosin heavy chain 9
    MYH9 gene
myiasis
    cutaneous m.
    facial m.
    gastric m.
    genitourinary m.
    intestinal m.
    nasal m.
    sanguivorous m.
myitis (*var. of* myositis)
Mylar capacitor

MYO
    myoglobin
myoadenylate
    m. deaminase
    m. deaminase deficiency
myoarchitectonic
myoatrophy
myoblast
myoblastoid carcinoma
myoblastoma
    granular cell m.
myoblastomatoid carcinoma
myocardia (*pl. of* myocardium)
myocardial
    m. anoxia
    m. bridge
    m. damage
    m. depressant factor (MDF)
    m. disease
    m. disease of unknown origin
      (MDUO)
    m. endocrine cell
    m. infarction (MI)
    m. infarction in dumbbell form
    m. infarction in H-form
    m. ischemia
    m. scarring
myocarditis
    acute isolated m.
    bacterial m.
    drug-induced m.
    Fiedler m.
    fragmentation m.
    fulminant m.
    giant cell m.
    hypersensitivity m.
    idiopathic m.
    indurative m.
    infectious m.
    Löffler m.
    rheumatic m.
    toxic m.
    viral m.
myocardium, pl. **myocardia**
    fragmentation of the m.
    hibernating m.
    stunned m.
myocardosis
myocele
myocelialgia
myocelitis
myocellulitis

M

NOTES

myocerosis
myochondroblast
myoclonica
    dyssynergia cerebellaris m.
myoclonic epilepsy
myocyte
    Anitschkow m.
    cardiac m.
    m. disarray
    Purkinje m.
    m. stretch
myocytolysis of heart
myocytoma
MyoD
    myogenic regulatory
    MyoD family of genes
    MyoD gene family
    MyoD protein
MyoD1
    MyoD1 immunostaining
    MyoD1 regulatory gene
myodegeneration
myodemia
myodiastasis
myoelastic
myoendocarditis
myoepithelial
    m. carcinoma
    m. cell
    m. sialadenitis (MESA)
myoepithelioma
    malignant m.
myoepithelium
    neoplastic m.
myofascial syndrome
myofascitis
myoferlin
myofiber
myofibril
    intracellular m.
    m. necrosis
myofibrilla, pl. myofibrillae
myofibrillar
myofibrillary hypertrophy
myofibroblast
    stromal m.
myofibroblastic
    m. differentiation
    m. immunophenotype
    m. lesion
    m. mammary stromal tumor
    m. proliferation
myofibroblastoma
myofibrohistiocytic
myofibroma
myofibromatosis
    infantile m.
myofibrosis cordis
myofibrositis

myofilament
    thick m.
    thin m.
myogenesis
myogenetic
myogenic
    m. cell
    m. paralysis
    m. regulatory (MyoD)
myogenin protein
myogen marker
myogenous
myoglobin (Mb, MYO)
    m. A, B, C, D, E, G, H
    carbon dioxide m. (MbCO)
    m. cardiac diagnostic test
    m. clearance test
    m. identification method
    m. stain
myoglobinemia
myoglobinuria
    acute paroxysmal m.
myoglobinuric
    m. nephropathy
    m. nephrosis
myoglobulin
myoglobulinuria
myohemoglobin
myoid
    m. cell
    m. marker
    m. marker expression
myointimal
    m. hyperplasia
    m. proliferation
myoischemia
myokerosis
myokinase
myolemma
myolipoma
myolysis
    cardiotoxic m.
myoma
myomalacia
myomatous polyp
myomelanosis
myometrial
myometrial hypertrophy (IMH)
myometritis
myometrium
myomitochondrion
myon
myonecrosis
    clostridial m.
    m., myoglobinuria, renal failure
myoneme
myoneural junction
myoneuroma
myonosus

myopachynsis
myopathic
myopathy
    alcoholic m.
    carcinomatous m.
    centronuclear m.
    congenital m.
    corticosteroid m.
    distal m.
    endocrine m.
    inflammatory m.
    mitochondrial m.
    myotubular m.
    nemaline m.
    rod m.
    thyrotoxic m.
myopericarditis
myopericytoma
myoperitonitis
myophagocytosis
myophosphorylase deficiency glycogenosis
myoplasm
myopodin gene
myorrhexis
myosalpingitis
myosarcoma
myosclerosis
myosin
    m. binding protein C
    m. cross-bridge
    m. filament
    m. heavy chain 9 (MYH9)
    m. phosphatase
    skeletal-muscle m.
myosis
    endolymphatic stromal m.
myositic
myositis, myitis
    acute disseminated m.
    clostridial m.
    epidemic m.
    m. fibrosa
    inclusion body m. (IBM)
    infectious m.
    interstitial m.
    multiple m.
    m. ossificans (MO)
    m. ossificans circumscripta
    m. ossificans progressiva
    ossifying interstitial m.
    proliferative m.
    m. sine dermatitides

myospherulosis
myostroma
myotenositis
myotonia
myotonic dystrophy (DM)
myotonin protein kinase gene
myotube
myotubular myopathy
myotubule
Myoviridae
myriapod
Myriapoda
myringa
myringitis
    bullous m.
myringomycosis
myrinx
Myriodontium
myristic acid
Myrmecia
myrmecia
Myrothecium
mysophilia
MYST
    mediastinal yolk sac tumor
mystax
    Ascaris m.
    Toxocara m.
myxadenitis
myxadenoma
myxedema
    m. heart
    idiopathic m.
    infantile m.
    pituitary m.
    pretibial m.
myxedematoid
myxedematosus
    lichen m.
myxedematous
myxemia
myxochondrofibrosarcoma
myxochondroid matrix
myxochondroma
Myxococcaceae
Myxococcales
Myxococcidium stegomyiae
myxocollagenous matrix
myxocyte
myxofibroma
myxofibrosarcoma
myxohyaline degeneration

NOTES

M

myxoid
    m. change
    m. cyst
    m. degeneration
    m. fibroma
    m. liposarcoma
    m. matrix
    m. mesenchyme
    m. neurofibroma
    m. stroma
    m. synovial sarcoma
myxolipoma
myxoliposarcoma
myxoma, pl. **myxomas, myxomata**
    atrial m.
    cardiac m. (CM)
    cystic m.
    m. enchondromatosum
    endochondromatous m.
    erectile m.
    m. fibrosum
    infectious m.
    lanceolate m.
    m. lipomatosum
    lipomatous m.
    nerve sheath m. (NSM)
    odontogenic m.
    m. sarcomatosum
    sinonasal m.
    vascular m.

myxomatodes
    carcinoma m.
    fibroma m.
    lipoma m.
myxomatosis
    cardiac valve m.
    m. virus
myxomatous degeneration
myxomycete
Myxomycetes
myxoneuroma
myxopapillary ependymoma
myxopapilloma
myxosarcoma
Myxospora
myxospore
Myxosporea
Myxosporidia
Myxotrichum
myxovirus
Myxozoa
Myzomyia
Myzorhynchus
MZ
    marginal zone
MZBCL
    marginal zone B-cell lymphoma
MZL
    mantle zone lymphoma
    marginal zone cell lymphoma

N
asparagine
newton
normal
N antigen
N0
no lymph nodes containing cancer cells
N5 submicron particle size analyzer
NA
nasopharyngeal angiofibroma
neutralizing antibody
nodular amyloidoma
NAAK
nerve agent antidote kit
nabothian
n. cyst
n. follicle
N-acetylaspartate acid
N-acetyl-B-hexosaminidase
N-acetylcysteine
N-acetylgalactosamine
N-acetylgalactosamine-4-sulfatase
N-acetylgalactosamine-6-sulfatase
N-acetylglucosamine
N-acetylglucosamine-6-sulfatase
N-acetylmannosamine
N-acetylmuramic acid
N-acetylneuraminic
NaCN
sodium cyanide
nacreous ichthyosis
N-acylsphingosine
NADH, NAD
nicotinamide adenine dinucleotide
NADH dehydrogenase
NADH methemoglobin reductase
nadir
Nadi reaction
NADP, NADPH
nicotinamide adenine dinucleotide
phosphate
intracellular NADP
Nadsonia
Naegeli (*var. of* Nägeli)
Naegleria fowleri
Naemacyclus
Naemospora
naeslundii
Actinomyces n.
NAF
neutrophil activating factor
Naffziger syndrome
NAFLD
nonalcoholic fatty liver disease
nagana

naganoensis
Leifsonia n.
Nagao enzyme
nagasakiensis
Thermaerobacter n.
Nägele pelvis
Nägeli, Naegeli
N. syndrome
N. type of monocytic leukemia
nagelii
Lactobacillus n.
Nageotte cell
Nagler reaction
nail
n. bomb
cornified layer of n.
germinative layer of n.
n. horn
horny layer of n.
n. plate
shell n.
sinus of n.
yellow n.
nail-patella syndrome
Nairobi
N. sheep disease
N. sheep disease virus
Nairovirus
NAIT
neonatal alloimmune thrombocytopenia
naive cell
Nakamurellaceae
Nakamurella multipartita
Nakanishi stain
naked virus
Nalgene
N. capsule filter
N. freezer storage rack
N. PETG media bottle
nalidixic acid
NAME
nevi, atrial myxoma, myxoid
neurofibroma, and ephelides
NAME syndrome
name
generic n.
Namibia
sulfur pearl of N.
namibiensis
Actinomadura n.
Gordonia n.
Thiomargarita n.
nana
Hymenolepis n.

N

NANB
non-A, non-B
NANB hepatitis
nanism
Nannizzia
NanoChip
N. molecular biology workstation
N. test for factor V Leiden single-
nucleotide polymorphism
nanocurie (nCi)
**Nanoduct neonatal sweat analysis
system**
nanoemulsion
surfactant n.
nanofarad (nF)
nanogram (ng)
nanoliter (nL)
nanomelia
nanometer (nm)
nanomole (nmol)
nanoparticle
MgO n.
Nanophyetus salmincola
nanoprobe
Nanoprobes
N. GoldEnhance reagent
N. Nanogold reagent
nanosecond (ns, nsec)
Nanovirus
nanukayami
nanum
Microsporum n.
NAP
neutrophil activating protein
nucleic acid panel
NAP bacteria differentiation test
NAP hepatitis B virus quantitative
panel
NAP modified LRP assay
nape nevus
naphtha
coal tar n.
naphthalenivorans
Polaromonas n.
naphthalenovorans
Paenibacillus n.
naphthol
alpha n.
n. ASBI phosphate stain
n. AS-D chloracetate (NASDCA)
beta n.
n. poisoning
n. pyronine
n. yellow S
**naphthol-AS-D-chloracetate esterase
(NASDCE)**
naphthophila
Thermotoga n.
Napier formol-gel test

napierian logarithm
napkin ring tumor
NAPP
nerve agent pyridostigmine pretreatment
NAPP tablet set
narcosis
carbon dioxide n.
nitrogen n.
narcotic
n. antagonist
n. blockade
NARES
nonallergic rhinitis with eosinophilia
naris, pl. nares
nares swab anthrax spore test
Narnavirus
NARP
neurogenic muscle weakness, ataxia, and
retinitis pigmentosa
narugense
Thermodesulfobium n.
nasal
n. allergic disorder
n. angiocentric T-cell lymphoma
(NATL)
n. cytology
n. gland
n. glioma
n. myiasis
n. polyp
n. smear
n. T/NK-cell lymphoma
nasales
glandulae n.
NASBA
nucleic acid sequence based amplification
nucleic acid sequence based analysis
nascent
NaSCN
sodium thiocyanate
NaSCN exchange assay
nasdae
Brevundimonas n.
NASDCA
naphthol AS-D chloracetate
NASDCE
naphthol-AS-D-chloracetate esterase
NASDCE stain
NASH
nonalcoholic steatohepatitis
nasi
cancrum n.
granulosis rubra n.
mucosae n.
tunica mucosa n.
nasicola
Actinomyces n.
Nasik vibrio

nasimurium
    Rothia n.
nasiphocae
    Arthrobacter n.
Naskapi
    albumin N.
nasogastric
nasolabial cyst
nasooral leishmaniasis
nasopalatal
nasopalatine duct cyst
nasopharyngeal (NP)
    n. aspirate
    n. carcinoma (NPC)
    n. culture
    n. leishmaniasis
    n. swab
nasopharyngitis
nasopharynx
nasosinusitis
nasus
NAT
    nucleic acid amplification test
    NAT for HCV and HIV-1 in
      blood donation
    minipool NAT
    MP NAT
natalensis
    Mastomys n.
natans
    Sphaerotilus n.
national
    N. Accrediting Agency for Clinical
      Laboratory Sciences
    N. Biomonitoring Program (NBP)
    N. Cancer Institute (NCI)
    N. Committee for Clinical
      Laboratory Standards (NCCLS)
    N. Council of Health Laboratory
      Services (NCHLS)
    N. Electronic Disease Surveillance
      System (NEDSS)
    n. examination
    N. Immunization Program (NIP)
    N. Institute for Occupational Safety
      and Health (NIOSH)
    N. Institutes of Health (NIH)
    n. laboratory
    N. Notifiable Diseases Surveillance
      System (NNDSS)
    N. Pharmaceutical Stockpile (NPS)
    N. Registry of Microbiologists

native albumin
NATL
    nasal angiocentric T-cell lymphoma
NATO
    North Atlantic Treaty Organization
    NATO code
    NATO code for arsine (SA)
    NATO code for chloracetophenone
      (CS)
    NATO code for 1-
      chloroacetophenone (CN)
    NATO code for cyanogen chloride
      ($CNCl_2$) (CK)
    NATO code for cyclosarin (GF)
    NATO code for dibenz(b,f)-1:4-
      oxazepine (CR)
    NATO code for
      diphenylaminearsine (adamsite)
      (DM)
    NATO code for
      diphenylaminochloroarsine
      (adamsite) (DM)
    NATO code for distilled (neat)
      sulfur mustard (HD)
    NATO code for an extremely
      toxic persistent nerve agent (no
      common chemical name) (VX)
    NATO code for HCN (AC)
    NATO code for impure sulfur
      mustard (H)
    NATO code for lewisite (L)
    NATO code for military obscurant
      smoke (zinc oxide and
      hexachloroethane, grained
      aluminum) (HC)
    NATO code for nerve agent
      cyclohexyl
      methylphosphonofluoridate (GF)
    NATO code for nerve agent
      isopropyl ethylphosphonofluoridate
      (GE)
    NATO code for nerve agent O-
      ethyl S-[2-(diethylamino)ethyl]
      ethylphosphonothioate (VE)
    NATO code for nerve agent O-
      ethyl S-[2-(diethylamino)ethyl]
      methylphosphonothioate (VM)
    NATO code for nerve agent O,O-
      diethyl S-[2-(diethylamino)ethyl]
      phosphonothioate (VG)
    NATO code for nitrogen mustard
      (HN)

N

NOTES

NATO (continued)
    NATO code for nitrogen mustard 1 (HN1)
    NATO code for nitrogen mustard 2 (HN2)
    NATO code for nitrogen mustard 3 (HN3)
    NATO code for nonpersistent nerve agent
    NATO code for o-chlorobenzylidene malononitrile (CS)
    NATO code for persistent nerve agent
    NATO code for phosgene (choking gas) (CG)
    NATO code for phosgene oxime (CX)
    NATO code for QNB (BZ)
    NATO code for riot control agent bromobenzylcyanide (CA)
    NATO code for sarin (GB)
    NATO code for soman (GD)
    NATO code for tabun (GA)
natremia, natriemia
Natrialba
    N. aegyptia
    N. chahannaoensis
    N. hulunbeirensis
    N. taiwanensis
Natrinema versiforme
natriuresis
natriuretic
    n. agent
Natronobacterium nitratireducens
natronolimnaea
    Dietzia n.
Nattrassia mangiferae
natural
    n. agglutinin
    n. antibody
    n. death
    n. dye
    n. focus of infection
    n. hemolysin
    n. host
    n. immunity
    n. killer cell (NK)
    n. killer cell leukemia
    n. killer cell lymphoma
    n. killer cell-stimulating factor (NKSF)
    n. selection
naturally occurring plague
Naucoria
nausea
    epidemic n.
Nauta stain
Nautiliaceae

Nautiliales
Nautilia lithotrophica
navarrensis
    Roseospira n.
navicular
    n. arthritis
    n. cell
navicularis
    fossa n.
NB
    neuroblastoma
NBC
    nuclear, biological, chemical (mass-casualty weapon)
NBCCG
    National Bladder Cancer Collaborative Group
NBCCS
    nevoid basal cell carcinoma syndrome
NBP
    National Biomonitoring Program
NBS
    Nijmegen breakage syndrome
    normal blood serum
NBT
    nitroblue tetrazolium
    NBT dye
    NBT reduction assay
    NBT test
NBTE
    nonbacterial thrombotic endocarditis
NC
    neural crest
n:c
    nuclear-to-cytoplasmic ratio
NCA
    nonspecific cross-reacting antigen
N-cadherin
    N-c. marker
NCCLS
    National Committee for Clinical Laboratory Standards
NCDB
    National Cancer Data Base
NCF
    neutrophil chemotactic factor
NCHLS
    National Council of Health Laboratory Services
NCI
    National Cancer Institute
nCi
    nanocurie
NCL-ARm monoclonal antibody
NCL-ARp polyclonal antibody
NCL-ER-LH2 monoclonal antibody
NCL-PCR monoclonal antibody
ND
    neonatal death

nondisabling
  ND virus
NDA
  no data available
  no demonstrable antibodies
NDFP
  nodular and diffuse fibrous proliferation
NDI
  nephrogenic diabetes insipidus
NDP
  net dietary protein
NDV
  Newcastle disease virus
Ne
  norepinephrine
nealsonii
  Bacillus n.
neapolitanus
  Halothiobacillus n.
neavei
  Simulium n.
Nebraska calf scours virus
nebulizer
  ultrasonic n. (USN)
nebulous urine
Necator americanus
necatoriasis
necessitatis
  empyema n.
neck
  buffalo n.
  bull n.
  Madelung n.
  potato tumor of n.
  radiation-induced sarcoma of the head and n. (RISHN)
  n. of spermatozoon
  TFL of head and n.
  webbed n.
necrobiosis
  n. lipoidica
  n. lipoidica diabeticorum
  superficial ulcerating rheumatoid n.
necrobiotic
  n. granuloma
  n. xanthogranuloma
necrocytosis
necrogenica
  verruca n.
necrogenic wart
necrogenous
necrogranulomatous

necrolysis
  toxic epidermal n. (TEN)
necrolytic migratory erythema
necroparasite
necropathy
necrophilic
necrophorum
  Fusobacterium n.
necrophorus
  Actinomyces n.
  Bacillus n.
  Fusiformis n.
  Sphaerophorus n.
necropolis
  Virgibacillus n.
necropsy
necroscopy
necrose
necrosis
  acidophilic n.
  acute inflammatory n.
  acute massive liver n.
  acute tubular n. (ATN)
  aseptic n.
  avascular n.
  bile duct n.
  bone aseptic n.
  bridging hepatic n.
  cardiac cell n.
  caseation n.
  caseous n.
  central n.
  central hemorrhagic n. (CHN)
  centrilobular n.
  cheesy n.
  coagulation n.
  coagulative n.
  colliquative n.
  comedo n.
  confluent hepatic n.
  contraction band n.
  cortical n.
  cystic medial n. (CMN)
  cytodegenerative n.
  cytotoxic n.
  diffuse n.
  dirty n.
  ductular piecemeal n.
  enzymatic fat n.
  epiphysial aseptic n.
  fat n.
  fibrinoid n.

NOTES

necrosis *(continued)*
    focal n.
    gangrenous n.
    geographic n.
    hepatocellular n.
    hyaline n.
    inflammatory n.
    intestinal n.
    intra vitam n.
    ischemic n.
    lamellar n.
    laminar cortical n.
    liquefaction n.
    liquefactive n.
    liver cell n.
    massive hepatic n. (MHN)
    medial cystic n.
    medullary n.
    midzonal n.
    moist n.
    mummification n.
    myofibril n.
    papillary n.
    peripheral n.
    periportal n.
    piecemeal n.
    postpartum pituitary n.
    progressive emphysematous n.
    pseudolaminar n.
    radiation n.
    radium n.
    renal cortical n.
    renal medullary n.
    renal papillary n.
    satellite cell n.
    sclerosing hyaline n.
    septic n.
    simple n.
    spotty lobular n.
    subcutaneous fat n. of newborn
    submassive confluent n.
    suppurative n.
    tissue n.
    total n.
    tumor n.
    n. tumor
    villous ischemic n.
    Zenker n.
    zonal n.
    zone of n.
necrospermia
necrosteon
necrosteosis
necrotic
    n. adipocyte
    n. cirrhosis
    n. cyst
    n. focus
    n. inflammation

    n. pseudoxanthomatous nodule
    (NPN)
necroticans
    enteritis n.
necrotisans
    phlebitis nodularis n.
necrotizing
    n. angiitis
    n. arteriolitis
    n. bronchopneumonia
    n. encephalitis
    n. encephalomyelopathy
    n. enterocolitis
    n. factor
    n. fasciitis
    n. funisitis
    n. glomerulonephritis
    n. granulomatous inflammation
    n. lobar pneumonia
    n. pancreatitis
    n. papillitis
    n. sialometaplasia
    n. ulcerative gingivitis (NUG)
    n. ulcerative gingivostomatitis
    n. vasculitis
necrotomy
Necrovirus
nectariphilum
    Catellibacterium n.
Nectria
Nectriopsis
NED
    no evidence of disease
NEDD8 gene
NEDSS
    National Electronic Disease Surveillance
    System
needle
    n. aspiration cytology
    Bard n.
    Becton-Dickinson n.
    n. core length in sextant biopsy
    Crown n.
    n. culture
    Jamshidi n.
    localization n.
    Manan n.
    Menghini n.
    Morrow Brown n.
    Surecut n.
    Tru-Cut n.
    Wang n.
    Wyeth bifurcated n.
Neer shoulder fracture I–III
Neethling virus
Neftel disease
neg
    negative
negative (neg)

n. anergy
n. assortative mating
n. base excess
beta-lactamase n.
n. catalyst
n. control enzyme induction
n. control repression
n. cytotaxis
D^u n.
false n.
n. neutrotaxis
n. phase
n. predictive value (NPV)
Rh n.
n. stain
n. strand virus
n. variation (NV)
negative-pressure room
negevensis
    Simkania n.
Negibacteria
Negishi virus
neglectum
    Mogibacterium n.
Negri
    N. body
    N. corpuscle
neidei
    Bacillus n.
Neisser
    diplococcus of N.
    N. stain
Neisseria
    anaerobic N.
    N. caviae
    N. flava
    N. flavescens
    N. gonorrhoeae
    N. gonorrhoeae culture
    N. gonorrhoeae smear
    N. lactamica
    N. meningitidis
    N. mucosa
    N. ovis
    N. perflava
    N. sicca
    N. subflava
Neisseriaceae
Neisser-Wechsberg phenomenon
Nelson
    N. syndrome
    N. tumor

Nelson-Salassa syndrome
nemaline
    n. myopathy
    n. rod
nemathelminth
Nemathelminthes
nematicidal
nematicide
nematization
nematoblast
nematocide
Nematoda
nematode
nematodiasis
Nematodirella
    N. longispiculata
    N. longissimespiculata
Nematodirus
nematoid
nematologist
nematology
Nematoloma
Nematomorpha
nematophilus
    Paenibacillus n.
nematosis
nematospermia
Nematospora
neoangiogenesis
neoantigens
Neoascaris vitulorum
neoautoimmune disease
Neobacteria
neocaledoniensis
    Nocardia n.
Neochlamydia hartmannellae
Neochordodes
Neocosmospora
neocyte
    donor n.
neocytosis
neoepitope
    cytokeratin n.
neoformans
    Cryptococcus n.
    Debaryomyces n.
    Filobasidiella n.
    Saccharomyces n.
neoformation
neoformative
neogenesis
Neohendersonia

N

NOTES

neomembrane
neomort
neomycin assay agar
neonatal
    n. alloimmune thrombocytopenia (NAIT)
    n. anemia
    n. apnea
    n. autoimmune thrombocytopenia
    n. biliary function
    n. bilirubin
    n. calf diarrhea virus
    n. cerebrovascular accident
    n. cholestasis workup
    n. CVA
    n. death (ND, NND)
    n. gastrointestinal hemorrhage
    n. hemochromatosis
    n. hepatitis
    n. herpes
    n. hypoglycemia
    n. isoerythrolysis
    isoimmune n.
    n. lupus
    n. necrotizing enterocolitis
    n. nesidioblastosis
    n. respiratory distress syndrome
    n. screening
    n. testing
    n. thymectomy
    n. thyroid-stimulating hormone
    n. thyroid-stimulating hormone test
neonatorum
    anemia n.
    anoxia n.
    atelectasis n.
    blennorrhea n.
    conjunctivitis n.
    dermatitis exfoliativa n.
    edema n.
    ichthyosis congenita n.
    impetigo n.
    mastitis n.
    ophthalmia n.
    pemphigus n.
    sclerema n.
neopathy
neoplasia
    cervical intraepithelial n. (CIN)
    ductal intraepithelial n. (DIN)
    gestational trophoblastic n.
    intraepithelial n.
    intratubular germ cell n. (IGCN)
    laryngeal intraepithelial n. (LIN)
    lobular n.
    lymphoreticular n.
    malignant intratubular germ-cell n. (MITGCN)
    mammary intraepithelial n.

    mesenchymal n.
    multiple endocrine n. (MEN)
    noninvasive lobular n.
    ocular surface squamous n.
    preinvasive urothelial n.
    prostatic intraepithelial n. (PIN)
    trophoblastic n.
    vaginal intraepithelial n.
    vulvar intraepithelial n. (VIN)
neoplasm
    adipocytic n.
    adnexal n.
    adrenal n.
    astrocytic n.
    B-cell n.
    benign n.
    clear cell n.
    epithelial n.
    epithelioid soft-tissue n. (ESTN)
    germ cell n.
    hematologic malignant n.
    histoid n.
    interdigitating papillary n.
    intraductal papillary mucinous n. (IPMN)
    lymphoid n.
    malignant n.
    metastatic n.
    nervous system n.
    oncocytic papillary n.
    pancreatic endocrine n. (PEN)
    papillary breast n. (PBN)
    papillary urothelial n.
    prostatic intraepithelial n. (PIN)
    renal epithelioid oxyphilic n. (REON)
    respiratory system n.
    Revised European-American Classification of Lymphoid N.'s
    sebaceous n.
    spinal n.
    sporadic ovarian n.
    stromal cell n.
    stromal-epithelial n.
    synchronous n.
    trophoblastic n.
    n. of uncertain behavior
    urothelial n.
    vascular n.
neoplastic
    n. arachnoiditis
    n. disease
    n. element
    n. epidermal cell
    n. epithelium
    n. hematopoietic tissue
    n. lymphocyte
    n. meningitis
    n. myoepithelium

n. proliferation
n. theory
neoprecipitin test (NPT)
neopterin
Neorickettsia
   N. helmintheca
   N. risticii
   N. sennetsu
Neosartorya fischeri
Neospora caninum
neoteny
Neotestudina rosatii
neotissue
Neotrombicula autumnalis
neotype
neovascularization
   choroidal n. (CNV)
nepalensis
   Staphylococcus n.
nephelometer
nephelometric
   n. immunoassay
   n. inhibition assay (NIA)
nephelometry
   rate n.
nephradenoma
nephrectasia
nephrectasis
nephredema
nephrelcosis
nephridium
nephritic
   n. calculus
   n. factor
   n. syndrome
nephritis, pl. **nephritides**
   acute interstitial n. (AIN)
   allergic interstitial n. (AIN)
   analgesic n.
   antibasement membrane n.
   antikidney serum n.
   bacterial n.
   chronic interstitial n. (CIN)
   crescentic n.
   diffuse proliferative lupus n.
   Ellis types 1, 2 n.
   focal proliferative lupus n.
   glomerular n.
   n. gravidarum
   hemorrhagic n.
   hereditary n. (HN)
   immune complex n.

interstitial n.
lupus n. (LN)
membranous lupus n.
mesangial lupus n.
nephrotoxic n. (NTN)
nephrotoxic serum n. (NTSN)
radiation n.
salt-losing n.
scarlatinal n.
serum n.
shunt n.
subacute n.
suppurative n.
syphilitic n.
transfusion n.
tuberculous n.
tubulointerstitial n.
uranium n.
nephritogenic
nephroblastoma
   cystic partially differentiated n. (CPDN)
nephrocalcinosis
nephrocystosis
nephrogenic
   n. adenoma
   n. diabetes insipidus (NDI)
   n. rest (NR)
nephrogenous ascites
nephrohydrosis
nephrolith
nephrolithiasis
nephrolysin
nephrolysis
nephrolytic
nephroma
   congenital mesoblastic n. (CMN)
   cystic n.
   embryonal n.
   mesoblastic n.
nephromalacia
nephromegaly
nephron
nephronic loop
nephropathia epidemica
nephropathic
nephropathy
   acute uric acid n.
   Alport hereditary n.
   analgesic n.
   Balkan n.
   Bence Jones cast n.

N

NOTES

nephropathy *(continued)*
    chronic pyelonephritis/reflux n.
    C1q n.
    Danubian endemic familial n.
    diabetic n.
    gout n.
    gouty n.
    hemoglobinuric n.
    heroin-associated n.
    human immunodeficiency virus-associated n. (HIVAN)
    hyperuricemic n.
    hypokalemic n.
    IgA n.
    IgM n.
    immune complex n.
    lead n.
    membranous n.
    mesangial IgA n.
    myeloma cast n.
    myoglobinuric n.
    reflux n.
    sickle cell n.
    thin basement membrane n.
    tubulointerstitial n. (TIN)
nephrophthisis
    familial juvenile n. (FJN)
nephroptosis, nephroptosia
nephropyelitis
nephrosclerosis
    arterial n.
    arteriolar n.
    benign n. (BNS)
    hyaline n.
    hyperplastic n.
    intercapillary n.
    malignant n.
    senile n.
nephrosclerotic
nephrosis, pl. **nephroses**
    acute n.
    amyloid n.
    bile n.
    cholemic n.
    familial n.
    hemoglobinuric n.
    hypokalemic n.
    hypoxic n.
    lipid n.
    lipoid n. (LN)
    lower nephron n.
    myoglobinuric n.
    osmotic n.
    toxic n.
    tubular n.
    vacuolar n.
nephrospasia
nephrospasis

nephrostogram
nephrotic syndrome (NS)
nephrotoxic
    n. antibody (NTAB)
    n. nephritis (NTN)
    n. serum
    n. serum nephritis (NTSN)
nephrotoxin
nephrotuberculosis
Nepovirus
neptunia
    Halomonas n.
neptuniae
    Devosia n.
neptunius
    Vibrio n.
Nernst equation
nerve
    n. agent
    n. agent antidote kit (NAAK)
    n. agent pyridostigmine pretreatment (NAPP)
    Auerbach n.
    n. cell
    n. cell body
    n. ending
    n. fascicle
    n. fiber
    n. ganglion
    ganglionic layer of optic n.
    n. growth factor (NGF)
    n. growth factor antiserum
    intersheath space of optic n.
    least splanchnic n.
    lesser splanchnic n.
    lipomatosis of n.
    myelinated n.
    myenteric n.
    obturator n.
    n. papilla
    peripheral n.
    postganglionic sympathetic n.
    n. root
    rootlet of spinal n.
    n.'s synapsing
nervea
    tunica n.
nervi (*pl. of* nervus)
nervosa
    anorexia n.
    foramina n.
    mycetism n.
    rhinitis n.
nervosum
    vaccinia n.
nervosus
    lobus n.

nervous
>n. system neoplasm
>n. tissue

nervus, pl. **nervi**
nesidioblast
nesidioblastoma
nesidioblastosis
>neonatal n.

nesidiodysplasia
nesslerization
nesslerize
Nessler reaction
nest
>Brunn epithelial n.
>cell n.
>cribriform n.
>epithelial n.
>isogenous n.
>tumor n.
>von Brunn n.

Nesterenkonia
>*N. halotolerans*
>*N. lacusekhoensis*
>*N. xinjisis*

NET
>neuroendocrine tumor

net
>Chiari n.
>chromidial n.
>n. dietary protein (NDP)
>n. protein ratio (NPR)
>n. protein utilization (NPU)

Netherton syndrome
N-ethylmaleimide-sensitive-factor (NSF)
N-ethylmaleimide-sensitive fusion protein
N-ethyl-N-(2-hydroxy-3-sulfopropyl)-3, 5-dimethoxyaniline (DAOS)
nettle gas
network
>chromatin n.
>Cooperative Human Tissue N.
>cytokine n.
>Health Alert N. (HAN)
>intercommunicating n.
>Laboratory Response N. (LRN)
>linin n.
>neural n. (NN)
>neurokeratin n.
>peritarsal n.
>probabilistic neural n. (PNN)
>Purkinje n.

>subpapillary n.
>trabecular n.

Neubauer hemocytometer
Neufeld
>N. capsular swelling
>N. reaction

Neumann
>N. cell
>N. disease
>N. sheath

neu-oncogene
neural
>n. crest (NC)
>n. crest cell
>n. cyst
>n. inclusion (NI)
>n. layer of retina
>n. rosette
>n. tube defect

neuralgic amyotrophy
neuraminic acid
neuraminidase digestion
neuraminoglycoprotein
>alpha-2 n.

neurapraxia
neurasthenia
neuraxis
neuraxon
neuregulin (NRG)
>n. 1 (protein) (NRG1)
>n. 2 (protein) (NRG2)
>n. 3 (protein) (NRG3)
>n. 4 (protein) (NRG4)

neurepithelium
neuridine
neurilemma, neurolemma
>n. cell

neurilemmitis
neurilemmoma
>acoustic n.
>ameloblastic n.
>Antoni type A, B n.
>malignant n.

neurilemosarcoma
neurility
neurimotility
neurimotor
neurinoma
>acoustic n.

neurite
>dystrophic n.

NOTES

N

neuritic
    n. atrophy
    n. plaques
neuriticum
    atrophoderma n.
neuritis
    adventitial n.
    allergic n.
    branchial n. (BN)
    experimental allergic n. (EAN)
    optic n.
    paralytic brachial n. (PBN)
neuroallergy
neuroarthropathy
neuroastrocytoma
neuroblast
    sympathetic n.
neuroblastic
neuroblastoma (NB)
    olfactory n. (ONB)
neuroborreliosis
    Lyme n.
neurocalcin immunoreactive neuron
neurochitin
neurochoroiditis
neurocognition
neurocristic hamartoma
neurocristopathy
neurocutaneous
    n. melanosis
    n. phacomatosis syndrome
neurocyte
neurocytology
neurocytolysis
neurocytoma
    central n.
neuroD
    transcription factor n.
neurodegeneration
neurodegenerative disorder
neurodendrite
neurodendron
neurodermatitis
neuroectodermal tumor
neuroectoderm-derived cell
neuroencephalomyelopathy
neuroendocrine
    n. differentiation
    n. ductal carcinoma in situ
    n. marker
    n. transducer cell
    n. tumor (NET)
neuroendocrine-type feature in adrenal cortical adenoma
neuroendocrinology
neuroepidemiology
neuroepithelial
    n. body

    n. cell
    n. layer of retina
neuroepithelioma
neuroepithelium
    n. of ampullary crest
    n. of macula
neurofiber
neurofibril in cytoplasm
neurofibrillar
neurofibrillary
    n. degeneration (tau)
    n. tangle
neurofibroma
    myxoid n.
    plexiform n.
    storiform n.
neurofibromatosis (NF)
    abortive n.
    central type n.
    incomplete n.
neurofibromin gene
neurofibrosarcoma
neurofilament
    n. protein (NFP)
    n. triplet polypeptide (NFP)
neuroganglion
neurogenesis
neurogenic
    n. arthropathy
    n. bladder
    n. inhibition
    n. muscle weakness, ataxia, and retinitis pigmentosa (NARP)
    n. muscular atrophy (NMA)
    n. sarcoma
    n. shock
neuroglia
    n. cell
    nuclei of n.
    Weigert stain for n.
neurogliacyte
neuroglial cell
neurogliomatosis
neurohemal
neurohistology
neurohormone
neurohumoral factor
neurohypophysial hormone
neurohypophysis
neuroid melanocytic structure
neuroimaging
neuroinflammation
neurokeratin
    n. network
    n. network of dissolved myelin
neurolemma (*var. of* neurilemma)
neuroleptic malignant syndrome
neuroleukin
neurological cell

neurolymphomatosis gallinarum
neurolysin
neuroma
    acoustic n.
    amputation n.
    n. cutis
    false n.
    fibrillary n.
    Morton n.
    mucosal n.
    pancinian n.
    plexiform n.
    n. telangiectodes
    traumatic n.
    Verneuil n.
neuromalacia
neuromatosa
    elephantiasis n.
neuromatosis
neuromedin B
neuromelanin
neuromelaninogenesis
neuromesenchyme
neuromuscular
    n. choristoma
    n. junction
    n. junction testing
    n. spindle
    n. system disease
neuromyelitis
neuromyopathy
    carcinomatous n.
neuromyositis
neuron
    alpha motor n.
    autonomic motor n.
    balloon n.
    bipolar n.
    n. cell adhesion molecule
    cytoplasm of n.
    dopaminergic n.
    fetal n.
    gamma motor n.
    ganglionic motor n.
    intercalary n.
    internuncial n.
    lower motor n.
    magnocellular hypothalamic n.
    motor n.
    multipolar motor n.
    n. of myenteric nerve plexus
    neurocalcin immunoreactive n.

    nucleus of motor n.
    parvocellular n.
    peptidergic n.
    POMC n.
    postganglionic motor n.
    preganglionic motor n.
    pseudounipolar n.
    quisqualate activated n.
    red n.
    somatic motor n.
    survival motor n. (SMN)
    tangle-bearing n.
    tangle-free n.
    unipolar n.
    upper motor n.
    vicinal n.
    visceral motor n.
neuronal
    n. cell intoxication
    n. choristoma
    n. chromatolysis
    n. hyperplasia
    n. intermediate filament inclusion disease (NIFID)
    n. intestinal dysplasia
    n. intranuclear inclusion
    n. Nissl substance
    n. nodular heterotopia
    n. perikarya
neuron-associated class III beta-tubulin
neurone
neuronevus
neuronophage
neuronophagia
neuron-specific
    n.-s. enolase (NSA, NSE)
    n.-s. esterase (NSE)
neurooncology
neuroparalytic illness
neuropathic
    n. albuminuria
    n. arthritis
neuropathologist
neuropathology (NP)
neuropathy
    amblyopia n.
    amyloid n.
    diabetic n.
    dysproteinemic n.
    entrapment n.
    hereditary sensory radicular n.
    hypertrophic interstitial n.

N

NOTES

neuropathy *(continued)*
   Leber hereditary optic n. (LHON)
   Nigerian nutritional ataxic n.
   organophosphate-induced delayed n.
      (OPIDN)
   paraproteinemic n.
   peripheral n. (PN)
   retrobulbar n.
   subacute myelooptic n. (SMON)
   n. target esterase (NTE)
   tropical ataxic n. (TAN)
   vincristine n.
   vitamin B12 n.
neuropeptide
   substance P n.
neurophysin
neuropil
neuropilin
neuroplasm
neuroplasticity
neuroplexus
neuropodion, pl. **neuropodia**
neuroprogenitor cell
neuroretinitis
neuroretinopathy
neurosarcocleisis
neurosarcoidosis
neurosarcoma
neuroschwannoma
neurosclerosis
neurosecretion
neurosecretory
   n. cell
   n. granule
   n. material (NSM)
   n. substance
neurospongium
Neurospora
neurosyphilis
neurotendinous
   n. organ
   n. spindle
neurothekeoma
   cellular n.
neurothekoma
neurothele
neurotica
   lipomatosis n.
neurotization
neurotome
neurotoxin
   Clostridium botulinum n. type A,
      B, C1, D, E, F, G
   human botulinum n. type A, B, E,
      F
   potent protein n.
neurotransmitter
neurotransporter receptor
neurotrauma

neurotrophic
   n. atrophy
   n. factor
   n. tyrosine kinase receptor, type 1
      (NTRK1)
neurotrophin
neurotropic virus
neurotubule
neurovaccine
neurovascular hamartoma
neurovirus
neurovisceral storage disorder
Neusser granule
neutral
   n. buffered formalin fixative
   n. lipid storage disease
   n. protamine Hagedorn (NPH)
   n. red
   n. stain
neutralization
   n. test (NT)
   viral n.
neutralizing antibody (NA)
neutrinimicus
   Streptacidiphilus n.
neutriphila
   Halorhodospira n.
neutron
   n. exposure
   n. meter
   n. personnel dosimeter
   slow n.
   n. source
   thermal n.
neutropenia
   cyclic n.
   drug-induced n.
   familial cyclic n.
   periodic n.
neutropenic angina
neutrophil, neutrophile
   n. activating factor (NAF)
   n. activating protein (NAP)
   band n.
   n. chemotactant factor
   n. chemotactic factor (NCF)
   filamented n.
   n. functional disorder
   giant n.
   n. granule
   granules of developing n.'s
   hereditary hypersegmentation of n.'s
   hypersegmented n.
   immature n.
   juvenile n.
   n. killing activity
   mature n.
   polymorphonuclear n. (PMN)
   rod n.

segmented n. (segs)
stab n.
transmigration n.
neutrophilia
giant n.
physiologic n.
neutrophilic
n. chemotactic factor
n. cryptitis
n. dermatosis
n. eccrine hidradenitis
n. hyperplasia
n. infiltrate
n. inflammation
n. leukemia
n. leukocyte
n. leukocytosis
n. leukopenia
n. lymphocytosis
n. marrow
n. metamyelocyte
n. myelocyte
n. pleocytosis
n. promyelocyte
neutrophilopenia
neutrophilous
neutrotaxis
indifferent n.
negative n.
nevi (*pl. of* nevus)
nevocarcinoma
nevocellular nevus
nevocyte
nevocytic nevus
nevoid
n. basal cell carcinoma syndrome (NBCCS)
n. elephantiasis
n. hypertrichosis
nevolipoma
nevomelanocyte
nevous, nevose
nevoxanthoendothelioma
Nevskiaceae
nevus, pl. **nevi**
acquired n.
acral n.
agminate n.
n. anemicus
n. angiomatodes
apocrine n.
n. arachnoideus

n. araneus
nevi, atrial myxoma, myxoid neurofibroma, and ephelides (NAME)
atypical melanocytic n. (AMN)
balloon cell n.
basal cell n.
bathing trunk n.
Becker n.
Blitz nevi
blue rubber bleb n.
capillary n.
n. cavernosus
n. cell
cellular blue n. (CBN)
Clark n.
comedo n.
n. comedonicus
compound n.
congenital melanocytic nevi (CMN)
connective tissue n.
deep penetrating n. (DPN)
dysplastic n.
n. elasticus of Lewandowski
epidermic-dermic n.
epithelioid cell n.
faun tail n.
flame n.
n. flammeus
n. follicularis keratosis
giant blue n.
giant hairy n.
giant pigmented n.
halo n.
inflammatory linear verrucous epidermal n. (ILVEN)
intradermal n.
Ito n.
Jadassohn n.
Jadassohn-Tièche n.
junction n.
junctional n.
lentigines, atrial myxoma, mucocutaneous myxomas, and blue nevi (LAMB)
n. lipomatodes
n. lipomatosus
lymphatic n.
n. lymphaticus
melanocytic n.
nape n.
nevocellular n.

N

NOTES

nevus *(continued)*
　　nevocytic n.
　　nodal n.
　　organoid n.
　　Ota n.
　　pigmented hair epidermal n.
　　n. pigmentosus
　　n. pilosus
　　sebaceous n.
　　spider n.
　　n. spilus
　　spindle cell n.
　　Spitz n.
　　spongy n.
　　strawberry n.
　　Sutton n.
　　systematized n.
　　n. unius lateris
　　UV-irradiated n.
　　vascular n.
　　n. venosus
　　verrucous n.
new
　　n. fuchsin
　　n. growth
　　n. methylene blue
　　N. World hookworm
　　N. World screwworm
　　N. Zealand mice
newborn
　　ABO hemolytic disease of the n.
　　alloimmune hemolytic disease of n.
　　n. aspiration
　　bullous impetigo of n.
　　n. crossmatch
　　hemolytic anemia of n.
　　n. hemolytic disease
　　hemolytic disease of n. (HDN)
　　hemorrhagic disease of n.
　　n. hemorrhagic disease
　　hyaline membrane disease of n.
　　icterus gravis of n.
　　leukocytosis of the n.
　　Parrot atrophy of the n.
　　n. pneumonitis virus
　　respiratory distress syndrome of n.
　　n. respiratory syndrome
　　n. screen
　　subcutaneous fat necrosis of n.
Newcastle
　　N. disease
　　N. disease virus (NDV)
　　N. virus disease (NVD)
Newcastle-Manchester bacillus
Newcomer fixative
newly formed vessel
neworleansense
　　Mycobacterium n.

newport
　　Salmonella enteritidis serotype *n.*
newton (N)
　　N. law of cooling
nexin
nexin-II
　　protease n.-II
nexus
Nezelof
　　N. syndrome
　　N. type of thymic alymphoplasia
NF
　　neurofibromatosis
nF
　　nanofarad
NF-1 gene
NFA-I
　　normal fecal antigen
NFB
　　nonfermentative bacillus
NF-kappa B protein
N_5-**formyl FH$_4$**
N-**formyl methionine**
NFP
　　neurofilament protein
　　neurofilament triplet polypeptide
ng
　　nanogram
NGC
　　nongynecologic cytopathology
NGF
　　nerve growth factor
　　　　NGF antiserum
NGU
　　nongonococcal urethritis
NHC
　　nonhistone chromosomal
　　　　NHC protein
NHL
　　non-Hodgkin lymphoma
NHPA
　　no histopathologic abnormality
NHS
　　normal horse serum
　　normal human serum
NI
　　neural inclusion
Ni
　　nickel
NIA
　　nephelometric inhibition assay
niacin test
niche
　　ecologic n.
　　enamel n.
Nichols
　　N. method
　　N. reagent
nickel (Ni)

n. dermatitis
n. grid
Raney n.
Nickerson
    N. medium
    N. medium smear
Nickerson-Kveim
    N.-K. test
    N.-K. test reaction
Nicklès test
Nicolas-Favre disease
Nicolle
    Novy, MacNeal, and N. (NNN)
    N. stain for capsules
    N. white mycetoma
nicolli
    Spelotrema n.
Nicol prism
Nicotiana
nicotinamide
    n. adenine dinucleotide (NADH, NAD)
    n. adenine dinucleotide phosphate (NADP, NADPH)
nicotine test
nicotinic acid
nidal
NIDDM
    noninsulin-dependent diabetes mellitus
nidi (*pl. of* nidus)
Nidoko disease
nidulans
    Aspergillus n.
    Emericella n.
nidus, pl. **nidi**
Nieden disease
Niemann disease
Niemann-Pick
    N.-P. cell
    N.-P. disease (NPD)
    N.-P. lipid
    N.-P. type of histiocyte
Niemann±Pick disease type C, tau pathology class I
Niesslia
NIFID
    neuronal intermediate filament inclusion disease
niger
    Aspergillus n.
    locus n.
    nucleus n.

    Peptococcus n.
    Rhizopus n.
Nigerian nutritional ataxic neuropathy
nighttime salivary cortisol test
nigra
    cataracta n.
    dermatosis papulosa n.
    pityriasis n.
    substantia n.
nigrescens
    Mermis n.
nigricans
    acanthosis n.
    Corynebacterium n.
    keratosis n.
    pseudoacanthosis n.
    Rhizopus n.
nigrificans
    Desulfotomaculum n.
nigripalpus
    Culex n.
nigrities
nigromaculis
    Aedes n.
nigrosin, nigrosine
nigrosperma
    Monodictys n.
Nigrospora sphaerica
nigrum
    pigmentum n.
    tapetum n.
NIH
    National Institutes of Health
nihonkaiense
    Diphyllobothrium n.
niigatensis
    Kitasatospora n.
    Nocardia n.
Nijmegen breakage syndrome (NBS)
Nikiforoff method
Nikolsky sign
Nikon microprocessor-controlled camera
nil
    n. disease
    n. lesion
Nile
    N. blue
    N. blue A
    N. blue fat stain
nilotica
    Limnatis n.

N

NOTES

NIN
    nuclear excision repair instability
ninhydrin reaction
ninhydrin-Schiff
    n.-S. reaction
    n.-S. stain for proteins
NIOSH
    National Institute for Occupational Safety
    and Health
NIOX nitric oxide monitoring system
NIP
    National Immunization Program
nipple
    n. adenoma
    n. arranged in a ring
    n. discharge cytology
    erosive adenomatosis of n.
nipponica
    Entamoeba n.
nipponicum
    Gnathostoma n.
Nippostrongylus
Nipride
NIS
    sodium-iodine symporter
NISH
    nonisotopic in situ hybridization
nishinomiyaensis
    Dermacoccus n.
nisin
Nissl
    N. body
    N. degeneration
    N. granule
    N. stain
    N. substance
    N. substance alteration
nit
Nitabuch
    N. fibrin
    N. layer
    N. membrane
    N. stria
nitida
    Gordonia n.
nitidus
    lichen n.
nitrate
    n. agar
    n. broth
    cold silver n.
    lanthanum n.
    peroxyacetyl n. (PAN)
    potassium n.
    n. reduction test
    silver n.
    sodium n.
    n. utilization test

nitratireducens
    Garciella n.
    Halobiforma n.
    Natronobacterium n.
    Thialkalivibrio n.
Nitratireductor aquibiodomus
nitratis
    Thialkalivibrio n.
nitrativorans
    Comamonas n.
nitrergic hyperinnervation
nitric
    n. acid
    n. acid test
    n. oxide (NO)
nitrifying bacterium
nitrile
    propane n.
nitrite
    sodium n.
    n. test
nitritireducens
    Stenotrophomonas n.
nitritoid reaction
nitrituria
nitroaniline poisoning
Nitrobacter
    N. hamburgensis
    N. vulgaris
Nitrobacteraceae
nitroblue
    n. tetrazolium (NBT)
    n. tetrazolium dye
    n. tetrazolium dye reduction assay
    n. tetrazolium stain
    n. tetrazolium test
nitrocellulose membrane
Nitrocystis
nitro dye
nitroferricyanide
    sodium n.
nitrogen
    alkali-soluble n. (ASN)
    alpha amino n.
    amino acid n. (AAN)
    n. balance
    blood urea n. (BUN)
    n. dilution
    n. distribution
    n. equivalent
    fecal n.
    n. lag
    n. narcosis
    nonprotein n. (NPN)
    partial pressure of n.
    n. partition
    serum urea n. (SUN)
    stool n.
    undetermined n.

urea n. (UN)
urinary n.
urine urea n. (UUN)
nitrogen-fixing
nitrogenous
nitroguajacolicus
    Arthrobacter n.
nitropropiol test
3-nitroproprionic acid (3NP)
nitroprusside
    sodium n.
    n. test
nitroreducens
    Diaphorobacter n.
nitrosa
    Nitrosomonas n.
nitrosamine
nitroso dye
nitroso-indole-nitrate test
Nitrosomonas
    N. aestuarii
    N. eutropha
    N. halophila
    N. marina
    N. nitrosa
    N. oligotropha
    N. ureae
nitrosothiol
nitrosourea agent
Nitrospina gracilis
Nitrospira moscoviensis
nitrous acid
nivalis
    Lanosa n.
niveiscabiei
    Streptomyces n.
niveum
    Trichophyton n.
NIXIE
    numeric indicator experimental number 1
    NIXIE tube
njovera
NK
    natural killer cell
    NK clonal diversity
    NK lymphoma
NK1-C3 antibody
NKH
    nonketotic hyperosmotic
NKHG
    nonketotic hyperglycinemia

NKSF
    natural killer cell-stimulating factor
nL
    nanoliter
NLH
    nodular lymphoid hyperplasia
N-linked glycosylation
NLT
    normal lymphocyte transfer test
NM
    not measurable
nm
    nanometer
NMA
    neurogenic muscular atrophy
NMDA
    N-methyl-D-aspartase
        NMDA receptor agonist
        NMDA receptor antagonist
***N*-methylacetamide**
N-methyl-D-aspartase (NMDA)
***N*-methylformamide**
N1-methylnicotinamide (NMN)
***N'*-methylnicotinamide**
NMID
    N-terminal mid fragment
N-MID
        N-MID osteocalcin ELISA
        N-MID osteocalcin ELISA test
NMN
    N1-methylnicotinamide
nmol
    nanomole
NMP
    nuclear matrix protein
NMP22
    NMP22 BladderChek test
NMRT
    National Medical Response Team
N-myc
    N-myc amplification
    N-myc oncogene
NN
    neural network
NND
    neonatal death
***N,N*-dimethylacetamide**
***N,N*-dimethylformamide**
NNDSS
    National Notifiable Diseases Surveillance
    System

N

NOTES

NNN
 Novy, MacNeal, and Nicolle
 NNN culture medium
NO
 nitric oxide
no
 no cancer spread to other organs (M0)
 no data available (NDA)
 no demonstrable antibodies (NDA)
 no evidence of disease (NED)
 no evidence of distant metastases (M0)
 no evidence of primary tumor (T0)
 no lymph nodes containing cancer cells (N0)
 no mineral component
 no reflow phenomenon
 no serious abnormality (NSA)
 no significant abnormality (NSA)
 no significant defect (NSD)
 no significant deviation (NSD)
 no significant difference (NSD)
 no significant disease (NSD)
Noack syndrome
Noble stain
Nocard bacillus
Nocardia
 N. abscessus
 N. africana
 N. alba
 N. asiatica
 N. asteroides
 N. beijingensis
 N. brasiliensis
 N. caishijiensis
 N. calcarea
 N. cerradoensis
 N. culture
 N. cummidelens
 N. cyriacigeorgica
 N. dacryolith
 N. farcinica
 N. fluminea
 N. ignorata
 N. inohanensis
 N. mediterranei
 N. minutissimum
 N. neocaledoniensis
 N. niigatensis
 N. nova
 N. orientalis
 N. otitidis-caviarum
 N. paucivorans
 N. pigrifrangens
 N. pseudovaccinii
 N. puris
 N. sienata
 N. soli

 N. tenerifensis
 N. testacea
 N. transvalensis
 N. veterana
 N. vinacea
 N. yamanashiensis
Nocardiaceae
nocardioform actinomycete
Nocardioidaceae
Nocardioides
 N. albus
 N. aquaticus
 N. aquiterrae
 N. ganghwensis
Nocardiopsaceae
Nocardiopsis
 N. aegyptia
 N. alkaliphila
 N. composta
 N. dassonvillei
 N. dassonvillei subsp. *albirubida*
 N. exhalans
 N. halotolerans
 N. kunsanensis
 N. metallicus
 N. salina
 N. trehalosi
 N. tropica
 N. umidischolae
 N. xinjiangensis
nocardiosis
nocere
 primum non n.
noctalbuminuria
nocturnal penile tumescence test
nodal
 n. involvement
 n. marginal zone B-cell lymphoma
 n. nevus
 n. tissue
NOD2/CARD15
 NOD2/CARD15 mutation
 PRO-GenoLogix NOD2/CARD15
node
 Auerbach n.
 Babès n.
 Bouchard n.
 n. of Cloquet
 cortex of lymph n.
 delphian n.
 Dürck n.
 germinal center of lymph n.
 Haygarth n.
 Heberden n.
 hemal n.
 hemolymph n.
 Hensen n.
 hilar n. (HN)
 hilum of lymph n.

lymph n. (LN)
medulla of lymph n.
Meynet n.
milker's n.'s
nonsentinel lymph n. (NSLN)
normal lymph n.
Osler n.
paraaortic lymph n.
portal lymph n.
n. of Ranvier
Ranvier n.
regional lymph n.
Rosenmüller n.
Rotter n.
SA n.
sentinel lymph n. (SLN)
shotty n.
signal n.
singer's n.
syphilitic n.
Troisier n.
Virchow n.

Nod factor
NOD2 gene
nodi (*pl. of* nodus)
nodosa
    arteritis n.
    arthritis n.
    periarteritis n.
    polyarteritis n. (PAN, PN)
    salpingitis isthmica n.
    trichorrhexis n.
    vasitis n.
nodose
    n. ganglion
    n. rheumatism
nodositas
nodosity
nodososetosus
    Arachnomyces n.
nodosum
    amnion n.
nodosus
    Bacteroides n.
    Dichelobacter n.
nodous
nodular
    n. adenosis
    n. amyloidosis
    n. arteriosclerosis
    n. blastema
    n. body

n. calcific aortic stenosis
n. colloid goiter
n. embryo
n. fasciitis
n. glomerulosclerosis
n. hidradenoma
n. histiocytic lymphoma
n. hyperplasia of prostate
n. hyperplastic goiter
n. leprosy
n. lymphocyte-rich Hodgkin disease
n. lymphoid hyperplasia (NLH)
n. melanoma
n. mesoneuritis
n. mesothelial hyperplasia
n. myofibroblastic stromal
  hyperplasia of the mammary
  gland
n. nonsuppurative panniculitis
n. non-X histiocytosis
n. palmar fibromatosis
n. panencephalitis
n. paragranuloma (NP)
n. poorly differentiated lymphocyte
  (NPDL)
n. prurigo
n. regenerative hyperplasia (NRH)
n. sclerosing Hodgkin disease
  (NSHD)
n. sclerosis (NS)
n. subepidermal fibrosis
n. syphilid
n. transformation of the liver
n. tuberculid
n. vasculitis (NV)
nodulare
    Trichophyton n.
    Trichophyton mentagrophytes var. *n.*
nodularis
    prurigo n.
nodulate
nodulation
nodule
    adenomatoid cystic papillary n.
    aggregated lymphatic n.
    apple jelly n.
    Arantius n.
    Aschoff n.
    Babès n.
    Caplan n.
    cold n.
    Dalen-Fuchs n.

N

NOTES

nodule *(continued)*
    discrete n.
    dysplastic n.
    endometrial stromal n. (ESN)
    fibrocalcific n.
    fibrosiderotic n.
    fibrous n.
    Gamna-Gandy n.
    Gandy-Gamna n.
    gastric lymphoid n.
    germinal center of lymphatic n.
    Hoboken n.
    hot n.
    hypervascular n.
    intracystic papillary n.
    Jeanselme n.
    junctional expansion n.
    juxtaarticular n.
    Kimmelstiel-Wilson n.
    laryngeal n.
    Lisch n.
    Losch n.
    lymph n.
    lymphoid n.
    malpighian n.
    microglial n.
    milker's n.
    Morgagni n.
    mural n.
    necrotic pseudoxanthomatous n.
      (NPN)
    parenchymal n.
    primary n.
    reactive spindle cell n. (RSCN)
    rheumatic n.
    rheumatoid n.
    sarcoma-like mural n. (SLMN)
    satellite n.
    Schmorl n.
    secondary n.
    siderotic n.
    silicotic n.
    singer's n.
    Sister Mary Joseph n.
    splenic lymph n.
    subcutaneous n.
    vocal fold n.
noduli (*pl. of* nodulus)
Nodulisporium
nodulous
nodulus, pl. **noduli**
    n. caroticus
    n. lymphaticus
nodus, pl. **nodi**
    n. lymphaticus
    nodi lymphoidei axillares
    nodi lymphoidei coeliaci
    nodi lymphoidei inguinales profundi

    nodi lymphoidei inguinales
      superficiales
nogabecina
    Amycolatopsis keratiniphila subsp. *n.*
noggin protein inhibitor
noguchi
    Phlebotomus n.
Noguchia
    N. granulosis
    N. granulosus
Nomarski
    N. microscope
    N. optics
nomenclature
    binary n.
    binomial n.
    chromosome n.
    n. of tumor
nomogram
    acid-base n.
    Andrews n.
    blood volume n.
    cartesian n.
    Radford n.
    Rumack-Matthew n.
    Siggaard-Andersen alignment n.
nomograph
nonadherent cell
nonagglutinating vibrio
non-A hepatitis
nonalcoholic
    n. fatty liver disease (NAFLD)
    n. steatohepatitis (NASH)
nonallergic
    n. rhinitis
    n. rhinitis with eosinophilia
      (NARES)
non-Alzheimer dementia
nonanaplastic invasive meningioma
non-A, non-B (NANB)
    n.-A, n.-B hepatitis
nonbacterial
    n. gastroenteritis virus
    n. thrombotic endocarditis (NBTE)
    n. verrucous endocarditis
non-B hepatitis
nonbirefringent
nonbrisk infiltrate
nonbursate
noncardiogenic pulmonary edema
noncaseating granuloma
noncellular
nonchromaffin
    n. paraganglia
    n. paraganglioma
nonchromogenicum
    Mycobacterium n.

noncleaved
> n. follicular center cell
> large n. (LNC)

noncollagenous pneumoconiosis

noncommunicating hydrocephalus

noncompetitive
> n. assay
> n. heterogeneous enzyme
>   immunoassay
> n. inhibitor

nonconjugative plasmid

nonconsanguineous

noncornifying form

noncorrosive

noncystic mucinous carcinoma

nondiabetic glycosuric melituria

nondisabling (ND)
> nonsymptomatic, n. (NSND)

nondiscrete bands

nondisease

nondisjunction
> maternal meiotic n.
> meiotic n.

nondissecting aortic aneurysm

nonelectrolyte

nonenveloped RNA virus

**nonepidermotropic primary cutaneous
  T-cell lymphoma**

nonesterified fatty acid

nonexophytic lesion

non-FCC
> nonfollicular center cell

nonfermentative bacillus (NFB)

**nonfilament polymorphonuclear
  leukocyte**

nonfilarial chylothorax

nonflagellated vegetative cell

nonfluorescent acetoxymethyl ester

nonfollicular center cell (non-FCC)

nonfunctional factor VIII-related gene

nongermline band

nonglomerular hematuria

nongonococcal urethritis (NGU)

nongranular leukocyte

nongynecologic cytopathology (NGC)

non-heat-extracted antigen

nonhematogenous

nonhemolytic
> n. jaundice
> n. streptococcus

non-HFE-related hemochromatosis

nonhistone
> n. chromosomal (NHC)
> n. chromosomal protein

non-Hodgkin lymphoma (NHL)

nonideal solution

nonimmune
> n. agglutination
> n. fetal hydrops
> n. hemolysis
> n. hemolytic anemia
> n. serum

nonimmunity

noninfectious

noninfiltrating lobular carcinoma

noninflammatory edema

**noninsulin-dependent diabetes mellitus
  (NIDDM)**

noninvasive
> n. implant
> n. lobular lesion
> n. lobular neoplasia

nonionic detergent

nonisolated proteinuria

nonisotopic
> n. gel detection system
> n. in situ hybridization (NISH)

**nonkeratinized stratified squamous
  epithelium**

nonketotic
> n. hyperglycemia
> n. hyperglycinemia (NKHG)
> n. hyperosmolar syndrome
> n. hyperosmotic (NKH)

nonlactose-fermenting bacterium

nonlamellar bone

nonleukemic myelosis

nonleukoreduced red cell

nonlineage
> n. marker
> n. specific transmembrane
>   glycoprotein

nonlipid histiocytosis

nonliquefaciens
> *Moraxella n.*
> *Pseudomonas n.*

nonlymphocytic leukemia

non-MALT
> nonmucosa-associated lymphoid tissue
> non-MALT lymphoma

nonmedullated fiber

nonmegaloblastic anemia

nonmelanocytic pigmentation

N

NOTES

nonmelanosomal vesicle
nonmembrane-bound nucleolus
nonmotile
    n. bacteria
    n. leukocyte
    n. organism
nonmucinous adenocarcinoma
nonmucosa-associated lymphoid tissue
    (non-MALT)
nonmyelinated
nonmyloidotic fibrillary glomerulopathy
nonmyogenous tumor
nonnecrotizing
    n. granuloma
    n. granulomatous inflammation
Nonne-Milroy disease
Nonne-Milroy-Meige syndrome
nonneoplastic
    n. disease of bone
    n. mucinous hyperplastic epithelium
non-nephrotic range proteinuria
Nonne test
nonnucleated
nonobstructive jaundice
nonoccluded virus
nonodontogenic
    n. cyst
    n. lesion
nonoemulsion disinfectant
Nonomuraea
    N. dietziae
    N. roseoviolacea subsp. *carminate*
nonossifying fibroma
nonparametric
nonparatrabecular
nonpathogenic
nonpenicillinase-producing *Staphylococcus*
    epidermidis
nonpermissive culture medium
nonpersistent agent
nonphotochromogenic mycobacteria
nonprecipitable antibody
nonprecipitating antibody
nonprotein
    n. nitrogen (NPN)
    n. nitrogen test
nonradioisotopic immunoassay
nonrandom pattern
nonrapid eye movement (NREM)
nonreactive (NR)
    n. pattern
nonrelapsing
    n. colitis
    n. disease
nonrenal
    n. azotemia
    n. death (NRD)
nonreplicating cell
nonreplicative state

nonrespiratory alkalosis
nonresponder tolerance
nonrotation
    n. of intestine
    n. of kidney
nonsecretor
    para-Bombay n.
nonsecretory myeloma
nonseminomatous germ cell tumor
    (NSGCT)
nonsense
    n. mutation
    n. triplet
nonsentinel lymph node (NSLN)
nonseptate mycelium
nonsister chromatid
nonsmall
    n. cell cancer (NSCC)
    n. cell lung cancer (NSCLC)
nonspecific (NS)
    n. anergy
    n. bronchial reactivity (NSBR)
    n. cross-reacting antigen (NCA)
    n. esterase (NSE)
    n. granulomatous prostatitis
    n. hepatocellular abnormality
    n. immunity
    n. interstitial pneumonitis (NSIP)
    n. protein
    n. system
    n. therapy
    n. urethritis (NSU)
    n. viral syndrome
nonspore-forming bacterium
nonsteroidal antiinflammatory (NSAID)
nonstress test (NST)
nonstructural gene
nonstructural protein 3
nonsuppressible insulinlike activity
    (NSILA)
nonsymptomatic, nondisabling (NSND)
nonsyndromal dysplasia
nonsyndromic
nontoxic goiter (NTG)
nontransmural myocardial infarction
nontreponemal antibody test
nontropical sprue
nontuberculous mycobacteria (NTM)
nontyepable
nontyphoidal infectious colitis
nonulcer dyspepsia
nonunion fracture
nonvascular
nonviable
nonviral hepatitis
Noonan syndrome
NOR
    nucleolar organizing region

nucleolus organizing region
  NOR banding
Nora lesion
Nordau disease
norepinephrine (Ne)
  urine n.
norimbergensis
  Pandoraea n.
normal (N)
  n. animal
  n. anion gap acidosis
  n. antibody
  n. antithrombin
  n. antitoxin
  n. blood serum (NBS)
  n. body temperature
  n. cholesteremic xanthomatosis
  n. complement of cells
  diphtheria toxin n. (DTN)
  n. exocrine pancreas
  n. horse serum (NHS)
  n. human plasma
  n. human serum (NHS)
  n. human serum albumin
  n. lymph node
  n. lymphocyte transfer test (NLT)
  n. opsonin
  n. plasma (NP)
  n. pressure hydrocephalus (NPH)
  n. rabbit serum (NRS)
  n. RB protein
  n. reference serum (NRS)
  n. replication
  n. single dose (NSD)
  n. term pregnancy
  n. thymus
  n. toxin
  upper limits of n. (ULN)
  n. value
normal-AG metabolic acidosis
normetanephrine
  urine n.
normoblast
  acidophilic n.
  basophilic n.
  intermediate n.
  mitosis of n.
  orthochromatic n.
  orthochromatophilic n.
  polychromatic n.
  polychromatophilic n.
normoblastic

normoblastosis
normocalcemia
normocellular bone marrow specimen
normochromia
normochromic anemia
normocomplementemia
normocyte
normocytic
  n. anemia
  n. erythrocyte
normocytosis
normoerythrocyte
normoglycemia
normoglycemic glycosuria
normokalemia, normokaliemia
normokalemic periodic paralysis
normolipemic xanthoma planum
normoplasia
normotensive
normovolemia
Norovirus
Norris corpuscle
North
  N. American blastomycosis
  N. Atlantic Treaty Organization
    (NATO)
Northern
  N. blot analysis
  N. blot technique
  N. blot test
norvegicus
  Enterovibrio n.
Norwalk
  N. agent
  N. disease
  N. virus (*Norovirus*)
Norymberski procedure
NOS
  nitric oxide synthase
  not otherwise specified
nose
  cleft n.
  dog n.
  olfactory region of tunica mucosa
    of n.
  respiratory region of tunica mucosa
    of n.
Nosema corneum
Nosematidae
nosepiece
nosocomial
  n. anemia

N

NOTES

nosocomial *(continued)*
    n. infection
    n. pneumonia
nosocomialis
    phagedena n.
nosologic drift
nosomycosis
nosophyte
Nosopsyllus fasciatus
nosotoxic
nosotoxin
Nostocales
nostras
    elephantiasis n.
    piedra n.
nostrum
    elephantiasis verrucosa n.
not
    n. measurable (NM)
    n. otherwise specified (NOS)
    n. recorded (NR)
    n. resolved (NR)
    n. significant (NS)
    n. statistically significant (NSS)
    n. sufficient (NS)
    n. sufficient quantity (NSQ)
notanencephalia
notation
    scientific n.
notatum
    Penicillium n.
notch
    Hutchinson crescentic n.
    Kernohan n.
Notch3 gene polymorphism in ischemic cerebrovascular disease
Notch receptor
notencephalocele
notencephalus
Nothopanus
notification
    death n.
notochord
notochordal sheath
Notoedres cati
NoTox formalin substitute solution
Nottingham histologic grade
nova
    Nocardia n.
Nova Celltrak 12 hematology analyzer
novae-caledoniae
    Ascotricha n.-c.
novalis
    Bacillus n.
Novapath HIV-1 immunoblot tester
novel
    n. coronavirus
    n. microbiology test
    n. toxicology test

novella
    Starkeya n.
Novelli stain
noverca
    Opisthorchis n.
Novirhabdovirus
novobiosepticus
    Staphylococcus hominis n.
Novosphingobium
    N. aromaticivorans
    N. capsulatum
    N. hassiacum
    N. pentaromativorans
    N. rosa
    N. stygium
    N. subarcticum
    N. subterraneum
    N. tardaugens
Novy
    N., MacNeal, and Nicolle (NNN)
    N., MacNeal, and Nicolle (NNN)
    N. rat disease
novyi
    Clostridium n.
noxa
NP
    nasopharyngeal
    neuropathology
    nodular paragranuloma
    normal plasma
    nucleoplasmic index
    nucleoprotein
    NP antigen
3NP
    3-nitroproprionic acid
N+P
    STA Liatest control N+P
NPC
    nasopharyngeal carcinoma
NPD
    Niemann-Pick disease
NPDL
    nodular poorly differentiated lymphocyte
NPG
    BactiSwab NPG
NPH
    neutral protamine Hagedorn
    normal pressure hydrocephalus
NPI
    Nottingham Prognostic Index
NPN
    necrotic pseudoxanthomatous nodule
    nonprotein nitrogen
NPR
    net protein ratio
n-propanol
NPS
    National Pharmaceutical Stockpile

NPT
  neoprecipitin test
NPU
  net protein utilization
NPV
  negative predictive value
NR
  nephrogenic rest
  nonreactive
  not recorded
  not resolved
  nucleotide residue
N-ras gene
NRBC
  nucleated red blood cell
NRD
  nonrenal death
NREM
  nonrapid eye movement
NRG
  neuregulin
NRG1
  neuregulin 1 (protein)
    NRG1 alpha
    NRG1 beta
NRG2
  neuregulin 2 (protein)
    NRG2 alpha
    NRG2 beta
NRG3
  neuregulin 3 (protein)
NRG4
  neuregulin 4 (protein)
NRH
  nodular regenerative hyperplasia
NRS
  normal rabbit serum
  normal reference serum
NS
  nephrotic syndrome
  nerve sheath
  nevus sebaceus
  nodular sclerosis
  nonspecific
  not significant
  not sufficient
ns, nsec
  nanosecond
NSA
  neuron-specific enolase
  no serious abnormality
  no significant abnormality

NSAID
  nonsteroidal antiinflammatory
NSBR
  nonspecific bronchial reactivity
NSCC
  nonsmall cell cancer
NSCLC
  nonsmall cell lung cancer
NSD
  normal single dose
  no significant defect
  no significant deviation
  no significant difference
  no significant disease
NSE
  neuron-specific enolase
  neuron-specific esterase
  nonspecific esterase
    NSE stain
nsec (*var. of* ns)
NSF
  N-ethylmaleimide-sensitive-factor
NSG
  necrotizing sarcoid granulomatosis
NSGCT
  nonseminomatous germ cell tumor
NSGO
  nonspecific granulomatous orchitis
NSHD
  nodular sclerosing Hodgkin disease
NSILA
  nonsuppressible insulinlike activity
NSIP
  nonspecific interstitial pneumonia
  nonspecific interstitial pneumonia/fibrosis
  nonspecific interstitial pneumonitis
NSLN
  nonsentinel lymph node
    NSLN involvement
NSM
  nerve sheath myxoma
  neurosecretory material
NSND
  nonsymptomatic, nondisabling
NSQ
  not sufficient quantity
NSS
  not statistically significant
NST
  nonstress test
  no specific type

NOTES

NSU
  nonspecific urethritis
NT
  neutralization test
NTAB
  nephrotoxic antibody
Ntaya virus
NTE
  neuropathy target esterase
N-telopeptide (NTx)
  cross-linked N.-t.
N-terminal
  N-t. fragment
  N-t. mid fragment (NMID)
  N-t. prohormone brain natriuretic
    peptide (NT-proBNP)
n-**tetracosanoic acid**
NTG
  nontoxic goiter
NTM
  nontuberculous mycobacteria
NTN
  nephrotoxic nephritis
NT-proBNP
  N-terminal prohormone brain natriuretic
    peptide
NTRK1
  neurotrophic tyrosine kinase receptor,
    type 1
NTSN
  nephrotoxic serum nephritis
NTx
  N-telopeptide
nubecula
nubinhibens
  Roseovarius n.
nuchal
  n. fibrocartilaginous pseudotumor
  n. fibroma
  n. hemangioma
  n. rigidity
nuclear
  n. aggregate lipid
  n. antibody
  n. aplasia
  n. bag
  n. bag fiber
  n., biological, and chemical
  n., biological, chemical (mass-
    casualty weapon) (NBC)
  n. chain
  n. chain fiber
  chemical, biological, radiological
    or n. (CBRN)
  n. crystalline aggregate
  n. dust
  n. envelope
  n. envelope of spermatid
  n. excision repair instability (NIN)

  n. fast red stain
  n. groove
  n. heterochromatin
  n. hyaloplasm
  n. hyperchromasia
  n. inclusion body
  n. isomerism
  n. layer of retina
  n. lipid aggregate
  n. magnetic resonance spectroscopy
  n. matrix protein (NMP)
  n. membrane
  n. membrane alteration
  n. mitotic apparatus (NuMA)
  n. palisading
  n. polarity
  n. pore
  n. pore alteration
  n. pore complex
  n. profile diameter
  n. proliferation marker pKi67
  n. pseudoinclusion
  n. pseudostratification
  n. pyknosis
  n. sap
  n. sap alteration
  n. shape alteration
  n. signal
  n. size alteration
  n. spindle
  n. staining
  n. unrest
  n. vacuolization
  n. wreath cell
nuclear-cytoplasmic
  n.-c. ratio
  n.-c. ratio alteration
nucleated red blood cell (NRBC)
nucleation
  heterogeneous n.
nucleatum
  Fusobacterium n.
nuclei (*pl. of* nucleus)
nucleic
  n. acid amplification test (NAT)
  n. acid amplification testing
  n. acid chip technology
  n. acid detection
  n. acid hybridization
  n. acid panel (NAP)
  n. acid probe
  n. acid sequence based
    amplification (NASBA)
  n. acid sequencing
  n. acid test
nucleiform
nucleocapsid
nucleochylema
nucleochyme

nucleocytoplasmic fractionation
nucleoid
    Lavdovsky n.
nucleolar
    n. organizing region (NOR)
    n. pattern
    n. RNAs
nucleolar-associated chromatin
nucleolar-nuclear ratio
nucleoli (*pl. of* nucleolus)
nucleoliform
nucleolin
nucleoloid
nucleolonema
    wandering n.
nucleolus, pl. **nucleoli**
    nonmembrane-bound n.
    organization of the n.
    n. organizing region (NOR)
nucleomegaly
nucleomicrosome
Nucleophaga
nucleophagocytosis
nucleophile
nucleophosphoprotein
nucleoplasm
nucleoplasmic index (NP)
Nucleopolyhedrovirus
nucleoprotein (NP)
    peptidyl-prolyl isomerase n. (Pin1)
nucleoreticulum
Nucleorhabdovirus
nucleorrhexis
nucleosidase
nucleoskeleton
nucleosome
5′ nucleotidase
nucleotide
    cyclic n.
    diphosphopyridine n. (DPN, DPNH)
    n. polymerase
    pyridine n.
    n. sequencing
nucleotidylexotransferase
    DNA n.
nucleotidyltransferase
    DNA n.
    RNA n.
nucleotoxin

Nuclepore
    N. filter
    N. method
nucleus, pl. **nuclei**
    n. accumbens
    arcuate n.
    Balbiani n.
    band shaped n.
    n. basalis of Ganser
    Bekhterev n.
    Cajal interstitial n.
    caudate n.
    cerebriform n.
    nuclei of chondrocyte
    cigar-shaped n.
    Clarke dorsal n.
    n. containing predominantly
     euchromatin
    dentate n.
    diploid n.
    droplet nuclei
    eccentric n.
    Edinger-Westphal n.
    hobnail n.
    horseshoe-shaped n.
    hyperchromatic n.
    hypersegmentation of granulocyte
     nuclei
    Klein-Gumprecht shadow nuclei
    medial preoptic n.
    n. of motor neuron
    n. of muscle fiber
    nuclei of neuroglia
    n. niger
    oligodendroglial n.
    Orphan Annie eye n.
    palisade arrangement of nuclei
    paraventricular n.
    pleomorphic n.
    popcorn nuclei
    presegmented n.
    prominent n.
    raisinoid n.
    reniform n.
    Schwann n.
    segmentation n.
    shadow n.
    smudged n.
    sole n.
    sperm n.
    stripped n.
    supraoptic n.

NOTES

N

nucleus *(continued)*
    trophic n.
    vesicular n.
    wrinkled n.
nucleus-to-cytoplasm ratio
NucliSens
    N. CMV assay
    N. HIV-1 QT assay
Nuel space
NUG
    necrotizing ulcerative gingivitis
Nuhn gland
nuisance fistula
null
    n. allele
    n. cell
    n. cell adenoma
    n. cell lymphoblastic leukemia
    n. cell lymphoma
    n. cell population
    n. lymphocyte
    n. phenotype
    n. phenotype lesion
null-point potentiometer
null-type non-Hodgkin lymphoma
NuMA
    nuclear mitotic apparatus
    NuMA gene
number
    acid n.
    n. of add-on tests needed to obtain a diagnosis
    atomic n.
    Avogadro n.
    CI n.
    complex n.
    CT n.
    dibucaine n. (DN)
    diploid n.
    DNA copy n.
    fluoride n.
    haploid n.
    iodine n.
    line n.
    mass n.
    modal centromere copy n.
    numeric indicator experimental n. 1 (NIXIE)
    oxidation n.
    random n.
    real n.
    Reynolds n.
    turnover n.
    n.'s of unique patterns per crypt
    wave n.
numbering
    stereospecific n.

numerical
    n. aperture
    n. hypertrophy
    n. karyotype
    n. taxonomy
numeric indicator experimental number 1 (NIXIE)
numerous mucosal folds
nummiform
nummular
    n. dermatitis
    n. eczema
    n. sputum
nummulation
NuPAGE Bis-Tris gel
nurse cell
Nutiliaceae
nutmeglike appearance
nutmeg liver
nutricium
    foramen n.
nutricius
    canalis n.
nutrient
    n. agar
    n. broth
    n. canal
    n. foramen
    n. medium
    mineral n.
    vehiculated n.
nutrition
    total parenteral n. (TPN)
nutritional
    n. anemia
    n. cirrhosis
    n. recovery syndrome
Nuttallia
NV
    negative variation
    nodular vasculitis
NVD
    Newcastle virus disease
nyctalopia
Nyctotherus
nymph
nymphal
nymphearum
    Dichotomophthoropsis n.
nymphitis
nympholabial
nymphoncus
Nyssorhynchus
nystagmus
    periodic alternating n. (PAN)
    positional alcohol n. (PAN)
nystatin assay agar

O

O agglutination
O agglutinin
alkaline toluidine blue O
O antibody
O antigen
O colony
coriphosphine O
magenta O
toluidine blue O

OA

osteoarthritis

OAAD

ovarian ascorbic acid depletion
OAAD test

O-acyl-transferase

phosphatidylcholine-sterol O.-a.-t.

OAD

obstructive airway disease

OAF

osteoclast activating factor

o-aminoazotoluene

OAP

osteoarthropathy

oasthouse urine disease

oat

o. cell
o. cell carcinoma

oatmeal-tomato paste agar

OAV

oculoauriculovertebral
OAV dysplasia
OAV syndrome

OB

osteoblastoma

Obermayer test

Obermeier spirillum

Obermüller test

obesity

central o.
exogenous o.

Obesumbacterium proteus

obidoxime therapy

object

o. code
o. glass
o. program
test o.

objective

achromatic o.
aplanatic o.
apochromatic o.
dry o.
flat-field o.
fluorite o.

immersion o.
semiapochromatic o.

obligate

o. aerobe
o. anaerobe
o. autotroph
o. coccobacillus
o. osteogenic transcription factor
o. parasite

oblique

o. fiber of muscular layer of
  stomach
o. fracture

obliterans

arteriosclerosis o.
arteritis o.
balanitis xerotica o.
bronchiolitis fibrosa o.
endangiitis o.
endarteritis o.
pericarditis o.
thromboangiitis o. (TAO)

obliterating

o. arteritis
o. endarteritis

obliteration

fibrous o.

obliterative

o. arachnoiditis
o. bronchiolitis
o. bronchitis
o. endarteritis
o. hepatocavopathy
o. inflammation
o. pericarditis
o. pleuritis

obnubilate

obnubilation

oboediens

Gluconacetobacter o.

OBS

organic brain syndrome

observation

censored o.

obsolescent glomerulus

obstetric

o. catastrophe
o. panel

obstetrics

International Federation of
  Gynecology and O. (FIGO)

obstipation

obstructed testis

obstruction

ball-valve o.

O

obstruction *(continued)*
    biliary o.
    bladder neck o. (BNO)
    bronchiole o.
    chronic airway o. (CAO)
    closed-loop o.
    common bile duct o.
    complete o.
    extrahepatic o. (EHO)
    intestinal o. (IO)
    intrahepatic vascular o.
    mesenteric vascular o.
    partial o.
    renal o.
    salivary duct o.
    site of venous o.
    ureteropelvic junction o.
    ureterovesical o.
    urethral o.
    urinary o.
    vena cava o.

obstructive
    o. airway disease (OAD)
    o. appendicitis
    o. atelectasis
    o. cirrhosis
    o. diverticulitis
    o. emphysema
    o. hyperbilirubinuria
    o. jaundice
    o. lung disease
    o. sleep apnea
    o. uropathy

obstruent

OBT
    occult blood test
    FlexSure OBT

obtecta
    pelvis o.

obturating embolism

obturation

obturator
    o. artery
    o. canal
    o. crest
    o. foramen
    o. hernia
    o. nerve
    o. vein

obturbans
    Armigeres o.

obvelata
    Syphacia o.

obvelatus
    Cosmocephalus o.

OC
    oleoresin capsicum
    organ confined

occidentalis
    Dermacentor o.

occipitoatlantoaxial junction

occlude

occluded virus

occludens
    zonula o.

occludin
    hyperphosphorylation of o.

occlusion
    aortic o.
    o. of arteries
    carotid artery o.
    coronary o.
    internal carotid artery o. (ICAO)
    retinal artery o.
    thrombotic o.
    o. time (OT)
    venous o.

occlusive meningitis

occult
    o. bleeding
    o. blood
    o. blood loss
    o. blood test (OBT)
    o. carcinoma
    o. metastasis
    o. nodular heterotopia

occulta
    spina bifida o.

occupational
    o. hypersensitivity pneumonitis
    o. lung disease
    o. medicine
    O. Safety and Health Administration (OSHA)

occurrence
    multicentric o.

oceanense
    Desulfofrigus o.

Oceanibulbus indolifex

Oceanicaulis alexandrii

Oceanicola
    O. batsensis
    O. granulosus

Oceanimonas
    O. baumannii
    O. doudoroffii

Oceanisphaera litoralis

Oceanithermus
    O. desulfurans
    O. profundus

Oceanobacillus iheyensis

Oceanobacter kriegii

Oceanospirillum

ocellus

OCG
    oral cholecystogram

ochraceum
>*Haliangium o.*
>*Simulium o.*
>*Virgisporangium o.*

ochraceus
>*Aspergillus o.*
>*Bacteroides o.*

ochratoxin
ochre mutation
Ochrobactrum
>*O. gallinifaecis*
>*O. grignonense*
>*O. tritici*

Ochroconis
Ochromyia anthropophaga
ochronosis
ochronotic
>o. arthritis
>o. pigment

OCT
>ornithine carbamoyltransferase
>oxytocin challenge test

octal
octane
octanoic acid
octavius
>*Anaerococcus o.*

Octosporomyces
octreotide scintigraph
octulosonic acid
ocular
>o. cicatricial pemphigoid
>compensating o.
>o. cytology
>o. grid
>o. humor
>Huygens o.
>o. hypertelorism
>o. inflammatory disease (OID)
>o. larva migrans
>o. lymphomatosis
>o. melanoma
>o. micrometer
>o. muscle dystrophy (OMD)
>Ramsden o.
>o. reticle
>o. surface squamous neoplasia
>widefield o.

ocular-mucous membrane syndrome
oculi
>*Dracunculus o.*
>tapetum o.

>tunica albuginea o.
>tunica externa o.
>tunica vasculosa o.

oculoauriculovertebral (OAV)
>o. dysplasia

oculobuccogenital syndrome
oculocerebrorenal syndrome
oculocutaneous albinism
oculodentodigital (ODD)
>o. dysplasia
>o. syndrome

oculodermal melanosis
oculoencephalic angiomatosis
oculogenitalis
>*Chlamydia o.*

oculomandibulodyscephaly
oculomandibulomelic (OMM)
oculomycosis
oculovertebral
>o. dysplasia
>o. syndrome

OD
>optical density
>outside diameter

ODD
>oculodentodigital
>ODD dysplasia
>ODD syndrome

odditis
>foreign body o.
>primary o.
>stenosing o.

odds
>logarithm of o. (LOD)

Odland body
ODN
>oligodeoxynucleotide

odontoameloblastoma
odontoblast
>o. process

odontoblastic
>o. layer
>o. tissue

Odontobutis
odontoclast
odontogenesis
odontogenic
>o. cyst
>o. epithelium
>o. fibroma
>o. fibrosarcoma
>o. ghost cell tumor

NOTES

O

odontogenic *(continued)*
    o. keratocyst (OKC)
    o. lesion
    o. myxoma
odontology
    forensic o.
odontolyticus
    Actinomyces o.
odontoma
    ameloblastic o.
    complex o.
    compound o.
    fibroameloblastic o.
odorans
    Alcaligenes o.
odoratism
odorifer
    Paenibacillus o.
odoriferous gland
odorimutans
    Anaerovorax o.
odysseyi
    Bacillus o.
Oe
    oersted
oedematiens
    Bacillus o.
oedipodis
    Brackiella o.
Oedocephalum
Oerskovia
    O. enterophila
    O. jenensis
    O. paurometabola
oersted (Oe)
Oesophagostomum
    O. apiostomum
    O. bifurcum
    O. brevicaudum
    O. brumpti
    O. columbianum
    O. dentatum
    O. georgianum
    O. quadrispinulatum
    O. radiatum
    O. stephanostomum
    O. venulosum
Oestridae
oestrids
oestrosis
Oestrus
    O. hominis
    O. ovis
OF
    Ovenstone factor
    oxidation-fermentation
    OF medium

OFB
    oval fat body
    OFB cast
OFD
    oral-facial-digital
    orofaciodigital
    OFD syndrome 1–8
office
    O. of Emergency Preparedness
    Epidemiology Program O. (EPO)
    O. of National Statistics (ONS)
    Public Health Practice Program O.
      (PHPPO)
officer
    medical review o. (MRO)
    radiation protection o. (RPO)
officinalis
    poxvirus o.
Ofuji disease
Ogawa antigen
Ogilvie syndrome
O'Grady prognostic indices
OGTT
    oral glucose tolerance test
Oguchi disease
oguniense
    Pyrobaculum o.
Ohara disease
O₂Hb

O$_2$Hb
    oxyhemoglobin
    O$_2$Hb fraction
17-OH corticoid test
OHL
    oral hairy leukoplakia
"ωH-like viruses"
Ohm law
ohmmeter
ohne Hauch
Ohngren line
OHP
    oxygen under high pressure
OHS
    ovarian hyperstimulation syndrome
o-**hydroxyphenylacetic acid**
OIA
    Optical ImmunoAssay
      CdTOX A OIA
      Chlamydia OIA
      GC OIA
      Strep B OIA
OID
    ocular inflammatory disease
      GC OID
      RSV OID
oidia (*pl. of* oidium)
Oidiodendron cerealis
Oidiomycetes
oidiomycin
oidiomycosis

Oidium
oidium, pl. **oidia**
oid-oid disease
OIF
oil immersion field
oil
anise o.
bergamot o.
cedar o.
chenopodium o.
clove o.
croton o.
o. cyst
distilled o.
o. embolism
essential o.
ethiodized o.
eucalyptus o.
fatty o.
fixed o.
flaxseed o.
fog o. (SGF2)
o. gland
o. immersion
o. immersion field (OIF)
o. immersion lens
joint o.
origanum o.
PFAPE o.
red o.
o. red O stain
safflower o.
sandalwood o.
santal o.
sesame o.
silicone o.
o. tumor
turpentine o.
o. vaccine
volatile o.
water in o. (W/O)
o. in water (O/W)
oil-aspiration pneumonia
oil-water ratio (O:W)
oily granuloma
ointment
BAL o.
Okavirus
Okazaki segment
OKC
odontogenic keratocyst

okeanokoites
Planomicrobium o.
okhotskensis
Psychrobacter o.
Okibacterium
O. fritillariae
OKT
Ortho-Kung T cell
OKT-9 antibody
okuhidensis
Bacillus o.
OLB
open lung biopsy
OLC
oligodendroglia-like cell
old
o. infarct
o. myocardial infarction (OMI)
o. thrombus
o. tuberculin (OT)
O. World hookworm
O. World screwworm
oleaginous
oleandomycin
olearia
Petrotoga o.
olearium
Sporobacterium o.
oleate
Oleavirus
olecranarthropathy
olefin
oleic
o. acid
o. acid I 125
o. acid uptake test
Oleiphilaceae
Oleiphilus messinensis
Oleispira antarctica
oleivorans
Thalassolituus o.
oleogranuloma
oleoma
oleoresin
aspidium o.
o. capsicum (OC)
olfactoriae
glandulae o.
olfactorius
bulbus o.
olfactory
o. bulb

NOTES

O

olfactory *(continued)*
    o. epithelium
    o. esthesioneuroblastoma
    o. gland
    o. glomerulus
    o. membrane
    o. mucosa
    o. neuroblastoma (ONB)
    o. organ
    o. receptor cell
    o. region of tunica mucosa of nose
olfactus
    organum o.
OLGC
    osteoclast-like giant cell
OLH
    ovine lactogenic hormone
Oligella urethralis
oligemia, olighemia
oligemic
oligoadenylate synthetase
oligoastrocytoma
oligoclonal
    o. band
    o. banding
oligocystic
oligocythemia
oligodactyly
oligodendria
oligodendroblast
oligodendroblastoma
oligodendrocyte
oligodendrogenic cell
oligodendroglia
    o. cell
    o. stain
    o. staining
oligodendroglial
    o. nucleus
    o. tumor
oligodendroglia-like cell (OLC)
oligodendroglioma
    anaplastic o.
    pleomorphic o.
oligodeoxynucleotide (ODN)
oligodynamic
oligofermentans
    Streptococcus o.
oligo-1,6-glucosidase
oligohydramnios
oligomeganephronia
oligomenorrhea
oligomer
    allele-specific o.
    toxic soluble o.
oligomeric plasmid
oligomerization
oligonephronic hypoplasia

oligonucleotide
    allele-specific o.
    enzyme-labeled o.
    o. genomic array
    o. primer
    o. probe
oligonucleotide-primed
    degenerate o.-p. (DOP)
oligopeptide
oligophrenia
Oligoporus
oligosaccharide
oligospermatism
oligospermia
oligospora
    Arthobotrys o.
oligosynaptic
oligotropha
    Nitrosomonas o.
oligotrophic
oligotyping
oligozoospermatism
oligozoospermia
oliguria
olivapovliticus
    Alkalibacterium o.
olivary eminence
olivocerebellar atrophy
olivopontocerebellar atrophy
olleyana
    Shewanella o.
Ollier disease
Ollulanus tricuspis
Olmer disease
olomoucine
Olsenella
    O. profusa
    O. uli
olympian forehead
Olympus
    O. AU5200 cholesterol analyzer
    O. BH2 microscope
OM
    otitis media
OMD
    ocular muscle dystrophy
omega
Omegatetravirus
Omenn syndrome
omentitis
omentovolvulus
omentum
    greater o.
    lesser o.
OMI
    old myocardial infarction
omicron
omitis

OMM
oculomandibulomelic
OMM dysplasia
OMM syndrome
omnibus hypothesis
Omnifix
omnivorum
Flavobacterium o.
Omnivue illuminated magnifier
OMPA
otitis media, purulent, acute
omphalelcosis
omphalitis
omphalocele
omphalomesenteric duct remnant
omphalophlebitis
Omphalospora
Omphalotus illudens
Omsk
O. hemorrhagic fever
O. hemorrhagic fever virus
OMT
ovarian mucinous tumor
ONB
olfactory neuroblastoma
Onchocerca
O. caecutiens
O. cervicalis
O. lienalis
O. volvulus
onchocerciasis, onchocercosis
onchocerciasis-type filariasis
onchocercid
Onchocercidae
onchocercosis (*var. of* onchocerciasis)
Oncocerca
OncoChek immunoassay
oncocyte
oncocytic
o. adenoma
o. carcinoma
o. cell
o. epithelium
o. hepatocellular tumor
o. metaplasia
o. papillary cystadenoma
o. papillary neoplasm
o. transformation
oncocytoma
renal o.
oncofetal
o. activation

o. antigen
o. marker
o. protein
oncogene
Abelson o.
bcl-2 o.
c-abl o.
c-fos o.
c-kit o.
cyclin D1 o.
erb A o.
erb B, B-2 o.
fms o.
HER-2/neu o.
Ki-67 o.
K-ras o.
MIC2 o.
myc o.
N-myc o.
p16 o.
ras o.
retroviral o.
oncogenesis
oncogenic
o. human papillomavirus
o. virus
oncogenous
oncoides
oncologist
oncology
oncolysis
oncolytic
oncoma
Oncomelania
Oncometrics Imaging Cyto-Savant image analyzer
oncophora
Cooperia o.
oncoplastic carcinoma
oncoprotein
o. antigen
c-erb-B2 o.
c-myc o.
Oncor
O. antifade mounting solution
O. Inform HER2/neu gene
amplification detection system
Oncorhynchus
oncornavirus
oncosis
oncosphere
oncotic pressure

NOTES

O

oncotropic
Oncovirinae
oncovirus
on-demand system
one-sided alternative
one-stage
    o.-s. factor assay
    o.-s. prothrombin time
    o.-s. prothrombin time test
One-Step hCG combo test
one-step nested PCR (OSNP)
one-tailed test
one-tube nested PCR
onion
    o. body
    o. scale lesion
onionskin
    o. change
    o. lesion
o-nitrophenyl-beta-D-galactopyranoside (ONPG)
o-nitrophenyl beta galactosidase
onkinocele
Onnia
onocytoma
ONPG
    o-nitrophenyl-beta-D-galactopyranoside
    ONPG test
ONS
    Office of National Statistics
Onthophagus
ontogeny
OnTrak TestTcard drug testing device
onychatrophia
onychia, onychitis
Onychocola canadensis
onychoheterotopia
onycholysis
onychoma
onychomycosis
onychoosteodysplasia
onychophosis
onychorrhexis
O'nyong-nyong
    O.-n. fever
    O.-n. fever virus
onyx (*var. of* unguis)
onyxitis
OO
    osteoid osteoma
OOC
    orthokeratinized odontogenic cyst
oocyst
oocyte
    integer o.
oogenesis
oogonium, ovogonium
ookinete
oolemma

oomycosis
oophoritic cyst
oophoritis
oophorocystosis
oophoroma
oophoron
oophorosalpingitis
oophorus
    cumulus o.
oosome
Oospora granulosa
oosporangium
oospore
Oosporidium
ootheca
ootid
ootype
OP
    osmotic pressure
    OP code
O&P
    ova and parasites
    O&P test
opacification of lens
opacity
    corneal o. (CO)
    ground glass o.
    lenticular o.
opalescent
opalgia
Opalski cell
opaque
    o. colony
    o. microscope
OPCP
    orthocresolphthalein complex
OPD4 antibody
open
    o. circuit
    o. lung biopsy (OLB)
    o. reading frame (ORF)
    o. tuberculosis
open-angle glaucoma
opera-glass hand
operating
    o. cycle
    o. system
    o. time
operation
    o. code
    comparison o.
    military o.
    parallel o.
    serial o.
    symmetry o.
    unattended laboratory o.
operational amplifier
operations
    morgue o.

operator
- o. certification
- o. gene

operculated

operculum, pl. **opercula**

operon
- arabinose o.
- lac o.
- tra o.

Ophiostoma

Ophiovirus

ophryogenes
- ulerythema o.

Ophryoscolecidae

ophthalmia
- gonococcal o.
- gonorrheal o.
- o. neonatorum
- spring o.
- sympathetic o.

ophthalmitis
- sympathetic o.

ophthalmobium
- *Agamodistomum o.*

ophthalmomandibulomelic dysplasia

ophthalmomycosis

ophthalmomyiasis

ophthalmopathy
- infiltrative o.
- thyroid o.

ophthalmoplegia

ophthalmoplegic-type progressive muscular dystrophy

ophthalmosteresis

ophthalmovascular choke

opiate
- o. assay
- Liquichek urine toxicology control C2, C3, S1, S2 low o.

OPIDN
- organophosphate-induced delayed neuropathy

opinion
- consensus pathology o.

opioid

opisthomastigote

opisthorchiasis

opisthorchid

Opisthorchiidae

Opisthorchioidea

Opisthorchis
- *O. felineus*
- *O. noverca*
- *O. sinensis*
- *O. viverrini*

opisthorchosis

opisthotonos

Opitutus terrae

Opitz
- O. disease
- O. GBBB syndrome

opium

Oppenheim
- O. disease
- O. syndrome

Oppenheim-Urbach disease

opportunistic
- o. infection
- o. mycosis
- o. pathogen

opsin

opsinogen

opsoclonus-myoclonus
- o.-m. diarrhea
- o.-m. syndrome

opsonic
- o. action
- o. index

opsonin
- bacterial o.
- common o.
- immune o.
- normal o.
- specific o.
- thermolabile o.
- thermostable o.

opsonization
- bacterial o.

opsonizing antibody

opsonocytophagic

opsonometry

opsonophilia

opsonophilic

optic
- o. atrophy
- o. nerve disease
- o. nerve glioma
- o. neuritis
- o. papillitis
- o. part of retina

optical
- o. activity
- o. allachesthesia
- o. density (OD)

O

NOTES

optical *(continued)*
    o. glass
    O. ImmunoAssay (OIA)
    o. isomer
    o. isomerism
    o. light scatter
    o. purity
    o. rotary dispersion (ORD)
    o. rotation
optici
    spatium intervaginale subarachnoidale nervi o.
    stratum ganglionare nervi o.
OptiClone monoclonal antibody
optics
    geometric o.
    Nomarski o.
    physical o.
OptiLyse lysing reagent
Optima
    O. L-XP, L-90 K, LE-80 K preparative ultracentrifuge
    O. Max, Max-E, TLX personal benchtop ultracentrifuge
optimal growth temperature
OptiMax immunostaining system
optimization
    automated assay o. (AAO)
    Sagian automated assay o.
optimized robot for chemical analysis (ORCA)
optimizing compiler
optimum temperature
Optochin susceptibility test
optomeninx
Opus cardiac troponin I assay
ora
    o. serrata
    o. serrata retinae
oral
    o. actinomycosis
    o. antibiotic
    o. cavity
    o. cavity cytology
    o. cholecystogram (OCG)
    o. flora
    o. glucose tolerance test (OGTT)
    o. hairy leukoplakia (OHL)
    o. infection
    o. lactose tolerance test
    o. pathology
    o. poliovirus vaccine
    o. smear
orale
    Desulfomicrobium o.
    Mycoplasma o.
oral-facial-digital (OFD)

oralis
    Bacteroides o.
    Prevotella o.
OralScreen
    O. 3-panel oral fluids test
    O. rapid oral fluid screening and test device
    O. 4 substance abuse test
oral-sinonasal melanoma
orange
    acridine o. (AO)
    ethyl o.
    o. G
    methyl o.
    o. peel corneal appearance
    Victoria o.
OraQuick rapid HIV-1 antibody test
OraSure HIV-1 oral specimen collection device
OraTest oral cancer test
orbiculare
    Pityrosporum o.
orbital
    o. abscess
    o. cellulitis
    o. cyst
    o. fracture
    o. hemangiopericytoma
    hybrid o.
    o. meningioma
    o. mucocele
    o. trauma
    o. tumor
orbitopathy
    thyroid o.
Orbivirus
ORCA
    optimized robot for chemical analysis
    ORCA Robot
orcein
    acetic o.
    acid o.
    o. stain
orchella
orchiatrophy
orchica
    adiposis o.
orchidic hormone
orchiditis
orchidoblastoma
orchidoptosis
orchiepididymitis
orchil
orchioblastoma
orchiocele
orchioncus
orchiopexy
orchitic

orchitis
 autoimmune o.
 granulomatous o.
 nonspecific granulomatous o.
  (NSGO)
orcini
 Diphyllobothrium o.
orcinol
 o. test
ORD
 optical rotary dispersion
order
 low o.
ordinal variable
ordinary smallpox
ordinate
orellanus
 Cortinarius o.
Orenia
 O. salinaria
 O. sivashensis
orexigenic factor
orexin A, B peptide
ORF
 open reading frame
orf infection
orf virus
organ
 accessory o.
 annulospiral o.
 Chievitz o.
 Corti o.
 o. culture
 digestive o.
 enamel o.
 end o.
 floating o.
 Golgi tendon o.
 gustatory o.
 lymphoid o.
 neurotendinous o.
 no cancer spread to other o.'s
  (M0)
 olfactory o.
 o. perfusion
 principal target o.
 ptotic o.
 reticular membrane of spinal o.
 sense o.
 o. of smell
 spiral o.
 subcommissural o.

 supernumerary o.
 target o.
 o. of taste
 tendon o.
 o. and tissue procurement
  organization
 o. tolerance dose (OTD)
 o. of touch
 vestibular o.
 wandering o.
 o. xenotransplantation
 Zuckerkandl o.
organa (*pl. of* organum)
organelle
 cell o.
 cytoplasmic o.
organic
 o. acid
 o. brain syndrome (OBS)
 o. cation
 o. chemistry
 o. chloroarsine
 o. contracture
 o. disease
 o. dust toxic syndrome
 o. lesion
 o. phosphate
 o. radical (R)
 o. solvent
organification defect
organism
 Arizona o.
 boxcar o.
 calculated mean o. (CMO)
 Campylobacter-like o. (CLO)
 catalase-negative o.
 catalase-positive o.
 o. characteristic
 demonstration of o.
 facultative o.
 hypothetical mean o. (HMO)
 indicator o.
 lepra cell o.
 nonmotile o.
 photosynthetic o.
 pleuropneumonia-like o. (PPLO)
 Ricketts o.
 Vincent o.
organivorans
 Halomonas o.
organization
 International Standards O. (ISO)

O

NOTES

organization *(continued)*
Joint Commission on Accreditation of Healthcare O.'s (JCAHO)
North Atlantic Treaty O. (NATO)
o. of the nucleolus
organ and tissue procurement o.
Professional Standards Review O. (PSRO)
World Health O. (WHO)

organized
o. hematoma
o. old thrombotic residue
o. pneumonia
o. thrombus

organizer
procentriole o.

organizing
o. inflammation
o. pneumonitis

organochlorine
o. insecticide
o. pesticide

organogenesis

organoid
o. arrangement
o. growth pattern
o. nevus
o. thymoma
o. tumor

organoma

organometallic compound

organophilum
Methylobacterium o.

organophosphate
o. compound
o. insecticide
o. pesticide

organophosphate-induced delayed neuropathy (OPIDN)

organophosphorous
toxic o.

organosilicon compound

organotaxis

organothiophosphate compound assay

organotroph

organotropic bacterium

organotropism, organotropy

organotypic feature

organ-specific antigen

organum, pl. **organa**
o. gustus
o. olfactus
organa sensuum
o. spirale
o. tactus

Oribacterium sinus

Oriboca virus

oricola
Actinomyces o.

Oriental
O. blood fluke
O. hemoptysis
O. lung fluke
O. lung fluke disease
O. ringworm
O. sore

orientalis
Acetobacter o.
Dermacentroxenus o.
Issatchenkia o.
Nocardia o.
Phlebotomus o.
Pseudomonas o.
Trichostrongylus o.

Orientia tsutsugamushi

orientis
Desulfosporosinus o.

orifice
golf hole ureteral o.

orificialis
tuberculosis cutis o.

origanum oil

origin
amyloid of immunoglobulin o. (AIO)
amyloid of unknown o. (AUO)
anomalous o.
arthritis of probable autoimmune o.
fever of undetermined o. (FUO)
fever of unknown o. (FUO)
hematopoietic cell o.
myocardial disease of unknown o. (MDUO)
ovarian sex cord-stromal o.
pyrexia of unknown o. (PUO)
tumor of germ cell o.

Orion
O. electrode
O. skin electrode for chloride

oris
Bacteroides o.
cancrum o.
Filaria hominis o.
glandulae o.
pachyderma o.
Prevotella o.
tunica mucosa o.

orisratti
Streptococcus o.

orleanensis
Acetobacter o.

Ormond disease

ornate

ornithine
o. aminotransferase
o. carbamoyltransferase (OCT)
o. carbamoyltransferase assay
o. carbamoyltransferase deficiency

o. decarboxylase
o. transcarbamoylase (OTC)
o. transcarbamoylase deficiency
ornithinemia
ornithine-oxo-acid aminotransferase
Ornithinimicrobium humiphilum
ornithinivorans
    Hongiella o.
ornithinolytica
    Raoultella o.
ornithinuria
Ornithobilharzia
Ornithodoros
    O. coriaceus
    O. erraticus
    O. hermsi
    O. lahorensis
    O. moubata complex
    O. pappilipes
    O. parkeri
    O. rudis
    O. savigni
    O. talaje
    O. tholozani
    O. turicata
    O. venezuelensis
    O. verrucosus
Ornithonyssus
ornithosis
    Miyagawanella o.
    o. virus
orodigitofacial dysostosis
orofaciodigital (OFD)
oropharyngeal
    o. anthrax
    o. tularemia
oropharynx
Oropouche virus
orosomucoid
orotate phosphoribosyltransferase
orotic
    o. acid
    o. aciduria
orotidine-5′-phosphate decarboxylase
orotidylate decarboxylase
Oroya fever
orphan
    O. Annie eye nucleus
    chicken embryo lethal o. (CELO)
    enteric cytopathogenic bovine o. (ECBO)
    enteric cytopathogenic human o. (ECHO)
    enteric cytopathogenic monkey o. (ECMO)
    enteric cytopathogenic swine o. (ECSO)
    enterocytopathogenic dog o. (ECDO)
    o. virus
orseillin BB
Ortalidae
Orth
    O. fixative
    O. fluid
    O. solution
    O. stain
orthoaminoazotoluene
Orthobunyavirus
orthochromatic
    o. megaloblast
    o. normoblast
orthochromatophilic normoblast
orthochromophil, orthochromophile
orthocresolphthalein complex (OPCP)
orthocytosis
orthodromic
Orthohepadnavirus
orthoiodohippurate
orthokeratinized odontogenic cyst (OOC)
orthokeratosis
orthokeratotic sparing
Ortho-Kung T cell (OKT)
Orthomune antibody
Orthomyxoviridae
orthomyxovirus
orthophosphoric
    o. acid
    o. ester monohydrolase
orthopnea
Orthopodomyia
Orthopoxvirus
Orthoptera
orthoptic transplantation
Orthoreovirus
Orthorrhapha
orthostatic
    o. albuminuria
    o. hypertension
    o. hypotension
    o. proteinuria
orthotolidine
orthotopic liver transplantation

O

NOTES

orthovanadate
    sodium o.
Ortolani sign
oryzae
    Azospira o.
    Helminthosporium o.
    Pyricularia o.
    Rhizopus o.
    Xanthomonas o.
Oryzavirus
OS
    osteosarcoma
    overall survival
Os
    osmium
osazone test
os (bone), gen. ossis, pl. ossa
OSBT
    ovarian serous borderline tumor
oscheitis
oschelephantiasis
oscheohydrocele
oscillation
oscillator
Oscillatoriales
Oscillochloridaceae
oscilloscope
    storage o.
Oscillospiraceae
osculum, pl. oscula
Osgood-Schlatter disease
OSHA
    Occupational Safety and Health
    Administration
Osler
    O. disease
    O. erythema
    O. node
Osler-Vaquez disease
Osler-Weber-Rendu
    O.-W.-R. disease
    O.-W.-R. syndrome
osloensis
    Moraxella o.
OSM
    oxygen saturation meter
Osm
    osmole
osmic
    o. acid
    o. acid fixative
osmicate
osmication
osmification
osmiophilic
    o. cell surface membrane
osmiophobic
osmium (Os)

o. tetroxide
o. tetroxide stain
osmolal
    o. clearance
    o. gap
osmolality
    calculated serum o.
    fecal o.
    stool o.
    urine o.
osmolar
    o. clearance (Cosm)
    o. gap
osmolarity
osmole (Osm)
osmometer
    freezing point depression o.
    vapor pressure depression o.
    Vapro vapor pressure o.
osmometry
osmophil
osmophilic
Osmoporus
osmoreceptor
osmosis
osmotic
    o. clearance
    o. coefficient
    o. diuretic
    o. fragility
    o. fragility test
    o. hemolysis
    o. nephrosis
    o. pressure (OP)
    o. shock
os (mouth), gen. oris, pl. ora
OSNP
    one-step nested PCR
ossa (*pl. of* os (bone))
ossea
ossei
    canales semicircularis o.
    labium limbi tympanicum laminae
     spiralis o.
    laminae spiralis o.
ossein
osseocartilaginous
osseomucin
osseous
    o. ankylosis
    o. cell
    o. hydatid
    o. hydatid cyst
    o. lacuna
    o. metaplasia
    o. polyp
    o. spiral lamina
    o. tissue

ossicle
    Andernach o.
ossicular
    o. chain disruption
    o. damage
ossiferous
ossificans
    lipoma o.
    myositis o. (MO)
    pelvospondylitis o.
ossification
    abnormal endochondral o.
    center of o.
    endochondral o.
    intramembranous o.
    membranous o.
    metaplastic o.
    point of o.
    primary center of o.
    primary point of o.
    secondary center of o.
    secondary point of o.
    zone of o.
ossificationis
    punctum o.
ossific center
ossiform
ossify
ossifying
    o. fibroma
    o. inflammation
    o. interstitial myositis
ossis (*gen. of* os (bone))
ossium
    fibrogenesis imperfecta o.
    fragilitas ossium
    medulla o.
    substantia compacta o.
    xanthoma generalisata o.
Ostase
    O. biochemical marker
    O. bone metabolism marker
osteal
ostealgia
osteanagenesis
osteanaphysis
ostein
osteitic
osteitis, ostitis
    caseous o.
    central o.
    o. condensans

    condensing o.
    cortical o.
    o. deformans
    dissecting o.
    o. fibrosa
    o. fibrosa circumscripta
    o. fibrosa cystica
    o. fibrosa disseminata
    hematogenous o.
    localized o. fibrosa
    multifocal o. fibrosa
    sclerosing o.
    o. tuberculosa multiplex cystica
ostemia
ostempyesis
osteoanagenesis
osteoarthritis (OA)
    hyperplastic o.
osteoarthropathy (OAP)
    hypertrophic pulmonary o.
    idiopathic hypertrophic o. (IHO)
    pneumogenic o.
    pulmonary o.
    secondary hypertrophic o. (SHO)
osteoblastic
    o. osteosarcoma
    o. response
osteoblastoma (OB)
osteoblast proliferation fluorometric assay
osteocalcin
osteocarcinoma
    central o.
osteocartilaginous exostosis
osteochondral
osteochondritis
    o. deformans juvenilis
    o. deformans juvenilis dorsi
    o. dissecans
    syphilitic o.
osteochondrodystrophia deformans
osteochondrodystrophy
osteochondrogenic cell
osteochondroma
    multiple o.'s
osteochondromatosis
    synovial o.
osteochondrosarcoma
osteochondrosis
osteochondrous
osteoclasia
osteoclasis

O

NOTES

osteoclast
> o. activating factor (OAF)
> bone-resorbing o.
> multinucleated o.

osteoclastic
> o. factor assay
> o. reaction
> o. resorption

osteoclast-like giant cell (OLGC)
osteoclastoma
osteocollagenous fiber
osteocystoma
osteocyte
osteodentin
osteodermatopoikilosis
osteodermatous
osteodermia
osteodiastasis
osteodysplasty
osteodystrophia
osteodystrophy
> Albright hereditary o.
> renal o.

osteoectasia
osteofibroma
osteofibrosis
osteofibrous dysplasia of Campanacci
osteogen
osteogenesis
> o. imperfecta
> o. imperfecta congenita
> o. imperfecta tarda

osteogenetic
> o. fiber
> o. layer

osteogenic
> o. cell
> o. sarcoma
> o. tissue

osteogenous
osteogeny
OsteoGram bone density test
osteohalisteresis
osteohypertrophy
osteoid
> o. matrix
> o. osteoma (OO)
> o. tissue

osteolathyrism
osteolipochondroma
osteolysis
osteolytic
osteoma
> o. cutis
> fibrous o.
> giant osteoid o.
> o. medullare
> osteoid o. (OO)

parosteal o.
> o. spongiosum

osteomalacia
> senile o.

osteomalacic pelvis
Osteomark NTx point-of-care device
osteomatoid
osteomesopyknosis
osteomyelitis
> Garré sclerosing o.
> pyogenic o.
> tuberculous o.

osteomyelodysplasia
osteomyelofibrotic syndrome
osteomyelosclerosis
osteon
osteoncus
osteonecrosis
osteonectin
osteoonychodysplasia
> hereditary o. (HOOD)

osteopathia
> o. condensans
> o. striata

osteopathy
> alimentary o.
> disseminated condensing o.
> myelogenic o.

osteopenia
osteoperiostitis
osteopetrosis
> o. acroosteolytica
> o. gallinarum

osteopetrotic
osteophage
osteophlebitis
osteophyma
osteophyte
osteoplaque
osteoplast
osteoplastic
osteoplastica
> tracheopathia o.

osteopoikilosis
osteopontin
osteoporosis
> o. circumscripta
> o. circumscripta cranii
> juvenile o.
> posttraumatic o.
> traumatic o.

osteoporotic
osteoprogenitor cell
osteopulmonary arthropathy
osteoradionecrosis
Osteosal osteoporosis test
osteosarcoma (OS)
> central o.
> chondroblastoma-like o.

extraskeletal o.
osteoblastic o.
parosteal o.
periosteal o.
telangiectatic o.
undifferentiated o. (UOS)
osteosclerosis congenita
osteosclerotic anemia
osteosis, ostosis
o. cutis
o. eburnisans monomelica
parathyroid o.
osteospongioma
osteosteatoma
osteothrombosis
Ostertagia
ostia (*pl. of* ostium)
ostiomeatal complex
ostitic
ostitis (*var. of* osteitis)
ostium, pl. **ostia**
Ostor study
ostosis (*var. of* osteosis)
ostracea
psoriasis o.
ostraceous
ostraviensis
Cellvibrio o.
Ostrum-Furst syndrome
Ostwald-Folin pipette
Ostwald viscosimeter
OT
occlusion time
old tuberculin
otalgia
Ota nevus
Ot antigen
OTC
ornithine transcarbamoylase
OTC deficiency
OTD
organ tolerance dose
otic abscess
otitic
o. abscess
o. meningitis
otitidis-caviarum
Nocardia o.-c.
otitis
Alloiococcus o.
o. desquamativa
o. diphtheritica

o. externa
o. labyrinthica
o. mastoidea
o. media (OM)
o. media, purulent, acute (OMPA)
o. mycotica
o. sclerotica
otoacariasis
otobiosis
Otobius
otocerebritis
otoconia
otocyst
Otodectes
otodectic
otoencephalitis
otolith
otolithic membrane
O-toluidine
otomandibular
o. dysostosis
o. syndrome
Otomyces
O. hageni
O. purpureus
otomycosis
otopharyngeal tube
otorrhagia
otorrhea
otosalpinx
otosclerosis
cochlear o.
ototoxic drug
ototoxicity
aminoglycoside o.
OTR
Ovarian Tumor Registry
Otto
O. disease
O. pelvis
Ottowia thiooxydans
Ouchterlony
O. double diffusion
O. immunodiffusion
O. method
O. technique
O. test
Oudemansiella
Oudin immunodiffusion
Ourmiavirus
outer
o. circumferential lamella

O

NOTES

outer *(continued)*
    o. dense fibers of spermatozoon
    o. hair cell
    o. leaflet
    o. longitudinal muscle layer
    o. margin
    o. mitochondrial membrane
    o. phalangeal cell
outlet
    pelvic o.
    right ventricle double o.
outlier
output
    basal acid o. (BAO)
    o. capacitor
    carbon dioxide o. ($\mathring{V}_{CO_2}$)
    CO_2 o.
    decreased cardiac o.
    o. impedance
    maximal acid o.
    peak acid o. (PAO)
outside diameter (OD)
ova (*pl. of* ovum)
oval
    o. corpuscle
    o. fat body (OFB)
    o. macrocyte
    o. subterminal spore
    o. window
ovalbumin
ovale
    anatomically patent foramen o.
    foramen o.
    functionally patent foramen o.
    incompetent valve foramen o.
    o. malaria
    patent foramen o.
    Pityrosporum o.
    Plasmodium o.
    prematurely closed foramen o.
    probe patent foramen o.
    Pseudeurotium o.
ovalis
    fenestra o.
    Malassezia o.
ovalocyte
ovalocytic anemia
ovalocytosis
oval-shaped goblet cell
ovaria (*pl. of* ovarium)
ovarian
    o. agenesis
    o. ascorbic acid depletion (OAAD)
    o. borderline tumor
    o. cancer
    o. cancer biomarker
    o. carcinoma
    o. cyst
    o. dysfunction

    o. failure
    o. follicle
    o. granulosa cell tumor
    o. hormone
    o. hyperstimulation syndrome
    (OHS)
    o. insufficiency
    o. masculinization
    o. mucinous tumor (OMT)
    o. pregnancy
    o. serous borderline tumor (OSBT)
    o. sex cord-stromal origin
    o. sex-cord tumor
    o. teratoma
    o. torsion
    o. tubular adenoma
    O. Tumor Registry (OTR)
    o. varicocele
ovaricus
    cumulus o.
ovarii
    cortex o.
    hilum o.
    Pseudomyxoma o.
    stratum granulosum o.
    stroma o.
    struma o.
ovarioabdominal pregnancy
ovarioncus
ovariosalpingitis
ovaritis
ovarium, pl. **ovaria**
ovary
    dermoid cyst of o.
    hilar cell tumor of o.
    hilum of o.
    inflammation of the o.
    polycystic o.
    rete cyst of o.
    stroma of o.
ovatum
    Loxotrema o.
ovatus
    Metagonimus o.
oven
    Bio-Rad H2500 microwave o.
Ovenstone factor (OF)
over
    unequal crossing o.
overall survival (OS)
overdominance
overexposure
    dental o.
overexpressing
overexpression
    HER-2/neu o.
    protein o.
overflow

overgrowth
>> adenocarcinoma of the uterus with sarcomatous o.
>> small intestine bacterial o.

overhydration

overlap
>> spectral o.
>> o. syndrome

overlapping inversion

overload
>> circulatory o.
>> dysmetabolic iron o.
>> iodine o.
>> iron o.

overpressure
>> peak o.

overshoot

overwhelming postsplenectomy sepsis

overwintering

ovigerous lamella

ovine
>> o. lactogenic hormone (OLH)
>> o. progressive pneumonia

ovinia

oviposit

oviposition

ovipositor

ovis
>> *Cysticercus o.*
>> *Neisseria o.*
>> *Oestrus o.*
>> *Streptococcus o.*
>> *Taenia o.*
>> *Tetratrichomonas o.*
>> *Trichomonas o.*

ovogonium (*var. of* oogonium)

ovoid bacterium

ovoides
>> *Trichosporon o.*

ovolarviparous

ovolyticum
>> *Tenacibaculum o.*

ovotestis

OvuKIT

ovula (*pl. of* ovulum)

ovular

ovulational sclerosis

ovulation test

ovule

ovulum, pl. **ovula**

ovum, pl. **ova**
>> blighted o.

>> cleavage of o.

ova and parasite examination

ova and parasites (O&P)

OvuQUICK

O/W
>> oil in water

O:W
>> oil-water ratio

Owen
>> contour line of O.
>> interglobular space of O.
>> O. line

owl
>> o. eye
>> o. eye appearance

Owren disease

oxalate
>> ammonium o.
>> calcium o. (CO)
>> o. calculus
>> double o.
>> potassium o.
>> urine o.

oxalatica
>> *Ralstonia o.*
>> *Wautersia o.*

oxalemia

oxalic
>> o. acid
>> o. acid assay
>> o. acid stain

Oxalicibacterium flavum

oxalism

oxaloacetate decarboxylase

oxaloacetic acid

oxalosis

oxaluria

oxazin, oxazine
>> o. dye

Oxford unit

ox heart

oxidant
>> o. stress
>> total o.

oxidase
>> aldehyde o.
>> coproporphyrinogen o.
>> cytochrome o.
>> D-amino acid o.
>> glucose o.
>> glycerol-3-phosphate o. (GOI)
>> homogentisate o.

O

NOTES

oxidase *(continued)*
 hydroxyproline o.
 L-amino acid o.
 p-hydroxyphenylpyruvate o.
 proline o.
 protoporphyrinogen o.
 o. reaction
 sulfite o.
 o. test
 xanthine o. (XO)
oxidase-induced acute hemolytic anemia
oxidation
 beta o.
 fatty acid o.
 o. number
 o. state
oxidation-fermentation (OF)
 o.-f. medium
 o.-f. test
oxidation-reducing potential
oxidation-reduction
 o.-r. indicator
 o.-r. reaction
oxidative
 o. energy
 o. phosphorylation
 o. phosphorylation inhibitor
 o. phosphorylation uncoupler
 o. stress
oxide
 aluminum o.
 ethylene o.
 magnesium o. (MgO)
 nitric o. (NO)
 sulfur o.
 vitamin K_1 o.
 zinc o.
oxidize
oxidized
 o. glutathione (GSSG)
 o. low density lipoprotein (oxLDL)
oxidizer
oxidizing
 o. agent
 o. detergent
 o. gas
oxidoreductase
 L-lysine:NAD^+ o.
oxime
 o. antidote
 NATO code for phosgene o. (CX)
oximeter
 AVOXimeter 4000 CO o.
 carbon monoxide o. (CO-oximeter)
oximetry
 arterial blood o.
 pulse o.
OXK
 lipopolysaccharide

oxLDL
 oxidized low density lipoprotein
OX2 lipopolysaccharide
OX19 lipopolysaccharide
oxo acid
oxobutyric acid
oxoglutarate dehydrogenase
oxoglutaric acid
oxoisovalerate dehydrogenase
oxolinic acid
oxonium ion
5-oxoproline
4-oxoproline reductase
oxoprolinuria
5-oxoprolinuria
oxosteroid reductase
ox-warble disease
oxyacoia
oxyaphia
oxybate
 sodium o.
oxybiotin
oxycephalic
oxycephaly, oxycephalia
oxychloride
 carbon o.
oxychromatic
oxychromatin
oxyclinae
 Desulfovibrio o.
oxygen
 o. acceptor
 o. affinity anoxia
 o. affinity hypoxia
 alveolar-arterial o.
 o. analyzer
 o. capacity of blood
 cerebral metabolic rate of o. (CMRO)
 concentration of total o. (CtO_2)
 o. consumption
 o. content of blood
 o. effect
 forced inspiratory o.
 fractional concentration of inspired o. (FiO_2)
 fraction of inspired o.
 o. half-saturation pressure of hemoglobin
 partial pressure of o. (P_{O_2})
 o. poisoning
 o. quotient (QO_2, qO_2)
 rapid recompression-high pressure o. (RR-HPO)
 o. saturation
 o. saturation measurement
 o. saturation meter (OSM)
 o. tension
 o. under high pressure (OHP)

o. uptake
o. utilization coefficient
oxygenase
heme o. (HO)
homogentisate o.
oxygenase-1
heme o. (HO 1)
oxygenated hemoglobin
oxygenation
extracorporeal membrane o.
(ECMO)
o. of tissue
oxygenator
oxygen-hemoglobin dissociation curve
oxygen-modified polystyrene
oxyhemoglobin (HbO$_2$, O$_2$Hb)
oxyhemogram
oxyhemograph
oxyntic
o. cell
o. gland
oxyntocardiac mucosa
oxyphil, oxyphile
o. adenoma
o. cell
o. chromatin
o. granule
o. inclusion body
oxyphilic
o. cell
o. endometrioid adenocarcinoma
o. leukocyte
o. papillary carcinoma
Oxyphotobacteria

oxypolygelatin
oxypurinol
Oxyspirura mansoni
oxytalan
o. fiber
o. fiber stain
oxytetracycline
oxytoca
Klebsiella o.
oxytocin
brain o.
o. challenge test (OCT)
synthesize o.
unit of o.
Oxytrema
Oxyurata
oxyuriasis
oxyuricide
oxyurid
Oxyuridae
Oxyuris
O. incognita
O. vermicularis
Oxyuroidea
ozaenae
Klebsiella pneumoniae subsp. *o.*
Oz antigen
ozone
ozonization
ozonolysis
Ozzard filaria
ozzardi
Mansonella o.

NOTES

O

φ

    φ 340, 350, 360, 390 benchtop pH/ISE meter
    φ 240, 250, 260 handheld pH/ISE meter
    φ 255, 265, 295 handheld waterproof pH/ISE meter
    φ 660, 690 high-performance pH/ISE meter

P

face of polyhedron
plasma
pressure
probability
    P antigen
    P blood group
    P cell
    P value

P_{O_2}

partial pressure of oxygen

p16

    p16 gene
    p16 oncogene

p24

    p24 HIV antigen
    p24 protein

p53

    p53 gene
    p53 immunohistochemical breast cancer analysis
    p53 mutation
    p53 tumor suppressor

P_1

parental generation

p15 gene
p16INK4A gene
"P1-like viruses"
"P22-like viruses"
p22phox gene
p27 antigen
"P2-like viruses"
"P4-like viruses"
P-50 blood gas
P54 antigen
p57 KIP^2 expression
P_{Na}

plasma sodium

p80NPM/ALK antibody
PA

pathology
pernicious anemia
phakic-aphakic
pleomorphic adenoma
protective antigen
    PA protein

Pa

pascal
protactinium

Paas disease
PAB, PABA

p-aminobenzoic acid
paraaminobenzoic acid

pacchionian

p. body
p. corpuscle
p. gland
p. granulation

pacefollower
pacemaker

p. check
p. twiddler's syndrome
wandering p.

P/ACE MDQ series capillary electrophoresis system
Pacheco parrot disease virus
pachnodae

Promicromonospora p.
Xylanimicrobium p.

pachometer
pachyacria
pachyblepharon
pachyblepharosis
pachycephalic, pachycephalous
pachycephaly, pachycephalia
pachycheilia
pachychromatic
pachydactylous
pachydactyly, pachydactylia
pachyderma

p. laryngis
p. lymphangiectatica
p. oris
p. verrucosa
p. vesicae

pachydermatis

Malassezia p.

pachydermatocele
pachydermatosis
pachydermatous
pachydermia
pachydermic
pachydermoperiostosis
pachyglossia
pachygyria
pachyhymenia
pachyhymenic
pachyleptomeningitis
pachylosis
pachymenia
pachymenic

P

pachymeningitis
    adhesive chronic p.
    chronic adhesive p.
    p. externa
    fibrous hypertrophic p.
    hemorrhagic p.
    hypertrophic cervical p.
    p. interna
    pyogenic p.
pachymeningopathy
pachymeter
pachynema
pachynsis
pachyntic
pachyonychia congenita
pachyperiostitis
pachyperitonitis
pachypleuritis
pachysalpingitis
pachysalpingoovaritis
Pachysolen tannophilus
pachysomia
pachytene
pachyvaginalitis
pachyvaginitis cystica
pacifica
    Cellulophaga p.
    Plesiocystis p.
    Rheinheimera p.
    Shewanella p.
pacificensis
    Psychrobacter p.
pacificum
    Carboxydibrachium p.
    Diphyllobothrium p.
pacificus
    Ignicoccus p.
    Ixodes p.
pacinian corpuscle
pacinii
    Vibrio p.
pacinitis
pack
    Vitros Immunodiagnostic Products
      anti-HBc reagent p.
package
    dual-in-line p.
    push p.
packed
    p. cell volume (PCV)
    p. human blood cells
    p. red blood cells
packet
packing ratio
paclitaxel
PACONA
    periodic acid-concanavalin A
    PACONA technique

pad
    Kendall Company Telfa p.
    periarterial p.
    protein p.
padenii
    Chlamydoabsidia p.
padwickii
    Trichoconis p.
Padykula-Herman stain for myosin ATPase
Paecilomyces lilacinus
paecilomycosis
Paederus
Paenibacillus
    P. agarexedens
    P. agaridevorans
    P. antarcticus
    P. azoreducens
    P. borealis
    P. brasilensis
    P. chinjuensis
    P. chitinolyticus
    P. cookii
    P. daejeonensis
    P. ehimensis
    P. favisporus
    P. glycanilyticus
    P. graminis
    P. granivorans
    P. jamilae
    P. koleovorans
    P. koreensis
    P. kribbensis
    P. lactis
    P. massiliensis
    P. naphthalenovorans
    P. nematophilus
    P. odorifer
    P. sanguinis
    P. stellifer
    P. terrae
    P. timonensis
    P. turicensis
PAF
    platelet-activating factor
    platelet-aggregating factor
    pulmonary arteriovenous fistula
PAF-AH
    platelet-activating factor acetylhydrolase
PAG
    protein A gold
    PAG complex
    PAG technique
Pagano-Levin medium smear
PAGE
    polyacrylamide gel electrophoresis
    2D PAGE
Paget
    P. cell

P. disease
P. disease of bone
P. disease of breast
P. test
Paget-Eccleston stain
pagetic
pagetoid
p. melanocytosis (PM)
p. reticulosis
p. spread
PAGMK
primary African green monkey kidney
PAH, PAHA
p-aminohippuric acid
paraaminohippuric acid
PAI
plasminogen activator inhibitor
pain
bone p.
crushing chest p.
metastatic p.
painful
p. bone
p. bruising syndrome
painless jaundice
painting
chromosome p.
pair
base p. (bp)
conjugate acid-base p.'s
conjugate redox p.
electron p.
ion p.
kilobase p. (kbp)
p. production
paired allosome
pairing
base p.
exchange p.
p. segment
somatic p.
PAIS
partial androgen insensitivity syndrome
pajaroello tick
Palaemonetes
Palaeococcus ferrophilus
palatal
p. cyst
p. enanthem
palate
cleft p.

inflammatory papillary hyperplasia
of the p. (IPHP)
isolated cleft p.
palaticanis
Gemella p.
palatina
tonsilla p.
palatinae
glandulae p.
palatine
p. gland
p. tonsil
palatitis
palatopharyngis
Amycolatopsis p.
pale
p. infarct
p. thrombus
palearctica
Yersinia enterocolitica subsp. *p.*
paleopathology
paleopneumoniae
Diplococcus p.
Peptostreptococcus p.
palindrome
palindromia
palindromic encephalopathy
palisade
p. arrangement of nuclei
p. formation
p. layer
palisaded
palisading
p. cell
p. granuloma
nuclear p.
palladium (Pd)
pallens
Enterococcus p.
Prevotella p.
palleroniana
Pseudomonas p.
pallescens
Curvularia p.
pallidipes
Glossina p.
pallidula
Glaciecola p.
pallidum
microhemagglutination assay-
Treponema p. (MHA-TP)
Treponema p.

NOTES

P

palm
  liver p.
palmar
  p. crease
  p. erythema
  p. fibromatosis
palmellin
Palmgren silver impregnation stain
palmitate
palmitatis
  Desulfuromonas p.
palmitic acid
palmitoleate
palmitoleic acid
palmitoyltransferase
  carnitine p. 2 (CPT2)
palmoplantar keratoderma
P.A.L.M. ultraviolet laser microbeam
palpalis
  Glossina p.
palpebral gland
palpebrarum
  tunica conjunctiva p.
  xanthelasma p.
  xanthoma p.
PALS
  periarterial lymphatic sheath
palsy
  bulbar p.
  cerebral p. (CP)
  facial p.
  progressive bulbar p.
  progressive dystonic p.
  progressive supranuclear p. (PSP)
  pseudobulbar p.
  Saturday night p.
paludal fever
paludicola
  Propionicimonas p.
Paludina
paludism
palustre
  Mycobacterium p.
palustris
  Trichococcus p.
PAM
  periodic acid-silver methenamine
  pulmonary alveolar macrophage
  pulmonary alveolar microlithiasis
  PAM method
p-aminobenzoate
  potassium *p*-a.
p-aminobenzoic acid (PAB, PABA)
p-aminodimethylaniline
p-aminohippurate
  p-a. clearance (C_{pah})
  p-a. clearance test
  sodium *p*-a.
p-aminohippuric acid (PAH, PAHA)

p-aminosalicylate
  potassium *p*-a.
  sodium *p*-a.
p-aminosalicylic acid (PAS)
PAMP
  pathogen-associated molecular pattern
pampiniform
pampinocele
PAN
  periodic alternating nystagmus
  peroxyacetyl nitrate
  polyarteritis nodosa
  positional alcohol nystagmus
panacinar emphysema
Panaeolina
Panaeolus
panagglutinable
panagglutination
panagglutinin
panamensis
  Leishmania braziliensis p.
panangiitis
panarteritis
panarthritis
panatrophy
pan-B
  p.-B antibody
  p.-B antigen
panbronchiolitis
  diffuse p. (DPB)
pANCA
  perinuclear antineutrophil cytoplasmic
    autoantibody
pancake
  p. kidney
  p. probe
pancarditis
pancervical smear
pancinian neuroma
Pancoast
  P. syndrome
  P. tumor
pancolitis
pancreas, pl. pancreata
  aberrant p.
  accessory p.
  alpha cell of p.
  amount of insulin extractable
    from p.
  annular p.
  p. antigen retrieval
  Baggenstoss change in p.
  beta cell of p.
  cystic fibrosis of p. (CFP)
  delta cell of p.
  exocrine p.
  fibrocystic disease of p.
  gamma cell of p.

islands of p.
normal exocrine p.
pancreatemphraxis
pancreatic
p. abscess
p. acinar metaplasia
p. amylase
p. ascites
p. calculus
p. cancer
p. carcinoma
p. cholera
p. colic
p. colipase
p. cyst
p. duct
p. duct-acinar-endocrine cell tumor
p. duct-endocrine cell tumor
p. encephalopathy
p. endocrine neoplasm (PEN)
p. exocrine function insufficiency
p. exocrine function test
p. fibrosis
p. gut hormone
p. islands
p. islet
p. islet cell antibody test
p. islet stain
p. juice
p. lipase
p. lithiasis
p. oncofetal antigen (POA)
p. polypeptide (PP)
p. pseudocyst
p. ribonuclease
ribonuclease (p.)
p. RNase
p. stress protein
pancreaticoduodenal endocrine cell
pancreaticum
Eurytrema p.
pancreaticus
ductus p.
hemosuccus p.
pancreatis
pars endocrina p.
pars exocrina p.
pancreatitis
acute hemorrhagic p.
calcifying p.
chronic fibrosing p.
hemorrhagic p.

necrotizing p.
relapsing p.
pancreatobiliary
pancreatoblastoma
pancreatography
pancreatolith, pancreolith
pancreatolithiasis
pancreatomegaly
pancreolith (*var. of* pancreatolith)
pancreoprivic
pancreozymin (PZ)
pancreozymin-cholecystokinin (PZ-CCK)
pancreozymin-secretin test
pancytokeratin immunostain
pancytopenia
autoimmune p.
congenital p.
Fanconi p.
pandemic
pandemicity
Pandoraea
P. apista
P. norimbergensis
P. pnomenusa
P. pulmonicola
P. sputorum
Pandy
P. reaction
P. test
panel
basic metabolic p. (BMP)
British Testicular Tumour P. (BTTP)
chemistry p. (chem)
p. FISH testing
lymphocyte subset p.
lymphocytic leukemia marker p.
NAP hepatitis B virus quantitative p.
nucleic acid p. (NAP)
obstetric p.
Profile-ER drugs of abuse screening p.
QuestTest diagnostic p.
Triage Cardiac p.
urine drug p. (UDP)
Panellus
panel-reactive antibody (PRA)
panencephalitis
nodular p.
subacute sclerosing p. (SSPE)
panenteroviral antibody

NOTES

P

735

Paneolus foenisicii
Paneth
>P. cell-like change
>P. cell metaplasia
>P. granular cell

Pangonia
panhyperemia
panhyperplasia
panhypopituitarism
>generalized p.
>postpubertal p.
>prepubertal p.

panic
>p. level
>p. value

Panicovirus
panimmunity
pankeratin antibody
panleukopenia
>p. virus (PLV)
>p. virus of cats

panlobular emphysema
panmacrophage marker
panmixis
pan-muscle actin
panmyelophthisis
panmyelosis
Panner disease
panniculitis, pl. **panniculitides**
>A1AT deficiency p.
>alpha$_1$ antitrypsin deficiency p.
>cytophagic histiocytic p.
>factitial p.
>lobular p.
>lupus p.
>mesenteric p.
>metastatic p.
>nodular nonsuppurative p.
>physical p.
>relapsing febrile nodular p.
>septal p.

panniculus, pl. **panniculi**
>p. carnosus

pannorus
>*Geomyces p.*

pannus
>degenerative p.
>p. degenerativus
>glaucomatous p.
>phlyctenular p.
>p. siccus
>p. trachomatosus

panophthalmitis
panoptic stain
pansclerosis
pansinusitis
panspermia
pansporoblast
pansporoblastic

PANSS
>positive and negative symptom scale

panstromal compartment
Panstrongylus
pan-T
>p.-T cell antigen
>p.-T marker

Panta antimicrobial agent
pantachromatic
pantaloon embolism
pantanencephaly
pantatrophia, pantatrophy
pantetheine
pantherina
>*Amanita p.*

pantheris
>*Lactobacillus p.*

pantomorphia
pantomorphic
pantothenic
>p. acid
>p. acid assay
>p. acid unit

pantropic virus
Panus
panzerherz
panzootic
PAO
>peak acid output

PAOD
>peripheral arterial occlusive disease
>peripheral arteriosclerotic occlusive disease

PAP
>peroxidase-antiperoxidase
>primary atypical pneumonia
>pulmonary alveolar proteinosis
>>PAP complex
>>PAP immunoperoxidase
>>PAP immunoperoxidase stain
>>PAP technique

Pap
>Papanicolaou
>>Pap examination
>>Pap method
>>Pap Plus HPV screen
>>Pap smear
>>Pap smear test
>>Pap stain

papain
>Wako 1% crude p.

Papanicolaou (Pap)
papatasii
>*Phlebotomus p.*

Papaver somniferum
papaya
>*Carica p.*

papayae
>*Erwinia p.*

paper
- alkannin p.
- azolitmin p.
- blue litmus p.
- p. capacitor
- chemical agent detector p.
- p. chromatography
- Congo red p.
- filter p.
- indicator p.
- Kuwabara p.
- litmus p.
- p. mill worker's disease
- probability p.
- p. radioimmunosorbent test (PRIST)
- red litmus p.
- test p.
- Whatman p.

papilla, gen. and pl. **papillae**
- acoustic p.
- circumvallate papillae
- clavate p.
- papillae conicae
- conical shaped filiform papillae
- p. of connective tissue
- papillae corii
- papillae of corium
- cribriform area of renal p.
- dermal p.
- p. dermatis
- p. duodeni major
- p. duodeni minor
- excavatio p.
- exophytic p.
- filiform p.
- papillae filiformes
- papillae foliatae
- foliate p.
- fungiform p.
- papillae fungiformes
- hair p.
- hypertrophic anal p.
- lenticular p.
- lingual p.
- p. lingualis
- major duodenal p.
- minor duodenal p.
- nerve p.
- parotid p.
- p. parotidea
- p. pili
- renal papillae
- papillae renalis
- tactile p.
- papillae vallatae
- vallate p.
- vascular p.
- p. of Vater

papillare
- corpus p.

papillaris
- foveola p.

papillar villous hyperplasia
papillary
- p. adenocarcinoma
- p. adenoma of large intestine
- p. adenomatous polyp
- p. breast neoplasm (PBN)
- p. cystadenoma
- p. cystadenoma lymphomatosum
- p. cystic adenoma
- p. duct
- p. ectasia
- p. endothelial hyperplasia (PEH)
- p. ependymoma
- p. excrescence
- p. foramina of kidney
- p. frond
- p. hidradenoma
- p. hyperplasia
- p. infolding
- p. intralymphatic angioendothelioma
- p. layer
- p., marginal, attached (PMA)
- p. muscle dysfunction
- p. muscle syndrome
- p. necrosis
- p. serous carcinoma of the peritoneum (PSCP)
- p. serous cystadenocarcinoma
- p. syringadenoma
- p. transitional cell carcinoma
- p. tumor
- p. urothelial neoplasm

papillary/verrucous architecture
papilledema
Papillibacter
- *P. cinnamivorans*

papilliferous
papilliferum
- syringocystadenoma p.

papilliform
papillitis
- anal p.

NOTES

737

papillitis *(continued)*
    chronic lingual p.
    necrotizing p.
    optic p.
papilloadenocystoma
papillocarcinoma
papilloma
    p. acuminatum
    basal cell p.
    p. canaliculum
    canine oral p.
    choroid plexus p.
    p. diffusum
    duct p.
    ductal p.
    p. durum
    fibroepithelial p.
    hard p.
    hyperkeratotic p.
    infectious p. of cattle
    p. inguinale tropicum
    intracystic p.
    intraductal p.
    inverted p.
    keratotic p.
    p. molle
    rabbit p.
    Shope p.
    soft p.
    squamous cell p.
    transitional cell p.
    urothelial p.
    p. venereum
    verrucous p.
    villous p.
    p. virus
papillomatosis
    p. of breast
    church spire p.
    confluent and reticulate p.
    p. cutis carcinoides
    florid oral p.
    intraductal p.
    juvenile p.
    laryngeal p.
    recurrent respiratory p. (RRP)
    subareolar duct p.
papillomatosus
    lupus p.
papillomatous
Papillomavirus
papillomavirus
    human p. (HPV)
    oncogenic human p.
Papillon-Léage and Psaume syndrome
Papillon-Lefèvre syndrome
papillula
papio
    herpesvirus p. 2

PAPI stain
PapNet Pap smear system
Papovaviridae
papovavirus
    lymphotropic p. (LPV)
PAPP-A
    pregnancy-associated plasma protein A
pappataci
    p. fever
    p. fever virus
PAPP-B
    pregnancy-associated plasma protein B
Pappenheim
    P. hemoblast
    lymphoid hemoblast of P.
    P. reagent
    P. stain
Pappenheimer body
pappilipes
    Ornithodoros p.
papula, pl. **papulae**
papular
    p. lesion
    p. mucinosis
    p. scrofuloderma
    p. stomatitis virus of cattle
    p. tuberculid
Papulaspora equi
papule
    demarcated raised p.
    Gottron p.
    moist p.
    mucous p.
    prurigo p.
papuliferous
papuloerythematous
papulonecrotic tuberculid
papulonodular lesion
papulonodule
papulopustule
papulosis
    bowenoid p. (BP)
    lymphomatoid p. (LyP)
    malignant atrophic p.
papulosquamous
papulovesicular
PAPVC
    partial anomalous pulmonary venous connection
papyraceous scar
PAR
    protease-activated receptor
paraaminobenzoic acid (PAB, PABA)
paraaminodimethylaniline
paraaminohippurate clearance
paraaminohippuric acid (PAH, PAHA)
para-**aminosalicylate**
    sodium *p.*-a.
para-**aminosalicylic acid (PAS)**

paraaortic
  p. body
  p. lymph node
paraaortica
  corpora p.
paraappendicitis
parabasal
  p. cell
  p. cell layer
parabiosis
parabiotic
parabola
paraboloid condenser
para-Bombay
  p.-B. nonsecretor
  p.-B. phenotype
Parabuthus
paracanthoma
paracanthosis
paracarcinomatous
  p. encephalomyelopathy
  p. myelopathy
paracarmine stain
paracasein
paracellular pathway
paracentesis
Parachlamydiaceae
paracholera vibrio
Parachordodes
parachordoma
parachromatopsia
parachute reflex
paracoagulation test
paracoccidioidal granuloma
Paracoccidioides brasiliensis
paracoccidioidin
paracoccidioidomycosis
Paracoccus
  P. haeundaensis
  P. seriniphilus
  P. yeei
  P. zeaxanthinifaciens
paracolic gutter
paracolitis
paracollinoides
  Lactobacillus p.
Paracolobactrum
  P. aerogenoides
  P. arizonae
  P. coliforme
  P. intermedium
paracolon bacillus

paracolpitis
paraconal fascia
paracortex
paracrine stimulation
paracusis of Willis
paracystitis
paracytic
paradenitis
paradental cyst
paradentium
paradidymis
paradimethylaminoazobenzene
paradoxa
  ectasia ventriculi p.
paradoxical
  p. embolism
  p. embolus
paradoxic embolism
paradoxus
  Thialkalivibrio p.
parafaecalis
  Alcaligenes faecalis subsp. *p.*
par. aff.
  part affected
paraffin
  bismuth iodoform p. (BIP)
  p. block
  p. cancer
  p. immunoperoxidase (PIP)
  p. miniblock
  p. section
  p. tumor
  p. wax
paraffin-embedded
  formalin-fixed p.-e. (FFPE)
  p.-e. tissue (PET)
  p.-e. tissue section
paraffinivorans
  Gordonia p.
paraffinoma
Parafilaria multipapillosa
paraflagellate
paraflagellum, pl. **paraflagella**
parafluorophenylalanine
parafollicular
  p. B-cell lymphoma (PBCL)
  p. cell
parafollicularis
  hyperkeratosis follicularis et p.
paraformaldehyde
Parafossarulus
parafrenal abscess

NOTES

P

739

parafuchsin
parafulva
    Pseudomonas p.
paraganglia
    nonchromaffin p.
paraganglioma
    aorticopulmonary p. (APPG)
    aorticosympathetic p.
    benign p. (BPG)
    chromaffin p.
    p. glomus
    malignant p. (MPG)
    nonchromaffin p.
    paravertebral p. (PVPG)
paraganglion
paraganglionic
    p. cell
    p. tissue
paragene
Paragon
    P. blue stain
    P. CZE 2000 capillary
    electrophoresis system
paragonimiasis
Paragonimus
    P. africanus
    P. caliensis
    P. heterotremus
    P. kellicotti
    P. mexicanus
    P. ringeri
    P. westermani
Paragordius
    P. cintus
    P. tricuspidatus
    P. varius
paragranuloma
    nodular p. (NP)
parahaemolyticus
    Haemophilus p.
    Vibrio p.
parahemophilia
parahormone
parahydroxyphenylpyruvic acid (PHPPA)
parahypophysis
paraimmunoblast cell
paraimmunoblastic lymphoma
parainfluenza
    p. antibody test
    p. viral serology
    p. virus antigen
    p. virus culture
    p. virus infection
    p. virus, types 1–4
parainfluenzae
    Haemophilus p.
parakeratosis
    p. pustulosa

    p. scutularis
    p. variegata
parakeratotic tiering
Paralactobacillus selangorensis
Paralaphostrongylus
paralbuminemia
paraldehyde
    p. assay
    p. poisoning
paraleprosis
paralimentarius
    Lactobacillus p.
Paraliobacillus ryukyuensis
parallel
    p. circuit
    p. grid
    p. operation
parallergic
paraluteal cell
paralysis, pl. paralyses
    acute atrophic p.
    Brown-Sequard p.
    Cruveilhier p.
    curariform p.
    Dejerine-Klumpke p.
    descending flaccid p.
    diaphragm p.
    fowl p.
    Gubler p.
    hypokalemic periodic p.
    immune p.
    immunological p.
    infectious bulbar p.
    Klumpke p.
    Kussmaul p.
    Kussmaul-Landry p.
    Lissauer p.
    Millard-Gubler p.
    myogenic p.
    normokalemic periodic p.
    periodic p.
    postdormital p.
    Pott p.
    Ramsay Hunt p.
    Remak p.
    rucksack p.
    tick p.
    Todd p.
    vasomotor p.
    vocal cord p.
    Volkmann ischemic p.
    Weber p.
    writer's p.
paralyssa
paralytic
    p. brachial neuritis (PBN)
    p. ileus
    p. syndrome
paralyzable detector

paramagnetic resonance of electrons
paramastigote
Paramax
    P. analyzer
    P. reagent
paramecium, pl. **paramecia**
Paramecium coli
paramesonephric rest
parameter
    immunohistochemical p.
    practice p.
paramethasone
parametric, parametritic
    p. abscess
parametritis
parametrium
Paramoeba
paramorphia
paramorphic
Paramphistomatidae
paramphistomiasis
Paramphistomum
paramyloidosis
paramyotonia congenita
Paramyxoviridae
Paramyxovirus
paramyxovirus
paraneoplasia
paraneoplastic
    p. acrokeratosis
    p. disorder
    p. encephalomyelopathy
    p. endocrine syndrome
    p. pemphigus (PNP)
paranephric
    p. abscess
    p. body
paranephros
paraneuron
paranuclear
    p. body
    p. cytoplasm
    p. whorl
paranucleate
paranucleolus
paranucleus
parapedesis
parapertussis
    Acinetobacter p.
    Bordetella p.
    Haemophilus p.
paraphilia

paraphimosis
paraphrophilus
    Haemophilus p.
paraphysial, paraphyseal
    p. cyst
paraplasm
paraplast
paraplastic
Paraplast Plus tissue embedding medium
paraplegia
Para 12 Plus Retics control
Paraponera
Parapoxvirus
paraproctitis
paraprostatitis
paraprotein
    monoclonal p.
paraproteinemia
paraproteinemic neuropathy
parapsilosis
    Candida p.
parapsoriasis
    p. en plaque
    p. guttata
    p. lichenoides
    p. lichenoides et varioliformis acuta
    p. varioliformis
paraputrificum
    Clostridium p.
paraquat assay
pararama
pararosanilin, pararosaniline
Parasa
Parasaccharomyces ashfordi
parasalpingitis
Parascardovia denticolens
Parascaris equorum
parascarlatina
parascrofulaceum
    Mycobacterium p.
paraseptal emphysema
parasite
    accidental p.
    duodenal p.
    extracellular p.
    facultative p.
    intermittent p.
    intestinal p.
    intracellular p.
    malarial p.
    metazoan p.

NOTES

P

parasite *(continued)*
    obligate p.
    ova and p.'s (O&P)
    periodic p.
    permanent p.
    protozoan p.
    p. screen
    smear preparation and staining for blood p.'s
    spurious p.
    string test for duodenal p.
    temporary p.
Parasitella
parasitemia
parasitic
    p. castration
    p. chylocele
    p. cyst
    p. ectopic pregnancy
    p. embolus
    p. fetus
    p. granuloma
    p. hemoptysis
    p. infestation
    p. leiomyoma
    p. thyroiditis
    p. twins
parasitica
    achromia p.
    Phialophora p.
parasiticidal
parasiticide
parasiticus
    Aspergillus p.
    dipygus p.
    epigastrius p.
    Rhizoglyphus p.
parasitism
parasitize
parasitocenose
parasitogenesis
parasitogenic
Parasitoidea
parasitoid mite
parasitologist
parasitology
parasitome
parasitosis
parasitotropic
parasitotropism
parasitotropy
parasitovorax
    Cheyletiella p.
paraspadias
Parasporobacterium paucivorans
Parastrongylus
parastruma

parasympathetic
    p. division
    p. stimulation
parasympathomimetic
parasynovitis
parasyphilis
paratenesis
paratenic host
paratenon
parathion
    methyl p.
parathormone (PTH)
parathyrin
parathyroid
    p. adenoma
    p. chief cell
    p. cyst
    p. disorder
    p. extract (PTE)
    p. gland
    p. hormone (PTH)
    p. hormone-related peptide (PTHrP)
    p. hormone-related protein (PTHrP)
    p. hormone secretion (PTHS)
    p. mass
    p. osteosis
    p. oxyphil cell
    p. transitional cell
    p. tumor
    p. wasserhelle cell
    water-clear cell of p.
parathyroidea
    glandula p.
parathyroidin
paratope
paratrophic
paratropicalis
    Haemophilus p.
paratuberculosis
    Mycobacterium p.
paratuberculous
    p. lymphadenitis
    p. pneumonia
paratyphi
    Salmonella p.
    Salmonella enteritidis serotype *p. A*
paratyphlitis
paratyphoid
    p. fever, types A, B, C
    p. immunization
paraurethral
    p. duct
    p. gland
paraurethrales
    ductus p.
paravaccinia virus
paravacuolar granule
paravaginitis
paraventricular nucleus

paravirus
Parazoa
parazoon
parcel bomb
parchment
    p. heart
    p. skin
Parechovirus
parectasis, parectasia
parencephalia
parencephalocele
parencephalous
parenchyma
    placental p.
parenchymal
    p. cell
    p. lesion
    p. nodule
parenchymatitis
parenchymatous
    p. cell of corpus pineale
    p. degeneration
    p. goiter
    p. keratitis
    p. mastitis
parent
    p. cell
    p. cyst
parentage
parental
    p. cell population
    p. generation (P_1)
parenteral
    transmitted via p.
paresis
    general p. (GP)
paresthesia
paries, pl. **parietes**
    p. tympanicus ductus cochlearis
    p. vestibularis ductus cochlearis
parietal
    p. cell
    p. cell antibody
    p. fistula
    p. thrombus
parietale
    peritoneum p.
parietes (*pl. of* paries)
parietotemporal
Parietti broth
Parinaud oculoglandular syndrome

Paris
    P. classification
    P. green
    P. line
    P. yellow
Paris-Trousseau platelet disorder
parity
    p. bit
    p. check
Park
    P. aneurysm
    hemoglobin M Hyde P.
parkeri
    Borrelia p.
    Ornithodoros p.
Parkinson
    P. disease (PD)
    P. facies
parkinsonian syndrome
parkinsonism
Park-Williams
    P.-W. bacillus
    P.-W. fixative
parmense
    Mycobacterium p.
parodontium
parodoxa
    Listerella p.
paromomycin
paromphalocele
Parona space
paronychia
    herpetic p.
parooensis
    Skermanella p.
paroophori
    ductuli p.
    tubuli p.
paroophoritic cyst
paroophoritis
parorchidium
parorchis
parosteal
    p. fasciitis
    p. osteoma
    p. osteosarcoma
parosteitis, parostitis
parosteosis, parostosis
parotid
    p. abscess
    p. duct

NOTES

P

parotid *(continued)*
   p. gland
   p. papilla
parotidea
   glandula p.
   papilla p.
parotideus
   ductus p.
parotidis
   socia p.
parotis
   glandula p.
parotitis, parotiditis
   epidemic p.'s
   postoperative p.
   punctate p.
   p. syndrome
   p. virus epidemic
parovaritis
paroxysm
paroxysmal
   p. aciduria
   p. atrial tachycardia
   p. cold hemoglobinuria (PCH)
   p. hypertension
   p. nocturnal hemoglobinemia
   p. nocturnal hemoglobinuria (PNH)
   p. supraventricular tachycardia
   p. ventricular tachycardia
parrot
   P. atrophy of the newborn
   P. disease
   p. fever
   p. virus
Parry disease
Parry-Romberg syndrome
pars, pl. partes
   p. amorpha
   p. compacta
   p. convoluta lobuli corticalis renis
   p. corneoscleralis reticuli
     trabecularis sclerae
   p. distalis adenohypophyseos
   p. endocrina pancreatis
   p. exocrina pancreatis
   p. fetalis placentae
   p. granulosa
   p. infundibularis
   p. intermedia
   p. nervosa hypophyseos
   p. optica retinae
   p. pharyngea hypophyseos
   p. radiata lobuli corticalis renis
   p. tuberalis
   p. uvealis reticuli trabecularis
     sclerae
Parson disease
part
   p. affected (par. aff.)

   infundibular p.
   intermediate p.
   malignant giant cell tumor of
     soft p.'s
   p.'s per million (ppm)
partes (*pl. of* pars)
parthenogenesis
parthenogenetic
   p. activation
   p. merogony
partial
   p. agglutinin
   p. androgen insensitivity syndrome
     (PAIS)
   p. anomalous pulmonary venous
     connection (PAPVC)
   p. antigen
   p. exchange transfusion
   p. identity pattern
   p. lesion
   p. lipoatrophy
   p. obstruction
   p. pressure
   p. pressure of carbon dioxide
     (PCO_2, pCO_2)
   p. pressure of nitrogen
   p. pressure of oxygen (P_{O_2})
   p. pressure of water vapor
   p. reaction of degeneration (PRD)
   p. remission (PR)
   p. thromboplastin time (PTT)
   p. thromboplastin time lupus
     anticoagulant (PTT-LA)
   p. thromboplastin time test
   p. trisomy
partially miscible
partial-thickness burn
particle
   p. agglutination test
   alpha p.
   beta p.
   bone marrow p.
   p. of bone marrow
   charged p.
   chromatin p.
   p. concentration fluorescence
     immunoassay (PCFIA)
   Dane p.
   defective interfering p.
   DI p.
   elementary p.
   gelatin sponge p.
   glycogen p.
   gold p.
   remanantlike lipoprotein p. (RLP)
   ridge of intramembranous p.
   stick-and-ball-shaped virion p.
   p. transport time (PTT)
   Zimmermann elementary p.

particle-enhanced turbidimetric inhibition immunoassay (PETINIA)
particulate
p. crystalline material
p. crystalline material deposition
settled p.
suspended p.
partition
p. coefficient
nitrogen p.
Partitivirus
parturition
parva
Emmonsia parva var. *p.*
parvalbumin protein
Parvibaculum lavamentivorans
parvilocular
p. cyst
p. cystoma
Parvobacteriaceae
parvocellular neuron
Parvoviridae
Parvovirus
parvovirus
p. B19 aplastic crisis
p. B19 infection
parvula
Veillonella p.
Parvularcula bermudensis
parvulus
Peptostreptococcus p.
parvum
Aquabacterium p.
Chlorobaculum p.
Chrysosporium p.
Corynebacterium p.
Cryptosporidium p.
Diphyllobothrium p.
Eubacterium p.
Haplosporangium p.
Roseospirillum p.
Treponema p.
Ureaplasma p.
parvus
Acinetobacter p.
Paryphostomum sufrartyfex
PAS
p-aminosalicylic acid
para-aminosalicylic acid
periodic acid-Schiff
pulmonary artery stenosis
PAS reaction

PAS stain
PAS technique
PAS test
pascal (Pa)
P. law
PASCC
pseudovascular adenoid squamous cell carcinoma
Paschen body
PASH
pseudoangiomatous stromal hyperplasia
PASM
periodic acid-silver methenamine
PAS-orange G stain
passage
blind p.
bouton en p.
damaged during p.
egg p.
serial p.
Passalurus ambiguus
passenger
p. cell
p. leukocyte effect
passive
p. agglutination
p. Arthus reaction
p. congestion
p. cutaneous anaphylactic reaction
p. cutaneous anaphylaxis (PCA)
p. cutaneous anaphylaxis test
p. epithelial displacement by needle biopsy
p. hemagglutination (PHA)
p. hemagglutination test
p. hemolysis
p. immunity
p. immunization
p. immunodiffusion immunoassay
p. medium
p. prophylaxis
p. sensitization
p. strangling
p. transfer
p. transport
Passovoy factor
passularum
Carpoglyphus p.
Pasteur
P. effect
P. pipette
P. vaccine

NOTES

P

Pasteurella
- *P. aerogenes*
- *P. enterocolitica*
- *P. haemolytica*
- *P. multocida*
- *P. pestis*
- *P. pneumotropica*
- *P. pseudotuberculosis*
- *P. septica*
- *P. skyensis*
- *P. tularensis*
- *P. ureae*

Pasteurellaceae
Pasteurelleae
pasteurellosis
Pasteuriaceae
pasteurianum
- *Clostridium p.*

pasteurianus
- *Streptococcus p.*
- *Streptococcus gallolyticus* subsp. *p.*

pasteurii
- *Sporosarcina p.*
- *Trichococcus p.*

pasteurization
pastorianus
- *Saccharomyces p.*

pastoris
- *Prochlorococcus marinus* subsp. *p.*

Patau syndrome
patch
- CF indicator system chloride p.
- Dacron p.
- gray p.
- herald p.
- Hutchinson p.
- MacCallum p.
- moth p.
- mucous p.
- Peyer p.
- salmon p.
- shagreen p.
- soldier's p.
- p. test
- p. testing
- white p.

patched hedgehog protein (PTCH)
patching capping
patch/plaque cell stage
patchy
- p. binding
- p. distribution

Patein albumin
Patella disease
patellae
- chondromalacia p.

patent
- p. blue V
- p. blue V dye

- p. ductus arteriosus
- p. foramen ovale

paternal imprint
paternity
- p. test
- p. testing

Paterson-Brown-Kelly syndrome
Paterson-Kelly syndrome
Paterson syndrome
path
- pathology

pathergy
pathoanatomic background
pathoanatomy
pathobiology
pathoclisis
pathogen
- antiplant p.
- class A, B, C, D p.
- foodborne p.
- mycelial p.
- opportunistic p.
- plant p.
- waterborne p.

pathogen-associated molecular pattern (PAMP)
pathogenesis
pathogenetic pathognomy
pathogen-free
- specific p.-f. (SPF)

pathogenic
pathogenicity
- bacterial p.
- p. island

pathognomonic
pathognomy
- pathogenetic p.

pathography
pathologic
- p. anatomy
- p. anthropology
- p. calcification
- p. cell
- characteristic p.
- p. diagnosis
- p. dislocation
- p. finding
- p. fracture
- p. glycosuria
- p. histology
- p. leukocytosis
- p. state

pathological anatomy
pathologist
- College of American P.'s (CAP)
- World Health Organization/International Society of Urologic P.'s (WHO/ISUP)

pathology (PA, path)

ageing (hippocampal region,
  patients over 75 years), tau p.
  class I
anatomic p.
anatomical p.
Armed Forces Institute of P.
  (AFIP)
cellular p.
clinical p.
comparative p.
dental p.
Down syndrome tau p.
experimental p.
functional p.
general p.
geographic p.
humoral p.
internal p.
International Society for
  Urological P. (ISUP)
medical p.
molecular p.
oral p.
posttransplant biopsy p.
Society for Pediatric P. (SPP)
solidistic p.
special p.
surgical p.
tau p. class I–IV
tau protein p.
World Association of Societies
  of P. (WASP)
pathomechanism
pathometric
pathometry
pathomorphism
pathonomia, pathonomy
pathophenotype
pathophysiologic
pathophysiology
pathotype
pathovar
PathVysion
  P. HER-2 DNA probe for breast
    cancer
  P. HER-2 DNA probe kit
pathway
  activation of the coagulation p.'s
  alternative complement p.
  amphibolic p.
  biosynthetic p.
  classical complement p.

coagulation p.
cortisol synthesis p.
critical p.
Embden-Meyerhof p.
Entner-Doudoroff p.
extrinsic p.
hexose monophosphate p.
internodal p.
intrinsic p.
lipoxygenase p.
Luebering-Rapaport p.
metabolic p.
paracellular p.
pentose phosphate p. (PPP)
phosphogluconate oxidative p.
polyol p.
reentrant p.
transcellular p.
tumor suppressor p.
ubiquitin-protease p.
wnt signaling transduction p.
patient
  adrenalectomized p.
  contaminated p.
  immobilized postoperative p.
  p. protective wrap (PPW)
Patois virus
pattern
  acinar p.
  angiocentric p.
  angiodestructive p.
  angled soot p.
  arborizing p.
  architectural p.
  basaloid growth p.
  basket-weave p.
  biphasic p.
  blue cell p.
  canalicular p.
  carcinoid-like architectural p.
  chicken-wire p.
  clear cell p.
  cribriform growth p.
  cross striation p.
  cytoplasmic p.
  diffuse p.
  double phenotypic p.
  euploid-polyploid p.
  fascicular p.
  filiform growth p.
  filigree p.
  finely stippled chromatin p.

NOTES

pattern (*continued*)
    fingerprint p.
    follicular p.
    full house p.
    fused glandular p.
    gel electrophoresis p.
    gene expression p.
    Gleason p.
    growth p.
    hemangiopericytomatous growth p.
    herringbone p.
    heterogeneous p.
    histological p.
    hyperploid p.
    identity p.
    immunohistochemical p.
    indeterminate p.
    Indian-file p.
    inheritance p.
    large glandular p.
    lobular p.
    lobulocentric p.
    luminal p.
    male sex chromatin p.
    membranous p.
    microacinar architectural p.
    microfollicular p.
    microglandular p.
    monoclonal B-cell p.
    mosaic p.
    moth-eaten p.
    multidot p.
    nonrandom p.
    nonreactive p.
    nucleolar p.
    organoid growth p.
    partial identity p.
    pathogen-associated molecular p.
      (PAMP)
    patternless p.
    perinuclear p.
    plasmalemmal p.
    plywood p.
    polka dot p.
    polyclonal p.
    protein expression p.
    pseudoalveolar p.
    pseudomantle zone p.
    pseudopapillary p.
    punctate p.
    quiltlike p.
    receptogram p.
    reticular growth p.
    rim p.
    scalloped p.
    Schmincke p.
    secretory p.
    Sertoli-like p.
    short fascicular growth p.

    single-dot p.
    skin reaction p.
    small glandular p.
    solid p.
    solid growth p.
    speckled p.
    spindle cell fascicular p.
    squamoid p.
    starburst p.
    storiform p.
    syringomatous growth p.
    targetoid p.
    trabecular p.
    tubulocystic growth p.
    tubulopapillary architectural p.
    vesicular chromatin p.
    whorled storiform p.
    XX/XY sex chromosome p.
    Zellballen p.

patternless pattern
patulous
patulum
    Penicillium p.
paucibacillary
paucicellular
    p. area
    p. collagen
pauciimmune
    p. crescentic and necrotizing
      glomerulonephritis
    p. glomerulonephritis
    p. RPGN
paucimobilis
    Pseudomonas p.
Paucimonas lemoignei
pauciseptate
paucisynaptic
paucity
paucivorans
    Brevibacterium p.
    Dolosicoccus p.
    Fusibacter p.
    Nocardia p.
    Parasporobacterium p.
paucula
    Wautersia p.
Paul
    P. reaction
    P. test
Paul-Bunnell-Barrett test
Paul-Bunnell heterophile antibody test
pauli
    Solirubrobacter p.
Pauly point
paurometabola
    Oerskovia p.
    Tsukamurella p.
paurometabolica
    Saccharomonospora p.

Pautrier
> P. abscess
> P. microabscess

Pauwel femoral neck fracture
Pauzat disease
pavement epithelium
Pavy disease
PAX2 gene
Paxillus involutus
Payr disease
PB
> protein binding

Pb
> barometric pressure

PBC
> primary biliary cirrhosis

PBCL
> parafollicular B-cell lymphoma

PBD
> proliferating bile ductules
> proliferative breast disease

PBG
> porphobilinogen

PBI
> protein-bound iodine
> > PBI test

PBL
> peripheral blood lymphocyte
> primary bone lymphoma

PBMC
> peripheral blood mononuclear cell

PBN
> papillary breast neoplasm
> paralytic brachial neuritis

PBP2′ rapid latex test for staphylococcus resistance
PBPC
> peripheral blood progenitor cell

PBS
> phosphate buffered saline

PBT4
> protein-bound thyroxine

PC
> phosphocreatine
> plasma cell
> platelet count

PCA
> passive cutaneous anaphylaxis
> prostatic adenocarcinoma

PCB
> polychlorinated biphenyl

PCC
> prothrombin complex concentration

PCD
> posterior corneal deposit

pCEA
> polyclonal carcinoembryonic antigen

PCFIA
> particle concentration fluorescence immunoassay

PCG
> plasma cell granuloma

PCH
> paroxysmal cold hemoglobinuria
> pulmonary capillary hemangiomatosis

PCHA
> proliferating cell nuclear antigen

PCHE
> pseudocholinesterase

PCI
> pneumatosis cystoides intestinalis

pCi
> picocurie

PCM
> protein-calorie malnutrition

PCNA
> proliferating cell nuclear antigen

PCNSL
> primary central nervous system lymphoma

PCO$_2$, pCO$_2$
> partial pressure of carbon dioxide

PCP
> pentachlorophenol

PCR
> plasma clearance rate
> polymerase chain reaction
> > allele-specific PCR (A-PCR)
> > DOP PCR
> > one-step nested PCR (OSNP)
> > one-tube nested PCR
> > PCR reaction testing
> > real-time reverse-transcriptase PCR
> > TaqMan real-time PCR
> > two-step nested PCR (TSNP)
> > two-tube nested PCR

PCr
> phosphocreatine

PCR-RFLP
> polymerase chain reaction-restriction fragment length polymorphism

NOTES

P

PCR-SSCP
  polymerase chain reaction-single-strand
    conformation polymorphism
PCT
  plasmacrit
  porphyria cutanea tarda
  prothrombin consumption time
PCV
  packed cell volume
  polycythemia vera
PCV-M
  myeloid metaplasia with polycythemia
    vera
PD
  Parkinson disease
  plasma defect
  poorly differentiated
Pd
  palladium
PDC
  pyruvate dehydrogenase complex
    PDC kinase molecule group
PDCD4
  programmed cell death 4 gene
PDGF
  platelet-derived growth factor
PDH
  phosphate dehydrogenase
***p*-dichlorobenzene**
PDLL
  poorly differentiated lymphocytic
    lymphoma
PDM
  polydimethylsiloxane
PE
  phycoerythrin
  pulmonary edema
  pulmonary embolism
PE-10 antibody
PE2100 spectroscope
peak
  absorption p.
  p. acid output (PAO)
  p. amplitude
  p. area
  biclonal p.
  p. broadening
  coincidence sum p.
  p. expiratory flow (PEF)
  p. expiratory flow rate (PEFR)
  p. height
  p. incidence
  p. inspiratory flow (PIF)
  p. inspiratory flow rate (PIFR)
  iodine escape p.
  kilovolt p. (kVp)
  p. kilovoltage
  monoclonal p.
  multimodal p.

  p. overpressure
  p. secretory flow rate (PSFR)
  p. transmittance
  unimodal p.
peak-and-trough level
peak-to-peak amplitude
peak-to-total ratio
pealeana
  Shewanella p.
peanut lectin
pearl
  amyl nitrite p.'s
  p. cell
  p. chain
  epidermic p.
  epithelial p.
  P. iron stain
  keratin p.
  Laënnec p.
  squamous p.
  p. tumor
pearl-worker's disease
peau d'orange
Pecluvirus
PEComa
  perivascular epithelioid cell tumor
pecorum
  Chlamydophila p.
pectenitis
pectenosis
pectin
pectinata
  Cooperia p.
  zona p.
pectinate
  p. body
  p. ligaments of iridocorneal angle
  p. ligaments of iris
  p. line
  p. zone
pectinatum
  ligamentum p.
Pectinibranchiata
pectinolytica
  Aeromonas salmonicida subsp. *p.*
pectinovorum
  Treponema p.
Pectobacterium
  P. atrosepticum
  P. betavasculorum
  P. carotovorum
  P. wasabiae
pectoral gland
pectoris
  angina p. (AP)
pectus
  p. carinatum
  p. excavatum

p. gallinatum
p. recurvatum
pedal system
pederin
pedes (*pl. of* pes)
Pediatric Oncology Group (POG)
Pedi-BacT
pedicel
pedicellate
pedicellation
Pedicinus ancoratus
pedicle
pedicular
pediculate
pediculation
pediculi (*pl. of* pediculus)
pediculicide
Pediculoides ventricosus
pediculosis ciliorum
pediculous
Pediculus
P. humanus
P. humanus capitis
P. humanus corporis
P. humanus humanus
P. humanus vestimentorum
P. inguinalis
P. pubis
P. vestimenti
pediculus, pl. pediculi
Rickettsia pediculi
pedigree chart
Pediococcus
pedis
dermatomycosis p.
tinea p.
Trichophyton p.
pedogenesis
pedrosoi
Acrotheca p.
Fonsecaea p.
Hormodendrum p.
peduncle
peduncular
pedunculate
pedunculated polyp
peenash
PEEP
positive end-expiratory pressure
PEF
peak expiratory flow
pefloxacin

PEFR
peak expiratory flow rate
peg
rete p.
wide rete p.
Pegohylemyia seneciella
PEH
papillary endothelial hyperplasia
PEI
phosphate excretion index
pekingensis
Rhodocista p.
PEL
permissible exposure limit
primary effusion lymphoma
pelagi
Fulvimarina p.
Pelamoviroid
Pel-Ebstein
P.-E. disease
P.-E. fever
P.-E. pyrexia
Pelecypoda
Pelger-Huët
P.-H. cell
P.-H. nuclear anomaly
peliosis
p. hepatis
p. hepatitis
p. lienalis
Pelizaeus-Merzbacher disease
pellagra preventive (PP)
Pellegrini disease
Pellegrini-Stieda disease
pellet
platelet p.
tissue p.
pelletieri
Actinomadura p.
Streptomyces p.
pellicle
pellicular
Pellicularia
pelliculous
Pellizzi syndrome
pellucid
pellucida
macula p.
zona p.
Pelodera
pelophilus
Geobacter p.

NOTES

P

751

pelophilus (continued)
    Propionibacter p.
    Propionivibrio p.
Pelospora glutarica
Pelotomaculum thermopropionicum
pelta
peltation
pelves (*pl. of* pelvis)
pelvic
    p. abscess
    p. cellulitis
    p. fracture
    p. infection
    p. inflammatory disease (PID)
    p. kidney
    p. outlet
    p. washing
pelvimetry
pelvirectal achalasia
pelvis, pl. **pelves**
    beaked p.
    caoutchouc p.
    frozen p.
    hardened p.
    kyphoscoliotic p.
    kyphotic p.
    lordotic p.
    Nägele p.
    p. obtecta
    osteomalacic p.
    Otto p.
    Prague p.
    pseudoosteomalacic p.
    rachitic p.
    Rokitansky p.
    rostrate p.
    rubber p.
    scoliotic p.
    spider p.
    split p.
    spondylolisthetic p.
    TCC of renal p.
pelvospondylitis ossificans
PEM
    polymorphic epithelial mucin
Pembrey method
pemphigoid
    benign mucosal p.
    Brunsting-Perry p.
    bulbous p.
    bullous p.
    cicatricial p.
    ocular cicatricial p.
pemphigosa
    variola p.
pemphigus
    p. antibody
    benign familial p.
    benign mucous membrane p.

    p. crouposus
    p. erythematosus
    familial benign p.
    p. foliaceous
    p. gangrenosus
    p. leprosus
    p. neonatorum
    paraneoplastic p. (PNP)
    p. vegetans
    p. vulgaris
PEN
    pancreatic endocrine neoplasm
pencil
    p. cell
    p. dosimeter
Pendred syndrome
pendulous heart
pendulum
    cor p.
penes (*pl. of* penis)
penetrability
penetrance
    complete p.
    incomplete p.
    reduced p.
penetrans
    Dermatophilus p.
    hyperkeratosis p.
    Pulex p.
    Sarcopsylla p.
    Tunga p.
penetrating
    p. radiation
    p. trauma
    p. ulcer
    p. wound
penetrometer
Penfield method
penicillamine
penicillate
penicillatum
    Trichosporon p.
penicillatus
    limbus p.
penicilli (*pl. of* penicillus)
penicillin
    p. allergy skin testing
    p. G
    potassium p. G
    potassium phenoxymethyl p.
    p., streptomycin, and tetracycline
     (PST)
    unit of p.
    p. V
penicillinase test
penicillin-fast
Penicilliopsis
penicilliosis

Penicillium
> P. *barbae*
> P. *bouffardi*
> P. fungus
> P. *minimum*
> P. *montoyai*
> P. *notatum*
> P. *patulum*
> P. *spinulosum*

penicilloyl polylysine
penicillus, pl. **penicilli**
penile
> p. blood flow
> p. cancer
> p. fibromatosis

Peniophora
peniplastica totalis
penis, pl. **penes**
> artery of the p.
> corpus spongiosum p.
> crura of the p.
> spongy body of p.
> trabeculae corporis spongiosi p.

penitis
pennivorans
> *Fervidobacterium p.*

penta
> p. X chromosomal aberration
> p. X syndrome

pentacarboxyporphyrin
> urine p.

pentacene
pentachlorophenol (PCP)
pentad
> Reynolds p.

pentaerythritol tetranitrate
pentafluoropropionic anhydride (PFP)
pentagastrin
> p. stimulated analysis
> p. test

pentalaminar granule
pentamer
pentamethyl violet
pentamidine
pentanoic acid
pentanucleotide
pentaromativorans
> *Novosphingobium p.*

Pentastoma
> P. *constrictum*
> P. *denticulatum*
> P. *taenioides*

pentastomiasis
Pentastomida
Pentatrichomonas hominis
pentatrichomoniasis
pentavalent
> p. botulinum toxoid vaccine
> p. gas gangrene antitoxin

pentene
pentobarbital
> sodium p.

penton antigen
pentose
> p. assay
> p. phosphate pathway (PPP)

pentosetest
> Bial p.

pentoside
pentosidine
pentosuria
> alimentary p.
> essential p.
> idiopathic p.
> primary p.

Pentra 60C+ analyzer
penumbra
PEP
> postexposure prophylaxis

peplomer
peplos
Pepper syndrome
pepsin
> proteolytic enzyme p.
> p. unit

pepsinogen assay
pepsinuria
peptic
> p. cell
> p. esophagitis
> p. gland
> p. ulcer (PU)

peptidase
peptide
> anionic neutrophil activating p.
> (ANAP)
> p. antibiotic
> antigenetic p.
> atrial natriuretic p. (ANP)
> p. bond
> C p.
> calcitonin gene-related p. (CGRP)
> cyclic citrullinated p. (CCP)
> gastric inhibitory p. (GIP)

NOTES

P

753

peptide *(continued)*
  gastrin releasing p. (GRP)
  p. group
  p. hormone
  human antimicrobial p.
  N-terminal prohormone brain
    natriuretic p. (NT-proBNP)
  p. nucleic acid (PNA)
  orexin A, B p.
  parathyroid hormone-related p.
    (PTHrP)
  phenylthiocarbamoyl p.
  POMC-derived anorexic p.
  prohormone B-type natriuretic p.
    (proBNP)
  proopiomelanocortin-related p.
  PTC p.
  p. regulatory factor (PRF)
  small p.
  trefoil p.
  vasoactive intestinal p. (VIP)
peptide-binding groove
peptide-loading compartment
peptidergic neuron
peptidivorans
  Clostridium p.
peptidoglycan
peptidolytica
  Pseudoalteromonas p.
peptidyl-prolyl isomerase nucleoprotein
  (Pin1)
Peptococcaceae
Peptococcus
  P. aerogenes
  P. anaerobius
  P. asaccharolyticus
  P. constellatus
  P. magnus
  P. niger
  P. prevotii
peptone shock
peptone-starch-dextrose (PSD)
Peptoniphilus
  P. asaccharolyticus
  P. harei
  P. indolicus
  P. ivorii
  P. lacrimalis
Peptostreptococcus
  P. anaerobius
  P. asaccharolyticus
  P. evolutus
  P. foetidus
  P. intermedius
  P. lanceolatus
  P. magnus
  P. micros
  P. morbillorum
  P. paleopneumoniae

  P. parvulus
  P. plagarumbelli
  P. prevotii
  P. productus
  P. putridus
PER
  protein efficiency ratio
peracetic
  p. acid
  p. acid-Schiff reaction
peracid
perambulating ulcer
perborate
  sodium p.
percent
  5 p. dextrose in water (D5W,
    D_5W)
  milligram p.
percentile
perchlorate
  p. discharge test
  potassium p.
  p. suppression test
perchloric acid
perchloroethylene
percolate
percolation
percreta
  placenta p.
percutaneous
  p. absorption
  p. allergy testing
  p. liver biopsy
  p. radiofrequency gangliolysis
  p. renal biopsy
  p. renal puncture
  p. transhepatic biliary drainage
  p. umbilical blood sampling
    (PUBS)
Peredibacter starrii
perencephaly
perester
perfect
  p. fungus
  p. stage
  p. state
  p. yeast
Perfectprep Plasmid 96 VAC direct
  bind purification system
perflava
  Neisseria p.
perfluoroalkylpolyether (PFAPE)
perfoliata
  Anoplocephala p.
perfoliatum
  Echinostoma p.
perforans
  Trichophyton tonsurans var.
    tonsurans p.

perforata
 zona p.
perforatae
 habenulae p.
perforated
 p. diverticulitis
 p. gastric ulcer
 p. layer of sclera
 p. viscus
perforating
 p. abscess
 p. fiber
 p. fiber of periodontal ligament and bone
 p. fibers of Sharpey
 p. ulcer
 p. wound
perforation
 bowel p.
 duodenal ulcer p. (DUP)
 esophageal p.
 inflammatory p.
perforin
perforin-dependent mechanism
performic
 p. acid
 p. acid reaction
 p. acid-Schiff (PFAS)
 p. acid-Schiff reaction
perfringens
 Clostridium p.
perfusate
perfuse
perfusion
 p. of alveoli
 Ca2+-free p.
 p. defect
 intervillous p.
 luxury p.
 organ p.
 p. pressure
 pulmonary p.
pergolide
periacinal
periadenitis
periampullary
perianal abscess
periangiitis, periangitis
periangiocholitis
periaortitis
periapical
 p. abscess

 p. cemental dysplasia
 p. granuloma
periappendiceal abscess
periappendicitis decidualis
periarterial
 p. lymphatic sheath (PALS)
 p. pad
periarteriolar lymphoid sheath
periarteritis
 p. gummosa
 p. nodosa
 syphilitic p.
periarticular abscess
periaxonal
peribiliary gland hamartoma
peribronchial cuffing
peribronchiolar
peribronchiolitis
peribronchitis
pericanalicular fibroadenoma
pericapillary cell
pericardia (*pl. of* pericardium)
pericardiac
pericardiaci
 villi p.
pericardial
 p. cyst
 p. effusion
 p. fluid examination
 p. friction rub
 p. serum
 p. tuberculosis
 p. villi
pericardii
 concretio p.
pericardiocentesis
pericarditic
pericarditis
 adherent p.
 adhesive p.
 bacterial p.
 carcinomatous p.
 chronic constrictive p.
 constrictive p.
 fibrinous p.
 fungal p.
 hemorrhagic p.
 idiopathic p.
 internal adhesive p.
 mediastinal p.
 p. obliterans
 obliterative p.

NOTES

P

pericarditis *(continued)*
    postmyocardial infarction p.
    postpericardiotomy p.
    posttraumatic p.
    purulent p.
    rheumatic p.
    serofibrinous p.
    p. sicca
    suppurative p.
    tuberculous p.
    uremic p.
    p. villosa
    viral p.
pericardium, pl. **pericardia**
    adherent p.
    bread-and-butter p.
    empyema of p.
    p. fibrosum
    p. serosum
    shaggy p.
pericellular fibrosis
pericemental attachment
pericentral fibrosis
pericentric inversion
pericholangitis
perichondral bone
perichondritis
    relapsing p.
perichondrium
perichoroidal
perichrome
pericolitis, pericolonitis
    p. dextra
    p. sinistra
pericolonic
pericolpitis
Periconia
pericorpuscular synapse
pericranitis
pericryptal
    p. fibroblast
    p. granuloma
pericrypt eosinophilic enterocolitis
pericystitis
pericystium
pericyte
    Rouget p.
    Zimmermann p.
    p. of Zimmermann
pericytial
pericytic venule
peridental
    p. ligament
    p. membrane
peridentium
periderm
peridermal
peridesmic
peridesmitis

peridesmium
perididymis
perididymitis
peridium
peridiverticulitis
periductal mastitis
periduodenitis
periecan
periencephalitis
perienteritis
periesophagitis
perifocal
perifollicular (PF)
    cutaneous p.
    p. hemorrhage
    p. stroma
perifolliculitis
periganglionic
perigastritis
perigemmal
periglandular collaring
periglandulitis
perihepatitis
perijejunitis
perikarya
    neuronal p.
perikaryal fluorescence
perikaryon
perikymata
perilesional ductule
periligamentous
perilobular
    p. mastitis
    p. stroma
periluminal lesion
perilymph, perilympha
perilymphangitis
perilymphatic duct
perilymphaticus
    ductus p.
perimeningitis
perimeter
perimetritis
perimetrium
perimortem artifact
perimuscular fibrosis
perimyelis
perimyelitis
perimyoendocarditis
perimyositis
perimysia (*pl. of* perimysium)
perimysial
perimysitis
perimysium, pl. **perimysia**
    p. externum
    p. internum
perinatal
    p. death
    p. mortality rate (PMR)

perinea (*pl. of* perineum)
perinecrotic zone
perineovaginal fistula
perinephric abscess
perinephritis
perineum, pl. **perinea**
    watering-can p.
perineural
    p. fibroblastoma
    p. invasion (PNI)
perineurial cell
perineurioma
perineurium
perineuronal
    p. satellite
    p. satellite cell
perinuclear
    p. cisterna
    p. halo
    p. hof
    p. pattern
    prominent p.
    p. space
period
    eclipse p.
    effective refractory p. (ERP)
    gap_0 p.
    gap_1 p.
    gap_2 p.
    incubation p. (IP)
    induction p.
    latency p. (LP)
    latent p.
    mitotic p.
    prepatent p.
    refractory p. (RP)
    relative refractory p. (RRP)
    synthesis p.
periodate-lysing-paraformaldehyde fixative
periodate-Schiff procedure
periodic
    p. acid
    p. acid-concanavalin A (PACONA)
    p. acid-Schiff (PAS)
    p. acid-Schiff method
    p. acid-Schiff reaction
    p. acid-Schiff test
    p. acid-silver methenamine (PAM, PASM)
    p. acid-silver methenamine stain
    p. alternating nystagmus (PAN)

    p. disease
    p. edema
    p. neutropenia
    p. paralysis
    p. parasite
    p. peritonitis
    p. polyserositis
    p. syndrome (PS)
    p. wave
periodicity
periodontal
    p. cyst
    p. disease
    p. ligament fiber
    p. membrane
periodontitis
periodontium, pl. **periodontia**
perioophoritis
perioophorosalpingitis
periorbital edema
periorchitis
    p. hemorrhagica
    meconium p.
periorificial lentiginosis
periost
periostea (*pl. of* periosteum)
periosteal
    p. bone
    p. chondroma
    p. fibroma
    p. fibrosarcoma
    p. ganglion
    p. implantation
    p. osteosarcoma
    p. sarcoma
periosteitis fibrosa
periosteoma
periosteomedullitis
periosteomyelitis
periosteophyte
periosteosis
periosteous
periosteum, pl. **periostea**
    alveolar p.
periostitis
periostoma
periostosis, pl. **periostoses**
periostosteitis
periovaritis
peripachymeningitis
peripancreatitis
peripartum cardiomyopathy

NOTES

P

peripheral
    p. ameloblastoma
    p. aneurysm
    p. arterial occlusive disease (PAOD)
    p. arteriosclerotic occlusive disease (PAOD)
    p. basophilia
    p. blood
    p. blood eosinophilia
    p. blood labeling index
    p. blood lymphocyte (PBL)
    p. blood lymphocytosis
    p. blood preparation
    p. blood progenitor cell (PBPC)
    p. blood smear
    p. blood stem cell infusion
    p. chemoreceptor
    p. circulatory failure
    p. dysostosis
    p. edema
    p. lesion
    p. lobule
    p. myelin protein 22 (PMP22)
    p. necrosis
    p. nerve
    p. neuroectodermal tumor (PNET)
    p. neuropathy (PN)
    p. odontogenic fibroma
    p. protein
    p. resistance unit (PRU)
    p. T-cell lymphoma (PTCL, PTL)
    p. total resistance (PTR)
    p. vascular disease (PVD)
    p. vein plasma (PVP)
    p. white count
    p. zone
    p. zone inflammation in chronic prostatitis
    p. zone of prostate
periphlebitic
periphlebitis
Periplaneta
periplasm
periplast
peripolar cell
peripolesis
periporitis
periportal
    p. cardiomyopathy
    p. fibrosis
    p. necrosis
    p. space of Mall
periproctitis
periprostatitis
peripylephlebitis
perirectal abscess
perirectitis

perirenal
    p. fascia
    p. insufflation
perisalpingo-oophoritis, perisalpingoovaritis
perisigmoiditis
perisinusoidal space
perispermatitis serosa
perisplanchnitis
perisplenitis
    hyaline p.
perispondylitis
peristalsis disorder
peristaltic hyperemia
peristasis
peristoma
peristome
periston
peristrumous
perisynovial
peritarsal network
peritendinitis
    p. calcarea
    p. serosa
peritenonitis
perithecium
perithelia (*pl. of* perithelium)
perithelial cell
perithelioma
perithelium, pl. **perithelia**
    Eberth p.
perithyroiditis
peritonea (*pl. of* peritoneum)
peritoneal
    p. borderline tumor
    p. cancer
    p. carcinomatosis
    p. exudate cell
    p. fluid examination
    p. gliomatosis
    p. hernia
    p. lavage
    p. melanosis
    p. mesothelium
    p. mucinous carcinoma (PMC)
    p. villi
peritoneales
    villi p.
peritonei
    gliomatosis p.
    Luteococcus p.
    pseudomyxoma p. (PP)
    tunica serosa p.
peritoneopathy
peritoneoscopy
peritoneum, pl. **peritonea**
    papillary serous carcinoma of the p. (PSCP)

p. parietale
p. viscerale
peritonitis
acute diffuse p.
adhesive p.
benign paroxysmal p.
bile p.
chemical p.
p. chronica fibrosa encapsulans
chyle p.
circumscribed p.
p. deformans
diaphragmatic p.
diffuse acute p.
p. encapsulans
feline infectious p.
fibrinohemorrhagic p.
fibrinous p.
fibrocaseous p.
p. fibroplastica encapsulatum
gas p.
general p.
gonococcal p.
localized p.
meconium p.
periodic p.
productive p.
secondary bacterial p.
septic p.
spontaneous bacterial p. (SBP)
tuberculous p.
peritonsillar abscess
peritrichal
Peritrichida
peritrichous
peritubular
p. capillary plexus
p. contractile cell
peritumoral
p. injection
p. tissue
periumbilical venous collateral
periungual fibroma
periureteral abscess
periureteritis plastica
periurethral
p. abscess
p. zone
periurethritis
perivaginitis
perivascular
p. cuff

p. cuffing
p. end feet
p. epithelioid cell
p. epithelioid cell tumor (PEComa)
p. fibrous astrocyte
perivasculitis
perivenular cell
perivesical
perivillitis
perivillous
p. fibrin
p. fibrin deposition
perivisceritis
Perkin-Elmer
P.-E. Cetus 480, 9600 DNA
Thermocycler
P.-E. DNA Thermal Cycler 480
perlatum
Lycoperdon p.
perlèche
perles
amyl nitrite p.
Perlman syndrome
Perls
P. Prussian blue stain
P. reaction
P. solution
P. test
permanent
p. cell
p. parasite
p. section
p. stained smear examination
permanganate
potassium p.
permeability
p. quotient (PQ)
p. of vacuum
vascular p.
permeability-inducing
bacterial permeability-inducing (BPI)
permeabilized
permeable
permease
permeation
permissible exposure limit (PEL)
permissive
p. culture medium
p. hypercapnia
permittivity of vacuum
Permount slide fixative
permutation

NOTES

P

759

Permutit
perniciosiform
perniciosus
> *Phlebotomus* p.

pernicious
> p. anemia (PA)
> p. anemia-type metarubricyte
> p. anemia-type prorubricyte
> p. anemia-type rubriblast
> p. malaria

pernio
> lupus p.

perniosis
perolens
> *Lactobacillus* p.

peromelia
> micrognathia with p.

peroneal muscular atrophy
per-operative approach
perosseous
peroxidase
> benzidine method for myoglobin p.
> concanavalin A-horseradish p.
> Dako Envision system p.
> endogenous p.
> glutathione p.
> horseradish p. (HRP)
> p. reaction
> s-ABC p.
> p. stain
> p. staining method

peroxidase-antiperoxidase (PAP)
> p.-a. complex

peroxidase-conjugated *Lotus tetragonolobus*
peroxidation
> lipid p.

peroxide
> acyl p.
> alkyl p.
> hydrogen p.

peroxisome
> p. proliferator-activated receptor (PPAR)

peroxyacetyl nitrate (PAN)
peroxyacylnitrate
peroxydisulfate
> ammonium p.

peroxynitrite formation
Perrin-Ferraton disease
persarum
> *Dracunculus* p.

Persephonella
> *P. guaymasensis*
> *P. hydrogeniphila*
> *P. marina*

Persian Gulf syndrome

persica
> *Borrelia* p.
> *Cellulomonas* p.

persicolor
> *Microsporum* p.
> *Trichophyton* p.

persicus
> *Argas* p.

persistence
> microbial p.

persistent
> p. agent
> p. chronic hepatitis
> p. filaria
> p. infection
> p. polyclonal B-cell lymphocytosis
> p. tolerant infection (PTI)
> p. truncus arteriosus (PTA)

persister
Persist skin prep swab
personal
> p. air sampler
> p. protection level A, B, C, D
> p. protective equipment (PPE)

personnel
perspiratory gland
perstans
> *Acanthocheilonema* p.
> acrodermatitis p.
> *Dipetalonema* p.
> erythema dyschromicum p.
> hyperkeratosis lenticularis p.
> *Mansonella* p.
> telangiectasia macularis eruptiva p.
> urticaria p.

persulcatus
> *Ixodes* p.

PERT
> program evaluation and review technique

pertactin
pertenue
> *Treponema* p.

Perthes disease
Pertik diverticulum
Pertofrane
perturbation
> cell-cycle p.

pertussis
> *Bacillus* p.
> *Bordetella* p.
> p. immune globulin
> p. immunoglobulin
> p. serology
> p. vaccine

peruana
> verruca p.
> verruga p.

peruensis
> *Lutzomyia* p.

peruviana
> *Leishmania p.*

peruzzii
> *Meningonema p.*

pes, pl. **pedes**
> p. febricitans

pessary
> p. cell
> p. corpuscle

pest
> fowl p.
> swine p.

Pestalotia

Pestalotiopsis

peste des petits ruminants

pesticemia

pesticide
> chlorinated hydrocarbon p.
> cyclodiene hydrocarbon p.
> organochlorine p.
> organophosphate p.

pestiferous

pestilence
> great p.

pestilential

pestis
> *Bacillus p.*
> *Pasteurella p.*
> *Yersinia p.*

Pestivirus

PET
> paraffin-embedded tissue
> predominantly epithelial thymoma
> preeclamptic toxemia
> pulmonary endodermal tumor

petechia, pl. **petechiae**
> pharyngeal p.
> Tardieu petechiae

petechial
> p. angioma
> p. hemorrhage

petechiasis

PETG
> polyethylene terephthalate

PETINIA
> particle-enhanced turbidimetric inhibition immunoassay

petiolate

petiole

petioled

petiolus

petit
> P. canal
> p. mal epilepsy

Petragnani medium

Petri
> P. dish
> P. dish culture
> P. test

Petriella

petriellidiosis

Petriellidium boydii

petrifaction

petrificans
> lipoma p.
> urethritis p.

petrii
> *Bordetella p.*

Petrobacter succinatimandens

Petroff-Hauser counting chamber

petroleum ether

Petromyces

petrophila
> *Thermotoga p.*

petrosal (*var. of* petrous)

petrositis, petrousitis

Petrotoga
> P. mexicana
> P. mobilis
> P. olearia

petrous, petrosal

petrousitis (*var. of* petrositis)

Pette-Döring disease

Petuvirus

Peutz-Jeghers
> P.-J. polyp
> P.-J. syndrome

Peutz syndrome

pexis

Peyer
> P. gland
> P. patch

peyerianum
> agmen p.

peyote

Peyronellaea

Peyronie disease

Pezicula

Peziza

Pezizella

PF
> perifollicular

NOTES

P

761

pF
  picofarad
PFA
  platelet function analyzer
    PFA 100
PFAPE
  perfluoroalkylpolyether
    PFAPE oil
PFAS
  performic acid-Schiff
Pfaundler-Hurler syndrome
PFC
  plaque-forming cell
Pfeiffer
    P. bacillus
    P. blood agar
    P. disease
    P. phenomenon
    P. syndrome
Pfeiffer-Comberg method
Pfeifferella anastipester
PFGC
  pseudofollicular growth center
PFGE
  pulsed field gradient gel electrophoresis
p-**fluorophenylalanine**
PFP
  pentafluoropropionic anhydride
  platelet-free plasma
PFT
  pulmonary function tests
PFU
  plaque-forming unit
PG
  prostaglandin
  proteoglycan
  pyoderma gangrenosum
PG1
  prostaglandin 1
PG2
  prostaglandin 2
PG3
  prostaglandin 3
pg
  picogram
PGD
  preimplantation genetic diagnosis
  pure gonadal dysgenesis
PGDR
  plasma glucose disappearance rate
PGH
  pituitary growth hormone
PGI
  potassium, glucose, and insulin
P-glycoprotein
PGP
  postgamma proteinuria
  protein gene product

PgR
  progesterone receptor
PGTR
  plasma glucose tolerance rate
PH
  prostatic hypertrophy
PH1
  primary hyperoxaluria, type 1
Ph
  phenyl
Ph1
  Philadelphia chromosome
pH
  hydrogen ion concentration
    pH alteration
    blood pH
    pH electrode
    fecal pH
    pH indicator
    pH meter
    scalp pH
    stool pH
PHA
  passive hemagglutination
  phytohemagglutinin
  pulse height analyzer
    PHA antigen
phacidiomorpha
    Didymella p.
Phacidium
phacoanaphylactic, phakoanaphylactic
    p. endophthalmitis
    p. uveitis
phacoanaphylaxis, phakoanaphylaxis
phacoma, phakoma
phacomalacia, phakomalacia
phacomatosis, phakomatosis
phacosclerosis, phakosclerosis
PHA-E
    Phaseolus vulgaris erythroglutinin
Phaenicia sericata
Phaeoannellomyces
    P. elegans
    P. werneckii
Phaeococcomyces catenatus
phaeohyphomycosis
phaeohyphomycotic cyst
Phaeolus
phaeomuriformis
    Sarcinomyces p.
phaeomycotic cyst
Phaeosclera dematioides
Phaeoscopulariopsis
phaeosporotrichosis
Phaeotheca
Phaeotrichoconis crotalariae
Phaeovirus
Phaffia

phage
    p. 1 artificial chromosome
    beta p.
    defective p.
    p. genetics
    temperate p.
phagedena
    p. gangrenosa
    p. nosocomialis
phagedenic ulcer
phage-resistant mutation
phagocyte
    alveolar p.
    p. dysfunction
    endothelial p.
    globuliferous p.
    melaniferous p.
    mononuclear p.
    sessile p.
phagocytic
    p. cell
    p. cell immunocompetence profile
    p. dysfunction disorder
      immunodeficiency
    p. function disorder
    p. histiocyte
    p. index
    p. macrophage
    p. pneumonocyte
phagocytin
phagocytize
phagocytoblast
phagocytolysis
phagocytolytic
phagocytophila
    Ehrlichia p.
phagocytophilum
    Anaplasma p.
phagocytose
phagocytosis
    p. assay
    frustrated p.
    induced p.
    macrophage p.
    spontaneous p.
    vacuole alteration p.
phagocytotic
phagolysis
phagolysosome
    acidified p.
    p. formation
phagolytic

phagosome
phagotype
phakic-aphakic (PA)
phakoanaphylactic (*var. of*
  phacoanaphylactic)
phakoanaphylaxis (*var. of*
  phacoanaphylaxis)
phakoma (*var. of* phacoma)
phakomalacia (*var. of* phacomalacia)
phakomatosis (*var. of* phacomatosis)
phakosclerosis (*var. of* phacosclerosis)
phalangeal
    p. cell
    p. cell of Deiters
phalanx, pl. **phalanges**
    tufted p.
phallitis
phalloides
    Amanita p.
phalloidin
phallolysin
phalloncus
phallus
Phanerochaete chrysosporium
phaneroplasm
Phaneropsolus bonnei
phanerosis
    fatty p.
phanerozoite
phantom
    p. cell
    p. corpuscle
    Hine-Duley p.
    tissue-compatible plastic p.
    p. tumor
pharmacodynamics
pharmacogenetics
pharmacokinetics
pharmacologic mediators of anaphylaxis
pharmacology
    p. of anticoagulant
    p. of immunosuppressive drug
    sympathetic p.
**PharmChek seat patch drug detection
test**
pharyngeal
    p. calculus
    p. gland
    p. hypophysis
    p. muscle disorder
    p. petechiae
    p. plague

NOTES

P

pharyngeal (*continued*)
    p. pouch syndrome
    p. tonsil
pharyngeales
    glandulae p.
pharyngealis
    tonsilla p.
pharyngis
    tunica mucosa p.
pharyngitic
pharyngitis
    atrophic p.
    croupous p.
    follicular p.
    gangrenous p.
    glandular p.
    granular p.
    p. herpetica
    p. hypertrophica lateralis
    membranous p.
    p. sicca
Pharyngobdellida
pharyngoconjunctival
    p. fever
    p. fever virus
pharyngoesophageal diverticulum
pharyngokeratosis
pharyngolaryngitis
pharyngolith
pharyngomycosis
pharyngopalatine
pharyngorhinitis
pharyngoscleroma
pharyngotonsillitis
pharyngotympanic tube
phase
    p. I immunoglobulin A antibody
    p. II antibody
    aqueous p.
    blastic p.
    catabolic flow p.
    cell cycle S p.
    continuous p.
    disperse p.
    ebb p.
    eclipse p.
    exponential p.
    G_0 p.
    G_1 p.
    G_2 p.
    inductive p.
    initial oliguric p.
    p. lag
    lag p.
    logarithmic p.
    M p.
    meiotic p.
    p. microscope
    mobile p.

    moving p.
    negative p.
    platelet p.
    positive p.
    previtellogenic p.
    proliferative p.
    radial melanoma growth p.
    S p.
    stationary p.
    synaptic p.
    synthesis p.
    vertical melanoma growth p.
phase-contrast
    p.-c. microscope
    p.-c. microscopy
phaseoliforme
    Trichophyton p.
***Phaseolus vulgaris* erythroglutinin (PHA-E)**
phasmid
Phasmidia
PHAT
    pleomorphic hyalinizing angiectatic tumor
Ph1$^+$ CML
    Philadelphia chromosome-positive chronic myelogenous leukemia
Phellinus
phenacetin breath test
phenacetolin
phenaceturic acid
phenanthrene
phenazopyridine hydrochloride
phencyclidine assay
phene
phenobarbital
    p. assay
    sodium p.
phenocopy
phenodeviant
phenogenetics
phenol
    p. assay
    p. coefficient
    p. sulfatase
phenolemia
phenolica
    Desulfobacula p.
    Pseudoalteromonas p.
phenolphthalein test
phenolsulfonphthalein (PSP)
    p. excretion
    p. test
phenoluria
phenom
    phenomenon
phenomenon, pl. phenomena (phenom)
    adhesion p.
    anarchic p.

Anderson p.
Arias-Stella p.
Arthus p.
atavistic p.
Azzopardi p.
Bordet-Gengou p.
cold-agglutination p.
Danysz p.
dawn p.
Debré p.
dedifferentiation p.
Denys-Leclef p.
d'Herelle p.
Donath-Landsteiner p.
Ehrlich p.
erythrocyte adherence p.
Felton p.
generalized Shwartzman p.
Gengou p.
halisteresis p.
Hamburger p.
Hektoen p.
Houssay p.
Huebener-Thomsen-Friedenreich p.
iceberg p.
immune adherence p.
Jod-Basedow p.
Kanagawa p.
Köbner p.
Koch p.
Koebner p.
LE p.
Lewis p.
Liacopoulos p.
Liesegang p.
Lucio leprosy p.
Mills-Reincke p.
Neisser-Wechsberg p.
no reflow p.
Pfeiffer p.
proliferation-dependent p.
prozone p.
quellung p.
Raynaud p.
reclotting p.
red cell adherence p.
Sanarelli p.
Sanarelli-Shwartzman p. (SSP)
satellite p.
Schultz-Charlton p.
second-set p.
Soret p.

Splendore-Hoeppli p.
Theobald Smith p.
Twort p.
Twort-d'Herelle p.
wavefront p.
phenone
phenothiazine
p. tranquilizer
p. tranquilizers assay
phenotype
adenocarcinoma p.
ayr p.
ayw p.
Bombay p.
endocrine p.
exocrine p.
Gerbich-negative p.
HLA-B8 p.
HLA-DR3 p.
lobular p.
McLeod blood p.
null p.
para-Bombay p.
prune belly p.
RER$^+$ p.
rhabdoid p.
secretor p.
phenotypic
p. adaptation
p. mixing
p. plasticity
p. variance
phenotypically manifest
phenotyping
alpha$_1$ antitrypsin p.
lipoprotein p.
phenoxypenicillin
phentolamine test
phenyl (Ph)
p. hydride
phenylacetica
Thauera p.
phenylacetic acid
phenylacetylglutamine
phenylalanine
p. agar
p. assay
formyl methionyl leucyl p. (fMLP, fMet-Leu-Phe)
p. hydroxylase
serum p.
p. test

NOTES

P

phenylalanine *(continued)*
    p. tolerance index
    urine p.
phenylalanine-free diet
phenylalanine-4-monooxygenase
phenylalanyl
phenylamine
phenylbutazone assay
phenylcarbinol
    benzoyl p.
phenylethyl alcohol blood agar
phenylethylbarbiturate
    sodium p.
phenylhydrazine
phenylhydrazone
    trifluorocarbonylcyanide p. (FCCP)
phenylketonuria (PKU)
    p. test
phenyllactic acid
phenylpyruvic
    p. acid
    p. acid test
    p. amentia
phenylpyruvica
    Moraxella p.
phenylpyruvicaciduria
phenylthiocarbamide (PTC)
phenylthiocarbamoyl peptide
phenylthiourea
phenytoin
    p. assay
    sodium p.
pheochrome cell
pheochromoblastoma
pheochromocyte
pheochromocytoma
    benign p. (BPC)
    malignant primary p. (MPPC)
    metastatic malignant p. (MMPC)
pheomelanin
pheomelanogenesis
pheomelanosome
pheresis
    granulocyte p.
pheromone
PHG
    pulmonary hyalinizing granuloma
Phialemonium
phialide
phialoconidium
Phialophora
    P. parasitica
    P. richardsiae
    P. verrucosa
Phialophore-type conidiophore
phialospore
Philadelphia
    P. chromosome (Ph1)
    P. translocation

Philip gland
philippina
    Taenia p.
philippinensis
    Capillaria p.
Philips 301 electron microscope
philomiragia
    Francisella p.
Philophthalmus
Philopia casei
phimosis
PHLA
    postheparin lipolytic activity
phlebarteriectasia
phlebectasia
phlebectomy
phlebectopia, phlebectopy
phlebemphraxis
phlebeurysm
Phlebia
Phlebiopsis
phlebismus
phlebitic
phlebitis
    adhesive p.
    p. nodularis necrotisans
    puerperal p.
    septic p.
    sinus p.
phlebography
phlebolith
phlebolithiasis
phlebometritis
phlebomyomatosis
phlebosclerosis
    idiopathic mesenteric p.
    mesenteric p.
phlebostenosis
phlebothrombosis
Phlebotominae
phlebotomine
phlebotomist
phlebotomize
phlebotomum
    Bunostomum p.
Phlebotomus
    P. argentipes
    P. chinensis
    P. flaviscutellatus
    P. intermedius
    P. longipalpis
    P. macedonicum
    P. major
    P. noguchi
    P. orientalis
    P. papatasii
    P. perniciosus
    P. sergenti

P. *verrucarum*
P. *vexator*
phlebotomus
    p. fever
    p. fever virus
phlebotomy
Phlebovirus
phlegm
phlegmasia
    p. alba dolens
    cellulitic p.
    p. cerulea dolens
    p. malabarica
    thrombotic p.
phlegmon
    diffuse p.
    emphysematous p.
    gas p.
phlegmonous
    p. abscess
    p. adenitis
    p. cellulitis
    p. enteritis
    p. gastritis
    p. mastitis
    p. ulcer
phlei
    Mycobacterium p.
phlogistica
    crusta p.
phlogocyte
phlogocytosis
phlogogenic
phlogogenous
phlogosin
phlogotherapy
phloridzin, phlorhizin, phlorizin
    p. diabetes
    p. glycosuria
phloroglucin, phloroglucinol
phloroglucol
phloxine
phloxine-tartrazine stain
phlyctenular
    p. conjunctivitis
    p. keratoconjunctivitis
    p. pannus
phlyctenule
phlyctenulosis
Phobetron
phocae
    Atopobacter p.

Phocanema decipiens
Phocas disease
Phocoenobacter uteri
phocomelia
phocomelic dwarfism
phoeniculicola
    Enterococcus p.
Pholioata mutabilis
Pholiota terrestris
Pholiotina
Phoma hibernica
Phomatospora minutissima
Phomopsis
phophoinositide turnover
phorate
phorbol myristate acetate
phoresy
Phoridae
Phormia regina
phorozoon
phosgene
    NATO code for p. (choking gas)
    (CG)
phosphatase
    acid p. (ACP)
    alkaline p. (alk phos, AP)
    alkaline phosphatase antialkaline p.
    (APAAP)
    bisphosphoglycerate p.
    cupric ion-inhibited acid p.
    diphosphoglycerate p.
    leukocyte alkaline p. (LAP)
    myosin p.
    placental alkaline p. (PLAP)
    prostate specific acid p. (PSAP)
    serine/threonine protein p.
    serum alkaline p. (SAP)
    tartrate inhibited acid p.
    tartrate resistant acid p. (TRAcP,
    TRAP)
    p. and tensin homolog
    p. test
    tissue-nonspecific alkaline p.
    (TNAP)
    total serum prostatic acid p.
    (TSPAP)
    p. unit
phosphate
    acid p.
    adenosine 3′,5′-cyclic p. (cAMP)
    aluminum p.
    ammonium magnesium p.

NOTES

P

767

phosphate *(continued)*
  p. assay
  basic calcium p. (BCP)
  p. buffer
  p. buffered formalin
  p. buffered saline (PBS)
  calcium p.
  carbamyl p.
  creatine p.
  p. dehydrogenase (PDH)
  deoxyguanosine p.
  deoxyuridine p.
  dibasic potassium p.
  dihydroxyacetone p. (DAP)
  diisopropyl p. (DIP)
  dimethyldichlorovinyl p. (DDVP)
  dolichol p.
  dried sodium p.
  effervescent sodium p.
  p. excretion index (PEI)
  p. group transfer potential
  guanosine 3′,5′-cyclic p.
  high-energy p.
  p. imbalance
  inorganic p.
  Krebs-Ringer p. (KRP)
  magnesium ammonium p.
  4-methylumbelliferyl p. (MUP)
  monobasic potassium p.
  monobasic sodium p.
  nicotinamide adenine dinucleotide p.
    (NADP, NADPH)
  organic p.
  potassium dihydrogen p.
  primaquine p.
  sodium acid p.
  sodium cellulose p.
  tartrate resistant acid p.
  tribasic potassium p.
  tricresyl p.
  tri-*o*-cresyl p.
  triple p.
  undecaprenol p.
phosphatemia
phosphatidalcholine
phosphatidalethanolamine
phosphatidate
phosphatid histiocytosis
phosphatidic acid
phosphatid-type histiocytosis
phosphatidylcholine
  amniotic fluid desaturated p.
  desaturated p. (DSPC)
phosphatidylcholine-cholesterol
  acyltransferase
phosphatidylcholine-sterol O-acyl-
  transferase
phosphatidylethanolamine
phosphatidylglycerol

phosphatidylinositide
phosphatidylinositol (PI)
  p. glycan linkage (PIG)
phosphatidylserine (PS)
phosphaturia, phosphoruria,
  phosphuresis, phosphuria
phosphide
  zinc p.
phosphine
phosphitoxidans
    Desulfotignum p.
phosphoadenosine diphosphosulfate
3′-phosphoadenosine 5′-phosphosulfate
phosphocholine
phosphocreatine (PC, PCr)
phosphodiesterase
  sphingomyelin p.
phosphoenolpyruvate
phosphoethanolamine
  urine p.
phosphofluoridate
  diisopropyl p.
6-phosphofructokinase
phosphofructokinase deficiency
phosphoglucomutase
phosphogluconate
  p. dehydrogenase
  p. dehydrogenase assay
  p. oxidative pathway
6-phospho-D-gluconate
phosphogluconic acid
6-phospho-D-gluconolactone
3-phosphoglyceraldehyde
2-phospho-D-glycerate
3-phospho-D-glycerate
phosphoglycerate kinase
phosphoglyceride
phosphoglyceromutase
phosphoguanidine
phosphohexokinase
phosphohexose isomerase deficiency
phosphoimager
phosphokinase
  creatine p. (CPK)
  serum creatine p. (SCPK)
phospholipase A₂, B, C
phospholipid (PL)
  amniotic fluid primary p.
  p. assay
  p. molecule
  p. staining
  p. test
  p. type anticoagulant
  p. vesicle
phosphomannosyl recognition marker
phosphomevalonic acid
phosphomolybdic
  p. acid
  p. acid stain

phosphomonoesterase
phosphonoacetic acid
phosphonothioate
> NATO code for nerve agent O,O-diethyl S-[2-(diethylamino)ethyl] p. (VG)

4′-phosphopantetheine
phosphoprotein
phosphopyridoxal
phosphorescence
phosphorescent
phosphoreum
> *Photobacterium p.*

phosphoribomutase (PRM)
5-phosphoribosyl-1-amine
phosphoribosyltransferase
> hypoxanthine p. (HPRT)
> hypoxanthine guanine p. (HGPRT)
> orotate p.

phosphoric
> p. acid
> p. acid test
> p. monoester hydrolase

phosphor image analysis
PhosphorImager
phosphoruria (*var. of* phosphaturia)
phosphorus
> p. assay
> red p. (RP)
> white p. (WP)
> yellow p.

phosphorus-32
phosphorylase
> p. deficiency
> glycogen p.
> inosine p.
> p. kinase
> purine nucleoside p. (PNP)

phosphorylated
> p. protein expression
> p. thiamine

phosphorylation
> oxidative p.
> substrate level p.
> tyrosine p.

phosphorylation-dependent/independent neurofilament epitope
phosphorylation-independent NF-H/M epitope
3-phosphoserine

5′-phosphosulfate
> 3′-phosphoadenosine 5′-p.

phosphotransferase (PT)
phosphotungstic
> p. acid (PTA)
> p. acid hematoxylin (PTAH)
> p. acid hematoxylin stain

phosphuresis (*var. of* phosphaturia)
phosphuria (*var. of* phosphaturia)
phot
photo
> gamma p.

photoaging
photoallergic sensitivity
photoallergy
photoautotroph
photoautotrophic
Photobacteria
Photobacterium phosphoreum
photobleaching
photocatalysis
photocatalyst
photocell
photochemical
> p. reaction
> p. smog

photochemistry
photochromogen
photochromogenicity
photochromogenic mycobacteria
photocoagulation
photoconductive cell
photocontact dermatitis
photocytometry
photodecomposition
photodecontamination
photodermatitis
photodetector
photodiode
photodissociation
photodistribution
photodynamic
> p. sensitization
> p. therapy

photoelectric effect
photoelectrometer
photoelectron
photogenesis
photogenic
photograph
> forensic p.

photographic effect

NOTES

P

photoheterotroph
photoheterotrophic
photoisomerization
photolithotroph
photolithotrophic
photoluminescence
photoluminescent
photolysis
photolytic
photomacrography
photometer
  double-beam p.
  filter p.
  flame p.
photometric
  p. accuracy
  p. linearity
  p. reproducibility
photometry
  flame p.
photomicrograph
  selected p.
photomicrography
  digital p.
  through-the-eyepiece p.
photomicroscope
photomicroscopy
photomultiplier tube
photomyoclonic response
photon counting
photoorganotroph
photoorganotrophic
photo-patch test
photopeak detection efficiency
photophoresis
  extracorporeal p.
photophthalmia
photoprotein aequorin
photopsin
photoreaction
photoreactivation
photoreceptor
  p. cell
  p. layer
  p. membrane (PRM)
photoresistor
photoretinitis
Photorhabdus
  P. asymbiotica subsp. *australis*
  P. luminescens subsp. *kayaii*
  P. luminescens subsp. *thracensis*
photosensitive porphyria
photosensitivity
photosensitization
photostable
photosynthesis
photosynthetic organism
phototaxis

phototoxic
  p. contact dermatitis
  p. sensitivity
phototoxicity
phototransistor
phototrophic
phototropism
phototube
photovoltaic cell
photuria
PHP
  pseudohypoparathyroidism
  pyridoxalated hemoglobin-
    polyoxyethylene
PHPPA
  parahydroxyphenylpyruvic acid
PHPPO
  Public Health Practice Program Office
phrenoptosia
phrenosin
phrygian cap
pH-stat titration application kit
phthalein test
phthalic acid
phthalocyanine dye
phthalylsulfathiazole
phthinoid
phthiriasis
Phthirus, Pthirus
  P. pubis
phthisic, phthisical
phthisis
Phycobacteria
phycoerythrin (PE)
Phycomyces
Phycomycetes
phycomycetosis
phycomycosis
p-hydroxybenzoic acid
p-hydroxyphenyllactic acid
p-hydroxyphenylpyruvate
  p-h. dioxygenase
  p-h. oxidase
p-hydroxyphenylpyruvic acid
phyla (*pl. of* phylum)
phylacagogic
phylactic
phylaxis
phyllode
  cystosarcoma p. (CP)
phyllodes tumor
phylloquinone
Phyllosticta
phylogeny
phylum, pl. phyla
phyma
phymatoid
phymatorrhysin
phymatosis

phymatum
> *Burkholderia p.*

P16-hypermethylation

Physa

Physalia

physaliferous (*var. of* physaliphorous)

physalifora
> ecchordosis p.

physaliform

physaliphore

physaliphorous, physaliferous
> p. cell

physalis

Physaloptera
> *P. caucasica*
> *P. mordens*

physalopteriasis

Physalopteridae

Physalospora

Physarum pusillum

physellae
> *Trichobilharzia p.*

physical
> p. adsorption
> p. allergy
> p. anthropology
> p. chemistry
> p. diagnosis
> p. half-life
> p. optics
> p. panniculitis
> p. record

physician assisted suicide

Physick pouch

physicochemical

physicochemically

physics
> health p.

physiochemical

physiologic
> p. albuminuria
> p. anemia
> p. chemistry
> p. equilibrium
> p. excavation
> p. hypertrophy
> p. hypogammaglobulinemia
> p. incompatibility
> p. leukocytosis
> p. neutrophilia
> p. saline solution

> p. sclerosis
> p. unit

physiological saline solution (PSS)

physiolysis

physis

physisorption

Physocephalus sexalatus

physocephaly

Physopsis

Physosporella Höhn

physostigmine salicylate

phytanic acid

phytate
> sodium p.

phytic acid

phytin

phytoagglutinin

Phytobdella

phytobezoar

phytofermentans
> *Clostridium p.*

Phytoflagellata

phytohemagglutinin (PHA)
> p. assay

phytoid

phytol

phytolectin

Phytomastigina

Phytomastigophora

Phytomastigophorasida

Phytomastigophorea

phytomitogen

phytophotodermatitis

Phytophthora infestans

phytopneumoconiosis

Phytoreovirus

phytotoxic

phytotoxin

PI
> phosphatidylinositol
> proliferative index
> propidium iodine
> protease inhibitor
> pulmonary incompetence
> pulmonary infarction

pi
> p. bond
> p. cell

PIA
> plasma insulin activity

pia-arachnitis

pial-glial membrane

NOTES

P

771

pia mater
Piazza test
pica
Picchini syndrome
Picci grading system
Piccolo blood chemistry analyzer
Pichia membranaefaciens
picipes
    Melanolestes p.
Pick
    P. atrophy
    P. bundle
    P. cell
    P. disease
    P. disease, tau pathology class III
    P. inclusion body
    P. syndrome
    P. tubular adenoma
picket cell
pickettii
    Ralstonia p.
pickwickian
    p. disease
    p. syndrome
picloram
picocurie (pCi)
picofarad (pF)
picogram (pg)
picometer (pm)
picopicogram (ppg)
Picornaviridae
picornavirus
picosecond (psec)
picramic acid
picrate test
picric
    p. acid
    p. acid fixative
    p. stain
picrocarmine stain
picroformol fixative
picroindigocarmine stain
picro-Mallory trichrome stain
picronigrosin stain
Picrophilaceae
Picrophilales
Picrophilea
picrosirius red technique
picrotoxin
pictor
    Aspergillus p.
picturae
    Brevibacterium p.
    Virgibacillus p.
PID
    pelvic inflammatory disease
    plasma iron disappearance
PIDT
    plasma iron disappearance time

PIE
    pulmonary infiltration and eosinophilia
    pulmonary interstitial emphysema
    PIE syndrome
piebald skin
piece
    end p.
    Fab p.
    Fc p.
    middle p.
    principal p.
piecemeal necrosis
piedra
    black p.
    p. nostras
    white p.
Piedraia hortae
pieds terminaux
Pierce Micro BCA Assay kit
Pierini
    atrophoderma of Pasini and P.
Pierre Robin syndrome
piezo-actuated microinjection
piezoelectric effect
piezogenic
piezophila
    Colwellia p.
PIF
    peak inspiratory flow
    prolactin-inhibiting factor
    proliferation inhibitory factor
pifanoi
    Leishmania mexicana p.
PIFR
    peak inspiratory flow rate
PIG
    phosphatidylinositol glycan linkage
pig
    virus pneumonia of p.'s
PIG-A gene
pigeon
    p. breast
    p. breeder disease
pigeon-breast deformity
piger
    Desulfovibrio p.
pigment
    accumulation of p.
    anthracotic p.
    bile p.
    bilharzial deposition p.
    brown hemoglobin-derived p.
    calculous p.
    p. calculus
    p. cast
    p. cell
    p. cell of iris
    p. cell of retina
    p. cell of skin

ceroid p.
cirrhosis p.
epithelial p.
p. epithelium
formalin p.
p. granule
hematogenous p.
hepatogenous p.
incontinence of p.
p. induration of the lung
lipid p.
lipochrome p.
lipofuscin p.
malarial deposition p.
melanotic p.
ochronotic p.
pseudomelanosis p.
respiratory p.
urine blood p.
wear-and-tear p.
yellow-brown wear and tear p.

pigmentary
p. cirrhosis
p. degeneration
p. dermatosis
p. dysplasia

pigmentation
arsenic p.
bismuth p.
exogenous p.
hematin p.
hematoidin p.
hemofuscin p.
hemoglobin p.
lead p.
lipochrome p.
melanin p.
nonmelanocytic p.
porphyrin p.
wear-and-tear p.

pigmented
p. ameloblastoma
p. cast
p. dermatofibrosarcoma
p. dermatofibrosarcoma protuberans
p. epulis
p. hair epidermal nevus
p. layer of ciliary body
p. layer of iris
p. layer of retina
p. pilocytic astrocytoma
p. purpuric lichenoid dermatitis

p. skin lesion (PSL)
p. villonodular synovitis (PVNS)
p. villonodular tenosynovitis

pigmenti
incontinentia p.

Pigmentiphaga
P. kullae

pigmentolysin

pigmentosa
dermatopathia p.
morphea p.
neurogenic muscle weakness, ataxia, and retinitis p. (NARP)
retinitis p.
urticaria p.

pigmentosum
atrophoderma p.
xeroderma p. (XDP, XP)

pigmentosus
nevus p.

pigmentum nigrum

pigrifrangens
Nocardia p.

PII
plasma inorganic iodine

Pike streptococcal broth

Pilaira

pilar
p. cyst
p. sheath acanthoma
p. tumor of scalp

pilaris
p. keratosis
pityriasis rubra p. (PRP)

pile
sentinel p.

pileous gland

pili (*pl. of* pilus)

piliate

Pilidae

piliferous cyst

piliform

pilimiction

pilin

pillar
p. cell
p. cell of Corti
Corti p.
p. of iris

pill esophagitis

pill-induced esophagitis

Pilobolus

NOTES

P

pilocarpine nitrate iontophoresis
pilocystic
pilocytic astrocytoma
Piloderma
piloid astrocytoma
pilomatricoma
pilomatrix carcinoma
pilomatrixoma
pilomotor fiber
pilonidal
    p. cyst
    p. fistula
    p. sinus
pilorum
    cruces p.
pilosa
    Cavernicola p.
pilosebaceous
pilosus
    nevus p.
pilus, pl. **pili**
    bulbus pili
    collum folliculi pili
    cuticula vaginae folliculi pili
    F pili
    folliculus pili
    papilla pili
    R p.
    radix pili
    sex pili
    type I–IV pili
PiMM genotype
PiMZ genotype
PIN
    prostatic intraepithelial neoplasia
    prostatic intraepithelial neoplasm
PIN 1
    prostatic intraepithelial neoplasia, mild
      dysplasia or low grade
PIN 2
    prostatic intraepithelial neoplasia,
      moderate dysplasia or high grade
PIN 3
    prostatic intraepithelial neoplasia, severe
      dysplasia or high grade
Pin1
    peptidyl-prolyl isomerase nucleoprotein
pinacyanol
pinch
    devil's p.
Pindborg tumor
pineal
    p. body
    p. cell
    p. cyst
    p. germinoma
    p. gland
    p. secretory rate

pineale
    chief cell of corpus p.
    corpus p.
    parenchymatous cell of corpus p.
pinealocyte
pinealoma
    ectopic p.
    extrapineal p.
pinealopathy
pineapple test
pineoblastoma
pineocytoma
pineocytomatous rosette
pine wood test
ping-pong
    p.-p. bone
    p.-p. mechanism
pinguecula
pink
    p. bread mold
    p. cytoplasm
    p. puffer (PP)
    p. puffer emphysema
pinkeye
Pinkus disease
pinnipedialis
    Jeotgalicoccus p.
pinnipedii
    Mycobacterium p.
pinocyte
pinocytosis
    mass p.
pinocytotic
    p. vesicle
    p. vessel
pinosome
pinpoint hemorrhage
pinta
pinus
pinworm preparation
pioepithelium
pion
Piophila casei
PIP
    paraffin immunoperoxidase
    proximal interphalangeal
pipe
    p. bomb
    light p.
piperatus
    Boletus p.
piperazine
pipe-smoker's cancer
pipestem
    p. artery
    p. cirrhosis
    p. fibrosis
pipette, pipet
    air-displacement p.

blowout p.
Eppendorf Repeater Pro p.
graduated p.
HandyStep electronic repeating p.
Labpette FX p.
measuring p.
Mohr p.
Ostwald-Folin p.
Pasteur p.
positive-placement p.
serologic p.
SoftGrip p.
TC p.
TD p.
transfer p.
volumetric p.
washout p.

pipiens
    Culex p.
Piptocephalis
Piptoporus
Pirenella
Piricauda
piriform, pyriform
    p. sinus carcinoma
Piroplasma
Piroplasmida
piroplasmosis
Pirquet
    P. cutaneous tuberculin test
    P. reaction
PIS
    pulmonary intimal sarcoma
Pisano method
pisciphila
    Exophiala p.
Piscirickettsia salmonis
pisiform
pisiformis
    Taenia p.
Pisolithus
pisotriquetral
pistol
    starter p.
PIT
    plasma iron turnover
pit
    central p.
    gastric p.
    Mantoux p.
    shuffle p.
    tubular p.

pit-1 protein
pitcher's elbow
pitch wart
pitch-worker's cancer
pith
Pithoascus langeronii
Pithomyces
PITR
    plasma iron turnover rate
Pitres section
pitting edema
Pitt-Rogers-Danks syndrome
pittsburgensis
    Legionella p.
Pittsburgh
    P. pneumonia
    P. pneumonia agent
pituicyte
pituicytoma
pituitaria
    glandula p.
pituitary
    p. adamantinoma
    p. adenoma
    p. ameloblastoma
    p. basophilia
    p. basophilism
    p. dwarf
    p. dwarfism
    p. dysfunction
    p. endocrine disorder
    p. function test
    p. gland
    Glenner-Lillie stain for p.
    p. glycoprotein hormone
    p. gonadotropic failure
    p. gonadotropin
    p. growth hormone (PGH)
    hyaline body of p.
    p. lactotroph
    lyophilized anterior p. (LAP)
    p. membrane
    p. microprolactinoma
    p. myxedema
    posterior p.
    p. stalk
    p. stalk section
    p. tumor
pituitary-like
    anterior p. (APL)

NOTES

P

pituitosa
>   membrana p.
>   *Sphingomonas p.*

pityriasic

pityriasis
>   p. alba
>   p. capitis
>   p. lichenoides chronica
>   p. lichenoides et varioliformis acuta (PLEVA)
>   p. nigra
>   p. rosea
>   p. rubra
>   p. rubra pilaris (PRP)
>   p. versicolor

Pityrosporum
>   *P. furfur*
>   *P. orbiculare*
>   *P. ovale*
>   *P. versicolor*

PIVKA
>   protein induced by vitamin K antagonist

pivotal transcription factor

pixel

pizza lung

Pizzolato peroxide-silver method

PK
>   Prausnitz-Küstner
>   pyruvate kinase
>>   PK deficiency
>>   PK reaction

PK110 centrifuge

PKC
>   protein kinase C
>>   PKC isoenzyme

PKD
>   polycystic kidney disease
>   proteinase K digestion

pKi67
>   nuclear proliferation marker p.

PKU
>   phenylketonuria
>>   PKU test

PL
>   phospholipid
>   placebo
>   placental lactogen

PLA2
>   agonist-induced activation of PLA2

PLAC coronary heart disease test

placebo (PL)

placei
>   *Haemonchus p.*

placenta, gen. and pl. **placentae**, pl. **placentas**
>   ablatio placentae
>   abruptio placentae
>   p. accreta
>   battledore p.

bilobate p.
p. circummarginata
circummarginate p.
circumvallate p.
dichorionic diamniotic p.
duplex p.
p. fenestrata
fenestrated p.
p. increta
mature abnormal p.
p. membranacea
monochorionic diamniotic p.
monochorionic monoamniotic p.
multilobate p.
p. multipartita
pars fetalis placentae
p. percreta
premature abnormal p.
prematurely separated p.
premature separation of p.
p. previa
p. previa abortion
p. spuria
p. succenturiata
p. triloba
trilobate p.
p. tripartita
twin p.
p. twins

placental
>   p. abruption
>   p. alkaline phosphatase (PLAP)
>   p. barrier
>   p. biopsy
>   p. disc margin
>   p. dysfunction
>   p. dysmaturity
>   p. and fetoplacental function tests
>   p. hemangioma
>   p. hormone
>   p. lactogen (PL)
>   p. malperfusion
>   p. membrane
>   p. parenchyma
>   p. polyp
>   p. residual blood volume (PRBV)
>   p. site nodule and plaque (PSNP)
>   p. site trophoblastic tumor (PSTT)
>   p. steroid sulfatase deficiency
>   p. thrombosis
>   p. transmogrification
>   p. tuberculosis

placentation
>   p. bleeding
>   circumvallate p.
>   extrachorial p.

placentitis

placentoma

placentomegaly

plagarumbelli
  Diplococcus p.
  Peptostreptococcus p.
plagiocephaly
Plagiorchiidae
Plagiorchioidea
Plagiorchis
plague
  p. aerosol
  p. bacillus
  black p.
  bubonic p.
  cattle p.
  cellulocutaneous p.
  duck p.
  fowl p.
  hemorrhagic p.
  p. meningitis
  naturally occurring p.
  pharyngeal p.
  pneumonic p.
  primary septicemic p.
  rabbit p.
  septicemic p.
  p. serum
  sylvatic p.
  urban p.
  p. vaccine
plague-infected flea
plakins
plakoglobin
plamare
  xanthoma striatum p.
plan
  Bioterrorism Readiness P.
  Bioterrrorism Readiness P.
plana (*pl. of* planum)
planar impact
Planck (*h*)
  P. constant (h)
  P. radiation law
Planctobacteria
Planctomycea
Planctomycetaceae
Planctomycetales
plane
  cleavage p.
  focal p.
  Meckel p.
  symmetry p.
  tangential p.
  p. wart

planimeter
  manual optic p.
plankter
plankton
planktonic
Planktothricoides raciborskii
planocellular
Planococcaceae
Planococcus
  P. alkanoclasticus
  P. antarcticus
  P. maitriensis
  P. maritimus
  P. psychrophilus
  P. rifietoensis
Planomicrobium
  P. koreense
  P. mcmeekinii
  P. okeanokoites
Planomonospora
planopilaris
  lichen p.
Planorbarius
planorbid
Planorbidae
Planorbis
plant
  p. agglutinin
  p. antitoxin
  p. estrogen
  p. indican
  p. pathogen
  p. protease test (PPT)
  p. toxin
  p. virus
Plantago major
plantar
  p. fascia fibromatosis
  p. wart
plantaris
  ichthyosis palmaris et p.
  keratoderma palmaris et p.
  keratosis palmaris et p.
  pustulosis palmaris et p.
  tylosis palmaris et p.
  verruca p.
plantarum
  Lactobacillus p.
Plantibacter
  P. flavus

NOTES

P

planticola
  Raoultella p.
planum, pl. **plana**
  coxa plana
  p. semilunatum
  verruca plana
  xanthoma p.
planuria
planus
  atrophic lichen p.
  bullous lichen p.
  hypertrophic lichen p.
PLAP
  placental alkaline phosphatase
plaque
  p. adhesion
  amyloid p.
  atheromatous p.
  attachment p.'s
  bacterial p.
  beta-amyloid p.
  cerebellar amyloid p.
  dental p.
  desmoplastic p.
  endocardial p.
  fibrofatty p.
  Hollenhorst p.'s
  hyaline p.
  island-sparing p.
  kuru p.
  mucous p.
  multiple red-to-purple skin p.
  neuritic p.'s
  parapsoriasis en p.
  placental site nodule and p.
    (PSNP)
  pleural p.
  Redlich-Fisher miliary p.'s
  p. rupture
  senile p.'s
  talc p.'s
  p. technique
plaque-forming
  p.-f. cell (PFC)
  p.-f. cell assay
  p.-f. unit (PFU)
plaque-stage cutaneous T-cell lymphoma
plasm
plasma (P)
  p. accelerator globulin
  p. activation
  adsorbed p.
  p. amino acid screening
  p. ammonia
  antihemophilic p.
  antihemophilic p. human
  antilymphocyte p. (ALP)
  anti-*Pseudomonas* human p.
  p. atrial natriuretic factor

p. bicarbonate
blood p.
p. blood cell
p. calcitonin
p. cell angiofollicular lymph node
  hyperplasia
p. cell antigen
p. cell dyscrasia
p. cell hepatitis
p. cell infiltrate
p. cell leukemia
p. cell mastitis
p. cell mucositis
p. cell pneumonia
p. cell vulvitis
p. clearance
p. clearance rate (PCR)
p. clot solubility assay
p. clotting factor
p. clotting time
p. colloid oncotic pressure
p. cortisol test
cryoprecipitate-depleted p.
p. defect (PD)
p. depletion
p. DNA
p. exchange
p. factor X
p. fibronectin
fresh frozen p. (FFP)
frozen p. (FP)
p. glucagon
p. glucose disappearance rate
  (PGDR)
p. glucose tolerance rate (PGTR)
p. hemoglobin test
p. inorganic iodine (PII)
p. insulin activity (PIA)
p. iodoprotein disorder
p. iron disappearance (PID)
p. iron disappearance time (PIDT)
p. iron turnover (PIT)
p. iron turnover rate (PITR)
p. kallikrein
p. kinin
p. labile factor
p. layer
p. luteinizing hormone
lymphoid p. (LP)
p. marinum
p. membrane
p. membrane bleb
normal p. (NP)
normal human p.
p. oncotic pressure (POP)
peripheral vein p. (PVP)
platelet-free p. (PFP)
platelet-poor p. (PPP)
platelet-rich p. (PRP)

p. progesterone
p. protein
p. protein fraction (PPF)
p. protein profile
psoralen-treated pooled p.
p. renin activity (PRA)
salted p.
SD p.
single-donor p.
p. sodium (P_{Na})
p. stain
p. substitute
p. therapy
p. thrombin clot method
p. thrombin time
p. thromboplastin antecedent (PTA)
p. thromboplastin antecedent
  deficiency
p. thromboplastin component (PTC)
p. thromboplastin factor (PTF)
p. thromboplastin factor B
p. triglyceride
ultrafiltrate of the blood p.
p. volume (PV)
p. volume expander
plasma-acetaminophen level
plasmablast
plasma-cell
  p.-c. labeling index
  p.-c. myeloma
plasmacrit (PCT)
  p. test
plasmacyte
plasmacytic
  p. blood cell
  p. infiltrate
  p. leukemia
  p. myeloma
plasmacytoblast
plasmacytoid
  p. differentiation
  p. lymphocyte
  p. lymphoma
  p. monocyte
plasmacytoma
  extramedullary solitary p. (EMP)
  extraosseous p.
  p. on tissue biopsy
plasmacytosis
plasmagene
**plasma glucose disappearance rate
  (PGDR)**

plasmalemma
plasmalemmal
  p. invagination
  p. pattern
plasmalogen
plasmal reaction
plasmapheresis
plasmarrhexis
plasmatic
  p. insudation
  p. stain
plasmatogamy (*var. of* plasmogamy)
Plasmavirus
plasmic stain
plasmid
  bacteriocinogenic p.
  conjugative p.
  F p.
  p. fingerprinting
  infectious p.
  p. integration
  nonconjugative p.
  oligomeric p.
  R p.
  resistance p.
  rough p.
  p. transfer
  transmissible p.
  p. vector
plasmin
  p. coagulation
  p. prothrombin conversion factor
  (PPCF)
plasminogen
  p. activator
  p. activator deficiency
  p. activator inhibitor (PAI)
  p. activator inhibitor assay
  p. activator inhibitor I, II
plasminokinase
plasminoplastin
plasmocrine vacuole
plasmocyte
plasmocytic leukemoid reaction
plasmodia (*pl. of* plasmodium)
plasmodial
Plasmodiidae
Plasmodium
  P. aethiopicum
  P. berghei
  P. brazilianum
  P. cynomolgi

NOTES

Plasmodium (*continued*)
    P. falciparum
    P. knowlesi
    P. kochi
    P. malariae
    P. ovale
    P. pleurodyniae
    P. vivax
    P. vivax minuta
plasmodium, pl. **plasmodia**
    p. embolism
    exoerythrocytic p.
Plasmodromata
plasmogamy, plasmatogamy, plastogamy
plasmogen
plasmoid humor
plasmolysis
plasmolytic
plasmolyze
plasmon
plasmoptysis
plasmorrhexis
plasmoschisis
plasmosin
plasmotomy
plasmotropic
plasmotropism
plasmotype
plasmozyme
plastic
    p. bronchitis
    p. corpuscle
    p. induration
    p. lymph
    p. pleurisy
    p. section stain
plastica
    linitis p.
    periureteritis p.
plasticity
    adult stem cell p.
    phenotypic p.
plasticizer
plastid
    blood p.
plastogamy (*var. of* plasmogamy)
plate
    Abbé test p.
    blood agar p. (BAP)
    chorionic p.
    colorimetric microtiter p. (CMP)
    cough p.
    counting p.
    Covalink MicroElisa culture p.
    p. culture
    decidual p.
    ductal p.
    DyNA block 1000 microtiter p.
    Dynex Immulon 1B microtiter p.

    end p.
    epiphysial p.
    flood p.
    foot p.
    growth p.
    Hospidex microtiter p.
    Kühne terminal p.
    lateral cartilaginous p.
    lawn p.
    Lowenstein-Jensen p.
    Maxisorp microtiter p.
    medial cartilaginous p.
    metaphase p.
    microtiter p.
    motor end p.
    nail p.
    polar p.'s
    pour p.
    Pro-Bind U-Bottom microfilter p.
    Sensititre *Streptococcus pneumoniae* HPB susceptibility p.
    spiral p.
    spread p.
    streak p.
    tarsal p.'s
    theoretical p.
    p. thrombosis
platelet
    acquired qualitative disorders of p.'s
    p. actomyosin
    p. adhesion test
    p. adhesiveness test
    p. agglutination
    p. agglutinin
    p. aggregation
    p. aggregation test
    p. antiaggregant
    p. antibody
    apheresis p.
    p. autoantibody
    Bizzozero p.
    p. cofactor
    p. concentrate
    p. count (PC)
    p. defect (PLD)
    p. factor 1–4
    p. function analyzer (PFA)
    p. function test
    giant p.
    p. GPIIb/IIIa
    hemolysis, elevated liver enzymes, and low p.'s (HELLP)
    p. isoantibody
    leukocyte-reduced p.'s
    p. membrane glycoprotein
    p. neutralization procedure
    p. pellet
    p. phase

p. phospholipid complex
p. plug
p. retention test
p. satellitism
single-donor p.'s
p. sizing
spent p.
splenic sequestration of p.'s
p. survival test
p. thrombosis
p. thrombus
p. tissue factor
p. transfusion
vacuolated p.
in vivo adhesive p. (IVAP)
platelet-activating
p.-a. factor (PAF)
p.-a. factor acetylhydrolase (PAF-AH)
platelet-aggregating factor (PAF)
platelet-associated bacteremia
platelet-derived growth factor (PDGF)
platelet-free plasma (PFP)
plateletpheresis
platelet-poor
p.-p. blood (PPB)
p.-p. plasma (PPP)
platelet-refractory state
platelet-rich plasma (PRP)
platelet-type von Willebrand disease
platelike
PlateTrak automated microplate processing system
platform
Rapid Analyte Measurement P. (RAMP)
plating density
platinosis
platinum group
platybasia
platycyte
platyhelminth
Platyhelminthes
platykurtic
Platynosomum fastosum
platys
Anaplasma p.
PLC
pleomorphic lobular carcinoma
PLCIS
pleomorphic lobular carcinoma in situ of the breast

PLD
platelet defect
pleated sheet
plebeius
Vaginulus p.
plecoglossicida
Pseudomonas p.
plectonemic coil
Plectosphaerella cucumerina
Plectrovirus
Pleiochaeta
pleiomorpha
Acrocarpospora p.
pleiotropic mutation
pleiotropy
Pleistophora
pleocellular
pleochroic
pleochroism
pleochromatic
pleochromatism
pleocytosis
neutrophilic p.
pleokaryocyte
pleomorpha
Cryptomyces p.
pleomorphic
p. adenoma (PA)
p. binucleated giant cell
p. fibroma
p. leiomyosarcoma
p. lipoma
p. lobular carcinoma in situ of the breast (PLCIS)
p. mononucleated giant cell
p. nucleus
p. oligodendroglioma
p. rhabdomyosarcoma
p. sarcoma
p. xanthoastrocytoma (PXA)
pleomorphism
cytonuclear p.
pleonosteosis
Leri p.
Pleospora herbarum
plerocercoid
plerocercus
Plesiocystis pacifica
Plesiomonas shigelloides
pleural
p. biopsy
p. calculus

NOTES

P

pleural *(continued)*
- p. effusion
- p. fibrin ball
- p. fibroma
- p. fibrosis
- p. fluid
- p. fluid examination
- p. friction rub
- p. mesothelioma
- p. plaque
- p. tuberculosis
- p. villi

pleurales
- villi p.

pleurisy
- adhesive p.
- benign dry p.
- costal p.
- diaphragmatic p.
- dry p.
- encysted p.
- epidemic benign dry p.
- epidemic diaphragmatic p.
- fibrinous p.
- hemorrhagic p.
- interlobular p.
- plastic p.
- productive p.
- proliferating p.
- pulmonary p.
- purulent p.
- sacculated p.
- serofibrinous p.
- serous p.
- suppurative p.
- visceral p.
- wet p.
- p. with effusion

pleuritic
pleuritis
- acute fibrinous p.
- lupus p.
- obliterative p.
- reactive eosinophilic p. (REP)

pleuritogenous
Pleurocapsales
Pleuroceridae
pleurodesis
pleurodynia
- epidemic p.

pleurodyniae
- *Plasmodium p.*

pleurogenous
pleurohepatitis
pleurolith
pleuropericarditis
Pleurophoma pleurospora
Pleurophragmium

pleuropneumonia
- contagious bovine p.

pleuropneumonia-like organism (PPLO)
pleuropulmonary blastoma
pleurorrhea
pleurospora
- *Pleurophoma p.*

Pleurotellus
Pleurotus
PLEVA
- pityriasis lichenoides et varioliformis acuta

plexiform
- p. fibrohistiocytic tumor of childhood
- p. layer
- p. layer of cerebral cortex
- p. layer of retina
- p. lesion
- p. neurofibroma
- p. neuroma
- p. schwannoma
- p. unicystic ameloblastoma

Plexiglas
plexitis
- brachial p.

plexogenic
- p. pulmonary
- p. pulmonary arteriopathy

plexopathy
- idiopathic brachial p.

plexosarcoma
plexus, pl. **plexus, plexuses**
- Auerbach p.
- Batson p.
- choroid p.
- Henle p.
- Meissner p.
- myenteric p.
- neuron of myenteric nerve p.
- peritubular capillary p.

PLGA
- polymorphous low-grade adenocarcinoma

PLH
- pulmonary lymphoid hyperplasia

plica, pl. **plicae**
- plicae ciliares
- plicae circulares
- plicae circulares intestini tenuis
- spiral p.

plicate
plicatilis
- *Spirochaeta p.*

Plicatura
Plimmer body
PLL
- prolymphocytic leukemia

PLNR
- perilobar nephrogenic rest

ploidy
   p. analysis
   DNA p.
plot
   Scatchard p.
   time-series p.
Ploton staining method
plotter
PLP
   pyridoxal-5'-phosphate
PLS
   prostaglandin-like substance
PLT
   psittacosis-lymphogranuloma venereum
   trachoma
   PLT group virus
plucked chicken appearance
plug
   adherent p.
   carpet tack follicular keratotic p.
   Dittrich p.
   Ecker p.
   fibrous p.
   mucous p.
   platelet p.
   Traube p.
plumbism
plumboporphyria
Plummer
   P. adenoma
   P. disease
Plummer-Vinson syndrome
plumose
plump cell
pluranimalium
   Arcanobacterium p.
pluricentric blastoma
pluriglandular adenomatosis
plurihormonal adenoma
plurilobulated shape
plurilocular
plurinuclear
pluriorificialis
   ectodermosis erosiva p.
pluripotent
   p. hematopoietic stem cell
   p. myeloid stem cell
   p. primitive mesodermal cell
pluripotential
   p. basal cell
   p. hemopoietic stem cell
   p. stromal cell

pluriresistant
plus
   Decal P.
   p. strand
Pluteus
plutonium
PLV
   panleukopenia virus
plymuthica
   Serratia p.
plywood pattern
PLZF
   promyelocytic leukemia zinc finger
PM
   pagetoid melanocytosis
   polymorph
   postmortem
pm
   picometer
"φM1-like viruses"
PMA
   papillary, marginal, attached
PMB
   polymorphonuclear basophil
PMC
   peritoneal mucinous carcinoma
   pseudomembranous colitis
PMD
   primary myocardial disease
   progressive muscular dystrophy
PMDS
   persistent müllerian duct syndrome
PME
   polymorphonuclear eosinophil
***p*-methoxyamphetamine assay**
PMF
   progressive massive fibrosis
PMI
   postmortem interval
PML
   progressive multifocal
   leukoencephalopathy
   promyelocytic leukemia protein
PMLS
   primary mediastinal large cell lymphoma
   with sclerosis
PMMA
   polymethylmethacrylate
PMN
   polymorphonuclear neutrophil

NOTES

P

PMP
postmenopausal
PMP woman
PMP22
peripheral myelin protein 22
PMP22 gene
PMR
perinatal mortality rate
polymorphic reticulosis
proportionate morbidity ratio
proportionate mortality ratio
PMS
postmitochondrial supernatant
pregnant mare serum
PMS-1, -2 gene
PMSG
pregnant mare serum gonadotropin
PMT
pseudosarcomatous myofibroblastic
tumor
PN
peripheral neuropathy
pneumonia
polyarteritis nodosa
pyelonephritis
PNA
peptide nucleic acid
PNA probe
PNEC
pulmonary neuroendocrine cell
PNET
peripheral neuroectodermal tumor
primitive neuroectodermal tumor
pneumarthrosis
pneumatic
pneumatization
pneumatocele
pneumatoides
cystitis p.
pneumatosis
p. cystoides intestinalis (PCI)
p. intestinalis cystica
pneumaturia
pneumobacillus
Friedländer p.
pneumocephalus
pneumococcal
p. pneumonia
p. polysaccharide
p. vaccine
pneumococcemia
pneumococci (*pl. of* pneumococcus)
pneumococcidal
pneumococcolysis
pneumococcosuria
pneumococcus, pl. **pneumococci**
pneumoconiosis, pneumonoconiosis,
pl. **pneumoconioses**
antimony p.

bauxite p.
coal worker's p. (CWP)
endogenous p.
fuller's earth p.
graphite p.
hematite p.
kaolin p.
mica p.
mixed dust p.
noncollagenous p.
polyvinyl chloride p.
rheumatoid p.
p. siderotica
talc p.
titanium dioxide p.
tungsten carbide p.
pneumocystiasis
Pneumocystis
P. carinii
P. carinii pneumonia
P. fluorescence
P. pneumoniae
pneumocystosis
pneumocyte
granular p.
pneumoderma
pneumogenic osteoarthropathy
pneumohemopericardium
pneumohemothorax
pneumohydroperitoneum
pneumohydrothorax
pneumohypoderma
pneumolith
pneumolithiasis
pneumomalacia
pneumomediastinum
pneumomycosis, pneumonomycosis
pneumonectomy evaluation
pneumonia (PN)
Acinetobacter p.
acute gelatinous p.
acute interstitial p. (AIP)
alcoholic p.
anaerobic p.
anthrax p.
aspiration p.
atypical primary p.
Bacteroides p.
bronchial p.
bronchiolitis obliterans organizing p.
(BOOP)
Candida p.
caseous p.
central p.
chemical p.
chlamydial p.
chronic eosinophilic p. (CEP)
confluent p.
core p.

cryptogenic organizing p. (COP)
desquamative interstitial p. (DIP)
diffuse interstitial p.
p. dissecans
double p.
Eaton agent p.
Enterobacter p.
eosinophilic p.
Escherichia coli p.
exogenous lipid p.
focal p.
Friedländer bacillus p.
fungal p.
gangrenous p.
giant cell interstitial p. (GIP)
glanders p.
Haemophilus influenzae p.
Hecht p.
hospital-acquired gram-negative p.
hypostatic p.
inhalation p.
p. interlobularis
p. interlobularis purulenta
interstitial giant cell p.
interstitial plasma cell p.
Klebsiella p.
lipid p.
lipoid p.
lobar p.
lobular p.
Louisiana p.
lymphocytic interstitial p. (LIP)
lymphoid interstitial p. (LIP)
p. malleosa
measles virus p.
metastatic p.
migratory p.
moniliasis p.
mycoplasmal p.
necrotizing lobar p.
nonspecific interstitial p. (NSIP)
nosocomial p.
oil-aspiration p.
organized p.
ovine progressive p.
paratuberculous p.
Pittsburgh p.
plasma cell p.
pneumococcal p.
Pneumocystis carinii p.
primary atypical p. (PAP)
primary influenza virus p.

Proteus p.
pseudomonal p.
Q fever p.
rheumatic p.
secondary eosinophilic p.
septic p.
severe atypical p.
staphylococcal p.
streptococcal p.
suppurative p.
tularemia p.
p. tularemia
tularemic p.
unresolved lobar p.
uremic p.
usual interstitial p. (UIP)
ventilator-associated p.
viral p.
p. virus of mice (PVM)
virus p. of pigs
wandering p.
white p.
woolsorter's p.

pneumoniae
Bacillus p.
Chlamydia p.
Chlamydophila p.
Diplococcus p.
Klebsiella p.
Miyagawanella p.
Mycoplasma p.
Pneumocystis p.
Streptococcus p.

pneumonia/fibrosis
nonspecific interstitial p./f. (NSIP)

pneumonic
p. plague
p. tularemia

pneumonitis
Ascaris p.
aspiration p.
chemical p.
desquamative interstitial p. (DIP)
eosinophilic p.
herpes p.
hypersensitivity p.
interstitial p.
lymphocytic interstitial p. (LIP)
measles p.
nonspecific interstitial p. (NSIP)
occupational hypersensitivity p.
organizing p.

NOTES

P

pneumonitis *(continued)*
    pulmonary p.
    radiation p.
    rheumatic p.
    uremic p.
    usual interstitial p. (UIP)
    p. virus
pneumonoconiosis *(var. of* pneumoconiosis)
pneumonocyte
    granular p.
    phagocytic p.
pneumonomoniliasis
pneumonomycosis *(var. of* pneumomycosis)
Pneumonyssus simicola
pneumoparotitis
pneumoperitoneum
pneumoperitonitis
pneumophila
    Legionella p.
pneumopleuritis
pneumoretroperitoneum
pneumoscrotum
pneumoserothorax
pneumosintes
    Bacteroides p.
    Dialister p.
pneumothorax (PT, Px)
    spontaneous p.
    therapeutic p.
pneumotropica
    Pasteurella p.
Pneumovirus
pneumovirus
PNH
    paroxysmal nocturnal hemoglobinuria
PNI
    perineural invasion
p-nitro-alpha-acetylamino-beta-hydroxy-propiophenone
p-**nitrophenylic acid**
p-**nitrosulfathiazole**
PNN
    probabilistic neural network
pnomenusa
    Pandoraea p.
PNP
    paraneoplastic pemphigus
    purine nucleoside phosphorylase
    PNP deficiency
PNST
    peripheral nerve sheath tumor
PNU
    protein nitrogen unit
P:O
    ratio of number of ATPs produced to number of atmospheric oxygen molecules converted to water

Po
    polonium
POA
    pancreatic oncofetal antigen
poae
    Leifsonia p.
POC
    point of care
PocketChem
    P. UA
    P. UA analyzer
pocket dosimeter
pocketed calculus
POCT
    point-of-care testing
poculum
podagra
podarthritis
podedema
poditis
podocyte foot process
podophyllin resin
podoplanin
    p. expression
    p. staining
Podospora
Podoviridae
poeciloides
    Eubacterium p.
POEMS
    polyneuropathy, organomegaly, endocrinopathy, monoclonal gammopathy, and skin changes
    POEMS syndrome
POES
    polyoxyethylene stearate
    POES additive
POG
    Pediatric Oncology Group
    POG surgicopathologic staging system
Pogonomyrmex
POGTD
    primary ovarian gestational trophoblastic disease
pOH
    hydroxyl concentration
poietin
poik
    poikilocyte
poikiloblast
poikilocyte (poik)
    tail p.
poikilocythemia
poikilocytosis
poikiloderma
    p. atrophicans and cataract
    p. atrophicans vasculare

p. of Civatte
p. congenitale
poikilodermatomyositis
poikilothrombocyte
point
Boas p.
boiling p. (bp)
p. of care (POC)
p. of care INR testing
clinical end p.
cold rigor p.
p. counting method
p. de repere (point of reference)
end p.
equivalence p.
p. estimate
freezing p. (FP)
Griffith p.
growing p.
ice p.
ignition p.
p. of inflection
isoelectric p.
isosbestic p.
Krafft p.
McEwen p.
melting p. (MP)
p. mutation
p. of ossification
Pauly p.
radix p.
Ramond p.
Robson p.
set p.
Staller p.
Sudeck p.
thermal death p.
triple p.
pointed
p. condyloma
p. wart
pointer variable
pointes
torsade de p.
point-of-care testing (POCT)
Poirier gland
poise
Poiseuille
P. law
P. space
poison
P. Control Center

industrial p.
mitotic p.
poisoning
acetanilid p.
amobarbital p.
antimony p.
arsenic p.
aspirin p.
benzene p.
blood p.
carbon disulfide p.
carbon monoxide p.
carbon tetrachloride p.
chloroform p.
cyanide p.
desquamative interstitial p.
enzymatic p.
ethyl alcohol p.
cthylcne glycol p.
food p.
heavy metal p.
lead p.
manganese p.
mercury p.
methanol p.
methotrexate p.
methyl alcohol p.
mushroom p.
naphthol p.
nitroaniline p.
oxygen p.
paraldehyde p.
salmonella p.
scombroid p.
systemic p.
tetrachloroethane p.
thallium p.
Poisson distribution
Poisson-Pearson formula
poker spine
pokeweed mitogen (PWM)
Poland syndrome
polar
p. anemia
p. body
p. cell
p. compound
p. coordinates
p. globule
p. lesion
p. plates
polarimeter

NOTES

P

polarimetry
polaris
    Glaciecola p.
    Kocuria p.
polarity
    cell p.
    nuclear p.
polarizability
polarization fluoroimmunoassay
polarize
polarized
    p. light
    p. microscopy
polarizer
polarizing microscope
polarogram
polarography
Polaromonas naphthalenivorans
polecki
    Entamoeba p.
Polerovirus
pol gene
Polhemus-Schafer-Ivemark syndrome
policeman
    p. glass stirring rod
    rubber p.
    p. tip
    p. transfer tool
polio
    poliomyelitis
polioclastic
poliodystrophia cerebri progressiva infantilis
poliodystrophy
    progressive cerebral p.
polioencephalitis infectiva
poliomyelitis (polio)
    acute anterior p.
    acute bulbar p.
    anterior acute p.
    chronic anterior p.
    p. I–III titer
    p. immune globulin (human)
    immunization reaction p.
    p. immunoglobulin
    late effect p.
    p. vaccine
    virus p.
    p. virus
poliovirus
    p. hominis
    p. vaccine
Polistes
polka
    p. dot pattern
    p. fever
polkissen of Zimmermann
Pollacia

pollen
    p. antigen
    p. extract
Pollenia
pollinosis
polocyte
polonica
    Bilharziella p.
polonium (Po)
polster
    Sanderson p.
poly
    polymorphonuclear leukocyte
polyA
    polyadenylic acid
    polyA tail
polyacrylamide
    p. gel
    p. gel electrophoresis (PAGE)
polyadenitis
polyadenopathy
polyadenosis
polyadenylate tail
polyadenylation
polyadenylic acid (polyA)
poly-ADP-ribose-polymerase enzyme
polyagglutination
polyamide
polyamine
polyamine-methylene resin
polyanetholsulfonate
Polyangiaceae
polyangiitis
    microscopic p.
polyanion
polyarteritis nodosa (PAN, PN)
polyarthritis
    p. chronica
    p. chronica villosa
    epidemic p.
    migratory p.
    p. rheumatica acuta
    vertebral p.
polybasic acid
polyblast
polyC
    polycytidylic acid
polycarbonate
polycationic dye
polycentric
Poly-Chem automated chemistry-immunoassay system
polychlorinated
    p. biphenyl (PCB)
    p. biphenyl assay
polychondritis
    chronic atrophic p.
    relapsing p.
polychromasia

polychromatia
polychromatic
 p. cell
 p. normoblast
polychromatocyte
polychromatocytosis
polychromatophil, polychromatophile
 p. cell
polychromatophilia
polychromatophilic
 p. erythroblast
 p. megaloblast
 p. normoblast
 p. rubricyte
polychromatosis
polychrome
 p. methylene blue
 p. methylene blue stain
polychromemia
polychromia
polychromophil
polychromophilia
polyclave
polyclonal
 p. activator
 p. anticarcinoembryonic antigen
 p. antiplacental antibody
 p. anti-S-100 protein
 p. gammopathy
 p. hypergammaglobulinemia
 p. lymphoid proliferation
 p. pattern
 p. prolactin antibody
 p. tumor
polyclonality
polycomb group
polycyclic aromatic hydrocarbon
polycystic
 p. change
 p. disease of kidney
 p. liver
 p. liver disease
 p. ovary
 p. ovary disease
 p. ovary syndrome
 p. renal disease
polycystin-1
Polycytella hominis
polycythemia
 absolute p.
 compensatory p.
 familial p.

 p. hypertonica
 myelopathic p.
 relative p.
 p. rubra
 p. rubra vera
 secondary p.
 smoker's p.
 splenomegalic p.
 p. vera (PCV, PV)
polycythemica
 hypertonia p.
 polyemia p.
polycytidylic acid (polyC)
polycytokeratin
polycytosis
polydactyly
polydeoxyribonucleotide synthetase
polydermatomyositis
Polydesmus
polydimethylsiloxane (PDM)
polydysplasia
polydystrophia
polydystrophic dwarfism
polydystrophy
 pseudo-Hurler p.
polyelectrolyte
polyembryony
polyemia
 p. aquosa
 p. hyperalbuminosa
 p. polycythemica
 p. serosa
polyendocrine
 p. adenomatosis
 p. autoimmune disease
polyendosporus
 Anaerobacter p.
polyene antibiotic
polyenoic acid
polyester resin
polyether sulfone filters
polyethylene
 p. glycol
 p. glycol precipitation assay
 p. terephthalate (PETG)
polygenic inheritance
polyglandular
polyglutamine
 p. disease
 p. expansion disorder
polygon
 frequency p.

NOTES

P

789

polygonal cell
polygyny
polygyria
polyhedral
    p. body
    p. cell
polyhedron
    face of p. (P)
polyhelminthism
PolyHeme blood substitute
polyhydramnios
    maternal p.
polyhydric alcohol
polyisoprenivorans
    Gordonia p.
polykaryocyte
    Warthin-Finkeldey-type p.
polykaryon
polyleptic fever
polylysine
    penicilloyl p.
polymastia
polymastigote
polymer
    addition p.
    condensation p.
    polymethylmethacrylate p.
    rod-shaped p.
    vinyl p.
polymerase
    p. chain reaction (PCR)
    p. chain reaction amplification
    p. chain reaction-based identity
      testing
    DNA p.
    nucleotide p.
    Promega Taq DNA p.
    RNA p.
    p. slippage
    p. slippage model
polymerization
    actin-filament p.
    cytoskeletal p.
polymerization-dependent amplification
polymerize
polymetaphosphate
polymethine dye
polymethylmethacrylate (PMMA)
    p. cement
    p. polymer
polymicrobial culture
polymicrogyria
polymicrolipomatosis
polymitus
polymorph (PM)
polymorpha
    Mima p.
polymorphe
    erythema p.

polymorphic
    p. B-cell lymphoma
    p. epithelial mucin (PEM)
    p. genetic marker
    p. light eruption
    p. reticulosis (PMR)
polymorphism
    balanced p.
    cleavase fragment length p. (CFLP)
    lipoprotein p.
    microsatellite p.
    NanoChip test for factor V Leiden
      single-nucleotide p.
    polymerase chain reaction-restriction
      fragment length p. (PCR-RFLP)
    polymerase chain reaction-single-
      strand conformation p. (PCR-
      SSCP)
    restriction fragment length p.
      (RFLP)
    single nucleotide p. (SNP)
    single-stranded conformation p.
      (SSCP)
polymorphocellular
polymorphocyte
polymorphocytic leukemia
polymorphonuclear
    p. basophil (PMB)
    p. eosinophil (PME)
    filament p.
    p. granulocyte
    p. leukocyte (poly)
    p. leukocytic infiltrate
    p. neutrophil (PMN)
    p. neutrophil chemotactic factor
polymorphonuclear-lymphocyte ratio
polymorphous
    p. dermatitis
    p. eruption
    p. layer
    p. low-grade adenocarcinoma
      (PLGA)
    p. low-grade carcinoma of salivary
      gland
    p. lymphoid infiltrate
polymyalgia
    p. arteritica
    p. rheumatica
polymyopathy
    alcoholic p.
polymyositis
polymyxa
    Bacillus p.
polymyxin
    p. B sulfate
    p. E
    p. test agar
polynesic

polynesiensis
    Aedes p.
polyneural
polyneuritic-type hypertrophic muscular atrophy
polyneuritiformis
    heredopathia atactia p. (HAP)
polyneuritis
    acute idiopathic p.
    idiopathic p.
    infectious p.
polyneuropathy
    chronic inflammatory
        demyelinating p. (CIDP)
    p., organomegaly, endocrinopathy,
        monoclonal gammopathy, and skin
        changes (POEMS)
polynuclear leukocyte
polynucleate
polynucleolar
polynucleosis
polynucleotide ligase
polyol
    p. dehydrogenase
    p. pathway
polyolefin
Polyomavirus
polyoma virus
polyoncosis, polyonchosis
    cutaneomandibular p.
polyorchism
polyostotic fibrous dysplasia
polyovular ovarian follicle
polyoxyethylene stearate (POES)
polyp
    adenomatous p.
    aural p.
    bladder p.
    bleeding p.
    bronchial p.
    cardiac p.
    cellular p.
    cervical p.
    choanal p.
    cholesterol p.
    cloacogenic p.
    cockscomb p.
    colon p.
    colorectal p.
    Cronkhite-Canada p.
    cystic p.
    decidual p.

endometrial p.
familial juvenile p. (FJP)
fibrinous p.
fibroepithelial p.
fibrous p.
fleshy p.
gallbladder p.
gastric p.
gelatinous p.
granulomatous p.
hamartomatous p.
hydatid p.
hyperplastic p.
inflammatory p.
juvenile p.
laryngeal p.
lipomatous p.
lymphangiomatous p. (LAP)
lymphoid p.
metaplastic p.
mucous p.
multiple adenomatous p.'s
myomatous p.
nasal p.
osseous p.
papillary adenomatous p.
pedunculated p.
Peutz-Jeghers p.
placental p.
postinflammatory p.
regenerative p.
retention p.
serrated colorectal p.
sessile p.
small intestine p.
sporadic adenomatous p. (SAP)
umbilical p.
vascular p.
villous p.
vocal fold p.
Polypaecilum insolutum
polyparasitism
polypeptide
    adrenocorticotropic p. (ACTP)
    p. coding
    gastric inhibitory p. (GIP)
    keratin p.
    neurofilament triplet p. (NFP)
    pancreatic p. (PP)
    TnC p.
    TnI p.

NOTES

P

polypeptide *(continued)*
   TnT p.
   vasoactive intestinal p. (VIP)
polyphaga
   Acanthamoeba p.
polyphase
polyphasic wave
polyphemus
   Limulus p.
polyphenism
polyphenotypia
polyphenotypic profile
polypheny
polyphosphoric acid
polyphyletic theory
polyphyletism
polypi (*pl. of* polypus)
polypiform
polyplasmia
Polyplax
Polyplis
polyploid
polyploidy
polypnea
polypoid
   p. adenocarcinoma
   p. adenoma
   p. cystitis
   p. excrescence
   p. hyperplasia
   p. intraluminal projection
polyporous
Polyporus
polyposa
   enteritis p.
   gastritis cystica p.
polyposis
   attenuated familial adenomatous p.
   p. coli
   familial adenomatous p. (FAP)
   familial intestinal p.
   lymphomatoid p.
   multiple intestinal p.
   multiple lymphomatous p.
polypous
   p. endocarditis
   p. gastritis
polypropylene
polyptychial
polypus, pl. **polypi**
polypyrrylmethane
polyradiculitis
polyradiculoneuritis
polyradiculoneuropathy
polyradiculopathy
polyribosome
   disaggregation of membrane-
    bound p.'s

polysaccharide
   cryptococcal p.
   pneumococcal p.
   specific soluble p.
polysaccharolyticum
   Thermoanaerobacterium p.
polyserositis
   familial paroxysmal p.
   familial recurrent p.
   periodic p.
polysialic acid
polysinusitis
polysomaty
polysome
polysomic
polysomy
polysorbate
polyspermy
Polysphondylium
polysplenia syndrome
Polystictus
polystyrene
   oxygen-modified p.
polysynaptic
Polytech 2000 laboratory information system
polytendinitis
polytene chromosome
polyteny
polytetrafluoroethylene
polytopic effect
polytoxicomania
polytoxicomaniac syndrome
polytypic
polyU
   polyuridylic acid
polyunsaturated fatty acid (PUFA)
polyunsaturated-to-saturated fatty acids ratio (P:S)
polyurethane (PU)
polyuric
polyuridylic acid (polyU)
polyvalent
   p. allergy
   p. antiserum
   p. serum
   p. vaccine
polyvesicular
   p. vitelline
   p. vitelline tumor
polyvinyl
   p. alcohol (PVA)
   p. alcohol fixative method
   p. chloride
   p. chloride pneumoconiosis
polyvinylpyrrolidone
polyvisceral echinococcosis
polyzoic
Pomatiopsis

pombe
>Schizosaccharomyces p.

POMC
>proopiomelanocortin
>POMC neuron

POMC-derived anorexic peptide

pomeroyi
>Silicibacter p.
>Vibrio p.

pomorum
>Alicyclobacillus p.

Pomovirus

Pompe disease

ponceau de xylidine

Poncet disease

Ponfick shadow

ponos

Pontamine sky blue stain

Pontiac fever

pontiacus
>Sulfitobacter p.

pontine
>p. angle tumor
>cerebellar p.

pontis
>basis p.

pontomedullary

pool
>circulating granulocyte p. (CGP)
>gene p.
>marginal granulocyte p. (MGP)
>metabolic p.
>rapidly miscible p. (RMP)
>total blood granulocyte p. (TBGP)
>vaginal p.

pooled
>p. blood serum
>p. estimate

poorly
>p. compliant bladder
>p. differentiated carcinoma
>p. differentiated lymphocytic
>lymphoma (PDLL)

POP
>plasma oncotic pressure

popcorn
>p. cell
>p. nuclei

popliteal aneurysm

pop-off technique

popper
>amyl nitrite p.

population
>p. biology
>p. cytogenetics
>disomic p.
>p. dispersion
>p. genetics
>null cell p.
>parental cell p.
>p. sample (PS)
>tumor cell p.

por1 adenocarcinoma

por2 adenocarcinoma

porcelain gallbladder

porcina
>Hespellia p.

porcine
>p. adenovirus
>p. hemagglutinating
>encephalomyelitis virus
>p. transmissible gastroenteritis

porcinum
>Bifidobacterium thermacidophilum
>subsp. p.

porcinus
>Enterococcus p.

porcupine skin

pore
>alveolar p.
>gustatory p.
>interalveolar p.
>Kohn p.
>nuclear p.
>slit p.
>sweat p.
>taste p.

porencephalic

porencephalitis

porencephalous

porencephaly

Porges-Meier test

Porges-Salomon test

pori (*pl. of* porus)

Poria

Porifera

pork tapeworm

porocarcinoma

porocele

porocephaliasis

Porocephalidae

Porocephalus
>P. armillatus
>P. clavatus

NOTES

P

Porocephalus (continued)
  P. constrictus
  P. denticulatus
poroconidium
porokeratosis
  actinic p.
  disseminated superficial actinic p.
    (DSAP)
  Mibelli p.
poroma
  eccrine p.
Poronia
porosis, pl. **poroses**
  cerebral p.
porosity
porospore
porotic
porous
porphin
porphobilinogen (PBG)
  p. deaminase
  p. deaminase deficiency
  p. synthase
  p. synthase assay
  p. synthase deficiency
  p. test
  urine p.
porphyria
  acquired hepatic p.
  acute intermittent p. (AIP)
  chemical p.
  congenital erythropoietic p. (CEP)
  p. cutanea tarda (PCT)
  p. cutanea tarda hereditaria
  erythrohepatic p.
  erythropoietic p.
  familial-type symptomatic p.
  hepatic p.
  hepatoerythropoietic p. (HEP)
  hereditary coproporphyria (HCP)
  latent p.
  photosensitive p.
  protoporphyria
  South African-type p.
  symptomatic p.
  variegate p.
porphyrin
  alpha p.
  p. assay
  erythropoietic p.
  fecal p.
  fractionated erythrocyte p.
  p. pigmentation
  stool p.
  p. synthesis
  p. test
  urine p.
porphyrinuria

Porphyrobacter
  P. cryptus
  P. sanguineus
Porphyromonas
  P. asaccharolytica
  P. catoniae
porrigo
  p. favosa
  p. furfurans
  p. lupinosa
  p. scutulata
porta, pl. **portae**
  p. lienis
  p. pulmonis
  p. renis
portable magnifier lab lamp
portal
  p. canal
  p. cirrhosis
  p. fibrosis
  p. hypertension
  p. lobule of liver
  p. lymph node
  p. pyemia
  p. system
  p. tract
  p. tract lesion
  p. triad
  p. vein
  p. vein thrombosis (PVT)
  p. venous pressure
portal-systemic encephalopathy (PSE)
Porter-Silber (PS)
  P.-S. chromogen (PSC)
  P.-S. chromogen test
  P.-S. reaction
Porteus maze test
Porthetria
portion
  epithelium-lined ductal p.
  excretory p.
  secretory p.
Portland
  P. cell
  hemoglobin P.
Portmann classification
Portuguese man-o'-war
portulacae
  Dichotomophthora p.
port-wine
  p.-w. mark
  p.-w. stain
porus, pl. **pori**
  p. gustatorius
  p. sudoriferus
Posada disease
Posadasia
Posada-Wernicke disease
Posibacteria

positional
- p. alcohol nystagmus (PAN)
- p. asphyxia

position isomerism

positive
- p. anergy
- p. assortative mating
- beta-lactamase p.
- p. cell
- p. control enzyme induction
- p. control repression
- p. cytotaxis
- cytotoxicity negative, absorption p. (CYNAP)
- D^u p.
- p. end-expiratory pressure (PEEP)
- false p.
- p. and negative symptom scale (PANSS)
- p. neutrotaxis
- p. phase
- predictive value p. (PVP)
- p. predictive value (PPV)
- p. pressure
- Rh p.
- p. stain
- uniformly p. (UP)
- variably p. (VP)
- weakly p. (WP)
- p. whiff test

positive-placement pipette

positive-pressure test

positivity/negativity

positron
- p. annihilation
- p. beta decay

Pospiviroid

post
- postmortem
- status post (s/p)

postabsorptive
- p. hypoglycemia
- p. state

postatrophic hyperplasia

postauricular

postcapillary
- high endothelial p.
- p. venule

postchromation

postchroming

postcolectomy ileitis

postcurettage reparative change

postdiction

postdormital paralysis

postductal coarctation of aorta

posteencephalitic parkinsonism, tau pathology class I

posterior
- p. cell
- p. centriole
- p. corneal deposit (PCD)
- p. dislocation injury
- p. elastic layer
- p. incisural space
- p. iridolenticular synechiae
- lamina elastica p.
- p. limiting layer of cornea
- p. lobe of hypophysis
- p. nerve root
- p. pituitary
- p. pituitary hormone
- p. semicircular canal
- sinus intercavernosi anterior et p.
- p. spinal sclerosis
- p. subcapsular cataract (PSC)
- p. urethritis
- p. wall infarct (PWI)

posteriores
- cellulae ethmoidales p.

post-event vaccination

postexposure
- p. immunization
- p. isolation
- p. prophylaxis (PEP)

postgamma proteinuria (PGP)

postganglionic
- p. motor neuron
- p. sympathetic nerve

postgastrectomy dumping syndrome

postgonococcal urethritis

posthemorrhagic anemia

postheparin lipolytic activity (PHLA)

posthepatitic cirrhosis

posthitis

postholith

posthypocapnia

Postia

postinfectious
- p. allergic encephalitis
- p. encephalomyelitis
- p. glomerulonephritis
- p. myelitis

postinflammatory
- p. polyp

NOTES

P

795

postinflammatory *(continued)*
    p. pseudotumor
    p. pulmonary fibrosis
postmaturity
postmenopausal (PMP)
    p. atrophy
    p. bleeding
    p. syndrome
postmitochondrial supernatant (PMS)
postmitotic cell
postmordant
postmordanting
postmortem (PM, post)
    p. aerosol-producing procedure
    p. angiography
    p. autolysis
    p. bleeding
    p. clot
    p. dental x-ray
    p. examination
    p. hypostasis
    p. imaging
    p. interval (PMI)
    p. livedo
    p. lividity
    p. pustule
    p. rigidity
    p. specimen
    p. suggillation
    p. thrombus
    p. tubercle
    p. wart
postmyocardial
    p. infarction
    p. infarction pericarditis
postnecrotic cirrhosis
postobstructive diuresis
postoperative
    p. clipped aneurysm
    p. congestion
    p. infection
    p. parotitis
    p. repair
postpartum (PP)
    p. hemorrhage (PPH)
    p. pituitary necrosis
    p. thyroiditis
postpericardiotomy pericarditis
postprandial (PP)
    p. blood sugar (PPBS)
    p. glucose
    p. hypoglycemia
    p. lipemia
postprimary tuberculosis
postpubertal
    p. hyperpituitarism
    p. panhypopituitarism
postpump syndrome (PPS)

postpyknotic
postradiation dysplasia (PRDX)
postrema
    area p.
postremoval and postfixation shrinkage
postrenal
    p. albuminuria
    p. azotemia
postrubella syndrome
postsclerotic hyperplasia
poststenotic dilatation
poststorage leukoreduction
poststreptococcal glomerulonephritis (PSGN)
postsynaptic membrane
postthymic
postthymic malignancy
posttransfusion
    p. hepatitis (PTH)
    p. mononucleosis (PTM)
    p. purpura (PTP)
posttransplant
    p. biopsy pathology
    p. lymphoproliferative disease (PTLD)
    p. lymphoproliferative disorder (PTLD)
posttraumatic
    p. epilepsy
    p. leptomeningeal cyst
    p. osteoporosis
    p. pericarditis
postulate
    Ehrlich p.
    Koch p.
postulated pathogenetic factor
postural
    p. albuminuria
    p. proteinuria
posture
    minimum mission-oriented protective p. (MOPP)
postvaccinal
    p. encephalitis
    p. myelitis
postvaccination
    p. allergic encephalitis
    p. encephalomyelitis (PVEM)
postvaccinial lymphadenitis
postvagotomy syndrome
potable
Potamidae
Potamon
potassium (K)
    p. acetate
    p. acidosis
    p. acid tartrate
    p. alkalosis
    p. alum

p. *p*-aminobenzoate
p. *p*-aminosalicylate
p. aspartate and magnesium
  aspartate
p. assay
p. bicarbonate
p. bichromate
p. bisperoxo oxovanadate V
p. bitartrate
p. bromide
p. carbonate
p. chlorate
p. chloride (KCl)
p. citrate
p. cyanide (KCN)
p. dichromate
p. dihydrogen phosphate
p. EDTA (K3 EDTA)
fecal p.
p. ferricyanide
p. glucaldrate
p. gluconate
p., glucose, and insulin (PGI)
glucose, insulin, and p. (GIK)
p. glycerophosphate
p. guaiacolsulfonate
p. hydroxide (KOH)
p. hydroxide test
p. imbalance
p. iodate
p. mercuric iodide
p. metabisulfate stain
p. metaphosphate
p. nitrate
p. oxalate
p. penicillin G
p. perchlorate
p. permanganate
p. permanganate stain
p. phenoxymethyl penicillin
p. simplex optimized medium
  (KSOM)
p. sodium tartrate
p. sorbate
stool p.
p. sulfate
p. thiocyanate
total body p. (TBK)
urine p.
potassium-42
potassium-sparing diuretic

potato
p. dextrose agar
p. tumor of neck
potato-blood agar
Potebniamyces
potential
amyloidogenic p.
atypical polypoid adenomyofibroma
  of low malignant p. (APA-LMP)
cervical somatosensory evoked p.
decomposition p.
diffusion p.
Donnan p.
electric p.
electrode p.
p. energy
fast action p.
giant cell tumor of low
  malignant p. (GCT-LMP)
half-wave p.
junction p.
liquid-liquid junction p.
low malignant p. (LMP)
membrane p.
muscle action p.
oxidation-reducing p.
phosphate group transfer p.
redox p.
reduction p.
resting membrane p.
smooth muscle tumor of uncertain
  malignant p. (SMTUMP)
standard electrode p.
standard reduction p.
undetermined malignant p. (UMP)
visual evoked p.
zeta p.
zoonotic p.
potentiation
long-term p. (LTP)
potentiometer
direct-reading p.
null-point p.
slide-wire p.
potentiometric titration
potentiometry
potent protein neurotoxin
Potexvirus
potomania
beer drinker's p.
Pott
P. abscess

NOTES

P

Pott (*continued*)
    P. aneurysm
    P. disease
    P. paralysis
Potter
    P. disease
    P. facies
    P. syndrome
Potter-Bucky grid
Potter-Elvehjem handheld tissue grinder
potter's asthma
Potyvirus
pouch
    p. culture
    p. of Douglas
    endodermal pharyngeal p.
    Hartmann p.
    Physick p.
    Rathke p.
    p. syndrome
pouchitis
    diversion p.
    preclosure p.
    short-strip p.
Poulet disease
poultry handler's disease
pounds per square inch (psi)
pour plate
povidone
povidone-iodine
Powassan
    P. encephalitis
    P. virus
powder
    black p.
power
    p. amplifier
    apparent p.
    carbon dioxide combining p.
    p. resistor
    resolving p.
    p. supply
PowerPlex 1.2 genetic identification kit
pox
    Kaffir p.
    sheep p.
Poxviridae
poxvirus officinalis
PP
    pancreatic polypeptide
    pellagra preventive
    pink puffer
    postpartum
    postprandial
    prothrombin-proconvertin
    protoporphyrin
    pseudomyxoma peritonei

P&P
    prothrombin and proconvertin
        P&P test
PPA
    primary pulmonary adenoma
PPAR
    peroxisome proliferator-activated receptor
        PPAR gamma protein
PPB
    platelet-poor blood
PPBS
    postprandial blood sugar
PPCA
    proserum prothrombin conversion
    accelerator
PP-CAP
    PP-CAP H. pylori IgA assay
    PP-CAP IgA enzyme immunoassay
        test
PPCF
    plasmin prothrombin conversion factor
PPD
    purified protein derivative
        PPD skin test
PPD-S
    purified protein derivative-standard
PPE
    personal protective equipment
PPF
    plasma protein fraction
ppg
    picopicogram
PPH
    postpartum hemorrhage
    primary pulmonary hypertension
PPHP
    pseudopseudohypoparathyroidism
PPHT
    primary plexogenic hypertension
PPLO
    pleuropneumonia-like organism
ppm
    parts per million
PPNAD
    primary pigmented nodular adrenocortical
    disease
pPNET
    primitive peripheral neuroectodermal
    tumor
^{32}P-postlabeling assay
PPP
    pentose phosphate pathway
    platelet-poor plasma
PPR
    Price precipitation reaction
PPRE
    putative peroxisome proliferator response
    element

PPS
postpump syndrome
PPT
plant protease test
ppt
precipitate
PPV
positive predictive value
PPW
patient protective wrap
PQ
permeability quotient
PR
partial remission
progesterone receptor
protein
Pr
prism
PRA
panel-reactive antibody
plasma renin activity
progesterone receptor assay
practice parameter
PRAD1 gene
Prader bead standard
Prader-Willi syndrome
P-radiolabeled DNA probe fragment
praeacuta
Tissierella p.
praeacutus
Bacteroides p.
praecox
dementia p.
icterus p.
lymphedema p.
macrogenitosomia p.
Prague pelvis
prairie itch
pralidoxime chloride
praseodymium
Prasinovirus
PRA-Stat enzyme linked immunosorbent assay
pratensis
Agreia p.
Subtercola p.
Prauserella
P. alba
P. halophila
P. rugosa

prausnitzii
Faecalibacterium p.
Prausnitz-Küstner (PK)
P. antibody
P. reaction
P. test
prazosin hydrochloride
PRBV
placental residual blood volume
PRCA
pure red cell aplasia
PRCC
papillary renal cell carcinoma
PRD
partial reaction of degeneration
PRDX
postradiation dysplasia
preadaptation
preadenomatous
preadipocyte factor (Pref-1)
prealbumin
p. test
thyroxine-binding p. (TBPA)
preamplifier
preanalytic error
pre-B cell
prebetalipoprotein
precancer
precancerosa
melanosis circumscripta p.
precancerous
p. dysplasia
p. lesion
p. melanosis of Dubreuilh
precatorius
Abrus p.
precaution
barrier isolation p.
precautions
droplet p.
universal p.
prechroming
preChx
preoperative chemotherapy
precipitant
precipitate (ppt)
alum p.
keratitic p. (KP)
precipitated
precipitating antibody
precipitation
double antibody p.

NOTES

799

precipitation (*continued*)
    hapten inhibition of p.
    immune p.
    p. test
    tuberculin p. (TP)
precipitin
    p. curve
    p. reaction
    p. test
    tube p. (TP)
precipitinogen, precipitogen
precipitinogenoid
precipitoid
precipitophore
precision
    P. QI-D handheld blood glucose test
    p. resistor
Precision-G handheld blood glucose test
preclosure pouchitis
precocious
    p. adrenarche
    p. pseudopuberty
    p. puberty
precocity
precollagenous fiber
preconfluent cell
precore mutant
precornified cell
precursor
    abnormally localized immature p. (ALIP)
    alkaline phosphatase, tissue-nonspecific isozyme protein p. (AP-TNAP)
    p. cell
    erythroid p.
    p. lesion
    megakaryocytic p.
precursory cartilage
predaceous mite
predecidual alteration
predeposit autologous transfusion
prediabetes
prediction
    antibody specificity p. (ASP)
predictive
    p. value
    p. value of negative test
    p. value positive (PVP)
    p. value of positive test
predictor of patient survival
PredictRx metabolites
predilection
    host of p.
predispose
predisposing
    p. cause
    p. factor

predisposition
    rhabdoid p.
prednisone
predominant
    p. cell
    lymphocyte p. (LP)
preductal coarctation of aorta
preeclampsia
preeclamptic toxemia (PET)
preeruptive
pre-event vaccination
preexisting actinic keratosis
preexposure immunization
Pref-1
    preadipocyte factor
preferential lysis
preformativa
    membrana p.
preganglionic motor neuron
Pre-Gen 26 colorectal cancer test
pregnancy
    aborted ectopic p.
    acute fatty liver of p.
    p. cell
    cornual p.
    corpus luteum of p.
    p. cycle
    ectopic p. (EP)
    exochorial p.
    extrauterine p.
    hydatid p.
    p. luteoma
    macrocytic anemia of p.
    mask of pregnancy
    megaloblastic anemia of p. (MAP)
    membranous p.
    molar p.
    normal term p.
    ovarian p.
    ovarioabdominal p.
    parasitic ectopic p.
    ruptured ectopic p.
    p. test
    toxemia of p.
    tubal p.
    p. urine (PU)
    voluntary interruption of p. (VIP)
pregnancy-associated plasma protein A (PAPP-A)
pregnancy-associated plasma protein B (PAPP-B)
pregnanediol
    p. assay
    urine p.
pregnanetriol
    urine p.
pregnant
    p. mare serum (PMS)

p. mare serum gonadotropin (PMSG)
pregnenolone
pregranulosa cell
prehepatic hypoproteinemia
prehormone
prehyoid gland
preictal
preimplantation genetic diagnosis (PGD)
preinvasive urothelial neoplasia
Preiser disease
Preisz-Nocard bacillus
prekallikrein
P-related blood group
preleukemia
prelymphoma
prelytic sphere
premalignant epidermal lesion
premammary abscess
premature
p. abnormal placenta
p. infant
p. rupture
p. rupture of (fetal) membranes (PROM)
p. senility syndrome
p. separation of placenta
prematurely
p. closed foramen ovale
p. separated placenta
prematurity
fetal p.
retinopathy of p. (ROP)
premeal glucose
premelanosome
premonocyte
premorbid
premunition
premunitive
premutation allele
premyeloblast
premyelocyte
prenatal
p. diagnosis
p. screening
prenecrotizing phagocytic lesion
preneoplastic
prenyl group
preoperative
preosteoblast
preovulatory

prep
preparation
prepare
wet prep
preparation (prep)
allergenic protein p.
biomechanical p.
broken cell p.
cell block p.
cervicovaginal smear p.
commercial insulin p.
corrosion p.
cytologic filter p.
heart-lung p.
impression p.
Institute of Virus P.'s
intraoperative touch p.
peripheral blood p.
pinworm p.
ThinPrep cytologic p.
touch p.
Trichomonas p.
wet p.
preparative
p. immunofiltration
p. ultracentrifugation
prepare (prep)
preparedness
Office of Emergency P.
prepatent period
PrepPlus[7] series workstation
preproprotein
prepubertal
p. hyperpituitarism
p. panhypopituitarism
preputial
p. calculus
p. gland
preputiale
sebum p.
preputiales
glandulae p.
preputii
smegma p.
prepyloric atresia
prerenal
p. albuminuria
p. azotemia
preRx
preoperative radiotherapy
presacral insufflation
presbycardia

NOTES

P

presbyopia
presegmented nucleus
presenile
    p. dementia with tangles and calcifications
    p. spontaneous gangrene
presentation
    antigen p.
    compound p.
preservative
PreservCyt fixative
prespermatogonia
pressor
    p. amine
    p. base
    p. substance
pressure (P)
    altered intravascular hydrostatic p.
    altered intravascular osmotic p.
    arterial p.
    p. atrophy
    barometric p. (Pb)
    blood p. (BP)
    p. catapulting
    central venous p.
    cerebrospinal fluid p.
    colloidal osmotic p. (COP)
    colloid oncotic p. (COP)
    continuous distending p. (CDP)
    p. differential
    end-systolic p. (ESP)
    hydrostatic p.
    maximum inspiratory p. (MIP)
    oncotic p.
    osmotic p. (OP)
    oxygen under high p. (OHP)
    partial p.
    perfusion p.
    plasma colloid oncotic p.
    plasma oncotic p. (POP)
    portal venous p.
    positive p.
    positive end-expiratory p. (PEEP)
    pulmonary p.
    pulse p.
    screen filtration p. (SFP)
    selection p.
    standard temperature and p.
    standard temperature and p., dry (STPD)
    systemic arterial p. (SAP)
    p. urticaria
    vapor p.
    venous p.
pressure-demand SCBA
pressure-volume curve
prestomal ileitis
prestorage leukoreduction

presumptive
    p. diagnosis
    p. heterophil test
    p. testing
presuppurative
presynaptic
    p. membrane
    p. vesicle
presyncope
prethymic lymphoblastic lymphoma
pretibial myxedema
pretoriensis
    Amycolatopsis p.
pretreatment
    nerve agent pyridostigmine p. (NAPP)
Preussia
prevalence rate
prevention
preventive
    p. medicine
    pellagra p. (PP)
    p. treatment
previa
    placenta p.
    vasa p.
previous value check
previtellogenesis
previtellogenic phase
Prevotella
    P. bivia
    P. denticola
    P. disiens
    P. enoeca
    P. heparinolytica
    P. intermedia
    P. melaninogenica
    P. oralis
    P. oris
    P. pallens
    P. salivae
    P. shahii
    P. tannerae
prevotii
    Anaerococcus p.
    Peptococcus p.
    Peptostreptococcus p.
PreVue *Borrelia burgdorferi* antibody detection assay
prezone
PRF
    peptide regulatory factor
    prolactin-releasing factor
PRFM
    prolonged rupture of fetal membranes
PRH
    prolactin-releasing hormone
priapism
priapitis

Price-Jones curve
Price precipitation reaction (PPR)
prickle
    p. cell
    p. cell layer
    intercellular p.
prick test
primaquine
    p. phosphate
    p. sensitivity
primaquine-sensitive anemia
primarium
    punctum ossificationis p.
primarius
    folliculus ovaricus p.
primary
    p. acquired melanosis
    p. active transport
    p. adrenal insufficiency
    p. African green monkey kidney (PAGMK)
    p. agammaglobulinemia
    p. amebic meningoencephalitis
    p. amenorrhea
    p. amyloidosis (AL)
    p. atelectasis
    p. atypical pneumonia (PAP)
    p. biliary cirrhosis (PBC)
    p. blast injury
    p. bone lymphoma (PBL)
    p. bone tumor
    p. bubo
    p. cardiomyopathy
    p. cementum
    p. center of ossification
    p. coccidioidomycosis
    p. coil
    p. cold agglutinin disease
    p. color
    p. complex
    p. constriction
    p. contamination
    p. cutaneous anaplastic large cell lymphoma
    p. cutaneous CD30+ large T-cell lymphoma
    p. effusion lymphoma (PEL)
    p. embryonic cell
    p. endocardial sclerosis
    p. erythroblastic anemia
    p. explant culture
    p. fibrinogenolysis syndrome

    p. fibrinolysis
    p. fibromyalgia syndrome
    p. gastric lymphoma
    p. glaucoma
    p. granule
    p. herpetic stomatitis
    p. hyperaldosteronism
    p. hyperoxaluria, type 1 (PH1)
    p. hyperparathyroidism
    p. hyperplasia
    p. hypoadrenocorticism
    p. hypodipsia
    p. hypogammaglobulinemia
    p. immune response
    p. influenza virus pneumonia
    p. irritant
    p. Ki-1 lymphoma of brain
    p. lesion
    p. lymphedema
    p. lymphoid follicle
    p. lysosome
    p. mammary mucinous cystadenocarcinoma
    p. mediastinal large cell lymphoma with sclerosis (PMLS)
    p. methemoglobinemia
    p. myelofibrosis
    p. myeloid metaplasia
    p. myocardial disease (PMD)
    p. nodule
    p. odditis
    p. ossification center
    p. ovarian follicle
    p. ovarian gestational trophoblastic disease (POGTD)
    p. pentosuria
    p. pigmented nodular adrenocortical disease (PPNAD)
    p. point of ossification
    p. pulmonary adenoma (PPA)
    p. pulmonary hypertension (PPH)
    p. pulmonary lobule
    p. pyoderma
    p. reaction
    p. reference material
    p. refractory anemia
    p. rejection
    p. renal calculus
    p. renal tubular acidosis
    p. repair
    p. salivary CCC
    p. sclerosing cholangitis (PSC)

NOTES

primary *(continued)*
    p. septicemic plague
    p. sequestrum
    p. sex character
    p. spermatocyte
    p. standard
    p. structure
    p. thrombocythemia
    p. transcript
    p. trisomy
    p. trisomy 18
    p. tuberculosis
    (p.) tumor, (regional lymph) nodes, (remote) metastases (TNM)
    p. union
primatum
    Mycoplasma p.
primed lymphocyte typing
primer
    oligonucleotide p.
    semi-nester p.
primerite
primidone assay
priming
    T-cell p.
primite
primitia
    Treponema p.
primitive
    p. erythroblast
    p. mesoblast
    p. neuroblastic cell
    p. neuroectodermal tumor (PNET)
    p. peripheral neuroectodermal tumor (pPNET)
    p. reticular cell
    p. small-cell thoracopulmonary tumor
primitive-looking cell
primordial
    p. cyst
    p. dwarf
    p. germ cell
    p. ovarian follicle
    p. sex cell
primordium, pl. primordia
primulin
primum non nocere
principal
    p. cell
    p. focus
    p. piece
    p. piece of spermatozoon
    p. target organ
principle
    antianemic p.
    Bernoulli p.
    Fick p.
    follicle-stimulating p.

    hematinic p.
    immediate p.
    luteinizing p.
    prothrombin-converting p.
    proximate p.
    ultimate p.
    uncertainty p.
Pringle disease
print culture
printed circuit
Prinzmetal angina
prion
    p. disease
    p. protein (PrPSc)
    p. protein cerebral amyloid angiopathy
Prions
    Fungal P.
    Mammalian P.
prion-transmitted disease
Prionurus
prism (Pr)
    adamantine p.
    enamel p.
    Nicol p.
prisma, pl. prismata
    prismata adamantina
prismatic
    p. follicular cell
PRIST
    paper radioimmunosorbent test
pristanic acid
private antigen
privileged site
PRL
    prolactin
PRM
    phosphoribomutase
    photoreceptor membrane
proaccelerin
proacrosomal granule
proactivator
    C3 p.
proatherogenic capacity
probability (P)
    conditional p.
    p. distribution
    p. paper
    significance p.
probable error
probacteriophage
    defective p.
proband
probe
    alpha p.
    amplified p.
    antisense p.
    ASO p.
    biotin-labeled p.

biotinylated DNA p.
CD44v6-specific p.
centromere enumeration p. (CEP)
chemiluminescent p.
cycling p.
cytochemical p.
direct p.
DNA p.
dual color p.
fluorescent p.
genomic p.
hybridized p.
immunogold p.
nucleic acid p.
oligonucleotide p.
pancake p.
p. patent foramen ovale
PNA p.
radioactive p.
reverse line p.
sequence specific oligonucleotide p.
  (SSOP)
Vidas p.
viral p.
Vysis p.
YAC p.
Pro-Bind U-Bottom microfilter plate
probiosis
probiotic
probit transformation
proBNP
  prohormone B-type natriuretic peptide
Probstymayria vivipara
procainamide assay
procaine hydrochloride
procalcitonin
Procandida
procapsid
Procarbazine
Procaryotae
procaryote (*var. of* prokaryote)
procaryotic (*var. of* prokaryotic)
procedure
  Bradford microassay p.
  Cherry-Crandall p.
  Clontech gene expression
    profiling p.
  concentration p.
  Cryptosporidium diagnostic p.
  falling drop p.
  flow cytometric platelet counting p.
  Gomori-Takamatsu p.

helminth identification p.
hydroxyapatite exchange p.
hypophysis staining p.
Jatlow-Nadim p.
Kjeldahl p.
loop electrosurgical excisional p.
Mantel-Cox p.
Merfiluor DFA
  Cryptosporidium/Giardia
  detection p.
multirule Shewhart p.
Norymberski p.
periodate-Schiff p.
platelet neutralization p.
postmortem aerosol-producing p.
protein A-Sepharose column p.
salting-out p.
Sheather sugar flotation p.
standard operating p. (SOP)
Tiselius p.
TTI p.
Vindelov p.
Westgard multirule p.
procentriole organizer
procercoid
Procerovum varium
process
  apical p.
  apoptotic p.
  astrocytic foot p.
  axonal p.
  p. control
  cytoplasmic p.
  dendritic cytoplasmic p.
  epithelial foot p.
  evidence gathering p.
  filiform p.
  foot p.
  fractured transverse p.
  granulomatous p.
  immune-mediated p.
  iterative p.
  Lenhossek p.
  lookback p.
  Löwenstein p.
  odontoblast p.
  podocyte foot p.
  psoralen-mediated p.
  styloid p.
  ThinPrep slide p.
  Tomes p.
  vasculoocclusive p.

NOTES

P

processing
  antigen p.
  automatic tissue p.
  interactive p.
  RNA p.
  tissue p.
processor
  Sakura Finetek Tissue-Tek VIP
    300E automatic tissue p.
  ThinPrep p.
processus ferreini
Prochloraceae
Prochlorales
Prochlorococcus
  P. marinus subsp. *marinus*
  P. marinus subsp. *pastoris*
Prochlorotrichaceae
procidentia
Procleix HIV-1/HCV Assay
procoagulant platelet-derived
  microparticle
procollagen alpha1(I) gene
proconvertase
proconvertin
  prothrombin and p. (P&P)
proctatresia
proctectasia
proctencleisis, proctenclisis
proctitis
  allergic p.
  chronic ulcerative p.
  idiopathic p.
proctocele
proctocolitis
  diversion p.
proctodeal
proctodeum
proctopolypus
proctoptosis
proctosigmoiditis
proctostenosis
procyonis
  Baylisascaris p.
prodigiosin
prodromal stage
prodrome
product
  advanced glycation end p. (AGE)
  anthrax-contaminated animal p.
  B-domain-deleted rFVIII p.
  cleavage p.
  concentration-time p. (Ct)
  contact activation p.
  cross p.
  decay p.
  dot p.
  end p.
  ERGIC-53 gene p.
  fibrin breakdown p.

  fibrin degradation p. (FDP)
  fibrin/fibrinogen degradation p.
    (FDP)
  fibrinogen breakdown p. (FBP)
  fibrinogen degradation p. (FDP)
  fibrinogen split p. (FSP)
  fibrinolytic split p. (FSP)
  fibrin-split p.
  fission p.
  gene p.
  Pro-PredictRx diagnostic p.
  protein gene p. (PGP)
  scalar p.
  solubility p.
  spallation p.
  substitution p.
  vector p.
  waste p.
production
  p. of aqueous humor
  carbon dioxide p.
  CO_2 p.
  ectopic hormone p.
  excessive heat p. (EHP)
  pair p.
  purulent sputum p.
production-defect anemia
productive
  p. inflammation
  p. peritonitis
  p. pleurisy
productus
  Peptostreptococcus p.
proenzyme
proerythroblast
proerythrocyte
Professional Standards Review
  Organization (PSRO)
Profeta law
profibrinolysin
Profichet
  P. disease
  P. syndrome
proficiency
  p. sample
  p. survey
  p. testing
profile
  Astra blood chemistry p.
  biochemical p.
  biophysical p.
  cell volume p. (CVP)
  chemistry p. (chem)
  fatty acid p.
  fetal biophysical p.
  p. of gene expression
  kidney p.
  liver p.

phagocytic cell
immunocompetence p.
plasma protein p.
polyphenotypic p.
test p.

Profile-ER
P.-E. drugs of abuse screening
panel
P.-E. one-step qualitative drug test

Profile-II ER drug screening device
profiling
gene expression p.
transcriptional p.

profluens
hydrops tubae p.

profound hypoglycemia
profunda
colitis cystica p.
gastritis cystica p.
jejunitis cystica p.
miliaria p.
Moritella p.
Psychromonas p.

profundi
nodi lymphoidei inguinales p.

profundus
Caminibacter p.
lupus erythematosus p.
morphea p.
Oceanithermus p.

profusa
Olsenella p.

Progen antibiotic solution
progenitalis
herpes p.

progenitor
p. cell
p. marker

PRO-GenoLogix NOD2/CARD15
progeny
progeria
p. with cataract
p. with microphthalmia

progeroid
progestagenic change
progestational
p. agent
p. hormone

progesteroid
progesterone
plasma p.
p. receptor (PgR, PR)

p. receptor assay (PRA)
p. unit

progestin
progestogen
proglottid
proglottis
prognathism
prognosis
loss of expression and p.

prognostic
p. criteria
p. factor
p. role

prognosticator
progonoma
p. of jaw
melanotic p.

program
Bioterrorism Preparedness and
Response P.
CAP sweat analysis proficiency
testing p.
p. evaluation and review technique
(PERT)
infection surveillance and
control p. (ISCP)
National Biomonitoring P. (NBP)
National Immunization P. (NIP)
object p.
Q-Probes p.
Q-Tracks p.
safety p.
Shelf-Life Extension P. (SLEP)
survey p.

programmed
p. cell death
p. cell death 4 gene (PDCD4)

programming
temperature p.

progranulocyte
progranulocytic leukemia
progravid
progressiva
fibrodysplasia ossificans p.
myositis ossificans p.

progressive
p. bacterial synergistic gangrene
p. bulbar palsy
p. cerebellar dyssynergia
p. cerebral poliodystrophy
p. cleavage
p. contraction of wound

NOTES

P

807

progressive *(continued)*
    dyssynergia cerebellaris p.
    p. dystonic palsy
    p. emphysematous necrosis
    p. hypocythemia
    p. impairment of renal function
    p. lipodystrophy
    p. massive fibrosis (PMF)
    p. multifocal leukoencephalopathy (PML)
    p. muscular dystrophy (PMD)
    p. pigmentary dermatosis
    p. pneumonia virus
    p. spinal muscular atrophy
    p. staining
    p. subcortical encephalopathy
    p. supranuclear palsy (PSP)
    p. supranuclear palsy, tau pathology class II
    p. systemic sclerosis (PSS)
    p. transformation of germinal center (PTGC)
    p. vaccinia
prohormone B-type natriuretic peptide (proBNP)
proinflammatory
    p. cytokine
    p. signal
proinsulin
project
    Chempack P.
    Early Surveillance P. (ESP)
projectile
    exiting p.
    fragmenting p.
    p. impact
    yawing p.
projection
    cytoplasmic p.
    Fischer p.
    hair-like filamentous p.
    intraductal papillary p.
    polypoid intraluminal p.
    transmandibular p.
    p. x-ray microscope
Prokaryotae
prokaryote, procaryote
prokaryotic, procaryotic
prolactin (PRL)
    p. cell
    chorionic growth hormone p. (CGP)
    human p. (hPrL)
    p. receptor
    p. release-inhibiting hormone
    p. test
    p. unit
prolactin-inhibiting factor (PIF)
prolactinoma

prolactin-producing adenoma
prolactin-releasing
    p.-r. factor (PRF)
    p.-r. hormone (PRH)
prolapse
    mitral valve p. (MVP)
    Morgagni p.
prolapsed umbilical cord
proleukocyte
proliferans
    endarteritis p.
    retinitis p.
    Trichophyton p.
proliferate
proliferating
    p. cell nuclear antigen (PCHA, PCNA)
    p. endarteritis
    p. focus
    p. pillar tumor
    p. pleurisy
    p. systematized angioendotheliomatosis
    p. thymolipoma
    p. trichilemmal cyst
proliferation
    bizarre parosteal osteochondromatous p. (BPOP)
    cell p.
    p. center
    cholangiolar p.
    p. cyst
    diffuse mesangial p.
    p. of fibroblast
    glandular p.
    inflammatory myofibrohistiocytic p.
    p. inhibitory factor (PIF)
    lobular p.
    p. marker
    myofibroblastic p.
    myointimal p.
    neoplastic p.
    nodular and diffuse fibrous p. (NDFP)
    polyclonal lymphoid p.
    pseudosarcomatous myofibroblastic p.
    reactive ductal p.
    T-cell p.
    tumor-assisted lymphoid p. (TALP)
proliferation-dependent phenomenon
proliferative
    p. activity
    acute p.
    p. breast disease (PBD)
    p. bronchiolitis
    p. chronic arthritis
    p. cyst
    p. disorder

p. endometrium
p. fasciitis
p. glomerulonephritis
p. glomerulopathy
p. index (PI)
p. inflammation
p. intimitis
p. mixoploid
p. myositis
p. phase
p. stage
p. synovitis
p. verrucous leukoplakia (PVL)
proliferous cyst
proliferum
    Sparganum p.
prolificans
    Scedosporium p.
proligerous
p. disc
p. membrane
proligerus
discus p.
proline
p. dehydrogenase
p. hydroxylase
p. oxidase
urine p.
proline-2-oxoglutarate dioxygenase
prolinemia
prolinuria
prolixus
    Rhodnius p.
prolongation
APTT p.
prolonged
p. alcohol intake
p. bleeding time
p. coagulation time
p. estrogen stimulation
p. rupture of fetal membranes (PRFM)
prolyl 4-hydroxylase
prolymphocyte cell
prolymphocytic leukemia (PLL)
PROM
premature rupture of (fetal) membranes
promastigote
promegakaryoblast
promegakaryocyte
promegaloblast
Promega Taq DNA polymerase

prometaphase banding
promethium
Promicromonospora
    P. aerolata
    P. pachnodae
    P. vindobonensis
Promicromonosporaceae
prominent
p. nuclear hof
p. nucleus
p. perinuclear
p. splenomegaly
promiscuous antigen receptor gene rearrangement
promoblast
promonocyte
promoter
cancer p.
eosinophil stimulation p. (ESP)
p. insertion
tumor p.
promoting agent
promotion
promotor region
prompt zinc insulin
promyelocyte
basophilic p.
eosinophilic p.
neutrophilic p.
promyelocytic
p. leukemia
p. leukemia zinc finger (PLZF)
Pronase antigen
pronephros
glomerulus of p.
pronormoblast
pronucleus
proof
constructive p.
existence p.
proopiomelanocortin (POMC)
proopiomelanocortin-related peptide
propagating
p. nuclear reaction
p. thrombosis
propagation
propagule
propane nitrile
propanoic acid
1-propanol
2-propanol
proparathyroid hormone

NOTES

P

propenal
propepsin
proper
    esophageal gland p.
    p. substance
properdin
    p. assay
    p. deposit
    p. factor A, B, D, E
    p. system
property
    aerobiological p.
prophage
    defective p.
prophase
prophlogistic
prophobilinogen
prophylactic
    p. membrane
    p. serum
    p. treatment
prophylaxis, pl. prophylaxes
    active p.
    chemical p.
    passive p.
    postexposure p. (PEP)
propidium
    p. iodide
    p. iodide solution
    p. iodine stain
propionate
    p. carboxylase
    p. metabolism
    sodium p.
Propionibacteriaceae
propionibacterial DNA in sarcoidosis
Propionibacterineae
Propionibacterium
    P. acnes
    P. australiense
    P. avidum
    P. freudenreichii
    P. granulosum
    P. jensenii
    P. lymphophilum
    P. microaerophilum
    P. propionicus
Propionibacter pelophilus
propionic
    p. acid
    p. acidemia
    p. aciduria
propionica
    Arachnia p.
    Smithella p.
Propionicimonas paludicola
propionicus
    Propionibacterium p.
Propionimicrobium lymphophilum

Propionispira arboris
Propionispora
    P. hippei
    P. vibrioides
propionitrile
Propionivibrio
    P. limicola
    P. pelophilus
propionyl-CoA carboxylase
proplasia
proplasmacyte
proportional
    p. count
    p. counter
proportionate
    p. morbidity ratio (PMR)
    p. mortality ratio (PMR)
propositus, pl. propositi
propoxur
propoxyphene assay
propranolol assay
Pro-PredictRx
    P.-P. diagnostic product
    P.-P. diagnostic test
    P.-P. Enzact
    P.-P. metabolite
    P.-P. TPMT
propria
    gastric lamina p.
    lamina p.
    tunica p.
proprioceptor
proprius
    sacculus p.
proprotein
proptosis
propyl alcohol
propylene glycol
prorubricyte
    pernicious anemia-type p.
proscolex
proscription
Pro-Scrub
    Zila P.-S.
prosecretion granule
prosection
prosector's
    p. tubercle
    p. wart
proserum prothrombin conversion accelerator (PPCA)
prosodemic
p-rosolic acid
prosopalgia
prosopectasia
prosoplasia
ProSpec
    BN P.

ProSpecT *Clostridium difficile* **toxin A microplate assay**
prospective study
prostacyclin
prostaglandin (PG)
    p. 1 (PG1)
    p. 2 (PG2)
    p. 3 (PG3)
    p. A, B
    p. D_2
    p. E_1, E_2
    p. endoperoxide
    p. F_1 alpha
    p. F_2 alpha
    p. G_2
    p. H_2
    p. I_2
    J-series p.
    p. test
prostaglandin-like substance (PLS)
prostanoic acid
prostanoid
prostata
prostatae
    substantia glandularis p.
    substantia muscularis p.
prostate
    amyloid body of p.
    bladder neck margin of the p.
    p. cancer
    p. gland
    p. gland biopsy
    glandular substance of p.
    p. hyperplasia
    muscular substance of p.
    p. needle core biopsy
    nodular hyperplasia of p.
    peripheral zone of p.
    p. seed
    p. stem cell antigen (PSCA)
    transurethral resection of p. (TURP)
prostate-specific
    p.-s. antigen (PSA)
    p.-s. membrane antigen (PSMA)
prostatic
    p. adenoma
    p. calculus
    p. duct
    p. ductule
    p. fluid
    p. hypertrophy (PH)

    p. intraepithelial neoplasia (PIN)
    p. intraepithelial neoplasm (PIN)
    p. tumor
prostatica
    glandula p.
prostatici
    ductuli p.
    ductus p.
prostatitic
prostatitis
    allergic granulomatous p.
    bacterial p.
    mycotic p.
    nonspecific granulomatous p.
    peripheral zone inflammation in chronic p.
    tuberculous p.
    xanthogranulomatous p.
prostatocystitis
prostatolith
prostatomegaly
prostatovesiculitis
Prosthenorchis elegans
prosthesis, pl. **prostheses**
    Bjork-Shiley mitral p.
    p. rupture
prosthetic group
Prosthodendrium molenkampi
Prosthogonimus macrorchis
prosurvival protein
prot
    protein
protactinium (Pa)
Protac venom
protamine
    p. sulfate
    p. sulfate assay
    p. sulfate test
    p. titration test
    p. zinc insulin
protanomaly
protanopia
Protargol stain
proteamaculans
    Serratia p.
protean
protease
    binding protein p. (BPP)
    calcium-activated neutral p.
    calpain family of p.
    CD p.
    p. inhibitor (PI)

NOTES

P

protease *(continued)*
    lysosomal p.
    MBL-associated serine p. (MASP)
    p. nexin-II
    regeneration-associated muscle p. (RAMP)
    slow-moving p. (SMP)
    tricorn p.
protease-activated receptor (PAR)
protect
    DNA/RNA P.
protected catheter brush
protectin
protection
    critical infrastructure p. (CIP)
    radiation p.
    p. test
protective
    p. antigen (PA)
    p. osmatic barrier
    p. protein
protector
    LATS p.
Proteeae
protein (PR, prot)
    p. A
    A68 p.
    p. absorption
    accumulation of p.
    activator p. 1 (AP1)
    acute phase p.
    acyl carrier p.
    ADAM p.
    ADAMTS 13 p.
    p. A gold (PAG)
    p. A gold complex technique
    AL p.
    ALK p.
    alpha fodrin p.
    amyloid beta p.
    amyloid precursor p. (APP)
    androgen-binding p. (ABP)
    antiapoptotic p.
    anti-S-100 p.
    antiviral p.
    p. A-Sepharose column procedure
    band 3 p.
    Bax p.
    bcl-2 p.
    bcl-X_L p.
    BCR-ABL hybrid p.
    Bence Jones p.
    p. binding (PB)
    BJ p.
    BPI p.
    p. breakdown
    p. buffer
    p. C
    calbindin p.

    calcium-sensing receptor p. (CASR)
    Caldesmon cell p.
    cAMP response element binding p. (CREB)
    carbonic anhydrase-related p. (CA-RP)
    carrier p.
    caspase p.
    p. catabolism
    catabolite activator p.
    CD p.
    cell-cycle inhibitory p.
    cell-surface p.
    cell-to-cell adherent p.
    cerebrospinal fluid myelin basic p.
    cerebrospinal fluid total p.
    channel-forming integral p. (CHIP-1)
    p. characterization system
    conjugated p.
    constitutive p.
    copper storage p.
    corticosteroid-binding p.
    C-reactive p. (CRP)
    CREB binding p. (CBP)
    cullin family p.
    cyclin D1 p.
    cyclin-dependent p.
    cytochrome C p.
    cytoskeletal p.
    cytoskeleton-associated p.
    cytotoxic p.
    death-associated p. (DAP)
    p. defect
    p. deficiency anemia
    p. denaturation
    derived p.
    dietary p.
    dipeptidyl peptidase IV p. (DPPIV)
    doppel p.
    EF p.
    p. efficiency ratio (PER)
    elastin-binding p.
    p. electrolyte
    p. electrophoresis
    endothelial immunoglobin family adhesion p.
    enhanced green fluorescent p. (EGFP)
    eosinophilic cationic p. (ECP)
    estrogen receptor p. (ERP)
    excitotoxin p.
    p. expression pattern
    extracellular matrix p.
    FAA p.
    FAC p.
    F-actin binding p.
    FAS-associated death domain p. (FADD)

Fas-Fas ligand p.
F-box p.
p. fever
FHIT p.
fibrinolytic p.
fibrous p.
FLICE-like inhibitory p. (FLIP)
foreign p.
p. fractionation
fusion p.
G p.
GCDFP-15 p.
p. gene product (PGP)
glial fibrillary acidic p. (GFAP)
gliofibrillary acidic p.
globular p.
GPT-binding p.
green fluorescence p. (GFP)
gross cystic disease fluid p. (GCDFP)
p. G Sepharose
GTPase-activating p.
guanyl-nucleotide-binding p.
hamartin p.
HDJ1 p.
heart fatty acid binding p. (H-FABP)
heat-labile p.
heat shock p. (HSP)
helicase p.
helix-loop-helix p.
HER-2 p.
HER-2/neu p.
heterologous p.
high p. (HP)
histidine-rich matrix p.
homeodomain p.
p. hormone
human liver-type fatty acid-binding p. (hL-FABP)
huntingtin p.
p. hydrolysate
immune p.
immunoglobulin family adhesion p.
p. induced by vitamin K antagonist (PIVKA)
integral p.
intermediate filament p.
iron p.
iron-sulfide p.
Ki-67 p.
p. kinase A

p. kinase C (PKC)
p. kinase C isoenzyme
kinase inhibitory p. (KIP)
Kolmer test with Reiter p. (KRP)
Kunitz domain-containing p.
latent membrane p. (LMP)
lenticular p.
leptin p.
LF p.
low p. (LP)
lysosomal-associated membrane p. (LAMP)
lysosomal trafficking regulator p. (LYST)
M p.
macrophage inflammatory p. (MIP)
major basic p. (MBP)
major outer membrane p. (MOMP)
membrane p.
microtubule-associated p. (MAP)
midkine p.
mild silver p.
minichromosome maintenance p.
mitogen-activated p. (MAP)
mitotic control p. (MCP)
MK p.
monoclonal p.
monocyte chemoattractant p. (MCP)
monocyte chemoattractant p. 1 (MCP 1)
monocyte chemotactic p. 1 (MCP 1)
multidrug resistance p. (MRP)
muscle contractile p.
myelin basic p. (MBP)
myeloblastic p.
myeloma p.
MyoD p.
myogenin p.
net dietary p. (NDP)
N-ethylmaleimide-sensitive fusion p.
neurofilament p. (NFP)
neutrophil activating p. (NAP)
NF-kappa B p.
NHC p.
ninhydrin-Schiff stain for p.'s
p. nitrogen unit (PNU)
nonhistone chromosomal p.
nonspecific p.
normal RB p.
nuclear matrix p. (NMP)
oncofetal p.

NOTES

P

protein *(continued)*
p. overexpression
p24 p.
PA p.
p. pad
pancreatic stress p.
parathyroid hormone-related p. (PTHrP)
parvalbumin p.
patched hedgehog p. (PTCH)
PcG p.
peripheral p.
peripheral myelin p. 22 (PMP22)
pit-1 p.
plasma p.
polyclonal anti-S-100 p.
PPAR gamma p.
pregnancy-associated plasma p. A (PAPP-A)
pregnancy-associated plasma p. B (PAPP-B)
prion p. (PrPSc)
promyelocytic leukemia p. (PML)
prosurvival p.
protective p.
p. purification
p. quotient
R p.
RanBP p.
Rb tumor suppressor p.
reactive p. (RP)
respiratory p.
retinoblastoma p.
retinol-binding p. (RBP)
rgp120 p.
rhoptry p.
ribonuclear p. (RNP)
p. S
S-100 p.
SAA p.
SCA p. (SCA)
scaffolding p.
selenium binding p. (SBP)
p. separation method
p. S-free kit
SHH p.
sHLA p.
p. shock
p. shock therapy
simple p.
sodium-iodide transport p.
soluble HLA p.
soluble NSF attachment p. (SNAP)
sterol carrier p.
stress p.
structural p.
surivivin p.
survivin p.
synaptosomal p. of 25 kDa

p. synthesis
Tamm-Horsfall p.
tau p.
p. test
thrombus precursor p.
thyroxine-binding p. (TBP)
total p. (TP)
total serum p. (TSP)
transmembrane p.
tropomyosin-binding p.
p. truncation assay
p. truncation test
tumor-suppressor p.
p. turnover
p. tyrosine kinase activity
unwinding p.
Vav1 signal transducer p.
vinculin p.
virus VP1 capsid p.
vitamin K dependent plasma p.
whey acidic p.
Wiskott-Aldrich syndrome p. (WASP)
WRN p.
p. X-PO4
Y-box binding p. (YB1)
zinc finger p.
ZO-1 p.

protein-1
lysosomal-associated membrane p.-1 (LAMP-1)
protein-2
lysosomal-associated membrane p.-2 (LAMP-2)
proteinaceous fluid
proteinase
aspartic p.
Bothrops atrox serine p.
p. inhibitor
p. K
p. K buffer
Sigma Tween p.
Staphylococcus aureus neutral p.
protein-binding
competitive p. (CPB)
protein-bound
p.-b. iodine (PBI)
p.-b. iodine assay
p.-b. iodine test
p.-b. iodine-131 test
p.-b. thyroxine (PBT4)
protein-calorie malnutrition (PCM)
ProteinChip
P. Biomarker DU, PA system
P. System Series 4000 biomarker/assay system
P. test
proteinemia
Bence Jones p.

protein-losing enteropathy
proteinosis
    alveolar p.
    lipid p.
    lipoid p.
    pulmonary alveolar p. (PAP)
protein-protein binding assay
proteinuria
    Bence Jones p.
    gestational p.
    isolated p.
    nonisolated p.
    non-nephrotic range p.
    orthostatic p.
    postgamma p. (PGP)
    postural p.
Proteobacteria
proteoglycan (PG)
    p. aggregate
    chondroitin sulfate p. (CSPG)
    heparan sulfate p.
    human stromelysin aggregated p.
    (H-SLAP)
proteolipid
proteolysis
proteolytic
    p. degradation
    p. digestion
    p. enzyme
    p. enzyme pepsin
proteolytica
    Pseudomonas p.
proteolyticum
    Trichosporon p.
proteolyticus
    Psychrobacter p.
    Vibrio p.
proteome analysis
ProteomeLab
    P. DU, PA 800 protein
    characterization system
    P. PF 2D protein fractionation
    system
    P. XL-A, XL-I protein
    characterization system
proteomic
proteomics
Proteomyces
Proteomyxidia
proteose
proteosome
proteosuria

Proteus
    P. inconstans
    P. mirabilis
    P. morganii
    P. OX2 antigen
    P. OX19 antigen
    P. OXK antigen
    P. pneumonia
    P. rettgeri
    P. stuartii
    P. urinary tract infection
    P. vulgaris
proteus
    Amoeba p.
    Bacillus p.
    p. group
    Obesumbacterium p.
prothionamide
prothoracicotropic hormone
prothrombase
prothrombin
    p. accelerator
    p. complex
    p. complex concentration (PCC)
    component A of prothrombin
    p. consumption test
    p. consumption time (PCT)
    p. deficiency
    p. G20210A mutation
    p. gene
    p. gene 20210A
    p. II mutation
    p. and proconvertin (P&P)
    p. and proconvertin test
    p. time (protime, PT)
    p. time test
prothrombinase
prothrombin-converting principle
prothrombinogen
prothrombinopenia
prothrombin-proconvertin (PP)
prothrombokinase factor
prothrombotic
proticity
protic solvent
ProTime
    P. INR test device
    P. microcoagulation system
    P. prothrombin time test system
protime
    prothrombin time
protirelin

NOTES

P

815

protist
Protista
protistologist
protistology
protium (^{1}H)
Protoarchaea
Protobacterieae
protobe
protobiology
protocol
    heat antigen retrieval p.
    Malmö p.
    standardized p.
    telomerase repeat amplification p.
    (TRAP)
    telomeric repeat amplification p.
    (TRAP)
protocoproporphyria hereditaria
Protoctista
Protocult test
protodiastolic
protoerythrocyte
protofibril
protofilament
protogonoplasm
protoleukocyte
protomerite
protometrocyte
protomyofibroblast
proton
    p. acceptor
    p. acid
    p. donor
    p. pump
    p. spectroscopy
    p. tautomer
protonephridium
proton-motive hypothesis
protonophore FCCP
protooncogene
    bcl-2 p.
    c-erb-B2 p.
    c-kit p.
    erb B p.
    kit p.
    myc p.
proto-oncogene
protoplasm
    totipotential p.
protoplasmic, protoplasmatic
    p. astrocyte
    p. astrocytoma
protoplasmolysis
protoplast fusion
protoporphyria
    erythropoietic p. (EPP)
protoporphyrin (PP)
    p. assay
    erythrocyte zinc p.

    p. test
    zinc p. (ZPP)
protoporphyrinogen
    p. oxidase
    p. oxidase deficiency
protoporthyrinuria
protospore
Protostrongylus rufescens
Prototheca
    P. ciferrii
    P. filamenta
    P. segbwema
    P. stagnora
    P. wickerhamii
    P. zopfii
protothecosis
prototrophic
prototype
Protozoa
protozoa (*pl. of* protozoon)
protozoal dysentery
protozoan parasite
protozoiasis
protozoicide
protozoologist
protozoology
protozoon, pl. protozoa
protozoophage
protransglutaminase
protriptyline assay
protrusio acetabulum
protrusion
    synovial villus p.
protuberance
    Rokitansky p.
protuberans
    dermatofibrosarcoma p. (DFSP)
    fibrosarcomatous variant of
      dermatofibrosarcoma p. (FS-DFSP)
    fibrous dysplasia p.
    pigmented dermatofibrosarcoma p.
protumorigenic
proud flesh
proventriculus
Providencia
    P. alcalifaciens
    P. providenciae
    P. rettgeri
    P. stuartii
    P. urinary tract infection
provirus
provisional
    p. callus
    p. cortex
provitamin
provocation
    subcutaneous/sublingual p.
    p. typhoid

provocative
  p. chelation test
  p. diagnosis
  p. Wassermann test
Prowazek-Greeff body
prowazeki
  Copromastix p.
prowazekii
  Rickettsia p.
Prower factor
Prower-Stuart factor
proximal
  p. centriole
  p. femur
  p. interphalangeal (PIP)
proximate
  p. cause
  p. principle
prozone
  p. phenomenon
  p. reaction
PRP
  pityriasis rubra pilaris
  platelet-rich plasma
PrPSc
  prion protein
PRU
  peripheral resistance unit
pruinosum
  Sporotrichum p.
prune
  p. belly
  p. belly phenotype
  p. belly syndrome
  p. juice expectoration
  p. juice sputum
prurigo
  p. aestivalis
  p. agria
  Besnier p.
  p. chronica multiformis
  p. ferox
  p. gestationis
  p. of Hebra
  melanotic p.
  p. mitis
  nodular p.
  p. nodularis
  p. papule
  p. simplex
pruritus
Prussak fiber

Prussian
  P. blue
  P. blue iron stain
prussiate
prussic acid
Prymnesiovirus
PS
  periodic syndrome
  phosphatidylserine
  population sample
  Porter-Silber
  pyloric stenosis
P:S
  polyunsaturated-to-saturated fatty acids
  ratio
PSA
  prostate-specific antigen
  complexed PSA
  Immulite 2000 free PSA
  Immulite 2000 third-generation PSA
  PSA index
  PSA IRMA kit
PSAD
  PSA density
psalterial cord
psammocarcinoma
  serous p.
Psammolestes
psammoma
  p. body
  Virchow p.
psammomatous
  p. calcification
  p. meningioma
psammomatous-melanotic schwannoma
psammous
PSAP
  prostate specific acid phosphatase
PSC
  Porter-Silber chromogen
  posterior subcapsular cataract
  primary sclerosing cholangitis
PSCA
  prostate stem cell antigen
PSCP
  papillary serous carcinoma of the
  peritoneum
PSCT
  peripheral stem cell transplant
PSD
  peptone-starch-dextrose

NOTES

P

PSE
    portal-systemic encephalopathy
psec
    picosecond
Pselaphephilia
pseudacromegaly
pseudalbuminuria
Pseudallescheria boydii
pseudallescheriasis
Pseudaminobacter
    P. defluvii
    P. salicylatoxidans
Pseudamphistomum truncatum
pseudarthrosis
Pseudeurotium ovale
pseudinoma
pseudoacanthosis nigricans
pseudoachondroplasia
pseudoachondroplastic spondyloepiphysial
   dysplasia
pseudoacinus, pl. pseudoacini
pseudoagglutination
pseudoainhum
pseudoalbuminuria
pseudoalcaligenes
    Pseudomonas p.
pseudoaldosteronism
pseudoallele
Pseudoalteromonadaceae
Pseudoalteromonas
    P. agarivorans
    P. aliena
    P. distincta
    P. elyakovii
    P. issachenkonii
    P. maricaloris
    P. mariniglutinosa
    P. peptidolytica
    P. phenolica
    P. ruthenica
    P. sagamiensis
    P. tetraodonis
    P. translucida
    P. ulvae
pseudoalveolar pattern
pseudoanaphylactic shock
pseudoanaphylaxis
pseudoanemia
pseudoaneuploidy
pseudoaneurysm
pseudoangiomatous
    p. hyperplasia
    p. stromal hyperplasia (PASH)
pseudoangiosarcoma
    Masson p.
pseudoangiosarcomatous carcinoma
Pseudoarachniotus
pseudoarthrosis
pseudobacillus

pseudobacterium
pseudobile canaliculus
pseudobowenoid change
pseudobulbar palsy
Pseudobutyrivibrio
    P. ruminis
    P. xylanivorans
pseudocapillarization
pseudocarcinomatous
    p. change
    p. hyperplasia
pseudocartilage
pseudocartilaginous
pseudocast
pseudocelom
Pseudochaetosphaeronema
pseudocholesteatoma
pseudocholinesterase (PCHE)
    p. deficiency
pseudochromhidrosis
pseudochylothorax
pseudochylous ascites
pseudocirrhosis
Pseudoclavibacter helvolus
Pseudoclitocybe
pseudoclonality
Pseudococcidioides
Pseudocochliobolus
pseudocolloid of lips
pseudocowpox virus
pseudocoxalgia
pseudo-Cushing state
pseudocyesis
pseudocylindroid
pseudocyst
    pancreatic p.
pseudodecidual
pseudodiphtheria
pseudodiphtheriticum
    Corynebacterium p.
pseudodiploid
pseudodiverticulum
pseudodysentery
pseudoepitheliomatous
    p. change
    p. hyperplasia
pseudoepithelium
pseudoerysipelas
pseudoexfoliation
pseudo-Felty syndrome
pseudofollicle
pseudofollicular
    p. appearance
    p. proliferation center
Pseudofusarium
pseudo-Gaucher cell
pseudogland
pseudoglanders

pseudoglandular phase of lung development
pseudoglomerulus
pseudoglucosazone
pseudogout
pseudo-Graefe sign
pseudo-gunpowder stippling
pseudogynecomastia
Pseudohansfordia
Pseudohazis
pseudohematuria
pseudohermaphrodite
    female p.
    male p.
pseudohermaphroditism
    dysgenetic male p. (DMPH)
pseudohernia
pseudoheterotopia
pseudo-Hurler polydystrophy
pseudohydrocephaly
pseudohydronephrosis
pseudohyperkalemia in specimen hemolysis
pseudohyperparathyroidism
pseudohyperplasia
pseudohypertrophic
pseudohypertrophy
pseudohypha
pseudohypoglycemia
pseudohypokalemia
pseudohyponatremia
pseudohypoparathyroidism (PHP)
pseudoinclusion
    nuclear p.
pseudointraligamentous
pseudoinvasion
pseudoinvasive appearance
pseudoisochromatic
pseudo-Kaposi lesion
pseudolaminar necrosis
pseudolepromatous leishmaniasis
pseudoleukemica
    anemia infantum p.
pseudolipoblast
pseudolipoma
pseudolipomatosis
pseudolithiasis
pseudolobule
pseudolymphocyte
pseudolymphocytic choriomeningitis virus
pseudolymphoma
    cutaneous p.

    Saltzstein p.
    Spiegler-Fendt p.
    p. of Spiegler-Fendt
pseudolymphomatous folliculitis
pseudolysogenic strain
pseudolysogeny
pseudomalignancy
pseudomallei
    Actinobacillus p.
    Bacillus p.
    Burkholderia p.
    Malleomyces p.
    Pseudomonas p.
pseudomamma
pseudomantle zone pattern
pseudomelanosis
    p. coli
    p. duodeni
    p. pigment
pseudomembrane
    fibrinous p.
pseudomembranous
    p. acute inflammation
    p. bronchitis
    p. colitis (PMC)
    p. enterocolitis
    p. gastritis
pseudometaplasia
pseudometastatic
Pseudomicrodochium
pseudomonad
Pseudomonadaceae
Pseudomonadales
Pseudomonadeae
Pseudomonadineae
pseudomonal pneumonia
Pseudomonas
    P. acidovorans
    P. aeruginosa
    P. alboprecipitans
    P. alcaligenes
    P. alcaliphila
    P. brassicacearum
    P. brenneri
    P. cannabina
    P. cedrina
    P. cepacia
    P. chloritidismutans
    P. congelans
    P. costantinii
    P. cremoricolorata
    P. diminuta

NOTES

P

Pseudomonas (continued)
- P. *extremorientalis*
- P. *fluorescens*
- P. *fragi*
- P. *frederiksbergensis*
- P. *grimontii*
- P. *indica*
- P. *jinjuensis*
- P. *kilonensis*
- P. *koreensis*
- P. *lini*
- P. *lutea*
- P. *maltophilia*
- P. *mandelii*
- P. *marina*
- P. *mediterranea*
- P. *meridiana*
- P. *mesophilica*
- P. *methanolica*
- P. *mosselii*
- P. *multiresinivorans*
- P. *nonliquefaciens*
- P. *orientalis*
- P. *palleroniana*
- P. *parafulva*
- P. *paucimobilis*
- P. *plecoglossicida*
- P. *proteolytica*
- P. *pseudoalcaligenes*
- P. *pseudomallei*
- P. *psychrophila*
- P. *psychrotolerans*
- P. *putida*
- P. *rhizosphaerae*
- P. *salomonii*
- P. selective agar
- P. *stutzeri*
- P. *syncyanea*
- P. *testosteroni*
- P. *thermotolerans*
- P. *thivervalensis*
- P. *trivialis*
- P. *umsongensis*
- P. urinary tract infection
- P. *vesicularis*

Pseudomonilia
pseudomosaicism
pseudomucinous
- p. cyst
- p. cystadenocarcinoma
- p. cystadenoma
- p. degeneration

pseudomyasthenic syndrome
pseudomycelium
Pseudomycoderma
pseudomyiasis
Pseudomyxoma ovarii
pseudomyxoma peritonei (PP)
Pseudonectria

pseudoneoplasm
pseudoneuroma
pseudoneutrophilia
Pseudonocardia
- P. *alaniniphila*
- P. *alni*
- P. *antarctica*
- P. *aurantiaca*
- P. *benzenivorans*
- P. *chloroethenivorans*
- P. *kongjuensis*
- P. *spinosispora*
- P. *xinjiangensis*
- P. *yunnanensis*
- P. *zijingensis*

Pseudonocardiaceae
Pseudonocardineae
pseudoosteomalacia
pseudoosteomalacic pelvis
pseudopalisading
pseudopapillary pattern
pseudoparakeratosis
pseudoparasite
pseudoparenchyma
pseudo-Pelger-Huët change
pseudoperiodic
pseudoperoxidation
- metal-catalyzed p.

Pseudophaeotrichum
pseudophlegmon
- Hamilton p.

pseudophyllid
Pseudophyllidea
pseudophyllidean
pseudoplatelet
pseudopod flow
pseudopodium, pl. pseudopodia
pseudopolycythemia
pseudopolydystrophy
pseudopolyp
pseudopolyposis
pseudoprecocious puberty
pseudoprecocity
- isosexual p.

pseudopseudohypoparathyroidism (PPHP)
pseudopseudolymphoma
pseudopuberty
- precocious p.

pseudopunctipennis
- *Anopheles* p.

pseudopyloric metaplasia
pseudorabies virus
Pseudoramibacter alactolyticus
pseudoreaction
pseudoreplica
pseudorheumatism
Pseudorhodobacter ferrugineus
pseudorosette
pseudorubella

pseudosarcoma botryoides
pseudosarcomatous
    p. carcinoma
    p. cell
    p. fasciitis
    p. fibromyxoid tumor
    p. myofibroblastic proliferation
    p. myofibroblastic tumor (PMT)
    p. stroma
pseudosclerosis
    Jakob-Creutzfeldt p.
    Westphal-Strümpell p.
pseudoscutellaris
    Aedes scutellaris p.
pseudoseizure
pseudoseptum, pl. **pseudosepta**
pseudosmallpox
pseudospiralis
    Trichinella p.
Pseudospirillum japonicum
Pseudostertagia bullosa
pseudostoma, pl. **pseudostomas,**
  pseudostomata
pseudostratification
    nuclear p.
pseudostratified columnar epithelium
pseudosynovium
pseudotattooing
Pseudoterranova decipiens
pseudothalidomide syndrome
Pseudothelphusa
pseudothrombocytopenia
    EDTA-dependent p.
pseudotortuosum
    Eubacterium p.
pseudotrichinosis
pseudotropicalis
    Candida p.
pseudotruncus arteriosus
pseudotubercle
pseudotuberculosis
    p. bacillus
    Corynebacterium p.
    Pasteurella p.
    Yersinia p.
pseudotubular degeneration
pseudotumor
    calcifying fibrous p.
    cerebri p.
    fibrous p.
    inflammatory p.
    nuchal fibrocartilaginous p.

    postinflammatory p.
    spindle cell p.
    xanthomatous p.
pseudo-Turner syndrome
pseudounipolar
    p. cell
    p. neuron
pseudouridine excretion
pseudovaccinii
    Nocardia p.
pseudovacuole
pseudovariola
pseudovascular adenoid squamous cell
  carcinoma (PASCC)
pseudoventricle
Pseudovirus
pseudo-von Willebrand disease
pseudoxanthoma
    p. cell
    p. elasticum (PXE)
pseudoxanthomatous transformation
Pseudoxanthomonas
    P. broegbernensis
    P. taiwanensis
Pseudozyma
PSFR
    peak secretory flow rate
    PSFR assay
PSGN
    poststreptococcal glomerulonephritis
psi
    pounds per square inch
PSI chromosome analysis system
Psilobotrys
psilocin
Psilocybe
psilocybin
Psilorchis hominis
psittaci
    Chlamydia p.
    Chlamydophila p.
    Lactobacillus p.
    Miyagawanella p.
psittacicida
    Volucribacter p.
psittacosis
    p. inclusion body
    p. titer
    p. virus
psittacosis-lymphogranuloma
    p.-l. venereum trachoma (PLT)
    p.-l. venereum-trachoma group

NOTES

P

PSL
  pigmented skin lesion
PSMA
  prostate-specific membrane antigen
PSNP
  placental site nodule and plaque
psoas abscess
psoralen-mediated process
psoralen-treated pooled plasma
psorelcosis
psorenteritis
Psorergates
psoriasiform dermatitis
psoriasis
  p. arthropica
  Barber p.
  buccal p.
  exfoliative p.
  generalized pustular p. of
    Zambusch
  p. ostracea
  pustular p.
  rupioides p.
  von Zumbusch p.
  p. vulgaris
psoriatic arthritis
Psorophora
Psoroptes
PSP
  phenolsulfonphthalein
  progressive supranuclear palsy
PSRO
  Professional Standards Review
    Organization
PSS
  physiological saline solution
  progressive systemic sclerosis
PST
  penicillin, streptomycin, and tetracycline
PSTT
  placental site trophoblastic tumor
Psychoda alternata
Psychodidae
psychogenic
  p. purpura
  p. seizure
psychogeriatric
psychological autopsy
psychomotor epilepsy
psychosine
psychraerophilum
  Bifidobacterium p.
psychralcaliphila
  Dietzia p.
Psychrobacter
  P. arenosus
  P. faecalis
  P. fozii

  P. jeotgali
  P. luti
  P. marincola
  P. maritimus
  P. okhotskensis
  P. pacificensis
  P. proteolyticus
  P. submarinus
psychrodurans
  Bacillus p.
Psychroflexus
  P. gondwanensis
  P. torquis
  P. tropicus
Psychromonadaceae
Psychromonas
  P. antarctica
  P. arctica
  P. kaikoae
  P. marina
  P. profunda
psychrophila
  Desulfotalea p.
  Pseudomonas p.
  Sporosarcina p.
psychrophile
psychrophilic bacterium
psychrophilum
  Clostridium p.
  Cryobacterium p.
psychrophilus
  Jeotgalicoccus p.
  Planococcus p.
psychrotolerans
  Bacillus p.
  Mycobacterium p.
  Pseudomonas p.
psyllium hydrophilic mucilloid
PT
  phosphotransferase
  pneumothorax
  prothrombin time
PTA
  persistent truncus arteriosus
  phosphotungstic acid
  plasma thromboplastin antecedent
  PTA deficiency
  PTA stain
PTAH
  phosphotungstic acid hematoxylin
  PTAH stain
PTC
  papillary thyroid carcinoma
  phenylthiocarbamide
  plasma thromboplastin component
  primary thymic carcinoma
  PTC deficiency
  PTC peptide

PTCH
> patched hedgehog protein
>> PTCH receptor

PTCL
> peripheral T-cell lymphoma
> postthymic T-cell lymphoma

PTE
> parathyroid extract
> pulmonary thromboembolism

PTED
> pulmonary thromboembolic disease

PTEN tumor suppressor gene

pteridine

pterin

pteroic acid

pteronyssinus
>> *Dermatophagoides p.*

pteroylglutamic acid

pteroylpolyglutamate

pterygium
> congenital p.
> p. syndrome

Pterygodermatites dipodomis

pterygoid chest

Pterygota

PTF
> plasma thromboplastin factor

PTGC
> progressive transformation of germinal
> center

PTH
> parathormone
> parathyroid hormone
> posttransfusion hepatitis
>> PTH assay

Pthirus (*var. of* *Phthirus*)

PTHrP
> parathyroid hormone-related peptide
> parathyroid hormone-related protein

PTHS
> parathyroid hormone secretion

PTI
> persistent tolerant infection

PTL
> peripheral T-cell lymphoma

PTLD
> posttransplant lymphoproliferative
> disease
> posttransplant lymphoproliferative
> disorder

PTM
> posttransfusion mononucleosis

pTNM
> pathologic tumor-node metastasis

ptomaine, ptomatine

ptomainemia

ptosed

ptosis, pl. **ptoses**

ptotic organ

PTP
> posttransfusion purpura

PTR
> peripheral total resistance

p-(trifluoromethoxy)phenylhydrazone
>> carbonyl cyanide p. (FCCP)

PTT
> partial thromboplastin time
> particle transport time

PTT-LA
> partial thromboplastin time lupus
> anticoagulant
>> PTT-LA reagent

ptyalocele

Ptychogaster

ptyocrinous

PU
> peptic ulcer
> polyurethane
> pregnancy urine

puberty
> delayed p.
> precocious p.
> pseudoprecocious p.

pubic
> p. louse
> p. tuberosity

pubis
>> *Pediculus p.*
>> *Phthirus p.*

public
> p. antigen
> p. health bacteriology
> p. health laboratory
> P. Health Practice Program Office
> (PHPPO)

PUBS
> percutaneous umbilical blood sampling

Puccinia
> *P. glumarum*
> *P. graminis*

Puchtler
> P. alkaline Congo red method
> P. Sirius red method

NOTES

P

Puchtler-Sweat
    P.-S. stain
    P.-S. stain for basement
      membranes
    P.-S. stain for hemoglobin and
      hemosiderin
PUE
    pyrexia of unknown etiology
puerperal
    p. eclampsia
    p. fever
    p. hematoma
    p. infection
    p. mastitis
    p. phlebitis
    p. septicemia
    p. thrombosis
puerperium
PUFA
    polyunsaturated fatty acid
puffball
puffer
    pink p. (PP)
pulcherrima
    Capronia p.
pulchrum
    Gongylonema p.
Pulex
    P. cheopis
    P. fasciatus
    P. irritans
    P. penetrans
    P. serraticeps
pulicicide
Pulicidae
pullulans
    Aureobasidium p.
    Pullularia p.
    Trichosporon p.
Pullularia pullulans
pullulate
pullulation
pulmolith
pulmonale
    cor p.
    glomus p.
pulmonalis
    Trichomonas p.
pulmonary
    p. accumulation
    p. acinus
    p. adenomatosis
    p. agent
    p. alveolar macrophage (PAM)
    p. alveolar microlithiasis (PAM)
    p. alveolar proteinosis (PAP)
    p. alveolus
    p. angiomyolipoma
    p. anthrax

p. arteriovenous fistula (PAF)
p. artery hypertension
p. artery stenosis (PAS)
p. aspergillosis
p. atresia
p. blast injury
p. blastoma
p. blastomycosis
p. blood flow
p. bulla
p. capacity test
p. capillary blood volume
p. capillary hemangiomatosis (PCH)
p. dirofilariasis
p. distomiasis
p. docimasia
p. dysmaturity syndrome
p. edema (PE)
p. embolism (PE)
p. eosinophilia
p. fibrosis
p. function tests (PFT)
p. glomangiosis
p. hamartoma
p. heart disease
p. hemosiderosis
p. hypersensitivity
p. hypostasis
p. incompetence (PI)
p. infarct
p. infarction (PI)
p. infection
p. infiltrate
p. infiltration and eosinophilia
  (PIE)
p. infundibular stenosis
p. insufficiency
p. interstitial emphysema (PIE)
p. interstitial lymphocytic
  infiltration
p. LAM
p. lymphangioleiomyomatosis
p. lymphangiomatosis
p. lymphoid hyperplasia (PLH)
p. MALT lymphoma
p. mucormycosis
p. neuroendocrine cell (PNEC)
p. osteoarthropathy
p. perfusion
p. pleurisy
plexogenic p.
p. pneumonitis
p. pressure
p. resistance (Rp)
p. sarcoidosis
p. surfactant
p. thromboembolic disease (PTED)
p. thromboembolism (PTE)
p. trunk

p. tuberculosis
p. vascular disease
p. venous congestion (PVC)
pulmonary-renal syndrome
pulmonicola
    Pandoraea p.
pulmonis
alveoli p.
hilum p.
Mycoplasma p.
porta p.
Tsukamurella p.
pulmonitis
pulp
artery of p.
dental p.
dentinal p.
putrescent p.
red p.
splenic p.
splenic red p.
tooth p.
white p.
pulpa
p. dentis
p. lienis
p. splenica
pulpar cell
pulpefaction
pulpiform
pulpitis
putrescent p.
pulposus
herniated nucleus p. (HNP)
pulpy
pulsating
p. empyema
p. metastasis
pulse
electromagnetic p. (EMP)
p. height analyzer (PHA)
p. oximetry
p. pressure
pulsed
p. field gel electrophoresis
p. field gradient gel electrophoresis (PFGE)
pulseless disease
pulsellum
pulsion diverticulum
pultaceous

pulverulenta
cataracta centralis p.
pulvinar
p. gliosis
p. sign
pumilum
    Mogibacterium p.
pumilus
    Bacillus p.
pump
chloroquine p.
proton p.
punch
p. biopsy
replicate p.
punched
p. out lytic bone lesion
p. out osteolytic lesion
p. out space
puncta (*pl. of* punctum)
punctata
Aeromonas p.
chondrodysplasia p.
chondrodystrophia congenita p.
Cooperia p.
dysplasia epiphysialis p.
keratosis p.
punctate
p. abrasion
p. basophilia
p. hemorrhage
p. keratoderma
p. nitrate residue
p. parotitis
p. pattern
punctation
punctiform
punctum, pl. **puncta**
p. luteum
p. ossificationis
p. ossificationis primarium
p. ossificationis secundarium
p. vasculosum
puncture
femoral p.
lumbar p.
lymph node p.
percutaneous renal p.
transethmoidal p.
punicea
    Glaciecola p.

NOTES

P

puniciscabiei
>*Streptomyces p.*

Punjab
>hemoglobin D P.

punjatensis
>*Ceratophyllus p.*

Puntius

PUO
>pyrexia of unknown origin

pupa, pl. **pupae**

pupil
>Adie p.
>Argyll Robertson p.
>Hutchinson p.

pupilla, pl. **pupillae**
>dilator pupillae

pupillaris
>membrana p.

pupiparous

pure
>p. antiandrogen
>chemically p. (CP)
>p. culture
>p. leukocytosis
>p. red cell agenesis
>p. red cell anemia
>p. red cell aplasia (PRCA)
>p. tumor

Puregene DNA isolation kit

purification
>immunoaffinity p.
>protein p.
>Wizard MagneSil plasmid p.
>Wizard SV 96 plasmid p.

purified
>affinity p.
>p. protein derivative (PPD)
>p. protein derivative skin test
>p. protein derivative-standard (PPD-S)
>p. protein derivative of tuberculin

puriform

purine
>p. bodies test
>p. nucleoside phosphorylase (PNP)
>p. nucleoside phosphorylase deficiency
>p. and pyrimidine bases

purinemia

purinergic receptor translocation assessment

puris
>liquor p.
>*Nocardia p.*

purity
>optical p.
>radiochemical p.
>radionuclidic p.

Purkinje
>P. cell
>P. cell layer
>P. corpuscle
>P. fiber
>P. myocyte
>P. network
>P. system

puromucous

purple
>bromcresol p.

purpura
>allergic p.
>anaphylactoid p.
>p. angioneurotica
>p. annularis
>p. annularis telangiectodes
>autoimmune thrombocytopenic p.
>cachectic p.
>p. of Doucas
>fibrinolytic p.
>p. fulminans
>p. hemorrhagica
>Henoch p.
>Henoch-Schönlein p. (HSP)
>hyperglobulinemic p.
>idiopathic thrombocytopenic p. (ITP)
>immune thrombocytopenic p.
>isoimmune neonatal p.
>Kapetanakis p.
>Majocchi p.
>posttransfusion p. (PTP)
>psychogenic p.
>Schönlein p.
>thrombocytopenic p. (TP)
>thrombotic thrombocytopenic p. (TTP)
>Waldenström p.

purpurascens
>*Epicoccum p.*

purpurea
>*Claviceps p.*
>*Digitalis p.*
>*Lamprocystis p.*
>*Micromonospora p.*

purpureus
>*Otomyces p.*
>*Rhinoestrus p.*

purpuric

purpurin
>alizarin p.

purpurinuria

purpuriparous

Purtscher disease

purulence

purulency

purulent
>p. debris

p. encephalitis
p. hypophysitis
p. inflammation
p. pericarditis
p. pleurisy
p. sputum production
p. synovitis

purulenta
pneumonia interlobularis p.
thromboarteritis p.

puruloid

purvisi
Cyclodontostomum p.

pus
anchovy sauce p.
blue p.
burrowing p.
p. cell
cheesy p.
p. corpuscle
curdy p.
green p.
ichorous p.
laudable p.
sanious p.
p. tube

pushchinoensis
Anoxybacillus p.

push package
push-pull amplifier
push-wedge method

pusilla
Terasakiella p.

pusillum
Physarum p.

pustular
p. bacterid
p. inflammation
p. psoriasis
p. vasculitis

pustule
anthrax malignant p.
p.'s of Kogoj
malignant p.
postmortem p.
shotty p.
spongiform p. of Kogoj

pustulosa
parakeratosis p.

pustulosis
p. palmaris et plantaris
p. vacciniformis acuta

putative
p. leukemia
p. peroxisome proliferator response element (PPRE)

putida
Pseudomonas p.

putidum
Treponema p.

Putnam-Dana syndrome

putredinis
Alistipes p.
Bacteroides p.

putrefaciens
Alteromonas p.

putrefaction

putrescent
p. pulp
p. pulpitis

putrescentiae
Tyrophagus p.

putrescine

putrid throat

putridus
Peptostreptococcus p.

putterlickiae
Kitasatospora p.

putty kidney

PUVA
P. lentigo
P. treatment

puzzle
blood p.

PV
plasma volume
polycythemia vera

PVA
polyvinyl alcohol
PVA fixative
PVA fixative method
PVA lacto-phenol medium

PVC
pulmonary venous congestion

PVD
peripheral vascular disease

PVEM
postvaccination encephalomyelitis

PVL
proliferative verrucous leukoplakia

PVM
pneumonia virus of mice
PVM virus

NOTES

P

827

PVNS
pigmented villonodular synovitis
PVOD
pulmonary veno-occlusive disease
PVP
peripheral vein plasma
predictive value positive
PVPG
paravertebral paraganglioma
PVT
portal vein thrombosis
PWI
posterior wall infarct
PWM
pokeweed mitogen
Px
pneumothorax
PXA
pleomorphic xanthoastrocytoma
PXE
pseudoxanthoma elasticum
pyarthrosis
Pycnidiella
Pycnoporus
pycnus
Bacillus p.
pyelectasis, pyelectasia
pyelitic
pyelitis
p. cystica
p. glandularis
pyelocaliectasis
pyelocystitis
pyelography
retrograde p.
pyelonephritic kidney
pyelonephritis (PN)
acute p.
ascending p.
chronic p. (CPN)
diffuse p.
xanthogranulomatous p. (XPN)
pyelonephrosis
pyeloureterectasis
pyemia
cryptogenic p.
portal p.
pyemic
p. abscess
p. embolism
Pyemotes tritici
Pyemotidae
pyencephalus
pyesis
Pygidiopsis summa
pygomelus
pygopagus
pyknocyte
pyknodysostosis

pyknometer
pyknometry
pyknomorphous
pyknosis
nuclear p.
pyknotic
p. cell
p. index
p. nucleus with irregular membrane
Pyle disease
pylemphraxis
pylephlebectasis, pylephlebectasia
pylephlebitic abscess
pylephlebitis
pylethrombophlebitis
pylethrombosis
pylori
Acceava *Helicobacter p.*
Campylobacter (Helicobacter) p.
coccoid *Helicobacter p.*
Helicobacter p.
pyloric
p. gland
p. gland metaplasia
p. stenosis (PS)
pyloricae
glandulae p.
pyloritis
pyloroduodenitis
pyloroptosis, pyloroptosia
pylorostenosis
Pym fever
pyocele
pyocelia
pyocephalus
circumscribed p.
external p.
internal p.
pyocin
pyocolpos
pyocyanase
pyocyaneus
Bacillus p.
pyocyanic
pyocyanin
pyocyanogenic
pyocyanolysin
pyocyst
pyocyte
pyoderma
chancriform p.
p. gangrenosum (PG)
primary p.
secondary p.
p. vegetans
pyodermatitis
pyodermatosis
pyogen

pyogenes
  Corynebacterium p.
  Staphylococcus p.
  Streptococcus p.
pyogenesis
pyogenetic
pyogenic
  p. abscess
  p. bacterium
  p. cholangitis
  p. fever
  p. granuloma
  p. infection
  p. membrane
  p. meningitis
  p. osteomyelitis
  p. pachymeningitis
  p. salpingitis
pyogenicum
  granuloma p.
pyogenous
pyogranulomatous
pyohemia
pyoid
pyometra
pyometritis
pyometrium
pyomyositis
pyonephritis
pyonephrolithiasis
pyonephrosis
pyopericarditis
pyopericardium
pyoperitoneum
pyoperitonitis
pyopoiesis
pyopoietic
pyopyelectasis
pyorrhea
pyosalpinx
pyosemia
pyosepticemia
pyosis
pyospermia
pyostatic
pyostomatitis vegetans
pyothorax
pyothorax-associated lymphoma
pyoureter
pyoverdin
pyoxanthin
pyoxanthose

pyramid
  Ferrein p.
pyramidal
  p. cell
  p. cell layer
  p. disease
pyran
pyranose
pyranoside
pyrazinamide
Pyrazus
pyrenemia
Pyrenochaeta romeroi
pyrenoid
Pyrenophora
pyrethrin
pyrethrum
pyrexia
  Pel-Ebstein p.
  p. of unknown etiology (PUE)
  p. of unknown origin (PUO)
Pyricularia oryzae
pyridine
  alum-precipitated p. (APP)
  p. nucleotide
pyridinivorans
  Rhodococcus p.
pyridoxalated
  p. hemoglobin-polyoxyethylene (PHP)
  p. stroma-free hemoglobin solution
pyridoxal-5′-phosphate (PLP)
pyridoxamine
pyridoxic acid
pyridoxine
pyridoxine-responsive anemia
pyriform (*var. of* piriform)
pyriformis
  Tetrahymena p.
pyrimethamine assay
pyrimidine
  p. base
  p. dimerization
Pyrobaculum
  P. arsenaticum
  P. oguniense
pyroborate
  sodium p.
pyrocarbonate
  diethyl p. (DEPC)
Pyrodictiaceae
pyrogallol

NOTES

P

pyrogallolphthalein
pyrogen
pyrogenic toxin
pyroglobulin
pyroglobulinemia
pyroglutamase
pyroglutamate hydroxylase
pyroglutamicaciduria
pyrolysis
pyronin B, G, Y
pyronine
    naphthol p.
pyroninophilia
pyroninophilic blast cell
pyrophosphatase
    inorganic p.
pyrophosphate
    coenzyme thiamine p.
    inorganic p.
    sodium p.
pyrophosphohydrolase
    ATP p.
    ectonucleotide p.
pyrophosphoric acid
pyropoikilocytosis
    hereditary p. (HPP)
pyroracemic acid
pyrosequencing
pyrosulfite
    sodium p.
pyrotoxin

pyrrol
    p. blue
    p. blue stain
    p. cell
pyrrole
pyrrolidone carboxylate
pyrroline-5-carboxylate
    p.-c. dehydrogenase
    p.-c. reductase
pyruvate
    p. carboxylase
    p. dehydrogenase complex (PDC)
    p. kinase (PK)
    p. kinase assay
    p. kinase deficiency
pyruvativorans
    Eubacterium p.
pyruvic
    p. acid
    p. acid assay
Pythium insidiosum
pythogenesis
pythogenic
pythogenous
pyuria
    sterile p.
PZ
    pancreozymin
PZ-CCK
    pancreozymin-cholecystokinin

Q

Q band
Q banding
Q beta replicase
Q disc
Q fever
Q fever endocarditis
Q fever pneumonia
Q fever titer

Q$_{10}$

temperature coefficient

Q$_B$

total body clearance

QA

quality assurance

Qa antigen
Q-banding stain
Q-band technique
Q-beta replicase system
QC

quality control

Q-enzyme
QF

quality factor

QFD

quartz fiber dosimeter

Q-FISH

quantitative fluorescence in situ
hybridization

QI

quality improvement

QIAamp DNA blood biorobot kit
Qiagen QIAquick gel extraction kit
QIAquick PCR 96 purification kit
QNB

3-quinuclidinyl benzilate
NATO code for QNB (BZ)

QNS

quantity not sufficient

QO$_2$, qO$_2$

oxygen quotient

QP

quanti-Pirquet reaction

Q-Prep workstation
Q-Probes program
QS

quantitation standard

Q-Tracks program
quadrant

4 q. biopsy
right lower q.

quadrata

Haloarcula q.

quadratic function

quadratum

caput q.

Quadricoccus australiensis
quadrigeminal
quadrilobata

Taenia q.

quadrimaculatus

Anopheles q.

quadriplegia

areflexic q.

quadripolar
quadriradial
quadrispinulatum

Oesophagostomum q.

quadrivalent
quail bronchitis virus
qualitative

q. analysis
q. fecal fat test
q. immunohistology
Q. Platform Immunoassay Device
  (QuPID)
q. staging of breast cancer
q. urine myoglobin dipstick test

quality

q. assurance (QA)
q. control (QC)
q. control chart
q. control serum
q. factor (QF)
q. improvement (QI)
q. of life

quanta

Q. Lite ANA ELISA test kit
Q. Lite CCP ELISA kit
Q. Lite ELISA autoimmune kit

quantasome
quantatrope
QuantiFERON-TB test
quantile
quantimeter
quanti-Pirquet reaction (QP)
quantitation

HIV q.
q. standard (QS)
q. test

quantitative

q. analysis
q. flow cytometric
  immunophenotyping
q. fluorescence in situ hybridization
  (Q-FISH)
q. hypertrophy
q. immunoglobulin
q. immunohistology

quantitative *(continued)*
    q. inheritance
    q. trait
quantity
    not sufficient q. (NSQ)
    q. not sufficient (QNS)
quantum, pl. **quanta**
    q. limit
    q. yield
Quaranfil virus
quarantine
quark
quarta
    crista q.
quartan
    q. fever
    q. malaria
quarti
    tela choroidea ventriculi q.
quartile
quartum
    Eubacterium q.
quartz fiber dosimeter (QFD)
quasicontinuous inheritance
quasidiploid
quasidominance
quasidominant inheritance
quasispecies
quaternary
    q. blast injury
    q. structure
    q. syphilis
Quebec platelet disorder
Queckenstedt test
Queensland tick fever
quellung
    q. phenomenon
    q. reaction
    q. test
quenching
    fluorescence q.
quercetin
quercicolus
    Dendrosporobacter q.
QuestDirect direct to consumer laboratory
question
    agent in q.
QuestTest diagnostic panel
queue
Queyrat
    erythroplasia of Q.
Quicgel method
Quick
    Q. method
    Q. Slide automated stainer
    Q. tourniquet test
quick-cool option on the cryostat

QuickVue
    Q. Advance *Gardnerella vaginalis* test
    Q. Advance pH and amines test
    Q. *Chlamydia* test
    Q. *H. pylori* gII test
    Q. influenza test
    Q. 1 step *Helicobacter pylori* test
    Q. UrinChek 10+ urine test
QuickVue+
    Q. infectious mononucleosis test
    Q. One-Step hCG Combo
quiet hip disease
quiltlike pattern
Quilty lesion
quinacrine
    q. banding
    q. chromosome banding stain
    q. hydrochloride
quinaldine red
Quincke
    Q. disease
    Q. edema
quinckeanum
    Trichophyton mentagrophytes var. *q.*
quinhydrone electrode
quinidine assay
quinine
    q. assay
    q. carbacrylic resin
    q. carbacrylic resin test
quinivorans
    Serratia q.
Quinlan test
quinoline dye
quinolinic acid
quinolinium dye
quinone
quinovose
Quinquaud disease
quinquefasciatus
    Culex q.
quinquevalent
quinsy
quintana
    Bartonella q.
    Rochalimaea q.
quintum
    Eubacterium q.
3-quinuclidinyl benzilate (QNB)
quisqualate activated neuron
quisquiliarum
    Cerasibacillus q.
quotidian
    q. fever
    q. malaria
quotient
    albumin q.
    blood q.

caloric q.
cerebral glucose oxygen q.
  (CG:OQ)
circadian q. (CQ)
oxygen q. (QO_2, qO_2)
permeability q. (PQ)
protein q.

rachidean q.
reaction q.
respiratory q.
QuPID
  Qualitative Platform Immunoassay
  Device
  QuPID pregnancy test

NOTES

R

Behnken unit
organic radical
Réaumur scale
regression coefficient
Rinne test
rough
    R antigen
    R banding
    R colony
    R determinant
    R factor
    R pilus
    R plasmid
    R protein

2R

chromotrope 2R

R-250

Coomassie brilliant blue R-250

RA

ragocyte
rheumatoid arthritis
    RA cell
    RA latex fixation test

rabbit

r. aorta-contracting substance
r. blood agar
r. fever (tularemia)
r. fibroma
r. fibroma virus
r. kidney
r. papilloma
r. plague
r. test

rabbitpox virus
rabid
rabies

r. immune globulin
r. immunoglobulin
r. vaccine
r. virus

raccoon's eye
RACE

rapid antigen uptake into the cytosol
    enterocytes
    RACE cell

racemase
racemate
racemic

r. aerosol
r. mixture
r. modification

racemization
racemosa

livedo r.

racemose

r. aneurysm
r. gland
r. hemangioma

racemosum

angioma venosum r.
Syncephalastrum r.

racemosus

Mucor r.

rachidean quotient
rachischisis
rachitic

r. pelvis
r. rosary

rachitis

r. fetalis
r. fetalis annularis
r. fetalis micromelica
r. intrauterina
r. uterina

raciborskii

Planktothricoides r.

rack

Nalgene freezer storage r.

racquet

r. hypha
r. shaped

RAD

radian
right axis deviation

rad

radiation absorbed dose

Radford nomogram
radial

r. aplasia-thrombocytopenia
r. aplasia-thrombocytopenia
    syndrome
r. diffusion
r. immunodiffusion (RID)
r. melanoma growth phase
r. scar
r. sclerosing lesion
r. styloid tendovaginitis
r. symmetry

radian (RAD)
radiant energy
radiata

corona r.

radiate

r. crown
r. layer of tympanic membrane

radiation

r. absorbed dose (rad)
alpha r.
r. anemia

radiation (*continued*)
    background r.
    beta r.
    braking r.
    Bremsstrahlung r.
    r. chimera
    r. colitis
    r. counter
    r. cystitis
    r. damage
    r. dermatitis
    r. dermatosis
    r. dispersal device (RDD)
    r. effect
    electromagnetic r.
    r. emergency area (REA)
    r. enteritis
    r. enterocolitis
    r. fibroblast
    r. gastritis
    general r.
    r. hazard
    r. injury
    ionizing r.
    r. measuring unit
    r. necrosis
    r. nephritis
    penetrating r.
    r. pneumonitis
    r. protection
    r. protection officer (RPO)
    r. sickness
    r. survey
    r. therapy
    ultraviolet r.
radiative capture
radiatum
    Oesophagostomum r.
radiatus
    Strongylus r.
radical
    cyanide r. (CN-)
    free r.
    hydroxyl r.
    organic r. (R)
    r. scavenger
radices (*pl. of* radix)
radicidentis
    Actinomyces r.
radicular cyst
radiculitis
    cervical r.
radiculoganglionitis
radiculomeningomyelitis
radiculomyelopathy
radiculoneuropathy
radiculopathy
    lumbosacral r.

radii lentis
radioactive
    r. challenge
    r. concentration
    r. constant
    r. decay
    r. drug
    r. equilibrium
    r. fibrinogen uptake test
    r. iodide (RAI)
    r. iodide uptake test
    r. iodinated human serum albumin (RIHSA)
    r. iodinated serum albumin (RISA)
    r. iodine (RAI)
    r. iodine uptake (RAIU, RIU)
    r. iodine uptake test
    r. label
    r. probe
    r. waste
radioactivity
    unknown r.
radioallergosorbent
    r. assay
    r. assay test (RAST)
radioassay
    C1q r.
radioautography
radiobacter
    Rhizobium r.
radiobiology
radiocalcium uptake
radiochemical purity
radiochromatogram
radiocolloid tracer
radiodense
radiodensity
radiodermatitis
radioenzymatic assay (REA)
radiofrequency
    high-energy r. (HERF)
radiography
    body-section r.
    breast specimen r.
    chest r.
    mass miniature r. (MMR)
    specimen r.
    stereoscopic r.
radiohumeral bursitis
radioimmunoassay (RIA)
    r. automation
    sandwich r.
    solid-phase r.
radioimmunodiffusion
radioimmunoelectrophoresis
radioimmunoprecipitation (RIP)
    r. assay (RIPA)
radioimmunosorbent test (RIST)

radioiodinated
r. fatty acid (RIFA)
r. serum albumin
radioiodination
lactoperoxidase r.
radioisotope
r. liver-lung scan for subdiaphragmatic abscess
r. renal excretion test
radioisotopic
r. culture
r. immunoassay
radiolabeled
radiolatum
Trichophyton r.
radioligand assay
radiological
r. agent
chemical, biological, and r. (CBR)
radiologic honeycombing
radiology
forensic r.
medical r.
radiolucency
central r.
soap-bubble r.
radiolysis
radiometer
radiometric antibody detection
Radiomyces
radionecrosis
radionucleotide ventriculography
radionuclide
r. body burden
transuranic r.
radionuclidic purity
radiopaque medium
radiopharmaceutical
radioreceptor assay (RRA)
radioresistant
radioresistens
Acinetobacter r.
radioresponsiveness
radiosensitivity
r. of specialized cell
r. test (RST)
radiostable water
radiostrontium
radiotherapy
chemotherapy and r. (chemrad)
preoperative r. (preRx)

radiotolerans
Kineococcus r.
Methylobacterium r.
radium necrosis
radius
r. of resolution
thrombocytopenia-absent r. (TAR)
r. of view
radix, pl. **radices**
r. pili
r. point
radon
RADS
reactive airways dysfunction syndrome
RAE
right atrial enlargement
RAEB
refractory anemia with excess of blasts
RAEBT
refractory anemia with excess blasts in transition
Raeder paratrigeminal syndrome
RAF
rheumatoid arthritis factor
Raffaelea
raffinose
ragocyte (RA)
r. cell
RAG-1, -2 recombinase enzyme system
RAH
regressing atypical histiocytosis
right atrial hypertrophy
RAI
radioactive iodide
radioactive iodine
RAI test
Rai
R. classification of chronic lymphocytic leukemia
R. classification of CLL
R. staging
Raillietiella
Raillietina
R. celebensis
R. demerariensis
raillietiniasis
rain
yellow r.
Rainier
hemoglobin R.
raised colony
raisinoid nucleus

NOTES

837

RAIU
> radioactive iodine uptake

Raji
> R. cell
> R. cell line
> R. cell radioimmune assay

Ralstonia
> R. *campinensis*
> R. *insidiosa*
> R. *mannitolilytica*
> R. *metallidurans*
> R. *oxalatica*
> R. *pickettii*
> R. *respiraculi*
> R. *syzygii*
> R. *taiwanensis*

RAM
> right anterior measurement

Raman
> R. microprobe
> R. spectroscopy

Ramaria
ramblicola
> *Idiomarina r.*

Rambourg
> R. chromic acid-phosphotungstic acid stain
> R. periodic acid-chromic methenamine-silver stain

ramex
rami (*pl. of* ramus)
Ramichloridium
ramification
ramify
Ramlibacter
> R. *henchirensis*
> R. *tataouinensis*

Ramond point
ramosa
> *Absidia r.*

ramose
ramosum
> *Clostridium r.*

RAMP
> Rapid Analyte Measurement Platform
> regeneration-associated muscle protease
> RAMP anthrax test
> RAMP biological test system
> RAMP botulinum toxin test
> RAMP heart attack test
> RAMP myoglobin test
> RAMP ricin test
> RAMP smallpox test

Ramsay
> R. Hunt paralysis
> R. Hunt syndrome

Ramsden
> R. eyepiece
> R. ocular

Ramularia destructiva
ramus, pl. **rami**
ranae
> *Aeromonas hydrophila* subsp. *r.*

ranarum
> *Basidiobolus r.*

Ranavirus
RanBP protein
rancid
rancidification
rancidity
random
> r. access immunoassay system
> r. amplified polymorphic DNA analysis (RAPD)
> r. coil
> r. error
> r. genetic drift
> r. mating
> r. number
> r. number generator
> r. plasma glucose test
> r. sample
> r. urine specimen
> r. variable

random-donor platelet concentrate
randomization
randomize
Raney nickel
range
> r. of fire
> r. of motion (ROM)
> semiinterquartile r.

rangeli
> *Trypanosoma r.*

Rangoon beggar's disease
Ranikhet disease
Rank
> Rankine temperature scale

rank
> r. correlation coefficient
> r. sum test

ranked data
Ranke formula
Rankine
> R. temperature scale (Rank)
> R. thermometer

RANKL
> receptor activator of nuclear factor kappa B ligand

Ranson
> R. acute pancreatitis criteria
> R. pyridine silver stain

RANTES
> regulated on activation, normal T expressed and secreted
> RANTES cycle

ranular cyst

Ranvier
>   R. cross
>   R. disc
>   node of R.
>   R. node
>   R. segment

Raoultella
>   *R. ornithinolytica*
>   *R. planticola*
>   *R. terrigena*

Raoult law

RAPD
>   random amplified polymorphic DNA
>   analysis

raphe

Raphidascaris

rapid
>   r. ACTH test
>   R. Analyte Measurement Platform
>   (RAMP)
>   r. antigen uptake into the cytosol
>   enterocytes (RACE)
>   r. corticotropin test
>   r. drug screen multiple drug screen
>   standard kit
>   r. drug screen on-site drug
>   screening
>   r. frozen section technique
>   r. grower
>   r. intraoperative quantitative RT-
>   PCR assessment of tumor marker
>   r. microsatellite analysis
>   R. One single dipstick system
>   R. One single drug screen dipstick
>   r. on-site specimen cytologic
>   evaluation
>   r. plasma reagin (RPR)
>   r. plasma reagin circle card test
>   (RPR-CT)
>   r. recompression-high pressure
>   oxygen (RR-HPO)
>   r. serum amylase test
>   r. susceptibility assay (RSA)
>   r. urease test (RUT)

RapID ANA II test

rapidly
>   r. miscible pool (RMP)
>   r. progressive glomerulonephritis
>   (RPGN)

rapid-lysis mutation

**RapidVUE particle shape and size
analyzer**

RapiTex
>   R. ASO latex agglutination test
>   R. Hp test

Rapoport test

Rappaport
>   R. acinus
>   R. classification

Rapp-Hodgkin syndrome

rapture of the deep

rara
>   lamina r.

rare
>   r. base cutters
>   r. clostridial strain of *Clostridium
>   argentinense*
>   r. clostridial strain of *Clostridium
>   baratii*
>   R. Donor File
>   r. earth element

rarefaction
>   bone r.

Rarobacteraceae

RARS
>   refractory anemia with ringed
>   sideroblasts
>   retinoic acid receptor

RAS
>   renal artery stenosis
>   reticular activating system

ras
>   r. cascade
>   r. gene
>   r. gene family
>   r. oncogene

rash
>   antitoxin r.
>   astacoid r.
>   black currant r.
>   butterfly r.
>   hydatid r.
>   malar r.
>   morbilliform r.
>   Murray Valley r.
>   serum r.
>   socks and gloves petechial r.

Rasmussen aneurysm

RAST
>   radioallergosorbent assay test
>   RAST inhibition

rat
>   black house r.
>   ship r.

NOTES

R

rat *(continued)*
    r. tapeworm
    r. unit (RU)
    r. virus (RV)
    Wistar r.

rat-bite
    r.-b. disease
    r.-b. fever

rate
    acid secretion r.
    adjusted r.
    age-adjusted r.
    age-specific r.
    albumin excretion r. (AER)
    aldosterone excretion r. (AER)
    aldosterone secretion r. (ASR)
    aldosterone secretory r. (ASR)
    amebic prevalence r. (APR)
    attack r.
    basal apoptotic r.
    basal metabolic r. (BMR)
    basal secretory flow r. (BSFR)
    bone formation r. (BFR)
    case fatality r.
    cause-specific death r.
    cerebral cortex perfusion r. (CPR)
    cerebral metabolic r. (CMR)
    cerebrospinal fluid IgG synthesis r.
    circulation r.
    r. constant
    corrected sedimentation r. (CSR)
    cortisol production r. (CPR)
    cortisol secretion r. (CSR)
    count r.
    crude r.
    decay r.
    dose r.
    error r.
    erythrocyte sedimentation r. (ESR)
    failure r.
    flotation r.
    flow r. (FR)
    glomerular filtration r. (GFR)
    incidence r.
    infant mortality r. (IMR)
    inspiratory flow r. (IFR)
    intrauterine growth r. (IUGR)
    maximal inspiratory flow r. (MIFR)
    maximal midexpiratory flow r.
      (MMEFR)
    maximal midflow r. (MMFR)
    maximum expiratory flow r.
      (MEFR)
    metabolic clearance r. (MCR)
    r. meter
    mitotic r.
    morbidity r.
    mortality r. (MR)
    mutation r.

    r. nephelometry
    peak expiratory flow r. (PEFR)
    peak inspiratory flow r. (PIFR)
    peak secretory flow r. (PSFR)
    perinatal mortality r. (PMR)
    pineal secretory r.
    plasma clearance r. (PCR)
    plasma glucose disappearance r.
      (PGDR)
    plasma glucose tolerance r. (PGTR)
    plasma iron turnover r. (PITR)
    prevalence r.
    reaction r.
    red cell iron turnover r.
    renin-release r. (RRR)
    Rourke-Ernstein sedimentation r.
    secondary attack r.
    secretion r. (SR)
    sedimentation r. (sed rate, SR)
    somnolent metabolic r. (SMR)
    specific r.
    standardized r.
    testosterone production r. (TPR)
    tumor mitotic r.
    Westergren sedimentation r.
    Wintrobe sedimentation r.
    work metabolic r. (WMR)
    zeta sedimentation r. (ZSR)

rate-controlling step

ratellina
    Grisonella r.

Rathayibacter
    R. caricis
    R. festucae

Rathke
    R. bundle
    R. cleft cyst
    R. pouch
    R. pouch tumor

rathouisi
    Fasciolopsis r.

rating
    reactivity hazard r.

ratio
    absolute terminal innervation r.
    acid-base r. (A:B)
    activity r.
    adenine-thymine/guanine-cytosine r.
      (AT:GC)
    adenosine 5′-diphosphate/adenosine
      triphosphate r. (ADP:ATP)
    AE1:AE3 antibody r.
    alanine aminotransferase:aspartate
      aminotransferase r. (ALT:AST)
    albumin-globulin r. (A:G)
    amniotic fluid
      lecithin/sphingomyelin r.
    amylase/creatinine clearance r.
      (A:C)

base r.
bile duct-to-portal space r. (BD/BS)
body hematocrit-venous
 hematocrit r. (BH:VH)
bound-free r. (B:F)
branching r.
BUN/creatinine r.
cell-fat r.
cholesterol/phospholipid r. (C:P)
common mode rejection r. (CMRR)
conversion r.
crude mortality r. (CMR)
cumula̗ed activity r.
cytoplasmic r.
de Ritis r.
desmin ensheathment r. (DER)
dextrose nitrogen r. (DN)
fluorescein-to-protein r. (F:P)
free T_4 r.
functional terminal innervation r.
glucose-nitrogen r. (G:N)
granulocyte/erythroid r. (G:E)
grid r.
hazard r. (HR)
helper/suppressor cell r.
IgG r.
IgG:albumin r.
inspiratory:expiratory phase r.
International Normalized R. (INR)
ketogenic/antiketogenic r.
lactate-pyruvate r. (L:P)
lecithin/sphingomyelin r. (L:S)
left-to-right r. (L:R)
mean diameter-thickness r. (MDTR)
monocyte-lymphocyte r. (M:L)
myeloid-erythroid r. (M:E)
net protein r. (NPR)
nuclear-cytoplasmic r.
nuclear-to-cytoplasmic r. (n:c)
nucleolar-nuclear r.
nucleus-to-cytoplasm r.
r. of number of ATPs produced
 to number of atmospheric oxygen
 molecules converted to water
 (P:O)
oil-water r. (O:W)
packing r.
peak-to-total r.
polymorphonuclear-lymphocyte r.
polyunsaturated-to-saturated fatty
 acids r. (P:S)
proportionate morbidity r. (PMR)

proportionate mortality r. (PMR)
protein efficiency r. (PER)
resin-uptake r. (RUR)
reversed albumin-globulin r.
r. scale
selectivity r.
signal to noise r. (S:N)
stalk to basilar artery r.
standard morbidity r. (SMR)
standard mortality r. (SMR)
stimulation r. (SR)
therapeutic r.
thyroid hormone binding r.
 (THBR)
thyroid-to-serum r. (TSR)
T_4/TBG r.
urine-plasma r. (U:P)
ventilation-perfusion r.

RatioVision
 AttoFluor R.
ratkowskyi
 Algoriphagus r.
rat-tail maggot
ratti
 Enterococcus r.
rattus
 Rattus r.
Rattus rattus
ratty edge of germinal center
raubitschekii
 Trichophyton r.
Rauscher leukemia virus
RAV
 Rous-associated virus
ray
 beta r.
 cathode r.
 corresponding r.
 delta r.
 gamma r.
 grenz r.
 medullary r.
Rayer disease
Raymond-Cestan syndrome
Raynaud
 R. disease (RD)
 R. phenomenon
RB
 RB gene
RB1
 retinoblastoma gene

NOTES

RB1 *(continued)*
    RB1 alteration
    RB1 protein transcription factor
RBA
    rose bengal antigen
R-banding stain
RBC
    red blood cell
RBC-ChE
    red blood cell cholinesterase
RBC/hpf
    red blood cells per high-power field
RBCM
    red blood cell mass
RBCs
    e-positive RBCs
RBCV
    red blood cell volume
RBE
    relative biological effectiveness
RBL
    Reid base line
RBP
    retinol-binding protein
Rb tumor suppressor protein
RC
    resistor capacitor
    RC circuit
RCBV
    regional cerebral blood volume
RCC
    red cell count
    renal cell carcinoma
RCC-CC
    clear cell renal cell carcinoma
RCF
    red cell folate
    relative centrifugal force
RCM
    red cell mass
RcoF
    ristocetin cofactor
    RcoF unit
RCS
    reticulum cell sarcoma
RCV
    red cell volume
RD
    Raynaud disease
    resistance determinant
    reticular dysgenesis
Rd
    rutherford
RDD
    radiation dispersal device
    Rosai-Dorfman disease
RDE
    receptor-destroying enzyme

RDI
    rupture-delivery interval
rDNA
    recombinant DNA
    ribosomal DNA
RDS
    respiratory distress syndrome
RDW
    red cell distribution width
RDWr
    reticulocyte distribution width
RE
    regional enteritis
REA
    radiation emergency area
    radioenzymatic assay
    restriction endonuclease analysis
reabsorb
reabsorption
    tubular r.
Reach & Roll cart
reactance
    capacitive r.
    inductive r.
reactant
    acute phase r. (APR)
    limiting r.
reacting
    limes r. (Lr)
reaction
    accelerated r.
    acid r.
    acrosome r.
    acute hemolytic transfusion r.
    acute phase r.
    addition r.
    alkaline r.
    allergic transfusion r.
    alloxan-Schiff r.
    amphoteric r.
    anamnestic r.
    anaphylactic transfusion r.
    anaphylactoid r.
    anoxia r.
    antigen-antibody r.
    antigen-antiglobulin r.
    argentaffin r.
    Arias-Stella r. (ASR)
    Arthus r.
    Ascoli r.
    associative r.
    autoimmune r.
    azo coupling r.
    bacterial transfusion r.
    Bauer r.
    Bence Jones r.
    Berthelot r.
    biuret r.
    Bloch r.

R

blocking antibody r.
Bordet-Gengou r.
Burchard-Liebermann r.
Cannizzaro r.
capsular precipitation r.
Carr-Price r.
cell-mediated r.
r. center
chain r.
Chantemesse r.
chemical r.
chill-fever r.
chloroacetate esterase r.
cholera-red r.
CHR r.
Christeller r.
chromaffin r.
clot r.
cocarde r.
colloidal gold r.
competitive reverse transcription
  polymerase chain r. (cRT-PCR)
complement-fixation r.
constitutional r.
contrast media r.
cross r.
cutaneous r.
cytokeratin antigen-antibody r.
cytotoxic hypersensitivity r.
DAB r.
Dale r.
dark r.
decidual r.
degenerate oligonucleotide primed
  polymerase chain r. (DOP-PCR)
r. of degeneration (DeR, DR)
delayed hemolytic transfusion r.
delayed hypersensitivity r.
depot r.
dermotuberculin r.
diaminobenzidine r.
diazo r.
digitonin r.
diphtheria toxin immunization r.
Dold r.
dopa r.
early r.
Edman r.
Ehrlich benzaldehyde r.
Ehrlich diazo r.
elimination r.
endergonic r.

endogenous antigen cell-bound
  antibody r.
endogenous antigen-circulating
  antibody r.
endogenous antigen-transferred cell-
  bound antibody r.
enthalpy of r.
exergonic r.
false-negative r.
false-positive r.
febrile nonhemolytic transfusion r.
  (FNHTR)
Felix-Weil r. (FWR)
Fenton r.
Fernandez r.
ferric chloride r. of epinephrine
Feulgen r.
first-order r.
fixation r.
flocculation r. (FR)
focal r.
foreign body r.
Forssman antigen-antibody r.
Frei-Hoffmann r.
fuchsinophil r.
Fujiwara r.
furfural r.
galactose oxidase Schiff r.
gapped ligase chain r.
gel diffusion r.
Gell and Coombs r.
generalized Sanarelli-Shwartzman r.
  (GSSR)
generalized Shwartzman r. (GSR)
Gerhardt r.
giant cell r.
glycine-arginine r.
graft versus host r. (GVHR)
Grimelius argyrophil r.
group r.
Gruber-Widal r.
Haber-Weiss r.
hemoclastic r.
hemolytic transfusion r. (HTR)
Henle r.
Herxheimer r.
heterophil antigen r.
highly complex series of r.
hypersensitivity r., type I–IV
r. of identity
idiosyncratic r.
immediate hypersensitivity r.

NOTES

reaction *(continued)*
immune complex-mediated
  hypersensitivity r.
immune inflammatory r.
incompatible blood transfusion r.
inflammatory r.
intense inflammatory r.
r. intermediate
intracutaneous r.
intradermal r. (IDR)
iodate r. of epinephrine
iodine r. of epinephrine
irreversible r.
Jaffe r.
Jarisch-Herxheimer r.
Jones-Mote r.
Klebanoff r.
Langhans type of giant cell r.
late r.
Leder r.
lepromin r.
leukemoid r.
leukoerythroblastic r.
Liebermann-Burchard r.
ligase chain r. (LCR)
light r. (LR)
local r.
localized Schwartzman r.
Loewenthal r.
lymphocytic leukemoid r.
Marchi r.
Meinicke turbidity r. (MTR)
miostagmin r.
Mitsuda r.
mixed agglutination r.
mixed lymphocyte r. (MLR)
mixed lymphocyte culture r.
monocytic leukemoid r.
myelocytic leukemoid r.
Nadi r.
Nagler r.
Nessler r.
Neufeld r.
Nickerson-Kveim test r.
ninhydrin r.
ninhydrin-Schiff r.
nitritoid r.
osteoclastic r.
oxidase r.
oxidation-reduction r.
Pandy r.
r. of partial identity
PAS r.
passive Arthus r.
passive cutaneous anaphylactic r.
Paul r.
peracetic acid-Schiff r.
performic acid r.
performic acid-Schiff r.

periodic acid-Schiff r.
Perls r.
peroxidase r.
photochemical r.
Pirquet r.
PK r.
plasmal r.
plasmocytic leukemoid r.
polymerase chain r. (PCR)
Porter-Silber r.
Prausnitz-Küstner r.
precipitin r.
Price precipitation r. (PPR)
primary r.
propagating nuclear r.
prozone r.
quanti-Pirquet r. (QP)
quellung r.
r. quotient
r. rate
reagin r.
redox r.
repair chain r.
reversed Prausnitz-Küstner r.
reverse transcriptase polymerase
  chain r. (RT-PCR)
reverse transcription polymerase
  chain r.
rheumatoid factor r.
Sakaguchi r.
Sanarelli-Shwartzman r.
Schmorl r.
Schultz r.
Schultz-Charlton r.
Schultz-Dale r.
second-order r.
sedimentation r.
Selivanoff r.
serum r.
Shwartzman r.
sigma r. (SR)
skin r.
so-called false-positive r.
specific r.
streptococcal toxin immunization r.
substitution r.
symptomatic r.
Szent-Györgyi r.
tetanus toxin immunization r.
thermoprecipitin r.
r. time (RT)
transcription-based chain r.
transferred antigen-cell-bound
  antibody r.
transferred antigen-transferred
  antibody r.
transfusion r.
Treponema pallidum
  immobilization r.

triketohydrindene r.
Trinder r.
tuberculin r.
tuberculin-type r.
type I–IV delayed-type r.
type I–IV hypersensitivity r.
typhoid immunization r.
unpredictable hypersensitivity-like r.
vaccinoid r.
Voges-Proskauer r.
von Kossa r.
Wassermann r.
Weidel r.
Weil-Felix r. (WFR)
Weinberg r.
wheal-and-erythema r.
wheal-and-flare r.
Widal r.
Yorke autolytic r.
zero-order r.
Zimmermann r.

reactivate
reactivation
dark r.
reactive
r. airways dysfunction syndrome (RADS)
r. astrocyte
atypical favor r.
r. cell
r. change
r. ductal proliferation
r. eosinophilic pleuritis (REP)
r. follicular hyperplasia
r. hyperemia (RH)
r. hyperemia blood flow (RHBF)
r. lymphocytes
r. material
r. oxygen metabolite (ROM)
r. oxygen species (ROS)
r. perforating collagenosis (RPC)
r. protein (RP)
r. spindle cell nodule (RSCN)
r. thrombocytosis
weakly r. (WR)
reactivity
CK20 r.
r. hazard rating
juxtanuclear Golgi r.
nonspecific bronchial r. (NSBR)
reactone red test

reactor
biologic false-positive r. (BFR)
readability
reader
Affinity multimode plate r.
Bio-Tek EIx800 plate r.
Cardiac R.
mark sense r.
reading
albumin r.
r. frame
r. frame shift mutation
Readit SNP genotyping system
readout
readthrough
re-aerosolization
reagent
Advia Centaur anti-HBs r.
Advia Centaur HBc IgM r.
analyte-specific r. (ASR)
analytical r. (AR)
Benedict-Hopkins-Cole r.
Bial r.
CellProbe cytoenzymology r.
chlorous acid r.
Cleland r.
Coleman-Schiff r.
CRPH high-sensitivity C-reactive protein r.
diazo r.
DNA synthesis r.
Drabkin r.
Edlefsen r.
Ehrlich diazo r.
Elecsys RBC folate hemolyzing r.
Eosinofix r.
Esbach r.
Folin-Ciocalteu r.
Fouchet r.
FPN r.
Frohn r.
furfural r.
Girard r.
gold chloride r.
r. grade
Gram-Sure r.
Griess r.
Günzberg r.
Hahn oxine r.
Hammarsten r.
Hanker-Yates r.
Horm collagen r.

R

NOTES

reagent *(continued)*
    Ilosvay r.
    immunoassay r.
    immunochemistry r.
    immunohistochemistry r.
    IntraPrep permeabilization r.
    IOPath immunohistochemistry r.
    Kasten fluorescent Schiff r.
    KP1 immunohistochemical r.
    Life Technologies TRIzol r.
    LipoClear Plus lipemia clearing r.
    Lloyd r.
    lysing r.
    MAK6 immunohistochemical r.
    Mandelin r.
    Marme r.
    Marquis r.
    maximum impurities r.
    Mecke r.
    Millon r.
    Nanoprobes GoldEnhance r.
    Nanoprobes Nanogold r.
    Nichols r.
    OptiLyse lysing r.
    Pappenheim r.
    Paramax r.
    PTT-LA r.
    r. red blood cell
    Rosenthaler-Turk r.
    Sanger r.
    Schaer r.
    Scheibler r.
    Schiff r.
    Selivanoff r.
    Sickledex r.
    Stravigen immunohistochemical r.
    streptavidin-Nanogold r.
    r. strip
    Sulkowitch r.
    test r.
    TRIzol r.
    Vectabond r.
    Vectastain immunohistochemical r.
    Vector Elite r.

reagin
    atopic r.
    automated r.
    rapid plasma r. (RPR)
    r. reaction
    unheated serum r. (USR)

reaginic antibody

REAL
    Revised European-American Lymphoma
    REAL classification

real number

real-time
    r.-t. clock
    r.-t. reverse-transcriptase PCR

reanneal

rearrangement
    bcl-2 gene r.
    breakpoint cluster region r.
    clonal gene r.
    immunoglobulin gene r.
    promiscuous antigen receptor
      gene r.

reassignment
    gender r.

reassociation
    DNA r.

Réaumur
    R. scale (R)
    R. thermometer

rebiopsy
rebound thrombocytosis
Rebuck skin window technique
recalcification time
receiver operating characteristic (ROC)
recent
    r. embolus
    r. infarct
    r. thrombus

receptogram pattern
receptoma
receptor
    r. activator of nuclear factor kappa
      B ligand (RANKL)
    alpha adrenergic r.
    antiasialoglycoprotein r.
    antiestrogen r.
    antiprogesterone r.
    asialoglycoprotein r. (ASGPR)
    r. assay
    autocrine motility factor r. (AMFR)
    B-cell antigen r.
    beta adrenergic r.
    bombesin r.
    calcitonin receptor-like r.
    calcium-sensing r.
    cell surface r.
    c-kit r.
    c-mp1 r.
    complement r. (CR)
    complement r. 3 (CR3)
    discoidin domain r. (DDR)
    endothelin-A, -B r. ,
    epidermal growth factor r. (EGFR)
    estradiol r.
    estrogen r. (ER)
    Fc r.
    fMLP r.
    folic acid r.
    glucocorticoid r. (GR)
    glycoprotein r.
    G protein-linked r.
    hormonal r.
    hormone r.
    human epidermal growth r. 2

hyperactive glutamate r.
J r.
juxtapulmonary-capillary r.
kainate r.
kappa opioid r. (KOR)
killer immunoglobulin-like r. (KIR)
laminin r.
low-affinity nerve growth factor r.
 (LNGFR)
low density lipoprotein r.
lymphatic endothelial hyaluronan r.
 (LYVE1)
lymphocyte homing r.
mineralocorticoid r.
M3 muscarinic acetylcholine r.
muscarinic r.
neurotransporter r.
neurotrophic tyrosine kinase r.,
 type 1 (NTRK1)
Notch r.
peroxisome proliferator-activated r.
 (PPAR)
progesterone r. (PgR, PR)
prolactin r.
protease-activated r. (PAR)
PTCH r.
retinoic acid r. (RARS)
retinoid X r. (RXR)
ryanodine r.
scavenger r.
sensory r.
serotonergic r.
serum soluble transferrin r.
r. site
soluble interleukin-2 r.
soluble NSF-attachment protein r.
 (SNARE)
soluble transferrin r. (sTfR)
somatostatin r.
specific cell r.
steroid hormone r.
stretch r.
T-cell r. (TCR)
T-cell antigen r.
T-cell/E-rosette r.
thrombopoietin r.
transferrin r.
tumor necrosis factor r. (TNFR)
tyrosine kinase r.
r. tyrosine kinase

urokinase plasminogen activator r.
 (uPAR)
vitronectin r.
receptor-destroying enzyme (RDE)
receptor-mediated endocytosis
recessive
 autosomal r.
 r. character
 r. gene
 r. inheritance
recipient
reciprocal
 r. transfusion
 r. translocation
Recklinghausen
 R. disease
 R. disease of bone
 R. tumor
Recklinghausen-Applebaum syndrome
reclotting phenomenon
Reclus disease
recognition
 antigen r.
 r. of antigen
 r. factor
recombinant
 r. DNA (rDNA)
 r. erythropoietin
 r. human insulin-like growth factor
 (rhIGF)
 r. immunoblot assay (RIBA)
 r. platelet-derived growth factor
 (rPDGF)
 r. strain
 r. vaccine
 r. vector
recombination
 r. frequency
 genetic r.
 high-frequency r. (Hfr)
 homologous r.
 meiotic r.
 r. signal sequence (RSS)
RecombiPlasTin thromboplastin
reconditum
 Dipetalonema r.
reconfigurable
reconstruction
 Born method of wax plate r.
record
 dental identification r.
 logical r.

R

NOTES

record *(continued)*
  medical r.
  physical r.
recorded
  not r. (NR)
recorder
recording
  r. electrode
  r. thermometer
recovery
  detect, incident command, scene
    safety and security, assess hazard,
    support required, triage and
    treatment, evacuation, r.
    (DISASTER)
  granulocyte r.
  r. time
recrudescent
  r. typhus
  r. typhus fever
recruitment
  leukocyte r.
recta (*pl. of* rectum)
rectae
  arteriolae r.
  venae r.
rectal
  r. bleeding
  r. column
  r. corticosteroid
  r. shelf tumor
rectale
  Eubacterium r.
recti
  Alcaligenes r.
  folliculi lymphatici r.
  stratum circulare tunicae
    muscularis r.
  stratum longitudinale tunicae
    muscularis r.
  tubuli seminiferi r.
  tunica muscularis r.
rectification
rectifier
  bridge r.
  full-wave r.
  half-wave r.
  silicon-controlled r.
rectitis
rectivirgula
  Saccharopolyspora r.
rectocele
rectocolitis
rectolabial fistula
rectostenosis
rectourethral fistula
rectovaginal fistula
rectovesical fistula
rectovestibular fistula

rectovulvar fistula
rectum, pl. **recta, rectums**
  benign lymphoma of r.
  lymphatic follicle of r.
  vasa recta
rectus
  Campylobacter r.
  tubulus r.
recurrence
  local r.
  r. risk
recurrent
  r. albuminuria
  r. bacterial infection
  r. bouts of nephrotic syndrome
  r. carcinoma
  r. encephalopathy
  r. fetal loss (RFL)
  r. hepatitis C virus infection
  r. inflammation
  r. sinus and pulmonary infection
  r. upper respiratory tract infection
    (RURTI)
  r. vasospasm
recurrentis
  Borrelia r.
recurring digital fibroma of childhood
recursion
recursive
  r. definition
  r. subroutine
recurvatum
  Echinoparyphium r.
  pectus r.
red
  acid r. 87, 91
  alizarin r.
  alizarin r. S
  amidonaphthol r.
  r. atrophy
  Biebrich scarlet r.
  r. blood cell (RBC)
  r. blood cell cast
  r. blood cell cholinesterase (RBC-
    ChE)
  r. blood cell count
  r. blood cell enzyme deficiency
  r. blood cell injury
  r. blood cell mass (RBCM)
  r. blood cell morphology
  r. blood cells per high-power field
    (RBC/hpf)
  r. blood cell survival
  r. blood cell survival time
  r. blood cell volume (RBCV,
    VRBC)
  r. bone marrow
  brilliant vital r.
  calcium r.

r. cell adherence phenomenon
r. cell adherence test
r. cell aplasia
r. cell count (RCC)
r. cell destruction
r. cell diameter width
r. cell distribution width (RDW)
r. cell folate (RCF)
r. cell fragility
r. cell fragmentation syndrome
r. cell indices
r. cell iron turnover rate
r. cell lake
r. cell mass (RCM)
r. cell membrane protein defect
r. cell survival test
r. cell volume (RCV)
chlorophenol r.
chrome r.
Congo r.
r. corpuscle
cresol r.
Darrow r.
r. degeneration
r. eye syndrome
r. fiber
r. half-moon
r. hepatization
r. induration
r. infarct
r. litmus paper
medicinal scarlet r.
methyl r. (MR)
r. mite
r. muscle
r. neuron
neutral r.
r. nucleus of midbrain
r. oil
r. phosphorus (RP)
r. pulp
r. pulp cord
quinaldine r.
ruthenium r.
scarlet r.
scharlach r.
Sirius r.
r. squill
Sudan r. III
r. thrombus
toluylene r.
trypan r.

Turkey r.
r. venous blood (RVB)
vital r.
reddish-blue mottling
reddish-brown infarct
redia, pl. **rediae**
redistribution of body fat
Redlich-Fisher miliary plaques
redox
r. couple
r. indicator
r. potential
r. reaction
Redquant kit
reduce
reduced
r. enamel epithelium
r. Fhit protein expression
r. glutathione
r. hematin
r. hemoglobin (HHb)
r. nicotinamide-adenine dinucleotide
r. penetrance
reducing
r. agent
r. substances in urine
r. sugar
reductant
reductase
acetoacetyl-CoA r.
cytochrome b5 r.
dihydrofolate r. (DHFR)
dihydropteridine r.
epoxide r.
folate r.
glutathione r. (GR)
glyoxylate r.
L-xylulose r.
lysine ketoglutarate r.
lysine-2-oxoglutaryl r.
methemoglobin r.
methylenetetrahydrofolate r.
   (MTHFR)
NADH methemoglobin r.
4-oxoproline r.
oxosteroid r.
pyrroline-5-carboxylate r.
thioredoxin r. (TrxR)
reduction
r. division
r. potential
tetrazolium r. (TR)

NOTES

reduplication of meiotic chromosome
reduvid, reduviid
Reduviidae
Reduvius
redux
    chancre r.
redwater disease
Reed cell
Reed-Hodgkin disease
Reed-Sternberg
    R.-S. cell (RS)
    Hodgkin and R.-S. (HRS)
Reed-variant
    R.-v. cell
    mononuclear R.-v. (MRV)
reentrant pathway
Rees culture medium
Rees-Ecker
    R.-E. fluid
    R.-E. method
Reeve rest
REF
    renal erythropoietic factor
refect
refeeding syndrome
reference
    common r.
    r. distribution
    r. electrode
    r. interval (RI)
    laboratory r. (LR)
    r. laboratory
    r. material
    r. method
    point de repere (point of r.)
    r. strain
    r. value (RV)
Refetoff syndrome
reflectance spectrophotometry
reflecting microscope
reflection
    angle of r.
    diffuse r.
    specular r.
    total internal r.
reflective testing
reflex
    esophagosalivary r.
    gag r.
    Magnus and de Kleijn neck r.
    parachute r.
    Roger r.
    r. sympathetic dystrophy
    viscerotrophic r.
reflexa
    tunica r.
reflexus
    Argas r.

reflux
    biliary r.
    esophageal r.
    r. esophagitis
    r. gastritis
    gastroesophageal r.
    hepatojugular r.
    r. nephropathy
    ureteral r.
    vesicoureteral r.
refluxate
refracting medium
refraction
    angle of r.
    double r.
    index of r.
refractive index (RI)
refractometer
refractometry
refractory
    r. anemia with excess of blasts (RAEB)
    r. anemia with excess blasts in transformation
    r. anemia with excess blasts in transition (RAEBT)
    r. anemia with ringed sideroblasts (RARS)
    r. period (RP)
    r. sideroblastic anemia
refringens
    Borrelia r.
Refsum disease
Regan isoenzyme
Regaud
    R. fixative
    R. pattern of growth
    residual body of R.
regeneration
    atypical r.
    r. cell
    compensatory r.
    epimorphic r.
    morphallactic r.
regeneration-associated muscle protease (RAMP)
regenerative
    r. blood shift
    r. crypt
    r. endometrium
    r. medicine field of research
    r. micronodularity
    r. polyp
regia
    aqua r.
regina
    Phormia r.

regio
> r. olfactoria tunicae
> r. respiratoria tunicae mucosae

region
> abnormal banding r.
> antigen-binding r.
> argyrophilic nucleolar organizer r.
> (AgNOR)
> breakpoint r.
> C r.
> cell-cell contact r.
> centromeric r.
> complementarity determining r.
> (CDR)
> constant r.
> critical r.
> C-terminus r.
> D-loop r.
> hinge r.
> homogeneous staining r. (HSR)
> homology r.
> hypervariable r.
> I r.
> major breakpoint r. (MBR)
> midcervical r.
> midthoracic r.
> minor cluster r. (MCR)
> mutation cluster r. (MCR)
> nucleolar organizing r. (NOR)
> nucleolus organizing r. (NOR)
> promotor r.
> silver-stained nucleolar organizer r.
> (AgNOR)
> silver-stained nucleolar organizing r.
> (AgNOR)
> variable r.

regional
> r. cerebral blood volume (RCBV)
> r. colitis
> r. enteritis (RE)
> r. enterocolitis
> r. granulomatous lymphadenitis
> r. ileitis (RI)
> r. lymph node

register
> index r.
> shift r.

registry
> Agency for Toxic Substances &
> Disease R. (ATSDR)
> Ovarian Tumor R. (OTR)
> tumor r.

Regitine
regressing atypical histiocytosis (RAH)
regression
> absent r.
> r. coefficient (R)
> r. curve
> extensive r.
> focal r.
> least squares r.
> linear r.
> multivariate logistic r.

regressively
> r. transformed follicle
> r. transformed germinal center

regressive staining
regulated
> r. area
> r. on activation, normal T
> expressed and secreted (RANTES)

regulation
> genetic r.
> lipolysis r.

regulator
> autocrine-paracrine growth r.
> autoimmune r. (Aire)
> cell-cycle r.
> current r.
> cystic fibrosis transmembrane
> conductance r. (CFTR)
> r. gene
> r. of G protein signaling protein 5
> (RGS5)
> humoral r.
> r. of invasion
> voltage r.

regulatory
> r. albuminuria
> r. gene
> r. hormone
> myogenic r. (MyoD)
> r. sequence

regurgitation
> aortic r.
> cardiac valvular r.
> r. jaundice
> mitral r.
> tricuspid r.

rehydration
Reibachia agariperforans
Reichmann
> R. disease
> R. syndrome

NOTES

851

Reid
   R. base line (RBL)
   R. index
Reifenstein syndrome
Reinekea marinisedimentorum
reinfection tuberculosis
Reinke
   R. crystal
   R. crystalloid
reinnervation
reinoculation
Reinsch test
Reis-Bücklers corneal lattice dystrophy
Reisseisen muscle
Reissner membrane
Reiter
   R. disease
   R. protein complement-fixation
   (RPCF)
   R. syndrome
Reitland-Franklin (RF)
   R. unit
rejection
   accelerated r.
   acute cellular r.
   acute humoral r.
   acute vascular r.
   allograft r.
   antibody-mediated r.
   chronic allograft r.
   first-set graft r.
   graft r.
   homograft r.
   hyperacute r.
   kidney transplant r.
   primary r.
   second-set graft r.
   transplant r.
rejuvenescence
relapsing
   r. disease
   r. febrile nodular panniculitis
   r. fever
   r. pancreatitis
   r. perichondritis
   r. polychondritis
relation
   Duane-Hunt r.
   equivalence r.
relationship
   host-parasite r.
relative
   r. biological effectiveness (RBE)
   r. centrifugal force (RCF)
   r. erythrocytosis
   r. fluorescence (RF)
   r. hepatic dullness (RHD)
   r. immunity
   r. leukocytosis
   r. polycythemia
   r. refractory period (RRP)
   r. retention time
   r. risk
   r. sagittal depth (RSD)
   r. sensitivity
   r. specific activity (RSA)
   r. specificity
   r. standard deviation (RSD)
   r. value index (RVI)
relaxin
relay
   mercury-wetted r.
release
   clandestine aerosol r.
   renin r. (RR)
releasing
   r. factor (RF)
   r. hormone (RH)
REM
   reticular erythematous mucinosis
   REM syndrome
remains
   commingled r.
   disposition of victim r.
   human r.
Remak
   R. fiber
   R. paralysis
remanantlike lipoprotein particle (RLP)
remission
   partial r. (PR)
   spontaneous r.
remittent
   r. malaria
   r. malarial fever
remnant
   allantoic duct r.
   Cloquet canal r.
   mesonephric r.
   omphalomesenteric duct r.
   sinus venosus r.
remnantlike lipoprotein particles-cholesterol (RLP-C)
remodeling
remotely controlled bomb
removal
   adduct r.
   wax r.
renal
   r. abscess
   r. adenocarcinoma
   r. agenesis
   r. amyloidosis
   r. angiomyolipoma
   r. artery arteriosclerosis
   r. artery stenosis (RAS)
   r. atheroembolic disease
   r. azotemia

r. blockade
r. calculus
r. capsule
r. carbuncle
r. carcinosarcoma
r. cast
r. cell carcinoma (RCC)
r. clear cell carcinoma
r. colic
r. column
r. corpuscle
r. cortex
r. cortical adenoma
r. cortical lobule
r. cortical necrosis
r. cyst
r. cystic disease
r. diabetes
r. dysplasia complex
r. erythropoietic factor (REF)
r. failure
r. fascia
r. function study (RFS)
r. function test
r. glycosuria
r. hamartoma
r. hemangioma
r. hematuria
r. hemorrhage
r. hypertension
r. hypoplasia
r. infarction
r. insufficiency
r. labyrinth
r. medullary necrosis
r. obstruction
r. oncocytoma
r. osteodystrophy
r. papillae
r. papillary necrosis
r. plasma flow (RPF)
r. pressor substance (RPS)
r. rickets
r. schwannoma
r. shutdown
r. threshold
r. threshold for glucose
r. transplant
r. tuberculosis
r. tubular acidosis (RTA)
r. tubular epithelial (RTE)
r. tubular epithelial cell

r. tumor
r. uriniferous tubule
r. vascular resistance (RVR)
r. vein renin activity (RVRA)
r. vein renin concentration (RVRC)
r. vein thrombosis (RVT)
r. venous renin assay (RVRA)

renale
Corynebacterium r.
Dioctophyma r.

renales
columnae r.

renalis
area cribrosa papillae r.
cortex r.
fascia r.
hilum r.
lobulus corticalis r.
papillae r.

renal-retinal dysplasia
renaturation
DNA r.
Renaut body
Rendu-Osler-Weber
R.-O.-W. disease
R.-O.-W. syndrome
reniculus, pl. **reniculi**
reniform
r. nucleus
renin
r. assay
r. release (RR)
r. secreting tumor
r. stimulation test
renin-aldosterone axis
renin-angiotensin-aldosterone system
renin-release rate (RRR)
renis
arteriae arcuatae r.
capsula adiposa r.
corpusculum r.
ectopia r.
foramina papillaria r.
pars convoluta lobuli corticalis r.
pars radiata lobuli corticalis r.
porta r.
tunica fibrosa r.
venulae rectae r.
venulae stellatae r.
rennin
renomedullary interstitial cell tumor
renomegaly

NOTES

renovascular hypertension
Renpenning syndrome
Renshaw cell
REON
    renal epithelioid oxyphilic neoplasm
Reoviridae
Reovirus
reovirus-like agent
reovirus types 1, 2, 3
REP
    reactive eosinophilic pleuritis
repair
    r. chain reaction
    density-dependent r.
    DNA r.
    fibrous r.
    mismatch r. (MMR)
    postoperative r.
    primary r.
    secondary r.
    tendon r.
reparative giant cell granuloma
repeat
    dinucleotide r.
    interspersed r.'s
    inverted r.
    mononucleotide r.
    tandem trinucleotide r.
    trinucleotide r.
    triplet r.
    variable number of tandem r.'s
     (VNTR)
repeatability
    wavelength r.
repeated DNA sequence
repens
    Aspergillus r.
    dermatitis r.
    Dirofilaria r.
    erythema gyratum r.
reperfusion injury
repertoire
    HLA sequence in NK r.
    KIR sequence in NK r.
repetitive stimulation
replacement
    aortic valve r. (AVR)
    r. bone
    r. fibrosis
replenisher
replica
    freeze-fracture r.
    r. grating
replicase
    Q beta r.
replicate punch
replication
    r. bubble
    r. cycle

r. fork
local r.
normal r.
self-sustained sequence r. (3SR)
r. and transfer (RTF)
replicative
    r. form
    r. state
replicator
replicon
repolarization
repression
    catabolite r.
    end-product r.
    enzyme r.
    negative control r.
    positive control r.
repressor gene
reproducibility
    photometric r.
reproduction
    asexual r.
    sexual r.
reproductive cell
reptilase
    r. fibrin
    r. time
reptilase-R time
Reptilia
repullulation
repulsion
RER
    rough endoplasmic reticulum
RER⁺ phenotype
RES
    reticuloendothelial system
resazurin
rescue
    marker r.
research
    histocytologic r.
    regenerative medicine field of r.
resection
    laparoscopic renal r.
    surgical r.
    total gastric r.
reserve
    r. cell
    r. cell carcinoma
    r. cell hyperplasia
reservoir
    chromatin r.
    r. host
    r. of infection
    rodent r.
    r. of virus
resident cell
residua (*pl. of* residuum)

residual
r. abscess
r. air
r. body
r. body of Regaud
r. carcinoma
r. cleft
r. lumen
r. lung capacity (RLC)
r. urine
r. volume (RV)
residue
amino acid r.
gunshot r. (GSR)
methanol-extruded r. (MER)
nucleotide r. (NR)
organized old thrombotic r.
punctate nitrate r.
spill r.
residuum, pl. **residua**
gastric residua
resin
anion-exchange r.
cation exchange r.
Chelex r.
cholestyramine r.
Effapoxy r.
Epon-Araldite r.
epoxy r.
Harleco synthetic r.
ion-exchange r.
methacrylate r.
podophyllin r.
polyamine-methylene r.
polyester r.
quinine carbacrylic r.
Spurr r.
r. uptake
Resinicium
resin-uptake ratio (RUR)
resistance
activated protein C r. (APCR)
airway r.
APC r.
bacteriophage r.
cerebrovascular r. (CVR)
chemotherapy r.
r. determinant (RD)
r. factor
r. inducing factor (RIF)
insulin r.
internal r. (IR)

main site of airway r.
multidrug r. (MDR)
multiple drug r. (MDR)
PBP2′ rapid latex test for
 staphylococcus r.
peripheral total r. (PTR)
r. plasmid
pulmonary r. (Rp)
renal vascular r. (RVR)
systemic vascular r. (SVR)
r. thermometer
total peripheral r. (TPR)
total pulmonary vascular r. (TPVR)
r. transfer factor (RTF)
r. transferring episome
r. unit (RU)
vascular r. (VR)
r. to venous return (RVR)
resistivity
resistor
r. capacitor (RC)
carbon r.
carbon-film r.
r. color code
composition r.
power r.
precision r.
trimming r.
variable r.
wire-wound r.
resolution
energy r.
limit of r.
radius of r.
spectral r.
resolved
not r. (NR)
resolvent
resolving
r. power
r. time
resonance
electron paramagnetic r.
electron spin r. (ESR)
r. fluorescence
r. line
resorcin
resorcin-fuchsin
resorcinol
r. phthalic anhydride
r. test
resorcinolphthalein sodium

NOTES

resorption
    alveolar bone r.
    bone r.
    dissection r.
    r. lacunae
    lacunar r.
    osteoclastic r.
    widespread bone r.
resource
    R. Conservation and Recovery Act
    death investigation r.'s
respiraculi
    Ralstonia r.
    Wautersia r.
respiration
    aerobic r.
    anaerobic r.
    Biot r.
    cellular r.
    Kussmaul r.
    Kussmaul-Kien r.
respirator
    air-purifying r. (APR)
    r. brain
    supplied air r. (SAR)
respiratorii
    bronchioli r.
respiratory
    r. acid-base disorder
    r. acidosis
    r. alkalosis
    r. angiocentric lymphoma
    r. bronchiole
    r. bronchiolitis
    r. burst
    r. chain
    r. depression
    r. distress syndrome (RDS)
    r. distress syndrome of newborn
    r. enteric orphan virus
    r. epithelium
    r. exanthematous virus
    r. failure
    r. function
    r. illness (RI)
    r. infection virus
    r. inflammation
    r. insufficiency
    r. lobule
    r. mucosa
    r. pigment
    r. protein
    r. quotient
    r. region of tunica mucosa of
      nose
    r. scleroma
    r. syncytial (RS)
    r. syncytial virus (RSV)
    r. syncytial virus antibody test
    r. syncytial virus antigen
    r. syncytial virus antigen test
    r. syncytial virus infection
    r. syncytial virus nucleic acid
    r. syncytial virus serology
    r. system neoplasm
    Taiwan acute r. (TWAR)
    r. tract
    r. tract fluid (RTF)
    r. tuberculosis
    r. viral disease
Respirovirus
responder
    r. cell
    first r.
response
    anamnestic r.
    biphasic r.
    booster r.
    clinical r.
    concentration-dependent
      nanomolar r.
    delayed-phase skin r.
    dramatic r.
    early-phase r.
    galvanic skin r. (GSR)
    heat shock r.
    host r.
    humoral immune r.
    immediate-phase skin r.
    immune r. (Ir)
    isomorphic r.
    late-phase r.
    lymphoplasmacytic r.
    osteoblastic r.
    photomyoclonic r.
    primary immune r.
    reticulocyte r.
    secondary immune r.
    sensitization r. (SR)
    spectral r.
    stringent r.
    total r. (TR)
    visual evoked r.
responsibility
    safety r.
rest
    aberrant r.
    adrenal r.
    cartilaginous r.
    congenital r.
    embryonal r.
    epithelial r.
    Erdheim r.
    intralobar nephrogenic r. (ILNR)
    Marchand r.
    mesonephric r.
    müllerian r.
    nephrogenic r. (NR)

paramesonephric r.
perilobar nephrogenic r. (PLNR)
Reeve r.
Walthard cell r.
wolffian r.
restiform
resting
r. B cell
r. membrane potential
r. stage
r. wandering cell
restitope
restless legs syndrome
restricted
r. access laboratory
r. light chain
restriction
r. endonuclease
r. endonuclease analysis (REA)
r. enzyme
r. fragment length polymorphism
(RFLP)
r. map
MHC r.
restrictive
r. cardiomyopathy
r. lung disease
restrictus
Azovibrio r.
Dehalobacter r.
restructured cell
restuans
Culex r.
result
fast therapeutic turnaround time
of r.'s
macrophage presented antigen r.
r. of severe fracture
Surveillance, Epidemiology, and
End R.'s (SEER)
resultant distortion of structure
retained
r. foreign body (RFB)
r. placental fragment
r. products of conception
r. testis
retardation
familial mental r. (FMR)
growth r.
Wilms tumor, aniridia, genital
anomalies, mental r. (WAGR)
rete, pl. **retia**

r. cell tumor
r. cord
r. cutaneum corii
r. cyst of ovary
malpighian r.
r. peg
r. ridge
r. subpapillare
r. testis
retention
r. cyst
fluid r.
increased sodium r.
r. index
r. jaundice
mucus r.
r. polyp
r. time
urinary r.
r. volume
retial
retic
reticulocyte
Retic-Chex linearity assay
reticle
ocular r.
reticONE system
reticula (*pl. of* reticulum)
reticular
r. activating system (RAS)
r. cartilage
r. cell
r. degeneration
r. dermis
r. dysgenesis (RD)
r. erythematous mucinosis (REM)
r. fiber
r. fibers in wall of central vein
r. fiber in wall of sinusoid
r. formation
r. growth pattern
r. keratitis
r. lamina
r. layer of corium
r. membrane of spinal organ
r. substance
r. tissue
reticularis
angiitis livedo r.
r. cell
dermatopathia pigmentosa r.
fetal r.

R

NOTES

reticularis *(continued)*
   formatio r.
   livedo r.
   substantia r.
   zona r.
reticulate body
reticulated
   r. bone
   r. corpuscle
   r. erythrocyte
reticulating colliquation
reticulation
   intralobar r.
reticulatum
   atrophoderma r.
reticulatus
   Dermacentor r.
reticulin
   r. fiber
   marrow r.
   r. stain
   r. staining
reticuliscabiei
   Streptomyces r.
reticulocyte (retic)
   r. count
   r. distribution width (RDWr)
   hemoglobin content of r.'s
   r. mean corpuscular volume
      (MCVr)
   r. response
   shift r.
   r. staining
   stress r.
reticulocytic
   r. marrow
   r. production index (RPI)
reticulocytopenia
reticulocytosis
reticuloendothelial
   r. cell
   r. cell hyperplasia
   r. iron stores
   r. sarcoma
   r. system (RES)
reticuloendothelioma
reticuloendotheliosis
   avian r.
   leukemic r.
   systemic r.
reticuloendothelium
reticulofilamentosa
   substantia r.
reticulohistiocytic granuloma
reticulohistiocytoma
reticulohistiocytosis
   multicentric r.
reticuloid
   actinic r.

reticulopenia
reticulosis
   benign inoculation r.
   histiocytic medullary r.
   Ketron-Goodman pagetoid r.
   leukemic r.
   lipomelanic r.
   lipomelanotic r.
   medullary histiocytic r.
   midline malignant reticulosis r.
   myeloid r.
   pagetoid r.
   polymorphic r. (PMR)
   Sézary r.
   Woringer-Kolopp pagetoid r.
reticulum, pl. **reticula**
   agranular endoplasmic r.
   r. cell
   r. cell hyperplasia
   r. cell lymphosarcoma
   r. cell sarcoma (RCS, RSA)
   cistern of cytoplasmic r.
   Ebner r.
   endoplasmic r. (ER)
   Golgi internal r.
   granular endoplasmic r.
   Kölliker r.
   rough endoplasmic r. (RER)
   rough-surfaced endoplasmic r.
   sarcoplasmic r.
   smooth endoplasmic r.
   smooth-surfaced endoplasmic r.
   r. stain
   stellate r.
   trabecular r.
   r. trabeculare sclerae
retiform
   r. hemangioendothelioma
   r. Sertoli-Leydig cell tumor
retina, gen. and pl. **retinae**
   ablatio retinae
   cerebral layer of r.
   cone cell of r.
   ganglion cell of r.
   horizontal cell of r.
   layer of r.
   limiting membrane of r.
   macula retinae
   molecular layer of r.
   neural layer of r.
   neuroepithelial layer of r.
   nuclear layer of r.
   optic part of r.
   ora serrata retinae
   pars optica retinae
   pigment cell of r.
   pigmented layer of r.
   plexiform layer of r.
   rod cell of r.

strata nuclearia externa et interna retinae
stratum cerebrale retinae
stratum moleculare retinae
stratum neuroepitheliale retinae
stratum pigmenti retinae
sustentacular fiber of r.
retinaculum
retinae
retinal
r. anlage tumor
r. aplasia
r. artery occlusion
r. cone
r. detachment
r. disorder
r. embolism
r. microaneurysm
retinalis
lipemia r.
retinitis
r. pigmentosa
r. proliferans
retinoblastoma
r. gene (RB1)
r. protein
retinochoroiditis
r. juxtapapillaris
toxoplasmic r.
retinoic
r. acid
r. acid binding protein 1 gene
r. acid receptor (RARS)
retinoid
r. X receptor (RXR)
r. X receptor alpha
retinol
retinol-binding protein (RBP)
retinopathy
circinate r.
diabetic r. (DR)
r. of prematurity (ROP)
retoperithelium
retort
Retortamonas intestinalis
retothelioma
retractile testis
retraction
r. artifact
clot r.
massive vitreous r. (MVR)

retrieval
antigen r.
epitope r.
heat-induced epitope r. (HIER)
heat-mediated antigen r.
information r.
low-temperature antigen r. (LTAR)
low-temperature, heat-mediated
antigen r. (LTHMAR)
pancreas antigen r.
sonication-induced epitope r. (SIER)
retrobulbar
r. abscess
r. neuropathy
retrocardiac tumor
retrocecal abscess
retrocolic hernia
retroflexion
retrograde
r. chromatolysis
r. degeneration
r. embolism
r. intussusception
r. metamorphosis
r. pyelography
retrogression
retrolental fibroplasia (RLF)
retromammary mastitis
retromorphosis
retroperitoneal
r. fibromatosis
r. fibrosis
r. gas insufflation
retroperitoneum
retroperitonitis
idiopathic fibrous r.
retropharyngeal abscess
retroplacental hematoma
retroplasia
retrospective study
retrosternal
r. hernia
r. tumor
retroversion
retroviral oncogene
Retroviridae
retrovirus
AKT8 r.
jaagsiekte sheep r.
zoonotic r.
Retsch MM200 mixer mill
Rettgerella rettgeri

R

NOTES

rettgeri
  Proteus r.
  Providencia r.
  Rettgerella r.
Rett syndrome
return
  resistance to venous r. (RVR)
Retzius
  calcification line of R.
  R. fiber
  line of R.
  R. line
  R. parallel striae
  sheath of Key and R.
reuniens
  canaliculus r.
  canalis r.
  ductus r.
Reuss
  R. formula
  R. test
revaccination
reverse
  r. agglutination
  r. banding
  r. bias
  r. blood typing
  r. dot-blot
  r. genetics
  r. grouping
  r. hemolytic plaque assay
  r. immunoelectrophoresis
  r. line probe
  r. mutation
  r. passive hemagglutination
  r. passive latex agglutination
  (RPLA)
  r. T_3
  r. transcriptase
  r. transcriptase polymerase chain
  reaction (RT-PCR)
  r. transcription
  r. transcription polymerase chain
  reaction
  r. triiodothyronine (rT_3)
reversed
  r. albumin-globulin ratio
  r. passive anaphylaxis
  r. Prausnitz-Küstner reaction
reversible
  r. calcinosis
  r. change
  r. injury
reversion
revertant
review
  drug utilization r.

revised
  R. European-American Classification
  of Lymphoid Neoplasms
  R. European-American Lymphoma
  classification
revision
  fusiform skin r. (FSR)
Revival Menopause Home Test
revivescence
revolutions per minute (rpm)
revolutum
  Echinostoma r.
revolver
Rexed
  lamina of R.
Reye syndrome
Reynolds
  R. lead citrate
  R. number
  R. pentad
RF
  Reitland-Franklin
  relative fluorescence
  releasing factor
  rheumatic fever
  rheumatoid factor
RFB
  retained foreign body
RFL
  recurrent fetal loss
RFLA
  rheumatoid factor-like activity
RFLP
  restriction fragment length polymorphism
  RFLP Southern hybridization
  analysis
RFS
  renal function study
rgp120 protein
RGS5
  regulator of G protein signaling protein 5
RH
  reactive hyperemia
  releasing hormone
Rh
  rhesus
  Rh agglutinin
  Rh antibody
  Rh antigen
  Rh blocking test
  Rh blood group
  Rh factor
  Rh immunization
  Rh incompatibility
  Rh isoantigen
  Rh isoimmunization syndrome
  Rh negative
  Rh null syndrome
  Rh positive

Rh type
Rh typing
rh
rheumatic
Rhabdiasoidea
Rhabditida
rhabditiform
Rhabditis hominis
rhabdocyte
rhabdoid
r. cell
r. phenotype
r. phenotype of large-cell
carcinoma
r. predisposition
Rhabdomonas
rhabdomyoblast
rhabdomyoblastic differentiation
rhabdomyolysis
acute recurrent r.
familial paroxysmal r.
idiopathic paroxysmal r.
rhabdomyoma
rhabdomyosarcoma (RM, RMS)
alveolar r. (ARMS)
botryoid r.
embryonal r. (ERMS)
r. marker
pleomorphic r.
rhabdosarcoma
Rhabdoviridae
rhabdovirus
Rhadinovirus
rhagades
rhagadiform
rhagiocrine
r. cell
r. vacuole
RHBF
reactive hyperemia blood flow
RHD
relative hepatic dullness
rheumatic heart disease
Rh$_o$(D)
R. immune globulin
R. immunoglobulin
R. typing
Rh$_{null}$ disease
Rheinberg microscope
Rheinheimera
R. baltica
R. pacifica

rhenobacensis
Rhodopseudomonas r.
rheobase
Rheolog device
rheostat
rheostosis
rheotaxis
rheotropism
rhestocythemia
rhesus (Rh)
r. monkey kidney (RMK)
rheum
rheumatic
rheumatic (rh, rheum)
r. arteritis
r. arthralgia
r. carditis
r. endocarditis
r. fever (RF)
r. heart disease (RHD)
r. lung disease
r. myocarditis
r. nodule
r. pericarditis
r. pneumonia
r. pneumonitis
r. valvulitis
rheumatica
polymyalgia r.
rheumatid
rheumatism
articular r.
chronic r.
gonorrheal r.
inflammatory r.
Macleod r.
muscular r.
nodose r.
tuberculous r.
rheumatismal
rheumatoid
r. agglutinator
r. ankylosing spondylitis
r. aortitis
r. arteritis
r. arthritis (RA)
r. arthritis factor (RAF)
r. episcleritis
r. factor (RF)
r. factor-like activity (RFLA)
r. factor reaction
r. factor test

NOTES

rheumatoid *(continued)*
 r. heart disease
 r. lung
 r. neutrophilic dermatosis
 r. nodule
 r. pneumoconiosis
 r. synovitis
rhIGF
 recombinant human insulin-like growth
 factor
rhinaria
 Linguatula r.
rhinitis
 acute r.
 allergic r.
 atrophic r.
 atrophic r. of swine
 fetid r.
 r. nervosa
 nonallergic r.
 seasonal r.
 vasomotor r. (VMR)
rhinoantritis
rhinocerebral
 r. aspergillosis
 r. disease
 r. zygomycosis
Rhinocladiella
Rhinocladium
rhinocleisis
rhinoentomophthoromycosis
rhinoestrosis
Rhinoestrus purpureus
rhinolaryngitis
rhinomucormycosis
rhinomycosis
rhinonecrosis
rhinopharyngitis mutilans
rhinophycomycosis
rhinophyma
rhinopneumonitis
 equine r. (ERP)
rhinoscleroma bacillus
rhinoscleromatis
 Klebsiella pneumonia r.
rhinosporidiosis
Rhinosporidium seeberi
rhinotracheitis
 feline viral r.
 infectious bovine r. (IBR)
Rhinotrichum
Rhinovirus
rhinovirus
 bovine r.
 equine r.
Rhipicentor
rhipicephali
 Rickettsia r.
Rhipicephalus sanguineus

Rhizidiomyces
Rhizidiovirus
Rhizobiaceae
Rhizobieae
Rhizobium
 R. indigoferae
 R. japonicum
 R. larrymoorei
 R. loessense
 R. radiobacter
 R. rhizogenes
 R. rubi
 R. sullae
 R. undicola
 R. vitis
 R. yanglingense
Rhizoctonia
rhizogenes
 Rhizobium r.
Rhizoglyphus parasiticus
rhizoid
rhizomelia
Rhizomucor
rhizophila
 Kocuria r.
 Stenotrophomonas r.
rhizoplast
rhizopod
Rhizopoda
Rhizopodasida
Rhizopodea
rhizopodoformis
 Rhizopus r.
Rhizopus
 R. arrhizus
 R. equinus
 R. niger
 R. nigricans
 R. oryzae
 R. rhizopodoformis
Rhizosphaera
rhizosphaerae
 Pseudomonas r.
rhizosphaericus
 Streptomyces r.
rhizospherae
 Agromyces r.
rhodamine
 r. B
 lissamine r. B 200
 r. stain
rhodanate
rhodanic acid
rhodanile blue
Rhodanobacter lindaniclasticus
Rhodesian trypanosomiasis
rhodesianum
 Methylobacterium r.

rhodesiense
    Trypanosoma brucei r.
rhodina
    Botryosphaeria r.
rhodinum
    Methylobacterium r.
Rhodnius prolixus
Rhodobaca bogoriensis
Rhodobacteria
Rhodoblastus acidophilus
Rhodocista pekingensis
Rhodococcus
    R. *aetherivorans*
    R. *baikonurensis*
    R. *equi*
    R. *gordoniae*
    R. *jostii*
    R. *koreensis*
    R. *maanshanensis*
    R. *pyridinivorans*
Rhodoferax
    R. *antarcticus*
    R. *ferrireducens*
Rhodoglobus vestalii
Rhodomyces
rhodophylactic
rhodophylaxis
Rhodophyllus sinuatus
Rhodopirellula baltica
Rhodopseudomonas
    R. *faecalis*
    R. *rhenobacensis*
rhodopsin
Rhodospirillaceae
Rhodospirillales
Rhodosporidium
Rhodotorula
    R. *mucilaginosa*
    R. *rubra*
rhodotorulosis
rho factor
RhoGAM vaccine
rhombencephalitis
rhombic lip
rhombocele
rhomboidal sinus
Rhombomys
rhopheocytosis
rhoptry protein
Rhus
    R. *toxicodendron* antigen
    R. *venenata* antigen

rhusiopathiae
    Actinomyces r.
    Erysipelothrix r.
rhypophagy
rhysodes
    Acanthamoeba r.
rhythm
    circadian r.
    infradian r.
    isochronal r.
    metachronal r.
    ultradian r.
rhytidosis
RI
    reference interval
    refractive index
    regional ileitis
    respiratory illness
RIA
    radioimmunoassay
    CA15-3 RIA
rib
    beading of r.'s
RIBA
    recombinant immunoblot assay
    RIBA 1, 2, 3
Ribas-Torres disease
ribavirin
Ribbert theory
ribbon stool
riboflavin
    r. assay
    r. loading test
    r. unit
riboflavin-5′-phosphate
ribonuclear protein (RNP)
ribonuclease (RNase, RNAse)
    r. (pancreatic)
    pancreatic r.
    r. protection assay
    r. solution
ribonucleic acid (RNA)
ribonucleoprotein (RNP)
    r. antibody test
    r. complex
    small nuclear r.'s (SNRPs)
ribonucleoside
ribonucleoside-5′-phosphate
    thymine r.
ribonucleotide
riboprobe
    digoxigenin-labeled r.

NOTES

863

riboprobe *(continued)*
    EBER1 r.
    U6 r.
ribose
ribose-1-phosphate
ribose-5-phosphate
ribosomal
    r. ambiguity
    r. DNA (rDNA)
    r. RNA (rRNA)
ribosome
    disaggregated r.
    free r.
ribosome-lamella complex
ribosuria
ribothymidylic acid
ribotyping
ribovirus
ribulose
ribulose-5-phosphate
rice
    r. blast
    r. body
    r. starch
rice-flour breath test
rice-Tween agar
rice-water stools
Richard-Allan Scientific Ultrafast Papanicolaou stain
richardsiae
    Phialophora r.
Richards-Rundle syndrome
Richet aneurysm
Richter
    R. hernia
    R. syndrome
ricin A, B chain
ricinoleic acid
ricinus
    Ixodes r.
Ricinus communis
rickets
    acute r.
    adult r.
    celiac r.
    hemorrhagic r.
    hypophosphatemic r.
    renal r.
    vitamin-D-dependent r.
    vitamin-D-resistant r.
rickettsi
    Dermacentroxenus r.
Rickettsia
    R. *aeschlimannii*
    R. *africae*
    R. *akari*
    R. *australis*
    R. *conorii*
    R. *felis*

    R. *honei*
    R. *japonica*
    R. *massiliae*
    R. *montana*
    R. *pediculi*
    R. *prowazekii*
    R. *rhipicephali*
    R. *rickettsii*
    R. *sennetsu*
    R. *sibirica*
    R. *slovaca*
    R. *tsutsugamushi*
    R. *typhi*
Rickettsiaceae
Rickettsiales
rickettsial infection
rickettsialpox
rickettsia vaccine, attenuated
Rickettsieae
rickettsii
    Rickettsia r.
rickettsiosis
rickettsiostatic
Ricketts organism
RID
    radial immunodiffusion
    RID assay
Rida virus
Rideal-Walker
    R.-W. coefficient
    R.-W. method
ridge
    epidermal r.
    gonadal r.
    interpapillary r.
    r. of intramembranous particle
    mucosal r.
    rete r.
    skin r.
riding embolism
Riechert-Mundiger stereotactic device
Riedel
    R. disease
    R. struma
    R. thyroiditis
Rieder
    R. cell
    R. cell leukemia
    R. lymphocyte
Rieger syndrome
Riehl melanosis
RIF
    resistance inducing factor
RIFA
    radioiodinated fatty acid
rifamycinica
    Amycolatopsis r.
rifietoensis
    Planococcus r.

R

rifling impression
Rift
    R. Valley fever
    R. Valley fever virus
Riga-Fede disease
Rigg disease
right
    r. anterior measurement (RAM)
    r. atrial enlargement (RAE)
    r. atrial hypertrophy (RAH)
    r. axis deviation (RAD)
    deviation to the r.
    r. and left fibrous rings of heart
    r. lower quadrant
    r. ovarian vein syndrome
    shield to the r.
    shift to the r.
    r. ventricle double outlet
    r. ventricular dysplasia
    r. ventricular enlargement (RVE)
    r. ventricular failure
    r. ventricular hypertrophy (RVH)
    r. ventricular hypoplasia
right-handed alpha helix
right-sided lesion
right-to-know law
rigidity
    decerebrate r.
    lead-pipe r.
    muscular r.
    nuchal r.
    postmortem r.
rigor mortis
rigorous
RIHSA
    radioactive iodinated human serum
    albumin
Riley-Day syndrome
Riley-Smith syndrome
RIM
    RIM A.R.C. Mono test
rim
    abrasion r.
    r. pattern
    r. of scant cytoplasm
Rimini test
rinderpest virus
Rindfleisch cell
ring
    abrasion r.
    aromatic r.
    Balbiani r.

    Bandl r.
    Biondi r.
    r. chromosome
    connecting r.
    contractile r.
    corrin r.
    r. counter
    esophageal r.
    F-actin r.
    Fleischer r.
    r. form
    r. granuloma
    Kayser-Fleischer r.
    Liesegang r.
    lower r.
    mesangial r.
    r. mosaic
    nipple arranged in a r.
    r. precipitin test
    Schatzki r.
    signet r.
    vascular r.
    Waldeyer r.
ring-chain tautomer
ringed sideroblast
Ringer
    R. injection
    R. irrigation
    R. lactate solution (RLS)
    R. mixture
ringeri
    Paragonimus r.
ring-wall lesion
ringworm
    r. of beard
    black-dot r.
    r. of body
    crusted r.
    r. of foot
    r. of genitocrural region
    gray-patch r.
    honeycomb r.
    r. of nails
    Oriental r.
    r. of scalp
    scaly r.
    Tokelau r.
Rinkel test
Rinne test (R)
riot
    r. control
    r. control agent

NOTES

RIP
  radioimmunoprecipitation
RIPA
  radioimmunoprecipitation assay
ripening
ripple
    r. counter
    r. factor
    r. voltage
RISA
  radioactive iodinated serum albumin
  RISA test
RISHN
  radiation-induced sarcoma of the head
  and neck
risk
    CDC Category A biological agents
    (the highest r.)
    CDC Category B biological agents
    (next highest r.)
    CDC Category C biological agents
    (third highest r.)
    r. factor
    Gail index of breast cancer r.
    r. group stratification
    recurrence r.
    relative r.
risk-adapted therapy
RIST
  radioimmunosorbent test
risticii
    Ehrlichia r.
    Neorickettsia r.
ristocetin cofactor (RcoF)
Ritter disease
Ritter-Oleson (RO)
  R. technique
rittmannii
    Alicyclobacillus acidocaldarius
    subsp. *rittmannii*
**ritual ligature strangulation
  (incaprettamento)**
RIU
  radioactive iodine uptake
river blindness
Rivinus
    R. duct
    R. gland
rivolta
    Isospora r.
riziform
RLC
  residual lung capacity
RLF
  retrolental fibroplasia
RLP
  remanantlike lipoprotein particle

RLP-C
  remnantlike lipoprotein particles-
  cholesterol
**RLP-Cholesterol Immunoseparation
  Assay kit**
RLS
  Ringer lactate solution
RLT
  reactive lymphoid tissue
RM
  rhabdomyosarcoma
RMK
  rhesus monkey kidney
RMP
  rapidly miscible pool
RMS
  rhabdomyosarcoma
RMSF
  Rocky Mountain spotted fever
RNA
  ribonucleic acid
    chromosomal RNA (cRNA)
    Epstein-Barr encoded RNA (EBER)
    expressed RNA
    heterogeneous nuclear RNA
      (hnRNA)
    hMAM RNA
    nucleolar RNAs
    RNA nucleotidyltransferase
    RNA polymerase
    RNA processing
    ribosomal RNA (rRNA)
    short-interference RNA (siRNA)
    RNA splicing
    transfer RNA (tRNA)
    translation control RNA (tcRNA)
    RNA tumor virus
RNA-driven hybridization
RNA-RNA hybridization
RNase, RNAse
  ribonuclease
    RNase A
    alkaline RNase
    RNase I
    pancreatic RNase
RNase-free condition
RNAzol
    R. B RNA extraction method
    R. Reagent Extractor
RNP
  ribonuclear protein
  ribonucleoprotein
    RNP complex
RO
  Ritter-Oleson
Roaf syndrome
robertsiae
    Wingea r.
robertsonian translocation

Roberts syndrome
Robiginitalea biformata
Robin
    R. sequence
    R. syndrome
Robinow syndrome
Robinson disease
Roble disease
robot
    ORCA R.
Robson
    R. point
    R. stage I, II renal carcinoma
robustum
    Ketogulonicigenium r.
robustus
    Atrax r.
    Gordius r.
ROC
    receiver operating characteristic
    ROC curve
roccellin
Rochalimaea
    R. henselae
    R. quintana
Roche
    R. Septi-Chek blood culture system
    R. Sysmex hematology system
rocker microtome
rocket immunoelectrophoresis
rocking microtome
Rocky
    R. Mountain spotted fever (RMSF)
    R. Mountain spotted fever antibody
    test
    R. Mountain spotted fever serology
    R. Mountain spotted fever vaccine
rod
    anaerobic r.
    Auer r.
    r. cell of retina
    Corti r.
    r. disc
    enamel r.
    r. fiber
    r. granule
    motile r.
    r. myopathy
    nemaline r.
    r. neutrophil
    r. nuclear cell
    r. photoreceptor cell

    policeman glass stirring r.
    r. shaped bacterium
    slightly curved r.
    spore-forming r.
    straight r.
rodent
    r. reservoir
    r. ulcer
rodenticide
rodentium
    Veillonella parvula subsp. *r.*
Rodrigues aneurysm
rod-shaped
    r. polymer
    r. structure
roetheln
Roger
    R. disease
    maladie de R.
    R. reflex
    R. syndrome
Rohr stria
Rokitansky
    R. disease
    R. pelvis
    R. protuberance
Rokitansky-Aschoff sinus
Rokitansky-Küster-Hauser syndrome
rolandic epilepsy
Rolando
    R. cell
    R. fissure
    R. gelatinous substance
role
    prognostic r.
roll
    iliac r.
    scleral r.
    r. tube
    r. tube technique
rolled sample
Rollet stroma
rolling hernia
ROM
    range of motion
    reactive oxygen metabolite
    rupture of membranes
Romaña
    R. sign
    R. sign/trill
Roman bridge formation
Romano-Ward syndrome

NOTES

R

Romanowsky, Romanovsky
    R. blood stain
    R. type stain
Romanowsky-Giemsa stain
Romberg
    R. disease
    R. syndrome
    R. trophoneurosis
rombergism
romeroi
    Pyrenochaeta r.
Römer test
Rommelaere sign
ronds
    corps r.
ronnel
room
    cold r.
    decontaminating r.
    negative-pressure r.
    r. temperature (RT)
root
    axon of anterior r.
    dorsal nerve r.
    ganglion cell of dorsal spinal r.
    hair r.
    mandrake r.
    nerve r.
    posterior nerve r.
    r. sheath
rootlet of spinal nerve
root-mean-square
ROP
    retinopathy of prematurity
ropalocytosis
Ropes test
ropey collagen
ROS
    reactive oxygen species
rosa
    Novosphingobium r.
rosacea
    acne r.
rosacea-like tuberculid
Rosai-Dorfman disease (RDD)
rosanilin dye
rosaniline
rosary
    rachitic r.
    scorbutic r.
rosati
rosatii
    Neotestudina r.
rose
    r. bengal
    r. bengal antigen (RBA)
    r. bengal radioactive ^{131}I test
    r. bengal sodium
    r. cold

rosea
    pityriasis r.
Rose-Bradford kidney
Roseburia intestinalis
Roseibium
    R. denhamense
    R. hamelinense
roseiflava
    Sphingomonas r.
Roseiflexus
    R. castenholzii
Roseinatronobacter
    R. thiooxidans
Roseivivax
    R. halodurans
    R. halotolerans
Rosellinia
Rosenbach
    R. disease
    R. syndrome
    R. test
Rosenbach-Gmelin test
rosenbergii
    Hyphomonas r.
Rosen criteria for lymphovascular invasion
Rosenmüller
    R. gland
    R. node
Rosenow veal-brain broth
Rosenthal
    R. fiber
    R. syndrome
Rosenthaler-Turk reagent
Rosenthal-Kloepfer syndrome
Roseococcus thiosulfatophilus
roseola
    epidemic r.
    r. infantilis
    r. infantum virus
    r. vaccination
Roseolovirus
Roseomonas
    R. gilardii
    R. mucosa
roseosalivarius
    Hymenobacter r.
Roseospira
    R. marina
    R. navarrensis
Roseospirillum parvum
Roseovarius nubinhibens
Rose test
rosette
    erythrocyte r.
    Flexner-Wintersteiner r.
    Homer-Wright r.
    hyalinizing spindle cell tumor with giant r.'s

malarial r.
neural r.
pineocytomatous r.
r. test
T-lymphocyte r.
rosette-forming cell
rosetting
roseus
    Arthrobacter r.
    Muricoccus r.
Rose-Waaler test
Rosewater syndrome
Ross
    R. River fever
    R. River virus
Rossbach disease
Ross-Jones test
rostellum
rostrate pelvis
Rosys Plato Gene Machine
rot
    Barcoo r.
    liver r.
    r. value
rotamer
rotary microtome
rotation
    axis of r.
    optical r.
    specific r.
rotator
    r. cuff injury
    r. cuff tear
rotavirus
rotavirus serology
Rotazyme test
rotenone
Roth
    R. disease
    R. spot
    R. syndrome
Roth-Bernhardt
    R.-B. disease
    R.-B. syndrome
Rothera nitroprusside test
Rothia
    R. aeria
    R. amarae
    R. dentocariosa
    R. mucilaginosa
    R. nasimurium
Rothmann-Makai syndrome

Rothmund syndrome
Rothmund-Thomson syndrome
rotiferianus
    Vibrio r.
Rotor syndrome
Rotter
    R. node
    R. syndrome
    R. test
rotunda
    fenestra r.
Rouget
    R. cell
    R. muscle
    R. pericyte
Rouget-Neumann sheath
rough (R)
    r. bacterium
    r. colony
    r. determinant
    r. factor
    r. plasmid
rough-smooth variation
rough-surfaced endoplasmic reticulum
Roughton-Scholander
    R.-S. apparatus
    R.-S. syringe
Rougnon-Heberden disease
rouleau, pl. **rouleaux**
    r. formation
round
    r. atelectasis
    r. cell
    r. cell sarcoma
    high-velocity steel-core r.
    jacketed high-velocity r.
    lead core high-velocity r.
    r. secretory granule
    r. window
rounded
    r. atelectasis
    r. mononuclear cell
rounding
roundworm
Rourke-Ernstein sedimentation rate
Rous
    R. sarcoma
    R. sarcoma virus
    R. test
    R. tumor
Rous-associated virus (RAV)
Roussy-Dejerine syndrome

NOTES

Roussy-Lévy
R.-L. disease
R.-L. syndrome
routine
r. test dilution (RTD)
trace r.
Roux
R. bottle
R. spatula
R. stain
Rovsing syndrome
rowbothamii
Legionella r.
Rowntree and Geraghty test
RP
reactive protein
red phosphorus
refractory period
Rp
pulmonary resistance
RPC
reactive perforating collagenosis
RPCF
Reiter protein complement-fixation
RPCF test
rPDGF
recombinant platelet-derived growth
factor
RPF
renal plasma flow
RPGN
rapidly progressive glomerulonephritis
pauciimmune RPGN
RPI
reticulocytic production index
RPLA
reverse passive latex agglutination
RPLND
retroperitoneal lymph node dissection
rpm
revolutions per minute
RPMI 1640 medium
RPO
radiation protection officer
RPR
rapid plasma reagin
RPR test
RPR-CT
rapid plasma reagin circle card test
RPS
renal pressor substance
RR
renin release
RRA
radioreceptor assay
RR-HPO
rapid recompression-high pressure
oxygen

rRNA
ribosomal RNA
RRP
recurrent respiratory papillomatosis
relative refractory period
RRR
renin-release rate
RS
Reed-Sternberg cell
respiratory syncytial
RSA
rapid susceptibility assay
relative specific activity
reticulum cell sarcoma
RSCN
reactive spindle cell nodule
RSD
relative sagittal depth
relative standard deviation
RSS
recombination signal sequence
RST
radiosensitivity test
RSV
respiratory syncytial virus
RSV culture
RSV OID
Rs virus
RT
reaction time
room temperature
rT$_3$
reverse triiodothyronine
RTA
renal tubular acidosis
classic RTA
distal RTA
RTD
renal tubular dysgenesis
routine test dilution
RTE
renal tubular epithelial
RTE cell
RTE cell cast
RTF
replication and transfer
resistance transfer factor
respiratory tract fluid
RTK
rhabdoid tumor of the kidney
RT-PCR
reverse transcriptase polymerase chain
reaction
RU
rat unit
resistance unit
rub
pericardial friction r.
pleural friction r.

Rubarth
- R. disease
- R. disease virus

rubber
- r. pelvis
- r. policeman

rubeanic acid

rubella
- r. antibody test
- congenital r. syndrome
- r. HI test
- measles, mumps, and r. (MMR)
- r. serology
- r. virus (RV)
- r. virus culture
- r. virus vaccine, live

rubeola
- r. serology
- r. virus

ruber
- *Salinibacter* r.
- *Thermovibrio* r.
- *Vibrio* r.

rubescens
- *Amanita* r.

rubescent

rubi
- *Rhizobium* r.

rubida
- *Amycolatopsis* r.

rubidaea
- *Serratia* r.

rubidomycin

rubidus
- *Hyostrongylus* r.

Rubinstein syndrome

Rubinstein-Taybi syndrome

Rubin test

Rubivirus

Rubner test

rubor

rubra
- *Basipetospora* r.
- *Leifsonia* r.
- medulla ossium r.
- miliaria r.
- pityriasis r.
- polycythemia r.
- *Rhodotorula* r.
- trichomycosis r.

rubratoxin

rubredoxin

rubriblast
- pernicious anemia-type r.

rubricyte
- polychromatophilic r.

rubrifaciens
- *Acidisphaera* r.

Rubrimonas cliftonensis

Rubritepida
- R. *flocculans*

Rubrobacteraceae

Rubrobacterales

Rubrobacteridae

Rubrobacter taiwanensis

rubropertincta
- *Gordonia* r.

rubrum
- r. Congo
- r. scarlatinum
- *Trichophyton* r.

Rubulavirus

ruby spot

rucksack paralysis

rudimentary
- r. finger
- r. lung
- r. structure
- r. testis syndrome

rudis
- *Ornithodoros* r.

Rudivirus

rudongensis
- *Ancylobacter* r.

Rud syndrome

Ruegeria
- R. *algicola*
- R. *atlantica*
- R. *gelatinovorans*

ruestringensis
- *Muricauda* r.

rufescens
- *Protostrongylus* r.

Ruffini
- R. corpuscle
- flower-spray organ of R.

ruficornis
- *Sarcophaga* r.

Ruge solution

rugglesi
- *Simulium* r.

rugosa
- *Prauserella* r.

R

NOTES

rule
 Clark r.
 Goriaew r.
 two-cell type r.
Rumack-Matthew nomogram
ruminantium
 Cowdria r.
ruminants
 peste des petits r.
ruminicola
 Bacteroides r.
ruminis
 Pseudobutyrivibrio r.
Ruminococcus luti
Rummo disease
rump
 crown r. (CR)
Rumpel-Leede test
Rundles-Falls syndrome
Runeberg formula
Runella zeae
runt disease
runting syndrome
Runyon
 R. classification
 R. mycobacteria (group I–IV)
ruoffiae
 Ignavigranum r.
rupial syphilis
rupioides psoriasis
rupture
 esophageal r.
 focal plaque r.
 inflammatory r.
 r. of membranes (ROM)
 plaque r.
 premature r.
 prosthesis r.
 tendon r.
 traumatic r.
ruptured
 r. aneurysm
 r. ectopic pregnancy
 r. myocardial infarct
 r. papillary muscle
 r. umbilical cord
 r. viscera
rupture-delivery interval (RDI)
RUR
 resin-uptake ratio
RURTI
 recurrent upper respiratory tract infection
Rushton body
Russell
 R. body
 R. corpuscle
 R. double-sugar agar
 R. syndrome
 R. unit

 R. viper venom (RVV)
 R. viper venom time (RVVT)
Russell-Crooke cell
russellii
 Zobellia r.
russensis
 Dethiosulfovibrio r.
Russian
 R. autumn encephalitis
 R. autumn encephalitis virus
 R. spring-summer encephalitis virus
 R. tick-borne encephalitis
russicus
 Arthrobacter r.
russii
 Fusobacterium r.
Russula emetica
Rust
 R. disease
 R. syndrome
rusty sputum
RUT
 rapid urease test
ruthenica
 Pseudoalteromonas r.
ruthenium
 r. red
 r. red labeling
rutherford (Rd)
 r. scattering
rutidosis
Rutstroemia
Ruysch
 R. disease
 R. glomeruli
 R. membrane
RV
 rat virus
 reference value
 residual volume
 rubella virus
RVB
 red venous blood
RVE
 right ventricular enlargement
RVH
 right ventricular hypertrophy
RVI
 relative value index
RVR
 renal vascular resistance
 resistance to venous return
RVRA
 renal vein renin activity
 renal venous renin assay
RVRC
 renal vein renin concentration
RVT
 renal vein thrombosis

RVV
  Russell viper venom
RVVT
  Russell viper venom time
RXR
  retinoid X receptor
    RXR alpha
ryanodine receptor
ryanodine-sensitive calcium transient
Ryan stain

Rye
  R. classification of Hodgkin
    disease
  R. histopathologic Hodgkin disease
    classification
  R. modification
Rymovirus
Ryparobius
ryukyuensis
    Paraliobacillus r.

R

NOTES

S
serum
smooth
sulfur
supravergence
Svedberg unit of sedimentation
coefficient
synthesis
S antigen
S colony
S phase
S and s antigen
S unit of streptomycin
S-100
S-100 antibody
S-100 immunostain
S-100 marker
S-100 protein
S-100 protein antigen
S-100 protein immunopositivity
s
second
S100A gene
S100 calcium binding protein A1 gene
SA
NATO code for arsine
sarcoma
secondary amenorrhea
serum albumin
sinoatrial
Stokes-Adams
SA node
SA 3100 surface area and pore
size analyzer
SAA
serum amyloid A
SAA protein
SAAG
serum ascites albumin gradient
saalensis
Sedimentibacter s.
SAB
significant asymptomatic bacteriuria
streptavidin-biotin
s-ABC peroxidase
saber
s. shin
s. tibia
Sabethes
Sabhi agar
Sabia virus
Sabin-Feldman
S.-F. dye test
S.-F. syndrome
Sabin vaccine

sabot
coeur en s.
s. heart
saboteur
Sabouraud
S. dextrose and brain heart
infusion agar
S. medium
Sabouraudites
sabulous
sac
air s.
alveolar s.
aneurysmal s.
dental s.
tooth s.
sacbrood
saccate
saccharase
saccharephidrosis
sacchari
Amycolatopsis s.
Burkholderia s.
saccharic acid
saccharin
saccharobutylicum
Clostridium s.
saccharogenic assay
saccharoid
saccharolytica
Soehngenia s.
saccharolyticum
Thermoanaerobacterium s.
saccharometer
Saccharomonospora
S. halophila
S. paurometabolica
S. viridis
Saccharomyces
S. albicans
S. anginae
S. apiculatus
S. capillitii
S. carlsbergensis
S. cerevisiae
S. coprogenus
S. epidermica
S. galacticolus
S. glutinis
S. hominis
S. lemonnieri
S. mellis
S. mycoderma
S. neoformans
S. pastorianus

S

saccharomyces
> Busse s.

Saccharomycetaceae
Saccharomycetales
Saccharomycodes
Saccharomycopsis
saccharomycosis
saccharophilum
> *Halonatronum s.*

saccharopine dehydrogenase
saccharopinuria
Saccharopolyspora
> *S. flava*
> *S. rectivirgula*
> *S. thermophila*

saccharorrhea
saccharose-mannitol agar
Saccharospirillum impatiens
saccharosuria
Saccharothrix
> *S. albidocapillata*
> *S. algeriensis*
> *S. tangerinus*
> *S. violacea*

Saccomanno
> S. collection fluid
> S. fixative

saccular
> s. aneurysm
> s. bronchiectasis
> s. gland
> s. spot

sacculated
> s. aneurysm
> s. pleurisy

saccule
sacculotubular element
sacculus, pl. sacculi
> s. alveolaris
> s. communis
> macula sacculi
> s. proprius
> s. vestibuli

SACD
> subacute combined degeneration

sacelli
> *Brachybacterium s.*

Sachs disease
Sachs-Georgi (S-G)
> S.-G. test

sacrococcygeal
> s. chordoma
> s. teratoma

sacroiliitis
sacroplasmic cisternae
saddle embolism
S-adenosyl-L-homocysteine
S-adenosyl-L-methionine
Saemisch ulcer

Saenger macula
saerimneri
> *Lactobacillus s.*

Saethre-Chotzen syndrome
SafeCrit microhematocrit tube
Safetex tube
Safe-T Lance Plus lancet
safety
> s. glasses
> s. goggles
> s. pin shaped coccobacillus
> s. program
> s. responsibility
> s. shower

SAF fixative
safflower oil
safranin
> s. O
> s. stain

safranophil, safranophile
sagamiensis
> *Pseudoalteromonas s.*

SAGE
> serial analysis of gene expression

Sagian
> S. automated assay optimization
> S. 180 CO2 incubator

saginata
> *Taenia s.*

sagitta
> *Dipus s.*

sago spleen
Sagrahamala
SAH
> subarachnoid hemorrhage

saheli
> *Ensifer s.*

Sahli method
sailor's skin
Saint Anthony's fire
sairae
> *Shewanella s.*

Sakaguchi reaction
Sakamoto
> S. classification
> S. poorly differentiated carcinoma

sakazakii
> *Enterobacter s.*

Saksenaea vasiformis
sakuensis
> *Serratia marcescens* subsp. *s.*

Sakura
> S. Finetek Tissue-Tek VIP 300E automatic tissue processor
> S. Seiki Autosmear automatic smear machine

SAL
> synchronous airway lesion

salaam spasm

Sala cell
Salana multivorans
salegens
  Salegentibacter s.
Salegentibacter
  S. holothuriorum
  S. salegens
SalEst
  S. system
  S. test
salexigens
  Aestuariibacter s.
  Chromohalobacter s.
  Salibacillus s.
  Virgibacillus s.
Salibacillus
  S. marismortui
  S. salexigens
salicampi
  Lentibacillus s.
salicin fermentation
salicylamide
salicylate
  s. assay
  s. intoxication
  s. level
  physostigmine s.
  sodium s.
  s. toxicity
salicylatoxidans
  Pseudaminobacter s.
salicylic
  s. acid
  s. acid test
salicylism
salicylsalicylic acid
salicylsulfonic acid
salicyluric acid
salimeter
salina
  Enhygromyxa s.
  Nocardiopsis s.
  Streptomonospora s.
salinaria
  Orenia s.
salinarius
  Culex s.
  Halanaerobacter s.
saline
  s. agglutination test
  s. agglutinin
  citrate-buffered s. (CBS)

  s. infusion primary
    hyperaldosteronism test
  phosphate buffered s. (PBS)
  s. solution
  s. technique
  Tris-buffered s.
saline-agglutinating antibody
Salinibacterium amurskyense
Salinibacter ruber
Salinicoccus alkaliphilus
Salinisphaera shabanensis
Salinivibrio costicola subsp. *vallismortis*
salinus
  Halobacillus s.
Salipiger mucescens
Salisbury common cold virus
salitolerans
  Swaminathania s.
salivae
  Prevotella s.
saliva ovulation test
salivaria
  glandula s.
salivarium
  Mycoplasma s.
salivarius
  Lactobacillus s.
  Streptococcus s.
salivary
  s. amylase
  s. calculus
  s. corpuscle
  s. duct
  s. duct obstruction
  s. fistula
  s. gland
  s. gland angiosarcoma
  s. gland anlage tumor (SGAT)
  s. gland carcinoma
  s. gland tumor
  s. gland virus (SGV)
  s. gland virus disease
Salk vaccine
salmincola
  Nanophyetus s.
  Troglotrema s.
Salmonella
  S. arizonae
  S. bongori
  S. choleraesuis subsp. *arizona*
  S. cholerae suis var. *kuzendorf*
  S. enteritidis

S

NOTES

Salmonella (continued)
    S. enteritidis serotype *agona*
    S. enteritidis serotype *heidelberg*
    S. enteritidis serotype *hirschfeldii*
    S. enteritidis serotype *infantis*
    S. enteritidis serotype *montevideo*
    S. enteritidis serotype *newport*
    S. enteritidis serotype *paratyphi* A
    S. enteritidis serotype *schottmülleri*
    S. enteritidis serotype *typhimurium*
    S. paratyphi
    S. titer
salmonella, pl. **salmonellae**
    s. agglutinin
    s. group
    s. poisoning
Salmonella-Shigella (**SS**)
    S.-S. agar
Salmonelleae
salmonellosis
salmoneum
    Acrodontium s.
salmonicida
    Aeromonas s.
salmonis
    Piscirickettsia s.
salmon patch
salmositica
    Cryptobia s.
salomonii
    Pseudomonas s.
salpinges (*pl. of* salpinx)
salpingioma
salpingitis
    chronic interstitial s.
    follicular s.
    foreign body s.
    gonorrheal s.
    s. isthmica nodosa
    pyogenic s.
salpingo-oophoritis
salpingoperitonitis
salpinx, pl. **salpinges**
salsalate
salsilacus
    Loktanella s.
salt
    s. agglutination
    s. antagonism
    bile s.'s
    s. bridge
    diazonium s.
    s. dye
    hexazonium s.
    insoluble s.
    s. loading
    s. sensitivity
    tetrazonium s.
    trisodium foscarnet s.

    s. wasting
    water-soluble s.
saltans
    Bodo s.
    thrombophlebitis s.
saltation
Saltatoria
saltatory
    s. conduction
    s. spasm
salted
    s. plasma
    s. serum
Salter-Harris 1–5 fracture
salting-in
salting-out procedure
salt-losing
    s.-l. crisis
    s.-l. nephritis
    s.-l. syndrome
Saltzstein pseudolymphoma
saluresis
saluretic
salvage
    blood s.
    cell s.
    s. therapy
salvarsanized serum
Salvia
    S. horminium
    S. sclarea
Salzer-Kuntschik grading system
Salzman method
SAM
    sulfated acid mucopolysaccharide
samarium (Sm)
sample
    clinical s.
    s. distribution
    environmental s.
    formalin-fixed paraffin-embedded s.
    s. interaction
    multiple stage random s.
    population s. (PS)
    proficiency s.
    random s.
    rolled s.
    simple random s.
    s. steady state
sampler
    air s.
    personal air s.
sampling
    chorionic villus s. (CVS)
    inferior petrosal sinus s.
    inferior petrosal vein s.
    percutaneous umbilical blood s.
     (PUBS)

sentinel lymph node identification and s.
transabdominal chorionic villus s.
transcervical chorionic villus s.
Samsonia
   S. erythrinae
San
   S. Joaquin Valley fever
   S. Miguel sea lion virus
Sanarelli phenomenon
Sanarelli-Shwartzman
   S.-S. phenomenon (SSP)
   S.-S. reaction
Sanchez Salorio syndrome
sand
   s. body
   brain s.
   s. granule
   intestinal s.
   s. tumor
   urinary s.
sandal foot
sandalwood oil
Sanders disease
Sanderson polster
sandfly
   s. fever
   s. fever virus
Sandhoff disease
Sandison-Clark chamber
sandpaper gallbladder
sandramycini
   Kribbella s.
Sandström body
sandwich
   s. hybridization
   s. nucleic acid hybridization assay
   s. radioimmunoassay
sandworm
Sanfilippo syndrome
Sanford test
Sanger
   S. DNA sequencing method
   S. reagent
Sanguibacteraceae
sanguifacient
sanguiferous
sanguification
sanguinegens
   Sneathia s.

sanguineous
   s. cyst
   s. infiltration
sanguineus
   Allodermanyssus s.
   Porphyrobacter s.
   Rhipicephalus s.
   sudor s.
sanguinis
   Brevibacterium s.
   fragilitas s.
   Gemella s.
   Luteococcus s.
   Paenibacillus s.
   Turicibacter s.
sanguinolent
sanguinolentis
   fetus s.
sanguinopurulent
sanguis
   Streptococcus s.
Sanguisuga
sanguivorous myiasis
sanies
saniopurulent
sanioserous
sanious pus
sanitary bacteriology
sanitization
santal oil
santonin
Santorini
   S. canal
   S. duct
   S. fissure
   S. major caruncle
   S. minor caruncle
SAP
   serum alkaline phosphatase
   sporadic adenomatous polyp
   systemic arterial pressure
sap
   cell s.
   nuclear s.
saponifiable fraction
saponification
saponify
saponin
   hemolysin s.
   s. lysing reagent stock solution
   steroid s.
   triterpenoid s.

S

NOTES

Sapovirus
Sappinea diploidea
sapremia
saprobe
saprobic
saprogen
saprogenic
Saprolegnia
sapronosis
saprophilous
saprophilus
    Mycetocola s.
saprophyte
saprophytic infestation
saprophyticus
    Staphylococcus s.
Saprospira
saprozoic
saprozoonosis
SAR
    supplied air respirator
saramycetin
sarcina
Sarcina ventriculi
Sarcinomyces phaeomuriformis
Sarcinosporon inkin
sarcoblast
sarcocele
sarcocyst
sarcocystin
Sarcocystis
    S. *bovihominis*
    S. *fusiformis*
    S. *hominis*
    S. *lindemanni*
    S. *miescheriana*
    S. *suihominis*
    S. *tenella*
sarcocystosis
sarcocyte
sarcode
Sarcodina
Sarcodontia
sarcogenic cell
sarcoglia
sarcoglycan
sarcoid
    Boeck s.
    Darier-Roussy s.
    granuloma s.
    s. granuloma
    Schaumann s.
    Spiegler-Fendt s.
    verrucous s.
sarcoidal granuloma
sarcoidosis
    HHV 8 DNA in s.
    hypercalcemic s.
    mycobacterial DNA in s.

    propionibacterial DNA in s.
    pulmonary s.
sarcolemma
sarcolemmal
    s. folding
    s. integrity
sarcoma, pl. sarcomata, sarcomas (SA)
    AIDS-related Kaposi s. (AIDS-KS)
    alveolar soft-part s. (ASPS)
    ameloblastic s.
    angiolithic s.
    avian s.
    biphasic synovial s.
    botryoid s.
    s. botryoides
    cerebellar s.
    clear cell s.
    endometrial stromal s. (ESS)
    endothelial s.
    epithelioid s. (ES)
    Ewing s. (ES)
    fascicular s.
    fibromyxoid s.
    follicular dendritic cell s.
    granulocytic s. (GS)
    hemangioendothelial s.
    Hodgkin s.
    immunoblastic s.
    interdigitating cell s.
    interdigitating dendritic cell s.
      (IDCS)
    Jensen s.
    juxtacortical osteogenic s.
    Kaposi s.
    Kupffer cell s.
    leukocytic s.
    low-grade endometrial stromal s.
      (LGESS)
    low-grade fibromyxoid s.
    lymphangioendothelial s.
    lymphatic s.
    lymphosarcoma-reticulum cell s.
      (LSA/RCS)
    mast cell s.
    medullary s.
    meningeal s.
    mesothelial s.
    monophasic synovial s. (MSS)
    multiple idiopathic hemorrhagic s.
    myelogenic s.
    myeloid s. (MS)
    myxoid synovial s.
    neurogenic s.
    osteogenic s.
    periosteal s.
    pleomorphic s.
    pulmonary intimal s. (PIS)
    reticuloendothelial s.
    reticulum cell s. (RCS, RSA)

round cell s.
Rous s.
small cell s.
spindle cell s.
stromal s.
synovial s. (SS, SYS)
telangiectatic osteogenic s.
undifferentiated s.
Sarcomastigophora
sarcomatoid
s. carcinoma
s. mesothelioma
s. tumor
sarcomatosis
meningeal s.
sarcomatosum
myxoma s.
sarcomatous component
sarcomere
sarcomeric actin
sarconeme
Sarcophaga
S. *carnaria*
S. *dux*
S. *fuscicauda*
S. *haemorrhoidalis*
S. *ruficornis*
Sarcophagidae
sarcoplasm
sarcoplasmic reticulum
sarcoplast
Sarcopsylla penetrans
Sarcopsyllidae
Sarcoptes scabiei
sarcoptic mange
sarcoptid
Sarcoptidae
sarcoptidosis
sarcosine dehydrogenase
sarcosinemia
sarcosis
sarcosome
Sarcosporidia
sarcosporidiosis
sarcostosis
sarcotic
sarcotubule
sarcous
sardinae
Eimeria s.
sarin
NATO code for s. (GB)

SARS
severe acute respiratory syndrome
SARS-CoV
severe acute respiratory syndrome
coronavirus
antibody to SARS-CoV
SART
standard acid reflux test
SAS
supravalvular aortic stenosis
SAS Rota test
saskatchewanense
Mycobacterium s.
Sassone score
SAT
subacute thyroiditis
sat
saturated
saturation
satelles
Shuttleworthia s.
satellite
s. abscess
s. cell
s. cell necrosis
s. cell of skeletal muscle
s. colony
s. metastasis
s. nodule
perineuronal s.
s. phenomenon
s. vesicular lesion
satellite-rich heterochromatin
satellitism
platelet s.
satellitosis
Sattler elastic layer
saturated (sat)
ambient temperature and
pressure, s. (ATPS)
body temperature, ambient
pressure, s. (BTPS)
s. fatty acid
s. hydrocarbon
s. solution (SS)
s. solution of potassium iodide
(SSKI)
saturation (sat)
s. analysis
arterial oxygen s.
s. current
s. and displacement assay

S

NOTES

saturation *(continued)*
    s. hybridization
    s. index (SI)
    s. limit
    oxygen s.
    transferrin s.
Saturday night palsy
saturnina
    arthralgia s.
saturnine
    s. encephalopathy
    s. gout
saturnus
    Williopsis s.
saucerize
Saundby test
Saunders disease
sauriasis
sauriderma
sauriosis
sauroderma
    ichthyosis s.
sausage finger
saved
    years of life s. (YLS)
savigni
    Ornithodoros s.
Savill disease
sawing
    bone s.
sawtooth wave
saxitoxin
saxobsidens
    Blastococcus s.
Sayeed stain
SB
    serum bilirubin
    Southern blot
    stillbirth
SBB
    Sudan black B
SBE
    subacute bacterial endocarditis
SBF
    splanchnic blood flow
SBH
    sequencing by hybridization
SBI
    silicone breast implant
SBP
    selenium binding protein
    spontaneous bacterial peritonitis
SBR
    Scarf-Bloom-Richardson
        SBR tumor grading system
SBS
    shaken baby syndrome
SBT
    sequenced-based typing

    serous borderline tumor
    serum bactericidal test
SBTI
    soybean trypsin inhibitor
SC
    sickle cell
    subcutaneous
Sc
    scandium
SCA
    SCA protein
    single-chain antigen-binding
        SCA protein (SCA)
scabby mouth
scabiei
    Acarus s.
    Sarcoptes s.
scabies
scabrisporus
    Streptomyces s.
SCAD
    segmental colitis associated with
        diverticulosis
    spontaneous coronary artery dissection
scaffolding protein
scala
    Löwenberg s.
    s. media
    s. vestibuli
scalar product
scalded skin syndrome (SSS)
scale
    absolute temperature s.
    Bauermeister s.
    Baumé s. (B)
    Benoist s. (B)
    Bethesda Pap smear rating s.
    Bloom-Richardson s.
    Celsius temperature s. (C)
    centigrade temperature s. (C)
    s. crust
    customary temperature s.
    full s.
    Gaffky s.
    gray s.
    Hamilton Rating S. (HRS)
    hydrometer s.
    interval s.
    kelvin temperature s. (k)
    positive and negative symptom s.
     (PANSS)
    Rankine temperature s. (Rank)
    ratio s.
    Réaumur s. (R)
scalene node biopsy (SNB)
scalenus anticus syndrome
scaler
scaler-timer

scallop
flail s.
scalloped pattern
scalloping
endosteal s.
scalp
s. contusion
s. pH
pilar tumor of s.
scaly ringworm
scan
biliary s.
bilirubin s.
bone marrow s.
dot s.
duplex s.
indium leukocyte s.
s. information density
tomographic s.
scandium (Sc)
scanning
s. electron micrograph (SEM)
s. electron microscope (SEM)
s. electron microscopy (SEM)
s. probe microscopy (SPM)
s. sequence
s. transmission electron microscopy
s. tunneling microscopy (STM)
scaphohydrocephalus
scaphoid
s. facies
s. fracture
scapularis
Ixodes s.
scar
s. cancer
s. carcinoma
cigarette-paper s.
hypertrophic s.
papyraceous s.
radial s.
scleroelastotic s.
scarabiasis
Scardovia inopinata
scardovii
Bifidobacterium s.
Scarf-Bloom-Richardson (SBR)
scarification test
scarlatina
anginose s.
s. hemorrhagica

s. latens
s. maligna
s. rheumatica
s. simplex
scarlatinal nephritis
scarlatinella
scarlatiniform
scarlatinoid
scarlatinum
rubrum s.
scarless healing
scarlet
Biebrich s.
s. fever (SF)
s. fever antitoxin
s. fever erythrogenic toxin
s. red
s. red stain
s. red sulfonate
water-soluble s.
scarring
consequences of intrahepatic s.
myocardial s.
SCAT
sheep cell agglutination test
sickle cell anemia test
Scatchard
S. equation
S. plot
scatemia
scatologic
scatology
scatoma
scatophagy
scatophila
scatoscopy
scatter
s. diagram
forward s. (FSC)
optical light s.
scattergram
scattering
elastic s.
inelastic s.
rutherford s.
scatterplot
Scaurus
scavenger
s. cell
radical s.
s. receptor

NOTES

883

SCBA
self-contained breathing apparatus
pressure-demand SCBA
SCC
small cell cancer
squamous cell carcinoma
SCD
subacute combined degeneration
sudden cardiac death
sudden coronary death
Scedosporium
S. *apiospermum*
S. *inflatum*
S. *prolificans*
SCF
stem cell factor
SCG
serum chemistry graft
Schaedler blood agar
Schaeffer-Fulton stain
Schaer reagent
Schafer syndrome
Schaffer test
Schales and Schales method for chloride
Schallibaum solution
Schamberg
S. dermatitis
S. disease
Schanz
S. disease
S. syndrome
scharlach red
Schatzki ring
Schaudinn fixative
Schaumann
S. body
S. disease
S. lymphogranuloma
S. sarcoid
S. syndrome
Scheibler reagent
Scheie syndrome
Scheloribates
schematic
scheme
classification s.
decay s.
Facklam classification s.
Van Nuys s.
Schenck disease
schenckii
Sporothrix s.
Sporotrichum s.
Scheuermann disease
Schick
S. method
S. test
S. test toxin

Schiff
S. base
S. reagent
S. stain
Schilder disease
Schiller-Duval body
Schiller test
Schilling
S. band cell
S. blood count
S. classification
S. index
S. test
S. type of monocytic leukemia
Schimmelbusch disease
schindleri
Acinetobacter s.
Schirmer
S. syndrome
S. test
schistocelia
schistocystis
schistocyte, schizocyte
schistocytosis
schistorrhachis
Schistosoma
S. *haematobium*
S. *hematobium*
S. *intercalatum*
S. *japonicum*
S. *malayensis*
S. *mansoni*
S. *mattheei*
S. *mekongi*
schistosomal cystitis
Schistosomatidae
Schistosomatoidea
schistosome granuloma
schistosomiasis serological test
schistosomicidal
schistosomicide
schistosomule
schistosomulum
Schistotaenia srivastavai
schizaxon
schizencephalic microcephaly
schizencephaly
Schizoblastosporion
schizocyte (*var. of* schistocyte)
schizocytosis
schizogenesis
schizogonic cycle
schizogony
schizogyria
schizomycete
Schizomycetes
Schizonella
schizont
schizonticide

Schizophora
Schizophyllum commune
Schizopora
Schizosaccharomyces pombe
schizotonia
Schizotrypanum cruzi
schizozoite
Schlatter disease
Schlatter-Osgood disease
Schlegelella thermodepolymerans
schlegeliana
    Shewanella s.
Schlemm
    canal of S.
schlieren microscope
Schmid-Fraccaro syndrome
Schmidt
    S. syndrome
    S. test
Schmidt-Lanterman
    S.-L. cleft
    S.-L. incisure
Schmincke
    S. pattern
    S. pattern of growth
Schmitz bacillus
Schmorl
    S. bacillus
    S. body
    S. disease
    S. ferric-ferricyanide reduction stain
    S. mosaic
    S. nodule
    S. picrothionin stain
    S. reaction
Schnabel cavernous degeneration
Schneider carmine
schneideri
    Elaeophora s.
schneiderian
    s. carcinoma
    s. membrane
    s. papilloma
schoenbuchensis
    Bartonella s.
schoenleinii
    Trichophyton s.
Scholz disease
Schönbein test
Schönlein
    S. disease
    S. purpura

Schottmüller disease
schottmülleri
    Salmonella enteritidis serotype *s.*
Schreger line
Schridde
    S. cancer hair
    S. syndrome
Schroeder
    S. disease
    S. syndrome
schroeteri
    Kytococcus s.
Schüffner
    S. dot
    S. granule
Schüller
    S. disease
    S. duct
    S. syndrome
Schüller-Christian
    S.-C. disease
    S.-C. syndrome
Schultz
    S. disease
    S. reaction
    S. stain
    S. syndrome
Schultz-Charlton
    S.-C. phenomenon
    S.-C. reaction
Schultz-Dale
    S.-D. reaction
    S.-D. test
Schultze
    S. cell
    S. membrane
    S. test
Schultze-Chvostek sign
Schumm test
Schwalbe
    S. corpuscle
    S. space
Schwann
    S. cell
    S. nucleus
    sheath of S.
    white substance of S.
    S. white substance
schwannian
Schwanniomyces
schwannoma
    acoustic s.

NOTES

S

schwannoma *(continued)*
    ancient s.
    cellular s.
    glandular s.
    granular cell s.
    malignant s.
    melanotic s.
    plexiform s.
    psammomatous-melanotic s.
    renal s.
schwannosis
Schwartz-Bartter syndrome
Schwartz syndrome
Schwarz test
Schweigger-Seidel
    sheath of S.-S.
Schweninger-Buzzi
    S.-B. anetoderma
    S.-B. disease
SCI
    Sertoli cell index
Scianna blood group system
sciatica
SCID
    severe combined immunodeficiency
science
    mortuary s.
    National Accrediting Agency for Clinical Laboratory S.'s
scientific notation
scientist
    biomedical s.
scimitar sign
scintigraph
    octreotide s.
scintigraphy
scintillation
    s. camera
    s. count
    s. counter
    s. crystal
    s. technique
scintillator
    liquid s.
scirrhoid
scirrhosity
scirrhous
    s. adenocarcinoma
    s. carcinoma
scirrhus
SCIS
    surface carcinoma in situ
scissiparity
scissors
    mini s.
SCJ
    squamocolumnar junction
SCK
    serum creatine kinase

sclarea
    Salvia s.
SCLC
    small cell lung carcinoma
sclera, gen. and pl. **sclerae**
    corneoscleral part of trabecular tissue of s.
    lamina cribrosa sclerae
    lamina fusca sclerae
    pars corneoscleralis reticuli trabecularis sclerae
    pars uvealis reticuli trabecularis sclerae
    perforated layer of s.
    reticulum trabeculare sclerae
    substantia propria sclerae
scleradenitis
scleral roll
scleratogenous
scleredema adultorum
sclerema
    s. adiposum
    s. neonatorum
sclerencephaly
scleriasis
scleroatrophy
sclerocornea
sclerocorneal junction
sclerodactyly
scleroderma
    s. antibody
    limited s.
    localized s.
    s. renal crisis
    systemic s.
sclerodermatitis
sclerodermatous
scleroelastotic scar
sclerogenic
sclerogenous
scleroid
scleroma
    respiratory s.
scleromalacia
scleromyxedema
sclero-oophoritis
Sclerophoma
sclerosal
sclerose
sclerosing
    s. bronchioloalveolar carcinoma
    s. cholangitis
    s. epithelioid fibrosarcoma
    s. hemangioma
    s. hyaline necrosis
    s. inflammation
    s. keratitis
    s. mediastinitis
    s. osteitis

s. polycystic adenosis
s. sarcomatoid transitional cell carcinoma
s. Sertoli cell tumor
s. sialadenitis
s. sinusitis
sclerosis, pl. **scleroses**
s. adenosis
Alzheimer s.
amyotrophic lateral s. (ALS)
arterial s.
arteriocapillary s.
arteriolar s.
bone s.
Canavan s.
cardiac s.
central hyaline s.
combined s.
s. corii
s. cutanea
cutaneous systemic s.
diffuse infantile familial s.
disseminated s.
endocardial s.
focal segmental glomerular s. (FSGS)
glomerular s.
hippocampal s. (HS)
hyaline s.
insular s.
laminar cortical s.
lobar s.
mantle s.
menstrual s.
Mönckeberg medial calcific s.
multiple s. (MS)
nodular s. (NS)
ovulational s.
physiologic s.
posterior spinal s.
primary endocardial s.
primary mediastinal large cell lymphoma with s. (PMLS)
progressive systemic s. (PSS)
subacute combined s.
systemic s.
tuberous s.
tumor-induced stromal s.
unicellular s.
vascular s.
s. of white matter
sclerostenosis

Sclerostoma
sclerotia (*pl. of* sclerotium)
sclerotic
s. body
s. coat
s. gastritis
s. kidney
s. margin
s. stomach
s. stroma
sclerotica
otitis s.
tunica s.
Sclerotinia
Sclerotium
sclerotium, pl. **sclerotia**
sclerotylosis
sclerous
SCML
small cell malignant lymphoma
SCNB
stereotactic core-needle biopsy
SCNC
small cell neuroendocrine carcinoma
scoleces (*pl. of* scolex)
scoleciasis
scoleciform
Scolecobasidium
scolecoid
scolecology
scolex, pl. **scoleces**
scoliosis series
scoliotic pelvis
Scolopendra
scomber
Cystoopsis s.
scombroid poisoning
scop
scopolamine
scopiformis
Streptomyces s.
scopolamine (scop)
Scopulariopsis
S. americana
S. aureus
S. blochi
S. brevicaulis
S. cinereus
S. koningi
S. minimus
scopulariopsosis

S

NOTES

scorbutic
>s. dysentery
>s. gingivitis
>s. rosary

score
>CD44v6 s.
>Child-Turcotte-Pugh s.
>Gleason prostate carcinoma s.
>initial prognostic s. (IPS)
>International Prostate Symptom S.
> (IPPS)
>LAP s.
>leukocyte alkaline phosphatase s.
>LOD s.
>MSTS s.
>Sassone s.
>standard s.
>Z s.

scoring
>Barr body s.
>specific IgE antibody s.

Scorpiones
Scorpionida
Scotch tape method
scoticum
>*Diphyllobothrium s.*

Scotobacteria
scotochromogen
scotochromogenic mycobacteria
scotoma, pl. **scotomata**
scotopic
scotopsin
Scott
>S. syndrome
>S. tap water substitute

SCPK
>serum creatine phosphokinase

Scr
>concentration of creatinine in serum

scraper
>cervical s.

scrapie
scraping
>balloon s.

scratch-pad memory
scratch test
screen
>amino acid s.
>s. burn
>cold agglutinin s.
>cord blood s.
>drug abuse s.
>s. filtration pressure (SFP)
>fungal antibody s.
>glucose-6-phosphate
> dehydrogenase s.
>heavy metal s.
>hypercoagulable state coagulation s.

>infertility s.
>intravascular coagulation s.
>latex s.
>multiple marker s.
>Pap Plus HPV s.
>parasite s.
>stool s.
>substance abuse s.
>sugar water test s.
>T_4 newborn s.
>Triage Tox drug s.
>triple s.
>urine drug s. (UDS)
>volatile s.

screening
>amino acid s.
>antibody s.
>automated multiphasic s. (AMS)
>cytologic s.
>s. dipstick
>genetic s.
>multiphasic s.
>neonatal s.
>plasma amino acid s.
>prenatal s.
>rapid drug screen on-site drug s.
>s. test

screw artery
screw-cup container
screwworm
>New World s.
>Old World s.

scrobiculate
scrofula
scrofulaceum
>*Mycobacterium s.*

scrofuloderma
>s. gummosa
>papular s.
>tuberculous s.
>ulcerative s.
>verrucous s.

scrofulotuberculosis
scrofulous
scroll ear
scrota (*pl. of* scrotum)
scroti
>elephantiasis s.

scrotitis
scrotum, pl. **scrota, scrotums**
>lymph s.
>watering-can s.

scrub typhus
SCT
>sex chromatin test
>squamous cell carcinoma of the thyroid
>staphylococcal clumping test

scum

SCUNC
    small cell undifferentiated
      neuroendocrine carcinoma
scurvy
    land s.
scuta (*pl. of* scutum)
Scutigera
scutula (*pl. of* scutulum)
scutular
scutularis
    parakeratosis s.
scutulata
    ichthyosis s.
    porrigo s.
scutulum, pl. **scutula**
scutum, pl. **scuta**
scybalous stool
Scytalidium
SD
    septal defect
    serologically defined
    serum defect
    solvent detergent treatment
    spontaneous delivery
    stable disease
    standard deviation
      SD antigen
      SD plasma
SDA
    strand displacement amplification
SDG
    sucrose density gradient
SDS
    sodium dodecyl sulfate
    sudden death syndrome
      SDS gel electrophoresis
      SDS gel filtration chromatography
SDS-PAGE
    sodium dodecyl sulfate-polyacrylamide
      gel electrophoresis
SE
    standard error
Se
    selenium
sea
    s. anemone ulcer
    s. urchin granuloma
sea-blue
    s.-b. histiocyte
    s.-b. histiocyte disease
    s.-b. histocytosis

seal
    hermetic s.
sealed
    s. beta gamma source
    s. envelope technique
    s. radioactive source
sealing
    impulse s.
Seal Rock hemoglobin
seared
    s. skin
    s. wound margin
seasonal rhinitis
Seattle classification
seatworm
SEB
    staphylococcal enterotoxin B
sebacea
    ichthyosis s.
sebaceae
    glandulae s.
sebaceous
    s. adenocarcinoma
    s. adenoma
    s. carcinoma
    s. cyst
    s. epithelioma
    s. follicle
    s. gland
    s. horn
    s. miliaria
    s. neoplasm
    s. nevus
    s. tubercle
sebaceum
    adenoma s.
    tuberculum s.
sebaceus
    lupus s.
    nevus s. (NS)
Sebastian syndrome
sebi
    Wallemia s.
sebiagogic
sebiferous
sebiparous
sebolith
seborrhea
seborrheic
    s. dermatitis
    s. keratosis

NOTES

S

889

seborrheic *(continued)*
   s. verruca
   s. wart
seborrheica
   acanthoma verrucosa s.
Sebright bantam syndrome
sebum preputiale
SEC
   sertoliform endometrioid carcinoma
   subepidermal connective tissue
Secernentasida
Secernentia
Seckel syndrome
second (s)
   cycle per s. (cps)
   s. filial generation (F_2)
   forced expiratory time in s.'s (FETS)
   forced expiratory volume at 1 s. (FEV-1)
   kilocycles per s. (kcps)
   vibration s. (vs)
secondary
   s. active transport
   s. aerosolization
   s. agammaglobulinemia
   s. amenorrhea (SA)
   s. amyloidosis
   s. antibody deficiency
   s. antiphospholipid syndrome
   s. atelectasis
   s. attack rate
   s. bacterial peritonitis
   s. blast injury
   s. bleeding time
   s. buffer
   s. carcinoma
   s. cementum
   s. center of ossification
   s. coccidioidomycosis
   s. coil
   s. cold agglutinin disease
   s. constriction
   s. contamination
   s. culture
   s. degeneration
   s. dextrocardia
   s. encephalitis
   s. eosinophilic pneumonia
   s. fixation
   s. glaucoma
   s. granule
   s. hemochromatosis
   s. hyperaldosteronism
   s. hyperparathyroidism
   s. hyperplasia
   s. hypertrophic osteoarthropathy (SHO)
   s. hypoadrenocorticism

   s. hypogammaglobulinemia
   s. immune response
   s. immunodeficiency
   s. infection
   s. lymphoid follicle
   s. lysosome
   s. malignant neoplasm, lung
   s. methemoglobinemia
   s. mucinosis
   s. myeloid metaplasia
   s. nodule
   s. ovarian follicle
   s. point of ossification
   s. polycythemia
   s. pulmonary hemosiderosis (SPH)
   s. pulmonary lobule
   s. pyoderma
   s. reference materials
   s. refractory anemia
   s. renal calculus
   s. renal tubular acidosis
   s. repair
   s. sex character
   s. spermatocyte
   s. structure
   s. thrombus
   s. trisomy
   s. tuberculosis
   s. union
   s. viremia
   s. X zone
second-degree
   s.-d. burn
   s.-d. frostbite
   s.-d. heart block
   s.-d. radiation injury
second-order reaction
second-set
   s.-s. graft rejection
   s.-s. phenomenon
second-strain infection
Secrétan syndrome
secreted
   regulated on activation, normal T expressed and s. (RANTES)
   s. toxin
secretin
   s. pancreozymin test
   s. test for exocrine pancreatic function
secretin-cholecystokinin-pancreatozymin stimulation test
secreting hydrochloric
secretion
   aldosterone s.
   cervical s.
   corrosive gastric s.'s
   cytocrine s.
   eccrine sweat gland s.

gland of internal s.
luteinizing hormone s.
parathyroid hormone s. (PTHS)
s. rate (SR)
stimulate enzyme s.
transport and s.
tubular s.
secretogranin
secretor
s. factor
s. gene
s. phenotype
s. trait
secretory
s. acinar element
s. acinus
s. adenosis
s. canaliculus
s. carcinoma
s. cell
s. component
s. cyst
s. duct
s. endometrium
s. exhaustion
s. gland
s. granule
s. IgA
s. immunoglobulin
s. otitis media
s. pattern
s. portion
s. stage
section
attached cranial s.
capture cross s.
cardiac muscle in longitudinal s.
celloidin s.
coronal s.
cryostat s.
s. cutting
detached cranial s.
en face s.
eosin-stained microscopic s.
formalin-fixed tissue s.
s. freeze substitution technique
frozen s. (FS, FZ)
longitudinal s.
lung s.
microscopic s.
paraffin s.
paraffin-embedded tissue s.

permanent s.
Pitres s.
pituitary stalk s.
serial s.
thin s.
tuberculosis organisms in tissue s.
vibratome tissue s.
whole-mount s.
sectioning
Albert-Linder bone s.
lymph node s.
multiple level s.
step s.
tangential s.
secular equilibrium
secundarium
punctum ossificationis s.
Securline blood band
SED
spondyloepiphyseal dysplasia
Sed
sedimentation
**Sed-Chek 2 bilevel whole blood
reference control**
sediment
crystals in urine s.
spun urine s.
stained urinary s. (SUS)
s. tube
urinary s.
sedimentate
sedimentation (Sed)
s. coefficient
s. equilibrium
erythrocyte s.
s. index
s. rate (sed rate, SR)
s. rate test (SRT)
s. reaction
s. technique
s. time
s. tube
velocity-diffusion s.
s. velocity-diffusion
sedimentator
sedimented red cell (SRC)
Sedimentibacter
S. hydroxybenzoicus
S. saalensis
sedimentometer
sedimentum lateritium
sedoheptulose 7-phosphate

NOTES

sed rate
sedimentation rate
SEE
standard error of estimate
seeberi
Rhinosporidium s.
seed
s. agar
prostate s.
seeding
cell s.
metachronous s.
SEER
Surveillance, Epidemiology, and End Results
segbwema
Prototheca s.
segment
frame-scanning s.
initial s.
interannular s.
internodal s.
Lanterman s.
s. long-spacing (SLS)
Okazaki s.
pairing s.
Ranvier s.
segmental
s. colitis associated with diverticulosis (SCAD)
s. glomerulonephritis
segmentation
s. nucleus
s. sphere
segmented (segs)
s. cell
s. granulocyte
s. hyalinizing vasculitis
s. leukocyte (segs)
s. neutrophil (segs)
segmenter
Segmentina
Segmentininae
segmentum internodale
segnis
Haemophilus s.
segregation
HLA haplotype s.
segregator
Luys s.
segs
segmented
segmented leukocyte
segmented neutrophil
Séguin sign
SeHCAT test
Seibert tuberculin
Seitelberger disease
Seitz filter

seizure
psychogenic s.
selangorensis
Paralactobacillus s.
Selas filter
Seldinger technique
Select-a-Fuge microcentrifuge machine
selected photomicrograph
selectin
selection
s. against dominant mutations
s. against heterozygotes
s. against homozygotes
s. against recessive mutations
coefficient of s.
directional s.
natural s.
s. pressure
selective
s. affinity
s. deficiency
s. medium
s. stain
s. transport
selectivity ratio
Selenihalanaerobacter shriftii
selenite broth
selenite-cystine broth
selenitireducens
Bacillus s.
selenium (Se)
s. assay
s. binding protein (SBP)
selenium-75
selenocyte
selenoid body
Selenomonas
selenoprotein P gene
Selenotila
self-absorption
self-complementary DNA
self-contained breathing apparatus (SCBA)
self-dose
self-immolation
self-infection
selfing
self-limited
s.-l. colitis
s.-l. disease
self-nucleate
self-renewal
self-renewing cell
self-replication
self-sustained sequence replication (3SR)
Selivanoff, Seliwanow
S. reaction
S. reagent
S. test

sella
    empty s.
    s. turcica syndrome
Selter disease
Selye syndrome
SEM
    scanning electron micrograph
    scanning electron microscope
    scanning electron microscopy
    SEM freeze-fracture method
semelincident
semen
    acid phosphatase test for s.
    s. analysis
    s. examination
    hyaluronidase unit for s. (HUS)
semenuria
semialdehyde
    glutamate s.
semiapochromatic objective
semiautomated susceptibility testing
semiautomatic handgun
semicanal
semicanalis
semicarbazide hydrochloride
semicircular
    s. canal
    s. duct
semicirculares
    ductus s.
semicircularis
    epithelium ductus s.
    membrana basalis ductus s.
    membrana propria ductus s.
semiconductor
    s. device
    extrinsic s.
    intrinsic s.
semidominance
semiinterquartile range
semilethal mutation
semilunar
semilunatum
    planum s.
seminal
    s. coagulum
    s. colliculus
    s. fibrinolysin
    s. fluid
    s. granule
    s. vesical cyst

seminalis
    ductus excretorius vesiculae s.
semi-nester primer
seminiferous
    s. epithelium
    s. tubule
    s. tubule dysgenesis
seminis
    Allofustis s.
seminoma
    anaplastic s.
    immune rejection of s.
    spermacytic s.
    spermatocytic s.
    syncytiotrophoblastic cell of s.
seminomatous
seminuria
semipermeable membrane
Semi-Q hCG combo test
semiquantitative
    s. analysis
    s. viral culture
semiquinone
Semisulcospina
Semliki Forest virus
Semple vaccine
senagalensis
    Curvularia s.
sendaiensis
    Alicyclobacillus s.
Sendai virus
Senear-Usher
    S.-U. disease
    S.-U. syndrome
seneciella
    Pegohylemyia s.
seneciosis
senescence
    cellular s.
senile
    s. amyloidosis
    s. amyloidosis of heart
    s. arteriosclerosis
    s. atrophy
    s. degeneration
    s. dwarfism
    s. ectasia
    s. elastosis
    s. fibroma
    s. hemangioma
    s. hip disease
    s. involution

S

NOTES

senile *(continued)*
    s. keratoderma
    s. keratoma
    s. keratosis
    malum coxae s.
    s. nephrosclerosis
    s. osteomalacia
    s. plaques
    s. sebaceous hyperplasia
    s. wart
senilis
    arcus s.
    malum articulorum s.
    vaginitis s.
    verruca plana s.
sennetsu
    Ehrlichia s.
    Neorickettsia s.
    Rickettsia s.
sennoside
Sensa
    Hemoccult S.
sense
    s. organ
    s. strand
SensiCath system
Sensititre *Streptococcus pneumoniae* **HPB susceptibility plate**
sensitive membrane antigen rapid test (SMART)
sensitivity
    acquired s.
    analytical s.
    antibiotic s.
    antigen s.
    clinical s.
    contact s.
    culture and s. (C&S)
    diagnostic s.
    electrode s.
    s. to gluten
    idiosyncratic s.
    induced s.
    multiple chemical s.
    photoallergic s.
    phototoxic s.
    primaquine s.
    relative s.
    salt s.
sensitization
    active s.
    autoerythrocyte s.
    passive s.
    photodynamic s.
    s. response (SR)
sensitize
sensitized
    s. antigen

    s. cell
    s. culture
sensitizer
sensitizing
    s. dose
    s. injection
    s. substance
sensor
sensorineural
    lentigines (multiple), electrocardiographic abnormalities, ocular hypertelorism, pulmonary stenosis, abnormalities of genitalia, retardation of growth, and deafness (s.) (LEOPARD)
sensory
    s. crossway
    s. receptor
sensuum
    organa s.
sentinel
    s. animal
    s. case
    s. event
    s. gland
    s. laboratory
    s. lymph node (SLN)
    s. lymph node biopsy
    s. lymph node identification and sampling
    s. pile
    s. tag
SEOC
    serous epithelial ovarian carcinoma
seoi
    Gymnophalloides s.
seoulensis
    Fibricola s.
Sepacell RZ-2000 device
separating medium
separation
    immunomagnetic cell s.
    multiangle polarized scatter s. (MAPSS)
    solid-phase s.
separator
    Amicus s.
separatory funnel
Sepedonium
Sepharose
    protein G S.
Sepsidae
sepsis, pl. **sepses**
    Chlamydia s.
    intestinal s.
    s. lenta
    overwhelming postsplenectomy s.
    s. syndrome

tularemia s.
tularemic s.
SEPT9 gene
septa (*pl. of* septum)
septal
s. bone
s. cell
s. defect (SD)
s. fibrosis of liver
s. panniculitis
s. panniculitis without vasculitis
Septata intestinalis
septate mycelium
septectomy
septic
s. abortion
s. arthritis
s. disease
s. embolus
s. endocarditis
s. fever
s. infarct
s. intoxication
s. knee
s. necrosis
s. peritonitis
s. phlebitis
s. pneumonia
s. shock
septica
iridocyclitis s.
Pasteurella s.
septicemia
acute fulminating meningococcal s.
anthrax s.
cryptogenic s.
puerperal s.
typhoid s.
septicemic
s. abscess
s. anthrax
s. plague
Septi-Chek
S.-C. culture system
septicopyemia
septicopyemic
septicum
Clostridium s.
Mycobacterium s.
septin gene family
septique
Vibrion s.

Septobasidium cokeri
Septomyxa
septooptic dysplasia
septulum testis
septum, pl. **septa**
alveolar s.
anterior part of s.
atrial s.
connective tissue septa
deviated s.
fibrovascular s.
interalveolar s.
s. interalveolare
interlobular connective tissue s.
transverse s.
sequela, pl. **sequelae**
s. of chronic active hepatitis
s. of rheumatic fever
sequence
insertion s.
intervening s.
s. ladder
long terminal repeat s. (LTR)
recombination signal s. (RSS)
regulatory s.
repeated DNA s.
Robin s.
scanning s.
s. specific oligonucleotide probe (SSOP)
termination s.
unstable trinucleotide repeat s.'s
sequenced-based typing (SBT)
sequencer
amino acid s.
sequencing
direct s.
DNA s.
genome s.
s. by hybridization (SBH)
nucleic acid s.
nucleotide s.
sequential
s. access
s. analysis
s. multichannel autoanalyzer (SMA, SMAC)
s. multiple analyzer (SMA)
Sequenza immunostaining system
sequester
sequestered antigen
sequestra (*pl. of* sequestrum)

S

NOTES

sequestral
sequestrant
sequestration
    biochemical s.
    s. bronchopnemonia
    bronchopulmonary s.
    s. crisis
    s. cyst
    s. dermoid
    extralobar s.
    intralobar s.
Sequestrene iron chelate
sequestrum, pl. **sequestra**
    primary s.
Sequivirus
sequoiosis
sera (*pl. of* serum)
seralbumin
Sereny test
SEREX
    serological expression of cDNA
    expression
    SEREX method
sergenti
    Phlebotomus s.
serial
    s. analysis of gene expression
    (SAGE)
    s. cardiac isoenzyme assay
    s. data transmission
    s. dilution
    s. operation
    s. passage
    s. section
    s. thrombin time (STT)
serialis
    Coenurus s.
    Multiceps s.
sericata
    Lucilia s.
    Phaenicia s.
Sericopelma communis
series, pl. **series**
    Accurun 515 drug resistant mutant
    control s.
    arranged in s.
    s. circuit
    erythrocytic s.
    granulocytic s.
    homologous s.
    lymphocytic s.
    monohistiocytic s.
    myeloid s.
    scoliosis s.
    thrombocytic s.
serine
serine/threonine protein phosphatase
Serinicoccus marinus

seriniphilus
    Paracoccus s.
serocolitis
seroconversion
serocystic
serodiagnosis
    Leptospira s.
serodiagnostic test
seroenteritis
seroepidemiology
serofast
serofibrinous
    s. effusion
    s. inflammation
    s. pericarditis
    s. pleurisy
serogroup
serologic
    s. pipette
    s. test for syphilis (STS)
serological expression of cDNA
    expression (SEREX)
serologically
    s. defined (SD)
    s. defined antigen
serology
    AIDS s.
    Aspergillus s.
    bacterial s.
    blastomycosis s.
    diagnostic s.
    fungal s.
    Helicobacter pylori s.
    HIV-1 s.
    Lyme disease s.
    mumps s.
    Mycoplasma s.
    parainfluenza viral s.
    pertussis s.
    respiratory syncytial virus s.
    Rocky Mountain spotted fever s.
    rotavirus s.
    SLEV s.
    s. test
    s. test for syphilis (STS)
    trichinosis s.
seroma
seromucoid
    acid s.
    alpha s.
    alpha-1 s.
seromucosa
    glandula s.
seromucous
    s. cell
    s. gland
seronegative
seropedicae
    Herbaspirillum s.

serophilic
seropositive
seropurulent
seropus
seroreversion
serosa
    glandula s.
    membrana s.
    perispermatitis s.
    peritendinitis s.
    polyemia s.
    tunica s.
serosal surface
serosamucin
serosanguineous effusion
serositis
    multiple s.
serosity
serosum
    pericardium s.
serosynovial
serosynovitis
serotherapy
serothorax
serotonergic receptor
serotonin
    s. assay
    s. release assay (SRA)
serotype
    heterologous s.
    homologous s.
serous
    s. acinus
    s. acute inflammation
    s. acute synovitis
    s. atrophy
    s. carcinoma
    s. cell
    s. coat
    s. cyst
    s. cystadenocarcinoma
    s. cystadenofibroma
    s. cystadenoma
    s. cystoma
    s. demilune
    s. effusion
    s. epithelial ovarian carcinoma
    (SEOC)
    s. fluid
    s. gland
    s. membrane
    s. meningitis

    s. otitis media
    s. pleurisy
    s. psammocarcinoma
    s. tunic
serovaccination
serovar
    Mycobacterium avium s. 1–29
serozyme
serpens
    Bacteroides s.
serpent
    s. infection
    s. worm
serpentine
    s. aneurysm
    s. blastema
serpiginosa
    elastosis perforans s.
serpiginosum
    angioma s.
serpiginosus
    lupus s.
serpiginous
    s. keratitis
    s. ulcer
serpigo
Serpula
serrata
    Linguatula s.
    ora s.
serrate
serrated
    s. adenoma
    s. colorectal polyp
Serratia
    S. liquefaciens
    S. marcescens
    S. marcescens subsp. *sakuensis*
    S. plymuthica
    S. proteamaculans
    S. quinivorans
    S. rubidaea
    S. urinary tract infection
serraticeps
    Pulex s.
Serratieae
serration
Serres gland
serrulate
Ser-Thr kinase
Sertoli
    S. cell

S

NOTES

Sertoli *(continued)*
    S. cell only syndrome
    S. cell tumor
    S. column
    S. stromal cell tumor
sertoliform
    s. component
    s. endometrioid carcinoma (SEC)
Sertoli-Leydig cell tumor
Sertoli-like pattern
serum, pl. **serums, sera (S)**
    s. accelerator globulin
    s. accident
    acid phosphatase s.
    s. agar
    aged s.
    s. agglutinin
    s. albumin (SA)
    s. alkaline phosphatase (SAP)
    s. alkaline phosphatase test
    s. amylase
    s. amylase test
    s. amyloid A (SAA)
    anallergenic s.
    anticholera s.
    anticolibacillary s.
    anticomplementary s.
    antidiphtheric s.
    antiepithelial s.
    antihepatic s.
    antihuman lymphocyte s. (AHLS)
    antilymphocyte s. (ALS)
    antimacrophage s. (AMS)
    antimeningococcus s.
    antimouse lymphocyte s. (AMLS)
    antineutrophilic s. (ANS)
    antinsulin s. (AIS)
    antipertussis s.
    antiplague s.
    antiplatelet s.
    antipneumococcus s.
    antirabies s. (ARS)
    antireticular cytotoxic s. (ACS)
    antiscarlatinal s.
    antistaphylococcus s.
    antistreptococcus s.
    antitetanic s. (ATS)
    antithymocyte s. (ATS)
    antitoxic s.
    antityphoid s.
    antivenomous s.
    s. ascites albumin gradient (SAAG)
    s. bacterial test
    s. bactericidal test (SBT)
    bacteriolytic s.
    s. beta-2 microglobulin
    s. bicarbonate
    s. bilirubin (SB)
    s. bilirubin test

blood grouping s.
s. broth
s. calcium test
s. chemistry graft (SCG)
concentration of creatinine in s.
  (Scr)
concentration of sodium in s.
  (SNa)
convalescent s.
Coombs s.
s. creatine kinase (SCK)
s. creatine kinase test
s. creatine phosphokinase (SCPK)
s. creatinine clearance
s. creatinine test
s. defect (SD)
s. diagnosis
s. disease
dried human s.
s. drug level
s. electrolyte
endotheliolytic s.
s. enzyme
s. enzyme test
equine antihuman lymphoblast s.
  (EAHLS)
s. estriol
fetal bovine s. (FBS)
Flexner s.
foreign s.
s. globulin test
s. glutamic oxaloacetic transaminase
  (SGOT)
s. glutamic pyruvic transaminase
  (SGPT)
guinea pig s. (GPS)
guinea pig antiinsulin s. (GPAIS)
s. hepatitis (SH)
s. hepatitis virus
hereditary erythrocytic
  multinuclearity with positive
  acidified s. (HEMPAS)
s. HER-2/neu
heterologous s.
hog cholera s.
homologous s.
horse s. (HS)
human measles immune s.
human pertussis immune s.
human scarlet fever immune s.
s. hydroxybutyrate dehydrogenase
  (SHBD)
hyperimmune s.
immune s.
s. immunofixation electrophoresis
inactivated leukocytolytic s.
s. intoxication
s. iron (SI)
s. isocitric dehydrogenase (SICD)

s. lactate dehydrogenase (SLD, SLDH)
liquid human s.
Löffler blood s.
measles convalescent s.
motile s.
muscle s.
s. nephritis
nephrotoxic s.
nonimmune s.
normal blood s. (NBS)
normal horse s. (NHS)
normal human s. (NHS)
normal rabbit s. (NRS)
normal reference s. (NRS)
s. p24 antigen concentration
pericardial s.
s. phenylalanine
s. phosphorus test
plague s.
polyvalent s.
pooled blood s.
s. precipitable iodine (SPI)
pregnant mare s. (PMS)
prophylactic s.
s. protein-bound iodine (SPBI)
s. protein electrophoresis (SPE, SPEP)
s. protein electrophoresis test
s. prothrombin conversion
s. prothrombin conversion acceleration (SPCA)
s. prothrombin conversion accelerator (SPCA)
s. prothrombin conversion accelerator factor
s. prothrombin time
quality control s.
s. rash
s. reaction
salted s.
salvarsanized s.
s. shock
s. sickness
silver-acidified s. (Ag-AS)
s. soluble transferrin receptor
specific s.
streptococcus s.
s. therapy
s. thrombotic accelerator (STA)
thyrotoxic s.

s. thyroxine measured by column chromatography $(T_4(C))$
s. urea nitrogen (SUN)
s. uric acid (SUA)
veronal-buffered saline/fetal bovine s. (VBS/FBS)

serumal
serum amyloid A (SAA)
serum-fast
serum-neutralizing (SN)
serums (*pl. of* serum)
service
　Department of Health and Human S.'s (DHHS)
　morgue s.
　National Council of Health Laboratory S.'s (NCHLS)
servomechanism
servomotor
seryl
sesame oil
sesquiterpene
sessile
　s. hydatid
　s. phagocyte
　s. polyp
　s. serrated adenoma
set
　s. of idiotopes
　medical equipment s. (MES)
　NAPP tablet s.
　s. point
　Shamrock Safety Winged S.
seta, pl. **setae**
setaceous
Setaria
　S. cervi
　S. equina
setariasis
setiferous, setigerous
Setosphaeria
SETTLE
　spindle cell epithelial tumor with thymus-like differentiation
settled particulate
seven-segment display
severe
　s. acute respiratory syndrome (SARS)
　s. acute respiratory syndrome coronavirus (SARS-CoV)
　s. atypical pneumonia

S

NOTES

severe *(continued)*
s. combined immunodeficiency (SCID)
s. hemolytic anemia
s. protein deprivation
severely
s. malnourished alcoholic
s. subnormal (SSN)
Severinghaus electrode
severity
s. of fibrosis after lung injury
s. of illness
Sever syndrome
Sevier-Munger stain
sex
s. cell
s. chromatin
s. chromatin study
s. chromatin test (SCT)
s. chromosome
s. chromosome abnormality
s. cord
s. cord-stromal tumor
s. cord tumor with annular tubule
s. determination
s. differentiation
s. factor
heterogametic s.
homogametic s.
s. hormone (SH)
s. hormone-binding globulin
s. pili
sexalatus
Physocephalus s.
sex-conditioned character
sexivalent
sex-limited character
sex-linked
s.-l. character
s.-l. gene
s.-l. heredity
s.-l. inheritance
sex-reversed mutation
sextant
s. biopsy
s. site
sexual
s. gland
s. reproduction
sexually transmitted disease (STD)
Sézary
S. cell
S. count
S. erythroderma
S. reticulosis
S. syndrome (SS)
SF
scarlet fever

SFG
spotted fever group
SFP
screen filtration pressure
SFT
solitary fibrous tumor
S-G
Sachs-Georgi
SG
skin graft
specific gravity
SGAT
salivary gland anlage tumor
SGC
sweat gland carcinoma
SGD
single gene disorder
SGF2
fog oil
SGOT
serum glutamic oxaloacetic transaminase
SGPT
serum glutamic pyruvic transaminase
SGV
salivary gland virus
SH
serum hepatitis
sex hormone
sinus histiocytosis
shabanensis
Salinisphaera s.
shackletonii
Bacillus s.
shadow
s. cell
s. corpuscle
Gumprecht s.
mediastinal s.
s. nucleus
Ponfick s.
shadow-casting
Shaffer-Hartmann method
shaft
cortex of hair s.
medulla of hair s.
shaggy pericardium
shagreen
s. lesion
s. patch
s. skin
shahii
Leptotrichia s.
Prevotella s.
shake
s. culture
s. test
shaken
s. adult syndrome
s. baby syndrome (SBS)

900

s. impact syndrome
s. infant syndrome
Shamrock Safety Winged Set
Shandon
S. Cadenza immunostainer
S. Cytospin chamber
S. fixative
shape
flattened s.
plurilobulated s.
shared hallucination
Sharpey
S. fiber
perforating fibers of S.
shattering ability
shave biopsy
Shaver disease
SHb
sulfhemoglobin
SHBD
serum hydroxybutyrate dehydrogenase
SHBG
steroid hormone binding globulin
sheath
archnoid s.
caudal s.
cuticle of root s.
dentinal s.
dural s.
enamel rod s.
external root s.
giant cell tumor of tendon s.
  (GCTTS)
glissonian s.
Henle s.
Huxley s.
internal root s.
s. of Key and Retzius
Mauthner s.
medullary s.
mitochondrial s.
myelin s.
nerve s. (NS)
Neumann s.
notochordal s.
periarterial lymphatic s. (PALS)
periarteriolar lymphoid s.
root s.
Rouget-Neumann s.
s. of Schwann
s. of Schweigger-Seidel
synovial s.

tail s.
s.'s of vessels
sheathed
s. artery
s. microfilaria
Sheather
S. sugar flotation method
S. sugar flotation procedure
shedding
syncytial s.
virus s.
Sheehan syndrome
sheep
s. blood agar
s. cell agglutination test (SCAT)
s. liver fluke
s. pox
s. pox virus
s. red blood cell (SRBC)
sheet
beta-pleated s.
material safety data s. (MSDS)
pleated s.
sheeting
architectural s.
sheetlike aggregate
Shelf-Life Extension Program (SLEP)
shell
diffusion s.
s. nail
staining s.
Sherman-Bourquin unit of vitamin B$_2$
Sherman-Munsell unit
Sherman unit
Shewanella
S. *affinis*
S. *denitrificans*
S. *fidelis*
S. *gaetbuli*
S. *japonica*
S. *livingstonensis*
S. *marinintestina*
S. *olleyana*
S. *pacifica*
S. *pealeana*
S. *sairae*
S. *schlegeliana*
S. *waksmanii*
Shewanellaceae
SHH
sonic hedgehog

NOTES

S

SHH (continued)
- SHH gene
- SHH protein

Shichito disease

shield
- chloride s.
- face s.
- gonadal s.
- s. to the left
- s. to the right
- syringe s.
- tabletop s.

shielding

shift
- antigenic s.
- bathochromic s.
- chemical s.
- chloride s.
- colloid s.
- s. counter
- hyperchromic s.
- hypochromic s.
- hypsochromic s.
- isohydric s.
- s. to the left
- left s.
- midline s.
- regenerative blood s.
- s. register
- s. reticulocyte
- s. to the right
- Stokes s.

Shiga
- S. bacillus
- S. toxin

Shigalike toxin

Shigella
- S. arabinotarda
- S. boydii
- S. dysenteriae
- S. flexneri
- S. rapid latex test
- S. sonnei

shigelloides
- Aeromonas (Plesiomonas) s.
- Plesiomonas s.

shigellosis

Shiiki
- method of S.

Shikimate dehydrogenase

shilonii
- Vibrio s.

Shimada classification

Shimadzu hemoglobin determination

shimamushi disease

Shimoda blood group system

Shimosato-Mukai classification

shin
- saber s.
- s. splint

shingles

Shinowara-Jones-Reinhard (SJR)
- S.-J.-R. unit

shinshuensis
- Leifsonia s.

shiny surface colony

ship
- s. fever
- s. rat

shipping fever virus

shirt-stud abscess

shivering thermogenesis

sHLA protein

SHML
- sinus histiocytosis with massive lymphadenopathy

SHO
- secondary hypertrophic osteoarthropathy

shock
- anaphylactic s.
- anaphylactoid s.
- s. antigen
- s. artifact
- cardiogenic s.
- colloid s.
- endotoxic s.
- endotoxin s.
- faradic s.
- Forssman s.
- hemoclastic s.
- hemorrhagic s.
- histamine s.
- hypoglycemic s.
- hypovolemic s.
- insulin s.
- s. lung
- neurogenic s.
- osmotic s.
- peptone s.
- protein s.
- pseudoanaphylactic s.
- septic s.
- serum s.
- thyrotoxin s.
- toxic s.
- vasogenic s.

shocking dose

Shone anomaly

Shope
- S. fibroma
- S. fibroma virus
- S. papilloma
- S. papilloma virus

shored-exit wound

Shorr trichrome stain

short
> s. bowel syndrome
> s. circuit
> s. fascicular growth pattern
> s. increment sensitivity index (SISI)
> s. incubation hepatitis
> s. stature

shortened
> s. bleeding time
> s. coagulation time

shortening
> abnormal s.
> telomere s.

short-interference RNA (siRNA)
short-lived evidence
short-strip pouchitis
shottsii
> *Mycobacterium s.*

shotty
> s. breast
> s. node
> s. pustule

shoulder
> distended bursa, s.

showae
> *Campylobacter s.*

shower
> safety s.

showing
> fenestrated capillary s.

Shprintzen syndrome
shrapnel
shriftii
> *Selenihalanaerobacter s.*

shrinkage
> postremoval and postfixation s.

shuffle pit
Shulman syndrome
shunt
> s. determination
> hexose monophosphate s. (HMPS)
> Le Veen s.
> s. nephritis

shutdown
> renal s.

Shuttleworthia satelles
Shwachman-Diamond syndrome
Shwachman syndrome
Shwartzman reaction
Shy-Drager syndrome

SI
> International System of Units
> saturation index
> serum iron
> soluble insulin
> syncytium inducing
> > SI variant
> > SI variant of HIV

SIA
> slide immunoenzymatic assay

Siadenovirus
SIADH
> syndrome of inappropriate secretion of antidiuretic hormone

sialadenitis
> HIV s.
> myoepithelial s. (MESA)
> sclerosing s.

sialadenoncus
sialadenosis
sialectasis
sialic acid
sialidase digestion
sialoblastoma
sialocele
sialoglycoprotein
> homologous single-pass membrane s.

sialolithiasis
sialometaplasia
> necrotizing s.

sialomucin
sialoprotein
> bone s.

sialorrhea
Sialosyl-Tn antigen
sialyl
> s. Lewis X (SLex)
> s. moiety

siamense
> *Gnathostoma s.*

siamensis
> *Asaia s.*

Siamese twins
Siberian tick fever
sibericus
> *Dermacentroxenus s.*

Sibine
sibirica
> *Rickettsia s.*

NOTES

S

sibiricum
    Anoxynatronum s.
    Thialkalimicrobium s.
sibiricus
    Thermococcus s.
Sibirina
Sibley-Lehninger (SL)
    S. unit
sibling species
sibship
Sicard syndrome
Sicariidae
sicca
    bronchiectasia s.
    cholera s.
    s. complex
    keratoconjunctivitis s.
    Neisseria s.
    pericarditis s.
    pharyngitis s.
    s. syndrome
siccant
siccative
siccolabile
siccostabile, siccostable
siccus
    pannus s.
SICD
    serum isocitric dehydrogenase
sick
    s. building syndrome
    s. sinus syndrome
sickle
    s. cell (SC)
    s. cell anemia
    s. cell anemia test (SCAT)
    s. cell beta thalassemia
    s. cell crisis
    s. cell hemoglobin (HbS)
    s. cell hemoglobin C, D disease
    s. cell nephropathy
    s. cell test
    s. cell thalassemia disease
    s. cell trait
Sickle-Chex
sickled
    s. cell
    s. erythrocyte
Sickledex
    S. reagent
    S. test
sicklemia
Sicklequik test
sickling
    s. disorder
    s. hemoglobin
    s. test
sickness
    African horse s.

    African sleeping s.
    altitude s.
    decompensation s.
    decompression s.
    green s.
    Jamaican vomiting s.
    radiation s.
    serum s.
    sleeping s.
siculi
    Thermococcus s.
side-chain theory
sidedness
    membrane s.
side effect
sideramine
sideroachrestic anemia
sideroblast
    refractory anemia with ringed s.'s
      (RARS)
    ringed s.
sideroblastica
    anemia refractoria s.
sideroblastic anemia
Siderocapsa
Siderocapsaceae
siderochrome
Siderococcus
siderocyte stain
siderocytic granule
sideroderma
siderofibrosis
siderogenous
sideromycin
sideropenia
sideropenic
    s. anemia
    s. dysphagia
siderophage
siderophagocytosis
siderophil, siderophile
siderophilin
siderophilous
siderophore
siderosilicosis
siderosis
siderosome
siderotic
    s. granule
    s. nodule
siderotica
    granulomatosis s.
    pneumoconiosis s.
SIDS
    sudden infant death syndrome
sienata
    Nocardia s.
SIER
    sonication-induced epitope retrieval

sieve
    s. bone
    molecular s.
sievert (Sv)
sIg
    surface immunoglobulin
Siggaard-Andersen alignment nomogram
sigma
    s. bond
    S. Glycergel
    s. isoform
    s. reaction (SR)
    S. Tween proteinase
sigmoid
    s. colon
    s. shape of the curve
sigmoiditis
sigmoidovesical fistula
Sigmund gland
sign
    Amoss s.
    André Thomas s.
    Argyll Robertson pupil s.
    Arroyo s.
    Brudzinski meningeal s.
    Chvostek s.
    Chvostek-Weiss s.
    Coopernail s.
    Courvoisier s.
    crescent s.
    Crichton-Browne s.
    Cullen s.
    dimple s.
    Fajersztajn crossed sciatic s.
    Froment paper s.
    Grey Turner s.
    groove s.
    Hawkins s.
    Higoumenakia s.
    Kernig meningeal s.
    Krisovski s.
    lemon s.
    long tract s.
    Mendel-Bekhterev s.
    Mirchamp s.
    Nikolsky s.
    Ortolani s.
    pseudo-Graefe s.
    pulvinar s.
    Romaña s.
    Rommelaere s.
    Schultze-Chvostek s.

    scimitar s.
    Séguin s.
    sonographic Murphy s.
    string s.
    Vierra s.
    vital s.'s (VS)
signal
    s. amplification
    analog s.
    s. averaging
    common mode s.
    deflection s.
    insufficient s. (IS)
    s. level
    s. node
    s. to noise ratio (S:N)
    nuclear s.
    proinflammatory s.
    spatial syndromic s.
    s. transducer and activator of transcription (STAT)
    trophic s.
signaling
    suppressor of cytokine s. (SOCS)
signature
    gene expression s.
    immunophenotypic s.
    tumor s.
signed
    s. magnitude
    s. rank test
signet
    s. ring
    s. ring adenocarcinoma
    s. ring cell
    s. ring cell carcinoma
    s. ring cell ductal carcinoma in situ
significance
    atypical glandular cell of undetermined s. (AGUS)
    atypical glandular cell of unknown s. (AGUS)
    atypical squamous cells of undetermined s. (ASCUS)
    s. level
    monoclonal gammopathy of undetermined s. (MGUS)
    monoclonal gammopathy of unknown s. (MGUS)
    s. probability
    test of s. (t)

NOTES

significant
- s. asymptomatic bacteriuria (SAB)
- s. digit
- not s. (NS)
- not statistically s. (NSS)
- statistically s. (SS)

Signify
- S. DOA test
- S. ER drug screen test

sign/trill
- Romaña s.

SiHa cell

sihwensis
- *Gordonia s.*

SIL
- squamous intraepithelial lesion

silacea
- *Chrysops s.*

silanated slide
silane
silanization
Silastic
silencing
- epigenetic s.
- gene s.

silent
- s. gene
- s. mutation
- s. myocardial infarction
- s. thalassemia
- s. thyroiditis

Silferskiöld syndrome
silhouette
- cardiac s.

silica (SiO₂)
- s. gel
- s. granuloma

silicate
silicatosis
Silicibacter
- *S. lacuscaerulensis*
- *S. pomeroyi*

silicic acid
silicofluoride
- sodium s.

silicon-controlled
- s.-c. rectifier
- s.-c. switch

silicone
- s. dioxide (SiO₂)
- s. granuloma
- s. lymphadenopathy
- s. oil

siliconoma
silicon-oxygen (Si-O)
silicoproteinosis
silicosis
- complication of s.

silicotic nodule

silo-filler's
- s.-f. disease
- s.-f. lung

silver (Ag)
- argentum
- s. ammoniacal silver stain
- s. cell
- Grocott methenamine s. (GMS)
- s. impregnation
- methenamine s.
- s. nitrate
- s. nitrate stain
- s. nitrate with hematoxylin
- s. nitroprusside test
- s. protein stain
- S. syndrome

silver-acidified serum (Ag-AS)
Silver-Russell
- S.-R. dwarfism
- S.-R. syndrome

silver/silver chloride electrode
silver-stained
- s.-s. nucleolar organizer region (AgNOR)
- s.-s. nucleolar organizing region (AgNOR)

Silvestrini-Corda syndrome
Silvex
silylation
Simbu
- S. hepatitis
- S. virus

simiae
- *Aeromonas s.*
- Herpesvirus s.
- *Mycobacterium s.*
- *Trypanosoma s.*

simian
- s. crease
- s. immunodeficiency virus (SIV)
- s. sarcoma virus (SSV)
- s. vacuolating virus No. 40
- s. virus (SV)

simicola
- *Pneumonyssus s.*

simii
- *Trichophyton s.*

similarity
- antigenic s.

Simkaniaceae
Simkania negevensis
simkin
- simulation kinetics
- simkin analysis

Simmonds disease
Simmons citrate agar
Simonea folliculorum
Simons disease
Simon septic factor

Simonsiella
Simonsiellaceae
simple
- s. adenosis
- s. asphyxiant
- s. atrophy
- s. bone cyst
- s. branched gland
- s. ciliated cuboidal
- s. columnar epithelium
- s. cuboidal epithelium
- s. endometrial hyperplasia
- s. fracture
- s. goiter
- s. hypertrophy
- s. lymphangiectasis
- s. microscope
- s. necrosis
- s. protein
- s. pulmonary eosinophilia
- s. radiological device
- s. random sample
- s. renal cyst
- s. solitary cyst
- s. squamous epithelium
- s. ulcer
- s. urethritis

simplex
- adiposis tuberosa s.
- carcinoma simplex
- epidermolysis bullosa s.
- herpes s. (HS)
- ichthyosis s.
- lymphangioma superficium s.
- prurigo s.
- toxoplasmosis, rubella, cytomegalovirus, and herpes s. (TORCH)
- verruca s.
- xanthoma tuberosum s.

Simplexvirus
simplicissima
- Spicaria s.

Simplify D-dimer assay
Sims-Huhner test
simulans
- Corynebacterium s.
- Staphylococcus s.

simulated hypertrophy
simulated matrix reference materials
simulation
- s. kinetics (simkin)

Simuliidae
Simulium
- S. damnosum
- S. neavei
- S. ochraceum
- S. rugglesi

simultaneous multiple analyzer (SMA)
sincalide
Sindbis
- S. fever
- S. virus

sinensis
- Knoellia s.
- Opisthorchis s.
- Streptococcus s.

sinesedis
- Gordonia s.

sine wave
singaporensis
- Actinopolymorpha s.
- Desulforhopalus s.

singer's
- s. node
- s. nodule

singe-to-multiple layers of follicular cell
single
- s. breath carbon monoxide diffusing capacity
- s. breath nitrogen elimination
- s. copy gene
- s. copy gene marker
- s. diffusion
- s. (gel) diffusion precipitin test in one dimension
- s. (gel) diffusion precipitin test in two dimensions
- s. gene disorder (SGD)
- s. human leukocyte antigen
- s. immunodiffusion
- s. nucleotide change
- s. nucleotide polymorphism (SNP)
- s. nucleotide polymorphism scoring technology
- s. unit smooth muscle
- S. Use Diagnostic System (SUDS)
- s. vial fixative

single-agent kinetic enzyme assay
single-analyte
- s.-a. immunologic assay
- s.-a. molecular assay

single-chain antigen-binding (SCA)
single-diffusion radial immunodiffusion

S

NOTES

single-donor
> s.-d. plasma
> s.-d. platelets

single-dot pattern

single-phase

single-stranded
> s.-s. conformation polymorphism (SSCP)
> s.-s. DNA (SS-DNA)

Singleton-Merten syndrome

sinica
> *Borrelia s.*

sinistra
> pericolitis s.

sinistrocardia
> isolated s.

sink
> heat s.

sinoatrial (SA)

sinonasal
> s. myxoma
> s. smooth muscle cell tumor
> s. undifferentiated carcinoma (SNUC)

Sinorhizobium
> *S. kummerowiae*
> *S. morelense*

sinuatum
> *Entoloma s.*

sinuatus
> *Rhodophyllus s.*

sinus, pl. **sinus, sinuses**
> anal s.
> Aschoff-Rokitansky s.
> cavernous s.
> coronary s.
> s. cyst
> dermal s.
> ethmoidal s.
> s. ethmoidales
> s. histiocytosis (SH)
> s. histiocytosis with massive lymphadenopathy (SHML)
> s. intercavernosi anterior et posterior
> lactiferous s.
> s. lienis
> lymph s.
> lymphatic s.
> medullary s.
> s. mucocele
> s. of nail
> s. node dysfunction syndrome
> *Oribacterium s.*
> s. phlebitis
> pilonidal s.
> rhomboidal s.
> Rokitansky-Aschoff s.
> splenic s.

> superior sagittal s.
> s. unguis
> s. of Valsalva aneurysm
> s. venosus remnant
> venous s.

sinusarabici
> *Flexistipes s.*

sinusitis
> allergic fungal s.
> sclerosing s.

sinusoid
> blood s.
> hepatic s.
> reticular fiber in wall of s.

sinusoidal
> s. capillary
> s. dilatation
> s. endothelial cell
> s. foam cell cluster
> s. inflammation

Si-O
> silicon-oxygen

SiO₂
> silica
> silicone dioxide

Siphona irritans

Siphonaptera

siphonis
> *Aquicella s.*

Siphoviridae

Siphunculina

Sipple syndrome

siralis
> *Bacillus s.*

sirenomelia

Sirius red

siRNA
> short-interference RNA

siro
> *Acarus s.*
> *Tyroglyphus s.*

Sirobasidium

SIRS
> soluble immune response suppressor

SISI
> short increment sensitivity index
> SISI test

sister
> s. chromatid
> S. Mary Joseph nodule

Sistotrema

Sisyrosea

site
> s. of action potential generation
> allosteric s.
> antibody combining s.
> antigen-binding s.
> antigen-combining s.
> combining s.

extravascular s.
immunologically privileged s.
implantation s.
ligand-induced binding s. (LIBS)
privileged s.
receptor s.
sextant s.
small discrete s.
s. of venous obstruction
site-specific biopsy mapping
sitophila
    Chrysonilia s.
sitosterolemia
    beta s.
situ
adenocarcinoma in s. (AIS)
apocrine ductal carcinoma in s.
argyrophilic ductal carcinoma in s.
carcinoma in s. (CIS)
clinging ductal carcinoma in s.
comedo ductal carcinoma in s.
cystic hypersecretory ductal
  carcinoma in s.
ductal carcinoma in s. (DCIS)
endocrine ductal carcinoma in s.
  (E-DCIS)
endometrial carcinoma in s. (ECIS)
epidermoid carcinoma in s.
in s.
isolated gland carcinoma in s.
  (GCIS)
lobular carcinoma in s. (LCIS)
malignant melanoma in s.
melanoma in s.
neuroendocrine ductal carcinoma
  in s.
signet ring cell ductal carcinoma
  in s.
squamous cell carcinoma in s.
surface carcinoma in s. (SCIS)
situs inversus
SIUD
    sudden intrauterine unexplained death
SIV
    simian immunodeficiency virus
sivashensis
    Orenia s.
Siwe-Letterer disease
sixth venereal disease
size
laser diffraction particle s.
mean follicle s.

size-exclusion chromatography
sizing
    platelet s.
Sjögren
    S. antibody
    S. disease
    S. syndrome
Sjögren-Larsson syndrome
SJR
    Shinowara-Jones-Reinhard
    SJR unit
skagerrakense
    Tenacibaculum s.
skatole
skatoxyl
skein cell
skeinoid fiber
skeletal
    s. disease
    s. fluorosis
    s. muscle
    s. muscle antibody
    s. muscle component of cardiac
      isoenzymes (MM)
    s. muscle fiber
    s. muscle tissue
    s. survey
skeletal-muscle myosin
skeleti
    musculus s.
skeleton
    gel-embedded GA-fixed s.
    gill-arch s.
    s. hand
    membrane s.
Skene
    Bartholin, urethral, S. (BUS)
    S. gland
skeneitis, skenitis
Skermanella parooensis
Skevas-Zerfus disease
skew
skewed distribution
skewness
skin
    alligator s.
    s. biopsy
    s. carcinoma
    congenital localized absence of s.
      (CLAS)
    deciduous s.
    elastic s.

NOTES

S

skin *(continued)*
    farmer's s.
    fish s.
    s. fungus culture
    glabrous s.
    s. graft (SG)
    s. groove
    hyperextensible s.
    layer of s.
    loose s.
    lymphocytic infiltration of s.
    mixed tumor of s.
    s. mycobacteria culture
    parchment s.
    piebald s.
    pigment cell of s.
    porcupine s.
    s. puncture
    s. reaction
    s. reaction pattern
    s. ridge
    sailor's s.
    seared s.
    shagreen s.
    s. shave biopsy
    stippling of s.
    s. stone
    stretchable s.
    s. tag
    s. test dose (STD)
    s. test unit (STU)
    thick s.
    thin s.
    s. tumor
    washerwoman's s.
    s. window test
    yellow discoloration of s.
skinbound disease
Skinner classification
skin-puncture test
skin-reactive factor (SRF)
Skinsense gloves
skin-sensitizing antibody (SSA)
skin-specific histocompatibility antigen
skin-to-tumor distance (STD)
skip
    s. areae
    s. lesion
    s. metastasis
skip-segment Hirschsprung disease
skull
    cloverleaf s.
    maplike s.
    steeple s.
sky blue
skyensis
    Pasteurella s.
SL
    Sibley-Lehninger

    small lymphocyte
    SL unit
sl
    slyke
SLA
    slide latex agglutination
    soluble liver antigen
Slackia
    S. exigua
    S. heliotrinireducens
slant culture
slaty anemia
SLD, SLDH
    serum lactate dehydrogenase
SLE
    St. Louis encephalitis
    systemic lupus erythematosus
sleep
    s. apnea syndrome
    s. disorder
sleeping sickness
sleeve lobectomy
SLEP
    Shelf-Life Extension Program
SLEV
    SLEV serology
SLex
    sialyl Lewis X
    blood group antigen SLex
SLFIA
    substrate-labeled fluorescence
    immunoassay
    substrate-labeled fluorescent
    immunoassay
SLI
    somatostatin-like immunoreactivity
slide
    s. agglutination test
    aminopropyltriethyoxysilane-coated
    glass s.
    s. bile solubility test
    ChemMate capillary gap s.
    Colorfrost disposable microscope s.
    Colormark s.
    s. flocculation test
    Genta s.
    hydrogel coated s.
    s. immunoenzymatic assay (SIA)
    s. latex agglutination (SLA)
    s. micrometer
    s. platelet aggregation test (SPAT)
    silanated s.
    Superfrost Plus glass s.
    triethylenethiophosphoramide
    precoated s.
    Ventana silanized capillary gap s.
SlidePro slide heater
slide-wire potentiometer
sliding microtome

slightly
s. curved rod
s. yellow colony
sling fiber
slippage
polymerase s.
slit
filtration s.
s. lamp
s. pore
slitlike
s. margin
s. space
SLKC
superior limbic keratoconjunctivitis
SLL
small lymphocytic lymphoma
SLMN
sarcoma-like mural nodule
SLN
sentinel lymph node
SLO
streptolysin O
slope culture
slot-blot
slot exhaust
slough
sloughing
s. ulcer
slovaca
Rickettsia s.
slow
s. fever
s. hemoglobin
s. neutron
s. reacting factor of anaphylaxis (SRF-A)
s. reacting substance of anaphylaxis (SRS-A, SRSA)
s. virus
s. virus disease
s. vital capacity (SVC)
slow-moving protease (SMP)
slow-reacting
slow-reacting substance (SRS)
SLS
segment long-spacing
SLS collagen
Sluder syndrome
sludge
sludged blood
sluggish layer

slurry
SLVL
splenic lymphoma with villous lymphocyte
Sly
S. disease
S. syndrome
slyke (sl)
SM
splenomegaly
Sm
samarium
SMA
sequential multichannel autoanalyzer
sequential multiple analyzer
simultaneous multiple analyzer
small muscle atrophy
smooth muscle actin
smooth muscle antibody
spinal muscular atrophy
infantile SMA
juvenile SMA
SMA-12 profile test
SMAC
sequential multichannel autoanalyzer
SMAC 6, 7, 10, 12, 20
SMAC test
SMAF
specific macrophage-arming factor
small
s. artery
s. bowel biopsy
s. bowel ischemia
s. calorie (c, cal)
s. cell cancer (SCC)
s. cell lung carcinoma (SCLC)
s. cell sarcoma
s. cell tumor
s. cell undifferentiated neuroendocrine carcinoma (SCUNC)
s. cleaved cell
s. discrete site
s. glandular pattern
s. intestine bacterial overgrowth
s. intestine polyp
s. intestine tumor
s. lymphocytic lymphoma (SLL)
s. muscle atrophy (SMA)
s. noncleaved cell (SNCC)
s. nuclear ribonucleoproteins (SNRPs)

NOTES

small *(continued)*
    s. peptide
    s. round cell tumor (SRCT)
    s. vein
smallpox
    s. as biological weapon
    coherent s.
    confluent s.
    discrete s.
    flat s.
    fulminating s.
    hemorrhagic s.
    s. immunization
    inoculation s.
    malignant s.
    modified s.
    modified type s.
    ordinary s.
    s. vaccination
    s. vaccine
    s. virus
    West Indian s.
Sm antigen
SMART
    sensitive membrane antigen rapid test
SmartCycler realtime PCR system
smart terminal
SMC
    skeletal myxoid chondrosarcoma
    somatomedin C
SMCD
    systemic mast cell disease
smear
    acid-fast s.
    AFB s.
    air-dried s.
    alcohol fixed s.
    alimentary tract s.
    auramine-stained buffy coat s.
    s. background
    Bethesda Pap s.
    blood s.
    Breed s.
    broad s.
    bronchoscopic s.
    buccal s.
    buffy coat s.
    cervical s.
    colonic s.
    cul-de-sac s.
    s. culture
    cytologic s.
    cytopuncture s.
    cytospin slide centrifuge gram-stained s.
    Diff-Quik s.
    dried s.
    duodenal s.
    ectocervical s.

    endocervical s.
    endometrial s.
    esophageal s.
    fast s.
    FGT cytologic s.
    fungus s.
    gastric s.
    lateral vaginal wall s.
    Legionella pneumophila direct fA s.
    lower respiratory tract s.
    malaria s.
    nasal s.
    Neisseria gonorrhoeae s.
    Nickerson medium s.
    oral s.
    Pagano-Levin medium s.
    pancervical s.
    Pap s.
    peripheral blood s.
    s. preparation and staining for blood parasites
    sputum s.
    sputum tuberculosis acid-fast s.
    TB s.
    s. test
    Tzanck s.
    urinary s.
    vaginal irrigation s. (VIS)
    VCE s.
    VEE s.
SMECE
    sclerosing mucoepidermoid carcinoma with eosinophilia
smegma
    s. bacillus
    s. clitoridis
    s. embryonum
    s. preputii
smegmalith
smegmatis
    Mycobacterium s.
smell
    organ of s.
S-**methylmalonyl-CoA mutase**
Smith
    S. disease
    S. silver stain
Smithella propionica
Smith-Lemli-Opitz syndrome
Smith-Magenis syndrome
Smith-Riley syndrome
Smith-Strang disease
SMN
    survival motor neuron
        SMN telomeric gene
SMO
    smoothened
        SMO gene

smog
    photochemical s.
SMOH
    smoothened homolog
smoke
    NATO code for military obscurant s. (zinc oxide and hexachloroethane, grained aluminum) (HC)
smoke-producing munition
smoker's
    s. granule
    s. polycythemia
smoky
    s. melanin
    s. urine
smoldering
    s. form of ATLL
    s. leukemia
SMON
    subacute myelooptic neuropathy
S-Monovette blood collection system
smooth (S)
    s. bacterium
    s. colony
    s. endoplasmic reticulum
    s. leprosy
    s. muscle
    s. muscle actin (SMA)
    s. muscle antibody (SMA)
    s. muscle cell
    s. muscle marker
    s. muscle metaplasia
    s. muscle tissue
    s. muscle tumor (SMT)
    s. muscle tumor of uncertain malignant potential (SMTUMP)
smoothened (SMO)
    s. homolog (SMOH)
smoothing
smooth-rough variation
smooth-surfaced endoplasmic reticulum
smooth-walled cyst
SMP
    slow-moving protease
SMR
    somnolent metabolic rate
    standard morbidity ratio
    standard mortality ratio
SMT
    smooth muscle tumor

SMTUMP
    smooth muscle tumor of uncertain malignant potential
smudge cell
smudged
    s. cell
    s. nucleus
smut
    wheat s.
SMZL
    splenic marginal zone lymphoma
SN
    serum-neutralizing
S:N
    signal to noise ratio
SNa
    concentration of sodium in serum
snakebite
snake venom (SV)
SNAP
    soluble NSF attachment protein
SNAP-25
snap-freezing of tissue
snap-frozen specimen
SNARE
    soluble NSF-attachment protein receptor
snatching
    body s.
SNB
    scalene node biopsy
SNCC
    small noncleaved cell
Sneathia sanguinegens
Sneddon syndrome
Sneddon-Wilkinson disease
sneeze gas
Snell law
***S*-nitrosohemoglobin**
SNOMED
    systematized nomenclature of medicine
Snook reticulum stain
SNOP
    Systematized Nomenclature of Pathology
snout
    cytoplasmic s.
snowshoe hare virus
snowstorm
    lead s.
SNP
    single nucleotide polymorphism
    SNP scoring technology
SNPstream genotyping system

S

NOTES

SNRPs
> small nuclear ribonucleoproteins

snub-nose dwarfism

SNUC
> sinonasal undifferentiated carcinoma

soap
> SoftCIDE-EC antimicrobial hand s.
> SoftCIDE hand s.
> SoftCIDE-NA plain hand s.

soap-bubble radiolucency

Sobemovirus

sobria
> *Aeromonas s.*

so-called false-positive reaction

socia parotidis

society
> American Chemical S. (ACS)
> Musculoskeletal Tumor S. (MSTS)
> S. for Pediatric Pathology (SPP)

socket
> tooth s.

socks and gloves petechial rash

SOCS
> suppressor of cytokine signaling

Sodalis glossinidius

sodium
> s. acetarsol
> s. acetate
> s. acetazolamide
> s. acid citrate
> s. acid phosphate
> s. alginate
> s. alizarinsulfonate
> s. *p*-aminohippurate
> s. *para*-aminosalicylate
> s. amobarbital
> s. antimonyltartrate
> s. arsenate
> s. ascorbate
> s. aurothiomalate
> s. aurothiosuccinate
> s. aurothiosulfate
> s. azide
> s. benzoate
> s. benzosulfimide
> s. bicarbonate
> s. biphosphate
> s. bisulfite stain
> s. borate
> s. bromide
> s. butabarbital
> s. cacodylate
> s. calcium edetate
> s. caprylate
> carbenicillin indanyl s.
> s. carbonate
> s. caseinate
> s. cellulose phosphate
> s. chloride

s. chloride broth
s. chloride culture medium
s. chromate
s. clearance
colistimethate s.
s. cyanide (NaCN)
s. cyclamate
dextrothyroxine s.
s. diphenylhydantoin
s. dithionate
s. dodecyl sulfate (SDS)
s. dodecyl sulfate-polyacrylamide gel electrophoresis (SDS-PAGE)
exchangeable s.
fecal s.
fluorescein s.
s. fluoride
s. fluoroacetate
s. fluorosilicate
s. folate
fractional excretion of s. (FENa)
s. fusidate
s. glutamate
s. glycolate
s. hexafluorosilicate
s. hydrate
s. hydroxide stain
s. hypochlorite
s. hyposulfite
s. imbalance
s. indigotin disulfonate
s. iodide
s. lactate
s. lauryl sulfate
mercaptomerin s.
s. metabisulfite sickle hemoglobin test
s. monofluorophosphate
s. morrhuate
s. nitrate
s. nitrite
s. nitroferricyanide
s. nitroprusside
s. orthovanadate
s. oxybate
s. *p*-aminohippuric acid
s. *p*-aminosalicylate
s. pentobarbital
s. perborate
s. phenobarbital
s. phenylethylbarbiturate
s. phenytoin
s. phytate
plasma s. (P_{Na})
s. polyethylene sulfonate
s. and potassium assays
s. potassium sodium tartrate
s. propionate
s. pyroborate

s. pyrophosphate
s. pyrosulfite
resorcinolphthalein s.
rose bengal s.
s. salicylate
s. silicofluoride
s. stearate
s. stibocaptate
stool s.
s. succinate
s. sulfite
sulfobromophthalein s.
s. sulfoxone
s. taurocholate
s. test
s. tetraborate
s. tetradecyl sulfate
s. thiamylal
s. thiocyanate (NaSCN)
s. thiopental
s. thiosulfate stain
s. tolbutamide
s. trimetaphosphate
s. tungstoborate
tyropanoate s.
urine s.
s. warfarin
Yb-169 pentetate s.
sodium-iodide
sodium-iodine symporter (NIS)
s.-i. transport protein
Soehngenia saccharolytica
Soemmerring
S. ganglion
S. spot
soft
s. chancre
s. papilloma
s. sore
s. tissue calcification (STC)
s. tissue lipoma
s. tissue tumor
s. tubercle
s. ulcer
s. wart
Sof-Tact
S.-T. diabetes management system
S.-T. glucose monitor
SoftCIDE-EC antimicrobial hand soap
SoftCIDE hand soap
SoftCIDE-NA plain hand soap
SoftGrip pipette

SoftGUARD hand cream
soft-spin technique
software
CellQuest Pro 4.0 flow cytometry s.
Expo 32 flow cytometry s.
Sohval-Soffer syndrome
SOL
solution
space-occupying lesion
sol
metal s.
solid s.
solani
Kribbella s.
solanine
Solanum carolinense
solar
s. elastosis
s. fever
s. keratosis
s. lentigo
s. urticaria
solder spot
soldier's patch
solenocyte
solenoid
Solenopotes capillatus
Solenopsis
sole nucleus
sole-plate ending
solfataricum
Desulfotomaculum s.
soli
Bacillus s.
Fulvimonas s.
Nocardia s.
Weissella s.
solid
s. adenocarcinoma
s. ameloblastoma
s. angle
s. carbon dioxide
s. carcinoma
s. edema
s. growth pattern
s. masses of epithelial cell
s. pattern
s. phase fluorescence immunoassay (SPFIA)
s. phase immunoassay
s. pseudopapillary tumor

NOTES

solid *(continued)*
    s. sol
    s. state
    s. teratoma
    total s. (TS)
solidistic pathology
solid-phase
    s.-p. hybridization
    s.-p. radioimmunoassay
    s.-p. separation
Solirubrobacter pauli
solitarii
    folliculi lymphatici s.
solitary
    s. bone cyst
    s. fibrous tumor (SFT)
    s. follicle
    s. gland
    s. nodule of intestine
    s. osteocartilaginous exostosis
    s. rectal ulcer syndrome
solium
    Taenia s.
sollicitans
    Aedes s.
Solobacterium moorei
solochrome
    s. azurine staining method
    s. cyanine stain
solubility
    s. coefficient
    s. product
    s. test
solubilization defect
solubilize
solubilized hemoglobin
solubilizer
soluble
    s. HLA
    s. HLA protein
    s. human leukocyte antigen
    s. immune response suppressor
    (SIRS)
    s. insulin (SI)
    s. interleukin-2 receptor
    s. liver antigen (SLA)
    s. NSF attachment protein (SNAP)
    s. NSF-attachment protein receptor
    (SNARE)
    s. ribonucleic acid (sRNA)
    s. specific substance
    s. transferrin receptor (sTfR)
solute
    total body s. (TBS)
solution (SOL)
    ammoniacal silver s.
    anticoagulant heparin s.
    aqueous s.
    Atroxin s.

azeotropic s.
Balamuth buffer s.
balanced salt s. (BSS)
Belzer s.
Benedict s.
blocking s.
Bouin s.
buffered saline s. (BSS)
Burow s.
Cajal formol ammonium bromide s.
carrageenin s.
Celsior s.
cleaning s.
Coleman Feulgen s.
Cytyc CytoLyt preservative s.
Cytyc PreservCyt preservative s.
Dakin s.
Dako target retrieval s.
Delafield fixative s.
Denhardt s.
Diaphane s.
disclosing s.
Dragendorff s.
Earle s.
Fehling s.
Fonio s.
formaldehyde s.
formalin s.
Fowler s.
FU-48 Zenker fixative s.
Gallego differentiating s.
Gowers s.
Gram s.
Hartmann s.
Hayem s.
Hinfl s.
Histoclear slide processing s.
Hollande s.
Hucker-Conn crystal violet s.
s. hybridization
hydrogen peroxide s.
ideal s.
isotonic sodium chloride s.
Kaiserling s.
Karnovsky II s.
Krebs-Ringer s.
lactated Ringer s. (LRS)
Lange s.
Locke s.
Locke-Ringer s.
Lugol iodine s.
Lumi-Phos s.
Monsel s.
mordant s.
nonideal s.
NoTox formalin substitute s.
Oncor antifade mounting s.
Orth s.
Perls s.

physiological saline s. (PSS)
physiologic saline s.
Progen antibiotic s.
propidium iodide s.
pyridoxalated stroma-free
  hemoglobin s.
ribonuclease s.
Ringer lactate s. (RLS)
Ruge s.
saline s.
saponin lysing reagent stock s.
saturated s. (SS)
Schallibaum s.
sodium chloride-sodium citrate s.
  (SSC)
standard s.
TAC s.
Tellyesnicky fixative s.
test s. (TS)
tetrazolium salt s.
Toison s.
volumetric s. (VS)
Weigert iodine s.
Zamboni s.
Zenker s.
solvate
solvation
solvent
aprotic s.
s. detergent treatment (SD)
s. extraction
organic s.
protic s.
solvolysis
soma
somaliensis
Streptomyces s.
soman
NATO code for s. (GD)
somatic
s. agglutinin
s. antigen
s. cell
s. cell genetics
s. chromosome
s. death
s. motor neuron
s. mutation theory of cancer
s. pairing
s. point mutation
somatochrome

somatomammotropin
chorionic s. (CS)
human chorionic s. (hCSM)
immunoradioassayable human
  chorionic s. (IRHCS)
somatomedin C (SMC)
somatoplasm
somatosexual ambiguity
somatostatin-like immunoreactivity (SLI)
somatostatinoma
somatostatin-producing small cell
somatostatin receptor
somatotroph, somatotrope
s. adenoma
s. release inhibiting factor
somatotropic
s. adenoma
s. hormone (STH)
somatotropic hormone (STH)
somatotropin
somatotropin-releasing
s.-r. factor (SRF)
s.-r. hormone (SRH)
somerae
Cetobacterium s.
somni
Histophilus s.
somniferum
Papaver a.
somnolent metabolic rate (SMR)
Somogyi
S. effect
S. method
S. unit
sonicate
sonication
**sonication-induced epitope retrieval
  (SIER)**
sonic hedgehog (SHH)
sonification
sonifier
sonify
Sonne-Duval bacillus
Sonne dysentery
sonnei
Shigella s.
sonographic Murphy sign
sonorensis
Bacillus s.
soot wart
sooty capsule

NOTES

SOP
standard operating procedure
sorbate
potassium s.
sorbefacient
sorbent
sorbic acid
sorbitol dehydrogenase
sorbitol-MacConkey medium
Sordaria
sordellii
Clostridium s.
sordidicola
Burkholderia s.
sore
canker s.
Ceylon mouth s.
cold s.
fungating s.
hard s.
s. mouth
Oriental s.
soft s.
venereal s.
sorehead
soremouth virus
soremuzzle
Soret
S. band
S. effect
S. phenomenon
sorption
Sorsby syndrome
sorter
fluorescence-activated cell s.
(FACS)
SOS bacterial DNA repair system
Sotos syndrome of cerebral gigantism
soudanense
Trichophyton s.
souniana
Vulcanisaeta s.
source
alpha s.
flood s.
hidden radiation s.
neutron s.
sealed beta gamma s.
sealed radioactive s.
s. statement
unsealed beta gamma s.
unsealed radioactive s.
sourekii
Facklamia s.
South
S. African-type porphyria
S. American blastomycosis
Southern
S. blot (SB)

S. blot analysis
S. blot technique
S. blot test
souvenir knife
soybean
s. test
s. trypsin inhibitor (SBTI)
Soymovirus
s/p
status post
sp, pl. **spp.**
species
space
air-filled tubular s.
anterior incisural s.
Blessig s.
Bowman s.
canalicular s.
capillary-like s.
capsomer capsular s.
capsular s.
cartilage s.
cavernous s.
s. charge
corneal s.
Czermak s.
Disse s.
extravascular s.
filtration s.
Fontana s.
haversian s.
His perivascular s.
honeycomb-like s.
intercristal s.
interglobular s.
intervillous s.
intracisternal s.
intracristal s.
intramembranous s.
intravascular s.
s. of iridocorneal angle
Kiernan s.
labyrinthine s.
lymph s.
Max-Joseph s.
medium incisural s.
Nuel s.
Parona s.
perinuclear s.
perisinusoidal s.
Poiseuille s.
posterior incisural s.
punched out s.
Schwalbe s.
slitlike s.
subarachnoid s.
subchorial s.
Virchow-Robin s.

vitreous s.
zonular s.
space-occupying lesion (SOL)
spacer
spacing
   third s.
spade
   s. finger
   s. hand
SPAI
   steroid protein activity index
spallation product
spalling
Spanish influenza
spanius
   Achromobacter s.
Sparassis
sparganoma
sparganosis
sparganum
Sparganum proliferum
sparing
   orthokeratotic s.
sparteine
spasm
   s. of accommodation
   bladder s.
   cadaveric s.
   diffuse esophageal s.
   epidemic transient diaphragmatic s.
   esophageal s.
   salaam s.
   saltatory s.
spasmogen
spastic
   s. anemia
   s. colitis
   s. colon
   s. ileus
SPAT
   slide platelet aggregation test
spatial
   s. isomerism
   s. scan statistic
   s. syndromic signal
spatium, pl. **spatia**
   spatia anguli iridocornealis
   s. interglobulare
   s. intervaginale subarachnoidale
   nervi optici
   spatia zonularia

spatula
   Ayre s.
   Roux s.
spatulata
   Cooperia s.
SPB
   solitary plasmacytoma of bone
SPBI
   serum protein-bound iodine
SPCA
   serum prothrombin conversion
   acceleration
   serum prothrombin conversion
   accelerator
   SPCA deficiency
   SPCA factor
SPE, SPEP
   serum protein electrophoresis
Spearman rank correlation coefficient
special
   s. pathology
   s. reference method
specialist
   blood bank technology s.
   s. dissection technique
specialization
   globose s.
specialized
   s. epithelium
   s. transduction
speciation
species (sp)
   reactive oxygen s. (ROS)
   sibling s.
   type s.
species-specific antigen
specific
   s. absorptivity
   s. active immunity
   s. anergy
   s. antibody deficiency
   s. antigen
   s. antiserum
   s. autoantibody
   s. bactericide
   s. capsular substance
   s. cell receptor
   s. coagulation factor deficiency
   s. disease
   s. dynamic action
   s. gene
   s. granule

NOTES

specific (*continued*)
s. gravity (SG, sp gr)
s. gravity test
s. heat
s. heat capacity
s. hemolysin
s. IgE
s. IgE antibody scoring
s. IgE antibody testing
s. immune globulin (human)
s. ionization
s. macrophage-arming factor (SMAF)
s. opsonin
s. passive immunity
s. pathogen-free (SPF)
s. rate
s. reaction
s. rotation
s. serum
s. soluble polysaccharide
s. soluble substance (SSS)
s. soluble sugar
s. transduction
s. virologic diagnosis

specificity
analytical s.
anti-P blood group s.
diagnostic s.
HLA-C locus s.
kappa chain s.
lambda chain s.
relative s.
tumor s.

specified
not otherwise s. (NOS)

Speci-Gard specimen transport bag
specimen
bacteriologic s.
biopsy s.
brush s.
clean-catch urine s.
clean-voided s. (CVS)
clinical bacteriologic s.
cytologic s.
double-voided urine s.
EDTA contamination of s.
first morning urine s.
grab urine s.
mammary aspiration s. (MAS)
normocellular bone marrow s.
postmortem s.
s. radiography
random urine s.
snap-frozen s.
surgical s.
swab s.
touch-smear s.
trimmed s.

speckled pattern
spectra (*pl. of* spectrum)
spectral
s. color
s. interference
s. karyotype
s. karyotyping
s. overlap
s. resolution
s. response

spectrin
spectrofluorometer
spectrograph
mass s.

spectrometer
energy dispersive s. (EDS)
gamma s.
mass s.

spectrometry
clinical s.
gamma s.
gas chromatography-mass s. (GC-MS)
isotope dilution-mass s.
MALDI-TOF mass s.
mass s. (MS)
matrix-assisted laser desorption and ionization mass s. (MALDIMS)
tandem mass s.

spectrophotometer
atomic absorption s. (AAS)
Cary 100 UV-Vis s.
DU Series 500, DU 800 UV/Vis s.

spectrophotometric assay
spectrophotometry
atomic absorption s. (AAS)
flame emission s.
infrared s. (IRS)
reflectance s.
ultraviolet/visible s.

spectroscope
direct vision s.
PE2100 s.

spectroscopic test
spectroscopy
atomic absorption s.
clinical s.
emission s.
energy dispersive x-ray s. (EDS)
flame emission s. (FES)
fluorescence correlation s. (FCS)
infrared s.
mass s.
microabsorption s.
nuclear magnetic resonance s.
proton s.

Raman s.
vibrational s.
spectrum, pl. **spectra, spectrums**
absorption s.
s. action
action s.
s. analyzer
antimicrobial s.
atomic s.
band s.
broad s.
chemical s.
clinical s.
continuous s.
emission s.
excitation s.
fiber s.
fluorescence s.
gamma-ray s.
gaseous s.
line s.
toxin s.
wide s.
specular reflection
speed vacuum concentrator
Spegazzinia
speibonae
Streptomyces s.
spelencephaly
Spelotrema nicolli
Spencer disease
spencerii
Aedes s.
Spencer-Wells forceps
Spen syndrome
spent platelet
SPEP (*var. of* SPE)
sperm
s. agglutinating antibody
s. cell
s. crystal
muzzled s.
s. nucleus
s. penetration assay
spermacytic seminoma
spermagglutination
spermatic
s. duct
s. filament
s. fistula
spermatici
tunicae funiculi s.

spermatid
nuclear envelope of s.
spermatin
spermatoblast
spermatocele
spermatocyst
spermatocytal
spermatocyte
primary s.
secondary s.
spermatocytic
s. granuloma
s. seminoma
spermatocytogenesis
spermatogenesis
spermatogenetic
spermatogenic
s. granuloma
s. maturation arrest
spermatogenous
spermatogeny
spermatogone
spermatogonium, pl. **spermatogonia**
spermatoid
spermatology
spermatolysin
spermatolysis
spermatolytic
spermatophore
spermatopoietic
spermatoxin
spermatozoal
spermatozoon, pl. **spermatozoa**
end piece of s.
mature s.
middle piece of s.
neck of s.
outer dense fibers of s.
principal piece of s.
spermaturia
spermia
spermiation
spermidine
spermiduct
spermine crystal
spermiogenesis
spermium
spermolith
spermolysis
Spermophilus
Spermospora

S

NOTES

spermotoxin
sperm-ubiquitin tag immunoassay (SUTI)
SPF
    specific pathogen-free
SPFIA
    solid phase fluorescence immunoassay
SP-GCT
    soft parts giant cell tumor
sp gr
    specific gravity
SPH
    secondary pulmonary hemosiderosis
sphacelate
sphacelation
sphacelism
sphaceloderma
sphacelous
sphacelus
Sphaerella
Sphaeria
sphaerica
    Nigrospora s.
sphaericus
    Bacillus s.
Sphaerobacteraceae
Sphaerobacterales
Sphaerobacteridae
Sphaerobolus
Sphaerophorus necrophorus
Sphaeropsis subglobosa
sphaerospora
    Xylogone s.
Sphaerotilus natans
S-phase fraction
sphenisci
    Corynebacterium s.
spheniscorum
    Corynebacterium s.
sphenoides
    Clostridium s.
sphenoiditis
sphenooccipital synchondrosis
sphenopetrosal synchondrosis
sphere
    attraction s.
    embryonic s.
    Morgagni s.
    prelytic s.
    segmentation s.
    vitelline s.
spherical polar coordinates
spherocyte with no central pallor zone
spherocytic
    s. anemia
    s. hereditary elliptocytosis
    s. jaundice

spherocytosis
    congenital s.
    hereditary s. (HS)
spherophakia-brachymorphia syndrome
spheroplast
spherospermia
spherule
spherulin
spherulosis
    collagenous s.
sphincter
    urinary tract s.
sphincteral achalasia
sphincteric structure
sphincteritis
sphinganine
sphingenine
Sphingobacteria
Sphingobacteriaceae
Sphingobium
    S. amiense
    S. chlorophenolicum
    S. herbicidovorans
    S. yanoikuyae
sphingolipidosis, pl. **sphingolipidoses**
    cerebral s.
sphingolipid storage disease
sphingolipodystrophy
Sphingomonadaceae
Sphingomonas
    S. aerolata
    S. alaskensis
    S. aquatilis
    S. aurantiaca
    S. chungbukensis
    S. cloacae
    S. faeni
    S. koreensis
    S. melonis
    S. pituitosa
    S. roseiflava
    S. taejonensis
    S. wittichii
    S. xenophaga
    S. yanoikuyae
sphingomyelin
    s. lipidosis
    s. phosphodiesterase
sphingomyelinase
sphingomyelinosis
Sphingopyxis
    S. alaskensis
    S. chilensis
    S. macrogoltabida
    S. terrae
    S. witflariensis
sphingosine
SPI
    serum precipitable iodine

Spicaria simplicissima
spicheri
> *Lactobacillus s.*

spicifera
> *Bipolaris s.*

spicula (*pl. of* spiculum)
spicular
spiculated
> s. body
> s. edge

spicule
> s. of bone
> s. of calcified cartilage

spiculum, pl. spicula
spider
> s. angioma
> arterial s.
> black widow s.
> brown recluse s.
> s. burst
> s. cancer
> s. cell
> s. mole
> s. nevus
> s. pelvis
> s. telangiectasia
> vascular s.

spidery
Spiegler-Fendt
> pseudolymphoma of S.-F.
> S.-F. pseudolymphoma
> S.-F. sarcoid

Spielmeyer acute swelling
Spielmeyer-Stock disease
Spielmeyer-Vogt disease
SPIFE
> S. acid hemoglobin assay
> S. alkaline hemoglobin assay

spike
> s. and dome appearance
> M s.
> monoclonal M s.

spill
> cellular s.
> s. control
> s. control kit
> s. residue

spiloma
Spilopsyllus cuniculi
spilus
> nevus s.

spina, pl. spinae

s. bifida
s. bifida aperta
s. bifida cystica
s. bifida manifesta
s. bifida occulta
s. ventosa
spinal
> s. cord compression
> s. cord concussion
> s. cord demyelinization
> s. cord disease
> s. cord infection
> s. cord inflammation
> s. cord injury
> s. cord tumor
> s. cord vascular malformation
> s. embolism
> s. fluid
> s. fluid culture
> s. fluid leak
> s. fluid leukocyte count
> s. meningioma
> s. muscular atrophy (SMA)
> s. neoplasm
> s. stenosis

Spinchron DLX, 15 series centrifuge
spindle
> achromatic s.
> s. attachment
> barbiturate s.
> bipolar s.
> s. cell
> s. cell carcinoma
> s. cell component
> s. cell epithelial tumor with thymus-like differentiation (SETTLE)
> s. cell fascicular pattern
> s. cell lipoma
> s. cell melanoma
> s. cell nevus
> s. cell pseudotumor
> s. cell sarcoma
> s. cell thymoma
> s. cell tumor
> central s.
> cleavage s.
> s. fiber
> Krukenberg s.
> Kühne s.
> mitotic s.
> multipolar s.

S

NOTES

spindle *(continued)*
    muscle s.
    neuromuscular s.
    neurotendinous s.
    nuclear s.
spindle-celled layer
spindle-shaped neoplastic stromal cell
spindling
spindly squamoid cell
spine
    s. cell
    cleft s.
    dendritic s.
    poker s.
Spiniger
spiniger
    Heterodoxus s.
spinigera
    Haemaphysalis s.
spinigerum
    Gnathostoma s.
spinipalpis
    Ixodes s.
spinnbarkeit
spinner
    DiffSpin slide s.
spinosa
    ichthyosis s.
spinosispora
    Pseudonocardia s.
spinosum
    stratum s.
spinous layer
spinulosum
    Penicillium s.
spiracle
spiradenitis
spiradenoma
    eccrine s.
spiral
    s. artery
    s. crest
    Curschmann s.
    s. foraminous tract
    s. fracture
    Herxheimer s.
    s. hypha
    s. lamina
    s. ligament of cochlea
    s. membrane
    s. organ
    s. plate
    s. plica
    s. tubule
    s. visual field
    s. wound (SW)
spirale
    organum s.

spiralis
    Acuaria s.
    crista s.
    membrana reticularis organi s.
    Trichinella s.
    Trichurus s.
spiramycin
spirilla (*pl. of* spirillum)
Spirillaceae
Spirillales
spirillar dysentery
Spirilleae
spirillosis
Spirillum
    S. minus
    S. volutans
spirillum, pl. **spirilla**
    Obermeier s.
spirit lamp
Spirocerca lupi
Spirochaeta
    S. americana
    S. bajacaliforniensis
    S. eurystrepta
    S. pallida
    S. plicatilis
    S. stenostrepta
Spirochaetaceae
Spirochaetae
Spirochaetales
Spirochaetes
spirochetal
spirochete
    Becker stain for s.'s
    Dutton s.
spirochetemia
spirochetolysis
spirochetosis
    icterogenic s.
spirogram
    forced expiratory s. (FES)
Spirolate broth
Spirometra
    S. mansoni
    S. mansonoides
Spiromicrovirus
spironolactone test
Spiroplasmataceae
Spirosomaceae
Spirotrichum
Spirurata
Spirurida
Spiruridae
Spiruroidea
spiruroid larva migrans
Spitz-like melanoma
Spitz nevus
spitzoid melanocytic lesion

SPL
    spontaneous lesion
splanchnic
    s. blood flow (SBF)
    s. mesenchyme
splanchnicus
    Bacteroides s.
splanchnocystica
    dysencephalia s.
splanchnoptosis, splanchnoptosia
splanchnosclerosis
splatter
    back s.
    impact s.
splatter-borne agent
spleen
    accessory s.
    Banti s.
    diffuse waxy s.
    Gandy-Gamna s.
    hilum of s.
    lardaceous s.
    lymphoid follicles of the s.
    malpighian body of s.
    sago s.
    sugar-coated s.
    venae cavernosae of s.
    waxy s.
splen accessorius
splenauxe
splendens
    linea s.
Splendore-Hoeppli phenomenon
splenectopia
splenelcosis
splenemphraxis
splenic
    s. anemia
    s. anemia of infants
    s. cell
    s. cord
    s. corpuscle
    s. flexure
    s. hemangiosarcoma
    s. index
    s. leukemia
    s. lymph follicle
    s. lymph nodule
    s. lymphoma with villous lymphocyte (SLVL)
    s. marginal zone lymphoma (SMZL)

    s. pulp
    s. red pulp
    s. sequestration of platelets
    s. sinus
    s. tumor
splenica
    pulpa s.
splenicum
    hilum s.
splenis
    tunica fibrosa s.
splenitis
    acute s.
splenocele
splenogonadal fusion
splenohepatomegaly
splenoma
splenomalacia
splenomedullary
splenomegalic polycythemia
splenomegaly (SM)
    congestive s.
    Egyptian s.
    fibrocongestive s.
    hemolytic s.
    marked s.
    prominent s.
splenomyelogenous
splenomyelomalacia
splenoncus
splenosis
splenotoxin
spliceosome
splicing
    gene s.
    RNA s.
splint
    shin s.
split
    s. collection urine test
    s. gene
    s. pelvis
    s. renal function (SRF)
    s. renal function study (SRFS)
    s. renal function test
    s. tolerance
split-thickness skin graft (STSG)
splitting
    beam s.
split-virus vaccine
SPM
    scanning probe microscopy

NOTES

S

"SPO1-like viruses"
spodogenous
spodogram
spodography
spodophorous
Spondweni virus
spondylitis
    ankylosing s.
    rheumatoid ankylosing s.
    tuberculous s.
spondylocace
Spondylocladium
spondyloepiphyseal, spondyloepiphysial
    s. dysplasia (SED)
spondylolisthesis
spondylolisthetic pelvis
spondylolysis
spondylomalacia
spondylopathy
spondyloptosis
spondylopyosis
spondyloschisis
spondylosis
    cervical s.
    hyperostotic s.
    lumbar s.
spondylosyndesis
sponge disease
spongiform
    s. degeneration
    s. encephalopathy
    s. pustule of Kogoj
spongioblast
spongioblastoma
spongiocyte
spongioid
spongiosa
    substantia s.
spongiosi
    tunica albuginea corporis s.
spongiosis
spongiositis
spongiosum
    corpus s.
    fibrous tunic of corpus s.
    osteoma s.
    stratum s.
spongiosus
    status s.
spongiotic dermatitis
Spongipellis
Spongiporus
spongy
    s. body of penis
    s. bone
    s. degeneration of infancy
    s. degenerative-type leukodystrophy
    s. nevus

spontanea
    dactylolysis s.
spontaneous
    s. abortion
    s. agglutination
    s. amputation
    s. bacterial peritonitis (SBP)
    s. coagulation
    s. coronary artery dissection (SCAD)
    s. delivery (SD)
    s. generation
    s. lesion (SPL)
    s. mutation
    s. phagocytosis
    s. pneumothorax
    s. remission
sporadic
    s. adenomatous polyp (SAP)
    Alzheimer disease familial and s.
    s. diffuse goiter
    s. dysentery
    s. nodular goiter
    s. ovarian neoplasm
    s. papillary renal cell carcinoma
sporadin
Sporanaerobacter acetigenes
sporangia (*pl. of* sporangium)
sporangiophore
sporangiospore
sporangium, pl. sporangia
spore
    anthrax s.
    bacterial s.
    central s.
    drumstick s.
    s. form
    fungal s.
    midterminal s.
    oval subterminal s.
    s. strip
spore-forming rod
Sporendonema
Sporichthyaceae
sporicidal
sporicide
Sporidesmium
Sporidiobolus
sporidium
sporoagglutination
Sporobacterium olearium
sporoblast
Sporobolomyces
Sporocybe
sporocyst
Sporocystinea
sporodochium

sporogenes
    Caminicella s.
    Clostridium s.
sporogenesis
sporogenous
sporogeny
sporogony
Sporomusa aerivorans
sporont
sporophore
sporoplasm
Sporormiella
Sporosarcina
    S. aquimarina
    S. globispora
    S. macmurdoensis
    S. pasteurii
    S. psychrophila
sporotheca
Sporothrix schenckii
Sporotomaculum syntrophicum
sporotrichosis
    lymphocutaneous s.
    s. serology
sporotrichositic chancre
Sporotrichum
    S. beurmanni
    S. gougerotii
    S. pruinosum
    S. schenckii
Sporozoa
sporozoan, pl. **sporozoa**
Sporozoasida
Sporozoea
sporozoite
sporozooid
sporozoon
sports-related sudden death
sporular
sporulate
sporulation
sporule
spot
    acoustic s.
    ash-leaf s.
    Bitot s.
    blood s.
    blue s.
    café au lait s.
    cayenne pepper s.
    cherry red s.
    Christopher s.

    chromatin s.
    cold s.
    de Morgan s.
    dried blood s.
    electronic focal s.
    embryonic s.
    eye s.
    s. film
    fluorescence intensity of
      telomere s.
    Fordyce s.
    germinal s.
    hot s.
    intranuclear s.
    Koplik s.
    lance-ovate s.
    milk s.
    milky s.
    mongolian s.
    Roth s.
    S. RT Monochrome Kodak KAI-
      2000 CCD digital camera
    ruby s.
    saccular s.
    Soemmerring s.
    solder s.
    Stephen s.
    Tardieu s.
    tendinous s.
    s. test
    s. test for infectious mononucleosis
    utricular s.
    white s.
    yellow s. (YS)
spot-blot
spotted
spotted fever
spotty lobular necrosis
SPP
    Society for Pediatric Pathology
spp. (*pl. of* sp)
spray
    cryogenic s.
    Fisher Scientific Histo-freeze 2000
      freezing s.
Spray-Cyte slide fixative
spread
    pagetoid s.
    s. plate
spreading factor
spring
    s. catarrhal conjunctivitis

NOTES

S

spring *(continued)*
>> hemoglobin Constant S.
>> s. ophthalmia

Sprinz-Nelson syndrome

sprue
>> celiac s.
>> collagenous s.
>> nontropical s.
>> tropical s. (TS)

spruelike syndrome

spumae
>> *Tsukamurella s.*

Spumavirinae

spumicola
>> *Friedmanniella s.*

spun urine sediment

spur
>> s. cell
>> s. cell anemia

spuria
>> hemospermia s.
>> placenta s.

spurious
>> s. cast
>> s. parasite

Spurr resin

Spurway syndrome

sputa (*pl. of* sputum)

sputi
>> *Gordonia s.*

Sputolysin

sputorum
>> *Campylobacter s.*
>> *Pandoraea s.*
>> *Vibrio s.*

sputum, pl. **sputa**
>> s. aerogenosum
>> s. cytology
>> s. examination
>> s. fungus culture
>> globular s.
>> green s.
>> s. induction
>> s. mycobacteria culture
>> nummular s.
>> prune juice s.
>> rusty s.
>> s. smear
>> s. tube
>> s. tuberculosis acid-fast smear

SQ
> subcutaneous

SQC
> squamous cell carcinoma

squalene

squama, pl. **squamae**

squamate

squamatization

squame

squamocellular

squamocolumnar junction (SCJ)

squamoid pattern

squamous
>> s. alveolar cell
>> s. cell carcinoma (SCC, SQC)
>> s. cell carcinoma in situ
>> s. cell index
>> s. cell papilloma
>> s. dysplasia
>> s. eddy
>> s. epithelial cell
>> s. epithelium
>> s. intraepithelial lesion (SIL)
>> s. metaplasia
>> s. metaplasia of amnion
>> s. morule
>> s. odontogenic tumor
>> s. pearl
>> s. syringometaplasia

square wave

squarrose, squarrous

squill
> red s.

SR
> secretion rate
> sedimentation rate
> sensitization response
> sigma reaction
> stimulation ratio

3SR
> self-sustained sequence replication

Sr
> strontium

^{90}Sr
> strontium-90

sr
> steradian

SRA
> serotonin release assay

SRBC
> sheep red blood cell

SRC
> sedimented red cell

SRCT
> small round cell tumor

SRF
> skin-reactive factor
> somatotropin-releasing factor
> split renal function
> subretinal fluid

SRF-A
> slow reacting factor of anaphylaxis

SRFS
> split renal function study

SRH
> somatotropin-releasing hormone

srivastavai
>> *Schistotaenia s.*

sRNA
  soluble ribonucleic acid
SRS
  slow-reacting substance
SRS-A, SRSA
  slow reacting substance of anaphylaxis
SRT
  sedimentation rate test
SS
  Salmonella-Shigella
  saturated solution
  Sézary syndrome
  statistically significant
  subaortic stenosis
  supersaturated
  synovial sarcoma
SSA
  skin-sensitizing antibody
  sulfosalicylic acid
SS-A/Ro antigen
SS-B/La antigen
SSC
  sodium chloride-sodium citrate solution
  standard saline citrate
SSCP
  single-stranded conformation
    polymorphism
    SSCP assay
SSD
  sum of square deviations
SS-DNA
  single-stranded DNA
SSKI
  saturated solution of potassium iodide
SSN
  severely subnormal
SSOP
  sequence specific oligonucleotide probe
SSP
  Sanarelli-Shwartzman phenomenon
SSPE
  subacute sclerosing panencephalitis
ssRNA virus
SSS
  scalded skin syndrome
  specific soluble substance
***S*-sulfoglutathione**
SSV
  simian sarcoma virus
ST
  surface tension

St.
  Saint
    St. Anthony dance
    St. Guy dance
    St. John dance
    St. Jude pediatric oncology staging
    system
    St. Louis encephalitis (SLE)
    St. Louis encephalitis virus
STA
  serum thrombotic accelerator
    STA hemostasis system
    STA Liatest control N+P
    STA Liatest D-DI
      coagulation/inflammation test kit
stab
  s. cell
  s. culture
  s. neutrophil
  s. wound
stabilate
stabile
stabilis
  Burkholderia s.
stability
  genome s.
stable
  s. cell
  s. factor
  s. factor deficiency
  s. fly
stachybotryotoxicosis
Stachybotrys
Stachylidium
stachyose
Staclot
  S. LA
  S. Protein S test kit
STA-Compact hemostasis system
Stadie-Riggs microtome
staff cell
stage
  algid s.
  Arneth s.
  cold s.
  defervescent s.
  Dukes A, B, C tumor s.
  end s.
  imperfect s.
  incubative s.
  s. of invasion
  latent s.

S

NOTES

stage *(continued)*
    menstrual s.
    patch/plaque cell s.
    perfect s.
    prodromal s.
    proliferative s.
    resting s.
    secretory s.
    Tanner s.
    tumor s.
    vegetative s.
staghorn calculus
staging
    American Joint Committee on
      Cancer S. (AJCCS)
    Braak neurofibrillary tangle s.
    Butchart tumor s.
    cancer s.
    Clark malignant melanoma s.
    Dukes s.
    Durie and Salmon multiple
      myeloma clinical s.
    FAB tumor s.
    FIGO classification of tumor s.
    Jewett and Strong s.
    malignant melanoma s.
    molecular s.
    Rai s.
    TNM s.
    tumor s.
stagnant
    s. anoxia
    s. hypoxia
    s. loop syndrome
Stagnicola
stagnora
    Prototheca s.
stain
    acetoorcein s.
    Achucarro s.
    acid-fast s.
    acid phosphatase s.
    acid-Schiff s.
    acridine orange s.
    AE1 immunoperoxidase s.
    AFB s.
    Ag-AS s.
    Albert diphtheria s.
    Alcian blue s.
    alizarin red s.
    alkaline phosphatase s.
    alpha 3, 4, 5 chain collagen s.
    Altmann anilin-acid fuchsin s.
    Alzheimer s.
    3-amino-9-ethylcarbazole s.
    ammonium silver carbonate s.
    amyloid s.
    aniline blue modified trichrome s.
    antibody s.

    anticytokeratin s.
    antimony s.
    argentaffin s.
    argyrophil s.
    arsenic s.
    astrocyte s.
    ATPase s.
    auramine O fluorescent s.
    auramine-rhodamine s.
    azan s.
    azure-eosin s.
    azure II-methylene blue s.
    B72.3 s.
    bacterial s.
    basic fuchsin-methylene blue s.
    Bauer chromic acid leucofuchsin s.
    Becker s. for spirochetes
    Bennhold Congo red s.
    Ber-EP4 immunoperoxidase s.
    Berg s.
    Best carmine s.
    beta amyloid precursor protein
      immunohistochemical s.
    Betke s.
    Betke-Kleihauer s.
    Bielschowsky s.
    Biondi-Heidenhain s.
    bipolar s.
    Birch-Hirschfeld s.
    Bodian copper-PROTARGOL s.
    Bodian histochemical s.
    Borrel blue s.
    Bowie s.
    Brown-Brenn s.
    Brown-Hopp tissue Gram s.
    butyrate esterase s.
    Cajal astrocyte s.
    Cajal gold sublimate s.
    calcofluor white s.
    carbolfuchsin s.
    carbol-thionin s.
    C-banding s.
    CEA Gold-5 s.
    CEA immunoperoxidase s.
    centromere banding s.
    certified s.
    cervical Gram s.
    chloracetate esterase
      histochemical s.
    chlorazol black E s.
    chondroitin sulfate s.
    ChrA immunoperoxidase s.
    chrome alum hematoxylin-
      phloxine s.
    Churukian-Schenck s.
    chymotrypsin s.
    Ciaccio s.
    colloidal iron s.
    Congo red s.

contrast s.
cresyl blue brilliant s.
cresyl violet s.
crystal violet s.
cyclin D s.
Da Fano s.
Dane and Herman keratin s.
DAPI s.
Darrow red s.
Delafield hematoxylin s.
del Rio Hortega s.
deoxyribonucleic acid s.
diaminobenzidine s.
diastase-periodic acid-Schiff s.
Dieterle s.
differential s.
Diff-Quik histochemical s.
direct fluorescent antibody s.
DOPA s.
Dorner s.
double s.
D-PAS s.
Ehrlich acid hematoxylin s.
Ehrlich aniline crystal violet s.
Ehrlich triacid s.
Ehrlich triple s.
Einarson gallocyanin-chrome
  alum s.
elastica van Gieson s.
elastic fiber s.
elastin s.
en-bloc s.
eosin Y derivative of
  fluorescein s.
Eranko fluorescence s.
ethidium bromide s.
fast green FCF s.
fecal fat s.
ferric ammonium sulfate s.
Feulgen s.
fibrin histochemical s.
Field rapid s.
Fink-Heimer s.
Fite s.
Fite-Faraco s.
Flemming triple s.
fluorescence plus Giemsa s.
Fontana-Masson silver s.
Fontana methenamine silver s.
Foot reticulin impregnation s.
Fouchet s.
fuchsin s.

fungal s.
Fungalase-F s.
ganglioside GD2 s.
G-banding s.
Genta s.
gentian orange s.
gentian violet s.
Giemsa chromosome banding s.
Gill #2 hematoxylin blue s.
Gimenez s.
Glenner-Lillie s. for pituitary
glycogen s.
glycolipid s.
glycoprotein s.
GMS s.
Golgi s.
Gomori aldehyde fuchsin s.
Gomori chrome alum hematoxylin-
  phloxine s.
Gomori-Jones periodic acid-
  methenamine silver s.
Gomori methenamine silver s.
  (GMS stain)
Gomori nonspecific acid
  phosphatase s.
Gomori nonspecific alkaline
  phosphatase s.
Gomori one-step trichrome s.
Gomori silver impregnation s.
Gomori-Takamatsu s.
Goodpasture s.
Gordon and Sweets s.
Gram s.
Gram-chromotrope s.
Gram-Weigert s.
Gridley s.
Grimelius s.
Grocott-Gomori methenamine
  silver s.
Hale colloidal iron s.
Hansel s.
H&E s.
Heidenhain azan s.
Heidenhain iron hematoxylin s.
hematoxylin s.
hematoxylin-malachite green-basic
  fuchsin s.
hematoxylin-phloxine B s.
hemosiderin s.
heparan sulfate PG s.
heparan sulfate proteoglycan s.
HHF 35 s.

S

NOTES

stain *(continued)*
Hirsch-Peiffer s.
Hiss capsule s.
histochemical s.
Holmes s.
Hortega neuroglia s.
Hucker-Conn s.
immunoalkaline phosphatase s.
immunofluorescent s.
immunohistochemical s.
immunoperoxidase s.
India ink capsule s.
indigo-carmine s.
intravital s.
iodine s.
iron hematoxylin s.
Jenner s.
Jenner-Giemsa s.
Jones methenamine silver s.
Kasten fluorescent Feulgen s.
Kasten fluorescent PAS s.
keratin s.
Kinyoun carbolfuchsin s.
Kittrich s.
Kleihauer s.
Kleihauer-Betke s.
Klüver-Barrera Luxol fast blue s.
Kokoskin s.
Kossa s.
Kronecker s.
lactophenol cotton blue s.
LAP s.
Lawless s.
lead citrate s.
lead hydroxide s.
Leder s.
Leishman s.
Lendrum inclusion body s.
Lendrum phloxine-tartrazine s.
Lepehne-Pickworth s.
leukocyte acid phosphatase s.
Leukostat s.
LeuM1 immunoperoxidase s.
Leung s.
Levaditi s.
Levine alkaline Congo red s.
Lillie allochrome connective
   tissue s.
Lillie azure-eosin s.
Lillie ferrous iron s.
Lillie sulfuric acid Nile blue s.
lipase 105 s.
lipid s.
Liquichek reticulocyte control
   and s.
Lison-Dunn s.
Löffler caustic s.
Lugol s.
Luna-Ishak s.

Luxol fast blue s.
Macchiavello s.
MacNeal tetrachrome blood s.
malachite green s.
malarial pigment s.
Maldonado-San Jose s.
Mallory s. for *Actinomyces*
Mallory aniline blue s.
Mallory collagen s.
Mallory s. for hemofuchsin
Mallory iodine s.
Mallory phloxine s.
Mallory phosphotungstic acid
   hematoxylin s.
Mallory trichrome s.
Mallory triple s.
Mancini iodine s.
Mann methyl blue-eosin s.
Marchi s.
Masson argentaffin s.
Masson-Fontana ammoniacal
   silver s.
Masson-Fontana ammoniac silver s.
Masson trichrome s.
Mayer acid alum hematoxylin s.
Mayer hemalum s.
Mayer hematoxylin s.
Mayer mucicarmine s.
Mayer mucihematein s.
May-Grünwald s.
May-Grünwald-Giemsa s.
meconium s.
Meissel s.
Merck new fuchsin s.
metachromatic s.
methenamine silver s.
methylene blue s.
methyl green-pyronin s.
M'Fadyean s.
Milligan trichrome s.
modified acid-fast s.
modified Steiner s.
Movat pentachrome s.
Mowry colloidal iron s.
MSB trichrome s.
mucicarmine s.
mucopolysaccharide s.
multiple s.
Musto s.
MY-10 clone s.
myeloperoxidase s.
myoglobin s.
Nakanishi s.
naphthol ASBI phosphate s.
NASDCE s.
Nauta s.
negative s.
Neisser s.
neutral s.

Nile blue fat s.
Nissl s.
nitroblue tetrazolium s.
Noble s.
Novelli s.
NSE s.
nuclear fast red s.
oil red O s.
oligodendroglia s.
orcein s.
Orth s.
osmium tetroxide s.
oxalic acid s.
oxytalan fiber s.
Padykula-Herman s. for myosin
   ATPase
Paget-Eccleston s.
Palmgren silver impregnation s.
pancreatic islet s.
panoptic s.
Pap s.
PAPI s.
PAP immunoperoxidase s.
Pappenheim s.
paracarmine s.
Paragon blue s.
PAS s.
PAS-orange G s.
Pearl iron s.
periodic acid-silver methenamine s.
Perls Prussian blue s.
peroxidase s.
phloxine-tartrazine s.
phosphomolybdic acid s.
phosphotungstic acid hematoxylin s.
picric s.
picrocarmine s.
picroindigocarmine s.
picro-Mallory trichrome s.
picronigrosin s.
plasma s.
plasmatic s.
plasmic s.
plastic section s.
polychrome methylene blue s.
Pontamine sky blue s.
port-wine s.
positive s.
potassium metabisulfate s.
potassium permanganate s.
propidium iodine s.
Protargol s.

Prussian blue iron s.
PTA s.
PTAH s.
Puchtler-Sweat s.
Puchtler-Sweat s. for hemoglobin
   and hemosiderin
pyrrol blue s.
Q-banding s.
quinacrine chromosome banding s.
Rambourg chromic acid-
   phosphotungstic acid s.
Rambourg periodic acid-chromic
   methenamine-silver s.
Ranson pyridine silver s.
R-banding s.
reticulin s.
reticulum s.
rhodamine s.
Richard-Allan Scientific Ultrafast
   Papanicolaou s.
Romanowsky blood s.
Romanowsky-Giemsa s.
Romanowsky type s.
Roux s.
Ryan s.
safranin s.
Sayeed s.
scarlet red s.
Schaeffer-Fulton s.
Schiff s.
Schmorl ferric-ferricyanide
   reduction s.
Schmorl picrothionin s.
Schultz s.
selective s.
Sevier-Munger s.
Shorr trichrome s.
silver ammoniacal silver s.
silver-ammoniac silver s.
silver nitrate s.
silver protein s.
Smith silver s.
Snook reticulum s.
sodium bisulfite s.
sodium hydroxide s.
sodium thiosulfate s.
solochrome cyanine s.
Steiner s.
Stirling modification of Gram s.
stool fecal fat s.
Sudan black B fat s.
supravital s.

S

NOTES

stain *(continued)*
  synaptophysin s.
  Taenzer s.
  Taenzer-Unna s.
  Takayama s.
  telomeric R-banding s.
  tetrachrome s.
  Tetragonolobus purpureas lectin s.
  tetramethylbenzidine s.
  thiazin s.
  thioflavin T s.
  thionin s.
  thyroglobulin s.
  Tilden s.
  Tizzoni s.
  T method s.
  Toison s.
  toluidine blue s.
  TRAP s.
  trichrome s.
  Truant auramine-rhodamine s.
  trypsin G-banding s.
  Turnbull blue s.
  TWAR s.
  ultrafast Pap s.
  Unna s.
  Unna-Pappenheim s.
  Unna-Taenzer s.
  uranyl acetate s.
  urate crystal s.
  van Ermengen s.
  van Gieson s.
  Ventana ES s.
  Verhoeff elastic tissue s.
  Verhoeff-van Gieson elastin s.
  Victoria blue s.
  vimentin immunoperoxidase s.
  vital s.
  von Kossa calcium s.
  VVG s.
  Wachstein-Meissel s. for calcium-
    magnesium-ATPase
  Wade-Fite-Faraco s.
  Warthin-Starry silver s.
  Wayson s.
  Weber s.
  Weber-modified trichome s.
  Weigert s. for elastin
  Weigert s. for fibrin
  Weigert-Gram s.
  Weigert iron hematoxylin s.
  Weigert s. for myelin
  Weigert s. for neuroglia
  Weigert-Pal s.
  Weil myelin sheath s.
  Wilder s. for reticulum
  Williams s.
  Wright s.
  Wright-Giemsa s.

  Ziehl s.
  Ziehl-Neelsen s.
stainable
  s. hemosiderin
  s. iron
stained
  s. cortex
  s. urinary sediment (SUS)
stainer
  Code-On Immunoslide s.
  Hematek 2000 slide s.
  Midas II automated s.
  Quick Slide automated s.
  Ventana Medical Systems Techmate
    500 automated s.
stainer/cytocentrifuge
  Aerospray acid-fast bacteria
    slide s./c.
  Aerospray hematology slide s./c.
staining
  acid phosphatase s.
  alkaline phosphatase s.
  amyloid s.
  anti-GFAP s.
  astrocyte s.
  automated slide s.
  bacterial s.
  bipolar s.
  card-amplified nanogold-gold s.
  card-amplified nanogold-silver s.
  CD34 s.
  chondroitin sulfate s.
  cytoplasmic s.
  deoxyribonucleic acid s.
  enterochromaffin s.
  fat s.
  fibrin s.
  fluorescent s.
  fluoro jade s.
  fungus s.
  glycogen s.
  glycolipid s.
  glycophorin A s.
  glycoprotein s.
  Gordon-Sweet s.
  H and E s.
  hemosiderin s.
  histologic s.
  immunoenzymometric s.
  immunofluorescent s.
  immunogold-silver s. (IGSS)
  immunohistochemical s.
  iodine s.
  keratin s.
  maspin nuclear s.
  mast cell s.
  mucopolysaccharide s.
  nuclear s.
  oligodendroglia s.

phospholipid s.
podoplanin s.
progressive s.
regressive s.
reticulin s.
reticulocyte s.
s. shell
Steiner s.
supravital s.
surface marker s.
thioflavin S s.
vital s.

Stains-All
Staleya guttiformis
stalk
   s. to basilar artery ratio
   infundibular s.
   pituitary s.
Staller
   S. kit
   S. point
Stamey test
Stamnosoma
Stamper-Woodruff assay
stand
standard
   s. acid reflux test (SART)
   air quality s.
   s. bicarbonate
   certified s.
   s. curve
   s. deviation (SD)
   s. electrode potential
   s. enthalpy of formation
   s. error (SE)
   s. error of estimate (SEE)
   s. free energy
   gold s.
   s. hydrogen electrode
   internal s.
   internal telomerase s. (ITAS)
   s. method agar
   s. morbidity ratio (SMR)
   s. mortality ratio (SMR)
   National Committee for Clinical Laboratory S.'s (NCCLS)
   s. operating procedure (SOP)
   Prader bead s.
   primary s.
   quantitation s. (QS)
   s. reduction potential

S.'s for Reporting of Diagnostic Accuracy (STARD)
   s. saline citrate (SSC)
   s. score
   s. serologic test for syphilis
   s. solution
   s. state
   s. temperature and pressure
   s. temperature and pressure, dry (STPD)
   s. test for syphilis (STS)
   s. urea clearance
standardization
standardize
standardized
   s. protocol
   s. rate
standing plasma test
standstill
   cardiac s.
stannic
stannous
Stanton disease
staph
   staphylococcus
Staph-Ident test
Staph-Trac test
staphyline
staphylococcal
   s. clumping test (SCT)
   s. enteritis
   s. enterotoxin
   s. enterotoxin B (SEB)
   s. pneumonia
   s. protein A binding assay
   s. scalded skin syndrome
Staphylococceae
staphylococcemia
staphylococci (*pl. of* staphylococcus)
staphylococcin
staphylococcolysin
staphylococcolysis
Staphylococcus
   S. albus
   S. aureus nasopharyngeal culture
   S. aureus neutral proteinase
   S. aureus urinary tract infection
   S. citreus
   S. epidermidis
   S. equorum subsp. *linens*
   S. fleurettii
   S. haemolyticus

S

NOTES

935

Staphylococcus (continued)
- *S. hominis*
- *S. hominis novobiosepticus*
- methicillin-resistant *S. aureus* (MRSA)
- methicillin-resistant coagulase-negative *S.* (MRCNS)
- methicillin-susceptible *S. aureus* (MSSA)
- methicillin-susceptible coagulase-negative *S.* (MSCNS)
- *S. nepalensis*
- *S. pyogenes*
- *S. pyogenes albus*
- *S. pyogenes aureus*
- *S. saprophyticus*
- *S. septicemia*
- *S. simulans*
- *S. succinus* subsp. *casei*
- *S. viridans*
- *S. warneri*

staphylococcus, pl. **staphylococci (staph)**
- s. antitoxin
- s. vaccine

staphylohemia
staphylohemolysin
staphylokinase
staphylolysin
- alpha s.
- beta s.
- delta s.
- epsilon s.
- gamma s.

staphyloma
staphyloopsonic index
Staphylothermus hellenicus
staphylotoxin
star
- lens s.
- macular s.
- venous s.
- Verheyen s.
- Winslow s.

starburst pattern
starch
- s. hydrolysis test
- hydroxyethyl s.
- rice s.
- s. tolerance test

STARD
- Standards for Reporting of Diagnostic Accuracy

Stargardt disease
Starkeya novella
Starkeyomyces
Starling law
starrii
- *Bacteriovorax s.*
- *Peredibacter s.*

starry-sky
- s.-s. appearance
- s.-s. macrophage

STart 8 clot detection system
start codon
starter pistol
StarTox 5 drugs of abuse screening test
starvation-induced protein breakdown
starvation ketoacidosis
stasis, pl. **stases**
- bile s.
- s. cirrhosis
- s. dermatitis
- s. syndrome
- s. ulcer
- venous s.

Stasisia
STAT
- signal transducer and activator of transcription

Stat-60 centrifuge
state
- absorptive s.
- baseline steady s.
- carrier s.
- central excitatory s. (CES)
- central inhibitory s. (CIS)
- chronic carrier s.
- complement deficiency s.
- euthyroid sick s.
- excited s.
- fasted s.
- ground s.
- immunity deficiency s. (IDS)
- imperfect s.
- metastable s.
- nonreplicative s.
- oxidation s.
- pathologic s.
- perfect s.
- platelet-refractory s.
- postabsorptive s.
- pseudo-Cushing s.
- replicative s.
- sample steady s.
- solid s.
- standard s.
- steady s.
- transition s.

statement
- assignment s.
- source s.

static
- s. balance receptor cell
- s. gangrene
- s. pulmonary compliance
- s. storage allocation
- s. telepathology

statin
stationary phase
statistic
Mann-Whitney rank sum s.
Office of National S.'s (ONS)
spatial scan s.
test s.
Wilcoxon signed rank s.
statistically significant (SS)
statistical symbol
statoconia
statoconial membrane
statoconiorum
membrana s.
statolith
statosphere
Stat Profile pHOx blood gas analyzer
STAT-Site M Hgb test system
StatSpin
S. Express 2 centrifuge
S. MP centrifuge
stat test
stature
short s.
status
s. asthmaticus
s. choreicus
s. cribrosus
s. criticus
S. Cup Plus drug testing device
s. dysmyelinisatus
s. dysraphicus
s. epilepticus
s. hemicranicus
hormone receptor s.
Karnofsky s.
s. lacunaris
s. lymphaticus
s. marmoratus
s. nervosus
s. raptus
s. spongiosus
s. thymicolymphaticus
s. thymicus
Staub-Traugott effect
Staurophoma
staurosporine
STC
sarcomatoid thymic carcinoma
soft tissue calcification
STD
sexually transmitted disease

skin test dose
skin-to-tumor distance
steady state
steady-state condition
steam-fitter's asthma
steapsin
stearate
polyoxyethylene s. (POES)
sodium s.
stearic acid
stearin
stearothermophilus
Bacillus s.
Geobacillus s.
steatitis
steatocystoma multiplex
steatohepatitis
nonalcoholic s. (NASH)
steatolytic enzyme
steatomatosis
steatonecrosis
steatopyga, steatopygia
steatopygous
steatorrhea
steatosis
centrilobar s.
s. cordis
hepatic s.
macrovesicular s.
steatozoon
Steele-Richardson-Olszewski syndrome
Steenbock unit
steeple skull
Stefan-Boltzmann law
stege
stegnosis
Stegobium
Stegomyia
stegomyiae
Myxococcidium s.
Steinbrocker syndrome
Steiner
S. stain
S. staining
S. syndrome
Steinert disease
Stein-Leventhal syndrome
steinstrasse (cobbled street ureteric lumen)
Stelangium

NOTES

stella
    s. lentis hyaloidea
    s. lentis iridica
Stellantchasmus falcatus
stellata
    Hemispora s.
stellatae
    venae s.
stellate
    s. abscess
    s. cell
    s. cell of cerebral cortex
    s. cell of liver
    s. density
    s. fracture
    s. reticulum
    s. vein
    s. venule
stellate-cell lipidosis
stellifer
    Paenibacillus s.
stellipolaris
    Alteromonas s.
stelliscabiei
    Streptomyces s.
stellulae
    s. vasculosae
    s. verheyenii
    s. winslowii
stem
    s. cell
    s. cell assay
    s. cell factor (SCF)
    s. cell leukemia
    s. cell lymphoma
    s. cell renewal factor
    gliosis of brain s.
    infundibular s.
    s. kit CD34+HPC enumeration
      system
stemline
stemonitis
    Doratomyces s.
Stemonitis flavogenita
Stemphylium macrosporoidium
Stem-Trol control cell
Stender dish
Stenella araguata
Stenoglossa
stenosal
stenosed
stenosing odditis
stenosis, pl. stenoses
    aortic valvular s.
    buttonhole s.
    calcific bicuspid aortic valve s.
    calcific nodular aortic s.
    carotid artery s.
    cervical canal s.

    congenital pyloric s.
    coronary ostial s.
    discrete subaortic s.
    Dittrich s.
    hypertrophic muscular subaortic s.
      (HMSAS)
    hypertrophic pyloric s. (HPS)
    idiopathic hypertrophic subaortic s.
      (IHSS)
    infundibular s.
    internal carotid s.
    lumbar canal s.
    mitral incompetency and s.
    muscular subaortic s.
    nodular calcific aortic s.
    pulmonary artery s. (PAS)
    pulmonary infundibular s.
    pyloric s. (PS)
    renal artery s. (RAS)
    spinal s.
    subaortic s. (SS)
    subvalvar s.
    supravalvular aortic s. (SAS,
      SVAS)
    tricuspid s.
    valvular s.
    vascular s.
stenostrepta
    Spirochaeta s.
stenothermal
stenotic
Stenotrophomonas
    S. acidaminiphila
    S. maltophilia
    S. nitritireducens
    S. rhizophila
stenoxenous
Stensen duct
step
    s. function
    rate-controlling s.
    s. sectioning
step-down transformer
Stephanoascus ciferii
Stephanofilaria stilesi
Stephanosporium
stephanostomum
    Oesophagostomum s.
Stephanurus dentatus
stephensi
    Anopheles s.
Stephen spot
step-up transformer
steradian (sr)
stercobilin
stercobilinogen
stercolith
stercoraceous ulcer

stercoral
    s. abscess
    s. appendicitis
    s. fistula
    s. ulcer
stercoricanis
    Sutterella s.
stercorihominis
    Anaerofustis s.
stercoris
    Collinsella s.
stercorisuis
    Hespellia s.
stercoroma
Sterculia
stereochemical isomerism
stereochemistry
stereocilium, pl. **stereocilia**
stereognosis
stereoisomer
stereoisomerism
stereology
stereometer
stereometry
stereomicroscopic
stereophotomicrograph
stereoscope
stereoscopic
    s. microscope
    s. radiography
stereospecific numbering
stereotactic
    s. brain biopsy
    s. breast biopsy
stereotaxis
Stereum
steric hindrance
sterigma, pl. **sterigmata**
Sterigmatocystis
Sterigmatomyces
sterile
    s. abscess
    s. cyst
    s. pyuria
    s. stick
sterility
    s. culture
    s. test broth
sterilization
    discontinuous s.
    fractional s.
    intermittent s.

sterilize
sterilizer
    gas s.
sternal synchondrosis
Sternberg
    S. disease
    S. giant cell
Sternberg-Reed cell
Sterneedle tuberculin test
Sternheimer-Malbin positive cell
sterni
    mucro s.
sternocostale
    trigonum s.
sternocostal triangle
sternoglossal
steroid
    anabolic s.
    s. cell tumor
    s. fever
    s. hormone
    s. hormone binding globulin
    (SHBG)
    s. hormone receptor
    ketogenic s. (KGS)
    17-ketogenic s.
    s. protein activity index (SPAI)
    s. saponin
    s. sulfatase (STS)
    s. sulfatase gene
steroid-binding betaglobulin
steroid-21-hydroxylase
steroid-21-monooxygenase
steroidogenesis
steroidogenic hormone
steroid-receptor complex
sterol
    s. carrier protein
    s. glycoside
Sterolibacterium denitrificans
stetharteritis
stethomyositis
Stevens-Johnson syndrome
Stewart-Bluefarb syndrome
Stewart-Morel syndrome
Stewart-Treves syndrome
sTfR
    soluble transferrin receptor
STH
    somatotropic hormone
STI
    systolic time interval

NOTES

S

stibine
stibocaptate
    sodium s.
stichochrome cell
stick
    sterile s.
stick-and-ball-shaped virion particle
Sticker disease
sticklandii
    Clostridium s.
Stickler syndrome
Stictis
Stieda disease
stigma, pl. stigmas, stigmata
    follicular s.
    s. ventriculi
stigmataophilia
Stigonematales
stilbene dye
stilbestrol
Stilbospora
stilbospora
    Taeniolella s.
stilesi
    Stephanofilaria s.
still
    S. disease
    s. layer
stillbirth (SB)
    macerated s.
Still-Chauffard syndrome
Stilling
    S. canal
    S. gelatinous substance
    S. syndrome
Stilling-Turk-Duane syndrome
stimulate enzyme secretion
stimulation
    paracrine s.
    parasympathetic s.
    prolonged estrogen s.
    s. ratio (SR)
    repetitive s.
stimulator
    B lymphocyte s. (BLyS)
    s. cell
    long-acting thyroid s. (LATS)
stipple cell
stippled epiphysis
stippling
    basophilic s.
    gunpowder s.
    pseudo-gunpowder s.
    s. of skin
    Ziemann s.
Stirling modification of Gram stain
stitch abscess
STKS automated cell counting
  instrument

STM
    scanning tunneling microscopy
Stobo antigen
stochastic
stock
    s. culture
    s. strain
    s. vaccine
stockpile
    National Pharmaceutical S. (NPS)
stoichiology
stoichiometry
Stokes
    S. law
    S. shift
Stokes-Adams (SA)
    S. disease
    S. syndrome
Stokvis-Talma syndrome
Stokvis test
Stoll dilution egg count technique
stolon
stolpii
    Bacteriovorax s.
stoma, pl. stomata, stomas
stomach
    bilocular s.
    s. cancer
    s. carcinoma
    chief cell of s.
    drain-trap s.
    foveolar cell of s.
    gastric carcinoma of the inner s.
    hourglass s.
    leather-bottle s.
    malignant tumors of the s.
    oblique fiber of muscular layer
      of s.
    sclerotic s.
    surface mucous cell of s.
    theca cell of s.
    trifid s.
    s. tumor
    wallet s.
    watermelon s.
    water-trap s.
stomal ulcer
stomas (*pl. of* stoma)
stomata (*pl. of* stoma)
stomatitis, pl. stomatitides
    angular s.
    aphthous s.
    bovine papular s.
    gangrenous s.
    herpetic s.
    lead s.
    primary herpetic s.
    vesicular s.
    Vincent s.

Stomatococcus mucilaginosus
stomatocyte
stomatocytic hereditary elliptocytosis
stomatocytosis
>hereditary s.
stomodeal
>s. ectoderm
stomodeum
Stomoxys calcitrans
stone
>ammonium magnesium phosphate s.
>cystine s.
>s. heart
>skin s.
>vein s.
stonelike debris
stone-stripper's asthma
stool
>acholic s.
>s. analysis
>bloody s.
>s. carbohydrate
>chemical examination of s.
>s. chloride
>s. collection
>s. color
>s. consistency
>s. electrolytes
>s. examination
>fat in s.
>s. fecal fat stain
>s. fungus culture
>Gram stain of s.
>s. guaiac
>s. guaiac test
>s. leukocyte
>s. leukocyte count
>s. lipids
>melanotic s.
>microscopic examination of s.
>s. mucus
>s. muscle fiber
>s. mycobacteria culture
>s. nitrogen
>s. occult blood
>s. osmolality
>s. pH
>s. porphyrin
>s. potassium
>s. reducing substances test
>ribbon s.
>rice-water s.'s

>s. screen
>scybalous s.
>s. sodium
>tarry s.
>s. toxin assay
>s. trypsin
>s. urobilinogen
stopcock
stop codon
storage
>s. allocation
>autologous leukapheresis, processing, and s. (ALPS)
>s. capacity
>common s.
>compressed gas s.
>ether s.
>external s.
>glycogen s.
>internal s.
>s. limit
>s. location
>mass s.
>s. oscilloscope
>s. phosphor autoradiography
>s. pool disease
>transport and s.
stores
>bone marrow iron s.'s
>reticuloendothelial iron s.'s
storiform
>s. neurofibroma
>s. pattern
storm
>thyroid s.
Stormer viscosimeter
Stormorken syndrome
Stovall-Black method
STPD
>standard temperature and pressure, dry
>STPD conditions of gas
Strachan syndrome
straddling embolism
straight
>s. rod
>s. tubule
>s. venule of kidney
strain
>attenuated s.
>avirulent s.
>s. birefringence
>carrier s.

S

NOTES

941

strain *(continued)*
    cell s.
    clostridial s.
    HFR s.
    hypothetical mean s. (HMS)
    lysogenic s.
    McKrae herpes simplex virus s.
    Mycobacterium bovis BCG s.
    pseudolysogenic s.
    recombinant s.
    reference s.
    stock s.
    type s.
    virulent Schu S4 tularemia s.
stramonium
    Datura s.
strand
    complementary s.
    s. displacement amplification (SDA)
    leading s.
    minus s.
    plus s.
    sense s.
    viral s.
strandjordii
    Tsukamurella s.
strangling
    passive s.
strangulated hernia
strangulation
    incaprettamento (ritual ligature s.)
    ritual ligature s. (incaprettamento)
strap cell
Strassburg test
Strasseria
strata (*pl. of* stratum)
Stratagene CastAway sequencing device
stratification
    s. index
    risk group s.
stratified
    s. ciliated columnar epithelium
    s. cuboidal epithelium
    s. random sample
    s. squamous nonkeratinized
    epithelium
    s. thrombus
stratiform
Stratiomyidae
stratum, pl. **strata**
    s. aculeatum
    s. basale
    s. basale epidermidis
    s. cerebrale retinae
    s. circulare membranae tympani
    s. circulare tunicae muscularis recti
    s. circulare tunicae muscularis
    ventriculi
    s. compactum

    s. corneum
    s. corneum epidermidis
    s. corneum unguis
    s. cutaneum membranae tympani
    s. cylindricum
    s. disjunctum
    s. fibrosum capsulae articularis
    s. functionale
    s. ganglionare nervi optici
    s. germinativum
    s. germinativum unguis
    s. granulosum
    s. granulosum corticis cerebelli
    s. granulosum epidermidis
    s. granulosum folliculi ovarici
    vesiculosi
    s. granulosum ovarii
    s. longitudinale tunicae muscularis
    coli
    s. longitudinale tunicae muscularis
    intestini tenuis
    s. longitudinale tunicae muscularis
    recti
    s. longitudinale tunicae muscularis
    ventriculi
    s. lucidum
    malpighian s.
    s. malpighii
    s. moleculare
    s. moleculare corticis cerebelli
    s. moleculare retinae
    s. neuroepitheliale retinae
    strata nuclearia externa et interna
    retinae
    s. papillare corii
    s. pigmenti bulbi
    s. pigmenti corporis ciliaris
    s. pigmenti iridis
    s. pigmenti retinae
    s. radiatum membranae tympani
    s. reticulare corii
    s. reticulare cutis
    s. spinosum
    s. spinosum epidermidis
    s. spongiosum
    s. subcutaneum
    s. synoviale
Stratus II automatic analyzer
Strauss
    allergic granulomatosis of Churg
    and S.
Stravigen immunohistochemical reagent
strawberry
    s. birthmark
    s. gallbladder
    s. gums
    s. mark
    s. nevus
strawberry-cream blood

stray light
streak
    angioid s.
    s. culture
    fibrous s.
    s. gonad
    gonadal s.
    s. hyperostosis
    meningitic s.
    s. plate
streaming movement
street virus
Strengeria
strength
    dielectric s.
    ionic s.
    magnetic field s.
    tensile s.
strep
    streptococcus
    Strep A OIA Max
    Strep B OIA
    strep throat
Streptacidiphilus
    S. albus
    S. carbonis
    S. neutrinimicus
streptavidin
streptavidin-biotin (SAB)
    s.-b. peroxidase method
streptavidin-biotin-based detection system
streptavidin-biotin-complex technique
streptavidin-Nanogold reagent
strepticemia
Streptobacillus
    S. moniliformis
    S. pseudotuberculosis
streptocerca
    Acanthocheilonema s.
    Dipetalonema s.
    Mansonella s.
streptocerciasis
Streptococcaceae
streptococcal
    s. antigen test
    s. carditis
    s. cellulitis
    s. fibrinolysin
    s. infection
    s. pneumonia
    s. toxic shock syndrome
    s. toxin immunization reaction

streptococcemia
Streptococcus
    S. agalactiae
    S. anaerobius
    S. anginosus
    S. anginosus-constellatus
    S. australis
    S. bovis
    S. canis
    S. caprinus
    S. constellatus
    S. cremoris
    S. devriesei
    S. didelphis
    S. durans
    S. endocarditis
    S. entericus
    S. equi
    S. evolutus
    S. faecalis
    S. faecium
    S. gallinaceus
    S. gallolyticus subsp. *macedonicus*
    S. gallolyticus subsp. *pasteurianus*
    S. garvieae
    S. gordonii
    S. halichoeri
    S. infantarius
    S. infantarius subsp. *coli*
    S. infantarius subsp. *infantarius*
    S. intermedius
    S. lutetiensis
    S. M antigen
    S. minor
    S. mitis
    S. morbillorum
    S. mutans
    S. oligofermentans
    S. orisratti
    S. ovis
    S. pasteurianus
    S. pyogenes
    S. salivarius
    S. sanguis
    S. sinensis
    S. uberis
    S. urinalis
streptococcus, pl. **streptococci (strep)**
    alpha s.
    anaerobic s.
    anhemolytic s.
    Bargen s.

NOTES

streptococcus *(continued)*
    beta s.
    beta-hemolytic s. (BHS)
    s. erythrogenic toxin
    Fehleisen s.
    gamma s.
    group A *S.*
    group B *S.*
    group D *S.*
    group N *S.*
    hemolytic s.
    microaerophilic s.
    nonhemolytic s.
    s. serum
streptolysin
    s. O (SLO)
    s. O test
Streptomonospora
    S. alba
    S. salina
Streptomyces
    S. africanus
    S. albus
    S. annulatus
    S. asiaticus
    S. aureus
    S. avermectinius
    S. avermitilis
    S. beijiangensis
    S. cangkringensis
    S. drozdowiczii
    S. europaeiscabiei
    S. gibsonii
    S. hebeiensis
    S. indonesiensis
    S. javensis
    S. laceyi
    S. luridiscabiei
    S. luteireticuli
    S. madurae
    S. mexicanus
    S. niveiscabiei
    S. pelletieri
    S. puniciscabiei
    S. reticuliscabiei
    S. rhizosphaericus
    S. scabrisporus
    S. scopiformis
    S. somaliensis
    S. speibonae
    S. stelliscabiei
    S. thermocoprophilus
    S. thermospinosisporus
    S. yatensis
    S. yeochonensis
    S. yunnanensis
Streptomycetaceae
Streptomycetales
Streptomycetes

streptomycin
    s. assay agar with yeast extract
    G unit of s.
    L unit of s.
    S unit of s.
    s. unit
Streptomycineae
streptomycosis
streptosepticemia
Streptosporangiaceae
Streptosporangineae
Streptosporangium subroseum
Streptothrix
streptotrichosis
streptozyme test
stress
    s. erythrocytosis
    s. fiber
    fluid shear s.
    s. fracture
    oxidant s.
    oxidative s.
    s. protein
    s. reticulocyte
    s. ulcer
stretch
    carbon-hydrogen s.
    C-H s.
    s. device
    myocyte s.
    s. receptor
stretchable skin
stria, pl. **striae**
    Amici s.
    striae atrophicae
    striae atrophicae
    Baillarger s.
    brown striae
    striae cutis distensae
    striae gravidarum
    Langhans s.
    Monakow s.
    Nitabuch s.
    Retzius parallel striae
    Rohr s.
    s. vascularis ductus cochlearis
    Wickham striae
    striae of Zahn
striata
    area s.
    osteopathia s.
striate body
striated
    s. brush border
    s. duct
    s. muscle
striation
    basal s.
    cross s.

cytoplasmic s.
tabby cat s.
tigroid s.
striatonigral
s. degeneration
s. fiber
striatum
corpus s.
Corynebacterium s.
striatus
lichen s.
limbus s.
stricto
Borrelia burgdorferi sensu s.
stricture
biliary s.
esophageal s.
Hunner s.
urethral s.
stridor
Strigeata
strigiphila
Tetrameres s.
string
auditory s.
s. sign
s. test for duodenal parasite
stringency
stringent response
strip
Albustix reagent s.
Cardiac Reader IQC test s.
reagent s.
spore s.
Titan III H cellulose acetate s.
UrinChek 10+ urine test s.'s
stripe
Baillarger s.
Hensen s.
Kaes-Bekhterev s.
vascular s.
striped form of interstitial fibrosis
stripped nucleus
stripping
electrolytic s.
strobe light
strobila, pl. **strobilae**
strobilocercus
strobiloid
stroboscopic microscope
stroma, pl. **stromata**
amyloid-containing s.

s. cell
connective tissue s.
desmoplastic s.
fibrocollagenous s.
s. glandulae thyroideae
host s.
hyalinized s.
hypocellular s.
s. iridis
s. of iris
juxtatumoral s.
lymphatic s.
mesenchymal s.
mucinous s.
mucohyaline s.
myxoid s.
s. ovarii
s. of ovary
perifollicular s.
perilobular s.
pseudosarcomatous s.
Rollet s.
sclerotic s.
s. of thyroid gland
tumor s.
s. of vitreous
s. vitreum
stroma-free
s.-f. hemoglobin
s.-f. methemoglobin
stromal
s. cell neoplasm
s. collagen band
s. desmoplasia
s. edema
s. endometriosis
s. hyperplasia
s. hyperthecosis
s. invasion
s. luteoma
s. mucopolysaccharide
s. myofibroblast
s. sarcoma
stromal-epithelial neoplasm
stromata (*pl. of* stroma)
stromatin
Stromatinia
stromatolysis
stromatosis
endometrial s.
stromelysin
stromic

NOTES

stromomyoma
stromovascular hyperplasia
Strong bacillus
Strongylata
strongyle
Strongylidae
strongylina
    Ascarops s.
Strongyloidea
Strongyloides
    S. fuelleborni
    S. stercoralis
strongyloidiasis
Strongyloididae
strongyloidosis
strongylosis
Strongylus
    S. asini
    S. edentatus
    S. equinus
    S. radiatus
    S. ventricosus
    S. vulgaris
strontium (Sr)
strontium-90 (^{90}Sr)
Stropharia
structural
    s. collapse
    s. correlation
    s. gene
    s. isomerism
    s. lesion
    s. protein
structure
    analogous s.
    s. collapse
    dipolar s.
    fine s.
    gas-containing abdominal s.
    glandular s.
    homologous s.
    lentiginous melanocytic s.
    list s.
    maturation of gonadal s.
    neuroid melanocytic s.
    primary s.
    quaternary s.
    resultant distortion of s.
    rod-shaped s.
    rudimentary s.
    secondary s.
    sphincteric s.
    tertiary s.
    tuboreticular s.
struma, pl. strumae
    s. aberrata
    s. colloides
    cystic s.
    Hashimoto s.

ligneous s.
s. lymphomatosa
s. maligna
s. medicamentosa
s. ovarii
Riedel s.
strumal carcinoid
strumatosis
strumiform
strumipriva
    cachexia s.
strumitis
strumosis
strumous
Strümpell disease
Strümpell-Leichtenstern disease
Strümpell-Lorrain disease
Strümpell-Marie disease
Strümpell-Westphal disease
struvite calculus
strychnine assay
Stryker-Halbeisen syndrome
STS
    serologic test for syphilis
    serology test for syphilis
    standard test for syphilis
    steroid sulfatase
    STS gene
STSG
    split-thickness skin graft
STT
    serial thrombin time
STU
    skin test unit
Stuart
    S. broth
    S. factor
stuartii
    Providencia s.
Stuart-Prower factor
stubby microvillus
Student-Newman-Keuls test
Student test
studeri
    Bertiella s.
study
    blood chemistry s.
    cardiopulmonary sleep s.
    case-control s.
    clinicopathologic s.
    clonality s.
    cohort s.
    cytogenetic s.
    double-blind s.
    double-contrast s.
    dual-contrast s.
    electrophysiology s.
    enzyme s.
    erythrokinetic s.

esophageal motility s.
fat absorption s.
ferrokinetics s.
gastrointestinal bleed localization s.
gene arrangement s.
haplotype association s.
immunophenotypic s.
Johns Hopkins Center for Civilian Biodefense S.'s
National Wilms Tumor S.
Ostor s.
prospective s.
renal function s. (RFS)
retrospective s.
sex chromatin s.
split renal function s. (SRFS)
ultrastructural s.

stump
s. cancer
s. carcinoma

stunned myocardium

stunted
s. embryo
s. fetus

Sturge-Kalischer-Weber syndrome
Sturge syndrome
Sturge-Weber syndrome
stutzeri
Pseudomonas s.
STVA
subtotal villous atrophy
stye
meibomian s.
zeisian s.
stygium
Novosphingobium s.
stylet
Liberator universal locking s.
styloiditis
styloid process
stylosteophyte
Styloviridae
styptic
chemical s.
mechanical s.
vascular s.
Stypven
S. time
S. time test
styrene
styrone
Stysanus

SUA
serum uric acid
subacute
s. abscess
s. bacterial endocarditis (SBE)
s. bronchopneumonia
s. combined degeneration (SACD, SCD)
s. combined degeneration of spinal cord
s. combined sclerosis
s. cutaneous lupus
s. glomerulonephritis
s. granulomatous thyroiditis
s. hepatitis
s. inclusion body encephalitis
s. infective endocarditis
s. inflammation
s. meningitis
s. myelomonocytic leukemia
s. myelooptic neuropathy (SMON)
s. necrotizing encephalopathy
s. necrotizing myelitis
s. nephritis
s. sclerosing leukoencephalitis
s. sclerosing panencephalitis (SSPE)
s. spongiform encephalopathy
s. thyroiditis (SAT)
subadventitial fibrosis
subaortic stenosis (SS)
subarachnoid
s. hemorrhage (SAH)
s. space
subarcticum
Novosphingobium s.
subareolar duct papillomatosis
subcapsular
subcartilaginous
subcellular
subchondral
subchorial
s. lake
s. space
subchorionic
s. fibrin
fibrin, s.
subchoroidal
subclass
immunoglobulin s.
subclassification
Lukes-Butler histologic s.
subclavian steal syndrome

S

NOTES

947

subclinical coccidioidomycosis
subcommissural organ
subconjunctival
subcorneal
   s. pustular dermatitis
   s. pustular dermatosis
subcortical
   s. arteriosclerotic encephalopathy
   s. arteriosclerotic
     leukoencephalopathy
subcu, subq
   subcutaneous
subculture
subcutanea
   tela s.
subcutaneous (SC, SQ, subcu, subq)
   s. emphysema
   s. fat
   s. fat necrosis of newborn
   s. nodule
   s. tissue
subcutaneous/sublingual provocation
subcutaneum
   stratum s.
subcuticular
subcutis
   superficial s.
subdermal
subdermic
subdiaphragmatic abscess
subdural
   s. empyema
   s. hematoma
   s. hematorrhachis
   s. hygroma
subendocardial
   s. connective tissue
   s. layer
   s. myocardial infarction
subendothelial
   s. immune complex deposition
   s. layer
subendothelium
subependymal
   s. giant cell astrocytoma
   s. glioma
subependymoma
subepidermal
   s. abscess
   s. blister
   s. connective tissue (SEC)
   s. fibrosis
subepidermic bulla
subepithelial
   s. collagen
   s. collagen band
subepithelium
suberosis
suberyl arginine

subfamily
subflava
   Neisseria s.
subfolium
subgemmal
subgenus
subglobosa
   Sphaeropsis s.
subgranular
subgroup
   mucopolysaccharidosis s.
subhepatic abscess
subicteric
subinfection
subinflammatory
subintegumental
subintimal
subinvolution
subkingdom
sublabial adhesion
subleukemia
subleukemic
   s. granulocytic leukemia
   s. lymphocytic leukemia
   s. monocytic leukemia
   s. myelosis
sublimation
   heat of s.
sublingual
   s. cyst
   s. gland
sublingualis
   glandula s.
sublithincola
   Aequorivita s.
sublobular
subluxation
   atlantoaxial s.
sublymphemia
submammary mastitis
submandibular
   s. duct
   s. salivary gland
submandibularis
   ductus s.
   glandula s.
submarinus
   Desulfonauticus s.
   Psychrobacter s.
submassive confluent necrosis
submaxillaris
   ductus s.
submaxillary
   s. duct
   s. gland
   s. glycoprotein
submembranous
submetacentric
submicronic

submicroscopic
submorphous
submucosa
> duodenal gland in s.
> tela s.
> tunica s.

submucosal
submucous
subneural apparatus
subnitrate
> bismuth s.

subnormal
> severely s. (SSN)
> s. temperature

subnuclear vacuolated cell
subnucleus
suborder
subpapillare
> rete s.

subpapillary
> s. layer
> s. network

subpapular
subperitoneal appendicitis
subphrenic abscess
subphylum
subplacental
subplasmalemmal
> s. dense zone
> s. density
> s. microfilament

subpleural bleb
subq (*var. of* subcu)
subretinal fluid (SRF)
subroseum
> *Streptosporangium s.*

subrostratus
> *Felicola s.*

subroutine
> recursive s.

subsclerotic
subscripted variable
subserous
subset
> lymphocyte s.

subsinusoidal fibrosis
subspecies
substage
substance
> s. abuse screen
> alpha s.
> amount of s.

anterior pituitary-like s.
antidiuretic s. (ADS)
bacteriotropic s.
basophil s.
beta s.
blood group s.
blood group-specific s.'s A, B
cement s.
cementing s.
chromidial s.
chromophil s.
s. concentration
controlled s.
cortical s.
erythrocyte-sensitizing s. (ESS)
exophthalmos-producing s. (EPS)
fat-mobilizing s. (FMS)
filar s.
gelatinous s.
ground s.
group of activating s.
H s.
hazardous s.
hemolytic s.
immunity s.
interspongioplastic s.
medullary s.
methylene blue active s. (MBAS)
neuronal Nissl s.
neurosecretory s.
Nissl s.
s. P
s. P neuropeptide
pressor s.
proper s.
prostaglandin-like s. (PLS)
rabbit aorta-contracting s.
renal pressor s. (RPS)
reticular s.
Rolando gelatinous s.
Schwann white s.
sensitizing s.
slow-reacting s. (SRS)
soluble specific s.
specific capsular s.
specific soluble s. (SSS)
Stilling gelatinous s.
threshold s.
thromboplastic s.
tigroid s.
tumor polysaccharide s. (TPS)

S

NOTES

substance (*continued*)
    white s.
    zymoplastic s.
substantia, pl. **substantiae**
    s. adamantina
    s. alba
    s. basophilia
    s. compacta
    s. compacta ossium
    s. corticalis
    s. eburnea
    s. fundamentalis
    s. gelatinosa
    s. gelatinosa centralis
    s. glandularis prostatae
    s. intermedia centralis
    s. lentis
    s. medullaris
    s. metachromaticogranularis
    s. muscularis prostatae
    s. nigra
    s. ossea dentis
    s. propria of cornea
    s. propria corneae
    s. propria membranae tympani
    s. propria sclerae
    s. reticularis
    s. reticulofilamentosa
    s. spongiosa
    s. trabecularis
    s. vitrea
substernal goiter
substituent
substitute
    blood s.
    plasma s.
    PolyHeme blood s.
    Scott tap water s.
    volume s.
substitution
    generic s.
    s. product
    s. reaction
substrate
    defined s. (DS)
    s. level phosphorylation
substrate-labeled
    s.-l. fluorescence immunoassay
      (SLFIA)
    s.-l. fluorescent immunoassay
      (SLFIA)
substratum
substructure
subsurface
    s. basement membrane
    s. cisterna
subsynchronous vibration
subtegumental
subtelocentric

Subtercola
    S. boreus
    S. frigoramans
    S. pratensis
subterranea
    Knoellia s.
    Thermotoga s.
subterraneum
    Novosphingobium s.
    Sulfurihydrogenibium s.
subterraneus
    Bacillus s.
    Caldanaerobacter s.
    Caldanaerobacter s. subsp.
      subterraneus
    Geobacillus s.
    Hydrogenobacter s.
    Thermaerobacter s.
    Thermoanaerobacter s.
subtilis
    Bacillus s.
    Copromonas s.
subtotal villous atrophy (STVA)
subtraction
    immunofixation by s.
subtribe
subtype
    chondroblastic s.
    desmoplastic s.
subungual
    s. abscess
    s. melanoma
subunit
    four s.
    HCG alpha s.
    HCG beta s.
    s. vaccine
subvalvar stenosis
subvibrioides
    Brevundimonas s.
subvital mutation
succentorius
    lien s.
succenturiata
    placenta s.
succenturiate lobe
successional lamina
succinate
    s. dehydrogenase
    sodium s.
succinate-ubiquinone-oxidoreductase
succinatimandens
    Petrobacter s.
succinic acid
succiniciproducens
    Anaerobiospirillum s.
succinifaciens
    Treponema s.
Succinivibrio dextrinosolvens

Succinivibrionaceae
succinylcoenzyme A
succus
sucking louse
Sucquet canal
Sucquet-Hoyer canal
sucrase
sucrase-isomaltase
sucrose
>   s. alpha-ᴅ-glucohydrolase
>   s. density gradient (SDG)
>   s. density gradient analysis
>   s. density gradient
>   ultracentrifugation
>   s. hemolysis test
>   s. intolerance
>   s. pad nuclear exchange assay

sucrosemia
sucrosuria
suction method
suction-type biopsy
Suctoria
suctorial
SUD
>   sudden unexpected death
>   sudden unexplained death

Sudan
>   S. black
>   S. black B (SBB)
>   S. black B fat stain
>   S. black Bizzozero
>   black Bizzozero, S.
>   S. brown
>   S. red III
>   S. yellow
>   S. yellow G

sudanophil
sudanophilia
sudanophilic leukodystrophy
sudanophobic
>   s. unit
>   s. zone

sudden
>   s. cardiac death (SCD)
>   s. coronary death (SCD)
>   s. death syndrome (SDS)
>   s. infant death syndrome (SIDS)
>   s. intrauterine unexplained death
>   (SIUD)
>   s. unexpected death (SUD)
>   s. unexpected death in infancy
>   (SUDI)

>   s. unexpected, unexplained death
>   (SUUD)
>   s. unexplained death (SUD)
>   s. unexplained death in epilepsy
>   (SUDEP)
>   s. unexplained infant death (SUID)

Sudeck
>   S. atrophy
>   S. disease
>   S. point

Sudeck-Leriche syndrome
SUDEP
>   sudden unexplained death in epilepsy

SUDI
>   sudden unexpected death in infancy

sudomotor fiber
sudor
>   s. sanguineus
>   s. urinosus

sudoriferae
>   corpus glandulae s.
>   glandulae s.

sudoriferous
>   s. abscess
>   s. duct
>   s. gland

sudoriferus
>   ductus s.
>   porus s.

sudorikeratosis
sudoriparous abscess
SUDS
>   Single Use Diagnostic System
>   SUDS HIV-1 test

sueciensis
>   *Helcococcus s.*

sufentanil
sufficient
>   s. condition
>   not s. (NS)
>   quantity not s. (QNS)

suffocation
>   indirect s.

suffocative goiter
suffodiens
>   folliculitis abscedens et s.

suffusion
suffusus
>   *Centruroides suffusus s.*

sufrartyfex
>   *Paryphostomum s.*

NOTES

sugar
  s. acid
  s. assimilation assay
  blood s. (BS)
  s. broth
  capillary blood s. (CBS)
  fasting blood s. (FBS)
  s. fermentation assay
  invert s.
  postprandial blood s. (PPBS)
  reducing s.
  specific soluble s.
  s. tumor
  s. water test screen
Sugar-Chex II glucose control
sugar-coated spleen
sugar-icing liver
suggillation
  postmortem s.
suicide
  s. gene
  hot antigen s.
  s. machine
  s. methodology
  physician assisted s.
suicloacalis
  Atopostipes s.
suicordis
  Corynebacterium s.
SUID
  sudden unexplained infant death
suid herpesvirus
suihominis
  Sarcocystis s.
suillum
  Dechlorosoma s.
Suillus
suimastitidis
  Actinomyces s.
suipestifer
  Bacillus s.
Suipoxvirus
suis
  Balantidium s.
  Brucella s.
  Isospora s.
  Mycoplasma s.
  Trichomonas s.
  Trichuris s.
  Trypanosoma s.
suit
  chemical splash s.
sulcatum
  keratoderma plantare s.
  keratoma plantare s.
sulcular
  s. epithelium
  s. fluid
sulcus, pl. **sulci**

sulci cutis
  external spiral s.
  s. matricis unguis
  s. spiralis externus
sulfa
  s. drug
  s. film
sulfabenzamide
sulfacetamide
sulfadiazine
sulfaguanidine
sulfamerazine
sulfameter
sulfamethazine
sulfamethizole
sulfamethoxazole
sulfanilamide
sulfanilic acid
sulfapyridine
sulfatase
  iduronic s.
  L-sulfoiduronate s.
  phenol s.
  steroid s. (STS)
  sulfatide s.
sulfate
  1-adamantanamine s.
  ammonium s.
  chondroitin s.
  colistin s.
  copper s.
  dehydroepiandrosterone s. (DHEAS)
  dermatan s.
  diethyl s.
  dimethyl s.
  heparan s.
  indoxyl s.
  keratan s.
  polymyxin B s.
  potassium s.
  protamine s.
  sodium dodecyl s. (SDS)
  sodium lauryl s.
  sodium tetradecyl s.
sulfated acid mucopolysaccharide (SAM)
sulfatemia
sulfatiazole
sulfatidase
sulfatide
  cerebroside s.
  s. lipidosis
  s. sulfatase
sulfation factor
sulfexigens
  Desulfocapsa s.
sulfhemoglobin (HbS, SHb)
sulfhemoglobinemia
sulfhemoglobinuria
sulfhydryl group

sulfidaeris
    Halomonas s.
sulfide
    dichlorodiethyl s.
    Timm silver s.
sulfidifaciens
    Globicatella s.
sulfidophilum
    Heliobacterium s.
sulfindigotic acid
sulfinic acid
sulfinpyrazone
sulfinyl
sulfisoxazole
sulfite
    s. agar
    anhydrous sodium s.
    s. challenge
    exsiccated sodium s.
    s. oxidase
    s. oxidase deficiency
    sodium s.
Sulfitobacter
    S. brevis
    S. delicatus
    S. dubius
    S. mediterraneus
    S. pontiacus
sulfmethemoglobin
sulfobromophthalein sodium
sulfolipid
Sulfolobaceae
Sulfolobales
"Sulfolobus SNDV-like viruses"
Sulfolobus tokodaii
sulfomucin
sulfonamide
    s. antagonist
    s. assay
sulfonate
    alkylbenzene s. (ABS)
    scarlet red s.
    sodium polyethylene s.
sulfonation
sulfone
sulfonic acid
sulfonivorans
    Arthrobacter s.
    Hyphomicrobium s.
sulfonmethane
sulfonyl
sulfonylurea assay

sulfoprotein
sulforhodamine B
sulfosalicylic
    s. acid (SSA)
    s. acid turbidity test
sulfotransferase
sulfoxide
    dimethyl s.
sulfoxone
    sodium s.
sulfur (S)
    s. bacterium
    s. dioxide
    s. dye
    s. granule
    s. oxide
    s. pearl of Namibia
    s. trioxide
sulfur-containing amino acid
sulfuric acid
Sulfurihydrogenibium
    S. azorense
    S. subterraneum
Sulfurimonas autotrophica
Sulfurospirillum
    S. arsenophilum
    S. halorespirans
    S. multivorans
sulfurous acid
Sulfurovum lithotrophicum
sulfurreducens
    Geobacter s.
Sulkowitch
    S. reagent
    S. test
sullae
    Rhizobium s.
sulphureum
    Trichophyton s.
    Trichophyton tonsurans var. *s.*
sulphureus
    Laetiporus s.
Sulzberger-Garbe syndrome
summa
    Pygidiopsis s.
summer
    s. asthma
    s. prurigo of Hutchinson
sum of square deviations (SSD)
SUN
    serum urea nitrogen
sunburst form

S

NOTES

sundaicus
  Anopheles s.
sunstroke
sup
  superficial
superacidity
superantigen
supercooled
superdistention
superdominance
superfamily
superfemale
superficial (sup)
  s. burn
  s. cell
  s. implantation
  s. malignant fibrous histiocytoma
  s. multicentric basal cell carcinoma
  s. mycosis
  s. spreading melanoma
  s. subcutis
  s. ulcerating rheumatoid necrobiosis
  s. wound
superficiales
  nodi lymphoidei inguinales s.
superficialis
  colitis cystica s.
  lupus s.
Superfrost Plus glass slide
supergene
  immunoglobulin s.
superheated
superinduce
superinfection
superior
  ductulus aberrans s.
  s. limbic keratoconjunctivitis (SLKC)
  lipodystrophia progessiva s.
  s. pulmonary sulcus tumor
  s. sagittal sinus
  s. sulcus tumor
  tarsus s.
  tela choroidea s.
  s. vena caval syndrome
  s. vena cava syndrome
Supermount slide fixative
supernatant
  culture fluid s.
  hybridoma s.
  postmitochondrial s. (PMS)
supernate
supernumerary
  s. kidney
  s. marker
  s. organ
  s. segmental artery
superoxide
  s. anion

  s. assay
  s. dismutase
  s. dismutase gene
superparasite
superparasitism
superpictus
  Anopheles s.
superpigmentation
supersaturated (SS)
Super Sensitive kit multistep detection system
superstes
Superstitionia donensis
supervoltage
superwarfarin
supplemental inheritance
supplementary gene
supplied air respirator (SAR)
supply
  double blood s.
  endometrial blood s.
  power s.
support
  granulocyte transfusion s.
  s. medium
  s. zone
supporting cell
suppressibility
suppression
  bone marrow s.
  bystander s.
  s. of cell cycle
  s. subtractive hybridization
suppressor
  s. cell
  s. of cytokine signaling (SOCS)
  s. gene
  s. mutation
  p53 tumor s.
  soluble immune response s. (SIRS)
  s. T lymphocyte
  tRNA s.
suppressor-sensitive mutant
suppurant
suppurate
suppuration
suppurativa
  hidradenitis s.
suppurative
  s. acute appendicitis
  s. acute inflammation
  s. arthritis
  s. cerebritis
  s. cholangitis
  s. chronic inflammation
  s. chronic otitis media
  s. encephalitis
  s. granulomatous inflammation
  s. hepatitis

s. infection
s. keratitis
s. mastitis
s. necrosis
s. nephritis
s. pericarditis
s. pleurisy
s. pneumonia
s. synovitis
suprabasal
s. cell layer
s. clefting
suprahyoid gland
supranormal venous oxygen content
supranuclear
supraoptic nucleus
supraopticohypophysialis
tractus s.
supraopticohypophysial tract
suprapapillary
suprapubic
s. needle aspiration
s. puncture
suprarenal
s. body
s. capsule
s. cortex
s. gland
suprarenalis
cortex glandulae s.
glandula s.
macrogenitosomia praecox s.
medulla glandulae s.
suprasellar
s. cyst
s. meningioma
supravalvular aortic stenosis (SAS, SVAS)
supraventricular tachycardia
supravergence (S)
supravital
s. stain
s. staining
Supre-Heme buffer
suramin
Sure Blot membrane
Surecut needle
SureStep
S. Flexx professional blood glucose management system
S. Pro glucose analyzer

surface
abluminal s.
s. absorptive cell
s. antigen
apical s.
s. carcinoma in situ (SCIS)
cut s.
s. denudation
s. epithelial-stromal tumor
s. epithelium
s. expression
intimal s.
s. marker
s. marker staining
s. mucous cell
s. mucous cell of stomach
serosal s.
s. tension (ST)
surface-active agent
surface-barrier detector
surface-oriented pinocytic activity
surfactant
amniotic fluid s.
amniotic fluid pulmonary s.
s. nanoemulsion
s. protein A, B, C
pulmonary s.
surgery
bariatric s.
video-assisted transthoracic s. (VATS)
surgical
s. ciliated cyst
s. defect
s. emphysema
s. pathology
s. resection
s. specimen
s. wound
Surgicutt device
Surgipath Decalcifier I, II
surivivin protein
surnumerary chromosome
surra
surrogate
biofidelic human s.
surveillance
immune s.
immunological s.
syndromic s.
survey
cross-sectional s.

S

NOTES

survey *(continued)*
iodine-131 thyroid metastatic s.
metastatic bone s.
s. meter
proficiency s.
s. program
radiation s.
skeletal s.
survival
s. of cancer cell
chromium-51 red cell s.
disease-free s. (DFS)
disease-specific s.
metastasis-free s.
s. motor neuron (SMN)
s. motor neuron telomeric gene
overall s. (OS)
predictor of patient s.
red blood cell s.
s. time
survivin protein
SUS
stained urinary sediment
susceptibility
disease s.
electric s.
genetic s.
magnetic s.
s. test
s. testing
suspected diagnosis
suspended particulate
suspension
DNAzole cell s.
extended insulin zinc s.
suspensory ligament of lens
suspicious cell
sustentacular
s. cell
s. fiber of retina
SUTI
sperm-ubiquitin tag immunoassay
Sutterella
S. stercoricanis
S. wadsworthensis
Sutton
S. disease
S. nevus
S. ulcer
Suttonella indologenes
suture
s. granuloma
localization s.
SUUD
sudden unexpected, unexplained death
suum
Ascaris s.
Suzanne gland

SV
simian virus
snake venom
SV 40 T antigen
Sv
sievert
SV40-adenovirus hybrid
SVAS
supravalvular aortic stenosis
SVC
slow vital capacity
Svedberg
S. equation
S. unit of sedimentation coefficient (S)
SVR
systemic vascular resistance
SW
spiral wound
swab
nasopharyngeal s.
Persist skin prep s.
s. specimen
Swachman-Diamond syndrome
Swaminathania salitolerans
swamp
s. fever
s. fever virus
Swann antigen
swan-neck deformity
Sw^a antigen
swarming
sweat
s. chloride level
s. duct
s. duct adenoma
excretory duct of s.
s. gland
s. gland adenocarcinoma
s. gland adenoma
s. gland carcinoma (SGC)
s. gland tumor
s. pore
s. test
Sweat-Chek conductivity analyzer
Swediaur disease
Sweet
S. disease
S. method
S. syndrome
swelling
albuminous s.
brain s.
Calabar s.
cellular s.
cloudy s.
fugitive s.
high amplitude s.
hydropic s.

Neufeld capsular s.
Spielmeyer acute s.
Swift disease
Swift-Feer disease
swimmer's itch
swimming
s. pool conjunctivitis
s. pool granuloma
swine
atrophic rhinitis of s.
s. encephalitis virus
s. fever
s. fever virus
s. influenza
s. influenza virus
s. pest
s. rotlauf bacillus
s. vesicular disease
swinepox virus
swirling comet tail colony
SWI/SNF complex
Swiss
S. cheese endometrium
S. cheese hyperplasia
S. mouse leukemia virus
Swiss-type
S.-t. agammaglobulinemia
S.-t. hypogammaglobulinemia
switch
angiogenic s.
class s.
double-pole double-throw s.
double-pole single-throw s.
silicon-controlled s.
switching
class s.
isotype s.
swollen crista
Sx
symptoms
sycoma
sycosis
Sydenham
S. chorea
S. disease
Sydney
S. classification
S. classification for gastritis
S. classification system
Sydowia
sylvatic plague
Sylvest disease

Symbiobacterium
S. thermophilum
symbion, symbiont
symbiosis
symbiote
symbiotic
symblepharon
symbol
hazard s.
statistical s.
sym-**dichloroethylene**
Symmers
S. clay pipestem fibrosis
S. disease
symmetric
s. adenolipomatosis
s. distribution
symmetrica
keratoderma s.
symmetrical gangrene
symmetry
axis of s.
bilateral s.
s. element
s. group
icosahedral s.
s. operation
s. plane
radial s.
sympathetic
s. chain
s. formative cell
s. imbalance
s. neuroblast
s. ophthalmia
s. ophthalmitis
s. pharmacology
sympathetoblast
sympathetoblastoma
sympathicectomy
sympathicoblast
sympathicoblastoma
sympathicogonioma
sympathiconeuritis
sympathicopathy
sympathicotonia
sympathicotripsy
sympathicotropic cell
sympathoblast
sympathoblastoma
sympathochromaffin cell
sympathogonia

NOTES

sympathogonioma
sympathomimetic
sympathotropic cell
sympexis
symphysis, gen. symphyses
symplasmatic
Sympodiophora
symport
symporter
    human sodium/iodide s. (hNIS)
    sodium-iodine s. (NIS)
symptomatic
    s. fever
    s. myeloid metaplasia
    s. porphyria
    s. reaction
    s. ulcer
    s. varicocele
symptomatica
    livedo reticularis s.
symptomatology
symptomatolytic
symptoms (Sx)
SYN
    synaptophysin
synapse
    axoaxonic s.
    axodendritic s.
    axosomatic s.
    electrotonic s.
    pericorpuscular s.
synapsing
    nerves s.
synapsis
synaptic
    s. bouton
    s. cleft
    s. ending
    s. phase
    s. terminal
    s. trough
    s. vesicle
synaptinemal complex
synaptobrevin
synaptology
synaptonemal complex
synaptophysin (SYN)
    s. antibody
    s. stain
synaptopodin gene
synaptosomal protein of 25 kDa
synaptosome
synaptotagmin
Syncephalastrum racemosum
syncephalus
synchondrosis
    sphenooccipital s.
    sphenopetrosal s.
    sternal s.

Synchron
    S. CX9 ALX clinical system
    S. CX clinical chemistry system
    S. CX4, CX5, CX9, CX500, CX1000 PRO clinical system
    S. CX3, CX4, CX5 Delta clinical system
    S. CX4, CX5, CX7 Super clinical system
    S. LX clinical chemistry system
    S. LX20 clinical system
    S. LX4201 clinical system
    S. LXi 725 clinical system
    S. LX20, LX2000 PRO clinical system
synchronism
    developmental s.
synchronized culture
synchronous
    s. airway lesion (SAL)
    s. cancer
    s. counter
    s. data transmission
    s. mass lesion
    s. neoplasm
    s. peritoneal implant
Synchytrium endobioticum
Syncleistostroma
syncope
    vasovagal s.
syncyanea
    Pseudomonas s.
syncyanin
syncytia (*pl. of* syncytium)
syncytial
    s. alteration
    s. endometritis
    s. knot
    s. knotting
    s. morphology
    respiratory s. (RS)
    s. shedding
    s. trophoblast
syncytiotrophoblast
syncytiotrophoblastic
    s. cell
    s. cell of seminoma
syncytium, pl. syncytia
    s. inducing (SI)
syndactyly
syndecan
syndecan-1
syndesmitis
syndesmophyte
syndromal dysplasia
syndrome
    Aarskog s.
    Aarskog-Scott s.
    abdominal muscle deficiency s.

Abercrombie s.
Achard s.
Achard-Thiers s.
Achenbach s.
acquired immunodeficiency s. (AIDS)
acrofacial s.
acute coronary s. (ACS)
acute radiation s. (ARS)
acute respiratory distress s. (ARDS)
acute urethral s.
Adair-Dighton s.
addisonian s.
Adie s.
adrenal feminizing s.
adrenal gland virilizing s.
adrenogenital s. (AGS)
adult respiratory distress s. (ARDS)
Ahumada-Del Castillo s.
Aicardi s.
Alagille s.
Albright s.
Albright-McCune-Sternberg s.
Aldrich s.
Alezzandrini s.
Allen-Masters s.
Alport s.
Alström s.
amenorrhea-galactorrhea s.
amniotic band s.
Amsterdam s.
Andersen s.
Andrade s.
androgen insensitivity s. (AIS)
Angelman s.
Angelucci s.
angioosteohypertrophy s.
antibody deficiency s. (ADS)
antiphospholipid s. (APS)
antiphospholipid antibody s.
antisynthetase s.
Anton s.
apallic s.
aplastic anemia s.
Argonz-Del Castillo s.
Arias s.
Arndt-Gottron s.
Arnold-Chiari s.
Arnold nerve reflex cough s.
arthritis-dermatitis s.
Ascher s.

Asherman s.
ataxia telangiectasia s.
autoerythrocyte sensitization s.
Avellis s.
Axenfeld s.
Ayerza s.
Baastrup s.
Babinski s.
Babinski-Fröhlich s.
Babinski-Nageotte s.
Babinski-Vaquez s.
bacterial overgrowth s.
Bäfverstedt s.
Balint s.
Baller-Gerold s.
Bamberger-Marie s.
Banti s.
Bardet-Biedl s.
bare lymphocyte s.
Barlow s.
Barré-Guillain s.
Barrett s.
Bart s.
Bartter s.
basal cell nevus s.
base lymphocyte s. (BLS)
Bassen-Kornzweig s.
Bateman s.
Batten-Mayou s.
Bazex s.
Beau s.
Beckwith s.
Beckwith-Wiedemann s.
Behçet s.
Benedikt s.
Beradinelli s.
Berlin breakage s.
Bernard s.
Bernard-Horner s.
Bernard-Sergent s.
Bernard-Soulier s. (BSS)
Bernhardt-Roth s.
Bernheim s.
Bertolotti s.
Besnier-Boeck-Schaumann s.
Bianchi s.
Biemond s.
bile salt deficiency s.
Birt-Hogg-Dube s.
Björnstad s.
Blackfan-Diamond s.
black thyroid s.

S

NOTES

syndrome *(continued)*

Blatin s.
blind loop s.
Bloch-Sulzberger s.
Bloom s.
blue diaper s.
Blum s.
body of Luys s.
bodypacker s.
Boerhaave s.
Bonnet-Dechaume-Blanc s.
Bonnevie-Ullrich s.
Bonnier s.
Böök s.
Börjeson s.
Börjeson-Forssman-Lehmann s.
Bouillaud s.
Bouveret s.
bowel bypass s.
Brachmann-de Lange s.
brachymesomelia-renal s.
brain death s.
Brennemann s.
Briquet s.
Brissaud-Marie s.
Brissaud-Sicard s.
Bristowe s.
Brock s.
bronchiolitis obliterans s.
brown bowel s.
Brown-Séquard s.
Brugsch s.
Bruns s.
Brunsting s.
Buckley s.
Budd s.
Budd-Chiari s.
Bürger-Grütz s.
Burnett s.
Buschke-Ollendorf s.
Bywaters s.
Cacchi-Ricci s.
Caffey s.
Caffey-Silverman s.
Canada-Cronkhite s.
Capgras s.
Caplan s.
carcinoid s.
cardiolipin antibody s.
Carney s.
carotid sinus s.
carpal tunnel s.
Carpenter s.
Castleman s.
cat's cry s.
cat's eye s.
Ceelen-Gellerstedt s.
cellular immunity deficiency s.
  (CIDS)

cerebellomedullary malformation s.
cerebral salt-washing s.
cerebrohepatorenal s.
cervical disk s.
cervical rib s.
Cestan s.
Cestan-Chenais s.
Cestan-Raymond s.
chancriform s.
Charcot s.
Charcot-Weiss-Baker s.
CHARGE s.
Charlin s.
Chauffard s.
Chauffard-Still s.
Chédiak-Higashi s. (CHS)
Chédiak-Steinbrinck-Higashi s.
Cheney s.
Chiari-Arnold s.
Chiari-Budd s.
Chiari-Frommel s.
Chiari II s.
Chilaiditi s.
CHILD s.
childhood hemolytic uremic s.
Chinese restaurant s. (CRS)
choriodecidual inflammatory
  response s.
Chotzen s.
Christian s.
Christ-Siemens s.
Christ-Siemens-Touraine s.
chromosomal breakage s.
chromosomal deletion s.
chromosomal malformation s.
chromosome breakage s.
chronic brain s. (CBS)
chronic fatigue immune
  dysfunction s. (CFIDS)
chronic intestinal
  pseudoobstructive s. (CIPS)
Churg-Strauss s.
Citelli s.
Clarke-Hadfield s.
Claude Bernard-Horner s.
Clough-Richter s.
Clouston s.
Cockayne s.
Coffin-Lowry s.
Coffin-Siris s.
Cogan s.
cold agglutinin s. (CAS)
Collet s.
Collet-Sicard s.
coloboma s.
combined immunodeficiency s.
  (CIDS)
common variable
  immunodeficiency s.

compartment s.
compartmental s.
complete androgen insensitivity s.
  (CAIS)
congenital rubella s.
Conn s.
Cornelia de Lange s.
coronary insufficiency s.
Costello s.
Costen s.
Cotard s.
Courvoisier-Terrier s.
Cowden s.
Crandall s.
CREST s.
cri du chat s.
Crigler-Najjar s.
Cronkhite-Canada s.
Crouzon s.
Crow-Fukase s.
CRST s.
crush s.
Cruveilhier-Baumgarten s.
cryopathic hemolytic s.
cryptophthalmus s.
Curtis-Fitz-Hugh s.
Curtius s.
Cushing s.
cutaneomucouveal s.
CVID s.
Cyriax s.
DaCosta s.
Danbolt-Closs s.
Dandy-Walker s.
Danlos s.
Debré-Semelaigne s.
de Clerambault s.
defibrination s.
Degos s.
Dejerine s.
Dejerine-Klumpke s.
Dejerine-Roussy s.
Dejerine-Sottas s.
de Lange s.
del Castillo s.
dengue shock s.
Dennie-Marfan s.
Denys-Drash s.
de Sanctis-Cacchione s.
de Toni-Fanconi s.
Devon polyposis s.
dialysis dysequilibrium s.

Diamond-Blackfan s.
DiGeorge s.
Di Guglielmo s.
Donath-Landsteiner s.
Donohue s.
Down s. (DS)
Dresbach s.
Dressler s.
Duane s.
Dubin-Johnson s.
Dubin-Sprinz s.
Dubreuil-Chambardel s.
Duchenne s.
Duchenne-Erb s.
dumping s.
Duncan s.
Duplay s.
Dupré s.
Dyggve-Melchior-Clausen s.
Dyke-Davidoff-Masson s.
dysmyelopoietic s.
dysplastic nevus s.
dystrophy-dystocia s. (DDS)
dysuria-pyuria s.
Eagle s.
Eaton-Lambert s.
economy class s.
ectopic ACTH s.
Eddowes s.
Edwards s.
Edwards-Patau s.
Ehlers-Danlos s. (EDS)
Eisenlohr s.
Eisenmenger s.
Ekbom s.
Ellis-van Creveld s.
EMG s.
empty sella s.
endocrine polyglandular s.
eosinophilia-myalgia s. (EMS)
Epstein s.
Erb s.
erythrodysesthesia s.
Evans s.
excited skin s.
Faber s.
facet s.
Fallot s.
Fanconi s.
Fanconi-Zinsser s.
Farber s.
Farber-Uzman s.

S

NOTES

syndrome *(continued)*
fat embolism s.
Fechtner s.
Felty s.
fertile eunuch s.
fetal alcohol s.
fetal face s.
fetal hydantoin s.
fetal trimethadione s.
Feuerstein-Mims s.
fibrinogen-fibrin conversion s.
Fiessinger-Leroy-Reiter s.
Figueira s.
first arch s.
Fisher s.
Fitz s.
Fitz-Hugh and Curtis s.
Fleischner s.
Flynn-Aird s.
focal dermal hypoplasia s.
Foix s.
folded-lung s.
Forbes-Albright s.
Forney s.
Foster Kennedy s.
Foville s.
fragile X s.
Fraley s.
Franceschetti s.
Franceschetti-Jadassohn s.
François s.
Fraser s.
Freeman-Sheldon s.
Frenkel anterior ocular traumatic s.
Frey s.
Friderichsen-Waterhouse s.
Friedmann vasomotor s.
Fröhlich s.
Froin s.
Frommel-Chiari s.
Fryn s.
Fuchs s.
Furst-Ostrum s.
G s.
Gaisböck s.
Gamstorp s.
Ganser s.
Gardner s.
Gardner-Diamond s.
Gasser s.
gay lymph node s.
Gélineau s.
Gerhardt s.
Gerstmann s.
Gianotti-Crosti s.
giant platelet s.
Gilbert s.
Gilles de la Tourette s.
Gitelman s.

Glanzmann-Riniker s.
glomangiomatous osseous malformation s.
glutaric aciduria type 2 s.
Goldberg-Maxwell s.
Goldenhar s.
Goldz-Gorlin s.
Goltz s.
Good s.
Goodpasture s.
Gopalan s.
Gordon s.
Gorlin s.
Gorlin-Chaudhry-Moss s.
Gorlin-Goltz s.
Gorlin-Psaume s.
Gorman s.
Gougerot-Blum s.
Gougerot-Carteaud s.
Gowers s.
gracilis s.
Gradenigo s.
Graham Little s.
gray platelet s. (GPS)
Greig s.
Griscelli s.
Grönblad-Strandberg s.
Gruber s.
Gubler s.
Guillain-Barré s.
Gulf War s.
Gull-Sutton s.
Gunn s.
gustatory sweating s.
Haber s.
Haddad s.
Hadfield-Clarke s.
Hakim s.
Hallermann-Streiff s.
Hallermann-Streiff-François s.
Hallervorden s.
Hallervorden-Spatz s.
Hallgren s.
Hallopeau-Siemens s.
Hamman s.
Hamman-Rich s.
hand-foot s.
hand-foot-uterus s.
Hanhart s.
Hanot-Chauffard s.
hantavirus pulmonary s.
happy puppet s.
Harada s.
Hare s.
Harris s.
Hartnup s.
Hassin s.
Hayem-Widal s.
heart-hand s.

Heerfordt s.
Hegglin s.
Heidenhain s.
HELLP s.
Helweg-Larssen s.
hemangioma-thrombocytopenia s.
hemolytic-uremic s. (HUS)
hemophagocytic s. (HPS)
hemorrhagic colitis s.
hemorrhagic fever with renal s.
Hench-Rosenberg s.
Henoch-Schönlein s.
hereditary flat adenoma s. (HFAS)
hereditary mixed polyposis s.
Herlitz s.
Hermansky-Pudlak s.
herniated disc s. (HDS)
Herrmann s.
Hines-Bannick s.
Hirschowitz s.
Hoffmann-Werdnig s.
Holmes-Adie s.
Holt-Oram s.
Homén s.
Horner s.
Horton s.
Houssay s.
Hünermann s.
hungry bone s.
Hunt s.
Hunter s.
Hunter-Hurler s.
Hurler s. (HS)
Hutchinson s.
Hutchinson-Gilford s.
Hutchison s.
hypereosinophilic s.
hyper-IgE s.
hyper-IgM s.
hyperventilation s.
hyperviscosity s.
hypophysial s.
idiopathic nephrotic s. (INS)
idiopathic respiratory distress s. (IRDS)
Imerslund-Grasbeck s.
immotile cilia s.
immune dysfunction s.
immunodeficiency s.
impingement s.
inappropriate antidiuretic hormone s.

s. of inappropriate secretion of antidiuretic hormone (SIADH)
India rubber man s.
infection-associated hemophagocytic s. (IAHS)
intersex s.
iridocorneal endothelial s. (ICE)
irradiation CVS/CNS s.
irradiation hematopoietic s.
Irvine s.
Ivemark s.
Jaccoud s.
Jackson s.
Jacod s.
Jadassohn-Lewandowski s.
Jaffe-Campanacci s.
Jahnke s.
Jeghers-Peutz s.
Jervell and Lange-Nielsen s.
Jeune s.
Job s.
Johnson-Dubin s.
Joseph s.
juvenile polyposis s.
Kallmann s.
Kandinskii-Clerambault s.
Kanner s.
Kartagener s.
Kasabach-Merritt s.
Kast s.
Kearns s.
Kearns-Sayre s.
Kennedy s.
Kiloh-Nevin s.
Kimmelstiel-Wilson s.
Kinsbourne s.
Klauder s.
Kleine-Levin s.
Klinefelter s. (KS)
Klippel-Feil s. (KFS)
Klippel-Trenaunay s.
Klippel-Trenaunay-Weber s.
Klumpke-Dejerine s.
Klüver-Bucy s.
Kniest s.
Kocher-Debré-Semelaigne s.
Koenig s.
Koerber-Salus-Elschnig s.
Korsakoff s.
Kostmann s.
Krabbe s.
Krause s.

S

NOTES

syndrome *(continued)*
Kunkel s.
Kuskokwim s.
kwashiorkor-marasmus s.
Laband s.
Labbé neurocirculatory s.
Ladd s.
LAMB s.
Lambert-Eaton s.
Lambert-Eaton myasthenic s. (LEMS)
Landry s.
Landry-Guillain-Barré s.
Larsen s.
Launois s.
Launois-Bensaude s.
Launois-Cléret s.
Laurence-Biedl s.
Laurence-Moon s.
Laurence-Moon-Bardet-Biedl s.
Laurence-Moon-Biedl s.
Lawford s.
Lawrence-Seip s.
lazy leukocyte s.
Lennox s.
Lenz s.
LEOPARD s.
Leriche s.
Leri-Weill s.
Lermoyez s.
Lesch-Nyhan s.
Lévy-Roussy s.
Leyden-Möbius s.
Lhermitte-McAlpine s.
Libman-Sacks s.
Lichtheim s.
Liddle s.
Li-Fraumeni cancer s.
light chain Fanconi s.
Lightwood s.
Lignac s.
Lignac-Fanconi s.
linear sebaceous nevus s.
Lobstein s.
Löffler s. I, II
Looser-Milkman s.
Lorain-Lévi s.
Louis-Bar s.
Lowe s.
Lowe-Terrey-MacLachlan s.
Lown-Ganong-Levine s.
Lucey-Driscoll s.
Lutembacher s.
Luys body s.
Lyell s.
lymphadenopathy s.
lymphoproliferative s.
MacKenzie s.
Macleod s.

Maffucci s.
malabsorption s.
male Turner s.
malformation s.
Mali s.
malignant carcinoid s.
Malin s.
Mallory-Weiss s.
mandibulofacial dysotosis s.
mandibulooculofacial s.
Marañón s.
Marchesani s.
Marchiafava-Micheli s.
Marcus Gunn s.
Marfan s.
Margolis s.
Marie s.
Marie-Bamberger s.
Marie-Robinson s.
Marinesco-Garland s.
Marinesco-Sjögren s.
Maroteaux-Lamy s.
Marshall s.
Martorell s.
Mauriac s.
Mayer-Rokitansky-Küster s.
McCune-Albright s. (MAS)
Meckel s.
Meckel-Gruber s.
megacystic s.
Meigs s.
MELAS s.
Melchior s.
Melkersson s.
Melkersson-Rosenthal s.
Melnick-Needles s.
Ménétrier s.
Mengert shock s.
Ménière s.
Menkes s.
menopausal s.
MEN s., type 1, 2, 2a, 2b, 3
metabolic s.
metastatic carcinoid s.
methionine malabsorption s.
Meyenburg-Altherr-Uehlinger s.
Meyer-Betz s.
Meyer-Schwickerath and Weyers s.
microdeletion s.
middle lobe s.
Miescher s.
Mikulicz s.
milk-alkali s.
Milkman s.
Millard-Gubler s.
Miller-Dieker s.
minimal-change nephrotic s.
Minkowski-Chauffard s.
Minot-von Willebrand s.

Mirizzi s.
mixed cryoglobulin s.
Möbius s.
Monakow s.
Montreal platelet s. (MPS)
Moore s.
Morel s.
Morgagni s.
Morgagni-Adams-Stokes s.
Morgagni-Stewart-Morel s.
Morquio s.
Morquio-Brailsford s.
Morquio-Ullrich s.
Morris s.
Morton s.
Morvan s.
Mosse s.
Mounier-Kuhn s.
Mucha-Habermann s.
Muckle-Wells s.
mucocutaneous lymph node s.
mucosal neuroma s.
mucosal prolapse s.
Muir-Torre s.
multiple hamartoma s.
multiple lentigines s.
multiple mucosal neuroma s.
multiple organ dysfunction s.
Murchison-Sanderson s.
mycosis fungoides/Sézary s.
  (MF/SS)
myelodysplastic s. (MDS)
myeloproliferative s.
myofascial s.
Naffziger s.
Nägeli s.
nail-patella s.
NAME s.
Nelson s.
Nelson-Salassa s.
neonatal respiratory distress s.
nephritic s.
nephrotic s. (NS)
Netherton s.
neurocutaneous phacomatosis s.
neuroleptic malignant s.
nevoid basal cell carcinoma s.
  (NBCCS)
newborn respiratory s.
Nezelof s.
Nijmegen breakage s. (NBS)
Noack s.

nonketotic hyperosmolar s.
Nonne-Milroy-Meige s.
nonspecific viral s.
Noonan s.
nutritional recovery s.
OAV s.
ocular-mucous membrane s.
oculobuccogenital s.
oculocerebrorenal s.
oculodentodigital s.
oculovertebral s.
ODD s.
OFD s. 1–8
Ogilvie s.
Omenn s.
OMM s.
Opitz GBBB s.
Oppenheim s.
opsoclonus-myoclonus s.
organic brain s. (OBS)
organic dust toxic s.
Osler-Weber-Rendu s.
osteomyelofibrotic s.
Ostrum-Furst s.
otomandibular s.
ovarian hyperstimulation s. (OHS)
overlap s.
pacemaker twiddler's s.
painful bruising s.
Pancoast s.
papillary muscle s.
Papillon-Léage and Psaume s.
Papillon-Lefèvre s.
paralytic s.
paraneoplastic endocrine s.
Parinaud oculoglandular s.
parkinsonian s.
parotitis s.
Parry-Romberg s.
partial androgen insensitivity s.
  (PAIS)
Patau s.
Paterson s.
Paterson-Brown-Kelly s.
Paterson-Kelly s.
4p deletion s.
Pellizzi s.
Pendred s.
penta X s.
Pepper s.
periodic s. (PS)
Perlman s.

S

NOTES

syndrome *(continued)*
Persian Gulf s.
persistent müllerian duct s.
(PMDS)
Peutz s.
Peutz-Jeghers s.
Pfaundler-Hurler s.
Pfeiffer s.
pharyngeal pouch s.
Picchini s.
Pick s.
pickwickian s.
PIE s.
Pierre Robin s.
Pitt-Rogers-Danks s.
Plummer-Vinson s.
POEMS s.
Poland s.
Polhemus-Schafer-Ivemark s.
polycystic ovary s.
polysplenia s.
polytoxicomaniac s.
postgastrectomy dumping s.
postmenopausal s.
postpump s. (PPS)
postrubella s.
postvagotomy s.
Potter s.
pouch s.
Prader-Willi s.
premature senility s.
primary fibrinogenolysis s.
primary fibromyalgia s.
Profichet s.
prune belly s.
pseudo-Felty s.
pseudomyasthenic s.
pseudothalidomide s.
pseudo-Turner s.
pterygium s.
pulmonary dysmaturity s.
pulmonary-renal s.
Putnam-Dana s.
radial aplasia-thrombocytopenia s.
Raeder paratrigeminal s.
Ramsay Hunt s.
Rapp-Hodgkin s.
Raymond-Cestan s.
reactive airways dysfunction s.
(RADS)
Recklinghausen-Applebaum s.
recurrent bouts of nephrotic s.
red cell fragmentation s.
red eye s.
refeeding s.
Refetoff s.
Reichmann s.
Reifenstein s.
Reiter s.

REM s.
Rendu-Osler-Weber s.
Renpenning s.
respiratory distress s. (RDS)
respiratory distress s. of newborn
restless legs s.
Rett s.
Reye s.
Rh isoimmunization s.
Rh null s.
Richards-Rundle s.
Richter s.
Rieger s.
right ovarian vein s.
Riley-Day s.
Riley-Smith s.
Roaf s.
Roberts s.
Robin s.
Robinow s.
Roger s.
Rokitansky-Küster-Hauser s.
Romano-Ward s.
Romberg s.
Rosenbach s.
Rosenthal s.
Rosenthal-Kloepfer s.
Rosewater s.
Roth s.
Roth-Bernhardt s.
Rothmann-Makai s.
Rothmund s.
Rothmund-Thomson s.
Rotor s.
Rotter s.
Roussy-Dejerine s.
Roussy-Lévy s.
Rovsing s.
Rubinstein s.
Rubinstein-Taybi s.
Rud s.
rudimentary testis s.
Rundles-Falls s.
runting s.
Russell s.
Rust s.
Sabin-Feldman s.
Saethre-Chotzen s.
salt-losing s.
Sanchez Salorio s.
Sanfilippo s.
scalded skin s. (SSS)
scalenus anticus s.
Schafer s.
Schanz s.
Schaumann s.
Scheie s.
Schirmer s.
Schmid-Fraccaro s.

Schmidt s.
Schridde s.
Schroeder s.
Schüller s.
Schüller-Christian s.
Schultz s.
Schwartz s.
Schwartz-Bartter s.
Scott s.
Sebastian s.
Sebright bantam s.
Seckel s.
secondary antiphospholipid s.
Secrétan s.
sella turcica s.
Selye s.
Senear-Usher s.
sepsis s.
Sertoli cell only s.
Sever s.
severe acute respiratory s. (SARS)
Sézary s. (SS)
shaken adult s.
shaken baby s. (SBS)
shaken impact s.
shaken infant s.
Sheehan s.
short bowel s.
Shprintzen s.
Shulman s.
Shwachman s.
Shwachman-Diamond s.
Shy-Drager s.
Sicard s.
sicca s.
sick building s.
sick sinus s.
Silferskiöld s.
Silver s.
Silver-Russell s.
Silvestrini-Corda s.
Singleton-Merten s.
sinus node dysfunction s.
Sipple s.
Sjögren s.
Sjögren-Larsson s.
sleep apnea s.
Sluder s.
Sly s.
Smith-Lemli-Opitz s.
Smith-Magenis s.
Smith-Riley s.

Sneddon s.
Sohval-Soffer s.
solitary rectal ulcer s.
Sorsby s.
Sotos s. of cerebral gigantism
Spen s.
spherophakia-brachymorphia s.
Sprinz-Nelson s.
spruelike s.
Spurway s.
stagnant loop s.
staphylococcal scalded skin s.
stasis s.
Steele-Richardson-Olszewski s.
Steinbrocker s.
Steiner s.
Stein-Leventhal s.
Stevens-Johnson s.
Stewart-Bluefarb s.
Stewart-Morel s.
Stewart-Treves s.
Stickler s.
Still-Chauffard s.
Stilling s.
Stilling-Turk-Duane s.
Stokes-Adams s.
Stokvis-Talma s.
Stormorken s.
Strachan s.
streptococcal toxic shock s.
Stryker-Halbeisen s.
Sturge s.
Sturge-Kalischer-Weber s.
Sturge-Weber s.
subclavian steal s.
sudden death s. (SDS)
sudden infant death s. (SIDS)
Sudeck-Leriche s.
Sulzberger-Garbe s.
superior vena cava s.
superior vena caval s.
Swachman-Diamond s.
Sweet s.
Takayasu s.
Tapia s.
TAR s.
tarsal tunnel s.
Taussig-Bing s.
Terry s.
testicular feminization s. (Tfm, TFS)
testicular regression s.

S

NOTES

syndrome *(continued)*

thalassemia s.
Thibierge-Weissenbach s.
third and fourth pharyngeal pouch s.
thoracic outlet s. (TOS)
Thorn s.
thrombocytopenia with absent radii s.
thrombopathic s.
thrombotic thrombocytopenic purpura and hemolytic uremic s. (TTP-HUS)
Tietze s.
Timme s.
Tolosa-Hunt s.
TORCH s.
Torkelson s.
Tornwaldt s.
Torre s.
Torsten Sjögren s.
Touraine-Solente-Golé s.
toxic shock s.
Treacher Collins s.
triad s.
trichorhinophalangeal s.
triple X s.
trisomy 8,13,18,20,21,22 s.
Troisier s.
tropical splenomegaly s. (TSS)
Trousseau s.
tryptophan malabsorption s.
tumor lysis s. (TLS)
Turcot s.
Turner s.
twiddler's s.
twin-to-twin transfusion s.
twin-twin transfusion s. (TTTS)
type 1 bare lymphocyte s.
Uehlinger s.
Ullrich-Feichtiger s.
Ullrich-Turner s.
Ulysses s.
undifferentiated connective tissue s.
urogenital s.
Usher s.
uveoencephalitic s.
van Buchem s.
van der Hoeve s.
Van der Woude s.
vasculocardiac s. of hyperserotonemia
velocardiofacial s. (VCFS)
Verner-Morrison s.
Vernet s.
vertebral basilar artery s.
vertebral crush-fracture s.
Villaret s.
Vinson s.

virilizing s.
virus-associated hemophagocytic s. (VAHS)
Vogt s.
Vogt-Koyanagi s.
Vohwinkel s.
Volkmann s.
von Willebrand s.
Waardenburg s.
WAGR s.
Waldenström s.
Wallenberg s.
Ward-Romano s.
Warkany s.
wasting s.
Waterhouse-Friderichsen s.
WDHA s.
Weber s.
Weber-Cockayne s.
Weber-Dubler s.
Wegener s.
Weil s.
Weill-Marchesani s.
Wells s.
Wermer s.
Werner s.
Wernicke s.
Wernicke-Korsakoff s.
West s.
Weyers oligodactyly s.
Weyers-Thier s.
whistling face s.
white clot s.
Widal s.
Wiedemann-Beckwith s.
Wildervanck s.
Willebrand s.
Williams s.
Williams-Campbell s.
Wilson s.
Wilson-Mikity s.
Winter s.
Wiskott-Aldrich s. (WAS)
Witkop-Von Sallmann s.
Wolf s.
Wolff-Parkinson-White s.
Wolf-Hirschhorn s.
Wolfram s.
Wright s.
s. X
XLP s.
XO s.
XXY s.
XYZ s.
yellow nail s.
Young s.
Zellweger s.
Zieve s.

Zinsser-Cole-Engman s.
Zollinger-Ellison s. (ZES)
syndromic
    s. surveillance
    s. surveillance system
synechia, pl. **synechiae**
    s. pericardii
    posterior iridolenticular synechiae
synencephalocele
syneresis
synergism
    agent, state, body site, effects,
        severity, time course, other
        (diagnoses), s. (ASBESTOS)
synergist
synergistic
synergy
Syngamidae
Syngamus
    S. laryngeus
    S. trachea
syngamy
syngeneic
    s. graft
    s. transplantation
syngenesioplastic transplantation
syngenesioplasty
syngenesiotransplantation
syngenic
syngraft
synkaryon
synophthalmia
synorchism
Synosternus pallidus
synostosis
    tribasilar s.
synotus
synovia (*pl. of* synovium)
synovial
    s. cancer
    s. cavity
    s. cell
    s. chondromatosis
    s. crypt
    s. cyst
    s. fluid
    s. fluid analysis
    s. fluid examination
    s. fringe
    s. membrane
    s. membrane biopsy
    s. osteochondromatosis

s. sarcoma (SS, SYS)
s. sheath
s. tuft
s. tumor
s. villi
s. villus protrusion
synoviale
    stratum s.
synoviales
    villi s.
synovialis
    membrana s.
synoviocyte
    knee s.
synovioma
    malignant s.
synovitis
    acute serous s.
    dendritic s.
    lymphoplasmacytic s.
    pigmented villonodular s. (PVNS)
    proliferative s.
    purulent s.
    rheumatoid s.
    serous acute s.
    suppurative s.
    tendinous s.
    vaginal s.
    villonodular pigmented s.
synovium, pl. **synovia**
syntaxin
syntectic
syntenic
synteny
syntexis
synthase
    fatty acid s. (FAS)
    glycogen (starch) s.
    methionine s.
    nitric oxide s. (NOS)
    porphobilinogen s.
    thymidylate s.
    uroporphyrinogen I s.
synthesis, pl. **syntheses (S)**
    cellular immunodeficiency with
        abnormal immunoglobulin s.
    collagenase s.
    DNA s.
    endogenous s.
    fatty acid s.
    globin-chain s.
    glycogen s.

S

NOTES

synthesis *(continued)*
    lipid s.
    s. period
    s. phase
    porphyrin s.
    protein s.
    triacylglyceride s.
    urea s.
synthesize oxytocin
synthetase
    acetyl-CoA s.
    acyl-CoA s.
    alanyl-ribonucleic acid s.
    alanyl-RNA s.
    argininosuccinate s.
    carbamoyl phosphate s. (CPS)
    carbamyl phosphate s. (CPS)
    glutamine s.
    glutathione s.
    heme s. (HS)
    inducible nitric oxide s. (iNOS)
    methionyl-RNA s.
    oligoadenylate s.
    polydeoxyribonucleotide s.
    tyrosyl-RNA s.
    valyl-RNA s.
synthetic
    s. antigen
    s. dye
    s. lethal
syntrophicum
    Sporotomaculum s.
syntrophism
Syntrophomonadaceae
Syntrophomonas curvata
Syntrophothermus lipocalidus
Syntrophus aciditrophicus
syntropic
synuclein
    alpha s.
Syphacia obvelata
syphilemia
syphilid
    bullous s.
    gummatous s.
    nodular s.
syphilimetry
syphilis
    endemic s.
    hemagglutination treponemal test for s.
    quaternary s.
    rupial s.
    serologic test for s. (STS)
    serology test for s. (STS)
    standard test for s. (STS)
    tertiary s.
    s. test
    venereal disease-s. (VDS)

syphilitic
    s. abscess
    s. aneurysm
    s. aortitis
    s. fever
    s. gumma
    s. lymphadenopathy
    s. meningitis
    s. meningoencephalitis
    s. nephritis
    s. node
    s. osteochondritis
    s. periarteritis
    s. ulcer
syphiliticum
    tuberculum s.
syphiloma of Fournier
syphilomatous
syringadenoma
    papillary s.
syringe
    Luer lock glass s.
    Roughton-Scholander s.
    s. shield
syringeal
syringitis
syringoadenoma
syringobulbia
syringocarcinoma
syringocele
syringocystadenoma papilliferum
syringocystoma
syringoencephalomyelia
syringoid
syringoma
    chondroid s.
syringomatous
    s. adenoma
    s. growth pattern
    s. metamorphosis
syringomeningocele
syringometaplasia
    squamous s.
syringomyelia
syringomyelocele
syringopontia
Syringospora albicans
syrinx
Syrphidae
SYS
    synovial sarcoma
Sysmex
    S. CA-6000 coagulation instrument
    S. HS-330 robotic hematology system
    S. NE-8000 CBC analyzer
    S. R-1000 reticulocyte counter
    S. XE-2100 hematology analyzer

S. XT-2000i automated hematology analyzer
system
10-20 s.
ABC immunodetection s.
absolute s. of units
Access 2 immunoassay s.
ACIT s.
ACS 180 SE automated chemiluminescent immunoassay s.
Adeza TLi fetal fibronectin analysis s.
Advia 120 hematology s.
AEC detection s.
Aeroset clinical chemistry s.
Affymetrix GeneChip s.
Alpha Dx point-of-need test s.
Amersham International ECL gene detection s.
A2 MicroArray s.
Ann Arbor staging s.
API 20 Strep S.
Array 360, 360CE/CE-AL protein/drug/serology s.
ASAP biopsy s.
association s.
AutoCyte PREP s.
automated cellular imaging s. (ACIS)
autonomous detection s. (ADS)
avidin-biotin based detection s.
avidin-biotin complex immunodetection s.
BacT/Alert automated microbial detection s.
Bactec blood culture s.
Bactec 9000 MB s.
Batson s.
Bayer AG II chemistry analyzer s.
BD BBL CultureSwab Plus collection and transport s.
BD Phoenix automated microbiology s.
Bethesda s.
bicarbonate buffer s.
biohazard detection s. (BDS)
blood group s.'s
buffer s.
cardiovascular system and central nervous s. (CVS/CNS)
CAS 200 Image Analysis s.
catalyzed signal amplification s.

cell-free s.
CellPrep sample preparation s.
CenSlide 2000 urinalysis s.
centimeter-gram-second s.
central nervous s. (CNS)
Ceprate SC stem cell concentration s.
CEQ 8000, 8800 genetic analysis s.
CGS s.
ChemMate multistep detection s.
CHEMXpress s.
Christopherson nuclear grading s.
chromaffin s.
CipherGen Express software biomarker analysis s.
CoaguChek Pro/DM s.
Colormate Tlc.BiliTest s.
combined DNA index s. (CODIS)
complement s.
Coulter reticONE s.
Coulter tetraONE s.
countercurrent multiplier s.
Cryo-Vac-A cryostat vacuum s.
CX9 ALX clinical s.
CX4, CX5, CX9, CX500, CX1000 PRO clinical s.
CX3, CX4, CX5 Delta clinical s.
CX4, CX5, CX7 super clinical s.
CytoLite luminescence assay s.
Cytomics FC 500 series flow cytometry s.
CytoRich cervical cytology monolayer s.
Dako Fast Red Substrate S.
dichroic filter s.
Diego blood group s.
Difco ESP testing s.
diffuse neuroendocrine s.
DNA-Prep workstation & reagent s.
DSX automated ELISA s.
Duffy blood group s.
DxI 800 immunoassay s.
Early Aberration Reporting S. (EARS)
Edmondson tumor grading s.
Ehrenreich and Churg membranous nephropathy staging s.
Elecsys troponin T immunoassay s.
Electra 1400C, 1800C coagulation s.

S

NOTES

system *(continued)*

enteric nervous s. (ENS)
EnVision non-avidin-biotin
detection s.
Epics Altra cell sorting s.
Epics XL, XLMCL flow
cytometer s.
ES300-Cardiac T ELISA troponin
T immunoassay s.
ESP II s.
excurrent duct s.
extrinsic s.
FastPack blood analyzer s.
fibrinolytic s.
FiltraCheck-UTI colorimetric
filtration s.
FiltraCheck-UTI disposable
colorimetric bacteriuria
detection s.
FreeStyle blood glucose
monitoring s.
Fuhrman s.
gamma motor s.
GenomeLab SNPstream
genotyping s.
Gerbich blood group s.
glandular s.
S. Gold HPLC
Halon s.
haversian s.
hematopoietic s.
HemoCue hemoglobin test s.
His-Tawara s.
HmX H20 hematology s.
Huvos grading s.
Hybrid Capture s.
Hybritech PSA determination s.
hypophyseoportal s.
hypothalamohypophysial portal s.
hypothalamoneurohypophysial s.
ID-Micro typing s.
Immage immunochemistry s.
Immulite 1000, 2000, 2500
immunoassay s.
Immulite 2500 SMS
immunoassay s.
immune s.
ImmunoPrep reagent s.
Impact on-site drug and alcohol
test s.
In Charge diabetes control s.
indicator s.
Infectious Disease Surveillance
Information S. (ISIS)
Integrated Core s.
integumentary s.
Intercept platelet s.
intermediary s.

International Neuroblastoma
Staging S. (INSS)
intrinsic s.
Isolator blood culture s.
Isolex 300i magnetic cell
selection s.
I-TRAC Plus transfusion s.
Jass staging s.
kallikrein s.
Kell blood group s.
Kidd blood group s.
kinin s.
LaChrom HPLC s.
Leitz image analysis s.
LightCycler s.
linnaean s. of nomenclature
Lipoprint cholesterol subfraction
test s.
LSAB2 multistep detection s.
LS 6500 liquid scintillation
counting s.
Lutheran blood group s.
LX4201 clinical s.
LXi 725 clinical s.
LX20, LX200, LX2000 PRO
clinical s.
lymphoreticular s.
Macroduct collecting s.
s. of macrophages
s. of macrophases
male reproductive s.
Mammotome biopsy s.
Masaoka thymic cancer staging s.
MB-Redox s.
MDS s.
mesolimbic dopaminergic s.
meter-kilogram-second s.
metric s.
metropolitan medical response s.
(MMRS)
MFO s.
microbiology identification s.
microsomal enzyme s.
mixed function oxidase s.
MKS s.
modified Masaoka thymic cancer
staging s.
monocyte-macrophage s.
mononuclear phagocyte s. (MPS)
MSTS staging s.
Munich tumor classification s.
myeloperoxidase s.
myeloperoxidase H_2O_2 halide s.
Nanoduct neonatal sweat
analysis s.
National Electronic Disease
Surveillance S. (NEDSS)
National Notifiable Diseases
Surveillance S. (NNDSS)

NIOX nitric oxide monitoring s.
nonisotopic gel detection s.
nonspecific s.
Oncor Inform HER2/neu gene
amplification detection s.
on-demand s.
operating s.
OptiMax immunostaining s.
P/ACE MDQ series capillary
electrophoresis s.
PapNet Pap smear s.
Paragon CZE 2000 capillary
electrophoresis s.
pedal s.
Perfectprep Plasmid 96 VAC direct
bind purification s.
Picci grading s.
PlateTrak automated microplate
processing s.
POG surgicopathologic staging s.
Poly-Chem automated chemistry-
immunoassay s.
Polytech 2000 laboratory
information s.
portal s.
properdin s.
protein characterization s.
ProteinChip Biomarker DU, PA s.
ProteinChip System Series 4000
biomarker/assay s.
ProteomeLab DU, PA 800 protein
characterization s.
ProteomeLab PF 2D protein
fractionation s.
ProteomeLab XL-A, XL-I protein
characterization s.
ProTime microcoagulation s.
ProTime prothrombin time test s.
PSI chromosome analysis s.
Purkinje s.
Q-beta replicase s.
RAG-1, -2 recombinase enzyme s.
RAMP biological test s.
random access immunoassay s.
Rapid One single dipstick s.
Readit SNP genotyping s.
renin-angiotensin-aldosterone s.
reticONE s.
reticular activating s. (RAS)
reticuloendothelial s. (RES)
Roche Septi-Chek blood culture s.
Roche Sysmex hematology s.

SalEst s.
Salzer-Kuntschik grading s.
SBR tumor grading s.
Scianna blood group s.
SensiCath s.
Septi-Chek culture s.
Sequenza immunostaining s.
Shimoda blood group s.
Single Use Diagnostic S. (SUDS)
SmartCycler realtime PCR s.
S-Monovette blood collection s.
SNPstream genotyping s.
Sof-Tact diabetes management s.
SOS bacterial DNA repair s.
STA-Compact hemostasis s.
STA hemostasis s.
STart 8 clot detection s.
STAT-Site M Hgb test s.
stem kit CD34+HPC
enumeration s.
St. Jude pediatric oncology
staging s.
streptavidin-biotin-based detection s.
Super Sensitive kit multistep
detection s.
SureStep Flexx professional blood
glucose management s.
Sydney classification s.
Synchron CX9 ALX clinical s.
Synchron CX clinical chemistry s.
Synchron CX4, CX5, CX9,
CX500, CX1000 PRO clinical s.
Synchron CX3, CX4, CX5 Delta
clinical s.
Synchron CX4, CX5, CX7 Super
clinical s.
Synchron LX20 clinical s.
Synchron LX4201 clinical s.
Synchron LX clinical chemistry s.
Synchron LXi 725 clinical s.
Synchron LX20, LX2000 PRO
clinical s.
syndromic surveillance s.
Sysmex HS-330 robotic
hematology s.
T s.
TD glucose monitoring s.
TechMate 500 automated
immunohistochemical s.
tetraONE s.
The Bethesda S. (TBS)

S

NOTES

system *(continued)*
    TheraTest Laboratories EL-RF test kit s.
    TNM staging s.
    T-tubular s.
    Typenex blood-recipient identification s.
    ubiquitin-proteasome s. (UPS)
    Ultima II refrigerator s.
    UniCel Dxl 800 immunoassay s.
    Unopette s.
    UP*link* point of care sample testing s.
    Uriscreen bacteriuria detection s.
    Vectastain Elite ABC s.
    ViraType In Situ S.
    ViroSeq HIV-1 genotyping s.
    Wampole Isolater blood culture s.
    Whitmore-Jewett tumor staging s.
    Xga blood group s.
systema
systematic
    s. bacteriology
    s. error
systematized
    s. nevus
    s. nomenclature of medicine (SNOMED)
    S. Nomenclature of Pathology (SNOP)
systemic
    s. air embolism
    s. anaphylaxis
    s. arterial pressure (SAP)

    s. autoimmune disease
    s. calciphylaxis
    s. ʟ-carnitine deficiency
    s. chondromalacia
    s. familial primary amyloidosis
    s. febrile disease
    s. histiocytosis
    s. hyalinosis
    s. lesion
    s. lupus erythematosus (SLE)
    s. mast cell disease (SMCD)
    s. mycosis
    s. myelitis
    s. poisoning
    s. reticuloendotheliosis
    s. scleroderma
    s. sclerosis
    s. sclerosis with lung involvement
    s. vascular resistance (SVR)
systemoid
systolic
    s. hypertension
    s. murmur with a midsystolic click
    s. time interval (STI)
Syva EMIT-II assay
syzygial
syzygii
    Acetobacter s.
    Ralstonia s.
syzygium
syzygy
Szent-Györgyi reaction
szulgai
    Mycobacterium s.

T

temperature
tesla
    T agglutination
    T agglutinogen
    T antibody
    T antigen
    T banding
    T and B lymphocyte subset assay
    T (cell) cytolytic (Tc)
    T (cell) cytotoxic (Tc)
    T cytotoxic cell
    T factor
    T helper cell
    T lymphocyte
    T method stain
    T system
    T tubule
    T zone

$T\frac{1}{2}$

terminal half-life

T_3

triiodothyronine
    reverse T_3
    T_3 uptake
    T_3 uptake test

T_m

maximal tubular excretory capacity of kidneys

T_{max}

time of maximum concentration

T_{mg}

maximal tubular reabsorption of glucose

T0

no evidence of primary tumor

T4

levothyroxine

t

test of significance
    t test

"T1-like viruses"
"T4-like viruses"
"T5-like viruses"
"T7-like viruses"
TA

alkaline tuberculin
therapeutic abortion
titratable acid
toxin-antitoxin
tube agglutination

TA-4

tumor-antigen 4

TAB

typhoid, paratyphoid A, and paratyphoid B

TAB 250 antibody
TAB vaccine

tabacinasalis

Facklamia t.

tabanid
Tabanidae
Tabanus
tabby

t. cat heart
t. cat striation

tabescence
tabescent
tabes dorsalis
tabetic
tabetiform
table

anthropomorphic t.
contingency t.
decision t.
Gaffky t.
life t.
thickened subepithelial collagen t.
truth t.

tablet

graph t.
Ictotest reagent t.

tabletop shield
tabun

NATO code for t. (GA)

TAC

tetracaine, Adrenalin (epinephrine), and cocaine
TAC solution

Tac

Tac antigen

Tacaribe complex of viruses
tache

t. blanche
t. laiteuse

tachetic
tachycardia

paroxysmal atrial t.
paroxysmal supraventricular t.
paroxysmal ventricular t.
supraventricular t.
ventricular t.

tachyphylaxis
tachypnea
tachyzoite

extracellular t.

tacrolimus
tactile

t. cell
t. corpuscle
t. disc

T

tactile *(continued)*
    t. meniscus
    t. papilla
tactoid body
tactor
tactus
    corpusculum t.
    meniscus t.
    organum t.
TAD
    thoracic asphyxiant dystrophy
tadpole cell
taejonensis
    Sphingomonas t.
Taenia
    T. africana
    T. armata
    T. bremneri
    T. canina
    T. confusa
    T. crassicollis
    T. cucurbitina
    T. demerariensis
    T. dentata
    T. diminuta
    T. echinococcus
    T. equina
    T. hominis
    T. hydatigena
    T. lata
    T. madagascariensis
    T. mediocanellata
    T. minima
    T. multiceps
    T. murina
    T. nana
    T. ovis
    T. philippina
    T. pisiformis
    T. quadrilobata
    T. saginata
    T. solium
    T. taeniaeformis
taenia *(var. of* tenia)
taeniacide *(var. of* teniacide)
taeniaeformis
    Hydatigera t.
    Taenia t.
taenial *(var. of* tenial)
Taeniarhynchus
taeniasis *(var. of* teniasis)
taeniform *(var. of* teniform)
taeniid
Taeniidae
taenioid *(var. of* tenioid)
taenioides
    Diphyllobothrium t.
    Pentastoma t.

Taeniolella stilbospora
taeniorhynchus
    Aedes t.
Taenzer stain
Taenzer-Unna stain
TAF
    albumose-free tuberculin
    toxoid-antitoxoid floccule
    trypsin-aldehyde-fuchsin
    tumor angiogenic factor
TAG
    tumor-associated glycoprotein
tag
    anal skin t.
    hymenal t.
    sentinel t.
    skin t.
TAG-72 antigen
tagging
    COOH-terminal t.
T-agglutination
TAGVHD
    transfusion-associated graft-versus-host disease
Tahyna virus
tail
    cytoplasmic t.
    high degree of unsaturation of fatty acid t.
    t. poikilocyte
    polyA t.
    polyadenylate t.
    t. sheath
tailed red cell
tailing
tainanensis
    Chitinibacter t.
Taiwan acute respiratory (TWAR)
taiwanensis
    Chitinimonas t.
    Natrialba t.
    Pseudoxanthomonas t.
    Ralstonia t.
    Rubrobacter t.
    Wautersia t.
Takahara disease
Takara
    T. Biomedicals One-Step RNA PCR kit
    T. Biomedicals Suprec tube
Takata-Ara test
Takayama stain
Takayasu
    T. arteritis
    T. disease
    T. syndrome
TAL
    thymic alymphoplasia

talaje
>*Alectorobius* t.
>*Ornithodoros* t.

Talaromyces
talc
>t. crystal
>t. plaques
>t. pneumoconiosis

talcosis
Talerman classification
Talfan disease
T-ALL
>T-cell acute lymphoblastic leukemia

Talma disease
TALP
>tumor-assisted lymphoid proliferation

TAM
>toxoid-antitoxoid mixture

Tamm-Horsfall
>T.-H. mucoprotein (THM)
>T.-H. protein

tamponade
>cardiac t.

Tamulus
TAN
>tropical ataxic neuropathy

tandem
>t. mass spectrometry
>t. trinucleotide repeat

tandoii
>*Acinetobacter* t.

tangent
tangential
>t. plane
>t. sectioning

tangerinus
>*Saccharothrix* t.

Tangier disease
tangle
>neurofibrillary t.
>t. only dementia

tangle-bearing neuron
tangle-free neuron
tannate
>albumin t.

tanned
>t. red cell (TRC)
>t. red cell hemagglutination inhibition test

tannerae
>*Prevotella* t.

Tannerella forsythensis

Tanner stage
tannic acid
tannophilus
>*Pachysolen* t.

tanycyte
TAO
>thromboangiitis obliterans

tap
>dry t.

TAP1/TAP2 heterodimer
tapasin
tape
>chemical agent detector t.
>Dissolve-A-Way t.
>end of t.
>magnetic t.
>t. mark
>t. transport

tapetal cell
tapeticola
>*Halospirulina* t.

tapetum
>t. alveoli
>t. nigrum
>t. oculi

tapeworm
>beef t.
>broad fish t.
>dwarf t.
>fish t.
>pork t.
>rat t.

Taphrina
Tapia syndrome
Tapinella
tapir mouth
Taq
>T. DyeDeoxy Terminator Cycle Sequencing kit
>T. Master Mix kit

TaqI restriction digest
TaqMan real-time PCR
TAR
>thrombocytopenia-absent radius
>TAR syndrome

tar
>coal t.
>t. keratosis

TARA
>tumor-associated rejection antigen

tarantula

NOTES

tarda
> *Edwardsiella t.*
> osteogenesis imperfecta t.
> porphyria cutanea t. (PCT)

tardaugens
> *Novosphingobium t.*

Tardieu
> T. ecchymoses
> T. petechiae
> T. spot
> T. test

tare
target
> t. amplification
> t. cell
> t. cell anemia
> t. fiber
> t. gland
> t. lesion
> t. organ

targetoid
> t. hemosiderotic hemangioma
> t. pattern

Tarlov cyst
tarry
> t. cyst
> t. stool

tarsal
> t. coalition
> t. cyst
> t. gland
> t. plates
> t. tunnel syndrome

tarsales
> glandulae t.

tarsalis
> *Culex t.*

tarsi (*pl. of* tarsus)
tarsitis
tarsoepiphyseal aclasis
tarsomegaly
tarsophyma
tarsus, pl. **tarsi**
> t. inferior
> t. superior

tartaric acid
tart cell
tartrate
> t. inhibited acid phosphatase
> potassium acid t.
> potassium sodium t.
> t. resistant acid phosphate
> t. resistant leukocyte acid phosphatase
> sodium potassium sodium t.

tartrazine
TARU
> technical advisory response unit

Tarui disease

tasmaniensis
> *Vibrio t.*

taste
> t. bud
> t. bulb
> t. cell
> t. corpuscle
> t. hair
> organ of t.
> t. pore

TAT
> tetanus antitoxin
> thromboplastin activation test
> total antitryptic activity
> toxin-antitoxin
> treponemal antibody test
> turn-around time

TATA
> tumor-associated transplantation antigen

tataouinensis
> *Ramlibacter t.*

Tatlockia micdadei
tattoo
> dental amalgam t.

tattooing abrasion
tau
> neurofibrillary degeneration
> tau gene
> tau molecular marker
> tau pathology class I–IV
> tau protein
> tau protein pathology

tauopathy class I–IV
taurine
taurinensis
> *Legionella t.*

taurochenodeoxycholate
taurochenodeoxycholic acid
taurocholate
> sodium t.

taurocholemia
taurocholic acid
taurodeoxycholic acid
taurolithocholic acid
Taussig-Bing
> T.-B. disease
> T.-B. syndrome

tautomer
> keto-enol t.
> proton t.
> ring-chain t.
> valence t.

tautomeric fiber
taxis
taxon
taxonomic
taxonomy
> numerical t.

Tay disease

Taylor disease
Taylorella asinigenitalis
Tay-Sachs disease (TSD)
TB
    toluidine blue
    tubercle bacillus
    tuberculosis
        TB smear
TBA
    testosterone-binding affinity
    thiobarbituric acid test
    thyroxine-binding albumin
TBBx
    transbronchial lung biopsy
TBC
    tuberculosis
TBD
    total body density
TBF
    total body fat
TBG
    thyroid-binding globulin
    thyroxine-binding globulin
        TBG assay
        TBG cap
TBGP
    total blood granulocyte pool
TBH
    total body hematocrit
TBI
    thyroxine-binding index
    traumatic brain injury
TBII
    TSH binding inhibitory immunoglobulin
TBK
    total body potassium
TBLB
    transbronchial lung biopsy
T/B lymphocyte assay
TBM
    tuberculous meningitis
    tubular basement membrane
TBNA
    transbronchial needle aspiration
TBP
    thyroxine-binding protein
TBPA
    thyroxine-binding prealbumin
TB-RD
    tuberculosis-respiratory disease

TBS
    The Bethesda System
    total body solute
TBSAH
    traumatic basal subarachnoid hemorrhage
TBT
    tolbutamide test
TBV
    total blood volume
TBW
    total body water
    total body weight
TC
    to contain
    temperature compensation
    thermal conductivity
    tissue culture
    total cholesterol
        TC detector
        TC pipette
T$_4$(C)
    serum thyroxine measured by column chromatography
Tc
    T (cell) cytolytic
    T (cell) cytotoxic
    technetium
    transcobalamin
^{99m}Tc
    technetium-99m
        ^{99m}Tc labeled human serum albumin
        ^{99m}Tc labeled red blood cell
        ^{99m}Tc pentetic acid
TCA
    total colonic aganglionosis
    tricarboxylic acid
        TCA cycle
TCBS
    thiosulfate citrate-bile salts-sucrose
        TCBS agar
TCC
    transitional cell carcinoma
        high-grade TCC
        low-grade TCC
        TCC of renal pelvis
TCCA
    tissue culture cytotoxin assay
TCD
    tissue culture dose
TCD$_{50}$
    median tissue culture dose

NOTES

TCDD
2,3,7,8-tetrachlorodibenzo-p-dioxin
TCDD intoxication
T-cell
T-c. activation
T-c. ALL
T-c. antibody labeling
T-c. antigen
T-c. antigen receptor
T-c. chronic lymphocytic leukemia
T-c. disorder
T-c. growth factor (TGF)
T-c. growth factor-1
T-c. growth factor-2
T-c. immunodeficiency
T-c. lymphoma
T-c. marker
T-c. mediated disease
T-c. priming
T-c. proliferation
T-c. prolymphocytic leukemia (T-PLL)
T-c. receptor (TCR)
T-c. receptor complex
T-c. replacing factor (TRF)
T-c. restricted intracellular antigen (TIA)
T-c. rich B-cell lymphoma (TCRBCL)
T-c. turnover
T-cell/E-rosette receptor
TCF
tissue-coding factor
TCH
thiophen-2-carboxylic acid hydrazide
total circulating hemoglobin
TCI
transient cerebral ischemia
TCID
tissue culture infective dose
TCID$_{50}$
median tissue culture infective dose
TCIE
transient cerebral ischemic episode
TCM
tissue culture medium
TCPI Rapid HIV test
TCR
T-cell receptor
TCR complex
TCR Vgamma9 test
TCRBCL
T-cell rich B-cell lymphoma
tcRNA
translation control RNA
TCT
thrombin clotting time
thymic carcinoid tumor
thyrocalcitonin

TCV
tall cell variant
TD
to deliver
teratoma differentiated
tetanus-diphtheria
thymus-dependent
TD glucose monitoring system
TD pipette
TDA
TSH displacing antibody
TDE
tetrachlorodiphenylethane
T-dependent antigen
TDF
testis-determining factor
thoracic duct fistula
TDI
total-dose infusion
t **distribution**
TDLU
terminal duct lobular unit
TDM
therapeutic drug monitoring
TDP
thiamine diphosphate
TdT
terminal deoxynucleotidyltransferase
TDT immunostain
TDTH cell
TdT-mediated dUTP nick-end labeling (TUNEL)
TDxFlx analyzer
TE
tissue-equivalent
total estrogen (excretion)
Te
tellurium
team
Disaster Medical Assistance T. (DMAT)
Disaster Mortuary T. (DMORT)
Infectious Disease Death Review T. (IDDRT)
National Medical Response T. (NMRT)
tear
cruciate ligament t.
t. gas
Mallory-Weiss t.
meniscal t.
rotator cuff t.
tendon t.
triangular fibrocartilage complex t.
triangular-shaped skin t.
teardrop red cell
tearing
medial collateral ligament t.
teasing

tebenquichense
    Halorubrum t.
TeBG
    testosterone-estradiol binding globulin
TEC
    transient erythroblastopenia of childhood
TechMate
    T. 500 automated
      immunohistochemical system
    T. 1000 immunostainer
technetium (Tc)
technetium-99m (^{99m}Tc)
technical advisory response unit
  (TARU)
technician
    histologic t. (HT)
    medical laboratory t.
technique
    ABC t.
    alkaline phosphatase antialkaline
      phosphatase t.
    antibody-coated microprobe t.
    antibody panning t.
    antigen-retrieval t.
    APAAP t.
    avidin-biotin immunoperoxidase t.
    Brecher new methylene blue t.
    Brown-Brenn t.
    Carey Ranvier t.
    Cattoretti t.
    cellulose tape t.
    Corbin t.
    counterstaining t.
    Crocker silver impregnation t.
    crypt isolation t.
    cumulative-summation t. (cusum)
    cytoblock t.
    Dennis t.
    DGGE t.
    dilution-filtration t.
    direct fluorescent antibody t.
    DNA slot blot t.
    double antibody t.
    double-layer fluorescent antibody t.
    double staining t.
    Duhamel t.
    enzyme-assisted immunoassay t.
    enzyme-dependent colorimetric t.
    enzyme-multiplied immunoassay t.
      (EMIT)
    extracorporeal photophoresis t.
    FA t.

    Ficoll-Hypaque t.
    flotation t.
    fluorescent antibody t.
    freeze-fracture t.
    Gallyas silver staining t.
    general dissection t.
    glove juice t.
    Highman Congo red t.
    Hotchkiss-McManus PAS t.
    hybridoma t.
    immunofluorescence t.
    immunohistochemical t.
    immunoperoxidase t.
    Jerne t.
    Kato thick smear t.
    Knott t.
    Kohn one-step staining t.
    Laurell t.
    McMaster t.
    membrane filter t.
    micropore filter t.
    modified zinc sulfate centrifugal
      flotation t.
    multiblock t.
    Northern blot t.
    Ouchterlony t.
    PACONA t.
    PAG t.
    PAP t.
    PAS t.
    picrosirius red t.
    plaque t.
    pop-off t.
    program evaluation and review t.
      (PERT)
    protein A gold complex t.
    Q-band t.
    rapid frozen section t.
    Rebuck skin window t.
    Ritter-Oleson t.
    roll tube t.
    saline t.
    scintillation t.
    sealed envelope t.
    section freeze substitution t.
    sedimentation t.
    Seldinger t.
    soft-spin t.
    Southern blot t.
    specialist dissection t.
    Stoll dilution egg count t.
    streptavidin-biotin-complex t.

T

NOTES

technique *(continued)*
thin-layer cervical cytology t.
time diffusion t.
titration t.
trypsin digest t.
Western blot t.
wet scanning t.
whole blood lysis t.
zinc sulfate centrifugal flotation t.
technologic life
technologist
medical t. (MT)
technology
automated cell-counter t.
bioelectronic sensor t.
DNA microarray t.
FFF t.
gene chip t.
nucleic acid chip t.
single nucleotide polymorphism
scoring t.
SNP scoring t.
tissue microarray t. (TMA)
Up-Converting Phosphor t. (UPT)
tecta
zona t.
Tectiviridae
Tectivirus
tectorial membrane of cochlear duct
tectorium
TED
threshold erythema dose
thromboembolic disease
teeth (*pl. of* tooth)
TEF
tracheoesophageal fistula
TEG
thromboelastographic monitor device
TEG trace
Teichobacteria
Teichococcus
T. ludipueritiae
teichoic
t. acid
t. acid antibody
tela
t. choroidea
t. choroidea of fourth ventricle
t. choroidea inferior
t. choroidea superior
t. choroidea of third ventricle
t. choroidea ventriculi quarti
t. choroidea ventriculi tertii
t. conjunctiva
t. elastica
in t.
t. subcutanea
t. submucosa
Teladorsagia davtiani

telangiectasia
ataxia t.
calcinosis cutis, Raynaud
phenomenon, sclerodactyly, and t.
(CRST)
calcinosis, Raynaud phenomenon,
esophageal motility disorders,
sclerodactyly, and t. (CREST)
cephalooculocutaneous t.
essential t.
hereditary hemorrhagic t. (HHT)
t. lymphatica
t. macularis eruptiva perstans
spider t.
t. verrucosa
telangiectasis, pl. **telangiectases**
telangiectatic
t. angioma
t. angiomatosis
t. cancer
t. fibroma
t. glioma
t. lipoma
t. osteogenic sarcoma
t. osteosarcoma
t. wart
telangiectatica
livedo t.
telangiectaticum
granuloma t.
telangiectodes
elephantiasis t.
neuroma t.
purpura annularis t.
telangioma, pl. **telangiomata**
telangion
telecytology
telehealth journal
telemedicine
telencephalization
teleomorph
teleonomy
telepathology
dynamic real-time t.
static t.
television microscope
tellurate
tellurite
t. glycine agar
t. medium
tellurium (Te)
t. assay
Tellyesnicky fixative solution
telocentric
telodendron
telogen hair
teloglia
telolysosome

telomerase
- t. activity
- t. enzyme
- t. function
- t. repeat amplification protocol (TRAP)

telomere
- t. banding
- t. shortening

telomeric
- t. R-banding stain
- t. repeat amplification protocol (TRAP)
- t. repeat amplification protocol assay
- t. restriction fragment (TRF)

telopeptide

telophase

Telosporea

Telosporidia

TEM
- transmission electron microscope
- transmission electron microscopy

temperate
- t. bacteriophage
- t. phage
- t. virus

temperature (T)
- ambient t.
- annealing t.
- body t.
- t. coefficient (Q_{10})
- t. compensation (TC)
- corpse t.
- critical t.
- effective t. (ET)
- eutectic t.
- flash-point t.
- ignition t.
- increased t.
- maximal growth t.
- maximum t.
- melting t. (Tm)
- minimal growth t.
- minimum t.
- normal body t.
- optimal growth t.
- optimum t.
- t. programming
- room t. (RT)
- subnormal t.

- ultra low t. (ULT)
- wet bulb globe t. (WBGT)

temperature-gradient gel electrophoresis (TGGE)

temperature-sensitive
- t.-s. mutant
- t.-s. mutation

template
- t. bleeding time
- t. bleeding time method
- DNA t.

temporal
- t. arteritis
- t. cluster
- t. lobe epilepsy
- t. temperature gradient gel electrophoresis (TTGE)

temporary
- t. cartilage
- t. cavitation
- t. parasite

TEMT
- tubular epithelial-myofibroblast transdifferentiation

TEN
- toxic epidermal necrolysis

Tenacibaculum
- *T. amylolyticum*
- *T. maritimum*
- *T. mesophilum*
- *T. ovolyticum*
- *T. skagerrakense*

tenacious consistency colony

tenacity
- cellular t.

tenaculum

tenascin

tenascin-C

tenascin-X deficiency

tenase complex

tenax
- *Trichomonas* t.

tendency
- central t.

Tenderlett Plus finger-stick blood collection device

tender line

tendinea
- inscriptio t.
- intersectio t.
- macula t.

NOTES

T

983

tendinis
    theca t.
    vagina mucosa t.
    vagina synovialis t.
tendinitis, tendonitis
    hypertrophic infiltrative t. (HIT)
tendinopathy
tendinous
    t. inscription
    t. intersection
    t. spot
    t. synovitis
tendomucin
tendon
    t. bundle
    t. cell
    coronary t.
    t. entrapment
    t. injury
    mucous sheath of t.
    t. organ
    t. repair
    t. rupture
    t. tear
tendonitis (*var. of* tendinitis)
tendosynovitis
tendovaginitis
    radial styloid t.
Tenebrio
tenella
    Sarcocystis t.
Tenericutes
tenerifensis
    Nocardia t.
tenesmus
tengcongensis
    Caldanaerobacter subterraneus
      subsp. *t.*
    Thermoanaerobacter t.
tenia, taenia, pl. **teniae**
    teniae coli
teniacide, taeniacide
teniafuge
tenial, taenial
teniasis, taeniasis
teniform, taeniform
tenioid, taenioid
teniposide
Tenney change
tennis
    t. elbow
    t. racket cell
tenofibril
tenonitis, tenontitis
tenontolemmitis
tenontothecitis
tenophyte
tenoreceptor
tenositis

tenostosis
tenosynovial giant cell tumor
tenosynovitis
    t. crepitans
    de Quervain t.
    localized nodular t.
    pigmented villonodular t.
    villonodular pigmented t.
    villous t.
tenovaginitis
tensile strength
Tensilon test
tension
    carbon dioxide t.
    t. cyst
    t. cyst of breast
    end-tidal CO_2 t.
    t. headache
    oxygen t.
    surface t. (ST)
tenue
    Eubacterium t.
tenuicollis
    Cysticercus t.
tenuis
    Alternaria t.
    Dirofilaria t.
    plicae circulares intestini t.
    stratum longitudinale tunicae
      muscularis intestini t.
    Trichostrongylus t.
    tunica mucosa intestini t.
    tunica muscularis intestini t.
    tunica serosa intestini t.
Tenuivirus
Tephrocybe
tephromalacia
tepidarius
    Thermithiobacillus t.
Tepidibacter
    T. formicigenes
    T. thalassicus
Tepidimonas
    T. aquatica
    T. ignava
Tepidiphilus margaritifer
tepidum
    Chlorobaculum t.
    Haliangium t.
terahertz (THz)
terangae
    Ensifer t.
Terasakiella pusilla
teratoblastoma
teratocarcinoma
teratogen
teratogenesis
teratogenic
teratogenicity

teratoid tumor
teratology
teratoma
    adult cystic t.
    anaplastic malignant t.
    benign cystic t.
    cystic dermoid t.
    t. differentiated (TD)
    differentiated t.
    embryonal t.
    immature t.
    malignant trophoblastic t. (MTT)
    mature t.
    monodermal t.
    ovarian t.
    sacrococcygeal t.
    solid t.
    triphyllomatous t.
    trophoblastic malignant t.
    undifferentiated malignant t.
teratomatous cyst
teratospermia
Teredinibacter turnerae
terephthalate
    polyethylene t. (PETG)
terminal
    t. addition enzyme
    amino t.
    t. axolysis
    axon t.
    t. banding
    t. bar
    t. bouton
    t. bronchiole
    carboxyl t.
    t. cisterna
    t. deletion
    t. deoxynucleotidyltransferase (TdT)
    t. deoxyribonucleotidyl transferase
    t. differentiation
    t. duct adenocarcinoma
    t. duct carcinoma
    t. endocarditis
    graphic t.
    t. half-life (T½)
    t. hematuria
    t. ileitis
    t. ileum
    t. latency
    t. leukocytosis
    t. nerve corpuscle
    smart t.

    synaptic t.
    t. web
terminale
    filum t.
terminalia
    corpuscula nervosa t.
terminalization
terminally truncated variant
terminatio
termination
    t. codon
    t. factor
    t. sequence
terminator
    dideoxy t.
terminaux
    pieds t.
terminus
Termitomyces
termone
ternary acid
Ternidens deminutus
terpene
terrae
    Gordonia t.
    Janibacter t.
    Mycobacterium t.
    Opitutus t.
    Paenibacillus t.
    Sphingopyxis t.
terragena
    Demetria t.
Terranova decipiens
terrenus
    Ureibacillus t.
terrestre
    Halorubrum t.
    Trichophyton t.
terrestris
    Pholiota t.
terreus
    Aspergillus t.
terricola
    Burkholderia t.
terrigena
    Raoultella t.
territorial matrix
terrorism
    agricultural t.
    biological t.
    emergency response to t. (ERT)
Terry syndrome

NOTES

Terson gland
tertian
    t. fever
    t. malaria
tertiarism
tertiarismus
tertiary
    t. blast injury
    t. cortex
    t. hyperparathyroidism
    t. structure
    t. syphilis
    t. trisomy
tertii
    tela choroidea ventriculi t.
tertium
    Clostridium t.
Teschen
    T. disease
    T. virus
TESE
    testicular sperm extraction
tesla (T)
tessellated
test (*See also* assay, kit)
    AAN t.
    Abrams t.
    ACB t.
    Access AccuTnI t.
    Access Hybritech PSA t.
    Access Ostase t.
    AccuDx t.
    AccuTnI t.
    acetic acid-induced writhing t.
    acetic acid and potassium
      ferrocyanide t.
    acetoacetic acid t.
    acetoin t.
    acetone t.
    acetowhite t.
    acid challenge t.
    acid clearance t. (ACT)
    acid elution t.
    acid hemolysin t.
    acid hemolysis t.
    acidified serum lysis t.
    acidity reduction t.
    acid lability t.
    acidosis t.
    acid perfusion t.
    acid phosphatase t.
    acid phosphatase t. for semen
    acid reflux t.
    ACPA t.
    Actalyke t.
    ACTH stimulation t.
    activated partial thromboplastin
      substitution t.
    active rosette t.

Activin AB free beta-HCG
  ELISA t.
Adamkiewicz t.
AD7C Alzheimer t.
Addis t.
adhesion t.
Adler t.
adrenal ascorbic acid depletion t.
adrenal function t.
adrenaline t.
adrenocortical inhibition t.
adrenocorticotropic hormone
  suppression t.
Aeroset abused drugs/toxicology t.
AFP t.
agglutination t.
ALA t.
AlaSTAT latex allergy t.
albumin cobalt binding t.
albumin suspension t.
aldolase t.
aldosterone stimulation t.
aldosterone suppression t.
alizarin t.
alkali denaturation t.
alkaline phosphatase antialkaline
  phosphatase antibody t.
alkali tolerance t.
alkaloid t.
alkaptonuria t.
Allen t.
Allen-Doisy t.
allergen challenge t.
Almén t. for blood
alpha amino nitrogen t.
ALT t.
Ames t.
aminopyrine breath t.
ammoniacal silver nitrate t.
ammonium chloride loading t.
amniotic fluid fern t.
amniotic fluid foam stability t.
amniotic fluid shake t.
Amplicor CT/NG t.
Amplicor HIV-1 monitor t.
amylase t.
Anderson-Collip t.
Anderson and Goldberger t.
androstenedione t.
AneuVysion prenatal t.
angiotensin I, II t.
anion gap t.
antibiotic sensitivity t.
antibody screening t.
anti-*Chlamydia* antibody t.
antichymotrypsin t.
antideoxyribonuclease B titer t.
antiendomysial antibody t.
antiglobulin t. (AGT)

antihuman globulin t.
anti-LA/SS-B t.
anti-Rho-D titer t.
anti-Ro/SS-A t.
anti-Sm t.
antithrombin III t.
antitrypsin t.
Anton t.
APAAP t.
APC gene stool t.
Apt t.
APTT t.
arabitol t.
arginine insulin tolerance t. (AITT)
arginine stimulation t.
arginine tolerance t. (ATT)
Argo corn starch t.
arylsulfatase t.
ascariasis serological t.
Aschheim-Zondek pregnancy t.
Ascoli t.
ascorbate-cyanide t.
ascorbic acid t.
ASO t.
Aspergillus antibody t.
ASPIRINcheck urine t.
aspirin tolerance t.
AST t.
Astwood t.
atropine suppression t.
augmented histamine t. (AHT)
autohemolysis t.
Autolet blood glucose t.
automated reagin t. (ART)
Autopath QC t.
AxSYM free PSA t.
A-Z pregnancy t.
babesiosis serological t.
Babystart ovulation t.
Bachman t.
Bachman-Pettit t.
bacitracin disc t.
Baker acid hematein t.
Baker pyridine extraction t.
Bang t.
Barany caloric t.
barium t.
Barr body t.
basal gastric secretion t.
basal secretory flow rate t.
basophil degranulation t.
Bauer-Kirby t.

BCR-ABL protein t.
BD BeAware t.
Beard t.
bedtime salivary cortisol t.
BEI t.
Bence Jones protein t.
Benedict t.
Benedict t. for glucose
bentiromide t.
bentonite flocculation t. (BFT)
benzidine t.
Bernstein t.
Berson t.
beta galactosidase t.
beta-hCG t.
beta-lactamase t.
beta quick strep t.
Betke-Kleihauer t.
Bettendorff t.
Beutler t.
BG t.
Bial t.
bicarbonate titration t.
bicolor guaiac t. (BCG)
bile acid tolerance t.
bile esculin hydrolysis t.
bile pigment t.
bile salt breath t.
bile solubility t.
bilirubin tolerance t.
Binax Now *Legionella* urine
  antigen t.
Binax Now *Streptococcus*
  pneumoniae antigen t.
Binax Now urinary antigen t.
Binz t.
Biosafe TSH t.
BioStar Strep A OIA MAX
  Streptococcus A t.
biuret t.
bleeding time t.
blind t.
blood urea nitrogen t.
Bloor t.
blot t.
Blount t.
Bloxam t.
Boas t.
Bonanno t.
borderline glucose tolerance t.
  (BGTT)
Bordet-Gengou t.

T

NOTES

test *(continued)*

Bouchardat t.
BRACAnalysis genetic susceptibility breast and ovarian cancer t.
Bradshaw t.
breath analysis t.
BreathTek UBT *H. pylori* t.
bromocriptine suppression t.
bromphenol t.
bromsulphalein t.
bronchial challenge t.
Brucella agglutination t.
BSFR t.
BSP excretion t.
buffy coat smear t.
butanol-extractable iodine t.
calcium oxalate t.
Calmette t.
Cambridge Biotech HIV-1 urine Western blot t.
CAMP t.
Candida precipitin t.
candidiasis serologic t.
capillary fragility t.
capon-comb-growth t.
carbohydrate fermentation t.
carbohydrate identification t.
carbohydrate tolerance t.
carbohydrate utilization t.
carbon dioxide challenge t.
carbon dioxide combining power t.
carbon 13-labeled ketoisocaproate breath t.
carbon monoxide t.
carcinoembryonic antigen t.
Cardiac Reader D-Dimer t.
Cardiac Reader M myoglobin t.
Cardiac Reader T quantitative troponin-T t.
Cardiac STATus CK-MB t.
Cardiac STATus CK-MB/myoglobin panel t.
Cardiac STATus myoglobin/troponin I t.
Cardiac STATus rapid format troponin I panel t.
cardiolipin t.
cardiopulmonary stress t.
Carrell t.
Carr-Price t.
Casoni intradermal t.
Castellani t.
catatorulin t.
catecholamine t.
14C-cholylglycine breath excretion t.
CDC t.
CEA t.
CEDIA drug of abuse t.

cephalin-cholesterol flocculation t.
cephalin flocculation t.
cercaria-hullen reaction schistosomiasis t.
cercarien-hullen-reaktion t.
ceruloplasmin t.
cervical mucus sperm penetration t.
cetylpyridium chloride t.
CF t.
CFF t.
C-glycocholic acid breath t.
7C gold urine protein t.
Chagas disease serological t.
checkerboard microdilution t.
Chédiak t.
chemical inhibition isoamylase t.
chemiluminescence t.
Chemstrip BG t.
Chen t.
chenodeoxycholic acid t.
Cherry-Crandall serum lipase t.
Chick-Martin t.
Chlamydia trachomatis direct FA t.
Chlamydiazyme t.
chlormerodrin accumulation t. (CAT)
cholecystokinin t.
cholesterol t.
cholesterol-lecithin flocculation t.
cholinesterase blood t.
chorionic gonadotropin t.
chromaffin reaction t.
chromogenic cephalosporin t.
chromogenic enzyme substrate t.
cis/trans t.
citrate t.
CK-MB tandem t.
C lactose t.
Clark t.
Clauberg t.
ClearView C. Diff A t.
Clinitest stool t.
CLO t.
clomiphene t.
clonidine suppression t.
coagulase t.
coagulation time t.
Cobas Amplicor HIV-1 monitor t.
coccidioidin t.
$^{14}CO_2$-cholyl-glycine breath t.
cold agglutinin t.
cold hemolysin t.
colloidal gold t.
ColorPAC toxin A t.
Coloscreen Self t.
comb-growth t.
combined pituitary function t.
compatibility t.
competitive protein-binding t.

complement direct Coombs t.
complement-fixation t. (CFT)
complement lysis sensitivity t.
concentration and dilution t.
confirmatory t.
conglutinating complement
  absorption t. (CCAT)
Congo red t.
contraction stress t.
Coombs t. (CT)
copper-binding protein t.
copper reduction t.
copper sulfate t.
coproporphyrin t.
corneal impression t. (CIT)
Corner-Allen t.
cortisone-glucose tolerance t.
  (CGTT)
cortisone-primed oral glucose
  tolerance t. (COGTT)
cosyntropin t.
C-peptide t.
C-reactive protein t.
creatine kinase t.
creatinine clearance t.
cresol-ammonia spot t.
critical flicker fusion t.
^{51}Cr red cell survival t.
C&S t.
CSF glutamine t.
cutaneous tuberculin t.
cutireaction t.
^{14}C-xylose breath t.
cyanide-ascorbate t.
cyanide-nitroprusside t.
cyclic AMP t.
CYP2D6 drug screen t.
cysteine t.
cystic fibrosis t.
cystinuria t.
cytochrome oxidase t.
cytotropic antibody t.
Davidsohn differential absorption t.
Davidsohn modification of Paul-
  Bunnell heterophile antibody t.
Day t.
D-dimer t.
deferoxamine challenge t.
deferoxamine mesylate infusion t.
deoxycorticosterone t.
deoxycortisol t.
deoxyribonuclease t.

deoxyuridine suppression t.
dexamethasone suppression t. (DST)
dextrose t.
DFA t.
DFA-TP t.
DHEA t.
DHT t.
Diagnex Blue t.
Diatest diabetes breath t.
diazepam breath t.
Dick t.
differential renal function t.
differential ureteral catheterization t.
Digene hc2 high-risk HPV DNA t.
diluted whole blood clot lysis t.
dilution t.
dinitrophenylhydrazine t.
diphtheria t.
direct agglutination t. (DAT)
direct agglutination pregnancy t.
  (DAPT)
direct antiglobulin t. (DAGT,
  DAT)
direct bilirubin t.
direct Coombs t. (DCT)
direct fluorescent antibody t.
direct fluorescent antibody-
  Treponema pallidum t. (DFA-TP)
disaccharide tolerance t.
disc approximation synergy t.
disc diffusion t.
dithionite t.
Dixon t.
DNase t.
DNPH t.
Dold t.
Donath-Landsteiner t.
Donné t.
dot blot t.
double diffusion t.
double (gel) diffusion precipitin t.
  in one dimension
double (gel) diffusion precipitin t.
  in two dimensions
Dragendorff t.
DR-70 tumor marker t.
DRx quantitative hCG patient
  monitor t.
Ducrey t.
Duke bleeding time t.
Duncan multiple-range t.
Dunnett multiple component t.

NOTES

test *(continued)*
D-xylose absorption t.
D-xylose tolerance t.
dye exclusion t.
dye excretion t.
E t.
echinococcosis serological t.
edrophonium chloride t.
Ehrlich t.
Elecsys total PSA t.
electrophoresis t.
electrotransfer t.
Elek t.
Ellsworth-Howard t.
Emmens S/L t.
endocervical/transformation zone
  data on Pap t.
enzyme-linked antibody t.
enzyme-linked antiglobulin t.
  (ELAT)
EP t.
ergonovine provocation t.
E-rosette t.
erythrocyte adherence t.
erythrocyte fragility t.
erythrocyte protoporphyrin t.
erythropoietin t.
esculin hydrolysis t.
esophageal acid infusion t.
esterase t.
estradiol t.
estrogen stimulation t.
ethanol gelation t.
euglobulin clot t. (ECT)
euglobulin lysis t.
ExacTech blood glucose meter t.
exoantigen t.
EZ-HP *Helicobacter pylori* t.
factor V Leiden mutation t.
FANA t.
Farber t.
Farr t.
fat absorption t.
febrile agglutination t.
fecal fat t.
fecal occult blood t. (FOBT)
fecal reducing substances t.
Fehling t.
fermentation t.
fern t.
ferric chloride t.
ferric ferricyanide reduction t.
FertilMARQ fertility screening t.
fetal antigen t.
fetal hemoglobin t.
Feulgen t.
FFN t.
fibrinogen titer t.
fibrinopeptide t.

fibrin stabilizing factor t.
FIBROSpec t.
FiF t.
FIGLU excretion t.
filter paper microscopic t.
FiltraCheck-UTI t.
Finn chamber patch t.
First Check home-screening t.
Fischer exact t.
Fishberg concentration t.
Fisher exact t.
fixation t.
Fleitmann t.
flocculation t.
flotation t.
FLU OIA A/B rapid t.
fluorescent allergosorbent t. (FAST)
fluorescent antibody t. (FAT)
fluorescent antinuclear antibody t.
fluorescent treponemal antibody-
  absorption t.
fluoroscopic diaphragmatic paralysis
  sniff t.
foam/shake t.
foam stability t.
Folin t.
Folin-Ciocalteu t.
Folin-Looney t.
foodSCAN food allergy t.
formol-gel t.
Foshay t.
Fouchet t.
fragility t.
Francis skin t.
free beta t.
free protein S t.
free/total PSA ratio t.
free urinary cortisol t.
Frei t.
Friedman t.
frog t.
fructose t.
FTA-ABS t.
Gaddum and Schild t.
galactose breath t.
galactose tolerance t.
GASDirect t.
gastric acid stimulation t.
gastric function t.
gastrin-calcium infusion
  stimulation t.
gastrin-protein stimulation t.
gastrin-secretin stimulation t.
Gastroccult t.
gastrointestinal blood loss t.
gastrointestinal protein loss t.
gel diffusion precipitin t.
gel diffusion precipitin t. in one
  dimension

gel diffusion precipitin t. in two dimensions
Genetic Systems HIV-1 Western blot t.
Geraghty t.
Gerhardt t. for acetoacetic acid
Gerhardt ferric chloride t.
Gerhardt t. for urobilin in the urine
germination tube t.
germ tube t.
Gibson-Cooke sweat t.
globulin t.
glucagon response t.
glucose fingerstick t.
glucose insulin tolerance t. (GITT)
glucose oxidase t.
glucose oxidase paper strip t.
glucose-6-phosphate dehydrogenase t.
glucose suppression t.
glucose tolerance t. (GTT)
glutathione instability t.
glutathione stability t.
glycogen storage t.
glycolic acid t.
glycosylated hemoglobin t.
glycyltryptophan t.
glyoxylic acid t.
Gmelin t.
Gofman t.
gold sol t.
gonadotropin t.
gonadotropin-releasing hormone stimulation t.
Gordon t.
Göthlin capillary fragility t.
G6PD t.
Graham-Cole t.
Gravindex pregnancy t.
growth hormone suppression t.
GSR t.
guaiac t.
guaiac-based fecal occult blood t.
guinea pig kidney absorption t. (GPKA)
Gunning-Lieben t.
Günzberg t.
Guthrie t.
Gutzeit t.
Haagensen t.
Haenszel t.

HAIRscreen drug t.
Hamel t.
Hammarsten t.
Ham paroxysmal nocturnal hemoglobinuria t.
hamster egg penetration t.
Hanger t.
haptoglobin t.
Harrison t.
Harris and Ray t.
hatching t.
hc2 CMV DNA t.
hc2 HPV DNA t.
HealthCheck HDL home-screening t.
HealthCheck One-Step One Minute pregnancy t.
HealthCheck total cholesterol home-screening t.
heat coagulation t.
heat instability t.
heat precipitation t.
heat stability t.
heavy metal screening t.
Heinz body t.
Helicobacter pylori breath t.
Helicobacter pylori gII t.
Helisal rapid blood t.
hemadsorption inhibition t.
hemadsorption virus t.
hemagglutination t.
hemagglutination-inhibition t. (HIT)
hematein t.
Hematest reagent tablet t.
heme t.
heme-porphyrin fecal occult blood t.
Hemoccult fecal occult blood t.
Hemoccult II Sensa fecal occult blood t.
hemodilution t.
hemoglobin S t.
HemoQuant fecal blood t.
hemosiderin t.
hemosiderinuria t.
Henry fructose t.
hepatic function t.
hepatitis B surface antigen t.
HercepTest immunohistochemical t.
HER-2/neu serum t.
Herter t.
heterophil antibody t.

T

NOTES

test *(continued)*

Hickey-Hare t.
Hicks-Pitney thromboplastin generation t.
Hinton t.
hippuric acid excretion t.
Histalog t.
histamine flare t.
histamine stimulation t.
histidine loading t.
histoplasmin-latex t.
Hivagen t.
HIV antibody t.
Hoesch t.
Hoffman t.
Hofmeister t.
Hogben t.
Hollander t.
Home Access hepatitis C Check t.
homocystinuria t.
homogentisic acid t.
homovanillic acid t.
Hooker-Forbes t.
Hopkins-Cole t.
Hoppe-Seyler t.
2-hour postprandial blood sugar t.
2-hour postprandial plasma glucose t.
Howard t.
Howell prothrombin t.
Huddleston agglutination t.
Huhner t.
human chorionic gonadotropin injection t.
human erythrocyte agglutination t. (HEAT)
human growth hormone stimulation t.
HVA t.
Hybrid Capture 2 Chlamydia t.
Hybrid Capture 2 HPV DNA t.
Hybritech free PSA t.
Hybritech PSA blood t.
hydrostatic t.
hydroxybutyric t.
17-hydroxycorticosteroid t.
5-hydroxyindoleacetic t.
17-hydroxyprogesterone t.
IBD First Step t.
ice water calorics t.
ICG excretion t.
Icon 25 hCG t.
icterus index t.
Ide t.
IDI-Strep B t.
immune adhesion t.
immunoblot t.
ImmunoCard STAT! rotavirus t.

immunochemical fecal occult blood t.
ImmunoCyt cytopathology recurrent bladder cancer t.
ImmunoDip urinary albumin t.
immunofluorescence t.
immunoglobulin A, D, G, M t.
immunologic pregnancy t.
immunoperoxidase t.
implantation t. (IT)
IMViC t.
indican t.
indigo-carmine t.
indirect antiglobulin t.
indirect bilirubin t.
indirect Coombs t.
indirect fluorescent antibody t.
indirect hemagglutination t.
indirect immunofluorescence t.
indocyanine green t.
indophenol t.
influenza t.
ingestion challenge t.
inhibition t.
In-Line Strep A t.
inosithin neutralization t.
Instant-View fecal occult blood t.
insulin clearance t.
insulin-glucose tolerance t.
insulin hypoglycemia t.
insulin sensitivity t. (IST)
insulin tolerance t. (ITT)
interference t.
intracavernous injection t.
intradermal t. (IT)
intraesophageal pH t.
intravenous glucose tolerance t. (IVGTT)
intravenous tolbutamide tolerance t. (IVTTT)
invasive activity t. (IAT)
iodine t.
iodine-azide t. (IAT)
iodine-131 uptake t.
iron-binding capacity t.
islet cell antibody screening t.
isocitrate dehydrogenase t.
isoniazid phenotype t.
isopropanol precipitation t.
Ito-Reenstierna t.
^{131}I uptake t.
Ivy bleeding time t.
Jacquemin t.
Jaffe t.
Jaworski t.
Jolles t.
Jones-Cantarow t.
Kahn t.
Katayama t.

Keto-Diastix urine ketone and glucose t.
ketogenic corticoid t.
ketone body t.
KidneyScreen At·Home mail-in t.
Kirby-Bauer t.
Kleihauer t.
Kleihauer-Betke t.
Kober t.
KOH t.
Kolmer t.
Kowarsky t.
Krokiewicz t.
Kruskal-Wallis t.
Kunkel t.
Kurzrok-Ratner t.
Kveim t.
Kveim-Stilzbach t.
lactate dehydrogenase t.
lactic dehydrogenase t.
lactose tolerance t.
Ladendorff t.
LAL gram-negative bacteria t.
Lancefield precipitation t.
Landsteiner-Donath t.
Lang t.
Lange colloidal gold t.
LAP t.
latex agglutination t.
latex agglutination-inhibition t. (LAIT)
latex fixation t.
latex flocculation t. (LFT)
latex particle agglutination t.
latex slide agglutination t.
LATS t.
LE cell t.
Lee-White clotting t.
Legal t.
leishmaniasis serological t.
lepromin skin t.
leucine aminopeptidase t.
leucine tolerance t.
leukoagglutinin t.
leukocyte adherence assay t.
leukocyte bactericidal assay t.
leukocyte esterase t. (LET)
leukocyte histamine release t.
Levinson t.
levulose tolerance t.
LHMT t.
Liebermann-Burchard t.

limulus lysate t.
line t.
lipase t.
lipid t.
Lipoprint LDL subfraction t.
lipoprotein electrophoresis t.
liver flocculation t.
liver function t.'s (LFT)
Lowenthal t.
Lücke t.
lupus band t.
lymphocyte transfer t.
lymphocyte transformation t.
lysozyme t.
Machado-Guerreiro t.
macrophage migration inhibition t.
magnesium t.
mail-in microalbumin t.
malaria film t.
male frog t.
male toad t.
mallein t.
Malmejde t.
mammary aspiration specimen cytology t. (MASCT)
Mantoux skin t.
mast cell degranulation t.
Master 2-step t.
mastic t.
maximal Histalog t.
Mazzotti t.
McNemar t.
McPhail t.
t. meal
Meinicke t.
melanin t.
melanogen t.
menopause home t.
metabisulfite t.
metachromatic stain t.
metanephrine t.
methanol t.
methionine t.
methoxy-4-hydroxymandelic acid t.
methylene blue t.
methyl red t.
Metopirone t.
metrotrophic t.
metyrapone stimulation t.
MHA-TP t.
Micral urine dipstick t.
microalbumin t.

T

NOTES

test *(continued)*

microbore t.
Microflow t.
microhemagglutination-*Treponema pallidum* t.
microimmunofluorescence t.
microlymphocytotoxicity t.
microprecipitation t.
microsomal thyroid antibody t.
Middlebrook-Dubos hemagglutination t.
MIF t.
migration inhibition t.
migration-inhibitory factor t.
Millon-Nasse t.
minimum bactericidal concentration t.
mixed agglutination t.
mixed lymphocyte culture t.
MLC t.
mobilization t.
Molisch t.
Moloney t.
monocyte function t.
Mono-Diff t.
Monoscreen t.
monospecific direct Coombs t.
Monospot t.
Monosticon Dri-Dot t.
Mono-Vacc t.
Montenegro skin t.
Mörner t.
Mosenthal t.
motility t.
Motulsky dye reduction t.
mucin clot t.
mucopolysaccharide t.
mucoprotein t.
Mulder t.
multiple antigen stimulation t. (MAST)
multiple puncture tuberculin t.
multipuncture tuberculin skin t.
multithread allergosorbent t. (MAST)
mumps sensitivity t.
Murex *Candida albicans* CA50 t.
Murphy-Pattee t.
mutagenicity t.
MycoAKT latex bead agglutination t.
myoglobin cardiac diagnostic t.
myoglobin clearance t.
NAP bacteria differentiation t.
Napier formol-gel t.
nares swab anthrax spore t.
NBT t.
neonatal thyroid-stimulating hormone t.

neoprecipitin t. (NPT)
neutralization t. (NT)
niacin t.
Nickerson-Kveim t.
Nicklès t.
nicotine t.
nighttime salivary cortisol t.
nitrate reduction t.
nitrate utilization t.
nitric acid t.
nitrite t.
nitroblue tetrazolium t.
nitropropiol t.
nitroprusside t.
nitroso-indole-nitrate t.
N-MID osteocalcin ELISA t.
NMP22 BladderChek t.
nocturnal penile tumescence t.
Nonne t.
nonprotein nitrogen t.
nonstress t. (NST)
nontreponemal antibody t.
normal lymphocyte transfer t. (NLT)
Northern blot t.
novel microbiology t.
novel toxicology t.
nucleic acid t.
nucleic acid amplification t. (NAT)
OAAD t.
Obermayer t.
Obermüller t.
t. object
occult blood t. (OBT)
17-OH corticoid t.
oleic acid uptake t.
one-stage prothrombin time t.
One-Step hCG combo t.
one-tailed t.
ONPG t.
O&P t.
Optochin susceptibility t.
oral glucose tolerance t. (OGTT)
oral lactose tolerance t.
OralScreen 3-panel oral fluids t.
OralScreen 4 substance abuse t.
OraQuick rapid HIV-1 antibody t.
OraTest oral cancer t.
orcinol t.
osazone t.
osmotic fragility t.
OsteoGram bone density t.
Osteosal osteoporosis t.
Ouchterlony t.
ovulation t.
oxidase t.
oxidation-fermentation t.
oxytocin challenge t. (OCT)
Paget t.

p-aminohippurate clearance t.
pancreatic islet cell antibody t.
pancreozymin-secretin t.
Pandy t.
t. paper
paper radioimmunosorbent t.
  (PRIST)
Pap smear t.
paracoagulation t.
parainfluenza antibody t.
partial thromboplastin time t.
particle agglutination t.
PAS t.
passive cutaneous anaphylaxis t.
passive hemagglutination t.
patch t.
paternity t.
Paul t.
Paul-Bunnell-Barrett t.
Paul-Bunnell heterophile antibody t.
PBI t.
penicillinase t.
pentagastrin t.
perchlorate discharge t.
perchlorate suppression t.
periodic acid-Schiff t.
Perls t.
Petri t.
PharmChek seat patch drug
  detection t.
phenacetin breath t.
phenolphthalein t.
phenolsulfonphthalein t.
phentolamine t.
phenylalanine t.
phenylketonuria t.
phenylpyruvic acid t.
phosphatase t.
phospholipid t.
phosphoric acid t.
photo-patch t.
phthalein t.
Piazza t.
picrate t.
pineapple t.
pine wood t.
Pirquet cutaneous tuberculin t.
pituitary function t.
PKU t.
PLAC coronary heart disease t.
placental and fetoplacental
  function t.'s

plant protease t. (PPT)
plasma cortisol t.
plasmacrit t.
plasma hemoglobin t.
platelet adhesion t.
platelet adhesiveness t.
platelet aggregation t.
platelet function t.
platelet retention t.
platelet survival t.
Porges-Meier t.
Porges-Salomon t.
porphobilinogen t.
porphyrin t.
Porter-Silber chromogen t.
Porteus maze t.
positive-pressure t.
positive whiff t.
potassium hydroxide t.
P&P t.
PP-CAP IgA enzyme
  immunoassay t.
PPD skin t.
Prausnitz-Küstner t.
prealbumin t.
precipitation t.
precipitin t.
Precision-G handheld blood
  glucose t.
Precision QI-D handheld blood
  glucose t.
predictive value of negative t.
predictive value of positive t.
Pre-Gen 26 colorectal cancer t.
pregnancy t.
presumptive heterophil t.
prick t.
t. profile
Profile-ER one-step qualitative
  drug t.
prolactin t.
Pro-PredictRx diagnostic t.
prostaglandin t.
protamine sulfate t.
protamine titration t.
protection t.
protein t.
protein-bound iodine t.
protein-bound iodine-131 t.
ProteinChip t.
protein truncation t.
prothrombin consumption t.

T

NOTES

test *(continued)*

prothrombin and proconvertin t.
prothrombin time t.
Protocult t.
protoporphyrin t.
provocative chelation t.
provocative Wassermann t.
pulmonary capacity t.
pulmonary function t.'s (PFT)
purified protein derivative skin t.
purine bodies t.
qualitative fecal fat t.
qualitative urine myoglobin
  dipstick t.
QuantiFERON-TB t.
quantitation t.
Queckenstedt t.
quellung t.
Quick tourniquet t.
QuickVue Advance *Gardnerella vaginalis* t.
QuickVue Advance pH and
  amines t.
QuickVue *Chlamydia* t.
QuickVue *H. pylori* gII t.
QuickVue+ infectious
  mononucleosis t.
QuickVue influenza t.
QuickVue 1 step *Helicobacter pylori* t.
QuickVue UrinChek 10+ urine t.
quinine carbacrylic resin t.
Quinlan t.
QuPID pregnancy t.
rabbit t.
radioactive fibrinogen uptake t.
radioactive iodide uptake t.
radioactive iodine uptake t.
radioallergosorbent assay t. (RAST)
radioimmunosorbent t. (RIST)
radioisotope renal excretion t.
radiosensitivity t. (RST)
RAI t.
RA latex fixation t.
RAMP anthrax t.
RAMP botulinum toxin t.
RAMP heart attack t.
RAMP myoglobin t.
RAMP ricin t.
RAMP smallpox t.
random plasma glucose t.
rank sum t.
rapid ACTH t.
RapID ANA II t.
rapid corticotropin t.
rapid plasma reagin circle card t.
  (RPR-CT)
rapid serum amylase t.
rapid urease t. (RUT)

RapiTex ASO latex agglutination t.
RapiTex Hp t.
Rapoport t.
reactone red t.
t. reagent
red cell adherence t.
red cell survival t.
Reinsch t.
renal function t.
renin stimulation t.
resorcinol t.
respiratory syncytial virus
  antibody t.
respiratory syncytial virus
  antigen t.
Reuss t.
Revival Menopause Home T.
Rh blocking t.
rheumatoid factor t.
riboflavin loading t.
ribonucleoprotein antibody t.
rice-flour breath t.
RIM A.R.C. Mono t.
Rimini t.
ring precipitin t.
Rinkel t.
Rinne t. (R)
RISA t.
Rocky Mountain spotted fever
  antibody t.
Römer t.
Ropes t.
Rose t.
rose bengal radioactive ^{131}I t.
Rosenbach t.
Rosenbach-Gmelin t.
rosette t.
Rose-Waaler t.
Ross-Jones t.
Rotazyme t.
Rothera nitroprusside t.
Rotter t.
Rous t.
Rowntree and Geraghty t.
RPCF t.
RPR t.
rubella antibody t.
rubella HI t.
Rubin t.
Rubner t.
Rumpel-Leede t.
Sabin-Feldman dye t.
Sachs-Georgi t.
SalEst t.
salicylic acid t.
saline agglutination t.
saline infusion primary
  hyperaldosteronism t.
saliva ovulation t.

Sanford t.
SAS Rota t.
Saundby t.
scarification t.
Schaffer t.
Schick t.
Schiller t.
Schilling t.
Schirmer t.
schistosomiasis serological t.
Schmidt t.
Schönbein t.
Schultz-Dale t.
Schultze t.
Schumm t.
Schwarz t.
scratch t.
screening t.
secretin-cholecystokinin-
  pancreatozymin stimulation t.
secretin pancreozymin t.
sedimentation rate t. (SRT)
SeHCAT t.
Selivanoff t.
Semi-Q hCG combo t.
sensitive membrane antigen rapid t.
  (SMART)
Sereny t.
serodiagnostic t.
serology t.
serum alkaline phosphatase t.
serum amylase t.
serum bacterial t.
serum bactericidal t. (SBT)
serum bilirubin t.
serum calcium t.
serum creatine kinase t.
serum creatinine t.
serum enzyme t.
serum globulin t.
serum phosphorus t.
serum protein electrophoresis t.
sex chromatin t. (SCT)
shake t.
sheep cell agglutination t. (SCAT)
Shigella rapid latex t.
sickle cell t.
sickle cell anemia t. (SCAT)
Sickledex t.
Sicklequik t.
sickling t.
signed rank t.

t. of significance (t)
Signify DOA t.
Signify ER drug screen t.
silver nitroprusside t.
Sims-Huhner t.
single (gel) diffusion precipitin t.
  in one dimension
single (gel) diffusion precipitin t.
  in two dimensions
SISI t.
skin-puncture t.
skin window t.
slide agglutination t.
slide bile solubility t.
slide flocculation t.
slide platelet aggregation t. (SPAT)
SMAC t.
SMA-12 profile t.
smear t.
sodium t.
sodium metabisulfite sickle
  hemoglobin t.
solubility t.
t. solution (TS)
Southern blot t.
soybean t.
specific gravity t.
spectroscopic t.
spironolactone t.
split collection urine t.
split renal function t.
spot t.
spot t. for infectious mononucleosis
Stamey t.
standard acid reflux t. (SART)
standard serologic t. for syphilis
standing plasma t.
Staph-Ident t.
Staph-Trac t.
staphylococcal clumping t. (SCT)
starch hydrolysis t.
starch tolerance t.
StarTox 5 drugs of abuse
  screening t.
stat t.
t. statistic
Sterneedle tuberculin t.
Stokvis t.
stool guaiac t.
stool reducing substances t.
Strassburg t.
streptococcal antigen t.

NOTES

test *(continued)*

streptolysin O t.
streptozyme t.
Student t.
Student-Newman-Keuls t.
Stypven time t.
sucrose hemolysis t.
SUDS HIV-1 t.
sulfosalicylic acid turbidity t.
Sulkowitch t.
susceptibility t.
sweat t.
syphilis t.
t t.
Takata-Ara t.
tanned red cell hemagglutination inhibition t.
Tardieu t.
TCPI Rapid HIV t.
TCR Vgamma9 t.
Tensilon t.
tetrazolium t.
Thayer-Martin t.
thermostable opsonin t.
thiamine t.
thiobarbituric acid t. (TBA)
Thompson t.
Thormählen t.
Thorn t.
three-glass t.
thrombin time t.
thromboplastin activation t. (TAT)
thromboplastin generation t. (TGT)
Thudichum t.
thymol turbidity t.
thyroid antibody t.
thyroid function t. (TFT)
thyroid-stimulating hormone stimulation t.
thyroid suppression t.
thyroid uptake t.
thyrotropin-releasing hormone challenge t.
thyrotropin-releasing hormone stimulation t.
thyroxine-binding index t.
TIBC t.
time-kill kinetics t.
tine t.
tissue oxidase t.
tissue thromboplastin inhibition t. (TTIT)
titratable acidity t.
toad t.
tolbutamide t. (TBT)
tolbutamide tolerance t. (TTT)
Töpfer t.
total catecholamine t.
TPH t.

TPI t.
transaminase t.
transferrin t.
treponemal antibody t. (TAT)
treponemal immobilization t.
Treponema pallidum complement fixation t.
TRH stimulation t.
Triage BNP t.
triiodothyronine resin uptake t.
triiodothyronine suppression t.
Trinder t.
triple t.
Trousseau t.
trypsin t.
tryptophan challenge t.
tryptophan load t.
TSH stimulating t.
TSH stimulation t.
T_3U t.
t. tube
tube dilution t.
tubeless gastric analysis t.
tuberculin skin t.
tuberculosis skin t.
tubular reabsorption of phosphate t.
tumor marker t.
tumor skin t. (TST)
T_3 uptake t.
two-glass t.
two-stage PT t.
two-tail t.
typhus antibody t.
tyramine t.
tyrosine t.
Tzanck t.
Uffelmann t.
unheated serum reagin t.
Uni-Gold *H. pylori* t.
Uni-Gold Recombigen HIV t.
urea breath t. (UBT)
urea clearance t.
urea concentration t.
urea nitrogen t.
urease t.
Urecholine supersensitivity t.
uric acid t.
Uricult dipslide t.
urinary concentration t.
urine acetone t.
urine amylase excretion t.
urine myoglobin t.
urine spot t.
Uriscreen t.
UriSite microalbumin/creatinine urine t.
Uri-Test protein in urine t.
urobilinogen t.
uroporphyrin t.

UroVysion bladder cancer recurrence t.
UroVysion FISH t.
USR t.
Valentine t.
van Deen t.
van den Bergh t.
van der Velden t.
vanillylmandelic acid t.
Van Slyke t.
VAP cholesterol t.
varicella-zoster antibody t.
VDRL t.
Verdict-II drug screening t.
Vgamma9 t.
ViraPap t.
virus neutralization t.
visual fluorescent screening t.
vitamin A clearance t.
vitamin B_{12} absorption t.
in vivo compatibility t.
VMA t.
Voges-Proskauer t.
Volhard t.
Vollmer t.
t. volume
VP t.
Wagner t.
Waldenström t.
Wang t.
Wassén t.
Wassermann t.
water deprivation diabetes insipidus differentiation t.
water gurgle t.
water loading t.
Watson-Schwartz t.
Weber t.
Webster t.
Weil-Felix t.
Welcozyme HIV 1&2 ELISA antibody t.
Werner t.
Westergren sedimentation rate t.
Western blot electrotransfer t.
Western immunoblot t.
West Nile virus IgM capture t.
Wetzel t.
wheal-and-erythema skin t.
Wheeler-Johnson t.
whiff t.
Whipple t.

Widal serum t.
wire-loop t.
Wormley t.
Wurster t.
Xenopus laevis t.
xylose absorption t.
xylose concentration t.
Yvon t.
Zimmermann t.
zinc flocculation t.
zinc sulfate turbidity t.
Zollinger-Ellison t.
zona-free hamster egg penetration t.
Zsigmondy t.

testacea
    Nocardia t.
Testacealobosia
testcross
tester
    Novapath HIV-1 immunoblot t.
testes (*pl. of* testis)
testi
    tubuli seminiferi recti t.
testibumin
testicular
    t. agenesis
    t. cancer
    t. duct
    t. dysgenesis
    t. failure
    t. feminization
    t. feminization syndrome (Tfm, TFS)
    t. germ cell tumor (TGCT)
    t. hormone
    t. regression syndrome
    t. Sertoli cell tumor
    t. torsion
    t. tubular adenoma
testicular-splenic fusion
testing
    antibacterial agent susceptibility t.
    avidity t.
    bacterial susceptibility t.
    biochemical t.
    calcitonin t.
    cardiopulmonary exercise t.
    confirmatory t.
    Crithidia immunofluorescence t.
    direct immunofluorescence t.
    epicutaneous t.

NOTES

T

testing *(continued)*
   evocative t.
   forensic urine drug t. (FUDT)
   fungal skin t.
   histocompatibility t.
   homocysteine t.
   homocystine t.
   human genetic identity t.
   hypothesis t.
   Intercept oral fluid drug t.
   intracutaneous allergy t.
   intracutaneous tuberculin skin t.
   intradermal allergy t.
   minipool nucleic acid t.
   molecular resistance t.
   multiple puncture tuberculin skin t.
   neonatal t.
   neuromuscular junction t.
   nucleic acid amplification t.
   panel FISH t.
   patch t.
   paternity t.
   PCR reaction t.
   penicillin allergy skin t.
   percutaneous allergy t.
   point of care INR t.
   point-of-care t. (POCT)
   polymerase chain reaction-based identity t.
   presumptive t.
   proficiency t.
   reflective t.
   semiautomated susceptibility t.
   specific IgE antibody t.
   susceptibility t.
   thallium stress t.
testis, pl. **testes**
   t. abscess
   t. carcinoma
   cryptorchid t.
   ductuli efferentes t.
   dysgenetic testes
   ectopia t.
   ectopic t.
   t. inflammation
   interstitial cell tumor of t.
   inverted t.
   lobule of t.
   lobuli t.
   movable t.
   obstructed t.
   retained t.
   rete t.
   retractile t.
   septulum t.
   torsion of t.
   trabecula t.
   tubule of t.
   tunica albuginea t.

   tunica vaginalis t.
   tunica vasculosa t.
   undescended t.
testitis
testoid hyperthecosis
testosterone
   free t.
   t. production rate (TPR)
testosterone-binding affinity (TBA)
testosterone-estradiol binding globulin (TeBG)
testosteroni
   Pseudomonas t.
TestPackChlamydia
testudineum
   Mycoplasma t.
testudinoris
   Corynebacterium t.
tet
   tetralogy of Fallot
tetani
   Bacillus t.
   Clostridium t.
tetanizing
tetanolysin
tetanomorphum
   Clostridium t.
tetanospasmin
tetanotoxin
tetanus
   t. antibody
   t. antitoxin (TAT)
   t. antitoxin unit
   t. bacillus
   t. and gas gangrene antitoxins
   t. immune globulin
   t. immunoglobulin
   t. toxin
   t. toxin immunization reaction
   t. vaccine
tetanus-diphtheria (TD)
tetanus-perfringens antitoxin
tetany
Tete virus
Tetko nylon mesh filter
tetraborate
   sodium t.
tetrabrachius
   dicephalus dipus t.
tetracaine, Adrenalin (epinephrine), and cocaine (TAC)
tetracarcinoma cell
tetrachloride
   carbon t. (CCl4)
2,3,7,8-tetrachlorodibenzo-p-dioxin (TCDD)
tetrachlorodiphenylethane (TDE)
tetrachloroethane poisoning
tetrachloroethylene

tetrachrome stain
tetracycline
    penicillin, streptomycin, and t.
    (PST)
tetrad
tetradecapeptide
tetradius
    Anaerococcus t.
tetraethylammonium
tetragonolobus
    peroxidase-conjugated *Lotus t.*
Tetragonolobus purpureas lectin stain
tetrahedron chest
tetrahydrobiopterin
tetrahydrocannabinol (THC)
tetrahydrochloride
    diaminobenzidine t.
tetrahydrocortisol (THC)
tetrahydrocortisone (THE)
tetrahydrodeoxycorticosterone (THDOC)
tetrahydro-11-deoxycortisol
tetrahydrofolate dehydrogenase
tetrahydrofolic acid
tetrahydrofuran
tetrahydropteroylglutamate
  methyltransferase
Tetrahymena pyriformis
tetralogy
    t. of Eisenmenger
    t. of Fallot (tet, TF)
tetramastigote
tetramer analysis
Tetrameres
    T. strigiphila
tetramethyl acridine
tetramethylbenzidine
    t. chromogen
    t. stain
tetramethylcarbazole
tetra-methylrhodamine ethyl ester
  (TMRE)
tetramethylrhodamine isothiocyanate
  (XRITC)
Tetramitidae
tetranectin
tetranitrate
    pentaerythritol t.
tetranucleotide
tetraodonis
    Pseudoalteromonas t.
tetraONE system
tetraparesis

Tetrapetalonema
tetraplegia
Tetraploa aristata
tetraploidization
tetraploid tumor
tetraploidy
tetraptera
    Aspiculuris t.
tetrasomic
tetrasomy
Tetrasphaera
    T. australiensis
    T. elongata
    T. japonica
tetrathionate enrichment broth
Tetratrichomonas
    T. buccalis
    T. hominis
    T. ovis
tetravalent
tetra-X chromosomal aberration
tetrazole
tetrazolium
    nitroblue t. (NBT)
    t. reduction (TR)
    t. reduction inhibition (TRI)
    t. salt solution
    t. test
tetrazonium salt
tetrodotoxin
tetrose
tetroxide
    dinitrogen t.
    osmium t.
tetter
    honeycomb t.
textiform
textiloma
textural
texture
    fractal t.
    markovian t.
textus
TF
    tetralogy of Fallot
    thymol flocculation
    tissue-damaging factor
    transfer factor
    tuberculin filtrate
    tubular fluid
TFA
    total fatty acid

T

NOTES

TFAA
  trifluoroacetic anhydride
TFF
  trefoil family factor
TFI
  tubular-fertility index
TFL
  tumefactive fibroinflammatory lesion
    TFL of head and neck
Tfm
  testicular feminization syndrome
TFPI
  tissue factor pathway inhibitor
TFS
  testicular feminization syndrome
TFT
  thyroid function test
TG
  thyroglobulin
  toxic goiter
  triglyceride
TGA
  transposition of great arteries
TGase
  transglutaminase
Tg cell
TGCT
  testicular germ cell tumor
TGE virus
TGF
  T-cell growth factor
    TGF alpha
    TGF beta
TGGE
  temperature-gradient gel electrophoresis
TGT
  thromboplastin generation test
  thromboplastin generation time
TGV
  thoracic gas volume
  transposition of great vessels
TH
  thermite
  tyrosine hydroxylase
Th
  thorium
thailandensis
    Weissella t.
thalamic hyperesthetic anesthesia
thalassanemia
thalassemia
    alpha t.
    beta-delta t.
    delta t.
    F t.
    gamma t.
    hemoglobin SC-alpha t.
    heterozygous t.
    heterozygous alpha t. 1

  homozygous t.
  homozygous alpha t. 1, 2
  t. intermedia
  Lepore t.
  t. major
  t. minor
  mixed t.
  sickle cell beta t.
  silent t.
  t. syndrome
  t. trait
thalassemia-sickle cell disease
thalassicus
    Tepidibacter t.
Thalassolituus oleivorans
Thalassomonas
    T. ganghwensis
    T. viridans
Thalassospira lucentensis
thalidomide
thallic
thallitoxicosis
thallium (Tl)
    t. assay
    t. poisoning
    t. stress testing
    t. sulfate
Thallophyta
thallophyte
thallospore
thallus
Thamnidium
Thamnostylum
Thanatephorus
thanatophoric dwarfism
thanatopsy
thapsigargin
Thauera
    T. aminoaromatica
    T. chlorobenzoica
    T. phenylacetica
thaumatropy
Thaumetopoea
Thaumetopoeidae
Thayer-Martin
    T.-M. agar
    T.-M. medium
    T.-M. test
Thaysen disease
THBR
    thyroid hormone binding ratio
THC
    tetrahydrocannabinol
    tetrahydrocortisol
THDOC
    tetrahydrodeoxycorticosterone
THE
    tetrahydrocortisone

thebaine
The Bethesda System (TBS)
theca, pl. thecae
    t. cell-granuloma cell tumor
    t. cell of stomach
    t. cordis
    t. externa
    t. folliculi
    t. interna
    t. interna cell
    t. interna cone
    t. lutein cell
    t. lutein cyst
    t. lutein tumor
    t. tendinis
thecal abscess
thecitis
thecoma
thecomatosis
Theile gland
Theiler
    T. disease
    T. mouse encephalomyelitis virus
    T. original virus
theileri
    Trypanosoma t.
Theileria
theileriasis
Theileriidae
theileriosis
Thelazia
    T. californiensis
    T. callipaeda
thelaziasis
Thelebolus
theliolymphocyte
thelium, pl. thelia
theloncus
T-helper/inducer subset marker
Theobald Smith phenomenon
theobromae
    Botryodiplodia t.
theophylline
    AccuMeter t.
    t. assay
theorem
    Bayes t.
    Bernoulli t.
    central limit t.
theoretical plate
theory
    Altmann t.

    Arrhenius t.
    Arrhenius-Madsen t.
    cellular immune t.
    clonal deletion t.
    clonal selection t.
    Cohnheim t.
    deletion t.
    Ehrlich side-chain t.
    emigration t.
    fitter cell t.
    Frerichs t.
    gametoid t.
    germ t.
    hematogenous t. of endometriosis
    information t.
    instructive t.
    kern-plasma relation t.
    lymphatic dissemination t. of
      endometriosis
    Metchnikoff t.
    monophyletic t.
    myelostimulatory t.
    neoplastic t.
    polyphyletic t.
    Ribbert t.
    side-chain t.
    somatic mutation t. of cancer
    Warburg t.
thèque
therapeutic
    t. abortion (TA)
    t. cloning
    t. cytapheresis
    t. drug level
    t. drug monitoring (TDM)
    t. malaria
    t. phlebotomy
    t. plasma exchange
    t. pneumothorax
    t. ratio
therapia magna sterilisans
therapy
    allogeneic cellular immune t.
      (ACIT)
    alpha interferon t.
    anticoagulant t. (ACT)
    antimicrobial t.
    autoserum t.
    cancer management t.
    chelation t.
    corticosteroid t.
    cytoreductive t.

T

NOTES

therapy *(continued)*
  desensitization t.
  eradication t.
  fibrinolytic t.
  foreign protein t.
  gene t.
  glucocorticoid t.
  gold t.
  heterovaccine t.
  hormonal t.
  induction t.
  insulin coma t. (ICT)
  insulin shock t. (IST)
  L-asparaginase t.
  molecularly targeted t.
  myeloablative t.
  nonspecific t.
  obidoxime t.
  photodynamic t.
  plasma t.
  protein shock t.
  radiation t.
  risk-adapted t.
  salvage t.
  serum t.
  thrombolytic t.
  warfarin t.
TheraTest Laboratories EL-RF test kit system
Thermaceae
thermacidophilum
  Bifidobacterium thermacidophilum subsp. *t.*
Thermaerobacter
  T. nagasakiensis
  T. subterraneus
thermal
  t. conductivity (TC)
  t. conductivity detector
  t. death point
  t. death time
  t. equilibrium
  t. neutron
Thermales
Thermanaeromonas toyohensis
Thermanaerovibrio
  T. acidaminovorans
  T. velox
thermantarcticus
  Bacillus t.
thermautotrophica
  Carboxydocella t.
thermelometer
Thermicanus aegyptius
thermionic emission
thermistor
thermite (TH)
Thermithiobacillus tepidarius

Thermoactinomyces
  T. candidus
  T. sacchari
  T. vulgaris
thermo agent
Thermoanaerobacter
  T. subterraneus
  T. tengcongensis
  T. yonseiensis
Thermoanaerobacterium
  T. polysaccharolyticum
  T. saccharolyticum
  T. zeae
Thermoascus aurantiacus
Thermobacillus xylanilyticus
thermocatenulatus
  Geobacillus t.
Thermococcaceae
Thermococcales
Thermococci
Thermococcus
  T. acidaminovorans
  T. aegaeus
  T. alcaliphilus
  T. atlanticus
  T. barophilus
  T. gammatolerans
  T. sibiricus
  T. siculi
  T. waiotapuensis
thermocoprophilus
  Streptomyces t.
thermocouple thermometer
Thermocrinis albus
thermocycler
  GeneAmp PCR System 9600 t.
  Perkin-Elmer Cetus 480, 9600 DNA T.
thermodenitrificans
  Bacillus t.
  Geobacillus t.
thermodepolymerans
  Schlegelella t.
Thermodesulfatator indicus
Thermodesulfobacteria
Thermodesulfobacteriaceae
Thermodesulfobacteriales
Thermodesulfobacterium
  T. hveragerdense
  T. hydrogeniphilum
Thermodesulfobiaceae
Thermodesulfobium narugense
Thermodesulfovibrio islandicus
thermodilution method
Thermodiscus maritimus
thermoduric
thermodynamic equilibrium
thermodynamics

thermoferrooxidans
  Leptospirillum t.
Thermofilaceae
thermogenesis
  shivering t.
thermogenic action
thermoglucosidasius
  Geobacillus t.
thermograph
Thermohalobacter berrensis
thermohalophila
  Anaerophaga t.
thermolabile opsonin
thermolacticum
  Clostridium stercorarium subsp. t.
thermoleovorans
  Geobacillus t.
Thermolospora viridis
thermoluminescence
thermoluminescent
  t. detector
  t. dosimeter (TLD)
thermolysis
thermometer
  air t.
  alcohol t.
  Beckmann t.
  bimetal t.
  Celsius t.
  centigrade t.
  differential t.
  Fahrenheit t.
  gas t.
  kelvin t.
  liquid-in-glass t.
  maximum t.
  mercurial t.
  metallic t.
  metastatic t.
  minimum t.
  Rankine t.
  Réaumur t.
  recording t.
  resistance t.
  thermocouple t.
thermometry
Thermomicrobia
Thermomicrobiaceae
Thermomicrobiales
Thermomonas
  T. brevis
  T. fusca

  T. haemolytica
  T. hydrothermalis
Thermomonosporaceae
Thermomyces lanuginosus
thermophila
  Anaerolinea t.
  Hydrogenimonas t.
  Saccharopolyspora t.
thermophile
thermophilic
  t. actinomycete
  t. bacterium
thermophilum
  Caenibacterium t.
  Symbiobacterium t.
thermophilus
  Deferribacter t.
Thermoplasma acidophilum
Thermoplasmata
Thermoplasmataceae
Thermoplasmatales
thermoprecipitin reaction
thermopropionicum
  Pelotomaculum t.
Thermoproteaceae
Thermoproteales
Thermoprotei
Thermoproteus uzoniensis
thermoregulation
thermoresistant
thermosaccharolyticum
  Clostridium t.
Thermosipho
  T. geolei
  T. japonicus
thermosphaericus
  Ureibacillus t.
thermospinosisporus
  Streptomyces t.
thermostable
  t. alkaline phosphatase
  t. body
  t. opsonin
  t. opsonin test
thermosyntrophicum
  Desulfotomaculum thermobenzoicum
  subsp. t.
thermotaxis
thermoterrenum
  Anaerobaculum t.
Thermotoga
  T. lettingae

T

NOTES

Thermotoga (*continued*)
- *T. naphthophila*
- *T. petrophila*
- *T. subterranea*

Thermotogaceae
Thermotogae
Thermotogales
thermotolerans
- *Haloterrigena t.*
- *Lactobacillus t.*
- *Pseudomonas t.*

thermotropism
Thermovenabulum ferriorganovorum
Thermovibrio
- *T. ammonificans*
- *T. ruber*

Thermus
- *T. antranikianii*
- *T. aquaticus*
- *T. igniterrae*

thesaurismosis
- lipoid t.

thesaurocyte
theta
- t. antigen
- t. band

thetaiotamicron
- *Bacteroides t.*

THF
- humoral thymic factor

Thialkalicoccus limnaeus
Thialkalimicrobium
- *T. aerophilum*
- *T. cyclicum*
- *T. sibiricum*

Thialkalivibrio
- *T. denitrificans*
- *T. jannaschii*
- *T. nitratireducens*
- *T. nitratis*
- *T. paradoxus*
- *T. thiocyanoxidans*
- *T. versutus*

thiamine, thiamin
- t. assay
- t. chloride unit
- t. deficiency
- t. diphosphate (TDP)
- t. hydrochloride unit
- phosphorylated t.
- t. test

thiamphenicol assay
thiamylal
- sodium t.

Thiara
Thiaridae
thiazide diuretic

thiazin
- t. dye
- t. stain

thiazole dye
Thibierge-Weissenbach syndrome
thick
- t. fibrous band
- t. filament
- t. myofilament
- t. skin

thickened subepithelial collagen table
thickening
- concentric intimal t.
- fibrointimal t.
- hyaline t.
- trophoblast basement membrane t.

thickness
- Breslow t.
- mean corpuscular t. (MCT)

thiel
Thielavia
Thielaviopsis
Thiel-Behnke corneal lattice dystrophy
Thiemann disease
thiemia
Thiersch canaliculus
thimerosal
thin
- t. basement membrane disease
- t. basement membrane nephropathy
- t. elastic fiber
- t. filament
- t. myofilament
- t. section
- t. skin

thin-layer
- t.-l. cervical cytology technique
- t.-l. chromatography (TLC)
- t.-l. cytology
- t.-l. electrophoresis (TLE)
- t.-l. immunoassay

thin-needle biopsy
ThinPrep
- T. cytologic preparation
- T. cytology
- T. processor
- T. slide process

thioacetamide
thioaldehyde
Thioalkalispira microaerophila
Thiobaca trueperi
Thiobacilleae
Thiobacteria
thiobarbiturate
thiobarbituric acid test (TBA)
Thiocapsa
- *T. litoralis*
- *T. marina*

Thiocapsaceae

thiocarbonyl group
thiochrome
thioctic acid
thiocyanate
  potassium t.
  sodium t. (NaSCN)
thiocyanoxidans
  Thialkalivibrio t.
thiodismutans
  Desulfonatronum t.
thioester
thioethanolamine
thioether
thioflavin, thioflavine
  t. S staining
  t. T stain
thiogenes
  Trichlorobacter t.
thioglycolate
  t. broth
  t. medium
thioglycolic acid
thioketone
thiol
thiolaminopropionic acid
thiolase
  acetoacetyl-CoA t.
  alpha-methylacetoacetyl CoA t.
thiolysis
Thiomargarita namibiensis
thionine
thionin stain
thiooxidans
  Acidithiobacillus t.
  Limnobacter t.
  Roseinatronobacter t.
thiooxydans
  Ottowia t.
thiopental
  sodium t.
thiophen-2-carboxylic acid hydrazide
  (TCH)
thiophilus
  Geovibrio t.
thioredoxin
  t. reductase (TrxR)
  t. reductase gene
thioridazine assay
thiosulfate
  amyl nitrite, sodium nitrite, and
    sodium t.
  t. citrate-bile salts-sucrose (TCBS)

thiosulfatigenes
  Desulfonispora t.
thiosulfatiphilum
  Chlorobaculum t.
thiosulfatireducens
  Clostridium t.
thiosulfatophilus
  Roseococcus t.
thiothixene
Thiothrix
  T. disciformis
  T. flexilis
thiourea
  alpha-naphthol t.
thioxanthene tranquilizer
third
  t. corpuscle
  t. disease
  t. and fourth pharyngeal pouch
    syndrome
  t. pharyngeal pouch cyst
  t. spacing
  t. tonsil
third-degree
  t.-d. burn
  t.-d. frostbite
  t.-d. heart block
  t.-d. radiation injury
third-space fluid loss
thirdspacing
thistle seed agar
thivervalensis
  Pseudomonas t.
thixotropic
thixotropy
THM
  Tamm-Horsfall mucoprotein
Thogotovirus
tholozani
  Ornithodoros t.
Thoma
  T. counting chamber
  T. fixative
Thomas antigen
thomasii
  Anaerobiospirillum t.
Thominx aerophilus
Thompson test
Thomsen
  T. antibody
  T. disease
Thomsen-Friedenreich antigen

T

NOTES

Thoms method
thoracentesis
thoracic
t. actinomycosis
t. aneurysm
t. asphyxiant dystrophy (TAD)
t. duct fistula (TDF)
t. gas volume (TGV)
t. goiter
t. index (TI)
t. outlet syndrome (TOS)
thoracic-pelvic-phalangeal dystrophy
thorium (Th)
t. dioxide
Thormählen test
thorn
t. apple crystal
dendritic t.
T. syndrome
T. test
Thornwaldt (*var. of* Tornwaldt)
Thorotrast
Thr
threonine
thracensis
Photorhabdus luminescens subsp. *t.*
thread
mucous t.
threadworm
threatened abortion
three-day
t.-d. fever
t.-d. measles
three dimensional composition
three-glass test
three-part mitosis
three-phase current
three-point cross
threonine (Thr)
threonyl
threose
thresher's lung
threshold
t. body
t. erythema dose (TED)
t. limit value (TLV)
mean cell t.
median detection t. (MDT)
renal t.
t. substance
thrive
failure to t.
throat
t. culture
putrid t.
strep t.
thrombase
thrombasthenia
Glanzmann t.

Glanzmann-Naegeli t.
hereditary hemorrhagic t.
thrombi (*pl. of* thrombus)
thrombin
t. clotting time (TCT)
t. time (TT)
t. time test
thrombinogen
thrombinogenesis
thromboagglutinin
thromboangiitis obliterans (TAO)
thromboarteritis purulenta
thromboasthenia
thromboblast
thromboclasis
thrombocyst
thrombocystis
thrombocytapheresis
thrombocytasthenia
thrombocyte
thrombocythemia
essential t. (ET)
hemorrhagic t.
primary t.
thrombocytic
t. leukemia
t. series
thrombocytin
thrombocytopathy, thrombocytopathia
thrombocytopenia
alloimmune t.
amegakaryocytic t.
autoimmune neonatal t.
dilutional t.
drug-induced t. (DIT)
essential t.
heparin-associated t. (HAT)
heparin-induced t. (HIT)
idiopathic t.
immune t.
isoimmune neonatal t.
neonatal alloimmune t. (NAIT)
neonatal autoimmune t.
t. with absent radii syndrome
X-linked t. (XLT)
thrombocytopenia-absent
t.-a. radius (TAR)
thrombocytopenia-thrombosis
heparin-induced t.-t. (HITT)
thrombocytopenic
idiopathic thrombocytopenic purpura
(ITP)
t. purpura (TP)
thrombocytopoiesis
thrombocytopoietic
thrombocytosis
clonal t.
essential t.

reactive t.
rebound t.
thromboelastogram
thromboelastograph
thromboelastographic monitor device (TEG)
thromboembolic disease (TED)
thromboembolism
pulmonary t. (PTE)
thromboendarteritis
thromboendocarditis
thrombogen
thrombogene
thrombogenic hypothesis
thrombogenicity
thromboglobulin
beta t.
thromboid
thrombokatilysin
thrombokinase
thrombolic
thrombolus
thrombolymphangitis
thrombolysis
thrombolytic
t. agent
t. therapy
thrombometer
thrombomodulin glycoprotein (TM)
thrombon
thrombonecrosis
arteriolar t.
thrombopathic syndrome
thrombopathy
constitutional t.
thrombopenia
thrombopenic anemia
thrombophilia
hereditary t.
thrombophlebitis
t. migrans
migrating t.
t. saltans
thromboplastic
t. plasma component (TPC)
t. substance
thromboplastid
thromboplastin
t. activation test (TAT)
t. antecedent deficiency
automated activated partial t.
cofactor of t.

t. generation accelerator
t. generation test (TGT)
t. generation time (TGT)
RecombiPlasTin t.
t. substitution test
tissue t.
thromboplastinogen
thromboplastinogenase
thromboplastinogenemia
thrombopoiesis
thrombopoietin (TPO)
t. receptor
thromboresistance
endothelial t.
thrombosed
t. arteriosclerotic aneurysm
t. hemorrhoid
thrombosin
thrombosis, pl. thromboses
agonal t.
arterial t.
atrophic t.
cardiac t.
cavernous sinus t.
cerebral t. (CT)
coronary t. (CT)
deep vein t. (DVT)
dilatation t.
fetal stem artery t.
generalized activation of t.
hepatic vein t.
intracellular t.
marantic t.
marasmic t.
mesenteric t.
placental t.
plate t.
platelet t.
portal vein t. (PVT)
propagating t.
puerperal t.
renal vein t. (RVT)
traumatic t.
venous t.
thrombospondin
thrombostasis
thrombosthenin
Thrombotest
thrombotic
t. gangrene
t. infarct
t. microangiopathy (TMA)

T

NOTES

thrombotic *(continued)*
t. nonbacterial endocarditis
t. occlusion
t. phlegmasia
t. pulmonary hypertension
t. thrombocytopenic purpura (TTP)
t. thrombocytopenic purpura and hemolytic uremic syndrome (TTP-HUS)
thrombotonin
thromboxane A_2, B_2
thrombozyme
thrombus, pl. **thrombi**
agglutinative t.
agonal t.
antemortem t.
ball t.
ball-valve t.
bile t.
canalized t.
fibrin t.
globular t.
hyaline t.
infective t.
laminated t.
marantic t.
marasmic t.
mixed t.
mural t.
old t.
organized t.
pale t.
parietal t.
platelet t.
postmortem t.
t. precursor protein
recent t.
red t.
secondary t.
stratified t.
t. tumor
tumor t.
valvular t.
vascular t.
white t.
through-and-through myocardial infarction
through-the-eyepiece photomicrography
thrush
t. breast heart
t. fungus
vaginal t.
thrust culture
Thudichum test
thulium (Tm)
thumb
cortical t.
hitchhiker t.
thumbprinting

thuringiensis
Bacillus t.
Thy-1 antigen
Thygeson disease
thylacitis
thymectomy
adult t.
neonatal t.
thymi *(gen. and pl. of* thymus)
thymic
t. abscess
t. agenesis
t. alymphoplasia (TAL)
t. carcinoma
t. cell emperipolesis
t. corpuscle
t. cortex
t. dysplasia
t. epithelial cell
t. epitheliocyte
t. humoral factor
t. hypoplasia
t. leukemia
t. lymphopoietic factor
t. replacing factor
t. reticulum cell
thymica
mors t.
thymicolymphaticus
status t.
thymic-parathyroid aplasia
thymicus
status t.
thymidine
t. diphosphate (dTDP)
t. kinase
t. monophosphate
t. triphosphate
tritiated t. (TTH)
thymidine-5′-phosphate
thymidylate synthase
thymidylic acid
thymidylyl
thymin
thymine
t. dimer
t. ribonucleoside
t. ribonucleoside-5′-phosphate
thymine-2-deoxyriboside
thymitis
thymocyte
antimouse t.
thymocytotoxic autoantibody
thymofibrolipoma
thymol
t. blue
t. flocculation (TF)
t. turbidity (TT)
t. turbidity test

thymolipoma
 proliferating t.
thymoliposarcoma
thymolphthalein
thymoma
 cortical t.
 epithelial t.
 intrapulmonary spindle cell t.
 lymphocyte-predominant t. (LPT)
 lymphocytic t.
 malignant t.
 medullary t.
 microscopic t.
 organoid t.
 predominantly epithelial t. (PET)
 spindle cell t.
thymopathy
thymopoietin
thymosin
thymus, gen. and pl. **thymi**, pl. **thymuses**
 congenital aplasia of t.
 cortex of t.
 t. gland
 t. leukemia (TL)
 lobule of t.
 lobuli thymi
 normal t.
 t. nurse cell
thymus-dependent (TD)
 t.-d. antigen
 t.-d. cell
 t.-d. zone
thymus-derived cell
thymuses (*pl. of* thymus)
thymus-independent antigen
thymus-leukemia antigen
Thynnascaris
thyristor
thyroadenitis
thyrocalcitonin (TCT)
thyrocardiac disease
thyrocele
thyrocolloid
thyroglobulin (TG)
 t. antibody
 iodinated t.
 t. stain
thyroglossal
 t. duct cyst
 t. fistula
thyroid
 accessory t.

t. adenoma
t. antibody test
t. antimicrosomal antibody
t. antithyroglobulin antibody
t. biopsy
t. body
t. cachexia
t. carcinoma
t. colloid
t. crisis
t. cyst
t. endocrine disorder
t. follicle
t. function test (TFT)
t. gland
t. hormone binding ratio (THBR)
light cell of t.
t. lobule
medullary carcinoma of t.
t. microsomal antibody (TMAb)
t. ophthalmopathy
t. orbitopathy
squamous cell carcinoma of the t. (SCT)
t. storm
t. suppression test
t. transcription factor-1 (TTF-1)
t. tumor
t. uptake test
thyroidal clearance
thyroid-binding globulin (TBG)
thyroidea
 t. accessoria
 glandula t.
thyroideae
 folliculi glandulae t.
 lobuli glandulae t.
 stroma glandulae t.
thyroiditis
 acute t.
 autoimmune t.
 chronic atrophic t.
 de Quervain t.
 focal lymphocytic t.
 giant cell t.
 granulomatous t.
 Hashimoto t.
 induced t.
 invasive fibrous t.
 ligneous t.
 lymphocytic t.
 parasitic t.

T

NOTES

thyroiditis (continued)
- postpartum t.
- Riedel t.
- silent t.
- subacute t. (SAT)
- subacute granulomatous t.

thyroid-stimulating
- t.-s. hormone (TSH)
- t.-s. hormone assay
- t.-s. hormone-releasing factor (TSH-RF)
- t.-s. hormone stimulation test
- t.-s. immunoglobulin (TSI)

thyroid-to-serum ratio (TSR)
thyrolingual cyst
thyrolytic
thyromegaly
thyroptosis
thyrosis
thyrotoxic
- t. complement-fixation factor
- t. encephalopathy
- t. heart disease
- t. myopathy
- t. serum

thyrotoxicosis factitia
thyrotoxin shock
thyrotrope adenoma
thyrotroph hyperplasia
thyrotropic hormone (TTH)
thyrotropin-producing adenoma
thyrotropin-receptor antibody (TSHR)
thyrotropin-releasing
- t.-r. factor (TRF)
- t.-r. hormone (TRH)
- t.-r. hormone challenge test
- t.-r. hormone stimulation test

thyroxine
- t. assay
- t. and cortisol treatment
- free (unbound) t. (FT$_4$)
- protein-bound t. (PBT4)
- total t. (TT)

thyroxine-binding
- t.-b. albumin (TBA)
- t.-b. globulin (TBG)
- t.-b. globulin assay
- t.-b. index (TBI)
- t.-b. index test
- t.-b. prealbumin (TBPA)
- t.-b. protein (TBP)
- t.-b. protein electrophoresis

thyroxine-specific activity (T$_4$SA)
thyrse
- en t.

Thysanophora
Thysanosoma actinoides
Thysanotaenia congolensis

THz
- terahertz

TI
- thoracic index
- time interval
- tricuspid incompetence
- tricuspid insufficiency

TIA
- T-cell restricted intracellular antigen
- transient ischemic attack

TIA-1 antibody
Tiarosporella
TIBC
- total iron-binding capacity
  - TIBC test

tibetense
- *Halorubrum* t.

tibia, pl. **tibiae**
- saber t.

tibial
- t. cortical bone
- t. tuberosity

tibialis
- apophysitis t.

TIC
- trypsin-inhibitory capacity

ticarcillin
tic disorder
tick
- t. fever
- pajaroello t.
- t. paralysis

tick-borne
- t.-b. encephalitis (Central European subtype)
- t.-b. encephalitis (Eastern subtype)
- t.-b. encephalitis virus

ticket
- antibody-based lateral flow economical recognition t. (ALERT)

TID
- titrated initial dose

tidal
- t. air
- t. volume (TV, VT)

tide
- acid t.
- alkaline t.
- fat t.
- t. mark

TIE
- transient ischemic episode

Tiedemann gland
tiedjei
- *Desulfomonile* t.

Tieghemella
Tieghemiomyces
Tierfellnaevus

tiering
    parakeratotic t.
Tietze syndrome
Tietz-Fiereck method
tiger
    t. heart
    t. lily heart
tight
    t. contact wound
    t. junction (TJ)
tigroid
    t. body
    t. striation
    t. substance
TIL
    tumor-infiltrating lymphocyte
Tilachlidium
Tilden stain
Tillaux disease
Tilletia
Tilletiopsis
tilorone
tilt table evaluation
time
    absolute retention t. (ART)
    access t.
    activated clotting t. (ACT)
    activated coagulation t. (ACT)
    activated partial thromboplastin t.
    (APTT, aPTT)
    automated coagulation t.
    bleeding t. (BT)
    blood-clot lysis t. (BLT)
    calcium t.
    cell cycle t.
    circulation t. (CT)
    clot lysis t. (CLT)
    clot retraction t.
    clotting t. (CT)
    coagulation t. (CT)
    compile t.
    corrected retention t.
    dead t.
    decimal reduction t.
    t. diffusion technique
    doubling t.
    Duke method of bleeding t.
    electrode response t.
    euglobin lysis t.
    euglobulin clot lysis t. (ECLT)
    euglobulin lysis t. (ELT)
    execution t.

    fast turnaround t.
    filter bleeding t.
    t. of flight
    forced expiratory t. (FET)
    gastric emptying t. (GET)
    gastric emptying half t. (GET1/2)
    generation t.
    grain count halving t.
    half t.
    helium equilibration t. (HET)
    t. interval (TI)
    Ivy method of bleeding t.
    kaolin-clotting t.
    kaolin partial thromboplastin t.
    (KPTT)
    lag t.
    t. of maximum concentration (T_{max})
    mean circulation t. (MCT)
    mean generation t.
    Mielke bleeding t.
    occlusion t. (OT)
    one-stage prothrombin t.
    operating t.
    partial thromboplastin t. (PTT)
    particle transport t. (PTT)
    plasma clotting t.
    plasma iron disappearance t.
    (PIDT)
    plasma thrombin t.
    prolonged bleeding t.
    prolonged coagulation t.
    prothrombin t. (protime, PT)
    prothrombin consumption t. (PCT)
    reaction t. (RT)
    recalcification t.
    recovery t.
    red blood cell survival t.
    relative retention t.
    reptilase t.
    reptilase-R t.
    resolving t.
    retention t.
    Russell viper venom t. (RVVT)
    secondary bleeding t.
    sedimentation t.
    serial thrombin t. (STT)
    serum prothrombin t.
    shortened bleeding t.
    shortened coagulation t.
    Stypven t.
    survival t.
    template bleeding t.

T

NOTES

time (*continued*)
    thermal death t.
    thrombin t. (TT)
    thrombin clotting t. (TCT)
    thromboplastin generation t. (TGT)
    tissue thromboplastin inhibition t.
    turn-around t. (TAT)
    t. of vomiting following irradiation
    wash t.
    wheal reaction t.
    whole-blood clotting t.

timed
    t. 24-hour volume
    t. two-hour volume

time-domain
time-kill kinetics test
time-of-flight
    matrix-assisted laser desorption
      ionization t.-o.-f. (MALDI-TOF)

time-resolved
    t.-r. fluorescence (TRF)
    t.-r. fluorescence immunoassay
    t.-r. fluorometry (TRF)

time-series plot
time-tension index (TTI)
timidum
    Mogibacterium t.

Timme syndrome
Timm silver sulfide
timonensis
    Paenibacillus t.

timothy bacillus
TIMP
    tissue inhibitor of metalloproteinase

TIN
    tubulointerstitial nephropathy

Tinca
tinctable
tinction
tinctorial
tincture of iodine
Tindallia
    T. californiensis
    T. magadiensis

tinea
    t. amiantacea
    t. barbae
    t. capitis
    t. ciliorum
    t. circinata
    t. corporis
    t. cruris
    t. faciale
    t. favosa
    t. glabrosa
    t. imbricata
    t. inguinalis
    t. kerion
    t. manus

    t. manuum
    t. nigra
    t. pedis
    t. sycosis
    t. tonsurans
    t. tropicalis
    t. unguium
    t. versicolor

tine test
tingibility
tingible
    t. body
    t. body macrophage

tinnitus
tiny canaliculi
tip
    Aerosol Resistant T.'s (ART)
    policeman t.

TIS
    tumor in situ

Tiselius
    T. electrophoresis cell
    T. procedure

Tissierella praeacuta
tissue
    aberrant t.
    adenoid t.
    adipose t.
    adjacent interstitial t.
    archival brain t.
    areolar connective t.
    t. artifact
    t. basophil
    bile pigment demonstration in t.
    bilirubin demonstration in t.'s
    bone t.
    bronchus-associated lymphoid t.
      (BALT)
    brown adipose t.
    bursa-equivalent t.
    cancellous t.
    capsular t.
    cardiac muscle t.
    cartilaginous t.
    cavernous t.
    chondroid t.
    chromaffin t.
    colon glandular t.
    compression of t.
    connective t.
    crushing of t.
    t. culture (TC)
    t. culture cytotoxin assay (TCCA)
    t. culture dose (TCD)
    t. culture infective dose (TCID)
    t. culture medium (TCM)
    cutaneous t.
    dartoic t.

defective formation of
  mesenchymal t.
dense irregular connective t.
dense regular connective t.
diffuse lymphatic t.
t. displaceability
t. displacement
donor t.
ectopic pancreatic t.
ectopic thyroid t.
elastic t.
epithelial t.
t. equivalent
erectile t.
extrathymic t.
t. factor
t. factor pathway inhibitor (TFPI)
fatty intraosseous t.
fibroadipose t.
fibrohyaline t.
t. fibronectin
fibrous t. (FT)
t. fluid
formalin-fixed t.
gastrointestinal associated
  lymphoid t. (GALT)
gelatinous t.
gingival t.
t. glycogen
granulation t.
granule cell of connective t.
gut-associated lymphoid t. (GALT)
Haller vascular t.
hard t.
hematopoietic t.
hemoglobin demonstration in t.
hormone demonstration in t.
t. hypoperfusion
t. hypoxia
inflammation of connective t. (ICT)
t. inhibitor of metalloproteinase
  (TIMP)
interfascicular connective t.
interstitial t.
investing t.
islet t.
lead demonstration in t.
loose irregular connective t.
t. lymph
lymphatic t.
malignant rhabdoid tumor of
  soft t. (MRTS)

mesenchymal t.
mesonephric t.
metanephrogenic t.
t. microarray technology (TMA)
mucosa-associated lymphoid t.
  (MALT)
mucous connective t.
t. multiblock
multilocular adipose t.
muscular t.
myeloid t.
t. necrosis
neoplastic hematopoietic t.
nervous t.
nodal t.
nonmucosa-associated lymphoid t.
  (non-MALT)
odontoblastic t.
osseous t.
osteogenic t.
osteoid t.
t. oxidase test
oxygenation of t.
papilla of connective t.
paraffin-embedded t. (PET)
paraganglionic t.
t. pellet
peritumoral t.
t. plasminogen factor
t. processing
reactive lymphoid t. (RLT)
reticular t.
skeletal muscle t.
smooth muscle t.
snap-freezing of t.
subcutaneous t.
subendocardial connective t.
subepidermal connective t. (SEC)
t. thromboplastin
t. thromboplastin inhibition (TTI)
t. thromboplastin inhibition test
  (TTIT)
t. thromboplastin inhibition time
t. tolerance dose (TTD)
tuberculosis granulation t.
t. typing
venous blood and t.
white adipose t.
WHO classification of tumors of
  the lymphoid t.
tissue-coding factor (TCF, TSF)

T

NOTES

tissue-compatible plastic phantom
tissue-damaging factor (TF)
tissue-equivalent (TE)
tissue-nonspecific alkaline phosphatase (TNAP)
tissue-specific antigen
tissular
Tistrella mobilis
Titan
    T. III H cellulose acetate strip
    T. yellow
titanium dioxide pneumoconiosis
titer
    agglutination t.
    AH t.
    antibody t.
    anti-F1 antigen t.
    antihyaluronidase t. (AHT)
    anti-Rh t.
    antistreptolysin-O t.
    ASO t.
    California encephalitis virus t.
    CF antibody t.
    Chlamydia group t.
    cold agglutinin t.
    cryptococcal antigen t.
    Cryptococcus antibody t.
    cysticercosis t.
    differential agglutination t. (DAT)
    Eastern equine encephalitis virus t.
    fibrin t.
    HAI t.
    hemagglutination inhibition t.
    Image T.
    influenza A, B t.
    lymphogranuloma venereum t.
    mumps antibody t.
    poliomyelitis I–III t.
    psittacosis t.
    Q fever t.
    Salmonella t.
titrant
titratable
    t. acid (TA)
    t. acidity test
titrated initial dose (TID)
titration
    amperometric-coulometric t.
    coulometric t.
    potentiometric t.
    t. technique
titrator
    Cotlove t.
titrimetric
Tityus serrulatus
Tizzoni stain
TJ
    tight junction

tjernbergiae
    Acinetobacter t.
TL
    thymus leukemia
Tl
    thallium
        TL antigen
TLA
    total laboratory automation
TLC
    thin-layer chromatography
    total L-chain concentration
    total lung capacity
TLD
    thermoluminescent dosimeter
    tumor lethal dose
T/LD$_{100}$
    minimum dose causing death or malformation of 100% of fetuses
TLE
    thin-layer electrophoresis
T-lineage
TLR4
    toll-like receptor 4
TLS
    tumor lysis syndrome
TLV
    threshold limit value
T-lymphocyte rosette
TM
    thrombomodulin glycoprotein
Tm
    melting temperature
    thulium
        Tm cell
TMA
    thrombotic microangiopathy
    tissue microarray technology
    transcription-mediated amplification
TMAb
    thyroid microsomal antibody
TMIF
    tumor-cell migration-inhibition factor
TMPRSS3
    transmembrane protease serine 3
TMRE
    tetra-methylrhodamine ethyl ester
TMV
    tobacco mosaic virus
T2 mycotoxin
Tn antigen
TNAP
    tissue-nonspecific alkaline phosphatase
T-natural
    T-n. killer cell (TNK)
    T-n. killer cell lymphoma
TnC
    troponin C
    TnC polypeptide

T$_4$ newborn screen
TNF
    tumor necrosis factor
        TNF alpha
        TNF beta
TNFR
    tumor necrosis factor receptor
TnI
    troponin I
        TnI polypeptide
TNK
    T-natural killer
    T-natural killer cell
TNM
    (primary) tumor, (regional lymph) nodes,
      (remote) metastases
    tumor-node-metastasis
        TNM staging
        TNM staging system
T-nodule
TnT
    troponin T
        TnT polypeptide
TNTC
    too numerous to count
TO
    TO virus
to
    to contain (TC)
    to deliver (TD)
TOA
    tuboovarian abscess
toad
    t. test
    t. toxin
tobacco
    t. amblyopia
    t. mosaic virus (TMV)
Tobamovirus
Tobie, von Brand, and Mehlman
    diphasic medium
tobramycin
Tobravirus
tocainide
tocodynagraph
tocodynamometer
tocolytic agent
Todd
    T. body
    T. paralysis
    T. unit (TU)
Todd-Hewitt broth

toe
    clubbed t.
    Hong Kong t.
    webbed t.
toebii
    Geobacillus t.
Togaviridae
togavirus
Togobacteria
Toison
    T. solution
    T. stain
Tokelau ringworm
Toker clear cell
tokodaii
    Sulfolobus t.
tolaasinivorans
    Mycetocola t.
tolbutamide
    sodium t.
    t. test (TBT)
    t. tolerance test (TTT)
tolerance
    aspirin t.
    drug t.
    glucose t. (GT)
    high-dose t.
    immune t.
    immunological t.
    immunologic high-dose t.
    t. interval
    t. limit
    nonresponder t.
    split t.
tolerogen
tolerogenic
toll-like receptor 4 (TLR4)
Tolosa-Hunt syndrome
toluene 2,4-diisocyanate
toluic acid
toluidine
    t. blue (TB)
    t. blue O
    t. blue stain
toluol
toluolica
    Desulfobacula t.
toluvorans
    Azoarcus t.
toluylene red
Tolypocladium

T

NOTES

tolypomycina
>*Amycolatopsis t.*

tomato
>*Macrosporium t.*

tombstone-like dermis

Tombusvirus

Tomes
>T. fiber
>T. granular layer
>T. process

Tommaselli disease

tomographic scan

tongue
>bifid t.
>black hairy t.
>t. blanching
>cleft t.
>t. worm

tonicity

toning
>gold t.

tonofibril

tonofilament

tonometer

tonoplast

tonsil
>eustachian t.
>faucial t.
>Gerlach t.
>laryngeal t.
>lingual t.
>Luschka t.
>palatine t.
>pharyngeal t.
>third t.
>tubal t.

tonsilla
>t. intestinalis
>t. lingualis
>t. palatina
>t. pharyngealis
>t. tubaria

tonsillar crypt

tonsillaris
>crypta t.
>cynanche t.

tonsillitis
>acute necrotizing ulcerative t.

tonsurans
>*Trichophyton t.*

tool
>policeman transfer t.

too numerous to count (TNTC)

tooth, pl. **teeth**
>auditory teeth
>t. cement
>Corti auditory teeth
>T. disease
>Huschke auditory teeth

>Hutchinson teeth
>t. pulp
>t. sac
>t. socket

Töpfer test

tophaceous gout

tophus, pl. **tophi**
>gouty t.

topical
>t. calciphylaxis
>t. corticosteroid

Topocuvirus

topo-II-alpha
>topoisomerase II-alpha
>topo-II-alpha index

topoisomerase
>t. II-alpha (topo-II-alpha)
>t. II enzyme

topopathogenesis

TOPV
>trivalent oral poliovirus vaccine

TORCH
>toxoplasmosis, rubella, cytomegalovirus, and herpes simplex
>TORCH syndrome

torcular herophili

Torkelson syndrome

Tornwaldt, Thornwaldt
>T. abscess
>T. disease
>T. syndrome

torocyte membrane

torose

Torovirus

torque

torquis
>*Psychroflexus t.*

torr

Torre syndrome

torsade de pointes

torsion
>t. injury
>ovarian t.
>testicular t.
>t. of testis

Torsten Sjögren syndrome

torticollis
>congenital t.

tortuosum
>*Eubacterium t.*

tortuous

Torula
>*T. capsulatus*
>*T. histolytica*

torular meningitis

Torulaspora

toruloidea
>*Hendersonula t.*

toruloma

Torulomyces lagena
Torulopsis glabrata
torulopsosis
torulosis
TOS
    thoracic outlet syndrome
Tospovirus
tosylate
total
    t. acidity
    t. antitryptic activity (TAT)
    t. blood granulocyte pool (TBGP)
    t. blood volume (TBV)
    t. body clearance (Q_B)
    t. body density (TBD)
    t. body fat (TBF)
    t. body hematocrit (TBH)
    t. body potassium (TBK)
    t. body solute (TBS)
    t. body water (TBW)
    t. body weight (TBW)
    t. calcium assay
    t. carbon dioxide content
    t. catecholamine test
    t. cell count
    t. cholesterol (TC)
    t. circulating hemoglobin (TCH)
    t. colonic aganglionosis (TCA)
    complement t.
    t. estriol
    t. estrogen (excretion) (TE)
    t. exchangeable potassium measurement
    t. fatty acid (TFA)
    t. gastric resection
    t. hematuria
    t. hemoglobin
    t. hexosaminidase
    t. internal reflection
    t. iron-binding capacity (TIBC)
    t. laboratory automation (TLA)
    t. L-chain concentration (TLC)
    t. lesion
    t. lung capacity (TLC)
    t. necrosis
    t. oxidant
    t. parenteral nutrition (TPN)
    t. peripheral resistance (TPR)
    t. protein (TP)
    t. protein expression
    t. pulmonary vascular resistance (TPVR)

    t. response (TR)
    t. ridge count (TRC)
    t. serum bilirubin (TSB)
    t. serum IgE
    t. serum prostatic acid phosphatase (TSPAP)
    t. serum protein (TSP)
    t. solids (TS)
    t. thyroxine (TT)
    t. urinary gonadotropin (TUG)
    t. urine estrogen
total-dose infusion (TDI)
totalis
    peniplastica t.
totipotency
totipotent
    t. cell
    t. HSC
totipotential
    t. protoplasm
    t. stem cell
Totivirus
touch
    t. cell
    t. corpuscle
    t. imprint
    t. imprint cytology
    organ of t.
    t. preparation
touch-smear specimen
Touraine-Solente-Golé syndrome
Tourette disease
Touton giant cell
towelette
    mini Hype-Wipe bleach t.
Towne CMV low passage clinical isolate
towneri
    Acinetobacter t.
tox
    toxic
    toxicology
    toxin
    Wampole *Clostridium difficile* Tox A/B II
toxalbumin
toxanemia
toxaphene
Toxascaris leonina
toxemia, toxicemia
    preeclamptic t. (PET)
    t. of pregnancy

NOTES

toxemic jaundice
toxic (tox)
- t. adenoma
- t. anemia
- t. chemical agent
- t. chemical handling
- t. cirrhosis
- t. colitis
- t. cyanosis
- t. dermatitis
- t. epidermal necrolysis (TEN)
- t. equivalent
- t. erythema
- t. glycosuria
- t. goiter (TG)
- t. granulation
- t. granule
- t. hemoglobinuria
- t. idiopathy
- t. megacolon
- t. methemoglobinemia
- t. myocarditis
- t. nephrosis
- t. organophosphorous
- t. shock
- t. shock syndrome
- t. shock syndrome toxin (TSST1)
- t. soluble oligomer
- t. unit (TU)
- t. waste

toxicant
toxicemia (*var. of* toxemia)
toxicity
- acetaminophen hepatic t.
- aspirin t.
- delayed radiation t.
- EP t.
- immediate radiation t.
- manganese t.
- salicylate t.

toxicogenic conjunctivitis
toxicogenomics
toxicologic
toxicologist
toxicology (tox)
- analytical t.
- clinical t.
- environmental t.
- forensic t.
- industrial t.

toxicopathic
toxicosis
- triiodothyronine t.

toxidrome
toxigenic bacterium
toxigenicity
toxin (tox)
- animal t.
- anthrax t.

Bacillus anthracis t.
- bacterial t.
- bee venom t.
- botulinum t.
- botulinus t.
- cagA t.
- cholera t. (CTX)
- *Clostridium difficile* t.
- *Clostridium perfringens* alpha t.
- *Clostridium perfringens* beta t.
- *Clostridium perfringens* epsilon t.
- *Clostridium perfringens* iota t.
- Coley t.
- diagnostic diphtheria t.
- Dick test t.
- dinoflagellate t.
- diphtheria t.
- disease-associated bacterial t.
- epsilon clostridial t.
- erythrogenic t.
- extracellular t.
- intracellular t.
- mitochondrial t.
- normal t.
- plant t.
- pyrogenic t.
- scarlet fever erythrogenic t.
- Schick test t.
- secreted t.
- Shiga t.
- Shigalike t.
- t. spectrum
- streptococcus erythrogenic t.
- T2 t.
- tetanus t.
- toad t.
- toxic shock syndrome t. (TSST1)
- t. unit (TU)

toxin-antitoxin (TA, TAT)
toxinic
toxinogenic
toxinogenicity
toxinology
toxinosis
toxipathic
toxipathy
Toxocara
- *T. canis*
- *T. cati*
- *T. mystax*

toxocariasis
toxoid
- alum-precipitated t. (APT)

toxoid-antitoxoid
- t. floccule (TAF)
- t. mixture (TAM)

toxon
toxoneme
toxonosis

toxophil
toxophore
toxophorous
Toxoplasma
    T. gondii
    T. pyrogenes
Toxoplasmatidae
Toxoplasmea
toxoplasmic retinochoroiditis
toxoplasmin
toxoplasmosis
    acquired t. in adults
    congenital t.
    t., rubella, cytomegalovirus, and
      herpes simplex (TORCH)
    t. serology
Toynbee corpuscle
toyohensis
    Thermanaeromonas t.
TP
    thrombocytopenic purpura
    total protein
    tryptophan
    tube precipitin
    tuberculin precipitation
TPA
    Treponema pallidum agglutination
TPC
    thromboplastic plasma component
TPCF
    Treponema pallidum complement fixation
TPH
    transplacental hemorrhage
    treponemal hemagglutination
    Treponema pallidum hemagglutination
      TPH test
TPHA
    Treponema pallidum hemagglutination
      assay
TPI
    Treponema pallidum immobilization
      TPI assay
      TPI test
TPIA
    Treponema pallidum immobilization
      (immune) adherence
T-PLL
    T-cell prolymphocytic leukemia
TPMT
    Pro-PredictRx TPMT
TPN
    total parenteral nutrition

TPO
    thrombopoietin
TPR
    testosterone production rate
    total peripheral resistance
TPS
    tumor polysaccharide substance
TPVR
    total pulmonary vascular resistance
TQ-Prep workstation
TR
    tetrazolium reduction
    total response
    tuberculin R (new tuberculin)
Tr
    trace
TRA-1-60 human embryonal carcinoma
    marker antigen
TRA antigen
trabecula, pl. **trabeculae**
    arachnoid t.
    t. of bone
    trabeculae carneae of right and left
      ventricles
    connective tissue t.
    t. corporis spongiosi
    t. corporum cavernosorum
    t. testis
    trabeculae carneae
trabecular
    t. adenocarcinoma
    t. adenoma
    t. blood vessel
    t. bone
    t. carcinoma
    t. meshwork
    t. network
    t. pattern
    t. reticulum
    t. zone
trabecularis
    substantia t.
trabeculate
trabeculation
trace (Tr)
    t. alternant
    t. element
    t. routine
    TEG t.
tracer
    radiocolloid t.
trachea, pl. **tracheae**

T

NOTES

trachea *(continued)*
    tunica mucosa tracheae
    tunica muscularis tracheae
tracheal
    t. aspiration
    t. gland
tracheales
    glandulae t.
tracheitis
trachelematoma
trachelocystitis
trachelomyitis
trachelopanus
trachelophyma
tracheoaerocele
tracheobiliary fistula
tracheobronchial
    t. amyloidosis
    t. dyskinesia
    t. tree
tracheobronchitis
tracheobronchomegaly
tracheoesophageal fistula (TEF)
tracheomalacia
tracheomegaly
tracheopathia osteoplastica
tracheopathy
Tracheophilus cucumerinum
tracheostenosis
Trachipleistophora
trachitis
trachoma
    t. body
    t. gland
    psittacosis-lymphogranuloma
      venereum t. (PLT)
    t. virus
trachoma-inclusion conjunctivitis (TRIC)
trachomatis
    Chlamydia t.
trachomatosus
    pannus t.
Trachybdella bistriata
trachychromatic
tracking
    lymphatic t.
TRAcP
    tartrate resistant acid phosphatase
tract
    alimentary t.
    Arnold t.
    association t.
    benign mesothelioma of genital t.
    Bürdach t.
    census t. (CT)
    digestive t.
    female genital t. (FGT)
    hypothalamohypophysial t.
    long t.

    portal t.
    respiratory t.
    spiral foraminous t.
    supraopticohypophysial t.
    upper aerodigestive t. (UADT)
    uveal t.
tractellum
traction
    t. aneurysm
    t. atrophy
    t. diverticulum
tractus
    t. spiralis foraminosus
    t. supraopticohypophysialis
TRAF
    tumor receptor-associated factor
traffic
    cell t.
trafficking
    membrane t.
trait
    hemoglobin E t.
    hemoglobin G Philadelphia t.
    hemoglobin Lepore t.
    quantitative t.
    secretor t.
    sickle cell t.
    thalassemia t.
trajectory
TRALI
    transfusion-related acute lung injury
Trametes
tram-track appearance
tram-tracking
trance
    death t.
tranquilizer
    major t.
    minor t.
    phenothiazine t.
    thioxanthene t.
trans
    t. activation
    t. face
transabdominal
    t. chorionic villus sampling
    t. CVS
transaldolase
transaminase
    aspartate t.
    erythrocyte glutamic oxaloacetic t.
      (EGOT)
    glutamate-pyruvate t.
    glutamic-oxaloacetic t. (GOT)
    glutamic-pyruvic t. (GPT)
    hepatic t.
    serum glutamic oxaloacetic t.
      (SGOT)
    serum glutamic pyruvic t. (SGPT)

t. test
valine t.
transamination
transbronchial
t. needle aspiration (TBNA)
transcapsidation
transcarbamoylase
ornithine t. (OTC)
transcellular
t. fluid
t. pathway
transcervical
t. chorionic villus sampling
t. CVS
transcobalamin (Tc)
transconfiguration
transcortin
transcript
BCR-ABL t.
EWS-WT1 chimeric t.
primary t.
transcriptase
avian myeloblastosis leukemia virus reverse t. (AMLV-RT)
human telomerase reverse t.
reverse t.
transcription
t. factor
t. factor beta
t. factor Cbfa1/Runx2
t. factor neuroD
gene t.
inhibitor of t.
reverse t.
signal transducer and activator of t. (STAT)
t. unit
transcriptional profiling
transcriptional promoter
transcription-based chain reaction
transcription-dependent amplification
transcription-mediated amplification (TMA)
transcription/translation
in vitro t. (IVTT)
transcriptome analysis
transdifferentiation
tubular epithelial-myofibroblast t. (TEMT)
transduce
transducer cell
transductant

transduction
abortive t.
adenoviral t.
complete t.
general t.
generalized t.
high-frequency t.
insulin receptor and signal t.
low-frequency t.
specialized t.
specific t.
transepidermal water loss (TWL)
transethmoidal puncture
transfection
transfer
DNA t.
t. factor (TF)
fluorescence resonance energy t. (FRET)
fluorescent resonance energy t. (FRET)
t. function
t. gene
group t.
t. host
passive t.
t. pipette
plasmid t.
replication and t. (RTF)
t. RNA (tRNA)
transferase
adenylyl t.
catechol-O-methyl t. (COMT)
glucuronosyl t.
terminal deoxyribonucleotidyl t.
UDP-glucuronyl t.
transferred
t. antigen-cell-bound antibody reaction
t. antigen-transferred antibody reaction
transferrin
t. assay
t. receptor
t. saturation
t. test
transformant
transformation
asbestos t.
bacterial t.
blastic t.
cell t.

T

NOTES

transformation *(continued)*
　　globular-fibrous t.
　　human lymphocyte t. (hLT)
　　logit t.
　　lymphocyte t.
　　lymphocytic t.
　　malignant t.
　　nodular t. of the liver
　　oncocytic t.
　　probit t.
　　pseudoxanthomatous t.
　　refractory anemia with excess
　　　blasts in t.
transformation-sensitive
　　large external t.-s. (LETS)
transformed lymphocyte
transformer
　　high-voltage t.
　　step-down t.
　　step-up t.
　　voltage-regulating t.
transforming
　　t. agent
　　t. gene
　　t. growth factor X
　　t. virus
transfusion
　　t. adult committee
　　autologous t.
　　coagulation factor t.
　　cryoprecipitate t.
　　directed donor t.
　　exchange t. (ET)
　　granulocyte t.
　　t. hepatitis
　　incompatible blood t.
　　intrauterine fetal t. (IVT)
　　leukocyte t.
　　massive t.
　　t. nephritis
　　partial exchange t.
　　platelet t.
　　predeposit autologous t.
　　t. reaction
　　reciprocal t.
　　t. transmitted virus (TTV)
transfusion-associated graft-versus-host disease (TAGVHD)
transfusion-mediated viral hepatitis
transfusion-related
　　t.-r. acute lung injury (TRALI)
　　t.-r. alloimmunization
transgene
transgenic mice
transglutaminase (TGase)
trans-Golgi
transheterozygosity
transient
　　t. acantholytic dermatosis

　　t. agammaglobulinemia
　　t. albuminuria
　　t. cerebral ischemia (TCI)
　　t. cerebral ischemic episode (TCIE)
　　t. derepression
　　t. enzyme abnormality
　　t. equilibrium
　　t. erythroblastopenia of childhood (TEC)
　　t. hypogammaglobulinemia
　　t. hypogammaglobulinemia of infancy
　　t. ischemic attack (TIA)
　　t. ischemic episode (TIE)
　　t. myeloproliferative disorder
　　ryanodine-sensitive calcium t.
transistor
　　field effect t.
　　insulated gate field effect t.
　　junction field effect t.
　　metal oxide semiconductor field effect t.
　　unijunction t.
transition
　　G to A stage tumor t.
　　isomeric t. (IT)
　　t. mutation
　　refractory anemia with excess blasts in t. (RAEBT)
　　t. state
　　t. zone (TZ)
transitional
　　t. cell
　　t. cell carcinoma (TCC)
　　t. cell papilloma
　　t. cell tumor
　　t. epithelium
　　t. leukocyte
　　t. zone
transketolase
　　t. assay
　　erythrocyte t.
translation control RNA (tcRNA)
translator
translocation
　　autosome t.
　　balance t.
　　chromosome t.
　　t. factor
　　insertional t.
　　Philadelphia t.
　　reciprocal t.
　　robertsonian t.
　　t. trisomy
translucency
　　fetal nuchal t.
translucent
translucida
　　Pseudoalteromonas t.

transmandibular projection
transmembrane
    transmembrane protein
transmembrane protease serine 3 (TMPRSS3)
transmethylase
transmethylation
transmigration
    leukocyte t.
    t. macrophage
    t. neutrophil
transmissible
    t. dementia
    t. disease
    t. enteritis
    t. gastroenteritis
    t. gastroenteritis virus of swine
    t. mink encephalopathy
    t. plasmid
    t. spongiform encephalopathy (TSE)
    t. turkey enteritis virus
transmission
    asynchronous data t.
    t. electron microscope (TEM)
    t. electron microscopy (TEM)
    fecal-oral t.
    glutamatergic t.
    horizontal t.
    serial data t.
    synchronous data t.
    vertical t.
transmittance
    peak t.
transmitted via parenteral
transmitter-gated ion channel
transmogrification
    placental t.
transmogrify
transmural
    t. gradient
    t. lymphoid aggregate
    t. lymphoid hyperplasia
    t. myocardial infarction
transmutation
transnexus channel
transparent
transpeptidase
    gamma-glutamyl t. (GGTP)
    glutamyl t. (GT)
transphosphorylase
transplacental hemorrhage (TPH)

transplant
    bone marrow t.
    canalicular organic anion t.
    'peripheral stem cell t. (PSCT)
    t. rejection
    renal t.
    umbilical cord blood t.
    t. vascular disease
transplantation
    allogeneic t.
    allogeneic bone marrow t. (allo-BMT)
    t. antigen
    autologous blood and marrow t. (ABMT)
    autologous bone marrow t. (ABMT)
    autologous peripheral blood stem cell bone marrow t.
    bone marrow t. (BMT)
    hematopoietic progenitor cell t.
    heterotopic t.
    homotopic t.
    t. immunology
    orthoptic t.
    orthotopic liver t.
    syngeneic t.
    syngenesioplastic t.
    t. workup
transport
    active t.
    axoplasmic t.
    t. of cancer cell
    carrier-mediated t.
    direct t.
    t. disease
    effective oxygen t. (EOT)
    indirect t.
    t. medium
    membrane t.
    passive t.
    primary active t.
    t. protein defect
    secondary active t.
    t. and secretion
    selective t.
    t. and storage
    tape t.
transportation
    lysis, storage, and t. (LST)
transporter
    biliary acid t. (BAT)

T

NOTES

transporter *(continued)*
    canicular multispecific organic anion t. (CMOAT)
    Dura-Temp specimen t.
    MDR1 t.
transposable element
transpose
transposition
    corrected t. (CT)
    t. of great arteries (TGA)
    t. of great vessels (TGV)
transposon
transrectal
    t. ultrasonography
    t. ultrasound-guided sextant biopsy (TRUS)
transrectal ultrasound-guided sextant biopsy (TRUS)
transseptal fiber
transsynaptic
    t. chromatolysis
    t. degeneration
transthyretin (TTR)
transubstantiation
transudate
    acute inflammatory t.
transudation
    generalized t.
transudative
    t. inflammation
    t. pleural effusion
transuranic radionuclide
transurethral resection of prostate (TURP)
transvaalensis
    Alkaliphilus t.
transvalensis
    Nocardia t.
transvector
transverse
    t. disc
    t. ductules of epoophoron
    t. fracture
    t. myelitis
    t. myelopathy
    t. perineal muscle
    t. septum
transversion mutation
transversus
    tubulus t.
tra operon
TRAP
    tartrate resistant acid phosphatase
    telomerase repeat amplification protocol
    telomeric repeat amplification protocol
    TRAP assay
    TRAP stain
Trapp formula
Trapp-Häser formula

Traube
    T. corpuscle
    T. plug
trauma, pl. **traumata**
    blunt t.
    blunt force t. (BFT)
    laryngeal intubation t.
    t. MCI
    orbital t.
    penetrating t.
traumatic
    t. abnormality
    t. anemia
    t. aneurysm
    t. atrophy
    t. basal subarachnoid hemorrhage (TBSAH)
    t. bone cyst
    t. brain injury (TBI)
    t. chylothorax
    t. fever
    t. hemolysis
    t. herpes
    t. neuroma
    t. osteoporosis
    t. progressive encephalopathy
    t. rupture
    t. subarachnoid hemorrhage (TSAH)
    t. thrombosis
traveler's diarrhea
TRC
    tanned red cell
    total ridge count
Treacher Collins syndrome
treatment
    antiretroviral t. (ART)
    immunomodulatory t.
    isoserum t.
    preventive t.
    prophylactic t.
    PUVA t.
    solvent detergent t. (SD)
    thyroxine and cortisol t.
tree
    tracheobronchial t.
trefoil
    t. family factor (TFF)
    t. peptide
trehala
trehalose
trehalosi
    Nocardiopsis t.
Trematoda
trematode
    blood t.
Tremella
tremelloid
tremellose

tremens
    delirium t. (DT)
tremor
    epidemic t.
trench
    t. fever
    t. foot
    t. mouth
trephine biopsy
trephocyte
Treponema
    T. azotonutricium
    T. buccale
    T. calligyrum
    T. carateum
    T. cuniculi
    T. denticola
    T. genitalis
    T. hyodysenteriae
    T. macrodentium
    T. microdentium
    T. mucosum
    T. orale
    T. pallidum
    T. pallidum agglutination (TPA)
    T. pallidum complement fixation (TPCF)
    T. pallidum complement fixation test
    T. pallidum hemagglutination (TPH)
    T. pallidum hemagglutination assay (TPHA)
    T. pallidum immobilization (TPI)
    T. pallidum immobilization assay
    T. pallidum immobilization (immune) adherence (TPIA)
    T. pallidum immobilization reaction
    T. parvum
    T. pectinovorum
    T. pertenue
    T. pintae
    T. primitia
    T. putidum
    T. refringens
    T. scoliodontum
    T. succinifaciens
    T. vincentii
treponema-immobilizing antibody
treponemal
    t. antibody
    t. antibody test (TAT)

    t. hemagglutination (TPH)
    t. immobilization test
Treponemataceae
treponematosis
tresis
trevisanii
    Leptotrichia t.
Trevor disease
TRF
    T-cell replacing factor
    telomeric restriction fragment
    thyrotropin-releasing factor
    time-resolved fluorescence
    time-resolved fluorometry
TRH
    thyrotropin-releasing hormone
        TRH stimulation test
TRI
    tetrazolium reduction inhibition
triac
triacetate
    glyceryl t.
triacetin
triacetylglycerol
triacetyloleandomycin
triacsin C
triacylglyceride synthesis
triacylglycerol lipase
triad
    acute compression t.
    adrenomedullary t.
    Andersen t.
    Beck t.
    Charcot t.
    fragile histidine t. (FHIT)
    Hutchinson t.
    portal t.
    t. syndrome
    Virchow t.
    Whipple t.
triage
    T. BNP test
    T. Cardiac Panel
    t. delayed
    HPV t.
    t. immediate
    T. MeterPlus
    t. minimal
    T. Tox drug screen
trial
    clinical t.
triamcinolone

NOTES

triangle
 Alsberg t.
 gastrinoma t.
 sternocostal t.
triangular
 t. fibrocartilage complex tear
 t. lamella
 t. wave
triangular-shaped skin tear
triarylmethane dye
Triatoma
triatomae
 Trypanosoma t.
triatomic
triatomid
Triatominae
triatriatum
 cor t.
tribasic
 t. acid
 t. potassium phosphate
tribasilar synostosis
tribrachius
 dicephalus dipus t.
 dicephalus tripus t.
TRIC
 trachoma-inclusion conjunctivitis
tricarboxylic
 t. acid (TCA)
 t. acid cycle
Tricercomonas
trichangion
Trichaptum
trichatrophia
trichilemmal
 t. cyst
 t. cystic squamous cell carcinoma
trichilemmoma
Trichina
trichina
Trichinella
 T. pseudospiralis
 T. spiralis
trichinelliasis
Trichinellicae
Trichinelloidea
trichinellosis
trichiniasis
trichiniferous
trichinization
trichinoscope
trichinosis serology
trichinous embolism
trichite
trichitis
trichiura
 Trichuris t.
trichlorfon

trichloride
 acetylene t.
 antimony t.
 vinyl t.
trichloroacetic acid
Trichlorobacter
 T. thiogenes
1,1,1-trichloroethane
1,1,2-trichloroethane
trichloroethylene
trichlorophenoxy acetic acid
Trichobilharzia physellae
trichoblastoma
 desmoplastic t.
trichocephaliasis
Trichocephalus trichiura
trichochrome
Trichocladium asperum
Trichococcus
 T. collinsii
 T. palustris
 T. pasteurii
Trichoconis padwickii
trichocyst
Trichodectes
trichodectis
 Cryptocystis t.
Trichoderma
trichodes
 Lactobacillus t.
trichodiscoma
trichoepithelioma
 desmoplastic t.
 hereditary multiple t.
 t. papillosum multiplex
trichofolliculoma
trichohyalin
trichoid
trichoides
 Cladosporium t.
tricholemmoma
Tricholoma
 T. magnivelare
 T. pardinum
trichomanas vaginitis
Trichomaris invadens
Trichometasphaeria
trichomonacide
trichomonad
Trichomonadidae
Trichomonas
 T. buccalis
 T. foetus
 T. gallinarum
 T. hominis
 T. infestation
 T. intestinalis
 T. ovis
 T. preparation

T. *pulmonalis*
T. *suis*
T. *tenax*
T. urethritis
T. *vaginalis*
trichomoniasis
trichomycosis
  t. axillaris
  t. chromatica
  t. favosa
  t. rubra
trichonodosis
trichophytic
trichophytid
trichophytin
Trichophyton
  T. agar
  T. *ajelloi*
  T. *asteroides*
  T. *concentricum*
  T. *cruris*
  T. *dankaliense*
  T. *epilans*
  T. *equinum*
  T. *equinum*
  T. *equinum* var. *autotrophicum*
  T. *equinum* var. *equinum*
  T. *erinacei*
  T. *ferrugineum*
  T. *fischeri*
  T. *flavescens*
  T. *floccosum*
  T. *gallinae*
  T. *glabrum*
  T. *gloriae*
  T. *gourvilii*
  T. *granulare*
  T. *granulosum*
  T. *gypseum*
  T. *inguinale*
  T. *interdigitale*
  T. *intertriginis*
  T. *kanei*
  T. *krajdenii*
  T. *longifusum*
  T. *megninii*
  T. *mentagrophytes*
  T. *mentagrophytes* var. *erinacei*
  T. *mentagrophytes* var. *interdigitale*
  T. *mentagrophytes* var. *mentagrophytes*
  T. *mentagrophytes* var. *nodulare*

T. *mentagrophytes* var. *quinckeanum*
T. *niveum*
T. *nodulare*
T. *pedis*
T. *persicolor*
T. *phaseoliforme*
T. *proliferans*
T. *purpureum*
T. *radiolatum*
T. *raubitschekii*
T. *rosaceum*
T. *rubrum*
T. *sabouraudi*
T. *schoenleinii*
T. *simii*
T. *soudanense*
T. *sulphureum*
T. *terrestre*
T. *tonsurans*
T. *tonsurans* var. *sulphureum*
T. *tonsurans* var. *tonsurans* *perforans*
T. *vanbreuseghemii*
T. *verrucosum*
T. *violaceum*
T. *yaoundei*
trichophytosis
  t. barbae
  t. capitis
  t. corporis
  t. cruris
  t. unguium
Trichopleuris
Trichoprosopon
Trichoptera
trichorhinophalangeal syndrome
trichorrhexis nodosa
Trichosanthes cucumerina
trichosomatous
Trichosporon
  T. *asahii*
  T. *asteroides*
  T. *beigelii*
  T. *cutaneum*
  T. *faecale*
  T. *fuscans*
  T. *giganteum*
  T. *gracile*
  T. *granulosum*
  T. *inkin*
  T. *loboi*
  T. *mucoides*

NOTES

Trichosporon (continued)
   T. ovoides
   T. pedrosianum
   T. penicillatum
   T. proteolyticum
   T. pullulans
   T. variabile
Trichosporonoides
trichosporosis
trichostrongyle
trichostrongyliasis
Trichostrongylidae
Trichostrongyloidea
trichostrongylosis
Trichostrongylus
   T. axei
   T. brevis
   T. capricola
   T. colubriformis
   T. instabilis
   T. longispicularis
   T. orientalis
   T. probolurus
   T. tenuis
   T. vitrinus
trichothecene mycotoxin
Trichothecium roseum
trichotomy
trichotoxin
Trichovirus
trichrome stain
trichuriasis
Trichuris
   T. suis
   T. trichiura
   T. vulpis
Trichuroidea
Trichurus spiralis
tricorn protease
tricresol
tricresyl phosphate
Tricula
tricuspid
   t. atresia
   t. incompetence (TI)
   t. insufficiency (TI)
   t. regurgitation
   t. stenosis
   t. valve
   t. valve cleft leaflet
tricuspidatus
   Paragordius t.
tricuspis
   Ollulanus t.
trident hand
tridermoma
triethanolamine
triethylenethiophosphoramide precoated slide

trifid stomach
trifluoride-methanol
   boron t.
trifluoroacetic anhydride (TFAA)
trifluorocarbonylcyanide phenylhydrazone (FCCP)
triglyceride (TG)
   t. assay
   long-chain t. (LCT)
   medium-chain t. (MCT)
   plasma t.
trigona (*pl. of* trigonum)
trigonitis
trigonocephalum
   Bunostomum t.
Trigonopsis
trigonosporus
   Microascus t.
trigonum, pl. **trigona**
   t. sternocostale
trihexosidase
   ceramide t.
trihexoside
   ceramide t. (CTH)
trihydride
   arsenic t.
triiodide
   bismuth t.
triiodothyronine (T_3)
   t. assay
   free t. (FT_3)
   t. resin uptake (T_3RU)
   t. resin uptake test
   reverse t. (rT_3)
   t. by RIA
   t. suppression test
   t. toxicosis
   t. uptake (T_3U)
triketohydrindene reaction
trilaminar
trilineage dysplasia
trilinear maturation
triloba
   placenta t.
trilobate placenta
trilocular heart
trilogy
Trilone
trimastigote
trimer
trimetaphosphate
   sodium t.
trimethoprim
trimethoxyamphetamine
trimethylacetate
   desoxycorticosterone t. (DCTMA)
trimethylamine
trimethylaminuria
trimmed specimen

trimming resistor
trimorphic
trimorphism
trimorphous
Trinder
    T. reaction
    T. test
trinitrotoluene
trinocular microscope
trinucleotide
    t. repeat
    t. repeat disorder
tri-*o*-cresyl phosphate
Triodontophorus diminutus
triol
triolein I-131
triose
triosephosphate
    t. dehydrogenase
    t. isomerase
    t. isomerase assay
    t. isomerase deficiency
trioxide
    arsenic t. (As_2O_3)
2,6,8-trioxypurine
tripartita
    placenta t.
triphasic wave
triphenylacetate
    desoxycorticosterone t. (DCTPA)
triphenyl albumin
triphenylmethane dye
Triphleps insidiosus
triphosphatase
    adenosine t. (ATPase)
triphosphate
    adenosine t. (ATP)
    adenosine 5'-
      diphosphate/adenosine t.
    cytidine t. (CTP)
    cytosine t. (CTP)
    deoxythymidine t. (dTTP)
    deoxyuridine t. (DUTP)
    guanosine t. (GTP)
    inosine t.
    thymidine t.
    uridine t. (UTP)
triphyllomatous teratoma
triple
    t. bond
    t. phosphate
    t. phosphate crystal

    t. point
    t. screen
    t. sugar iron (TSI)
    t. sugar iron agar
    t. symptom complex
    t. test
    t. X syndrome
triple-blind
triplet
    t. code
    coding t.
    nonsense t.
    t. repeat
triple-X chromosomal aberration
triploblastic
triploid mosaicism
triploidy
trisacryl gelatin microsphere
Tris-buffered saline
triseriatus
    Aedes t.
Tris-HCl buffer
tris(hydroxymethyl) aminomethane
trisodium foscarnet salt
trisomic cell
trisomy
    t. 12
    chromosome t.
    complete t.
    double t.
    t. 8 mosaicism
    partial t.
    primary t.
    primary t. 18
    secondary t.
    t. 8,13,18,20,21,22 syndrome
    tertiary t.
    translocation t.
tristearin
trisymptome
trit
    triturate
triterpene
triterpenoid saponin
tritiated
    t. gas
    t. thymidine (TTH)
    t. water
triticeous
tritici
    Ochrobactrum t.
    Pyemotes t.

T

NOTES

Tritimovirus
Tritirachium
tritium (H3)
triton tumor
Triton-X 100
Tritrichomonas
triturate (trit)
trivalent oral poliovirus vaccine (TOPV)
triviale
    Mycobacterium t.
trivialis
    Pseudomonas t.
trivittatus
    Aedes t.
Trizma buffer concentrate
TRIzol reagent
trizonal
TRK-A gene expression
tRNA
    transfer RNA
    tRNA suppressor
Troglotrema salmincola
Troglotrematidae
Troisier
    T. ganglion
    T. node
    T. syndrome
troitsensis
    Arenibacter t.
Trojan horse inhibitor
troleandomycin
Tröltsch corpuscle
Trombicula
    T. akamushi
    T. alfreddugesi
    T. autumnalis
    T. deliensis
    T. pallida
    T. scutellaris
    T. tsalsahuatl
trombiculiasis
Trombiculidae
trombiculid mite
Trombidiidae
Trombidoidea
tromethamine
tropeolin
trophedema
Tropheryma whipplei
trophic
    t. gangrene
    t. lesion
    t. nucleus
    t. signal
    t. ulcer
trophoblast
    t. basement membrane thickening
    t. cell
    syncytial t.

trophoblastic
    t. cell membrane
    t. disease
    t. embolization
    t. malignant teratoma
    malignant teratoma, t. (MTT)
    t. neoplasia
    t. neoplasm
    t. tumor
trophoblastoma
trophochromatin
trophochromidia
trophocyte
trophoderm
trophodermatoneurosis
trophoneurosis
    facial t.
    Romberg t.
trophoneurotic leprosy
trophonucleus
trophoplasm
trophoplast
trophospongium, pl. trophospongia
trophotaxis
trophozoite
tropica
    Herpetomonas t.
    Leishmania t.
    Nocardiopsis t.
tropical
    t. abscess
    t. anemia
    t. ataxic neuropathy (TAN)
    t. bubo
    t. diarrhea
    t. disease
    t. eosinophilia
    t. mask
    t. measles
    t. splenomegaly syndrome (TSS)
    t. sprue (TS)
    t. typhus
tropicalis
    Acetobacter t.
    adenitis t.
    Candida t.
Tropicorbis
tropicum
    granuloma inguinale t.
    papilloma inguinale t.
tropicus
    Amphibacillus t.
    Psychroflexus t.
tropism
    viral t.
tropocollagen
tropoelastin
tropomyosin
    alpha t.

tropomyosin-binding protein
troponin
    t. C (TnC)
    t. I (TnI)
    t. T (TnT)
trough
    synaptic t.
Trousseau
    T. syndrome
    T. test
Trousseau-Lallemand body
TRU
    turbidity-reducing unit
T₃RU
    triiodothyronine resin uptake
Truant auramine-rhodamine stain
Tru-Cut, Tru-cut, Trucut
    T.-C. biopsy
    T.-C. needle
true
    t. aneurysm
    t. diverticulum
    t. hypertrophy
    t. mucosal margin
    T. test kit
trueperi
    Thiobaca t.
TruGene HIV-1 genotyping kit
Trump fixative
truncate
Truncatella
truncation
truncatum
    Pseudamphistomum t.
truncus
    t. arteriosus
    t. fascicularis atrioventricularis
trunk
    t. abscess
    t. of atrioventricular bundle
    t. duplication
    pulmonary t.
TRUS
    transrectal ultrasound-guided sextant
    biopsy
truth table
TrxR
    thioredoxin reductase
trypan
    t. blue
    t. red
trypanicidal

trypanicide
trypanid
trypanocidal
trypanocide
Trypanoplasma
Trypanosoma
    T. ariarii
    T. avium
    T. brucei brucei
    T. brucei gambiense
    T. brucei rhodesiense
    T. castellani
    T. congolense
    T. cruzi
    T. dimorphon
    T. equinum
    T. equiperdum
    T. escomelis
    T. evansi
    T. hominis
    T. lewisi
    T. melophagium
    T. nigeriense
    T. rangeli
    T. simiae
    T. suis
    T. theileri
    T. triatomae
    T. ugandense
    T. vivax
trypanosomatid
Trypanosomatidae
trypanosome
trypanosomiasis
    African t.
    American t.
    Brazilian t.
    East African (Rhodesian) t.
    Gambian t.
    Rhodesian t.
trypanosomic
trypanosomicidal
trypanosomicide
trypanosomid
tryparsamide
Trypetidae
trypomastigote
trypsin
    t. assay
    t. digest technique
    fecal t.
    t. G-banding stain

T

NOTES

trypsin *(continued)*
    t. inhibitor
    stool t.
    t. test
trypsin-aldehyde-fuchsin (TAF)
trypsin-inhibitory capacity (TIC)
trypsinization
trypsinogen
tryptamine
tryptase
    t. immunostain
    mast cell t.
tryptic
    t. activity
    t. soy agar
trypticase
    t. soy agar (TSA)
    t. soy with agar broth
    t. soy yeast (TSY)
tryptone
tryptonemia
tryptophan (TP)
    t. challenge test
    t. load test
    t. malabsorption syndrome
tryptophanemia
tryptophanuria
tryptophyl
TS
    test solution
    total solids
    tropical sprue
TSA
    trypticase soy agar
    tyramide signal amplification
T₄SA
    thyroxine-specific activity
TSAH
    traumatic subarachnoid hemorrhage
TSB
    total serum bilirubin
TSC
    tuberous sclerosis complex
TSC1 gene
TSC2 gene
TSD
    Tay-Sachs disease
TSE
    transmissible spongiform encephalopathy
tsetse fly
TSF
    tissue-coding factor
TSH
    thyroid-stimulating hormone
        TSH assay
        TSH binding inhibitory
            immunoglobulin (TBII)
        TSH displacing antibody (TDA)
        TSH releasing hormone

        TSH stimulating test
        TSH stimulation test
TSHR
    thyrotropin-receptor antibody
TSH-RF
    thyroid-stimulating hormone-releasing
        factor
TSI
    thyroid-stimulating immunoglobulin
    triple sugar iron
        TSI agar
t-s mutation
TSNP
    two-step nested PCR
TSP
    total serum protein
TSPAP
    total serum prostatic acid phosphatase
TSR
    thyroid-to-serum ratio
TSS
    tropical splenomegaly syndrome
TSST1
    toxic shock syndrome toxin
TST
    tumor skin test
TSTA
    tumor-specific transplantation antigen
T-strain mycoplasma
Tsukamurella
    T. inchonensis
    T. paurometabola
    T. pulmonis
    T. spumae
    T. strandjordii
    T. tyrosinosolvens
    T. wratislaviensis
Tsukamurellaceae
Tsunami laser
T-suppressor cell
T-suppressor/cytotoxic subset marker
tsuruhatensis
    Delftia t.
tsutsugamushi
    t. disease
    t. fever
    Orientia t.
    Rickettsia t.
TSY
    trypticase soy yeast
TT
    thrombin time
    thymol turbidity
    total thyroxine
        TT virus
T₄/TBG ratio
TTD
    tissue tolerance dose

TTF-1
thyroid transcription factor-1
TTGE
temporal temperature gradient gel
electrophoresis
TTH
thyrotropic hormone
tritiated thymidine
TTI
time-tension index
tissue thromboplastin inhibition
TTI procedure
TTIT
tissue thromboplastin inhibition test
**T/T Mega advanced multifunction
microwave labstation**
T2 toxin
TTP
thrombotic thrombocytopenic purpura
TTP-HUS
thrombotic thrombocytopenic purpura
and hemolytic uremic syndrome
TTR
transthyretin
TTT
tolbutamide tolerance test
TTTS
twin-twin transfusion syndrome
T-tubular system
TTV
transfusion transmitted virus
TU
Todd unit
toxic unit
toxin unit
tuberculin unit
T₃U
triiodothyronine uptake
T₃U test
tub1 adenocarcinoma
tub2 adenocarcinoma
tuba, pl. **tubae**
t. acustica
t. auditiva
t. auditoria
t. eustachiana
laciniae tubae
tubaeforme
Ancylostoma t.
tubal
t. abortion

t. air cell of pharyngotympanic
tube
t. infantilism
t. pregnancy
t. tonsil
tubaria
tonsilla t.
tubariae
glandulae t.
tube
t. agglutination (TA)
ampulla of uterine t.
auditory t.
Babcock t.
capillary t.
t. cast
cathode ray t.
t. cell
ClearCRIT microhematocrit t.
Corvac integrated serum
separator t.
Craigie t.
t. culture
digestive t.
t. dilution test
discharge t.
Durham t.
electron multiplier t.
Eppendorf t.
eustachian t.
fermentation t.
Ferrein t.
fimbriae of uterine t.
germ t.
gland of eustachian t.
glow modulator t.
Greiner Vacuette coagulation
plastic t.
Hamamatzu high-sensitivity
photomultiplier t.
Hemochron P214 glass-activated
ACT t.
indicator t.
Isolator lysis-centrifugation t.
lateral plate of cartilaginous
auditory t.
LipoClear reagent t.
Luki aspirating t.
medial plate of cartilaginous
auditory t.
Mett test t.
microfuge t.

NOTES

tube (*continued*)
 mucous gland of auditory t.
 mycobacteria growth indicator t.
  (MGIT)
 NIXIE t.
 otopharyngeal t.
 pharyngotympanic t.
 photomultiplier t.
 t. precipitin (TP)
 pus t.
 roll t.
 SafeCrit microhematocrit t.
 Safetex t.
 sediment t.
 sedimentation t.
 sputum t.
 Takara Biomedicals Suprec t.
 test t.
 tubal air cell of
  pharyngotympanic t.
 Unopette t.
 Vacuette blood sample t.
 vacuum t.
 Veillon t.
 voltage-regulator t.
 Wintrobe hematocrit t.
tubeless
 t. gastric analysis
 t. gastric analysis test
tuber
tuberalis
 pars t.
tubercle
 anatomic t.
 anatomical t.
 Babès t.
 t. bacillus (TB)
 caseous t.
 dissection t.
 fibrous t.
 Ghon t.
 Ghon-Sachs t.
 hard t.
 hyaline t.
 Montgomery t.
 mycobacteria other than t. (MOTT)
 postmortem t.
 prosector's t.
 sebaceous t.
 soft t.
tubercula
 t. dolorosa
tubercular
tuberculate
tuberculated
tuberculation
tuberculid
 nodular t.
 papular t.

 papulonecrotic t.
 rosacea-like t.
tuberculin
 albumose-free t. (TAF)
 alkaline t. (TA)
 Büchner t.
 t. filtrate (TF)
 Koch old t.
 old t. (OT)
 t. precipitation (TP)
 purified protein derivative of t.
 t. reaction
 t. R (new tuberculin) (TR)
 Seibert t.
 t. skin test
 t. unit (TU)
 vacuum t. (VT)
tuberculin-type
 t.-t. hypersensitivity
 t.-t. reaction
tuberculitis
tuberculization
tuberculochemotherapeutic
tuberculocidal
tuberculoderma
tuberculofibroid
tuberculoid
 t. granuloma
 t. leprosy
tuberculoid-type granuloma
tuberculoma
tuberculoopsonic index
tuberculoprotein
tuberculosis (TB, TBC)
 acute miliary t.
 adult t.
 anthracotic t.
 arrested t.
 attenuated t.
 Bacillus t.
 basal t.
 central nervous system t.
 cerebral t.
 childhood type t.
 cutaneous t.
 t. cutis
 t. cutis luposa
 t. cutis orificialis
 t. cutis verrucosa
 dermal t.
 disseminated t.
 endobronchial t.
 extrapulmonary t.
 gastrointestinal t.
 general t.
 generalized t.
 t. granulation tissue
 healed t.
 inactive t.

laryngeal t.
t. lymphadenitis
miliary t.
Mycobacterium t. (MTB)
open t.
t. organisms in tissue section
pericardial t.
placental t.
pleural t.
postprimary t.
primary t.
pulmonary t.
reinfection t.
renal t.
respiratory t.
secondary t.
t. skin test
t. ulcerosa
urinary t.
t. vaccine
tuberculosis-respiratory disease (TB-RD)
tuberculostat
tuberculostatic
tuberculostearic acid
tuberculostearicum
    Corynebacterium t.
tuberculosus
lupus t.
tuberculous
t. abscess
t. bronchopneumonia
t. cystitis
t. gumma
t. infiltration
t. lymphadenitis
t. meningitis (TBM)
t. nephritis
t. osteomyelitis
t. pericarditis
t. peritonitis
t. prostatitis
t. rheumatism
t. scrofuloderma
t. spondylitis
t. wart
tuberculum, pl. **tubercula**
t. arthriticum
tubercula dolorosa
t. sebaceum
t. syphiliticum
tuberiferous
tuberin

tuberoeruptive xanthoma
tuberosa
urticaria t.
tuberosity
ischial t.
pubic t.
tibial t.
tuberosum
xanthoma t.
tuberous
tuberous sclerosis
tuberum
    Burkholderia t.
tubi (*pl. of* tubus)
Tubifera ferruginosa
tubocurarine
tuboendometrioid
t. metaplasia
t. type
tuboovarian
t. abscess (TOA)
t. varicocele
tuboovaritis
tuboreticular structure
tubovillous adenoma
tubular
t. adenocarcinoma
t. adenoma
t. adenosis
t. aggregate
t. aneurysm
t. basement membrane (TBM)
t. carcinoma
t. cristae
t. cyst
t. epithelial-myofibroblast transdifferentiation (TEMT)
t. fluid (TF)
t. gland
t. infiltration
t. nephrosis
t. pit
t. reabsorption
t. reabsorption of phosphate test
t. secretion
t. visual field
tubule
Albarrán y Dominguez t.
aluminal t.
connecting t.
convoluted seminiferous t.
dental t.

NOTES

1037

tubule *(continued)*
    dentin t.
    dentinal t.
    discharging t.
    t. formation
    Henle t.
    mesonephric t.
    metanephric t.
    renal uriniferous t.
    seminiferous t.
    sex cord tumor with annular t.
    spiral t.
    straight t.
    T t.
    t. of testis
    typical seminiferous t.
    uriniferous t.
tubuli (*pl. of* tubulus)
tubuliform
tubulin
    beta t.
tubulitis
tubuloacinar gland
tubuloalveolar mucous gland
tubulocyst
tubulocystic growth pattern
tubulodermoid
tubulointerstitial
    t. lesion
    t. nephritis
    t. nephropathy (TIN)
tubulonecrosis
tubuloneogenesis
tubulopapillary
    t. architectural pattern
    t. carcinoma
tubuloracemose
tubuloreticular aggregate
tubulorrhexis
tubulous, tubulose
tubulovesicle
tubulovesicular
tubulus, pl. **tubuli**
    tubuli biliferi
    tubuli contorti
    tubuli dentales
    tubuli epoophori
    tubuli galactophori
    tubuli lactiferi
    tubuli paroophori
    t. rectus
    t. renalis contortus
    tubuli seminiferi recti
    tubuli seminiferi recti testi
    t. transversus
tubus, pl. **tubi**
    t. digestorius
tucumana
    Mansonella t.

tuffstone body
tuft
    enamel t.
    glomerular t.·
    malpighian t.
    synovial t.
tufted
    t. cell
    t. phalanx
tufting enteropathy
tuftsin deficiency
TUG
    total urinary gonadotropin
tularemia
    t. agglutinin
    deerfly fever (t.)
    enteric t.
    oculoglandular t.
    oropharyngeal t.
    t. pneumonia
    pneumonia t.
    pneumonic t.
    rabbit fever (t.)
    t. sepsis
    typhoidal t.
    ulceroglandular t.
tularemic
    t. chancre
    t. conjunctivitis
    t. pneumonia
    t. sepsis
tularense
    Bacillus t.
tularensis
    Pasteurella t.
tumefacient
tumefaction
tumefactive fibroinflammatory lesion (TFL)
tumefy
tumentia
tumescence
tumescent
tumeur d'emblée
tumid
tumor
    Abrikosov t.
    acellular t.
    acinar cell t.
    acinic cell t.
    acute splenic t.
    adenoid t.
    adenomatoid odontogenic t.
    adipose t.
    adrenal t.
    adrenocortical rest t.
    adult granulosa cell t. (AGCT)
    ameloblastic adenomatoid t.
    ampullary t.

amyloid t.
aneuploid t.
t. aneuploidy
t. angiogenesis
t. angiogenic factor (TAF)
angiomatoid t.
t. antigen
aortic body t.
Askin t.
astrocytic t.
atypical carcinoid t.
atypical teratoid t. (ATT)
atypical teratoid/rhabdoid t.
  (AT/RT)
basaloid t.
Bednar t.
benign epithelial breast t.
biphasic t.
bladder t. (BT)
blood t.
blue cell t.
t. blush
Bolande t.
bone t.
borderline ovarian t.
brain t. (BT)
brainstem t.
breast t.
Brenner t.
bronchogenic t.
Brooke t.
brown t.
Brown-Pearce t.
t. burden
Burkitt t.
burnt-out germ cell t.
Buschke-Löwenstein t.
calcifying epithelial odontogenic t.
  (CEOT)
t. of Capella
t. capsule
carcinoid t.
carotid body t.
t. cell
t. cell kinetics
t. cell motility
t. cell population
cellular t.
central nervous system t.
cerebellar t.
cerebellopontine angle t.
chemoreceptor t.

chiasmal t.
chondromatous giant cell t.
chromaffin t.
chromophobe t.
clear cell borderline t.
clear cell sugar t.
Codman t.
collision t.
colon t.
compound t.
connective t.
cutaneous neural t. (CNT)
Dabska t.
dendritic cell t.
dentigerous mixed t.
dermal duct t.
dermoid t.
desmoid t.
desmoplastic small round cell t.
  (DSRCT)
diploid t.
ductectatic-type mucinous cystic t.
ductus deferens t.
dysembryoplastic neuroepithelial t.
dysplastic neuroepithelial t. (DNET)
eccrine t.
ectomesenchymal chondromyxoid t.
  (ECT)
Ehrlich t.
eighth nerve t.
t. embolism
t. embolus
embryonal t.
embryonic t.
endobronchial t.
endocervical mucinous borderline t.
  (EMBLT, EMBT)
endodermal sinus t.
endometrioid t.
epithelial-stromal t.
Erdheim t.
esophageal t.
Ewing sarcoma family of t.'s
  (ESFT)
Ewing sarcoma/peripheral
  neuroectodermal t.
Ewing sarcoma/primitive
  neuroectodermal t. (EWS/PNET)
extracapsular t.
extragonadal germ cell t.
extrarenal rhabdoid t. (ERRT)

T

NOTES

tumor *(continued)*
extrauterine-extraovarian
  endometrioid stromal t.
exuberant t.
eye t.
fallopian tube t.
fecal t.
Fechner t.
feminizing t.
fibroid t.
Fuhrman grade t.
functional t.
gastric t.
gastrointestinal autonomic nerve t.
  (GANT)
gastrointestinal pacemaker cell t.
  (GIPACT)
gastrointestinal smooth muscle t.
gastrointestinal stromal t. (GIST)
G-cell t.
gemistocytic t.
germ cell t.
t. of germ cell origin
giant cell t.
giant cell t. of bone (GCTB)
giant cell t. of lung
giant cell t. of tendon sheath
  (GCTTS)
globoid encapsulated t.
glomus jugulare t.
Godwin t.
gonadal stromal t.
t. grading
granular cell t.
granulosa cell t.
granulosa-stromal cell t.
granulosa-theca cell t.
Grawitz t.
Gubler t.
hamartomatous t.
heart t.
hepatic t.
heterologous t.
hilar cell t. of ovary
histoid t.
homologous t.
Hürthle cell t.
hyalinizing trabecular t.
hylic t.
inflammatory fibromyxoid t.
inflammatory myofibroblastic t.
  (IMT)
innocent t.
interdigitating dendritic cell t.
interstitial cell t. of testis
intestinal mucinous borderline t.
  (IMBT)
intracranial t.

intraductal papillary mucinous t.
  (IPMT)
intratesticular t.
intravascular sclerosing
  bronchioloalveolar t. (IVBAT)
islet cell t.
juvenile granulosa cell t. (JGCT)
juxtaglomerular cell t. (JGCT)
Koenen t.
Krukenberg t.
lacrimal gland t.
lacrimal sac t.
Landschutz t.
large-cell calcifying Sertoli cell t.
  (LCCSCT)
t. lethal dose (TLD)
Lewis lung t.
Leydig cell t.
Leydig-Sertoli cell t.
Lindau t.
lipophyllodes t.
localized fibrous t. (LFT)
low-risk t. (LRT)
lung t.
luteinizing t.
Lynch syndrome t.
t. lysis syndrome (TLS)
malignant breast t.
malignant cartilaginous t.
malignant giant cell t. (MGCT)
malignant mixed t. (MMT)
malignant mixed mesodermal t.
  (MMMT)
malignant mixed müllerian t.
  (MMMT)
malignant peripheral nerve sheath t.
  (MPNST)
malignant plasma cell t.
malignant rhabdoid t. (MRT)
malignant triton t. (MTT)
malignant vascular t.
t. map
t. marker
t. marker test
Masson t.
mast cell t.
mediastinal yolk sac t. (MYST)
melanotic neuroectodermal t.
melanotic neuroectodermal t. of
  infancy
Merkel cell t.
mesenchymal t.
mesonephroid t.
metanephric stromal t.
metastatic t.
t. mitotic rate
mixed epithelial t.
mixed epithelial-mesenchymal t.
mixed germ cell t. (MGCT)

mixed mesodermal t.
mixed t. of salivary gland
mixed t. of skin
monoclonal t.
mucinous borderline t. (MBT)
mucinous cystic t. (MCT)
mucoepidermoid t.
müllerian t.
multiple t.
myofibroblastic mammary stromal t.
napkin ring t.
necrosis t.
t. necrosis
t. necrosis factor (TNF)
t. necrosis factor alpha (TNF alpha)
t. necrosis factor beta (TNF beta)
Nelson t.
t. nest
neuroectodermal t.
neuroendocrine t. (NET)
no evidence of primary t. (T0)
nomenclature of t.
nonmyogenous t.
nonseminomatous germ cell t. (NSGCT)
odontogenic ghost cell t.
oil t.
oligodendroglial t.
oncocytic hepatocellular t.
orbital t.
organoid t.
ovarian borderline t.
ovarian granulosa cell t.
ovarian mucinous t. (OMT)
ovarian serous borderline t. (OSBT)
ovarian sex-cord t.
Pancoast t.
pancreatic duct-acinar-endocrine cell t.
pancreatic duct-endocrine cell t.
papillary t.
paraffin t.
parathyroid t.
pearl t.
peripheral nerve sheath t. (PNST)
peripheral neuroectodermal t. (PNET)
peritoneal borderline t.
perivascular epithelioid cell t. (PEComa)
phantom t.

phyllodes t.
pilar t. of scalp
Pindborg t.
pituitary t.
placental site trophoblastic t. (PSTT)
pleomorphic hyalinizing angiectatic t. (PHAT)
polyclonal t.
t. polysaccharide substance (TPS)
polyvesicular vitelline t.
pontine angle t.
potato t. of neck
primary bone t.
(primary) t., (regional lymph) nodes, (remote) metastases (TNM)
primitive neuroectodermal t. (PNET)
primitive peripheral neuroectodermal t. (pPNET)
primitive small-cell thoracopulmonary t.
t. progression marker
proliferating pillar t.
t. promoter
prostatic t.
pseudosarcomatous fibromyxoid t.
pseudosarcomatous myofibroblastic t. (PMT)
pulmonary endodermal t. (PET)
pure t.
Rathke pouch t.
Recklinghausen t.
rectal shelf t.
t. registry
renal t.
renin secreting t.
renomedullary interstitial cell t.
rete cell t.
retiform Sertoli-Leydig cell t.
retinal anlage t.
retrocardiac t.
retrosternal t.
Rous t.
salivary gland t.
salivary gland anlage t. (SGAT)
sand t.
sarcomatoid t.
sclerosing Sertoli cell t.
serous borderline t. (SBT)
Sertoli cell t.
Sertoli-Leydig cell t.

T

NOTES

tumor *(continued)*
Sertoli stromal cell t.
sex cord-stromal t.
t. signature
sinonasal smooth muscle cell t.
t. in situ (TIS)
skin t.
t. skin test (TST)
small cell t.
small intestine t.
small round cell t. (SRCT)
smooth muscle t. (SMT)
soft parts giant cell t. (SP-GCT)
soft tissue t.
solid pseudopapillary t.
solitary fibrous t. (SFT)
t. specificity
spinal cord t.
spindle cell t.
splenic t.
squamous odontogenic t.
t. stage
t. stage at diagnosis
t. staging
steroid cell t.
stomach t.
t. stroma
sugar t.
superior pulmonary sulcus t.
superior sulcus t.
t. suppressor gene
t. suppressor pathway
surface epithelial-stromal t.
sweat gland t.
synovial t.
tenosynovial giant cell t.
teratoid t.
testicular germ cell t. (TGCT)
testicular Sertoli cell t.
tetraploid t.
theca cell-granuloma cell t.
theca lutein t.
thrombus t.
t. thrombus
thymic carcinoid t. (TCT)
t. of thymic epitheliocyte
thyroid t.
transitional cell t.
triton t.
trophoblastic t.
turban t.
ulcerogenic t.
urethral t.
uterine tumor resembling an
  ovarian sex-cord t. (UTROSCT)
vaginal t.
villous t.
t. virus
vulvar t.

Warthin t.
Wharton t.
WHO histologic classification of
  ovarian t.'s
Wilms t.
xenograft t.
xenografted t.
Yaba t.
yolk sac t.
Zollinger-Ellison t.
tumoraffin
tumoral calcinosis
tumor-antigen 4 (TA-4)
**tumor-assisted lymphoid proliferation
  (TALP)**
tumor-associated
t.-a. glycoprotein (TAG)
t.-a. rejection antigen (TARA)
t.-a. transplantation antigen (TATA)
**tumor-cell migration-inhibition factor
  (TMIF)**
tumorigenesis
foreign body t.
tumorigenic
tumorigenicity
tumor-induced stromal sclerosis
tumor-infiltrating lymphocyte (TIL)
tumorlet
tumor-like lesion
tumor-node-metastasis (TNM)
tumorous
**tumor-specific transplantation antigen
  (TSTA)**
tumor-suppressor protein
tundrae
Acetobacterium t.
TUNEL
TdT-mediated dUTP nick-end labeling
  TUNEL assay
Tunga penetrans
tungiasis
Tungidae
Tungrovirus
tungstate
lithium t.
tungsten
t. arc lamp
t. carbide pneumoconiosis
t. halogen lamp
tungstic acid
tungstoborate
sodium t.
tunic
Bichat t.
Brücke t.
circular layer of muscular t.
corneoscleral t.
longitudinal layer of muscular t.
mucosal t.

muscular t.
serous t.
tunica, pl. **tunicae**
   t. adventitia
   t. albuginea
   t. albuginea corporis spongiosi
   t. albuginea corporum cavernosorum
   t. albuginea oculi
   t. albuginea testis
   t. carnea
   t. conjunctiva
   t. conjunctiva bulbi
   t. conjunctiva palpebrarum
   t. dartos
   t. elastica
   t. externa
   t. externa oculi
   t. externa thecae folliculi
   t. extima
   t. fibrosa
   t. fibrosa bulbi
   t. fibrosa hepatis
   t. fibrosa lienis
   t. fibrosa renis
   t. fibrosa splenis
   t. interna thecae folliculi
   t. intima
   t. media
   t. media of arteriole
   t. mucosa
   t. mucosa bronchi
   t. mucosa cavitatis tympani
   t. mucosa coli
   t. mucosa ductus deferentis
   t. mucosa esophagi
   t. mucosa gastrica
   t. mucosa intestini tenuis
   t. mucosa laryngis
   t. mucosa linguae
   t. mucosa nasi
   t. mucosa oris
   t. mucosa pharyngis
   t. mucosa tracheae
   t. mucosa tubae auditivae
   t. mucosa tubae uterinae
   t. mucosa ureteris
   t. mucosa urethrae femininae
   t. mucosa uteri
   t. mucosa vaginae
   t. mucosa vesicae biliaris
   t. mucosa vesicae felleae
   t. mucosa vesicae urinariae

   t. muscularis
   t. muscularis bronchiorum
   t. muscularis coli
   t. muscularis ductus deferentis
   t. muscularis esophagi
   t. muscularis intestini tenuis
   t. muscularis recti
   t. muscularis tracheae
   t. muscularis tubae uterinae
   t. muscularis ureteris
   t. muscularis urethrae femininae
   t. muscularis uteri
   t. muscularis vaginae
   t. muscularis ventriculi
   t. muscularis vesicae biliaris
   t. muscularis vesicae felleae
   t. muscularis vesicae urinariae
   t. nervea
   t. propria
   t. propria corii
   t. propria lienis
   t. reflexa
   regio olfactoria tunicae
   t. sclerotica
   t. serosa
   t. serosa coli
   t. serosa hepatis
   t. serosa intestini tenuis
   t. serosa peritonei
   t. serosa tubae uterinae
   t. serosa uteri
   t. serosa ventriculi
   t. serosa vesicae biliaris
   t. serosa vesicae felleae
   t. serosa vesicae urinariae
   t. submucosa
   t. vaginalis
   t. vaginalis testis
   t. vasculosa
   t. vasculosa bulbi
   t. vasculosa lentis
   t. vasculosa oculi
   t. vasculosa testis
   t. vitrea
tunicae
   t. funiculi spermatici
tunnel
   t. cell
   Corti t.
turban
   t. growth
   t. tumor

NOTES

Turbatrix aceti
turbid
turbidimeter
turbidimetric
  t. aggregometry
  t. immunoassay
turbidimetry
turbidity
  thymol t. (TT)
turbidity-reducing unit (TRU)
turbinal varix
turcica
  Borrelia t.
Türck degeneration
Turcot syndrome
turgescence
turgescent
turgid
turicata
  Ornithodoros t.
turicatae
  Borrelia t.
turicensis
  Paenibacillus t.
Turicibacter sanguinis
Türk
  T. cell
  T. irritation leukocyte
turkey
  bluecomb disease of t.'s
  t. meningoencephalitis virus
  T. red
turkmenica
  Haloterrigena t.
Turlock virus
turn-around time (TAT)
Turnbull
  T. blue
  T. blue stain
turnerae
  Teredinibacter t.
Turner syndrome
turnover
  bone t.
  t. number
  phophoinositide t.
  plasma iron t. (PIT)
  protein t.
  T-cell t.
TURP
  transurethral resection of prostate
  TURP chip
turpentine oil
turricephaly
TV
  tidal volume
TWAR
  Taiwan acute respiratory
  TWAR stain

twiddler's syndrome
twig
  motor axon t.
twin
  t. cone
  conjoined t.'s
  corpora lutea t.'s
  t. crystal
  dichorionic placenta t.'s
  dizygotic t.'s
  fraternal t.'s
  heterokaryotic t.'s
  identical t.'s
  incomplete conjoined t.'s
  monoamniotic placenta t.'s
  monochorionic diamniotic
    placenta t.'s
  monozygotic t.'s
  parasitic t.'s
  t. placenta
  placenta t.'s
  Siamese t.'s
twin-to-twin transfusion syndrome
twin-twin transfusion syndrome (TTTS)
TWL
  transepidermal water loss
two-cell
  t.-c. wide vertical cord
two-cell type rule
two-dimensional (2D)
  t.-d. chromatography
  t.-d. gel electrophoresis
  t.-d. immunoelectrophoresis
  t.-d. polyacrylamide gel
    electrophoresis
two-glass test
two-parameter histogram
Twort-d'Herelle phenomenon
Twort phenomenon
two's complement
two-sided alternative
two-site immunoenzymometric assay
two-slide method
two-stage PT test
two-step nested PCR (TSNP)
two-tail test
two-tube nested PCR
Ty
  typhoid
TY1-S-33 medium
tylosis, pl. tyloses
  t. palmaris et plantaris
Tymovirus
tympani
  membrana t.
  stratum circulare membranae t.
  stratum cutaneum membranae t.
  stratum radiatum membranae t.

substantia propria membranae t.
tunica mucosa cavitatis t.

tympanic
t. body
t. cell
t. gland
t. lip of limbus of spiral lamina
t. membrane
t. wall of cochlear duct

tympanicae
cellulae t.

tympanosclerosis

tympanum
membrane of t.

Tyndall effect

tyndallization

type
t. II alveolar epithelial cell
t. II alveolar epithelial cell
adenocarcinoma
atypical melanocytic nevi of
genital t. (AMNGT)
t. 1 bare lymphocyte syndrome
B cell lymphoma of MALT t.
blood t.
t. I cell
t. C nevus cell
t. I–XX collagen
t. I collagen gene
t. culture
t. I–IV delayed-type reaction
t. 1–4 dextrocardia
Duffy blood antibody t.
t. I, II dysgammaglobulinemia
t. I, II error
t. V glycogenosis
hyperplasia of usual t. (HUT)
t. I–IV hypersensitivity reaction
hypertyrosinemia, Oregon t.
intratubular germ cell neoplasia,
unclassified t. (IGCNU)
Kell body antibody t.
Kidd blood antibody t.
Lutheran blood antibody t.
membrane t. 1–6
t. II membranoproliferative
glomerulonephritis
mixed epithelial papillary
cystadenoma of borderline
malignancy of müllerian t.
(MEBMM)
no specific t. (NST)

t. species
t. strain
tuboendometrioid t.
wild t.

Typenex blood-recipient identification system

typhi
Bacillus t.
Eberthella t.
Rickettsia t.

typhimurium
Salmonella enteritidis serotype *t.*

typhinia

typhlectasis

typhlitis

Typhlocoelum cucumerinum

typhlomegaly

typhlonius
Helicobacter t.

typhoid (Ty)
t. bacillus
t. bacteriophage
t. cholera
t. enteritis
t. fever
t. immunization reaction
t., paratyphoid A, and paratyphoid
B (TAB)
provocation t.
t. septicemia

typhoidal tularemia

typhoid-paratyphoid A and B vaccine

typholysin

typhosepsis

typhosus
Bacillus t.

typhous

typhus
t. antibody test
endemic murine t.
t. epidemic
epidemic louse-borne t.
louse-borne t.
mite t.
murine t.
recrudescent t.
scrub t.
tropical t.
t. vaccine

typical
t. seminiferous tubule
t. smooth muscle cell

T

NOTES

typing
> ABO t.
> ABO-Rh t.
> bacteriophage t.
> blood t.
> forward blood t.
> HLA t.
> molecular t.
> primed lymphocyte t.
> reverse blood t.
> Rh t.
> $Rh_o(D)$ t.
> sequenced-based t. (SBT)
> tissue t.

tyramide signal amplification (TSA)
tyramine test
Tyroglyphidae
Tyroglyphus
> *T. longior*
> *T. siro*

tyroid
tyroketonuria
tyroma
Tyromyces
tyropanoate sodium
Tyrophagus putrescentiae
tyrosinase deficiency
tyrosine
> t. assay

> t. crystal
> t. hydroxylase (TH)
> kinase t. (KIT)
> t. kinase receptor
> t. phosphorylation
> t. test

tyrosinemia
> hereditary t.

tyrosinosis
tyrosinosolvens
> *Tsukamurella t.*

tyrosinuria
tyrosis
tyrosyl
tyrosyl-RNA synthetase
tyrosyluria
tyrothricin
TYSGM-9 medium
Tyson gland
Tyzzer disease
Tyzzeria
TZ
> transition zone

Tzanck
> T. cell
> T. smear
> T. test

T-zone dysplasia

U
    unit
        U fiber
U6 riboprobe
UA
    uric acid
    urinalysis
    uterine aspiration
        PocketChem UA
UACL
    ulcer associated cell lineage
UADT
    upper aerodigestive tract
UBBC
    unsaturated vitamin B_{12}-binding capacity
uberis
        Streptococcus u.
UBF
    uterine blood flow
UBG
    urobilinogen
UBI
    ultraviolet blood irradiation
ubiq
    ubiquitin
ubiquinol
ubiquinone
ubiquitin (ubiq)
        u. C-terminal hydrolase
        u. ligase
ubiquitinated inclusion
ubiquitination
ubiquitin-protease pathway
ubiquitin-proteasome system (UPS)
ubisemiquinone
ubonensis
        Burkholderia u.
UBT
    urea breath test
UC
    ulcerative colitis
    ultracentrifugal
UcA
    urothelial carcinoma
U-cell lymphoma
UCG
    urinary chorionic gonadotropin
UCHL1 antibody
UCHL1ᵃ antibody
UCL3D3 antibody
UCP
    urinary coproporphyrin
Ucr
    concentration of creatinine in urine

UD
    urethral discharge
UDCA
    ursodeoxycholic acid
Udeniomyces
UDG
    uracil DNA glycosylase
UDP
    uridine diphosphate
    urine drug panel
UDP-*N*-acetyl-ᴅ-galactosamine
UDP-*N*-acetyl-ᴅ-glucosamine
UDP-galactose
UDP-glucose
UDP-glucose-hexose-1-phosphate
        UDP-g.-h.-p. uridylyltransferase
        UDP-g.-h.-p. uridylyltransferase
        assay
UDP-glucuronate
UDP-glucuronic acid
UDP-glucuronyl transferase
UDP-ʟ-iduronate
UDP-iduronic acid
UDP-xylose
UDS
    urine drug screen
UE
    Ulex europaeus
UEC
    uterine endometrial carcinoma
Uehlinger syndrome
UF
    ulcerating form
UFA
    unesterified fatty acid
Uffelmann test
U-fiber
        cortical U-f.
Uganda S virus
ugandense
        Trypanosoma u.
UGI
    upper gastrointestinal
Uhl anomaly
UIBC
    unsaturated iron-binding capacity
UIF
    undegraded insulin factor
UIP
    usual interstitial pneumonia
    usual interstitial pneumonitis
UJ127.11 antibody
UJ13A monoclonal antibody
UL
    undifferentiated lymphoma

U

ulcer
- acute hemorrhagic u.
- amebic u.
- amputating u.
- aphthous ileal u.
- u. associated cell lineage (UACL)
- Bairnsdale u.
- Barrett u.
- Buruli u.
- chancroidal u.
- chiclero u.
- chronic u.
- chronic decubitus u. zone I, II
- cockscomb u.
- cold u.
- constitutional u.
- corneal u.
- creeping u.
- Cruveilhier u.
- Curling u.
- Cushing u.
- decubitus u.
- diabetic u.
- diphtheritic u.
- discoid u.
- distention u.
- duodenal u.
- elusive u.
- Fenwick-Hunner u.
- focal u.
- gastric u. (GU)
- groin u.
- gummatous u.
- hard u.
- healed u.
- hemorrhagic u.
- herpetic u.
- Hunner u.
- indolent u.
- inflamed u.
- Kocher dilatation u.
- linear u.
- Lipschütz u.
- lupoid u.
- marginal u.
- Marjolin u.
- Meleney u.
- penetrating u.
- peptic u. (PU)
- perambulating u.
- perforated gastric u.
- perforating u.
- phagedenic u.
- phlegmonous u.
- rodent u.
- Saemisch u.
- sea anemone u.
- serpiginous u.
- simple u.
- sloughing u.
- soft u.
- stasis u.
- stercoraceous u.
- stercoral u.
- stomal u.
- stress u.
- Sutton u.
- symptomatic u.
- syphilitic u.
- trophic u.
- varicose u.
- venereal u.
- warty u.
- Zambesi u.

ulcera (*pl. of* ulcus)

ulcerans
- *Corynebacterium u.*
- *Mycobacterium u.*

ulcerate

ulceration
- aphthous u.
- crateriform u.
- diffuse u.

ulcerative
- u. colitis (UC)
- u. cystitis
- u. dermatosis
- u. inflammation
- u. scrofuloderma

ulcerogenic tumor

ulceroglandular tularemia

ulceromembranous

ulcerosa
- blepharitis u.
- tuberculosis u.

ulcerous

ULCL4D12 antibody

ulcus, pl. **ulcera**
- u. ambulans
- u. terebrans
- u. venereum
- u. vulvae acutum

ulegyria

ulerythema ophryogenes

Ulex
- *U. europaeus* (UE)
- *U. europaeus* agglutinin
- *U. lectin*

uli
- *Olsenella u.*

uliginosa
- *Cellulophaga u.*
- *Zobellia u.*

uliginosum
- *Clostridium u.*

Ullmann line

Ullrich-Feichtiger syndrome

Ullrich-Turner syndrome

ulmi
  Xylanibacterium u.
ULMS
  uterine leiomyosarcoma
ULN
  upper limits of normal
ulnar nerve entrapment
Ulocladium chartarum
ulodermatitis
uloid
ULT
  ultra low temperature
  -86C ULT freezer
Ultima II refrigerator system
ultimate principle
ultimobranchial body
ultimum moriens
ultracentrifugal (UC)
ultracentrifugation
  preparative u.
  sucrose density gradient u.
ultracentrifuge
  Airfuge u.
  analytic u.
  Discovery SE u.
  Optima L-XP, L-90 K, LE-80 K
   preparative u.
  Optima Max, Max-E, TLX
   personal benchtop u.
ultracytostome
ultradian rhythm
ultrafast Pap stain
ultrafilter
ultrafiltrate of the blood plasma
ultrafiltration hemodialyzer
ultrahigh vacuum
ultra low temperature (ULT)
ultramicroanalysis
ultramicroscope
ultramicroscopic
ultramicrotome
ultramicrotomy
ultrashort-segment Hirschsprung disease
ultrasonic
  u. cell disrupter
  u. microscope
  u. nebulizer (USN)
ultrasonication
ultrasonography
  endoscopic u.
  transrectal u.

ultrasound
  intravascular coronary u.
ultrastructural
  u. anatomy
  u. characteristic
  u. difference
  u. immunochemistry
  u. morphology of bone mineral
  u. study
ultrastructure
ultrathin section
ultra-trace element
ultraviolet
  u. blood irradiation (UBI)
  u. burn
  u. fluorescent dosimeter
  u. irradiation
  u. light
  u. light-induced mutation
  u. microscope
  u. radiation
ultraviolet/visible spectrophotometry
ultravirus
ultropaque method
ulvae
  Pseudoalteromonas u.
Ulvibacter litoralis
Ulysses syndrome
umbilical
  u. cord blood transplant
  u. cyst
  u. fistula
  u. hernia
  u. polyp
Umbravirus
umbrella cell
Umbre virus
umidischolae
  Nocardiopsis u.
UMP
  undetermined malignant potential
umsongensis
  Pseudomonas u.
UN
  urea nitrogen
UNa
  concentration of sodium in urine
unaggregated
unamae
  Burkholderia u.
unattended laboratory operation

U

NOTES

unbiased estimate
unbound thyroxine-binding globulin (UTBG)
unbranched simple tubular exocrine gland
uncal herniation
uncertainty principle
uncia
Uncinaria
    U. americana
    U. duodenalis
uncinariasis
uncinate epilepsy
Uncinocarpus
unclassified
    arbovirus group u.
    carcinoma in situ/intratubular germ cell neoplasia u. (CIS/ITGCNU)
uncoded amino acid
uncommon developmental disorder
uncompensated
    u. acidosis
    u. alkalosis
uncomplemented
unconditional jump
unconjugated
    u. bilirubin
    u. estriol
    u. hyperbilirubinemia
uncontained criticality
uncontrolled fission
uncoossified
uncoupler
    oxidative phosphorylation u.
unctuous
undae
    Exiguobacterium u.
undecaprenol phosphate
undegraded insulin factor (UIF)
underflow
underlying cause of death
underphosphorylated protein expression
understain
Underwood disease
undescended testis
undetermined
    u. nitrogen
undiagnosing consultation
undicola
    Rhizobium u.
undifferentiated
    u. adenocarcinoma
    u. cell
    u. cell adenoma
    u. connective tissue syndrome
    u. epidermoid carcinoma
    u. lymphoma (UL)
    u. malignant teratoma
    malignant teratoma, u. (MTU)

    u. osteosarcoma (UOS)
    u. sarcoma
    u. squamous cell carcinoma
    u. type fever
undifferentiation
undosum
    Heliobacterium u.
Undritz anomaly
undulans
    Entamoeba u.
undulant fever
undulate
undulating
    u. edges colony
    u. membrane
undulipodium
unequal
    u. crossing over
    u. crossing over model
unesterified fatty acid (UFA)
UNG
    uracil-N-glycosylase
unglycosylated
unguis, onyx, pl. **ungues,** pl. **onyches**
    sinus u.
    stratum corneum u.
    stratum germinativum u.
    sulcus matricis u.
    vallecula u.
unguium
    achromia u.
    dystrophia u.
unheated
    u. serum reagin (USR)
    u. serum reagin test
uniaxial
Unibacteria
Uniblue A
unicameral bone cyst
UniCel Dxl 800 immunoassay system
unicellular
    u. gland
    u. sclerosis
unicentral
unicentric blastoma
unicornis uterus
unicystic ameloblastoma
unidirectional
uniflagellate
UniFluidics
unifocal eosinophilic granuloma
uniforate
uniform
unigene database
uniglandular
Uni-Gold
    U.-G. *H. pylori* test
    U.-G. Recombigen HIV test
unijunction transistor

unilaminar primary follicle
unilateral renal agenesis
unilobar
unilocular
    u. echinococcosis
    u. fat
    u. hydatid cyst
unimodal peak
uninuclear
uninvolved artery
union
    faulty u.
    primary u.
    secondary u.
    vicious u.
unionized hemoglobin (HHb)
uniovular
unipapillary
uniparental disomy (UPD)
unipolar
    u. cell
    u. neuron
    u. neuron of dorsal root ganglion
uniport
unipotential
unirenicular
uniseptate
Unistat bilirubinometer
unit (U)
    absolute system of u.'s
    alexin u.
    Allen-Doisy u.
    alpha u.
    amboceptor u.
    androgen u.
    antigen u.
    antitoxin u. (AU)
    atomic mass u. (amu)
    atomic weight u. (awu)
    base u.
    Behnken u. (R)
    Bessey-Lowry u. (BLU)
    Bethesda u. (BU)
    biological standard u.
    bird u.
    BLB u.
    Bodansky u. (BU)
    Bowers-McComb u.
    British thermal u. (BTU)
    cat u.
    u. cell
    central processing u.

    CGS u.
    chlorophyll u.
    chorionic gonadotropin u.
    Clauberg u.
    colony-forming u. (CFU)
    complement u.
    Corner-Allen u.
    corpus luteum hormone u.
    Dam u.
    dial u.
    digitalis u.
    diphtheria antitoxin u.
    dog u.
    Ehrlich u. (EU)
    electromagnetic u. (emu)
    electrostatic u. (ESU)
    enzyme u. (EU)
    epidermal-melanin u.
    equine gonadotropin u.
    estradiol benzoate u.
    estrone u.
    Fishman-Lerner u.
    Florey u.
    flotation u.
    G u. of streptomycin
    Gutman u.
    Hazardous Materials Response U. (HMRU)
    heat u. (HU)
    hemagglutinating u. (HU)
    hemolysin u.
    hemolytic u.
    hemorrhagin u.
    heparin u.
    Holzknecht u. (H)
    Hounsfield u. (H)
    Howell u.
    hyperemia u. (HU)
    immunizing u. (IU)
    u. inheritance
    insulin u.
    u. of intermedin
    international u. (IU)
    International benzoate u. (IBU)
    International System of U.'s (SI)
    Jenner-Kay u.
    kallikrein-inhibiting u. (KIU)
    Karmen u. (KU)
    King u.
    King-Armstrong u. (KAU)
    L u. of streptomycin
    lung u.

U

NOTES

unit *(continued)*

u. of luteinizing activity
Mache u. (MU)
map u.
u. of mass
u. membrane
meter-kilogram-second u.
Mett u.
minimal hemolytic u.
MKS u.
mobile chilling u.
Montevideo u. (MU)
mouse u. (MU)
mouse uterine u. (MUU)
Oxford u.
u. of oxytocin
pantothenic acid u.
u. of penicillin
pepsin u.
peripheral resistance u. (PRU)
phosphatase u.
physiologic u.
plaque-forming u. (PFU)
u. of progestational activity
progesterone u.
prolactin u.
protein nitrogen u. (PNU)
radiation measuring u.
rat u. (RU)
RcoF u.
Reitland-Franklin u.
resistance u. (RU)
riboflavin u.
Russell u.
Sherman u.
Sherman-Bourquin u. of vitamin B$_2$
Sherman-Munsell u.
Shinowara-Jones-Reinhard u.
Sibley-Lehninger u.
SJR u.
skin test u. (STU)
SL u.
Somogyi u.
S u. of streptomycin
Steenbock u.
streptomycin u.
sudanophobic u.
technical advisory response u. (TARU)
terminal duct lobular u. (TDLU)
tetanus antitoxin u.
thiamine chloride u.
thiamine hydrochloride u.
u. of thyrotrophic activity
Todd u. (TU)
toxic u. (TU)
toxin u. (TU)
transcription u.
tuberculin u. (TU)

turbidity-reducing u. (TRU)
u. of vasopressin
vitamin A u.
vitamin B$_1$ hydrochloride u.
vitamin B$_2$ u.
vitamin B$_6$ u.
vitamin C u.
vitamin D u.
vitamin E u.
vitamin K u.
u. of wavelength
u. of weight
Wohlgemuth u.

unitarian hypothesis
United States Army Medical Research Institute of Infectious Disease (USAMRIID)
unit-erythroid

burst-forming u.-e. (BFU-E)
colony-forming u.-e. (CFU-E)

uniting

u. canal
u. cartilage
u. duct

unit-megakaryocyte

colony-forming u.-m. (CFU-Meg)

units/mL

colony-forming u./mL (CFU/mL)

unit-spleen

colony-forming u.-s. (CFU-S)

univalent antibody
univariate analysis
universal

u. donor
U. ISH detection kit
u. leukoreduction
u. precautions

universale

melasma u.

universalis

adiposis u.
alopecia u.
calcinosis u.

univitelline
unknown

u. etiology
u. radioactivity

unmasking

enzymatic antigen u.
epitope u.

unmedullated
unmyelinated

u. axon
u. fiber

Unna

U. cell
U. disease
U. mark
U. stain

Unna-Pappenheim stain
Unna-Taenzer stain
Unopette
    U. system
    U. tube
unorganized virus
unpredictable hypersensitivity-like
  reaction
unrearranged germline
unresolved
    u. hepatitis
    u. lobar pneumonia
unresponsiveness
    immunologic u.
unrest
    nuclear u.
unsaturated
    u. hydrocarbon
    u. iron-binding capacity (UIBC)
    u. vitamin B_{12}-binding capacity
    (UBBC)
unsealed
    u. beta gamma source
    u. radioactive source
unspun peripheral blood
unstable
    u. hemoglobin
    u. hemoglobin disease
    u. hemoglobin hemolytic anemia
    u. trinucleotide repeat sequences
unstriated muscle
ununited fracture
unusual isolates/fastidious organisms
Unverricht disease
unwinding protein
UOS
    undifferentiated osteosarcoma
UP
    uniformly positive
    uroporphyrin
U:P
    urine-plasma ratio
up
    colony stands up
UP1a uroplakin gene
UP1b uroplakin gene
UPII
    uroplakin II
      UPII gene
UPIII
    uroplakin III
      UPIII gene

uPA
    urokinase plasminogen activator
uPAR
    urokinase plasminogen activator receptor
Up-Converting Phosphor technology
  (UPT)
UPD
    uniparental disomy
UPEP
    urine protein electrophoresis
UPG
    uroporphyrinogen
UPI
    uteroplacental insufficiency
UP*link* point of care sample testing
  system
upper
    u. aerodigestive tract (UADT)
    u. anal canal
    u. gastrointestinal (UGI)
    u. limits of normal (ULN)
    u. motor neuron
    u. respiratory disease (URD)
    u. respiratory infection (URI)
    u. respiratory tract infection
    (URTI)
up-regulation
UPS
    ubiquitin-proteasome system
upsilon
upstream binding factor
UPT
    Up-Converting Phosphor technology
uptake
    absolute iodine u. (AIU)
    bipolar u.
    oxygen u.
    radioactive iodine u. (RAIU, RIU)
    radiocalcium u.
    resin u.
    T_3 u.
    triiodothyronine u. (T_3U)
    triiodothyronine resin u. (T_3RU)
uptime
urachal
    u. carcinoma
    u. cyst
    u. fistula
urachus
uracil DNA glycosylase (UDG)
uracil-N-glycosylase (UNG)
uracrasia

U

NOTES

uranin
uranium
    depleted u. (DU)
    u. nephritis
uranyl acetate stain
uraroma
urarthritis
urate
    u. calculus
    u. crystal
    u. crystal stain
    de Galantha method for u.'s
    monosodium u. (MSU)
uratemia
uratohistechia
uratoma
uratosis
uraturia
Urbach-Oppenheim disease
Urbach-Wiethe disease
urban plague
URD
    upper respiratory disease
urea
    u. agar
    u. breath test (UBT)
    u. clearance
    u. clearance test
    u. concentration test
    u. cycle
    u. nitrogen (UN)
    u. nitrogen assay
    u. nitrogen or plasma
    u. nitrogen test
    u. synthesis
ureae
    Nitrosomonas u.
    Pasteurella u.
urealyticum
    Ureaplasma u.
Ureaplasma
    U. parvum
    U. urealyticum
    U. urealyticum genital culture
ureapoiesis
urease
    u. enzyme
    Helicobacter pylori u.
    u. test
    u. test broth
urea-splitting bacterial infection
urecchysis
Urecholine supersensitivity test
uredema
Ureibacillus
    U. terrenus
    U. thermosphaericus
urelcosis

uremia
    hypercalcemic u.
uremic
    u. cachexia
    u. cardiomyopathy
    u. colitis
    u. coma
    u. eclampsia
    u. encephalopathy
    u. inflammation
    u. lung
    u. pericarditis
    u. pneumonia
    u. pneumonitis
uremigenic
ureolyticus
    Bacteroides u.
ureotelic
ureter
    bifid u.
ureteral
    u. atresia
    u. calculus
    u. carcinoma
    u. hyperperistalsis
    u. ileus
    u. peristalsis disorder
    u. reflux
ureterectasia
ureteris
    tunica mucosa u.
    tunica muscularis u.
ureteritis
    u. cystica
    u. glandularis
ureterocele
ureterocutaneous fistula
ureterohydronephrosis
ureterolith
ureterolithiasis
ureterolysis
ureteropelvic
    u. junction
    u. junction obstruction
ureteropyelitis
ureteropyelonephritis
ureteropyosis
ureterostenosis
ureterostoma
ureterovaginal fistula
ureterovesical obstruction
urethrae
    corpus cavernosum u.
urethral
    u. caruncle
    u. discharge (UD)
    u. diverticulum
    u. hematuria
    u. obstruction

u. stricture
u. tumor
urethralis
Oligella u.
urethratresia
urethrism
urethritis
follicular u.
granular u.
nongonococcal u. (NGU)
nonspecific u. (NSU)
u. petrificans
posterior u.
postgonococcal u.
simple u.
Trichomonas u.
urethrocele
urethrocystitis
urethrophyma
urethrostenosis
urethrovaginal fistula
URF
uterine-relaxing factor
urhidrosis
URI
upper respiratory infection
uric
u. acid (UA)
u. acid assay
u. acid calculus
u. acid crystal
u. acid infarct
u. acid test
uricacidemia
uricemia
uricolytic index
uricosuria
uricosuric
Uricult dipslide test
uridine
u. diphosphate (UDP)
u. monophosphate
u. triphosphate (UTP)
uridine-5′-phosphate
uridrosis
uridylic acid
uridyltransferase
galactose phosphate u. (GPUT)
galactose-1-phosphate u. (GALT)
hexose-1-phosphate u.
uridylyl

uridylyltransferase
UDP-glucose-hexose-1-phosphate u.
urinae
ardor u.
urinaehominis
Aerococcus u.
urinale
Actinobaculum u.
urinalis
Streptococcus u.
urinalysis (UA)
midstream u.
urinariae
tunica mucosa vesicae u.
tunica muscularis vesicae u.
tunica serosa vesicae u.
urinarius
Bodo u.
urinary
u. amylase
u. bladder fistula
u. bladder hernia
u. calculus
u. cast
u. catecholamine
u. chorionic gonadotropin (UCG)
u. concentration test
u. coproporphyrin (UCP)
u. cyst
u. estriol
u. free cortisol
u. frequency
u. hydroxyproline
u. incontinence
u. nitrogen
u. obstruction
u. retention
u. sand
u. sediment
u. smear
u. tract brush biopsy
u. tract disease
u. tract infection (UTI)
u. tract sphincter
u. tuberculosis
UrinChek 10+ urine test strips
urine
u. acetone test
alkalinization of u.
u. alpha hydroxybutyric acid
u. amino acid
ammoniacal u.

U

NOTES

urine *(continued)*
  u. amylase
  u. amylase excretion test
  u. argininosuccinic acid
  black u.
  u. blood pigment
  u. calcium
  u. catecholamines
  u. chloride
  chylous u.
  u. citrulline
  cloudy u.
  concentration of creatinine in u. (Ucr)
  concentration of sodium in u. (UNa)
  u. copper
  u. coproporphyrin
  u. creatinine
  crude u.
  u. crystals
  u. cystathionine
  u. cystine
  u. cytology
  diabetic u.
  u. 2,5-dihydroxyphenylacetic acid
  u. dopamine
  u. drug panel (UDP)
  u. drug screen (UDS)
  u. epinephrine
  u. estradiol fraction
  u. estriol fraction
  febrile u.
  feverish u.
  u. fungus culture
  Gerhardt test for urobilin in the u.
  u. glucose
  u. glycine
  gouty u.
  u. heptacarboxyporphyrin
  u. hexacarboxyporphyrin
  u. histidine
  u. homocystine
  u. homogentisic acid
  honey u.
  u. 5-hydroxyindoleacetic acid
  u. hydroxyproline
  u. isoleucine
  u. leucine
  u. leukocyte esterase
  u. lysozyme
  u. magnesium
  u. metanephrine
  u. microscopy
  milky u.
  u. mycobacteria culture
  u. myoglobin test
  nebulous u.
  u. norepinephrine
  u. normetanephrine
  u. osmolality
  u. oxalate
  u. pentacarboxyporphyrin
  u. phenylalanine
  u. phosphoethanolamine
  u. placental estriol
  u. porphobilinogen
  u. porphyrin
  u. potassium
  pregnancy u. (PU)
  u. pregnanediol
  u. pregnanetriol
  u. proline
  u. protein electrophoresis (UPEP)
  u. pyridinoline cross-link
  reducing substances in u.
  residual u.
  u. sediment crystal
  smoky u.
  u. sodium
  u. specimen collection
  u. spot test
  u. total estrogen
  u. urea nitrogen (UUN)
  u. uric acid
  u. urobilinogen (UU)
  u. uroporphyrin
  u. valine
  u. vanillylmandelic acid
urinemia
urine-plasma ratio (U:P)
uriniferous tubule
urinific
uriniparous
urinoma
urinometer
urinometry
urinoscopy
urinosus
  sudor u.
urinothorax
urinous
Uriscreen
  U. bacteriuria detection system
  U. test
UriSite microalbumin/creatinine urine test
Urisys 2400 urine analyzer
Uri-Test protein in urine test
uroammoniac
urobenzoic acid
urobilin assay
urobilinemia
urobilinogen (UBG)
  u. assay
  fecal u. (FU)
  increased urine u.
  stool u.

u. test
urine u. (UU)
urobilinogenuria
urobilinuria
urocanic acid
urocele
urocheras
urochrome
urocortisol
urocrisia
urocyanin
urocyanogen
urocyanosis
Urocystis
urocystitis
UROD
uroporphyrinogen decarboxylase
uroedema
uroerythrin
urofuscohematin
urogastrone
urogenital
u. disorder
u. fistula
u. syndrome
urogenitalis
Actinomyces u.
Amoeba u.
uroglaucin
urogram
excretory u. (XU)
urography
urogravimeter
urohemolytic coefficient
urokinase
u. plasminogen activator (uPA)
u. plasminogen activator receptor
(uPAR)
urolith
urolithiasis
urolithic
urometer
uromucoid assay
uroncus
Uronema caudatum
uronephrosis
uronic acid
uronophile
uronoscopy
uropathogen
uropathy
obstructive u.

uropepsin
uropepsinogen assay
urophanic
urophein
urophilia
uroplakin
u. II (UPII)
u. III (UPIII)
uroporphyria
uroporphyrin (UP)
u. assay
u. test
urine u.
uroporphyrinogen (UPG)
u. III cosynthase
u. III cosynthase deficiency
u. decarboxylase (UROD)
u. decarboxylase deficiency
u. I synthase
u. synthase deficiency
uroporphyrinuria
uropsammus
urorosein
urorubin
urorubrohematin
uroschesis
uroscopic
uroscopy
urosemiology
urosepsin
urosepsis
uroseptic
urothelial
u. carcinoma (UcA)
u. leiomyomatous hamartoma
u. neoplasm
u. papilloma
urothelium
urotoxic coefficient
uroureter
**UroVision bladder cancer recurrence
kit**
UroVysion
U. bladder cancer recurrence test
U. FISH test
uroxanthin
ursincola
Blastomonas u.
ursingii
Acinetobacter u.
ursodeoxycholic acid (UDCA)

U

NOTES

URTI
> upper respiratory tract infection

urticaria
>> aquagenic u.
>> cholinergic u.
>> cold u.
>> congelation u.
>> factitious u.
>> giant u.
>> u. gigantea
>> u. perstans
>> u. pigmentosa
>> pressure u.
>> solar u.
>> u. tuberosa

urticate

urticating
>> u. agent
>> u. caterpillar

Uruma virus

usage
> Working Formulation for Clinical U. (WF)

USAMRIID
> United States Army Medical Research Institute of Infectious Disease

USC
> uterine serous carcinoma

useful life

Usher syndrome

US-licensed formaldehyde-killed whole bacilli vaccine

USN
> ultrasonic nebulizer

USR
> unheated serum reagin
>> USR test

ustilaginism

Ustilago
>> *U. maydis*
>> *U. zeae*

usual
>> u. interstitial pneumonia (UIP)
>> u. interstitial pneumonitis (UIP)

uta

utahensis
>> *Halorhabdus u.*

UTBG
> unbound thyroxine-binding globulin

uteri
>> *Phocoenobacter u.*

uteri (*pl. of* uterus)

uterinae
>> ampulla tubae u.
>> fimbriae tubae u.
>> glandulae u.
>> tunica mucosa tubae u.
>> tunica muscularis tubae u.
>> tunica serosa tubae u.

uterine
>> u. aspiration (UA)
>> u. blood flow (UBF)
>> u. calculus
>> u. cancer
>> u. colic
>> u. descensus
>> u. endometrial carcinoma (UEC)
>> u. endometriosis
>> u. gland
>> u. granuloma
>> u. leiomyoma
>> u. serous carcinoma (USC)
>> u. surface carcinoma

uterine-relaxing factor (URF)

uteritis

utero
>> dead fetus in u. (DFU)
>> in u.

uterolith

uteroovarian varicocele

uteroperitoneal fistula

uteroplacental
>> u. fibrinoid layer
>> u. insufficiency (UPI)

uterus, pl. **uteri**
>> adenomyosis uteri
>> arcuatus u.
>> asymmetric u.
>> bicornuate u.
>> bifid u.
>> cervical gland of u.
>> coiled artery of the u.
>> glandulae cervicales uteri
>> gliosis uteri
>> ichthyosis uteri
>> male rudimentary u.
>> tunica mucosa uteri
>> tunica muscularis uteri
>> tunica serosa uteri
>> unicornis u.

UTI
> urinary tract infection

utilization
>> ketone body u.
>> net protein u. (NPU)

UTP
> uridine triphosphate

UTPC
> usual type papillary carcinoma

utricle

utricular
>> u. cyst
>> u. spot

utricularis
>> *Badhamia u.*

utriculi (*pl. of* utriculus)

utriculitis

utriculosaccular duct

utriculosaccularis
> ductus u.

utriculus, pl. **utriculi**
> macula utriculi

utrophin marker

UTROSCT
> uterine tumor resembling an ovarian sex-cord tumor

UU
> urine urobilinogen

UUN
> urine urea nitrogen

uvea

uveal
> u. melanoma
> u. tract

uveitis
> lens-induced u.
> phacoanaphylactic u.

uveoencephalitic syndrome

uveomeningitis

uveoparotid fever

uviform

uviofast

uvioresistant

uviosensitive

UV-irradiated nevus

Uvitex 2B

uvulitis

uzenensis
> *Geobacillus* u.

uzoniensis
> *Thermoproteus* u.

NOTES

U

V

 valine
 vanadium
 volt
  V agent
  V antigen

V̇$_{CO_2}$

 carbon dioxide output

VA

 vacuum aspiration
 volt-ampere

VACB

 vacuum-assisted core biopsy

vaccenic acid

vaccimaxillae

 Actinomyces v.

vaccina (*var. of* vaccinia)

vaccinal

vaccinate

vaccinated

 distantly v.

vaccination

 inactivated ricin toxoid v.
 post-event v.
 pre-event v.
 roseola v.
 smallpox v.

vaccinator

vaccinatum

 eczema v.

vaccine, vaccinum

 adjuvant v.
 aqueous v.
 attenuated v.
 autogenous v.
 BCG v.
 Brucella strain 19 v.
 Calmette-Guérin v.
 cholera v.
 Cox v.
 crystal violet v.
 diphtheria, tetanus, and pertussis v. (DTP)
 diphtheria toxoid, tetanus toxoid, and pertussis v.
 duck embryo origin v.
 Flury strain v.
 foot-and-mouth disease virus v.
 Haemophilus pertussis v. (HPV)
 Haffkine v.
 hepatitis B v.
 heterogenous v.
 high egg-passage Flury strain rabies v.
 hog cholera v.

 human diploid cell rabies v. (HDCV)
 inactivated poliovirus v. (IPV)
 influenza virus v.
 killed v. (KV)
 killed measles virus v. (KMV)
 live oral poliovirus v.
 low egg-passage v.
 v. lymph
 measles, mumps, and rubella v.
 measles virus v.
 multivalent v.
 mumps virus v.
 oil v.
 oral poliovirus v.
 Pasteur v.
 pentavalent botulinum toxoid v.
 pertussis v.
 plague v.
 pneumococcal v.
 poliomyelitis v.
 poliovirus v.
 polyvalent v.
 rabies v.
 recombinant v.
 RhoGAM v.
 rickettsia v., attenuated
 Rocky Mountain spotted fever v.
 rubella virus v., live
 Sabin v.
 Salk v.
 Semple v.
 smallpox v.
 split-virus v.
 staphylococcus v.
 stock v.
 subunit v.
 TAB v.
 tetanus v.
 trivalent oral poliovirus v. (TOPV)
 tuberculosis v.
 typhoid-paratyphoid A and B v.
 typhus v.
 US-licensed formaldehyde-killed whole bacilli v.
 v. virus
 whooping cough v.
 yellow fever v.

vaccinia, vaccina

 fetal v.
 v. gangrenosa
 generalized v.
 v. immune globulin (VIG)
 v. nervosum
 progressive v.

V

vaccinia *(continued)*
    variola v.
    v. virus
vaccinial
vacciniform
vaccinist
vaccinization
vaccinogen
vaccinogenous
vaccinoid reaction
vaccinostyle
vaccinum *(var. of* vaccine)
Vacuette blood sample tube
vacuo
    in v.
vacuolar
    v. degeneration
    v. interface dermatitis
    v. nephrosis
vacuolate
vacuolated
    v. cell
    v. cytoplasm
    v. lymphocyte
    v. platelet
vacuolating
    v. agent
    v. virus
vacuolation
vacuolatus
    Desulforhopalus v.
vacuole
    v. alteration phagocytosis
    autophagic v.
    condensing v.
    contractile v.
    cytoplasmic v.
    digestion v.
    heterophagic v.
    intracytoplasmic v.
    plasmocrine v.
    rhagiocrine v.
vacuolization
    cytoplasmic v.
    nuclear v.
vacuome
Vacutainer
vacuum
    v. aspiration (VA)
    v. breaker
    v. distillation
    v. flask
    v. gauge
    high v.
    permeability of v.
    permittivity of v.
    v. tube
    v. tuberculin (VT)

    v. tube voltmeter (VTVM)
    ultrahigh v.
vadensis
    Victivallis v.
vagabond's
    v. disease
    v. melanosis
vagale
    glomus v.
vagina, pl. **vaginae**
    v. cellulosa
    congenital absence of v. (CAV)
    v., ectocervix, endocervix (VCE)
    v. mucosa tendinis
    v. synovialis tendinis
    tunica mucosa vaginae
    tunica muscularis vaginae
vaginae
    v. vasorum
vaginal
    v. adenosis
    v. atresia
    v. cancer
    v. carcinoma
    v. clear cell adenocarcinoma
    v. epithelium
    v. gland
    v. intraepithelial neoplasia
    v. irrigation smear (VIS)
    v. leukocyte
    v. pool
    v. synovial membrane
    v. synovitis
    v. thrush
    v. tumor
vaginalis
    Anaerococcus v.
    Gardnerella v.
    Trichomonas v.
    tunica v.
vaginalitis
vaginate
vaginismus
vaginitis, pl. **vaginitides**
    adhesive v.
    bacterial v.
    v. cystica
    desquamative inflammatory v.
    v. emphysematosa
    emphysematous v.
    granular v.
    v. senilis
    trichomanas v.
vaginomycosis
Vaginulus plebeius
Vagitest
Vagococcus
    V. carniphilus
Vahlkampfia

VAHS
    virus-associated hemophagocytic
      syndrome
Val
    valine
valence
    v. electron
    v. tautomer
Valentin corpuscle
Valentine test
valerianellae
    Acidovorax v.
valeric acid
valgum
    genu v.
valgus deformity
validation
valine (V, Val)
    v. aminotransferase
    v. transaminase
    urine v.
valinemia
valinuria
vallatae
    papillae v.
vallate papilla
vallecula unguis
valley fever
vallismortis
    Salinivibrio costicola subsp. *v.*
vallum
valproic acid
Valsa
Valsalva maneuver
value
    absolute v.
    acetyl v.
    acid v.
    buffer v.
    buffer v. of the blood
    cot v.
    crisis v.
    D v.
    GC v.
    globular v.
    iodine v.
    negative predictive v. (NPV)
    normal v.
    P v.
    panic v.
    positive predictive v. (PPV)
    predictive v.

    reference v. (RV)
    rot v.
    threshold limit v. (TLV)
valva, pl. **valvae**
valvarum
    Cardiobacterium v.
valvate
valve
    Amussat v.
    atrioventricular v.
    Bianchi v.
    congenital v.
    v. of coronary vein
    damaged fibrotic v.
    incompetent foramen ovale v.
    Kerckring v.
    mitral v.
    tricuspid v.
valvula, pl. **valvulae**
    Amussat v.
    Gerlach v.
valvulae
    v. conniventes
valvular
    v. atresia
    v. disease of heart (VDH)
    v. endocarditis
    v. incompetence
    v. stenosis
    v. thrombus
    v. tissue embolus
valvulitis
    rheumatic v.
valvulotomy
valyl
valyl-RNA synthetase
Vampirolepis
van
    v. Bogaert disease
    v. Buchem syndrome
    v. Buren disease
    v. Deen test
    v. den Bergh test
    v. der Hoeve syndrome
    v. der Velden test
    v. der Waals equation
    v. der Waals forces
    V. der Woude syndrome
    V. Diest criteria
    v. Ermengen stain
    v. Gieson stain
    v. Hansemann cell

NOTES

van *(continued)*
    V. Nuys scheme
    V. Slyke apparatus
    V. Slyke and Cullen method
    V. Slyke formula
    V. Slyke test
vanadium (V)
vanbaalenii
    Mycobacterium v.
vanbreuseghemii
    Microsporum v.
    Trichophyton v.
vancomycin
vancomycin-insensitive *Staphylococcus aureus* **(VISA)**
vancomycin-resistant
    v.-r. enterococci assay
    v.-r. *Enterococcus* (VRE)
vancoresmycina
    Amycolatopsis v.
vanillic acid
vanillism
vanillylmandelic
    v. acid (VMA)
    v. acid test
VAP cholesterol test
vapor
    combustible v.
    partial pressure of water v.
    v. pressure
    v. pressure depression osmometer
vaporization
    heat of v.
vaporize
vapor-phase chromatography (VPC)
Vapro vapor pressure osmometer
Vaquez disease
Vaquez-Osler disease
var
    variant
variabile
    Cellulosimicrobium v.
    Trichosporon v.
variabilis
    Brevundimonas v.
    Dermacentor v.
    erythrokeratodermia v.
    Isoptericola v.
    Mesocestoides v.
variability
    interobserver v.
    intraobserver v.
variable
    v. autotransformer
    v. capacitor
    common v.
    dependent v.
    dichotomous v.
    double-precision v.

    dummy v.
    endogenous v.
    exogenous v.
    fixed-point v.
    floating-point v.
    independent v.
    label v.
    v. number of tandem repeats (VNTR)
    ordinal v.
    pointer v.
    random v.
    v. region
    v. resistor
    subscripted v.
variance
    analysis of v. (ANOVA)
    multivariate analysis of v. (MANOVA)
    phenotypic v.
varians
    Micrococcus v.
variant (var)
    aggressive follicular v.
    blastoid v.
    columnar cell v. (CCV)
    cribriform-morular v.
    diffuse follicular v.
    floral v.
    germline v.
    v. hemoglobin
    inherited albumin v.
    L-phase v.
    macrofollicular v.
    SI v.
    v. sickling hemoglobin anemia
    tall cell v. (TCV)
    terminally truncated v.
variate
    binary v.
variation
    alpha-beta v.
    coefficient of v. (CV)
    contingent negative v. (CNV)
    meristic v.
    microbial v.
    negative v. (NV)
    rough-smooth v.
    smooth-rough v.
Varibaculum cambriense
varication
variceal
varicella
    v. encephalitis
    v. virus
varicellation
varicella-zoster (VZ, V-Z)
    v.-z. antibody test

v.-z. virus (VZV)
v.-z. virus serology
varicelliform eruption
varicelloid
Varicellovirus
varices (*pl. of* varix)
variciform
varicocele
ovarian v.
symptomatic v.
tuboovarian v.
uteroovarian v.
varicoid
varicole
varicophlebitis
Varicosavirus
varicose
v. aneurysm
v. ulcer
v. vein
varicosis, pl. **varicoses**
varicosity
varicosum
lymphangioma capillare v.
varicule
variegata
parakeratosis v.
variegate porphyria
variegatum
Amblyomma v.
Hyalomma v.
variegatus
Aedes v.
variglandis
Austrobilharzia v.
Microbilharzia v.
variicola
Klebsiella v.
variola
v. benigna
v. hemorrhagica
v. major
v. maligna
v. miliaris
v. minor
v. pemphigosa
v. sine eruptione
v. vaccine
v. vera
v. verrucosa
v. virus
variolar

variolate
variolation
variolic
varioliform
varioliform gastritis
varioliformis
parapsoriasis v.
variolization
varioloid
variolous
variolovaccine
varium
Procerovum v.
varius
Paragordius v.
varix, pl. **varices**
v. anastomoticus
aneurysmal v.
cirsoid v.
esophageal varices
lymph v.
v. lymphaticus
turbinal v.
varus deformity
vas, pl. **vasa**
v. afferens
v. capillare
v. deferens
v. efferens
vasa
v. aberrantia
v. previa
v. recta
v. vasorum
vascular
v. addressin
v. anomaly
v. birthmark
v. bud
v. cell adhesion molecule-1 (VCAM-1)
v. cone
v. corrosion cast
v. dementia
v. density
v. disorder
v. dissection
v. ectasia
v. endothelial cadherin (VE-cadherin)
v. endothelial growth factor receptor 3 (VEGFR3)

V

NOTES

vascular *(continued)*
 v. gland
 v. hemophilia
 v. keratitis
 v. lacune
 v. lake
 v. layer
 v. layer of choroid coat of eye
 v. leakage
 v. leiomyoma
 v. malformation
 v. morphology
 v. myelopathy
 v. myxoma
 v. neoplasm
 v. nevus
 v. papilla
 v. permeability
 v. permeability factor
 v. polyp
 v. resistance (VR)
 v. ring
 v. sclerosis
 v. spider
 v. stenosis
 v. stripe
 v. styptic
 v. thrombus
vasculare
 poikiloderma atrophicans v.
vascularization
 corneal v.
vascularize
vasculature
 lesion of v.
vasculitis, pl. **vasculitides**
 Churg-Strauss v.
 cryoglobulinemic v.
 cutaneous v.
 hypersensitivity v.
 leukocytoclastic v.
 livedo v.
 lymphocytic v.
 lymphohistiocytic v.
 necrotizing v.
 nodular v. (NV)
 pustular v.
 segmented hyalinizing v.
 septal panniculitis without v.
vasculocardiac syndrome of hyperserotonemia
vasculomyelinopathy
vasculoocclusive process
vasculopathic
vasculosa
 Haller tunica v.
 tunica v.
vasculosae
 stellulae v.

vasculosi
 coni v.
vasculosum
 punctum v.
vasculosyncytial membrane
vasculotoxic
vasiformis
 Saksenaea v.
vasitis nodosa
vasoactive
 v. intestinal peptide (VIP)
 v. intestinal polypeptide (VIP)
 v. mediator
vasoconstriction
 hypoxic v.
vasodepressor material (VDM)
vasodilatation
vasoexcitor material (VEM)
vasoformative cell
vasoganglion
vasogenic shock
vasomotor
 v. hypotonia
 v. instability
 v. paralysis
 v. rhinitis (VMR)
vasoocclusive crisis
vasoparalysis
vasoparesis
vasopressin (VP)
 arginine v. (AVP)
 unit of v.
vasorum
 vaginae v.
 vasa v.
vasospasm
 recurrent v.
vasospastic
vasovagal
 v. attack
 v. syncope
VATER
 vertebral defects, anal atresia, tracheoesophageal fistula with esophageal atresia, and radial and renal anomalies
 VATER complex
Vater
 V. corpuscle
 papilla of V.
Vater-Pacini corpuscle
VATS
 video-assisted transthoracic surgery
Vav1 signal transducer protein
VBS/FBS
 veronal-buffered saline/fetal bovine serum

VCA
viral capsid antigen
VCA IgM
VCAM-1
vascular cell adhesion molecule-1
VCE
vagina, ectocervix, endocervix
VCE smear
VCFS
velocardiofacial syndrome
VD
venereal disease
VDBR
volume of distribution of bilirubin
VDEL
venereal disease experimental laboratory
VDG
venereal disease gonorrhea
VDH
valvular disease of heart
VDM
vasodepressor material
VDRL
Venereal Disease Research Laboratory
VDRL test
VDS
venereal disease-syphilis
VE
NATO code for nerve agent O-ethyl S-[2-(diethylamino)ethyl] ethylphosphonothioate
VE-cadherin
vascular endothelial cadherin
Vectabond reagent
Vectastain
V. ABC Elit kit
V. Elite ABC system
V. immunohistochemical reagent
V. Universal Elite ABC kit
V. Universal Quick kit
vection
vector
biological v.
cloning v.
electric field v.
V. Elite reagent
expression v.
V. Laboratories VectaShield antifading buffer
mechanical v.
V. MOM kit
plasmid v.

v. product
recombinant v.
vectorial
VEE
Venezuelan equine encephalomyelitis
VEE smear
VEE virus
vegetans
keratosis v.
pemphigus v.
pyoderma v.
pyostomatitis v.
vegetation
bacterial v.
verrucous v.
vegetative
v. anthrax bacilli
v. bacillus
v. bacteriophage
v. cell
v. endocarditis
v. multiplication
v. stage
VEGF
vascular endothelial growth factor
VEGFR3
vascular endothelial growth factor receptor 3
VEGFR3 marker
vehiculated nutrient
veil
aqueduct v.
v. cell
veiled cell
Veillonaceae
Veillonella
V. alcalescens subsp. *alcalescens*
V. alcalescens subsp. *dispar*
V. montpellierensis
V. parvula
V. parvula subsp. *atypica*
V. parvula subsp. *rodentium*
Veillonellaceae
Veillon tube
vein
arterialization of v.
capillary v.
external pudendal v.
key v.
Krukenberg v.
large v.
medium v.

NOTES

V

vein (*continued*)
    obturator v.
    portal v.
    reticular fibers in wall of
      central v.
    small v.
    stellate v.
    v. stone
    valve of coronary v.
    varicose v.
veined
veinlet
vein-to-vein anastomosis
Vejovis
vela (*pl. of* velum)
velamen, pl. **velamina**
    v. vulva
velamentous
    v. cord
    v. insertion
    v. vessel
velamentum, pl. **velamenta**
velamina (*pl. of* velamen)
Vel antigen
velar
veliform
vellicate
vellication
vellus
    v. anagen follicle
    v. hair
    v. hair cyst
    v. telogen follicle
velocardiofacial syndrome (VCFS)
velocity
    v. coefficient
    wave v.
velocity-diffusion
    sedimentation v.
    v. sedimentation
velogenic Newcastle disease
velopharyngeal insufficiency
velox
    Thermanaerovibrio v.
velum, pl. **vela**
VEM
    vasoexcitor material
vena cava obstruction
venae
    v. cavernosae of spleen
    v. centrales hepatis
    v. rectae
    v. stellatae
Ven antigen
venenata
    dermatitis v.
veneniferous
venenous

venereal
    v. disease (VD)
    v. disease experimental laboratory
      (VDEL)
    v. disease gonorrhea (VDG)
    v. disease-syphilis (VDS)
    v. lymphogranuloma
    v. sore
    v. ulcer
    v. wart
venerealis
    Campylobacter fetus subsp. *v.*
venereology
venereum
    lymphogranuloma v. (LGV)
    lymphopathia v.
    papilloma v.
veneris
    corona v.
venesect
Venezuelan
    V. equine A encephalomyelitis
      virus
    V. equine encephalitis
    V. equine encephalomyelitis (VEE)
    V. equine encephalomyelitis virus
venezuelensis
    Borrelia v.
    Leishmania mexicana v.
    Ornithodoros v.
venin
venipuncture
venofibrosis
venogram
venolymphatic
venom
    antisnake v. (ASV)
    cobra v.
    hymenoptera v.
    kokoi v.
    Malayan pit viper v.
    Protac v.
    Russell viper v. (RVV)
    snake v. (SV)
    viper v. (VV)
venoocclusive disease of the liver
venosclerosis
venostasis
venosus
    nevus v.
venous
    v. blood
    v. blood and tissue
    v. capillary
    v. claudication
    v. congestion
    v. embolism
    v. gangrene
    v. hematocrit (VH)

v. insufficiency
v. lake
mixed v.
v. occlusion
v. pressure
v. sinus
v. star
v. stasis
v. thrombosis
Ventana
V. alkaline phosphatase blue
detection kit
V. automated immunostainer
V. ES slide processor machine
V. ES stain
V. Medical Systems Techmate 500
automated stainer
V. NexES immunostainer
V. silanized capillary gap slide
V. TechMate 100 immunostainer
ventilation
v. defect
local exhaust v.
maximum voluntary v. (MVV)
mechanical v.
ventilation-perfusion ratio
ventilator-associated pneumonia
ventilatory failure
ventosa
spina v.
ventosae
Halomonas v.
ventral respiratory group
ventricle
tela choroidea of fourth v.
tela choroidea of third v.
trabeculae carneae of right and
left v.'s
ventricose
ventricosus
Haemodipsus v.
Pediculoides v.
Strongylus v.
ventricular
v. aneurysm
v. bigeminy
v. diverticulum
v. dysfunction
v. hypertrophy
v. layer
v. septal defect (VSD)
v. tachycardia

ventriculi
anadenia v.
descensus v.
Sarcina v.
stigma v.
stratum circulare tunicae
muscularis v.
stratum longitudinale tunicae
muscularis v.
tunica muscularis v.
tunica serosa v.
ventriculography
radionucleotide v.
ventriculonector
ventriculoradial dysplasia
ventriculus
ventroptosia
ventroptosis
Venturia
venula, pl. **venulae**
venulae rectae renis
venulae stellatae renis
venular
venule
high-endothelial v. (HEV)
pericytic v.
postcapillary v.
stellate v.
venulitis
cutaneous necrotizing v.
venulosum
Oesophagostomum v.
venulous
venustensis
Alcanivorax v.
vera
cutis v.
decidua v.
hemospermia v.
myeloid metaplasia with
polycythemia v. (PCV-M)
polycythemia v. (PCV, PV)
polycythemia rubra v.
verapamil
verbascose
Verdict-II
V.-II drug screening device
V.-II drug screening test
verdoglobin
verdohemochrome
verdohemoglobin
verdoperoxidase

V

NOTES

verge
  anal v.
vergeture
verheyenii
  stellulae v.
Verheyen star
Verhoeff elastic tissue stain
Verhoeff-van
  V.-v. Gieson (VVG)
  V.-v. Gieson elastin stain
veriformis
  Hartmannella v.
vermicidal
vermicide
vermicular
Vermicularia
vermicularis
  Enterobius v.
  Oxyuris v.
vermicule
vermiculous
vermiculus
vermiform
vermiformis
  appendix v.
  folliculi lymphatici aggregati
  appendicis v.
vermifugal
vermifuge
vermilion
  v. border
  v. zone
vermin
verminal
vermination
verminous
  v. abscess
  v. colic
vermis
verna
  Amanita v.
vernal
  v. conjunctivitis
  v. encephalitis
Verner-Morrison syndrome
Vernet syndrome
Verneuil
  V. disease
  hidradenitis axillaris of V.
  V. neuroma
vernier dial caliper
vernix caseosa
Verocay body
Vero cell
vero cytotoxin
Veronaea botryosa
veronal buffer
veronal-buffered saline/fetal bovine
  serum (VBS/FBS)

verotoxin
Verpa bohemica
verruca, verruga, pl. **verrucae**
  v. acuminata
  v. digitata
  v. filiformis
  v. glabra
  v. mollusciformis
  v. necrogenica
  v. peruana
  v. plana
  v. plana juvenilis
  v. plana senilis
  v. plantaris
  seborrheic v.
  v. seborrheica
  v. simplex
  v. virus
  v. vulgaris
verrucal
  v. atypical endocarditis
  v. nonbacterial endocarditis
verrucarum
  Phlebotomus v.
verruciform
verruciformis
  acrokeratosis v.
  epidermodysplasia v.
Verrucomicrobiaceae
Verrucomicrobiae
Verrucomicrobiales
verrucopapillary
  v. alteration
  v. external genital lesion
verrucosa
  Amoeba v.
  dermatitis v.
  pachyderma v.
  Phialophora v.
  telangiectasia v.
  tuberculosis cutis v.
  variola v.
verrucose
verrucosis
  lymphostatic v.
verrucosum
  eczema v.
  molluscum v.
  Trichophyton v.
verrucosus
  lupus v.
  Ornithodoros v.
verrucous
  v. acanthosis
  v. angiosarcoma
  v. carcinoma
  v. carditis
  v. endocarditis
  v. hyperplasia

v. melanoma
v. nevus
v. papilloma
v. sarcoid
v. scrofuloderma
v. vegetation
v. xanthoma
verruculosa
Curvularia v.
verruga (*var. of* verruca)
verruga peruana
Versant HCV RNA 3.0 assay
Verse disease
Versene
versican
versicolor
Aspergillus v.
membrana v.
pityriasis v.
Pityrosporum v.
versiforme
Natrinema v.
version
HD allele v.
versmoldensis
Lactobacillus v.
versutus
Thialkalivibrio v.
vertebral
v. arthritis
v. basilar artery syndrome
v. crush-fracture syndrome
v. polyarthritis
v. defects, anal atresia,
tracheoesophageal fistula with
esophageal atresia, and radial and
renal anomalies (VATER)
vertical
v. melanoma growth phase
v. transmission
verticil
verticillate
Verticillium alboatrum
Verticillium graphii
vertigo
verumontanitis
**verumontanum mucosal gland
hyperplasia**
very
v. large scale integration (VLSI)
v. late activation (VLA)
very-high-density lipoprotein (VHDL)

very-high frequency
very-low birth weight (VLBW)
very-low-density lipoprotein (VLDL)
vesica, pl. **vesicae**
bullous edema vesicae
ectopia vesicae
malacoplakia vesicae
pachyderma vesicae
vesical
v. blood fluke
v. calculus
v. diverticulum
v. dysplasia
v. endometriosis
v. fistula
v. gland
v. hematuria
vesicalis
anus v.
vesicant
vesicating agent
vesicle
acrosomal v.
air v.
Baer v.
clathrin-coated v.
coated electron-lucent v.
electron-lucent v.
excretory duct of seminal v.
germinal v.
internalized v.
matrix v.
micropinocytotic v.
nonmelanosomal v.
phospholipid v.
pinocytotic v.
presynaptic v.
synaptic v.
villous v.
vesicobullous
vesicocolic fistula
vesicocutaneous fistula
vesicointestinal fistula
vesicolithiasis
vesicopustular
vesicopustule
vesico-sphincter dyssynergia
vesicoureteral reflux
vesicouterine fistula
vesicovaginal fistula
vesicovaginorectal fistula
vesicula, pl. **vesiculae**

V

NOTES

vesicular
    v. acute inflammation
    v. chromatin pattern
    v. emphysema
    v. exanthema
    v. exanthema of swine virus
    v. granulomatous inflammation
    v. keratitis
    v. mole
    v. nucleus
    v. ovarian follicle
    v. stomatitis
    v. stomatitis virus (VSV)
vesicularis
    Brevundimonas v.
    Pseudomonas v.
vesiculate
vesiculated
vesiculation
vesiculiform
vesiculin
vesiculitis
vesiculocavernous
vesiculopapular
vesiculoprostatitis
vesiculopustular
vesiculose
vesiculosi
    stratum granulosum folliculi
      ovarici v.
vesiculosum
    eczema v.
    hydroa v.
vesiculosus
    folliculus ovaricus v.
vesiculous
Vesiculovirus
Vesivirus
vessel
    aberrant renal v.
    blood v.
    capillary v.
    chyle v.
    efferent lymphatic v.
    endothelial lining of v.
    great v.
    lacteal v.
    newly formed v.
    pinocytotic v.
    sheaths of v.'s
    trabecular blood v.
    transposition of great v.'s (TGV)
    velamentous v.
vestalii
    Rhodoglobus v.
vestfoldensis
    Loktanella v.
vestibular
    v. anus

    v. canal
    v. gland
    v. hair cell
    v. lip of limbus of spiral lamina
    v. membrane
    v. organ
    v. wall of cochlear duct
    v. window
vestibule
    fenestra of the v.
vestibuli
    aqueductus v.
    fenestra v.
    sacculus v.
    scala v.
vestigial
vestimenti
    Pediculus v.
vestimentorum
    Pediculus humanus v.
vestrisii
    Bosea v.
vesuvin
veterana
    Nocardia v.
veterinary vaccine Stern strain *Bacillus anthracis*
vexans
    Aedes v.
vexator
    Phlebotomus v.
VG
    NATO code for nerve agent O,O-diethyl S-[2-(diethylamino)ethyl] phosphonothioate
VGA
    villoglandular adenocarcinoma
Vgamma9 test
VH
    venous hematocrit
VHD
    viral hematodepressive disease
VHDL
    very-high-density lipoprotein
VHF
    viral hemorrhagic fever
VHL
    von Hippel-Lindau
      VHL gene
VI
    vascular invasion
Vi
    Vi agglutination
    Vi antibody
    Vi antigen
VIA
    virus-inactivating agent
viability
viable cell count

vial
vibration
    v. second (vs)
    subsynchronous v.
vibrational spectroscopy
vibratome tissue section
Vibrio
    V. aerogenes
    V. aestuarianus
    V. agarivorans
    V. alginolyticus
    V. brasiliensis
    V. calviensis
    V. chagasii
    V. cholerae
    V. cholerae biotype El Tor (El Tor
      vibrio)
    V. coralliilyticus
    V. cyclitrophicus
    V. fluvialis
    V. fortis
    V. furnissii
    V. gallicus
    V. group F (EF-6)
    V. hepatarius
    V. hispanicus
    V. hollisae
    V. kanaloae
    V. lentus
    V. metschnikovii
    V. mimicus
    V. neptunius
    V. pacinii
    V. parahaemolyticus
    V. pomeroyi
    V. proteolyticus
    V. proteus
    V. rotiferianus
    V. ruber
    V. shilonii
    V. sputorum
    V. tasmaniensis
    V. viscosus
    V. vulnificus
    V. wodanis
    V. xuii
vibrio
    Celebes v.
    cholera v.
    Nasik v.
    nonagglutinating v.
    paracholera v.

vibrioides
    Propionispora v.
Vibrionaceae
Vibrion septique
vibriosis
vicarious
    v. hemoptysis
    v. hypertrophy
Vi-CELL series cell viability analyzer
Vicia graminea
vicinal neuron
vicine
vicious union
victim identification
Victivallales
Victivallis vadensis
Victoria
    V. blue
    V. blue stain
    V. orange
Vidal disease
vidarabine
Vidas
    V. probe
    V. total PSA assay kit
vide infra
video time-lapse microscopy
Vielle menopause home test kit
Vierra sign
vietnamensis
    Desulfovibrio v.
view
    radius of v.
VIG
    vaccinia immune globulin
Vignal cell
Villaret syndrome
villi (*pl. of* villus)
villiform configuration
villin
villitis
villoglandular adenocarcinoma (VGA)
villoma
villonodular
    v. pigmented synovitis
    v. pigmented tenosynovitis
villorum
    Enterococcus v.
villosa
    pericarditis v.
    polyarthritis chronica v.
villose

V

NOTES

villositis
villosity
villous
  v. adenoma
  v. atrophy
  v. capillary hypervascularity
  v. carcinoma
  v. ischemic necrosis
  v. papilloma
  v. polyp
  v. tenosynovitis
  v. tumor
  v. vesicle
villus, pl. **villi**
  abnormal chorionic v.
  arachnoid v.
  chorionic v.
  intestinal v.
  villi intestinales
  mature abnormal chorionic v.
  molar villi
  villi pericardiaci
  pericardial villi
  peritoneal villi
  villi peritoneales
  pleural villi
  villi pleurales
  synovial villi
  villi synoviales
vimentin immunoperoxidase stain
VIN
  vulvar intraepithelial neoplasia
  warty VIN
vinacea
  Nocardia v.
vinaceus
  Actinomyces v.
Vincent
  V. angina
  V. bacillus
  V. disease
  V. organism
  V. stomatitis
  V. white mycetoma
vincentii
  Borrelia v.
vincristine neuropathy
vinculin protein
Vindelov procedure
vindobonensis
  Promicromonospora v.
vinegar acid
vinsonii
  Bartonella v.
Vinson syndrome
vinyl
  v. chloride
  v. chloride disease

  v. polymer
  v. trichloride
violacea
  Lentzea v.
  Saccharothrix v.
violaceinigra
  Duganella v.
violaceous
violaceum
  Cardiobacterium v.
  Chromobacterium v.
  Trichophyton v.
violet
  amethyst v.
  ammonium oxalate crystal v.
  aniline gentian v. (AGV)
  Bensley safranin acid v.
  Bernthsen methylene v.
  chrome v.
  cresyl v. (CV)
  cresylecht v.
  crystal v.
  gentian v. (GV)
  hexamethyl v.
  Hoffman v.
  Lauth v.
  methyl v.
  methylene v.
  pentamethyl v.
viomycin
viosterol
VIP
  vasoactive intestinal peptide
  vasoactive intestinal polypeptide
  voluntary interruption of pregnancy
viper
  v. venom (VV)
vipoma, VIPoma
viral
  v. capsid antigen (VCA)
  v. carcinogenesis
  v. culture
  v. dysentery
  v. encephalomyelitis
  v. envelope
  v. gastroenteritis
  v. genome
  v. genomic diversity
  v. hemagglutination
  v. hematodepressive disease (VHD)
  v. hemorrhagic fever (VHF)
  v. hemorrhagic fever virus
  v. hepatitis, types A–E
  v. hybrid capture
  v. inclusion
  v. load
  v. meningitis
  v. myocarditis
  v. neutralization

v. nucleic acid
v. pericarditis
v. pneumonia
v. probe
v. respiratory infection (VRI)
v. strand
v. tropism
v. wart
ViraPap test
ViraType In Situ System
Virchow
V. cell
V. corpuscle
V. crystal
V. disease
V. hydatid
V. law
V. node
V. psammoma
V. triad
Virchow-Hassall body
Virchow-Robin space
viremia
asymptomatic v.
secondary v.
vireti
Bacillus v.
Virgibacillus
V. carmonensis
V. marismortui
V. necropolis
V. picturae
V. salexigens
virginal hypertrophy
virgin B cell
virginity
Virgisporangium
V. aurantiacum
V. ochraceum
viricidal
viricide
viridans
Aerococcus v.
Carnobacterium v.
Staphylococcus v.
Thalassomonas v.
viridilutea
Actinomadura v.
viridis
Euglena v.
Saccharomonospora v.
Thermolospora v.

virilism
adrenal v.
congenital adrenal v. (CAV)
virilization
adrenal v.
virilizing syndrome
virion
virogene
viroid
virologist
virology laboratory
viropexis
ViroSeq HIV-1 genotyping system
Virotrol syphilis total control
virtual autopsy
virtually diagnostic
virucidal
virucide
virucopria
virulence factor
virulent
v. bacteriophage
v. Schu S4 tularemia strain
viruliferous
viruria
virus
2060 v.
Abelson murine leukemia v.
adeno-associated v. (AAV)
adenosatellite v.
African horse sickness v.
African swine fever v.
AIDS-related v. (ARV)
Akabane v.
AKT1 v.
Aleutian mink disease v.
amphotropic v.
animal v.
v. animatum
APC v.
apeu v.
Argentine hemorrhagic fever v.
attenuated v.
Aujeszky disease v.
Australian X disease v.
Australian X encephalitis v.
avian encephalomyelitis v.
avian erythroblastosis v.
avian infectious laryngotracheitis v.
avian influenza v.
avian leukosis-sarcoma v.
avian lymphomatosis v.

NOTES

virus *(continued)*

avian myeloblastosis v.
avian myelocytomatosis v. (AMV2)
avian neurolymphomatosis v.
avian pneumoencephalitis v.
avian sarcoma v.
avian viral arthritis v.
bacterial v.
Bittner v.
biundulant milk fever v.
BK v.
v. blockade
bluecomb v.
bluetongue v.
Borna disease v.
Bornholm disease v.
bovine leukemia v. (BLV)
bovine leukosis v.
bovine papular stomatitis v.
breakpoint cluster region-Abelson
  murine leukemia v. (BCR-ABL)
brick-shaped v.
v. bronchopneumonia
Brunhilde v.
Bunyamwera v.
Bwamba fever v.
C v.
CA v.
Cache Valley v.
California encephalitis v.
California myxoma v.
canarypox v.
canine distemper v.
Capim v.
Caraparu v.
cat distemper v.
cattle plague v.
Catu v.
CELO v.
Central European encephalitis v.
  (CEEV)
Central European tick-borne
  encephalitis v.
C group v.
Chagres v.
chicken embryo lethal orphan v.
chickenpox v.
chikungunya fever v.
"c2-like v.'s"
Coe v.
cold v.
Colorado tick fever v.
Columbia SK v.
common cold v.
contagious ecthyma (pustular
  dermatitis) v. of sheep
contagious pustular stomatitis v.
coryza v.
cowpox v.

Crimean-Congo hemorrhagic
  fever v.
Crimean hemorrhagic fever v.
croup-associated v.
cytomegalic inclusion disease v.
cytopathogenic v.
defective v.
delta v.
dengue v., types 1–4
diphasic meningoencephalitis v.
diphasic milk fever v.
distemper v.
DNA v.
dog distemper v.
double-stranded DNA v.
duck hepatitis v.
duck influenza v.
duck plague v.
Eastern equine encephalomyelitis v.
EB v.
Ebola v.
"Ebola-like v.'s"
ECBO v.
ECDO v.
ECHO v.
ECMO v.
ecotropic v.
ECSO v.
ecthyma infectiosum v.
ectromelia v.
EEE v.
EMC v.
emerging v.
encephalitis v.
encephalomyocarditis v.
enteric orphan v.
entomopox v.
enzootic encephalomyelitis v.
ephemeral fever v.
epidemic gastroenteritis v.
epidemic keratoconjunctivitis v.
epidemic myalgia v.
epidemic parotitis v.
epidemic pleurodynia v.
Epstein-Barr v. (EBV)
equine abortion v.
equine arteritis v.
equine coital exanthema v.
equine encephalomyelitis v.
equine infectious anemia v.
equine influenza v.
equine rhinopneumonitis v.
feline ataxia v. (FAV)
feline leukemia v. (FeLV)
feline panleukopenia v.
feline rhinotracheitis v.
fibrous bacterial v.
fifth disease v.
filamentous bacterial v.

filterable v.
fixed v.
Flury strain rabies v.
FMD v.
foamy v.
foot-and-mouth disease v.
fowl erythroblastosis v.
fowl lymphomatosis v.
fowl myeloblastosis v.
fowl neurolymphomatosis v.
fowl plague v.
fowlpox v.
fox encephalitis v.
Friend leukemia v.
GAL v.
gallus adenolike v.
gastroenteritis v. type A, B
Gauma v.
German measles v.
Germiston v.
Graffi v.
green monkey v.
Gross leukemia v.
group B arbor v.
Guama v.
Guanarito v.
Guaroa v.
hand-foot-and-mouth disease v.
Hantaan v.
hard pad v.
helper v.
hemadsorption v. type 1, 2
hepatitis v.
hepatitis A v. (HAV)
hepatitis B v. (HBV)
hepatitis C v. (HCV)
hepatitis D v. (HDV)
hepatitis delta v. (HDV)
hepatitis E v. (HEV)
"hepatitis E-like v.'s"
hepatitis G v. (HGV)
hepatitis GB v. (HGBV)
herpangina v.
herpes v.
herpeslike v. (HLV)
herpes simplex v. (HSV)
herpes-type v. (HTV)
herpes zoster v.
hog cholera v.
horsepox v.
human B lymphotropic v. (HBLV)
human immunodeficiency v. (HIV)

human T-cell leukemia-
lymphoma v. (HTLV)
human T-cell lymphotropic v. type
I (HTLV-I)
human T-cell lymphotropic v. type
II (HTLV-II)
human T-cell lymphotropic v. type
III (HTLV-III)
Ibaraki v.
IBR v.
"Ictalurid herpes-like v.'s"
IgM anti-hepatitis A v.
v. III of rabbits
Ilhéus v.
inadvertent inoculation of
vaccinia v.
inclusion conjunctivitis v.
infantile gastroenteritis v.
infectious arteritis v. of horses
infectious bovine rhinotracheitis v.
infectious bronchitis v. (IBV)
infectious ectromelia v.
infectious hepatitis v.
"infectious laryngo-tracheitis-
like v.'s"
infectious papilloma v.
infectious porcine
encephalomyelitis v.
influenza v.
insect v.
iridescent v.
Itaqui v.
Jamestown Canyon v.
Japanese B encephalitis v.
JC v.
JH v.
Junin v.
K v.
Kelev strain rabies v.
v. keratoconjunctivitis
Kilham rat v.
Kisenyi sheep disease v.
Koongol v.'s
Korean hemorrhagic fever v.
Kumba v.
Kyasanur Forest disease v.
La Crosse v.
lactate dehydrogenase v.
lactic dehydrogenase v. (LDV)
Lansing v.
Lassa v.
latent rat v.

NOTES

V

virus *(continued)*
   LCM v.
   Leon v.
   "λ-like v.'s"
   "φ29-like v.'s"
   louping ill v.
   Lucké v.
   Lunyo v.
   lymphadenopathy-associated v.
    (LAV)
   lymphocytic choriomeningitis v.
   lymphogranuloma venereum v.
   Machupo v.
   maedi v.
   Maloney leukemia v.
   mammary tumor v. (MTV)
   mammary tumor v. of mice
   Marburg v.
   "Marburg-like v.'s"
   Marek disease v.
   "Marek's disease-like v.'s"
   Marituba v.
   marmoset v.
   masked v.
   Mason-Pfizer monkey v.
   Mayaro v.
   measles v.
   Mengo v.
   milker's nodule v.
   mink enteritis v.
   MM v.
   Mokola v.
   molluscum contagiosum v. (MCV)
   molluscum sebaceum v.
   Moloney leukemogenic v. (MLV)
   Moloney sarcoma v. (MSV)
   monkey B v.
   monkeypox v.
   mouse encephalomyelitis v.
   mouse hepatitis v.
   mouse leukemia v. (MLV)
   mouse mammary tumor v.
    (MMTV)
   mouse parotid tumor v.
   mouse poliomyelitis v.
   mousepox v.
   mouse thymic v.
   mucosal disease v.
   "mu-like v.'s"
   mumps v.
   murine sarcoma v. (MSV)
   Murutucu v.
   MVE v.
   myxomatosis v.
   Nairobi sheep disease v.
   naked v.
   ND v.
   Nebraska calf scours v.
   Neethling v.

   negative strand v.
   Negishi v.
   neonatal calf diarrhea v.
   neurotropic v.
   v. neutralization test
   newborn pneumonitis v.
   Newcastle disease v. (NDV)
   nonbacterial gastroenteritis v.
   nonenveloped RNA v.
   nonoccluded v.
   Norwalk v. (*Norovirus*)
   Ntaya v.
   occluded v.
   "ωH-like v.'s"
   Omsk hemorrhagic fever v.
   oncogenic v.
   O'nyong-nyong fever v.
   orf v.
   Oriboca v.
   ornithosis v.
   Oropouche v.
   orphan v.
   Pacheco parrot disease v.
   panleukopenia v. (PLV)
   panleukopenia v. of cats
   pantropic v.
   papilloma v.
   pappataci fever v.
   papular stomatitis v. of cattle
   parainfluenza v., types 1–4
   paravaccinia v.
   parrot v.
   Patois v.
   pharyngoconjunctival fever v.
   phlebotomus fever v.
   plant v.
   "P1-like v.'s"
   "P2-like v.'s"
   "P4-like v.'s"
   "P22-like v.'s"
   PLT group v.
   "φM1-like v.'s"
   pneumonia v. of mice (PVM)
   v. pneumonia of pigs
   pneumonitis v.
   poliomyelitis v.
   v. poliomyelitis
   polyoma v.
   porcine hemagglutinating
    encephalomyelitis v.
   Powassan v.
   progressive pneumonia v.
   pseudocowpox v.
   pseudolymphocytic
    choriomeningitis v.
   pseudorabies v.
   psittacosis v.
   PVM v.
   quail bronchitis v.

Quaranfil v.
rabbit fibroma v.
rabbitpox v.
rabies v.
rat v. (RV)
Rauscher leukemia v.
reservoir of v.
respiratory enteric orphan v.
respiratory exanthematous v.
respiratory infection v.
respiratory syncytial v. (RSV)
Rida v.
Rift Valley fever v.
rinderpest v.
RNA tumor v.
roseola infantum v.
Ross River v.
Rous-associated v. (RAV)
Rous sarcoma v.
Rs v.
Rubarth disease v.
rubella v. (RV)
rubeola v.
Russian autumn encephalitis v.
Russian spring-summer
  encephalitis v.
Sabia v.
Salisbury common cold v.
salivary gland v. (SGV)
sandfly fever v.
San Miguel sea lion v.
Semliki Forest v.
Sendai v.
serum hepatitis v.
v. shedding
sheep pox v.
shipping fever v.
Shope fibroma v.
Shope papilloma v.
Simbu v.
simian v. (SV)
simian immunodeficiency v. (SIV)
simian sarcoma v. (SSV)
simian vacuolating v. No. 40
Sindbis v.
slow v.
smallpox v.
snowshoe hare v.
soremouth v.
"SPO1-like v.'s"
Spondweni v.
ssRNA v.

St. Louis encephalitis v.
street v.
"Sulfolobus SNDV-like v.'s"
swamp fever v.
swine encephalitis v.
swine fever v.
swine influenza v.
swinepox v.
Swiss mouse leukemia v.
Tacaribe complex of v.'s
Tahyna v.
temperate v.
Teschen v.
Tete v.
TGE v.
Theiler mouse encephalomyelitis v.
Theiler original v.
tick-borne encephalitis v.
"T1-like v.'s"
"T4-like v.'s"
"T5-like v.'s"
"T7-like v.'s"
TO v.
tobacco mosaic v. (TMV)
trachoma v.
transforming v.
transfusion transmitted v. (TTV)
transmissible gastroenteritis v. of
  swine
transmissible turkey enteritis v.
TT v.
tumor v.
turkey meningoencephalitis v.
Turlock v.
Uganda S v.
Umbre v.
unorganized v.
Uruma v.
vaccine v.
vaccinia v.
vacuolating v.
varicella v.
varicella-zoster v. (VZV)
variola v.
VEE v.
Venezuelan equine A
  encephalomyelitis v.
verruca v.
vesicular exanthema of swine v.
vesicular stomatitis v. (VSV)
viral hemorrhagic fever v.
visceral disease v.

V

NOTES

virus *(continued)*
    visna v.
    v. VP1 capsid protein
    VS v.
    WEE v.
    Wesselsbron disease v.
    Western equine encephalomyelitis v.
    West Nile encephalitis v.
    Willowbrook v.
    v. X disease
    xenotropic v.
    Yaba monkey v.
    yellow fever v.
    Zika v.
virus-associated hemophagocytic syndrome (VAHS)
virus-inactivating agent (VIA)
virus-neutralizing (VN)
virusoid
virus-transformed cell
VIS
    vaginal irrigation smear
VISA
    vancomycin-insensitive *Staphylococcus aureus*
viscera
viscera (*pl. of* viscus)
visceral
    v. disease virus
    v. inversion
    v. larva migrans
    v. leishmaniasis
    v. lymphomatosis
    v. motor neuron
    v. pleurisy
viscerale
    peritoneum v.
visceromegaly
visceroptosia
visceroptosis
viscerotomy
viscerotrophic reflex
viscid
viscidity
viscidosis
viscometer
viscosa
    Moritella v.
viscose
viscosimeter
    Ostwald v.
    Stormer v.
viscosimetry
viscosity
    absolute v.
    dynamic v.
    kinematic v.
viscosus
    Actinomyces v.

    Vibrio v.
    Xanthobacter v.
viscous
viscus, pl. **viscera**
    abdominal viscera
    perforated v.
    ruptured viscera
visible light
vision
    cribriform field of v.
VisionSaver lab lamp
Visiprep solid-phase extraction vacuum manifold
visna virus
visual
    v. evoked potential
    v. evoked response
    v. fluorescent screening test
    v. receptor cell
visualization
    computer graphics v.
vital
    v. dye
    v. red
    v. signs (VS)
    v. stain
    v. staining
vitamin
    v. A
    v. A_1
    v. A_1 aldehyde
    v. A_2
    v. A and carotene assays
    v. A clearance test
    v. A, D intoxication
    v. A unit
    v. B_1
    v. B_1 hydrochloride unit
    v. B_2
    v. B_2 unit
    v. B_3
    v. B_6
    v. B_7
    v. B_{12}
    v. $B12^a$
    v. B_{12} absorption test
    v. B_{12} assay
    v. B_{12} deficiency
    v. B12 neuropathy
    v. B_{12} unsaturated binding capacity
    v. B_6 assay
    v. B_c
    v. B complex
    v. B_6 unit
    v. B_x
    v. C unit
    v. D_3
    v. D assay
    v. deficiency anemia

v. D unit
v. E assay
v. E unit
v. K$_1$
v. K$_1$ oxide
v. K$_2$
v. K$_3$
v. K assay
v. K deficiency
v. K dependent plasma protein
v. K unit
microbial v.
water-soluble v.
vitamin-D-dependent rickets
vitamin-D-resistant rickets
vitaminoid action
Vitek GPI
vitellarium
Vitellibacter
   V. vladivostokensis
vitellin
vitellina
   membrana v.
vitelline
   polyvesicular v.
   v. sphere
vitellointestinal cyst
viterbiensis
   Caloramator v.
vitiation
vitiliginous
vitiligo, pl. **vitiligines**
   circumnevic v.
vitiligoidea
vitis
   Rhizobium v.
Vitivirus
vitrea
   lamina v.
   membrana v.
   substantia v.
   tunica v.
Vitreoscillaceae
vitreous
   v. body
   v. cavity
   v. cell
   v. humor
   v. lamella
   v. membrane
   v. space
   stroma of v.

vitreum
   corpus v.
   stroma v.
vitreus
   humor v.
vitrinus
   Trichostrongylus v.
vitro
   in v.
vitronectin
   v. receptor
Vitros
   V. analyzer
   V. anti-HBs assay
   V. HBsAg assay
   V. HBsAg confirmatory kit
   V. Immunodiagnostic Products anti-HBc calibrator
   V. Immunodiagnostic Products anti-HBc reagent pack
Vittaforma
vituli
   Acholeplasma v.
vitulorum
   Neoascaris v.
vivax
   v. fever
   v. malaria
   Plasmodium v.
   Trypanosoma v.
viverrini
   Opisthorchis v.
vivipara
   Probstymayria v.
Viviparidae
viviparus
   Dictyocaulus v.
vivo
   ex v.
   in v.
vivum
   contagium v.
VLA
   very late activation
   VLA antigen
vladivostokensis
   Vitellibacter v.
VLBW
   very-low birth weight
VLDL
   very-low-density lipoprotein

NOTES

V

VLSI
　　very large scale integration
VM
　　NATO code for nerve agent O-ethyl S-
　　[2-(diethylamino)ethyl]
　　methylphosphonothioate
VMA
　　vanillylmandelic acid
　　　VMA test
VMR
　　vasomotor rhinitis
VN
　　virus-neutralizing
VNTR
　　variable number of tandem repeats
VOC
　　volatile organic compound
vocal
　　　v. cord disease
　　　v. cord paralysis
　　　v. fold nodule
　　　v. fold polyp
vogeli
　　　Echinococcus v.
Voges-Proskauer (VP)
　　　V.-P. broth
　　　methyl red, V.-P. (MR-VP)
　　　V.-P. reaction
　　　V.-P. test
Vogt-Koyanagi syndrome
Vogt-Spielmeyer disease
Vogt syndrome
Vohwinkel syndrome
voinovskiensis
　　　Anoxybacillus v.
volatile
　　　v. nerve agent
　　　v. oil
　　　v. organic substances assay
　　　v. screen
　　　v. substance inhalation
volatility
volatilization
vole
　　　v. bacillus
　　　field v.
Volhard test
Volkmann
　　　V. canal
　　　V. contracture
　　　V. disease
　　　V. ischemic paralysis
　　　V. membrane
　　　V. syndrome
Vollmer test
volt (V)
　　　ampere-second per v. (As/V)
　　　electron v. (eV)
　　　giga electron v. (geV)

　　　kiloelectron v. (keV)
　　　megaelectron v. (MeV)
　　　million electron v.'s (MeV)
voltage
　　　anode v.
　　　v. divider
　　　v. drop
　　　high v.
　　　v. regulator
　　　ripple v.
voltage-gated channel
voltage-regulating transformer
voltage-regulator tube
voltage-to-frequency converter
voltammetry
volt-ampere (VA)
voltmeter
　　　digital v.
　　　vacuum tube v. (VTVM)
volt-ohm-milliammeter (VOM)
Voltolini disease
Volucribacter
　　　V. amazonae
　　　V. psittacicida
volume
　　　amniotic fluid total v.
　　　blood v. (BV)
　　　cell v. (CV)
　　　central blood v. (CBV)
　　　circulating blood v. (CBV)
　　　v. coefficient
　　　v. conduction
　　　conductivity cell v. (CCV)
　　　corpuscular v. (CV)
　　　corrected blood v. (CBV)
　　　v. depletion
　　　v. of distribution of bilirubin
　　　　(VDBR)
　　　effective circulating v. (ECV)
　　　effective circulating blood v.
　　　　(ECBV)
　　　euvolemic v.
　　　v. expansion
　　　extracellular v. (ECV)
　　　extracellular fluid v. (ECFV, EFV)
　　　fluid v. (FV)
　　　v. index
　　　inspiratory reserve v. (IRV)
　　　intracellular fluid v. (IFV)
　　　intrathoracic gas v. (IGV)
　　　v. of isoflow
　　　maximum expiratory flow v.
　　　　(MEFV)
　　　mean cell v. (MCV)
　　　mean corpuscular v. (MCV)
　　　mean platelet v. (MVP)
　　　minute v. (MV)
　　　packed cell v. (PCV)
　　　v. of packed cells (VPC)

v. of packed red cells (VPRC)
placental residual blood v. (PRBV)
plasma v. (PV)
pulmonary capillary blood v.
red blood cell v. (RBCV, VRBC)
red cell v. (RCV)
regional cerebral blood v. (RCBV)
residual v. (RV)
retention v.
reticulocyte mean corpuscular v.
  (MCVr)
v. substitute
test v.
thoracic gas v. (TGV)
tidal v. (TV, VT)
timed 24-hour v.
timed two-hour v.
total blood v. (TBV)
weight per v. (w/v)
volumetric
v. flask
v. pipette
v. solution (VS)
**voluntary interruption of pregnancy
(VIP)**
volutans
  Spirillum v.
Volutella cinerescens
volutin
Volvariella
Volvox
volvulosis
volvulus
gastric v.
Onchocerca v.
VOM
volt-ohm-milliammeter
vomica
vomicose
vomiting
v. agent
epidemic v.
vomitoria
Calliphora v.
vomitoxin
vomitus
colonic v.
von
v. Apathy gum syrup medium
v. Bechterew disease
v. Brunn nest
v. Clauss method

v. Economo disease
v. Economo encephalitis
v. Gierke disease
v. Hansemann histiocyte
v. Hansemann macrophage
v. Hippel disease
v. Hippel-Lindau disease
v. Hippel-Lindau gene
v. Jaksch disease
v. Kossa calcium assay
v. Kossa calcium stain
v. Kossa method
v. Kossa reaction
v. Meyenburg complex
v. Meyenburg disease
v. Recklinghausen disease
v. Willebrand disease (VW)
v. Willebrand factor
v. Willebrand factor antigen
v. Willebrand factor assay
v. Willebrand factor multimer
  assay
v. Willebrand syndrome
v. Zumbusch psoriasis
Voorhoeve disease
vortex, pl. **vortices**
vortexing
Vorticella
vortices (*pl. of* vortex)
vorticose
VP
variably positive
vasopressin
Voges-Proskauer
  VP test
VPC
vapor-phase chromatography
volume of packed cells
VPRC
volume of packed red cells
V/Q mismatch
VR
vascular resistance
VRBC
red blood cell volume
VRE
vancomycin-resistant *Enterococcus*
VRI
viral respiratory infection
Vrolik disease
VS
vital signs

V

NOTES

VS *(continued)*
  volumetric solution
    VS virus
vs
  vibration second
VSD
  ventricular septal defect
VSMC
  vascular smooth muscle cell
    VSMC infolding
VSV
  vesicular stomatitis virus
VT
  tidal volume
  vacuum tuberculin
VTVM
  vacuum tube voltmeter
VUE
  villitis of unknown etiology
Vuilleminia
vulcanalis
  Alicyclobacillus v.
vulcani
  Bacillus v.
Vulcanisaeta
  V. distributa
  V. souniana
vulgare
  Ketogulonicigenium v.
vulgaris
  acne v.
  Cellvibrio v.
  ichthyosis v.
  lupus v.
  Nitrobacter v.
  pemphigus v.
  Proteus v.
  psoriasis v.
  Strongylus v.
  verruca v.
vulneris
  Escherichia v.
vulnificus
  Vibrio v.
vulpis
  Crenosoma v.
  Trichuris v.
vulva, gen. and pl. **vulvae**

  elephantiasis v.
  kraurosis vulvae
  leukoplakia v.
  lichen sclerosus of v.
  multinucleated atypia of the v.
    (MAV)
  velamen v.
vulvar
  v. cancer
  v. dystrophy
  v. intraepithelial neoplasia (VIN)
  v. squamous hyperplasia
  v. tumor
vulvitis
  chronic atrophic v.
  chronic hypertrophic v.
  leukoplakic v.
  plasma cell v.
vulvovaginal
  v. anus
  v. candidiasis
  v. gland
vulvovaginitis
  Candida v.
VV
  viper venom
VVG
  Verhoeff-van Gieson
    VVG stain
VW
  von Willebrand disease
Vw antigen
VX
  NATO code for an extremely toxic
    persistent nerve agent (no common
    chemical name)
Vysis probe
VZ, V-Z
  varicella-zoster
VZV
  varicella-zoster virus
    VZV culture

W
watt
W factor
Waardenburg syndrome
Wachstein-Meissel stain for calcium-magnesium-ATPase
Waddliaceae
Waddlia chondrophila
Wade-Fite-Faraco stain
wadei
Leptotrichia w.
wadsworthensis
Sutterella w.
wadsworthia
Bilophila w.
wadsworthii
Legionella w.
Wagner
W. disease
W. test
Wagner-Meissner corpuscle
WAGR
Wilms tumor, aniridia, genital anomalies, mental retardation
WAGR syndrome
WAIHA
warm autoimmune hemolytic anemia
Waikavirus
waiotapuensis
Thermococcus w.
Wako
W. 1% crude papain
W. NEFA test kit
waksmanii
Shewanella w.
Waldenström
W. disease
W. macroglobulinemia (WM)
W. purpura
W. syndrome
W. test
Waldermaria
Waldeyer
W. gland
W. ring
W. ring lymphoma
Walker
W. carcinoma
W. carcinosarcoma
wall
anterior w.
cell w.
cross w.
hypertrophy of chamber w.
Wallemia sebi

Wallenberg syndrome
wallerian degeneration (WD)
wallet stomach
Walsh average
Walthard
W. cell
W. cell rest
Walther
W. canal
W. duct
Waltomyces
Wampole
W. *Clostridium difficile* Tox A/B II
W. Isolater blood culture system
wandering
w. abscess
w. cell
w. goiter
w. liver
w. nucleolonema
w. organ
w. pacemaker
w. pneumonia
Wang
W. needle
W. test
Wangiella
W. dermatitidis
warble fly
Warburg theory
Wardomyces inflatus
Wardomycopsis
Ward-Romano syndrome
Wardrop disease
warfare
biological w. (BW)
chemical w. (CW)
chemical and biological w. (CBW)
warfarin
w. assay
w. dosing decision
sodium w.
w. therapy
Warkany syndrome
warm
w. agglutination
w. agglutinin
w. autoantibody
w. autoimmune hemolytic anemia (WAIHA)
w. hemagglutinin
w. reactive antibody
warm-and-cold-type autoimmune hemolytic anemia

W

warm-cold hemolysin
warming
> blood w.

warneri
> *Staphylococcus* w.

wart
> anatomic w.
> anatomical w.
> anogenital w.
> cattle w.
> common w.
> digitate w.
> fig w.
> filiform w.
> flat w.
> genital w.
> Hassall-Henle w.
> infectious w.
> moist w.
> mosaic w.
> necrogenic w.
> pitch w.
> plane w.
> plantar w.
> pointed w.
> postmortem w.
> prosector's w.
> seborrheic w.
> senile w.
> soft w.
> soot w.
> telangiectatic w.
> tuberculous w.
> venereal w.
> viral w.

Wartenberg disease
Warthin-Finkeldey multinucleate giant cell
Warthin-Finkeldey-type
> W.-F.-t. polykaryocyte

Warthin-Starry
> W.-S. method
> W.-S. silver stain

Warthin tumor
wartpox
warty
> w. carcinoma
> w. dyskeratoma
> w. horn
> w. ulcer
> w. VIN

WAS
> Wiskott-Aldrich syndrome

wasabiae
> *Pectobacterium* w.

wash
> Gravlee jet w.
> w. time
> Zila Pro-Wash antiseptic hand w.

washed
> w. out deposit
> w. platelet activation
> w. red blood cell
> w. red cell (WRC)

washerwoman's skin
washing
> bronchial w.
> w. cytology
> pelvic w.

washout pipette
Wasmann gland
WASP
> Wiskott-Aldrich syndrome protein
> World Association of Societies of Pathology

Wassén test
wasserhelle
> w. cell
> w. hyperplasia

Wassermann
> W. antibody
> W. antigen
> W. reaction
> W. test

Wassermann-fast
Wassilieff disease
waste
> chemical w.
> infectious w.
> w. product
> radioactive w.
> toxic w.

wasting
> w. disease
> salt w.
> w. syndrome

Watanabe silver impregnation
water
> w. aspirator
> w. bacterium
> w. balance
> w. bath
> w. clear cytoplasm
> w. conductivity
> DEPC-treated w.
> w. deprivation diabetes insipidus differentiation test
> dextrose in w. (percent) (D/W)
> extracellular w. (ECW)
> w. gas
> gentian aniline w.
> w. gurgle test
> heavy w.
> HPLC w.
> w. of hydration
> w. immersion
> interstitial w. (ISW)
> w. intoxication

intracellular w. (ICW)
light w.
w. loading test
oil in w. (O/W)
w. in oil (W/O)
5 percent dextrose in w. (D5W, D₅W)
radiostable w.
ratio of number of ATPs produced to number of atmospheric oxygen molecules converted to w. (P:O)
total body w. (TBW)
tritiated w.

waterborne pathogen
water-clear
  w.-c. cell
  w.-c. cell hyperplasia
  w.-c. cell of parathyroid
Waterhouse-Friderichsen syndrome
watering-can
  w.-c. perineum
  w.-c. scrotum
watermelon stomach
waterpox
water-soluble
  w.-s. salt
  w.-s. scarlet
  w.-s. vitamin
water-trap stomach
watery diarrhea, hypokalemia, achlorhydria (WDHA)
watsoni
  Cladorchis w.
  Watsonius w.
Watsonius watsoni
Watson-Schwartz test
watt (W)
Wautersia
  W. basilensis
  W. campinensis
  W. eutropha
  W. gilardii
  W. metallidurans
  W. oxalatica
  W. paucula
  W. respiraculi
  W. taiwanensis
wave
  acid w.
  alkaline w.
  w. amplitude
  w. analyzer

diphasic w.
monophasic w.
w. number
periodic w.
polyphasic w.
sawtooth w.
sine w.
square w.
triangular w.
triphasic w.
w. velocity
waveform
wavefront phenomenon
waveguide
wavelength
  w. accuracy
  w. repeatability
  unit of w.
wavy border colony
wax
  embedding w.
  grave w.
  paraffin w.
  w. removal
waxy
  w. degeneration
  w. finger
  w. kidney
  w. liver
  w. spleen
  w. urinary cast
Wayson stain
waywayandensis
  Lentzea w.
WB
  whole blood
Wb
  weber
WBC
  white blood cell
   WBC urinary cast
WBC/hpf
  white blood cells per high-power field
WBF
  whole-blood folate
WBGT
  wet bulb globe temperature
WBH
  whole-blood hematocrit
WC
  whole complement

NOTES

WCC
    white cell count
WD
    wallerian degeneration
    well-differentiated
    Wilson disease
WDCA
    well-differentiated carcinoma
WDFA
    well-differentiated fetal adenocarcinoma
WDHA
    watery diarrhea, hypokalemia,
      achlorhydria
      WDHA syndrome
WDLL
    well-differentiated lymphocytic
      lymphoma
WE
    Western encephalitis
    Western encephalomyelitis
weakly
    w. positive (WP)
    w. reactive (WR)
weakness
    congenital vascular w.
weapon
    aerosolized plague w.
    anthrax as biological w.
    antique w.
    biological w.
    bone w.
    CBRN w.
    w. grade
    mass-casualty w. (MCW)
    nuclear, biological, chemical (mass-
      casualty w.) (NBC)
    smallpox as biological w.
weaponized T2 mycotoxin
weapons-grade nuclear material
wear-and-tear
    w.-a.-t. pigment
    w.-a.-t. pigmentation
web
    actin-myosin w.
    cell w.
    esophageal w.
    laryngeal w.
    terminal w.
Webb antigen
webbed
    w. finger
    w. neck
    w. toe
webbing
weber (Wb)
    W. gland
    W. paralysis
    W. stain

    W. syndrome
    W. test
Weber-Christian disease
Weber-Cockayne syndrome
Weber-Dubler syndrome
Weber-modified trichome stain
Weber-Rendu-Osler disease
Webster test
weddellite calculus
WEE
    Western equine encephalomyelitis
    WEE virus
weed
    Jimson w.
Weeks bacillus
Weeksella zoohelcum
Wegener
    W. granulomatosis
    W. syndrome
Wegner
    W. disease
    W. line
Weibel-Palade body
Weichselbaum diplococcus
Weidel reaction
Weigert
    W. iodine solution
    W. iron hematoxylin
    W. iron hematoxylin stain
    W. stain for *Actinomyces*
    W. stain for elastin
    W. stain for fibrin
    W. stain for myelin
    W. stain for neuroglia
Weigert-Gram stain
Weigert-Pal stain
weighing
weight (wt)
    atomic w.
    fat-free dry w. (FFDW)
    fat-free wet w. (FFWW)
    gram molecular w. (GMW)
    high birth w. (HBW)
    high molecular w. (HMW)
    ideal body w. (IBW)
    low birth w. (LBW)
    low molecular w. (LMW)
    molar w.
    molecular w. (MW)
    w. per volume (w/v)
    total body w. (TBW)
    unit of w.
    very-low birth w. (VLBW)
weighted average
weihenstephanensis
    Bacillus w.
Weil
    W. basal layer
    W. basal zone

W. disease
W. myelin sheath stain
W. syndrome
Weil-Felix (WF)
W.-F. agglutinin
W.-F. reaction (WFR)
W.-F. test
Weill-Marchesani syndrome
Weinberg reaction
Weinman medium
Weir Mitchell disease
Weiss criteria
Weissella
W. cibaria
W. kimchii
W. koreensis
W. minor
W. soli
W. thailandensis
Welch bacillus
welchii
Bacillus w.
Welcozyme HIV 1&2 ELISA antibody test
welder's
w. conjunctivitis
w. lung
Welker method
well
alive and w. (A&W)
w. differentiated
worried w.
well-differentiated (WD)
w.-d. carcinoma (WDCA)
w.-d. lymphocytic lymphoma (WDLL)
Wells syndrome
welt
wen
Wenckebach disease
wenyonii
Mycoplasma w.
Wepfer gland
Werdnig-Hoffmann disease
Werlhof disease
Wermer syndrome
werneckii
Cladosporium w.
Exophiala w.
Hortaea w.
Phaeoannellomyces w.

Werner
W. syndrome
W. test
Werner-His disease
Werner-Schultz disease
Wernicke
W. encephalopathy
W. syndrome
Wernicke-Korsakoff (WK)
W. encephalopathy
W. syndrome
Wescor Sweat-Chek conductivity analyzer
Wesenberg-Hamazaki body
Wesselsbron
W. disease
W. disease virus
W. fever
West
W. African fever
W. Indian smallpox
W. Nile encephalitis virus
W. Nile fever
W. Nile virus IgM capture test
W. syndrome
Westerdykella
Westergren
W. sedimentation rate
W. sedimentation rate test
westermani
Paragonimus w.
Western
W. blot
W. blot analysis
W. blot electrotransfer test
W. blot technique
W. encephalitis (WE)
W. encephalomyelitis (WE)
W. equine encephalitis
W. equine encephalomyelitis (WEE)
W. equine encephalomyelitis virus
W. immunoblot test
W. subtype Russian spring-summer encephalitis
Western-type intestinal lymphoma
westfalica
Gordonia w.
Westgard
W. multirule procedure
W. selection grid
Westphal disease

W

NOTES

Westphal-Strümpell
  W.-S. disease
  W.-S. pseudosclerosis
wet
  w. beriberi
  w. bulb globe temperature (WBGT)
  w. gangrene
  w. mount
  w. pleurisy
  w. prep
  w. preparation
  w. scanning technique
wetting agent
Wetzel test
Weyers oligodactyly syndrome
Weyers-Thier syndrome
WF
  Weil-Felix
  Working Formulation for Clinical Usage
WFR
  Weil-Felix reaction
WGA
  wheat germ agglutinin
  whole genome amplification
    MDA in WGA
Wharton
  W. duct
  W. jelly
  W. tumor
whartonitis
Whatman paper
wheal-and-erythema
  w.-a.-e. reaction
  w.-a.-e. skin test
wheal-and-flare reaction
wheal reaction time
wheat
  w. broth
  w. germ agglutinin (WGA)
  w. smut
Wheatstone bridge
Wheeler-Johnson test
whetstone crystal
whewellite calculus
whey
  w. acidic protein
  litmus w.
whiff test
whiplash
Whipple
  W. disease
  W. method
  W. test
  W. triad
whipplei
  Tropheryma w.
whipworm infection
Whispovirus
whistling face syndrome

white
  w. adipose tissue
  w. bile
  w. blood cell (WBC)
  w. blood cell antibody
  w. blood cell cast
  w. blood cell count
  w. blood cells per high-power field (WBC/hpf)
  w. cell count (WCC)
  w. clot syndrome
  w. corpuscle
  W. disease
  w. of eye
  w. fat
  w. fiber
  w. gangrene
  w. graft
  w. infarct
  w. leg
  w. matter
  methylene w.
  w. muscle
  w. muscle disease
  w. patch
  w. phosphorus (WP)
  w. piedra
  w. pneumonia
  w. pulp
  w. spot
  w. spot disease
  w. substance
  w. substance of Schwann
  w. thrombus
whitehead
whitepox
whitlow
  herpetic w.
  melanotic w.
Whitmore
  W. bacillus
  W. disease
  W. fever
  W. melioidosis
Whitmore-Jewett tumor staging system
whitmori
  Bacillus w.
  Malleomyces w.
Whitten effect
WHO
  World Health Organization
    WHO classification of tumors of the lymphoid tissue
    WHO histologic classification of ovarian tumors
WHO/ISUP
  World Health Organization/International Society of Urologic Pathologists
    WHO/ISUP classification

whole
  w. blood (B, WB)
  w. blood lysis technique
  w. complement (WC)
  w. genome amplification (WGA)
  w. ragweed extract (WRE)
whole-arm fusion
whole-blood
  w.-b. clotting time
  w.-b. folate (WBF)
  w.-b. hematocrit (WBH)
  w.-b. mercury level
whole-body titration curve
whole-mount section
whooping
  w. cough
  w. cough vaccine
whorl
  bone w.
  keratin w.
  paranuclear w.
whorled
  w. appearance
  w. mass
  w. storiform pattern
whorling cell
whorl-like array
Whytt disease
WI-38 cell
Wickerhamia
Wickerhamiella
wickerhamii
  Prototheca w.
Wickersheimer medium
wick fixative
Wickham striae
Widal
  W. reaction
  W. serum test
  W. syndrome
wide
  w. rete peg
  w. spectrum
widefield
  w. capillary microscopy
  w. eyepiece
  w. ocular
wide-spectrum keratin
widespread bone resorption
WiDr human colorectal cancer cell line
width
  hemoglobin distribution w. (HDW)

  red cell diameter w.
  red cell distribution w. (RDW)
  reticulocyte distribution w. (RDWr)
Wiedemann-Beckwith syndrome
WIF
  wnt inhibitory factor
Wilcoxon signed rank statistic
wild
  w. type
  w. yeast
Wilder stain for reticulum
Wildervanck syndrome
wild-type
  w.-t. allele
  w.-t. gene
Wilkie disease
Wilkins-Chilgren agar
Willebrand syndrome
Willemze type A lymphocyte
Williams
  W. factor
  W. stain
  W. syndrome
Williams-Campbell syndrome
williamsi
  Iodamoeba w.
Williamsia maris
Williopsis saturnus
Willis
  W. cord
  W. disease
  paracusis of W.
willisii
  chordae w.
Willowbrook virus
Wilms
  W. tumor
  W. tumor, aniridia, genital
    anomalies, mental retardation
    (WAGR)
Wilson
  W. disease (WD)
  W. method
  W. syndrome
wilsonian fulminant hepatitis
Wilson-Mikity syndrome
Winckel disease
wind
  blast w.
  w. contusion
windage
Windelmann granuloma

W

NOTES

window
> cochlear w.
> w. frame appearance
> oval w.
> round w.
> vestibular w.

windpipe
Windscheid disease
wing cell
Wingea robertsiae
wingless signaling pathway in
Drosophila
Winiwarter-Buerger disease
Winkler disease
winogradskyi
> *Algoriphagus w.*

winslowii
> stellulae w.

Winslow star
winter
> w. dysentery of cattle
> w. itch
> W. syndrome

winthemi
> *Margaropus w.*

Winton disease
Wintrobe
> W. hematocrit tube
> W. and Landsberg method
> macromethod of W.
> W. sedimentation rate
> W. sedimentation rate method

wipe
> bullet w.
> decontamination w.

wire-like collagen
wire-loop
> w.-l. abnormality
> w.-l. lesion
> w.-l. test

wire-wound resistor
Wirsung
> W. canal
> W. duct

wiry
Wiskott-Aldrich
> W.-A. syndrome (WAS)
> W.-A. syndrome protein (WASP)

WISP1
> wnt-1-induced secreted protein 1

wispy
> w. adhesion
> w. intraluminal basophilic mucin

Wistar rat
witflariensis
> *Sphingopyxis w.*

withering crypt appearance
within normal limits (WNL)
Witkop disease

Witkop-Von Sallmann syndrome
wittichii
> *Sphingomonas w.*

Wizard
> W. MagneSil PCR cleanup
> W. MagneSil plasmid purification
> W. MagneSil sequencing cleanup
> W. SV 96 plasmid purification

WK
> Wernicke-Korsakoff

WM
> Waldenström macroglobulinemia

WMD
> weapon of mass destruction
> biologic WMD
> chemical WMD

WMR
> work metabolic rate

WNL
> within normal limits

wnt
> wnt inhibitory factor (WIF)
> wnt signaling transduction pathway

wnt-1-induced secreted protein 1
(WISP1)
W/O
> water in oil

wobble hypothesis
wodanis
> *Vibrio w.*

woesei
> *Conexibacter w.*

Wohlfahrtia
> *W. magnifica*
> *W. opaca*
> *W. vigil*

wohlfahrtiosis
Wohlfart-Kugelberg-Welander disease
Wohlgemuth unit
Wojnowicia
Wolbachieae
Wolfe breast carcinoma
Wolff-Chaikoff effect
wolffian
> w. cyst
> w. duct carcinoma
> w. rest

Wolff-Parkinson-White (WPW)
> W. syndrome

Wolf-Hirschhorn syndrome
wolfii
> *Mortierella w.*

Wolfiporia
Wölfler gland
Wolf-Orton body
Wolfram syndrome
Wolfring gland
Wolf syndrome
Wolhynia fever

Wolinella
Wolman
    W. disease
    W. xanthoma
woman
    PMP w.
Wood
    W. glass
    W. lamp
    W. light
woodcutter's encephalitis
Woodsholea
    W. maritima
woodworker's lung
Wookey skin flap
woolgathering
woolsorter's
    w. disease (anthrax)
    w. pneumonia
Woringer-Kolopp
    W.-K. disease
    W.-K. pagetoid reticulosis
Workcell
    LH 755 hematology W.
worker
    abattoir w.
working
    w. distance
    W. Formulation for Clinical Usage (WF)
    W. Group on Civilian Biodefense
work metabolic rate (WMR)
workstation
    Biomek 2000, 3000, FX, FX assay, NX laboratory automation w.
    Coulter Gen-S Cell hematology w.
    Coulter TQ-Prep w.
    NanoChip molecular biology w.
    PrepPlus^7 series w.
    Q-Prep w.
    TQ-Prep w.
workup
    neonatal cholestasis w.
    transplantation w.
World
    W. Association of Societies of Pathology (WASP)
    W. Health Organization (WHO)
    W. Health Organization/International Society of Urologic Pathologists (WHO/ISUP)

worm
    w. abscess
    adult w.
    Bancroft filarial w.
    dragon w.
    Eustoma rotundatum parasitic w.
    serpent w.
    tongue w.
Wormley test
worried well
wort broth
wound
    abraded w.
    w. aspiration
    avulsed w.
    w. botulism
    center-fire rifle w.
    close range entrance w.
    contact entrance w.
    contused w.
    cranial gunshot w.
    w. culture
    distant range entrance w.
    w. elasticity
    entrance w.
    entry w.
    exit w.
    w. fever
    forensic evaluation of handgun w.
    gunshot w.
    w. healing
    hesitation w.
    incised w.
    indeterminate range entrance w.
    intermediate range entrance w.
    lacerated w.
    long-range w.
    loose contact w.
    missile w.
    mutilating w.
    penetrating w.
    perforating w.
    progressive contraction of w.
    shored-exit w.
    spiral w. (SW)
    stab w.
    superficial w.
    surgical w.
    tight contact w.
    zone of antemortem w.
woven bone

W

NOTES

WP
   weakly positive
   white phosphorus
WPW
   Wolff-Parkinson-White
WR
   weakly reactive
Wr^a antigen
wrap
        patient protective w. (PPW)
wratislaviensis
        Tsukamurella w.
Wratten filter
Wr^b antigen
WRC
   washed red cell
WRE
   whole ragweed extract
Wright
        W. antigen
        W. stain
        W. syndrome
Wright-Giemsa
        W.-G. stain
        W.-G. stained touch imprint

wrinkled
        w. nucleus
        w. silk appearance
writer's paralysis
WRN
        WRN gene
        WRN protein
wt
   weight
wt1 gene
Wu
        Folin and W. (FW)
Wuchereria
        W. bancrofti
        W. malayi
        W. pacifica
wuchereriasis
Wurster test
wurstgift (sausage poison)
w/v
   weight per volume
Wyeomyia
Wyeth bifurcated needle

X

magnification
X chromatin
X chromatin body
X chromosome
compound X
X deletion
globulin X
histiocytosis X
X karyotype
monosomy X
plasma factor X
X zone

Xa

antifactor Xa

xanchromatic

xanthelasma

generalized x.
x. palpebrarum

xanthelasmoidea

xanthelasmoideum

lymphangioma x.

xanthematin

xanthemia

xanthene dye

xanthine oxidase (XO)

xanthinuria

xanthoastrocytoma

pleomorphic x. (PXA)

Xanthobacter

X. aminoxidans
X. viscosus

xanthochromatic

xanthochromia

xanthochromic

xanthocyte

xanthoderma

xanthoerythrodermia perstans

xanthogranuloma

adult-type x.
juvenile x. (JXG)
necrobiotic x.

xanthogranulomatous

x. bursitis
x. cholecystitis
x. prostatitis
x. pyelonephritis (XPN)

xanthoma

x. cell
x. disseminatum (XD)
fibrous x.
x. generalisata ossium
normolipemic x. planum
x. palpebrarum
x. planum

x. striatum plamare
tuberoeruptive x.
x. tuberosum
x. tuberosum simplex
verrucous x.
Wolman x.

xanthomatosis

biliary x.
cerebrotendinous x.
normal cholesteremic x.

xanthomatous

x. deposition
x. pseudotumor

Xanthomonas

X. cynarae
X. maltophilia
X. oryzae

Xanthophyllomyces

xanthopsia

xanthopsydracia

xanthopterin

xanthosine monophosphate

xanthosine-5′-phosphate

xanthosis

xanthous

xanthum

Flavobacterium x.

xanthurenic

x. acid
x. aciduria

xanthuria

xanthylic acid

x-axis

XD

xanthoma disseminatum

XDP

xeroderma pigmentosum

Xe

xenon

^{127}Xe

^{133}Xe

xenic culture

xenoantigen

xenobiotic

xenocytophilic antibody

xenodiagnosis

xenogeneic graft

xenogenic

xenogenous

xenograft

x. tumor

xenografted tumor

xenology

Xenomeris

xenon (Xe)

X

xenon-127
xenon-133
xenoparasite
xenophaga
    Sphingomonas x.
xenopi
    Mycobacterium x.
Xenopsylla
    X. astia
    X. brasiliensis
    X. cheopis
Xenopus
    X. laevis
    X. laevis test
xenotransplantation
    organ x.
xenotropic virus
xenovorans
    Burkholderia x.
xeransis
xerantic
Xerocomus
xerocytosis
xeroderma pigmentosum (XDP, XP)
xeronosus
xerophthalmia
xerosis
    Corynebacterium x.
xerostomia
xerotic
Xerula
Xga blood group system
Xg antigen
xiligouense
    Myceligenerans x.
X-inactivation
xinjiangense
    Flavobacterium x.
    Halorubrum x.
xinjiangensis
    Ensifer x.
    Nocardiopsis x.
    Pseudonocardia x.
xinjisis
    Nesterenkonia x.
xiphoiditis
XLA
    X-linked agammaglobulinemia
    XLA gene
XLD
    xylose-lysine-deoxycholate
    XLD agar
X-linked
    X-l. agammaglobulinemia (XLA)
    X-l. agammaglobulinemia of Bruton
    X-l. character
    X-l. dominant inheritance
    X-l. familial hypophosphatemia
    X-l. gene

X-l. heredity
X-l. ichthyosis
X-l. infantile
    hypogammaglobulinemia
X-l. lymphoproliferative (XLP)
X-l. lymphoproliferative disease
X-l. microthrombocytopenia
X-l. recessive disorder
X-l. recessive inheritance
X-l. thrombocytopenia (XLT)
XLP
    X-linked lymphoproliferative
    XLP gene
    XLP syndrome
XLT
    X-linked thrombocytopenia
XM
    crossmatch
XO
    xanthine oxidase
    XO gonadal dysgenesis
    XO karyotype
    XO syndrome
X-Omat AR film
XP
    xeroderma pigmentosum
XPN
    xanthogranulomatous pyelonephritis
X-PO4
    protein X-PO4
x-ray
    butterfly pattern on chest x-r.
    x-r. crystallography
    full-body x-r.
    x-r. microscope
    postmortem dental x-r.
XRITC
    tetramethylrhodamine isothiocyanate
XS
    excess
x-scanning
    fast x-s.
XU
    excretory urogram
Xu
    x-unit
xuii
    Vibrio x.
x-unit (Xu)
XX
    XX gonadal dysgenesis
    XX karyotype
XXX
    XXX disorder
    XXX karyotype
XXXX disorder
XXXXY disorder
XXXY disorder
XX/XY sex chromosome pattern

XXY
    XXY karyotype
    XXY syndrome
XXYY disorder
XY
    XY female
    XY gonadal dysgenesis
    XY karyotype
Xylanibacterium ulmi
xylanilytica
    Cellulomonas x.
xylanilyticus
    Thermobacillus x.
Xylanimicrobium pachnodae
Xylanimonas cellulosilytica
xylanivorans
    Pseudobutyrivibrio x.
xylanovorans
    Clostridium x.
Xylaria
xylene
    acetone, methylbenzoate, x.
    (AMeX)
    x. artifact
    modified acetone methylbenzoate x.
    (ModAMeX)

xylene-soluble mounting medium
xyli
    Leifsonia x.
    Leifsonia xyli subsp. *x.*
xylidine
    ponceau de x.
xylinus
    Acetobacter x.
xylitol dehydrogenase
Xylogone sphaerospora
Xylohypha
xyloketose
xylol
xylose
    x. absorption test
    x. concentration test
xylose-lysine-deoxycholate (XLD)
xylosuria
xylulose
xylulosuria
xysma
XYY karyotype
X-Y-Z beam scanning method
    coordinates
XYZ syndrome

NOTES

Y

Y body
Y cartilage
Y chromatin
Y chromosome
fragment Y

Yaba

Y. monkey virus
Y. tumor

YAC

yeast artificial chromosome
YAC probe

Yakima

hemoglobin Y.

yamanashiensis

Nocardia y.

yanglingense

Rhizobium y.

Yania halotolerans

yanoikuyae

Sphingobium y.
Sphingomonas y.

yaoundei

Trichophyton y.

Yarrowia
Yatapoxvirus
yatensis

Streptomyces y.

yawing projectile
yaws

crab y.
forest y.

y-axis
YB1

Y-box binding protein

Yb

ytterbium

Yb-169 pentetate sodium
Y-box binding protein (YB1)
years of life saved (YLS)
yeast

baker's y.
dried y.
y. extract agar
y. fungus
imperfect y.
y. peptone dextrose
perfect y.
trypticase soy y. (TSY)
wild y.

yeei

Paracoccus y.

yellow

acridine y.
alizarin y.

y. atrophy of liver
y. body
y. bone marrow
brilliant y.
butter y.
y. cartilage
chrome y.
y. corallin
corralin y.
y. discoloration of skin
fast y.
y. fat
y. fever
y. fever vaccine
y. fever virus
y. fiber
y. hepatization
hydrazine y.
Leipzig y.
martius y.
metaniline y.
methyl y.
y. nail
y. nail syndrome
naphthol y. S
Paris y.
y. phosphorus
y. rain
y. spot (YS)
Sudan y.
Titan y.

yellow-brown wear and tear pigment
yellowish

eosin y.
light green SF y.

yeochonensis

Streptomyces y.

Yersinia

Y. enterocolitica
Y. enterocolitica antibody
Y. enterocolitica subsp. *palearctica*
Y. frederiksenii
Y. intermedia
Y. kristensenii
Y. pestis
Y. pestis antibody
Y. pestis F1 capsular antigen
Y. pseudotuberculosis

Yersinia-**related enterocolitis**
Yersinieae
yield

quantum y.

y-intercept
YKL-40

Y

Y-linked
> Y-l. character
> Y-l. gene

YLS
> years of life saved

Yokogawa fluke

yokogawai
> *Metagonimus y.*

yolk
> y. cell
> y. membrane
> y. sac antigen
> y. sac carcinoma
> y. sac tumor

yonseiensis
> *Caldanaerobacter subterraneus*
> subsp. *y.*
> *Thermoanaerobacter y.*

Yorke autolytic reaction

young
> maturity onset diabetes of the y.
> (MODY)
> Y. syndrome

Yperite (mustard gas)

YS
> yellow spot

YSI 2300 STAT glucose and lactate analyzer

Yta antigen

ytterbium (Yb)

yuanmingense
> *Bradyrhizobium y.*

yunnanensis
> *Pseudonocardia y.*
> *Streptomyces y.*

Yvon test

Z

Z band
Z disc
Z filament
Z line
Z score

Z1, Z2 series Coulter counter
Z2 Coulter Counter
Zahn

Z. infarct
Z. line
lines of Z.
striae of Z.

Zahorsky disease
Zambesi ulcer
Zamboni

Z. fluid
Z. solution

Zambusch

generalized pustular psoriasis of Z.

ZAP-70 deficiency
Zappert counting chamber
zatmanii

Methylobacterium z.

Zavarzinia compransoris
z-axis
ZB4 antibody
Z/D

zero defects

Z-dependent protease inhibitor (ZPI)
ZE

Zollinger-Ellison

zeae

Runella z.
Thermoanaerobacterium z.
Ustilago z.

zeaxanthinifaciens

Paracoccus z.

zebra body
Zebrina
Zein agar
Zeis gland
zeisian stye
Zeiss

Z. Axiophot fluorescent microscope
Z. Axioplan microscope
Z. Axioskop microscope
Z. counting cell
Z. LSM-10 laser microscope
Z. transmission electron microscope

Zellballen pattern
zellen

helle z. (pale cells)

Zellweger syndrome

Zenker

Z. degeneration
Z. diverticulum
Z. dysplasia
Z. fixative
Z. fluid
Z. necrosis
Z. solution

zenkerize
zeolite
zero

absolute z.
z. defects (Z/D)
limes z. (L₀, Lo)

zero-order

z.-o. kinetics
z.-o. reaction

ZES

Zollinger-Ellison syndrome

zeta

z. isoform
z. potential
z. sedimentation rate (ZSR)

zetacrit
zidovudine
Ziehen-Oppenheim disease
Ziehl-Neelsen

Z.-N. carbolfuchsin
Z.-N. method
Z.-N. stain

Ziehl stain
Ziemann

Z. dot
Z. stippling

Zieve syndrome
ZIG

zoster immune globulin

zijingensis

Pseudonocardia z.

Zika

Z. fever
Z. virus

Zila

Z. Pro-Scrub
Z. Pro-Wash antiseptic hand wash

Zimmermann

Z. corpuscle
Z. elementary particle
Z. granule
Z. pericyte
pericyte of Z.
polkissen of Z.
Z. reaction
Z. test

Zimmermannella
    Z. *alba*
    Z. *bifida*
    Z. *faecalis*
    Z. *helvola*
zinc
    z. assay
    z. deficiency
    z. finger gene
    z. finger protein
    z. flocculation test
    z. formalin
    z. oxide
    z. phosphide
    z. protoporphyrin (ZPP)
    z. sulfate centrifugal flotation
        technique
    z. sulfate flotation concentration
    z. sulfate flotation method
    z. sulfate turbidity test
zincalism
zinc-containing endopeptidase
Zinn zonule
Zinsser-Brill disease
Zinsser-Cole-Engman syndrome
ziram
zirconium granuloma
Z-line
ZO-1 protein
Zobellia
    Z. *amurskyensis*
    Z. *galactanivorans*
    Z. *laminariae*
    Z. *russellii*
    Z. *uliginosa*
zobellii
    Idiomarina z.
zoite
Zollinger-Ellison (ZE)
    Z.-E. syndrome (ZES)
    Z.-E. test
    Z.-E. tumor
zombie cell
zona, pl. **zonae**
    z. arcuata
    z. ciliaris
    z. dermatica
    z. epithelioserosa
    z. facialis
    z. fasciculata
    z. glomerulosa
    z. ignea
    z. medullovasculosa
    z. ophthalmica
    z. pectinata
    z. pellucida
    z. perforata
    z. reticularis

    z. serpiginosa
    z. tecta
zona-free hamster egg penetration test
zonal
    z. aganglionosis
    z. centrifugation
    z. electrophoresis
    z. necrosis
zonary
zonate
zonation effect
zone
    androgenic z.
    z. of antemortem wound
    antibody excess z.
    arcuate z.
    basement membrane z.
    centrilobular z.
    ciliary z.
    decontamination z.
    z. electrophoresis
    entry z.
    ependymal z.
    epileptogenic z.
    equivalence z.
    z. of equivalence
    extranodal marginal z.
    fetal z.
    flame intensity z.
    focal z.
    Golgi z.
    grenz z.
    hemorrhoidal z.
    hot z.
    hyperesthetic z.
    mantle z.
    marginal z. (MZ)
    z. of necrosis
    z. of ossification
    pectinate z.
    perinecrotic z.
    peripheral z.
    periurethral z.
    secondary X z.
    spherocyte with no central
        pallor z.
    subplasmalemmal dense z.
    sudanophobic z.
    support z.
    T z.
    thymus-dependent z.
    trabecular z.
    transition z. (TZ)
    transitional z.
    vermilion z.
    Weil basal z.
    X z.
zoning

zonula
- z. adherens
- z. ciliaris
- z. occludens

zonular
- z. fiber
- z. keratitis
- z. space

zonulares
- fibrae z.

zonularia
- spatia z.

zonule
- ciliary z.
- Zinn z.

zooanthroponosis
zooblast
zoofulvin
Zoogloea
zoograft
zoohelcum
- *Weeksella* z.

zooid
Zoomastigina
Zoomastigophorasida
Zoomastigophorea
zoomylus
Zoon balanitis
zoonosis
- bacterial z.
- enteric helminthic z.

zoonotic
- z. disease
- z. infection
- z. potential
- z. retrovirus

zooparasite
zoophilic
zoophyte
zooprophylaxis
Zooshikella ganghwensis
zoospermia
zootoxin
Zopfia
zopfii
- *Prototheca* z.

zoster
- z. encephalomyelitis
- z. immune globulin (ZIG)

zosterae
- *Desulfovibrio* z.

ZPI
- Z-dependent protease inhibitor
  - ZPI deficiency

ZPP
- zinc protoporphyrin

Z-protein
Zsigmondy test
ZSR
- zeta sedimentation rate
  - ZSR method

ZstatFlu
- Z. rapid diagnostic test for influenza A and B
- Z. test kit

Zuberella
zuckergussleber
Zuckerkandl
- Z. body
- Z. organ

Zülch
- monstrocellular sarcoma of Z.

Zurich
- hemoglobin Z.

Zyderm collagen
ZYF gene
Zygoascus
Zygofabospora
Zygohansenula
Zygolipomyces
Zygomycetes
zygomycosis
- rhinocerebral z.

zygonema
Zygopichia
Zygorenospora
Zygorhynchus
Zygosaccharomyces
zygosperm
zygospore
Zygosporium mansonii
zygote
zygotene
zygotoblast
zygotomere
Zygowillia
Zymobacterium
Zymodebaryomyces
zymodeme
zymogen granule
zymogenic cell
zymogram
zymographic analysis

NOTES

Z

zymography
    gelatin z.
Zymomonas
Zymonema
Zymopichia

zymoplastic substance
zymosan
Zyplast implant
Zythia

Anatomical Illustrations

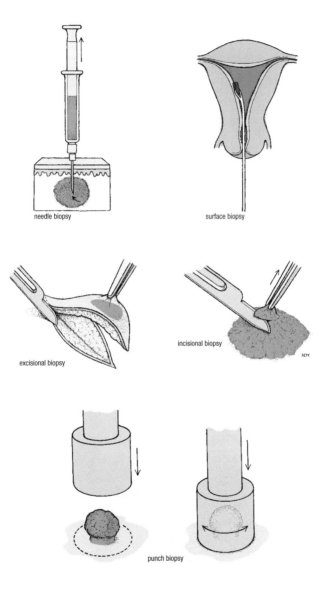

needle biopsy

surface biopsy

excisional biopsy

incisional biopsy

punch biopsy

biopsy techniques

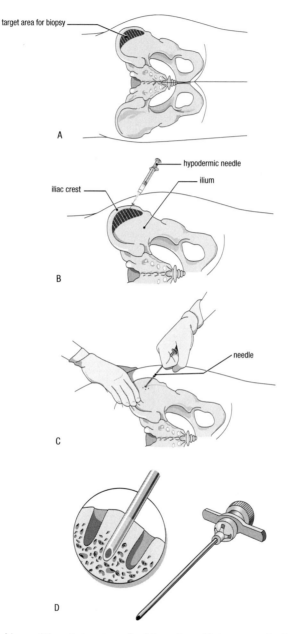

bone marrow biopsy: (A) posterior view of pelvic region with target area for bone marrow biopsy highlighted; (B) hypodermic needle penetrating skin at an angle to reach the ilium just below the iliac crest; (C) procedure used to obtain a bone marrow sample for biopsy from ilium by aspiration through needle; (D) close-up of aspiration technique and needle used for procedure

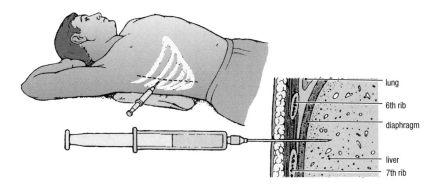

liver biopsy procedure

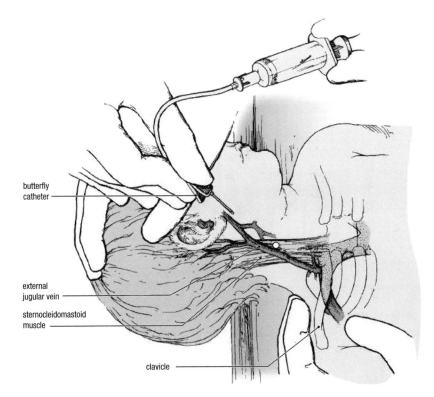

technique used in external jugular venipuncture: butterfly catheter is about to be inserted into external jugular vein of supine infant

A3

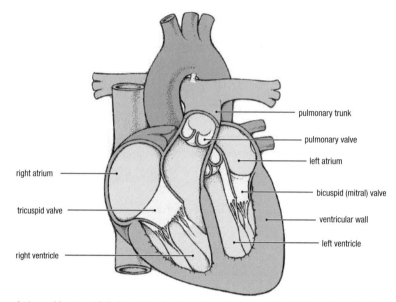

coronal view of heart with left ventricular hypertrophy: notice the thickened ventricular wall

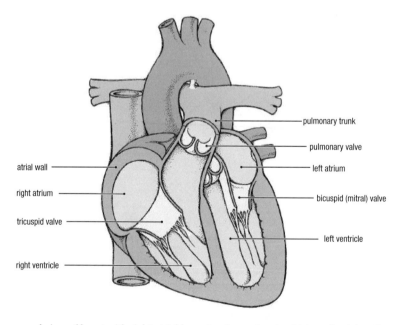

coronal view of heart with right atrial hypertrophy: notice the thickened atrial wall

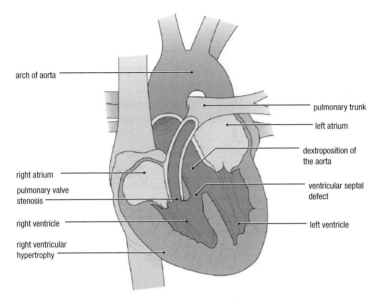

arch of aorta

pulmonary trunk

left atrium

dextroposition of
the aorta

right atrium

ventricular septal
defect

pulmonary valve
stenosis

right ventricle

left ventricle

right ventricular
hypertrophy

coronal view of heart in tetralogy of Fallot: characteristics include pulmonary valve stenosis, right ventricular hypertrophy, dextroposition of the aorta, and ventricular septal defect

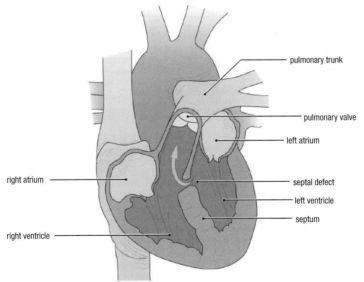

pulmonary trunk

pulmonary valve

left atrium

right atrium

septal defect

left ventricle

septum

right ventricle

coronal view of heart with a congenital ventricular septal defect: oxygenated blood is allowed to travel from the left to right ventricle into the pulmonary trunk

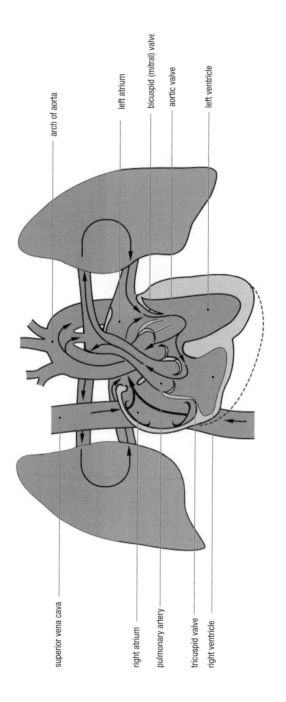

superior vena cava

right atrium

pulmonary artery

tricuspid valve

right ventricle

arch of aorta

left atrium

bicuspid (mitral) valve

aortic valve

left ventricle

coronal view of heart with tricuspid atresia: altered blood circulation due to a congenital lack of the tricuspid valve depicted

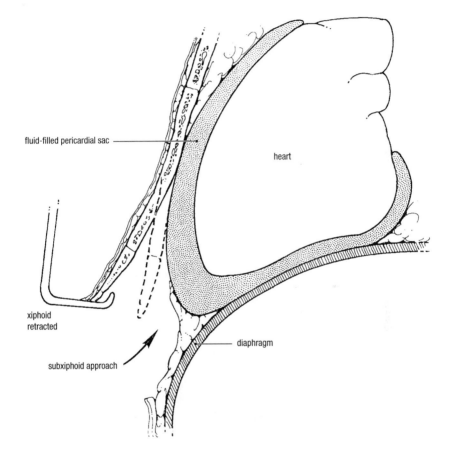

fluid-filled pericardial sac

heart

xiphoid
retracted

subxiphoid approach

diaphragm

cardiac tamponade: midsagittal view showing fluid-filled pericardial sac and subxiphoid surgical approach

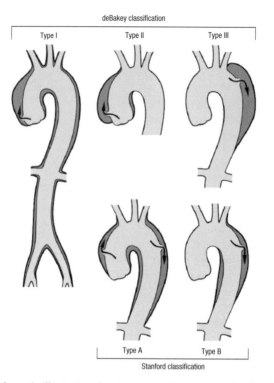

schematic illustration showing types of aneurysms affecting the aorta

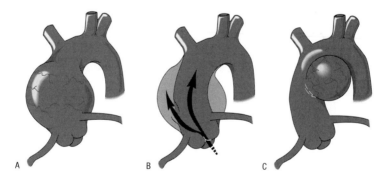

types of aortic aneurysms: (A) ascending aortic aneurysm; (B) aortic aneurysm; (C) aortic dissection

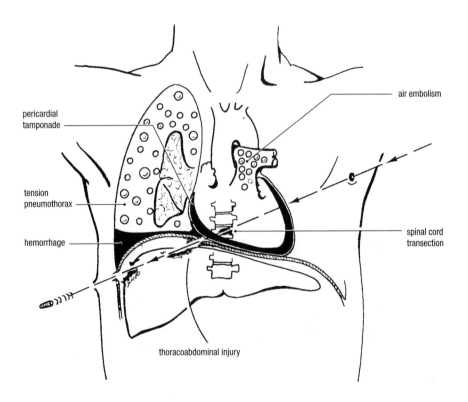

air embolism

pericardial
tamponade

tension
pneumothorax

hemorrhage

spinal cord
transection

thoracoabdominal injury

mechanisms of shock in penetrating thoracic trauma

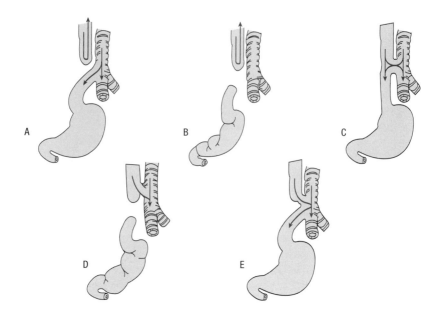

five variations of esophageal atresia: A) the most common is when the esophagus ends in a blind pouch; (B) both upper and lower segments end in blind pouches; (C) both upper and lower segments communicate with trachea; (D) very rarely, the upper segment ends in a blind pouch and communicates by a fistula to the trachea; (E) fistula connects to both upper and lower segments of the esophagus

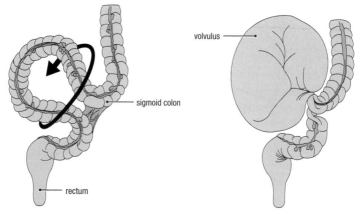

volvulus of sigmoid colon: the unattached loop of bowel twists (left), causing the bowel lumen to become obstructed (right), which leads to the inability of stool to pass and compression of the blood supply to the looped bowel segment

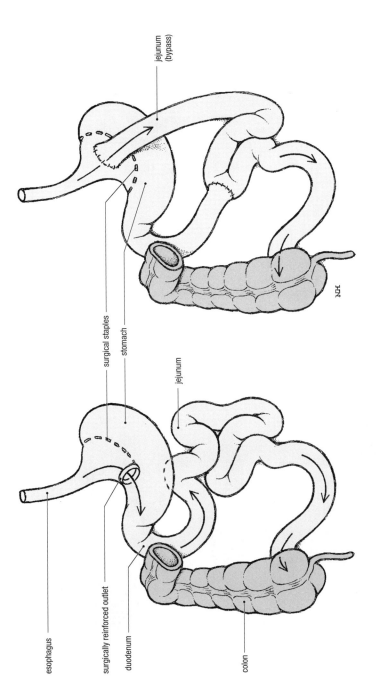

surgical procedures to control morbid obesity: (A) vertical banded gastroplasty; (B) gastric bypass (gastrojejunostomy); in both procedures, the reduction in gastric capacity leads to early satiety and, thus, favors consumption of smaller meals

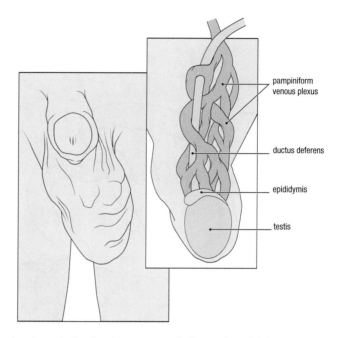

pampiniform
venous plexus

ductus deferens

epididymis

testis

varicocele: image of male genitalia showing anatomical abnormality of left scrotum ("bag of worms" appearance); insert shows internal anatomy of scrotum with abnormal dilation of the cremaster and pampiniform venous plexuses surrounding the spermatic cord

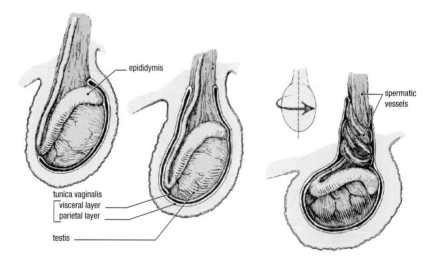

epididymis

spermatic
vessels

tunica vaginalis
visceral layer
parietal layer

testis

torsion: normal testicular anatomy (left); a bell-clapper deformity in the tunica vaginalis (middle), which can permit torsion of spermatic cord vessels (right)

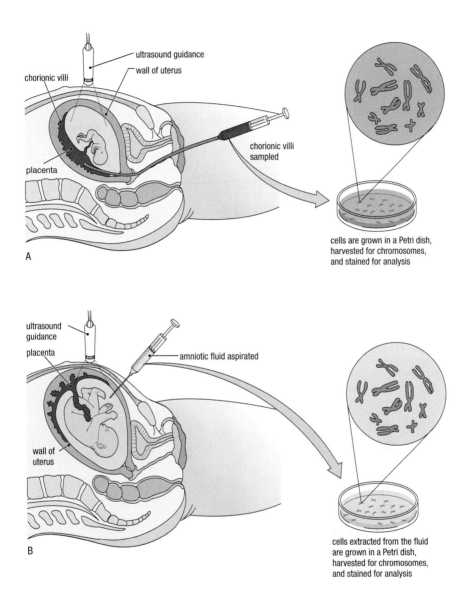

A

chorionic villi sampled

cells are grown in a Petri dish, harvested for chromosomes, and stained for analysis

B

amniotic fluid aspirated

cells extracted from the fluid are grown in a Petri dish, harvested for chromosomes, and stained for analysis

(A) chorionic villus sampling (9 to 11 weeks); (B) amniocentesis (15 to 18 weeks)

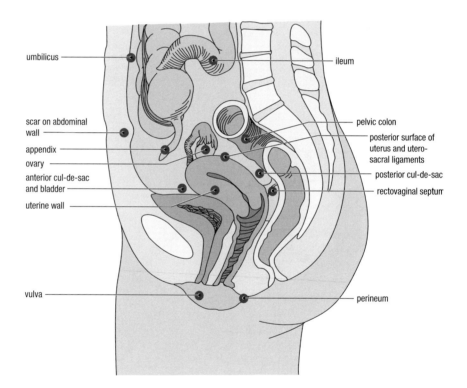

umbilicus

ileum

scar on abdominal
wall

pelvic colon

appendix

posterior surface of
uterus and utero-
sacral ligaments

ovary

anterior cul-de-sac
and bladder

posterior cul-de-sac

uterine wall

rectovaginal septum

vulva

perineum

sagittal view of female pelvic and abdominal regions showing common sites (dots) of endometriosis formation)

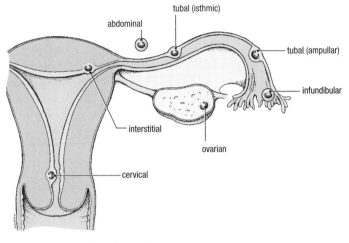

sites of ectopic pregnancy

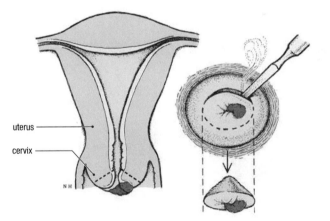

conization: neoplasm shown as darkest area, dashed line shows extent of resection

Appendix 1

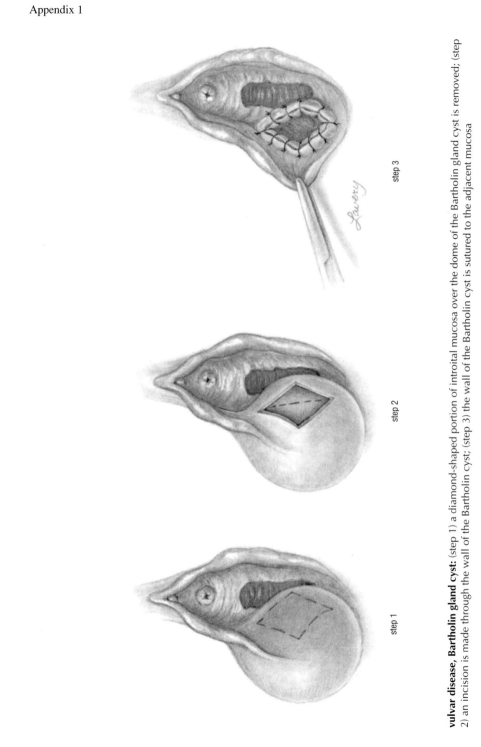

step 1   step 2   step 3

vulvar disease, Bartholin gland cyst: (step 1) a diamond-shaped portion of introital mucosa over the dome of the Bartholin gland cyst is removed; (step 2) an incision is made through the wall of the Bartholin cyst; (step 3) the wall of the Bartholin cyst is sutured to the adjacent mucosa

A16

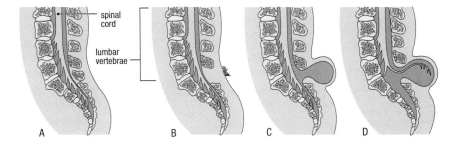

four degrees of spinal cord anomalies: (A) normal spinal cord; (B) spina bifida occulta; (C) meningo-cele; (D) myelomeningocele

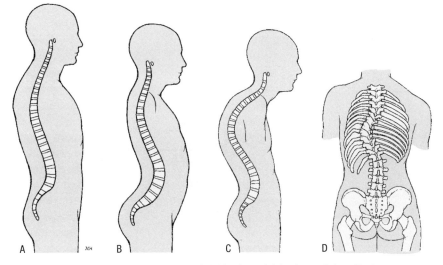

spinal curvatures: (A) normal; (B) lordosis; (C) kyphosis; (D) scoliosis

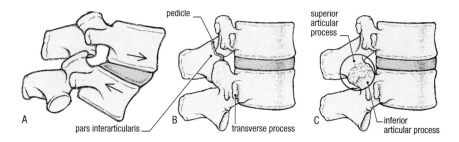

spondylolisthesis: (A) showing forward slippage of lumbar vertebra; spondylolysis: (B) showing fracture of pars interarticularis; spondylosis: (C) showing fixation of the articular processes

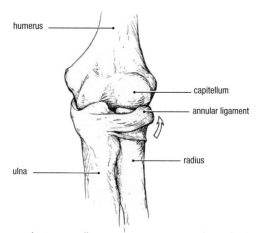

nursemaid's elbow: anatomy of injury to elbow joint; interposition of annular ligament between radial head and capitellum

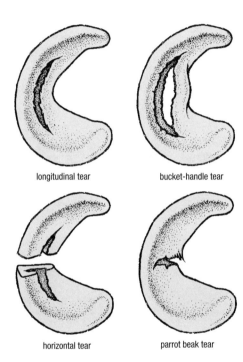

longitudinal tear

bucket-handle tear

horizontal tear

parrot beak tear

meniscal tears

Appendix 1

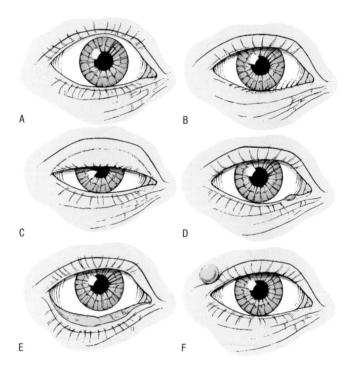

structural alterations and disorders of the eye: (A) exophthalmos; (B) entropion; (C) ptosis; (D) sty; (E) ectropion; (F) chalazion

(von) Apathy gum syrup medium
A1 broth, medium
acetamide nutrient broth
acetate agar
Acetobacter agar
acid broth
acriflavine-ceftazidime agar
actinomycete isolation agar
Aeromonas isolation agar base
agar No.1 bacteriological
agar No.2 bacteriological
agarose gel
algae culture agar, broth
Amies transport medium
Amies with charcoal
Amies without charcoal
AmnioMAX C-100 basal medium
anaerobe identification medium base
anaerobic agar, brewer's
anaerobic blood agar
anaerobic blood agar according to CDC
anaerobic egg agar base
antibiotic agar, broth
antibiotic broth
antibiotic medium 1 (See Penassay seed
    agar)
antibiotic medium 11 (See neomycin
    assay agar)
antibiotic medium 2 (See Penassay base
    agar)
antibiotic medium 3 (See Penassay
    broth)
antibiotic medium 5 (See streptomycin
    assay agar)
APT (all purpose Tween) agar
ascitic agar
aseptic commissioning broth
asparagine proline broth

Aspergillus differentiation agar base
ASS (antibiotic sulfonamide sensitivity)
    test agar
azide blood agar base
azide dextrose broth
azide glucose broth
Azotobacter agar glucose
Azotobacter agar mannitol
B12 assay broth USP
Bacillus cereus agar
Bacillus cereus egg yolk polymyxin
    agar base
Bacillus cereus selective agar
Bacillus medium
bacteriological peptone
Baird Parker agar, base, medium
Balamuth culture medium
Barnes agar
BBE (*Bacteroides* bile esculin) agar
BCYE (buffered charcoal yeast extract)
    agar
BDG (buffered deoxycholate glucose)
    broth
BDG (buffered deoxycholate glucose)
    broth, Hajna
beef extract dehydrated
beef heart infusion lactose agar
beef lactose agar
beta *Streptococcus* agar
BG (brilliant green)
BG (brilliant green) sulfa agar
BHI (brain-heart infusion) agar, broth
BHIS (brain heart infusion with fetal
    calf serum) broth
BiGGY (bismuth glycine glucose yeast)
    agar (See Nickerson agar)
bile broth
bile esculin agar

bile salt agar
bile salts brilliant green starch agar
biotin assay medium
biphasic broth medium
birdseed *(Guizotia abysinnica)* agar
BISC (bismuth iron sulfite cycloserine)
  medium
bismuth sulfite agar
bismuth sulphate sugar base A, base B
blood agar base
blood culture broth, medium
Boeck Drbohlav Locke egg serum
  medium
Bordet-Gengou medium
Bordet Gengou potato blood agar
boric acid broth
BPL (brilliant green, phenol red,
  lactose) agar according to Kauffmann
BPLS (brilliant green, phenol red,
  lactose, sucrose) agar
brain heart agar (See brain heart
  infusion agar)
Brazier CCEY (cefoxitin-cycloserine
  egg yolk) agar
Brettanomyces selective broth
brewer's anaerobic agar
BRILA (brilliant green bile lactose)
  broth
BRILA MUG (brilliant green bile,
  lactose, 4-methylumbelliferyl-B-D-
  glucuronide) broth
brilliant green 2%-bile broth
brilliant green agar modified
brilliant green agar with phosphates
brilliant green bile salt agar
BROLAC (bromothymol-blue, lactose)
  agar
BROLACIN (bromothymol-blue,
  lactose, cystine) agar
BROLACIN MUG(bromothymol-blue,
  lactose, cystine 4-methylumbelliferyl-
  B-D-glucuronide) agar
bromcresol purple lactose agar

bromocresol purple azide broth
Brucella agar
Brucella sheep blood agar
BSM (*Bifidus* selective medium) agar,
  broth, supplement
buffalo green monkey cells
buffered *Listeria* broth
buffered peptone water
buffered yeast agar (See yeast agar,
  buffered)
calcium caseinate agar
Campylobacter agar, broth
Campylobacter blood-free medium
Campylobacter selective agar according
  to Karmali (See Karmali
  Campylobacter agar)
Campylobacter selective supplement
CAN (colistin-nalidixic acid) agar
Candida Ident agar
carbohydrate broth
Cary Blair medium
casein agar
casein peptone lecithin polysorbate
  broth
casein peptone soybean flour peptone
  agar (See CASO agar or tryptic soy
  agar)
casein peptone soybean flour peptone
  broth (See CASO broth or tryptic soy
  broth)
casein soya broth (See tryptic soy broth
  or CASO broth)
casein-peptone dextrose yeast agar (See
  plate count agar)
casein-peptone dextrose yeast MUG(4-
  methylumbelliferyl-B-D-glucuronide)
  agar (See plate count MUG agar)
Casman broth
CASO (casein soy), salt broth (See
  tryptic soy salt broth)
CATC (citrate azide Tween carbonate)
  agar
cation-adjusted Mueller-Hinton broth

CB (chocolate blood) agar
CDC (Centers for Disease Control) anaerobic blood agar
CE (*Campylobacter* enrichment) broth
cetrimide agar
Chang complete medium
Chapman agar (*Staphylococcus* agar)
China Blue lactose agar
chlortetracycline selective supplement
chopped meat broth, medium
Christensen urea agar
CIN (cefsulodin-Irgasan-novobiocin) agar (See *Yersinia* agar)
citrate agar
citrate utilization test (See Simmons citrate agar)
citrate-citric acid buffer
clearing medium
CLED (cystine, lactose, electrolyte deficient) agar
CLED MUG (cystine, lactose, electrolyte deficient, 4-methylumbelliferyl-B-D-glucuronide) agar (See BROLACIN MUG agar)
clostridial differential broth
clostridial nutrient medium
Clostridium difficile agar base
Clostridium difficile supplement
coliform PA (presence absence) broth
Columbia agar base
Columbia blood agar
Columbia calcium nutrient agar
Columbia horse blood CAN (colistin-nalidixic acid) agar
Columbia medium
cooked meat broth, medium
cornmeal agar
Corynebacterium selective agar
CPC (cellobiose, polymyxin, colistin) agar, base
CPC (cellobiose, polymyxin, colistin) selective supplement
Cryo Gel embedding medium

CTA (cystine trypticase agar)
culture medium
CVS (chorionic villi) medium
cycloserine-cefoxitin-fructose agar
Czapek solution agar
Czapek Dox agar, medium
DCA (deoxycholate citrate agar)
DCA (deoxycholate citrate agar) Hynes modification
DCA (deoxycholate citrate agar) Leifson (See Leifson agar)
DCLS (deoxycholate, citrate, lactose, sucrose) agar
decarboxylase broth
deep agar
deoxycholate, desoxycholate agar
deoxycholate lactose agar
DEV Endo agar
DEV gelatin agar
DEV glucose broth
DEV glutamate broth
DEV lactose broth
DEV lactose peptone broth
DEV nutrient agar
DEV nutrient gelatin
DEV tryptophan broth
dextrose agar, broth
dextrose casein peptone agar
dextrose tryptone agar
DHL (deoxycholate hydrogen sulfide lactose) agar
DIASSALM (diagnostic semisolid *Salmonella*) agar
differential agar
differential medium
dispersive medium
DNase (deoxyribonuclease) agar, test agar
DRBC (dichloran rose bengal) agar
DRCM (See clostridial differential broth)
Drigalski LL (litmus lactose) agar
DTM (dermatophyte test medium)

DTM (dermatophyte test medium) agar
Duncan Strong broth, modified
Eagle basal medium
Easter and Gibson preenrichment broth
Easter and Gibson *Salmonella* medium
EC (*Escherichia coli*) broth, medium
ECD (*Escherichia coli* direct) agar
ECD MUG (*Escherichia coli* direct, 4-methylumbelliferyl-B-D-glucuronide) agar
EE (Enterobacteriaceae enrichment) broth (See Mossel broth)
egg yolk agar
egg yolk emulsion
egg yolk tellurite emulsion
Eijkman lactose broth
Elliker broth
Ellinghausen-McCullough/Johnson-Harris medium
EMB (eosin methylene blue) agar, base
EMEM (Eagle minimum essential medium)
Emmon modification of Sabouraud dextrose agar
Endo agar, medium
enriched medium
enrichment medium
Enterococcus selective agar
Escherichia coli MUG (4-methylumbelliferyl-B-D-glucuronide) agar
EVA (ethyl violet azide) broth
FAA (fastidious anaerobe agar)
FAB (fastidious anaerobe broth)
Farrant medium
FIL-IDF (Fédération Internationale de Laiterie, International Dairy Federation)
FDA (Federal Drug Administration)
fluid Sabouraud medium
fluid thioglycolate medium, USP
fluorescence agar
folic acid assay medium
formate ricinoleate broth

Fraser broth
Fraser broth base
FTM (fluid thioglycolate medium)
Gassner agar
GC (gonococcus) agar base
gelatin phosphate buffer
gelatin phosphate salt agar
germ count agar for foodstuffs
germ count agar sugar-free FIL-IDF
Giolitti Cantoni broth
glucose azide broth
glucose broth
glucose casein-peptone agar
glucose salt Teepol broth
glucose format broth
glycerin broth
glycerin potato broth
glycerol gelatin medium
GN (gram-negative) broth
GN (gram-negative) broth Hajna
GN (gram-negative) enrichment broth
GPS (gelatin phosphate salt) agar
GSP (glutamate starch phenol red) agar
Haemophilus medium
Halobacterium agar
Ham F-10 complete medium
Hanahan broth (See SOB broth)
HAT (hypoxanthine, aminopterin, and thymidine) medium
HBT (human blood Tween) agar
heart infusion agar
Hektoen enteric agar
Helicobacter pylori agar base
hippurate broth
HITES (hydrocortisone, insulin, transferrin, estradiol, and selenium) medium
Hoyle medium, base
IMA (inhibitory mold agar)
indole nitrate broth
inositol gelatin medium
iron broth
iron sulfite agar (See sulfite iron agar)

KAA (kanamycin aesculin azide) agar, broth
kanamycin agar for *Streptococcus*
kanamycin broth
Kaper agar
Karmali *Campylobacter* agar, base
KIA (Kligler iron agar)
King agar A, B
Kirchner TB (tuberculosis) medium
Koser citrate broth
KRANEP (potassium thiocyanate, actidione, sodium azide, egg-yolk, pyruvate) agar
Kundrat agar
KVLBA (kanamycin, vancomycin laked blood agar)
Lactobacillus agar according to DeMan, Rogosa and Sharpe (See MRS agar)
Lactobacillus broth (See Elliker broth)
Lactobacillus broth according to DeMan, Rogosa and Sharpe (See MRS broth)
Lactobacillus bulgaricus agar, base
Lactobacillus selective agar (See Rogosa agar)
lactose broth
lactose fuchsin sulfite agar (See DEV Endo agar)
lactose gelatin broth
Lambda medium
Lash casein hydrolysate serum medium
lauryl casein peptone broth (See lauryl sulfate broth)
lauryl sulfate broth
lauryl tryptose broth
LB (laked blood) agar, broth
LB (Luria Bertani) agar
LB top (Luria Bertani) agar
LDS (lysine decarboxylase sulfhydrase) test medium according to Costin
LE broth (*Listeria* enrichment)
LE/FDA broth (*Listeria* enrichment according to FDA/IDF-FIL)

lead broth
LEB (*Listeria* enrichment broth) according to FDA/IDF-FIL
Leifson agar (See DCA Leifson)
Letheen agar
Letheen agar base modified
Levine EMB (eosin methylene blue) agar
Lim broth
lipase-salt-mannitol agar
liquid Baird-Parker medium
Listeria broth
Listeria identification agar, PALCAM (See PALCAM Listeria selective agar)
Listeria identification broth, PALCAM (See L-PALCAM Listeria selective enrichment broth)
Listeria medium
Listeria Oxford medium (See Oxford agar)
Listeria selective agar
Listeria selective agar, Oxford (See Oxford agar)
Listeria selective enrichment supplement according to FDA
Listeria selective enrichment supplement according to IDF/FIL
litmus milk
liver broth
liver broth, starch
LL (lactose litmus) broth
LL (litmus lactose) agar according to Drigalski
Loeffler, Löffler agar
Loeffler, Löffler blood culture medium
Loeffler, Löffler coagulated serum medium
Loeffler, Löffler serum medium
Lowenstein-Jensen medium
L-PALCAM (*Listeria* polymixin, acriflavine, lithium chloride,

ceftazidine, aesculin, mannitol) selective enrichment broth

LPM (lithium chloride phenyl ethanol moxalactam) plating agar

LS (*Lactobacillus Streptococcus*) differential agar

LST (lauryl sulfate tryptose)

LST-MUG (lauryl sulfate tryptose 4-methylumbelliferyl-B-D-glucuronide) broth

lysine arginine iron agar

lysine decarboxylase salt broth

lysine iron agar

M (membrane filter) azide broth

M (membrane filter) broth

M (membrane filter) *Enterococcus* agar

M (membrane filter) *Enterococcus* agar, modified

M (membrane filter) standard methods broth

M 17 agar, broth

M BCG (membrane filter bromcresol green) yeast and mold broth

M Endo (membrane filter Endo) broth

MacConkey agar

MacConkey agar No. 3

MacConkey agar, sorbitol

MacConkey agar, with salt

MacConkey agar, without salt

MacConkey broth

MacConkey broth purple

MacConkey sorbitol agar

magnesium chloride malachite green broth (See RVS broth, modified)

malachite green broth

malonate phenylalanine broth

malt agar

malt extract agar, broth, powder

mammalian cells

mannitol salt agar

mannitol salt phenol red agar

mannitol, lysine, crystal violet, brilliant

mannitol-egg yolk-Polymyxin agar (See *cereus* selective agar)

Martin broth

Martin Lester agar, medium

maximal recovery diluent

McBride agar

McClung Toabe agar base

McCoy cells

m-CP (membrane filter *Clostridium perfringens*) agar base

meat liver agar

MEM alpha (minimum essential medium with alpha modification)

membrane filter rinse fluid, USP

M-HD (membrane filter Hajna Damon) Endo broth with brilliant green

MF (membrane filter) Endo broth

m-FC (membrane focal coli) broth with rosolic acid

M-H (Mueller-Hinton) agar, broth

M-Hajna Damon Endo broth with brilliant green

M-HD (membrane filter Hajna Damon) Endo broth

Middlebrook agar, broth, medium

milk agar

milk agar with cetrimide

milk agar, modified according to Brown & Scott

milk plate count agar

mineral modified glutamate broth, base, medium

Mitchison medium

MLS (membrane lauryl sulfate) broth

modified Holt-Harris & Teague medium

modified NYC (New York City) medium

modified Stuart medium

modified Thayer-Martin agar

modified Tinsdale agar

modified TSB for E. coli 0157

Mossel broth

motility medium

motility nitrate agar

MOX (magnesium oxalate) agar

MRS (deMan, Rogosa, Sharpe) agar, broth

MR-VP (methyl red and Voges-Proskauer) broth, medium

MSA (mannitol salt agar)

MSRV (modified semisold Rappaport-Vassiliadis) medium

Mucate broth

Mueller-Hinton agar, broth

Mueller-Kauffman tetra broth

MUG (4-methylumbelliferyl-B-D-glucuronide) agar

MUG (4-methylumbelliferyl-B-D-glucuronide) tryptone soya agar

MY (malt extract yeast extract) glucose agar

mycobiotic agar

neomycin assay agar

Neussel-Linzenmeier agar

niacin assay medium

Nickerson BiGGY agar (See BiGGY agar)

NIH (National Institutes of Health) thioglycolate broth

nitrate agar, broth

nonselective medium

Novy- McNeal-Nicolle medium

Nu Sens agar

nutrient agar

nutrient agar for oxidase

nutrient agar with NaCl

nutrient broth

nutrient broth E

nutrient broth No 2

nutrient broth without NaCl

nutrient gelatin

nutrient medium

oatmeal tomato paste agar

OF (oxidation fermentation) medium

OF (oxidation fermentation) basal medium

OF (oxidation fermentation) test nutrient agar

OGY (oxytetracycline glucose yeast) agar

OGYE (oxytetracycline, glucose, yeast extract) agar base

ÖNÖZ agar (*Salmonella* agar according to Önöz)

OPSP (oleandomycin, polymyxin, sulfadiazine *perfringens*) medium

orange serum agar, broth

Oxford agar base

Oxford *Listeria* selective agar

oxidative-fermentative-polymixin B-bacitracin-lactose agar

PA (presence absence) broth

Pai agar

PALCAM (polymixin, acriflavine, lithium chloride, ceftazidine, aesculin, mannitol) agar base

PALCAM (polymixin, acriflavine, lithium chloride, ceftazidine, aesculin, mannitol) *Listeria* selective *supplement* according to Van Netten et al.

pantothenate medium USP

Parietti broth

Park and Sanders enrichment broth (base)

Park and Sanders selective supplement I, II

passive medium

PBW (peptone water, phosphate-buffered)

PC (*Pseudomonas cepacia*) agar

PEA (phenylethyl alcohol) agar

PEA (phenylethyl alcohol) blood agar

Penassay base agar, broth

Penassay base agar, Grove and Randall antibiotic agar

Penassay broth, Grove and Randall antibiotic broth

Penassay seed agar

peptone proteose (See proteose-peptone)

peptone sorbitol bile broth

peptone water (See tryptone water)

peptone water tryptic digest (See tryptone water)

peptone water, phosphate-buffered

peptone yeast dextrose agar, broth (See YPD agar, broth)

peptone yeast extract agar (See YEPD agar)

peptone yeast extract iron citrate agar

peptonized milk agar

perfringens agar base (See OPSP)

perfringens selective agar according to Angelotti (See SPS agar)

perfringens supplement I, II

Petragnani medium

Pfeiffer blood agar

phenethyl alcohol agar

phenol red broth base

phenylalanine agar

phosphate gelatin buffer (See gelatin phosphate buffer)

Pike streptococcal broth

plant tissue culture media

plate count agar

plate count agar APHA

plate count agar with antibiotic free skim milk (See plate count skim milk agar)

plate count agar, special

plate count MUG (4-methylumbelliferyl-B-D-glucuronide) agar

plate count skim milk agar

PM (penicillin in milk) indicator agar

polysorbate 80 medium

potassium chlorate supplement

potassium tellurite solution

potassium thiocyanate actidione sodium azide egg-yolk pyruvate agar (See KRANEP agar)

potato dextrose (glucose) agar

potato flakes agar

potato glucose rose bengal agar, base

potato glucose sucrose agar

preenrichment broth

Preuss broth

Pril mannitol agar

Propionibacteria growth supplement

proteose-peptone

PRYES (pentachloro rose bengal yeast extract) agar

Pseudomonas agar (King agar B)

Pseudomonas agar base

Pseudomonas agar F

Pseudomonas agar F base

Pseudomonas agar P

Pseudomonas agar P base

Pseudomonas and *Aeromonas* selective agar according to Kielwein (See GSP agar)

Pseudomonas asparagine broth

Pseudomonas isolation agar

Pseudomonas selective agar base (See cetrimide agar)

purple carbohydrate fermentation broth (See bromocresol purple azide broth)

rabbit blood agar

Raka Ray broth

Rambach equivalent agar (See *Salmonella* Chromogen agar)

RBC (rose bengal chloramphenicol) agar, base

RC agar (*Clostridium* agar)

RCA (reinforced Clostridial agar)

RCM (reinforced clostridial medium) (See clostridial nutrient medium)

REA (rice extract agar)

Rees culture medium

refracting medium

Regan-Lowe charcoal agar

Regan-Lowe transport medium

rice Tween agar

Rogosa agar
Rogosa agar, modified
Rogosa SL agar
Rosenow veal brain broth
Roswell Park Memorial Institute
   medium
RVS (Rappaport Vassiliadis) broth,
   medium
RVS (Rappaport Vassiliadis) broth,
   modified
RVS (Rappaport Vassiliadis) enrichment
   broth
RVS (Rappaport Vassiliadis) semisolid
   medium
Sabhi agar, medium
Sabouraud 2% dextrose (glucose) agar
Sabouraud 4% dextrose (glucose) agar
Sabouraud agar modified
Sabouraud dextrose broth
Sabouraud glucose agar modified (See
   Sabouraud 2% glucose agar)
Sabouraud liquid medium USP
Sabouraud maltose agar, broth
Saccharomyces medium
salicin broth
Salmonella agar according to Önöz
Salmonella chromogen agar
Salmonella enrichment broth according
   to Rappaport and Vassiliadis (See
   RVS broth, modified)
salt meat broth
SBM (selenite brilliant green mannitol)
   enrichment broth
Schaedler blood agar
Schaedler medium
Schleifer-Kramer agar
SDA (Sabouraud dextrose agar)
selective agar for pathogenic fungi
selective blood agar
selective medium
selenite broth base
selenite cystine broth
selenite enrichment broth

sensitivity test agar
separating medium
serum agar, broth
SFP (sugar-free penicillin) agar
Shapton agar
sheep blood agar
Simmons citrate agar
single step *Staphylococcus* selective
   agar (4S medium)
skim milk agar
Slanetz and Bartley agar (See
   Enterococcus selective agar)
sodium biselenite
sodium chloride (6.5%) culture medium
sorbic acid agar, base
sorbitol-MacConkey agar
soy agar, broth
soybean casein digest agar (See CASO
   agar or tryptic soy agar)
soybean casein digest broth (See CASO
   broth or tryptic soy broth)
soybean casein digest MUG agar (See
   CASO MUG agar)
soybean casein digest salt broth (See
   tryptic soy salt broth)
SP4 medium
Spirolate broth
SPS (sulfite polymyxin sulfadiazine)
   agar, modified
SS (*Salmonella Shigella*) agar
standard II nutrient agar
standard methods agar (See plate count
   agar)
Staphylococcus agar, medium
Staphylococcus enrichment broth
   according to Giolitti and Cantoni
   (See Giolitti Cantoni broth)
Staphylococcus selective agar (See
   Baird Parker agar)
sterility test broth
Streptococcus agalactiae selective agar
   (See TKT agar)
Streptococcus selective agar

Streptococcus thermophilus isolation agar
Streptomyces medium
Streptomycin assay agar
Stuart broth
Stuart Ringertz agar
Stuart transport medium
sucrose broth
sucrose-phosphate-glutamate transport
  medium
sugar broth
sugar-free agar
sulfate reducing broth
sulfite iron agar
Superbroth agar
supplemented anaerobic blood agar
support medium
synthetic medium old tuberculin
  trichloroacetic acid (precipitated)
Tartoff-Hobbs broth, modified (See
  terrific broth, modified)
TAT broth base
TB (tetrathionate broth)
TB (tetrathionate broth) agar
TBG (tetrathionate, brilliant green, bile)
  enrichment broth
TBX (tryptone bile X-glucuronide) agar
TCBS (thiosulfate citrate bile salts
  sucrose) *cholerae* medium
TCBS (thiosulfate citrate bile sucrose)
  agar
tellurite glycine agar, base, medium
Tergitol-7 agar
terrific broth, modified (See Tartoff-
  Hobbs broth)
test agar for the residue test according
  to Kundrat (See Kundrat agar)
tetrathionate crystal violet enrichment
  broth according to Preuss (See Preuss
  broth)
tetrathionate enrichment broth
  according to Muller-Kauffmann
TG (thioglycolate) broth, medium

TG (thioglycolate) broth with
  Resazurine
TG (thioglycolate) 135C broth
Thermoacidurans agar
Ticarcillin supplement
tissue culture medium
TKT (thallium sulfate,crystal violet, B
  toxin blood) agar
TM (Thayer-Martin) agar, medium
TMAO (trimethylamine N-oxide) agar
Tobie, von Brand, and Mehlman
  diphasic medium
Todd-Hewitt agar, broth
tomato juice agar, broth
TPB (tryptone phosphate broth)
TPEY (tellurite polymyxin egg yolk)
  agar, base
transport medium
transport medium according to Stuart,
  modified by Ringertz (See Stuart
  Ringertz agar)
tributyrin agar
tryptic soy agar (See CASO agar)
tryptic soy broth (See CASO broth)
tryptic soy lecithin polysorbate broth
  (See casein peptone lecithin
  polysorbate broth)
tryptic soy MUG (4-methylumbelliferyl-
  B-D-glucuronide) agar (See CASO
  MUG agar)
tryptic soy salt broth
tryptic soy yeast extract broth
trypticase soy agar
trypticase soy with agar broth
tryptone agar
tryptone bile agar
tryptone bile glucuronide agar
tryptone glucose yeast extract agar (See
  plate count agar)
tryptone medium
tryptone phosphate water (See peptone
  water, phosphate-buffered)
tryptone soy agar USP

tryptone soy broth USP

tryptone soya agar (See tryptic soy agar or CASO agar)

tryptone soya broth (See tryptic soy broth or CASO broth)

tryptone soya lecithin polysorbate broth (See casein peptone lecithin polysorbate broth)

tryptone soya MUG (4 methylum-belliferyl-B-D-glucuronide) agar (See CASO MUG agar)

tryptone soya salt agar with magnesium sulfate

tryptone soya salt broth (See tryptic soy salt broth)

tryptone water (See also peptone water)

tryptone yeast extract agar

tryptose agar, broth

tryptose blood agar base

TSA (tryptic soy agar) (See CASO agar)

TSA (tryptic soy agar) blood agar base

TSAMS (See tryptone soya salt agar with magnesium sulfate)

TSB (trypticase soy broth)

TSC (tryptose sulfite cycloserine) agar (See *perfringens* agar)

TSI (triple sugar iron) agar

TT (tetrathionate) broth, base, enrichment broth

TTC (triphenyltetrazolium chloride) solution

TYC (trypticase, yeast extract, cystine) medium

Tyrobutyricum broth (base)

UB (universal beer) agar

urea agar base according to Christensen (See Christensen urea agar)

urea agar, base, broth

urea test agar (See Christensen urea agar)

urease test broth

USP (United States Pharmacopeia)

UVM (University of Vermont) broth base

UVM (University of Vermont) *Listeria* broth, medium

UVM (University of Vermont) *Listeria* selective enrichment broth, modified

V-8 agar for lactobacilli (See tomato juice agar, broth)

vaginalis agar

Vibrio selective agar (See TCBS agar)

vitamin B12 assay broth base, medium

vitamin biotin assay broth

vitamin folic acid assay broth base

vitamin nicotinic acid assay broth

vitamin pantothenic acid assay broth

VJ agar (Vogel-Johnson) agar

VP (Voges Proskauer) broth, modified

VP (Voges Proskauer) broth

VPSA (*Vibrio parahaemolyticus* sucrose agar)

VRB (violet red bile) agar

VRB MUG (violet red bile 4-methyl-umbelliferyl-B-D-glucuronide) agar

VRBD (violet red bile dextrose) agar

VRBG (violet red bile glucose) agar

Wadsworth *Brucella* blood agar

Wagatsuma agar

water agar

water blue metachrome-yellow lactose agar according to Gassner (See Gassner agar)

Weinman medium

Wesley broth

West-Wilkins medium

wheat broth

Wilkins-Chalgren agar, broth

Wilson Blair selective media (See bismuth sulfite agar)

WL (Wallerstein Laboratory) differential agar

WL (Wallerstein Laboratory) nutrient agar, medium

wort agar, broth

XLD (xylose-lysine-deoxycholate) agar
yeast agar, buffered
yeast and mold broth
yeast carbon base
yeast extract agar
yeast extract powder
yeast nitrogen base
yeast nitrogen base without amino acids
yeast nitrogen base without amino acids
    and ammonium sulfate
YEPD (yeast extract peptone dextrose)
    agar, broth (See YPD)
YER (yeast extract rose bengal) broth,
    base
Yersinia enrichment broth base
Yersinia isolation agar
Yersinia selective agar (See CIN)
YGC (yeast extract glucose
    chloramphenicol) agar
YM (yeast malt) agar, broth
YPD (yeast peptone dextrose) agar,
    broth (See YEPD)

Stains, Dyes, and Fixatives

Abbott stain
aceto orcein stain
acetic-lacmoid stain
Achúcarro stain
acid blue 45
acid dye
acid fuchsin stain
acid green 25
acid phosphatase stain
acid phosphatase stain with tartrate
acid phosphatase stain without tartrate
acid red 87
acid red 91
acid stain
acid methenamine silver stain
acid-Schiff stain
acridine dye
acridine orange stain
acridine yellow
acriflavine HCl
acriflavine neutral
acriflavine stain
ACS (amino-cupric-silver)
AFB (acid fast bacillus) stain
Ag-AS (silver-ammoniacal silver) stain
Albert diphtheria stain
Albert stain No. 1
Alcian blue 8GX
Alcian blue stain
Alcian yellow stain
alizarin
alizarin cyanin
alizarin cyanin BBS stain
alizarin purpurin
alizarin red
alizarin red S
alizarin red stain
alizarin yellow

alizarin yellow R
alizarin yellow R sodium salt
alkaline phosphatase stain
alkaline toluidine blue O
alpha-naphthyl esterase stain with or
    without fluoride
Altmann aniline acid fuchsin stain
alum carmine
Alzheimer stain
amaranth
amethyst violet
amido black 10B stain
amidonaphthol red
aminoanthraquinone dye
3 amino 9 ethylcarbazole stain
ammonium oxalate crystal violet
ammonium silver carbonate stain
amphoteric dye
aniline blue
aniline blue modified trichrome stain
aniline blue water soluble
aniline gentian violet
aniline xylene
anionic dye
anthracene blue
antimony stain
Archibald stain
argentaffin stain
argyrophil stain
arsenic stain
auramine O fluorescent stain
auramine-rhodamine stain
azan stain
azocarmine B stain
azovan blue
azure I, II
azure A, B, C stain
azure eosin stain

azure II-methylene blue stain
Baker Sudan black
basic fuchsin hydrochloride
basic fuchsin stain
basic fuchsin-methylene blue stain
Bauer chromic acid leucofuchsin stain
Becker stain
Belke-Kleihauer stain
Bennhold Congo red stain
Bensley aniline-acid fuchsin-methyl
    green
Bensley safranin acid violet
benzo fast pink 2BL
benzo sky blue method
benzopurpurin 4B
Berg stain
Berlin blue
Bernthsen methylene violet
Best carmine stain
beta-glucuronidase stain
Betke stain
Biebrich scarlet red
Biebrich scarlet water soluble
Biebrich scarlet-picroaniline blue
Bielschowsky stain
Biondi-Heidenhain stain
bipolar stain
Birch-Hirschfeld stain
Bismarck brown R
Bismarck brown stain
Bismarck brown Y stain
Bodian copper-Protargol stain
Borrel blue stain
Bowie stain
brilliant black BN
brilliant blue G250
brilliant blue R250
brilliant cresyl blue stain
brilliant crocein MOO
brilliant green
brilliant vital red
brilliant yellow
bromcresol purple

bromocresol green
bromocresol purple desoxycholate
bromphenol blue
bromthymol blue
Brown-Brenn stain
butyrate esterase stain
Cajal astrocyte stain
Cajal gold sublimate stain
calcium red
calcofluor white stain
carbolfuchsin stain
carbolfuchsin-methylene blue stain
carbol-thionin stain
carmine
carminic acid 50%
carminic acid 95%
C-banding stain
CEA gold-5 stain
CEA immunoperoxidase stain
celestine blue B
Chicago sky blue 6B
China blue
chlorazol black E stain
chlorophenol red
chocolate brown
chondroitin sulfate stain
ChrA (chromogranin A)
    immunoperoxidase stain
chromate stain
chrome alum carmine
chrome alum hematoxylin-phloxine
    stain
chrome azurol S
chrome red
chrome violet
chrome violet CG
chrome yellow
chromotrope 2B
chromotrope 2R
chromoxane cyanine R
chrysophenine
Churukian-Schenck stain
Ciaccio stain

Clayton yellow
cochineal red A
colloidal iron stain
colophonium alcohol
Congo Corinth
Congo red stain
contrast stain
Coomassie brilliant blue G-250
Coomassie brilliant blue R-250
cotton blue
cresol red
cresyl blue
cresyl blue brilliant
cresyl fast violet
cresyl violet
cresyl violet acetate
cresylecht violet
crocein scarlet 3B
crystal violet stain
curcumin
cyclin D stain
Da Fano stain
Dane and Herman keratin stain
Dane stain
DAPI (46'-diamidino-2-phenylindole-2
   HCl) dye, stain
Darrow red stain
del Rio-Hortega stain
Delafield hematoxylin stain
deoxyribonucleic acid stain
dextran blue
Diagnex Blue
diaminobenzidine stain
diazo blue B
diazo stain
dibromofluorescein
Dieterle stain
differential stain
Diff-Quik stain
diphenylmethane dye
direct fluorescent antibody stain
DOPA (dihydroxyphenylalanine) stain
Dorner stain

double stain
D-PAS (diastase-periodic acid-Schiff)
   stain
eau de Javelle
Ehrlich acid hematoxylin stain
Ehrlich aniline crystal violet stain
Ehrlich triacid stain
Ehrlich triple stain
Einarson gallocyanin-chrome alum stain
elastic fiber stain
elastica van Gieson stain
endolymphatic dye
eosin B spirit soluble
eosin B stain
eosin B water soluble
eosin stain
eosin Y free acid
eosin Y sodium salt
eosin Y stain
eosin-methylene blue
Eranko fluorescence stain
eriochrome black A
eriochrome black T reagent ACS
eriochrome blue black R
eriochrome cyanine R
erioglaucine
erythrosine B
erythrosine B free acid
ethidium bromide stain
ethyl eosin
ethyl green
ethyl orange
ethyl violet
Evans blue
Farrant medium
fast blue B stain
fast garnet GBC base, salt
fast green FCF
fast green stain
fast red B stain
fast sulphon black F
fast yellow stain
ferric ammonium sulfate stain

Feulgen stain (Schiff reagent)
Feulgen sulfurous acid solution
Field rapid stain
Fink-Heimer stain
Fite stain
Fite Faraco stain
Flemming triple stain
fluorescein alcohol soluble
fluorescein alcohol soluble USP
fluorescein stain
fluorescein water soluble
fluorescence plus Giemsa stain
fluorescent dye
fluorescent stain
fluorochrome stain
Fontana-Masson silver stain
Fontana methenamine silver stain
Fontana stain
Foot reticulin impregnation stain
Foot silver solution
formol-calcium
Fouchet stain
Fraser-Lendrum stain
fuchsin acid
fuchsin basic
fuchsin stain
fungal stain
Fungalase-F stain
gallamine blue
gallein
gallocyanine
ganglioside GD2 stain
G banding stain
Genta stain
gentian orange stain
gentian violet stain
Giemsa chromosome banding stain
Giemsa stain
Gill #2 hematoxylin blue stain
Gill hematoxylin stain
Gimenez stain
Glenner-Lillie stain
glycogen stain

glycolipid stain
glycoprotein stain
GMS (Gomori methenamine-silver) stain
Golgi stain
Gomori aldehyde fuchsin stain
Gomori chrome alum hematoxylin-phloxine stain
Gomori-Jones periodic acid-methenamine-silver stain
Gomori nonspecific acid phosphatase stain
Gomori nonspecific alkaline phosphatase stain
Gomori one-step trichrome stain
Gomori silver impregnation stain
Gomori Takamatsu stain
Gomori trichrome stain
Goodpasture stain
Gordon and Sweet stain
Gothard differentiator
Gram iodine stain
Gram stain
Gram-chromotrope stain
Gram-Weigert stain
Gridley stain
Grimelius argyrophil stain
Grimelius stain
Grocott-Gomori methenamine-silver stain
Grocott methenamine silver stain
guinea green B
Hale colloidal iron stain
Hansel stain
Harris hematoxylin
H&E (hematoxylin and eosin) stain
Heidenhain azan stain
Heidenhain iron hematoxylin stain
Heinz body stain
Helly fixative
hemalum
hematein
hematoxylin and eosin (H&E) stain

hematoxylin stain
hematoxylin, malachite green, basic
   fuchsin
hematoxylin-phloxine B stain
hematoxylin, phloxine, saffron
hemosiderin stain
heparan sulfate PG (proteoglycan) stain
hexamethyl violet
Highman Congo red
Hirsch-Peiffer stain
Hiss capsule stain
histochemical stain
Hoechst dye
Hoffman violet
Holmes stain
Hortega neuroglia stain
Hucker-Conn crystal violet solution
Hucker-Conn stain
hydrazine yellow
hydroxyketone dye
8-hydroxy-136-pyrenetrisulfonic acid
   trisodium salt
immunoalkaline phosphatase stain
immunofluorescent stain
immunogold-silver stain
immunohistochemical stain
immunoperoxidase stain
indamine dye
India ink capsule stain
India ink stain
indigo blue
indigo carmine
indigo synthetic
indigoid dye
indocyanine green
indophenol blue
indophenol dye
indulin water soluble
intravital stain
iodine stain
iodonitrotetrazolium
iron hematoxylin stain
iron stain

Isamine blue
isosulfan blue
Janus green B
Jenner Giemsa stain
Jenner stain
Jones methenamine silver stain
Jones stain
Kaiserling fixative
Kasten fluorescent Feulgen stain
Kasten fluorescent PAS (periodic acid-
   Schiff) stain
Kermes dye
ketonimine dye
Kinyoun acid-fast stain
Kinyoun carbolfuchsin stain
Kinyoun stain
Kittrich stain
Kleihauer stain
Kleihauer-Betke stain
Klinger-Ludwig acid-thionin stain
Klüver-Barrera Luxol fast blue stain
Kokoskin stain
Kossa stain
Kronecker stain
Kühne methylene blue
laccaic acid
lacmoid
lactone dye
lactophenol cotton blue stain
LAP (leukocyte alkaline phosphatase)
   stain
Lauth violet
Lawless stain
lead citrate stain
lead hydroxide stain
Leder stain
Leipzig yellow
Leishman stain
Lendrum inclusion body stain
Lendrum phloxine-tartrazine stain
Lepehne-Pickworth stain
leuco crystal violet
leuco patent blue

leucomethylene blue
leukocyte acid phosphatase stain
Leukostat stain
Leung stain
Levaditi stain
Levine alkaline Congo red stain
light green SF
light green SF yellowish
Lillie allochrome connective tissue stain
Lillie azure-eosin stain
Lillie ferrous iron stain
Lillie sulfuric acid Nile blue stain
Liquichek reticulocyte control and stain
Lison-Dunn stain
lissamine green B
lithium carmine
Loeffler, Löffler caustic stain
Loeffler, Löffler methylene blue
Loeffler, Löffler stain
Lugol stain
Luna-Ishak stain
Luxol fast blue stain
Macchiavello stain
MacNeal tetrachrome blood stain
malachite green
malachite green oxalate
malarial pigment stain
Maldonado-San Jose stain
Mallory aniline blue stain
Mallory collagen stain
Mallory iodine stain
Mallory phloxine stain
Mallory phosphotungstic acid
  hematoxylin
Mallory trichrome stain
Mallory triple stain
Mancini iodine stain
Mann methyl blue-eosin stain
Marchi stain
martius scarlet blue
martius yellow
Masson argentaffin stain
Masson trichrome stain

Masson-Fontana ammoniacal silver
  stain
Maximow stain
Mayer acid alum hematoxylin stain
Mayer hemalum stain
Mayer hematoxylin stain
Mayer mucicarmine stain
Mayer mucihematein stain
May-Grünwald stain
May Grünwald Giemsa stain
Meissel stain
mercurochrome 220
metachromatic dye
metachromatic stain
metanil yellow stain
methenamine silver stain
methine dye
methyl blue
methyl green
methyl green-pyronin
methyl green zinc chloride salt
methyl green pyronin stain
methyl orange
methyl orange reagent ACS
methyl red
methyl violet
methyl violet 2B
methyl yellow
methylene azure
methylene blue
methylene blue chloride
methylene blue dye
methylene blue stain
methylene green
methylene violet
methylene violet 3RAX
methylene white
methylthymol blue
Milligan trichrome stain
modified acid-fast stain
modified auramine-rhodamine stain
modified Kinyoun stain
modified Steiner stain

modified Ziehl-Nielsen stain

Morin (fluorescent) stain

Movat pentachrome stain

Mowry colloidal iron stain

MSB (martius scarlet blue) trichrome stain

mucicarmine stain

Musto stain

myeloperoxidase stain

n-propyl red

Nakanishi stain

naphthol-ASD chloroacetate esterase stain

naphthol green B

naphthol yellow S stain

natural dye

natural red Certistain

Nauta stain

NBT (nitroblue tetrazolium) dye, stain

negative stain

Neisser stain

neutral red

neutral stain

new coccine dye

new fuchsin

new methylene blue

new methylene blue N

Nicolle stain

night blue stain

nigrosin stain

nigrosin water soluble

nigrosin B alcohol soluble

Nile blue

Nile blue A

Nile blue A chloride

Nile blue A sulfate

Nile red

ninhydrin Schiff stain

Nissl stain

nitro dye

nitroso dye

Noble stain

Novelli stain

NSE (nonspecific esterase) stain

nuclear fast red stain

nuclear stain

oil red O stain

orange II, IV

orange IV

orange G stain

orcein stain

Orth lithium carmine stain

osmium tetroxide stain

oxalic acid stain

oxazin dye

oxytalan fiber stain

Padykula-Herman stain

Paget-Eccleston stain

Palmgren silver impregnation stain

panoptic stain

PAP (peroxidase-antiperoxidase) stain

Pap stain

paracarmine stain

Paragon blue stain

pararosaniline acetate

pararosaniline HCl

Paris green

Paris yellow

PAS (periodic acid-Schiff) stain

PAS-orange G stain

patent blue

patent blue A

patent blue V dye

patent blue VF

patent blue violet

Pearl iron stain

pentamethyl violet

periodic acid-silver methenamine stain

Perls Prussian blue stain

peroxidase stain

phenosafranin

4-(phenylazo)-1-naphthalenamine hydrochloride (Chrysoidin)

phloxine B stain

phloxine-tartrazine stain

phosphomolybdic acid stain

phthalocyanine dye
picric stain
picrocarmine stain
picroindigocarmine stain
picro Mallory trichrome stain
picronigrosin stain
Pizzolato peroxide-silver
plasmocorinth B
polychrome methylene blue stain
polymethine dye
Ponceau 3R
Ponceau 4R
Ponceau 6R stain
Ponceau G R 2R
Ponceau S
Pontamine sky blue stain
potassium metabisulfate stain
potassium permanganate stain
Procion blue HB
p-rosaniline acetate stain
p-rosaniline acetate powder
Protargol stain
Prussian blue iron stain
Prussian blue stain
PTA (phosphotungstic acid) stain
PTAH (phosphotungstic acid
  hematoxylin) stain
Puchtler alkaline Congo red
Puchtler Sirius red
Puchtler-Sweat stain
pyronin B
pyronin Y
pyrrol blue stain
Q-banding stain
quinacrine chromosome banding stain
quinaldine red
quinoline dye
quinoline yellow
quinoline yellow SS
Rambourg periodic acid, chromic acid,
  methenamine silver stain
Ranson pyridine silver stain

reactive red 4
rhodamine 6G
rhodamine B
rhodamine B base alcohol soluble
rhodamine B O
rhodamine blue
rhodamine stain
Romanowsky blood stain
Romanowsky stain
Romanowsky-Giemsa stain
rosaniline dye
rose bengal stain
rosolic acid
Roux stain
ruthenium red
Ryan stain
Sabin-Feldman dye
saffron
safranin O
safranin stain
salt dye
Sayeed stain
SBB (Sudan black B) stain
scarlet red stain
scarlet red sulfonate
Schaeffer-Fulton stain
scharlach red
Schiff stain
Schmorl ferric-ferricyanide reduction
  stain
Schmorl picrothionin stain
Schneider carmine
Schultz stain
selective stain
Sevier-Munger stain
Shorr trichrome stain
silver impregnation
silver nitrate stain
silver nitroprusside
silver protein stain
silver stain
silver-ammoniacal silver stain

Sirius red
Sirius red F3B
Smith silver stain
Snook reticulum stain
sodium bisulfite stain
sodium hydroxide stain
sodium thiosulfate stain
Steiner stain
Sternheimer-Malbin Sedi-stain
Sternheimer-Malbin stain
stilbene dye
stilbene yellow
Stirling modification of Gram stain
Sudan I, II, III, IV
Sudan black stain
Sudan brown
Sudan orange G
Sudan red 7B
Sudan red III
Sudan yellow
Sudan yellow G
sulfur dye
supravital stain
Susa fixative
synthetic dye
Taenzer stain
Taenzer Unna stain
Takayama stain
tartrazine stain
tetrachrome stain
tetramethylbenzidine stain
thiazin dye
thiazole dye
thioflavine S
thioflavine T, TG
thionin acetate
thionin stain
thymol blue
Tilden stain
Timm silver sulfide
titan yellow
Tizzoni stain
Toison stain

toluidine blue O
toluidine blue stain
toluylene red
TRAP (tartrate-resistant acid
    phosphatase) stain
triarylmethane dye
trichrome stain
triphenylmethane dye
tropaeolin O
Truant auramine-rhodamine stain
trypan blue
trypan red
Turk blood counting fluid
Turkey red
Turnbull blue stain
ultrafast Pap stain
ultramarine blue
Unna stain
Unna Pappenheim stain
Unna-Taenzer stain
uranyl acetate stain
urate crystals stain
van Ermengen stain
van Gieson stain
Ventana ES stain
Verhoeff elastic tissue stain
Victoria blue B
Victoria blue R
Victoria blue stain
Victoria orange
vimentin immunoperoxidase stain
vital dye
vital red
vital stain
von Kossa stain
VVG (Verhoeff-van Gieson) stain
Wachstein-Meissel stain
Wade-Fite-Faraco stain
Warthin-Starry silver stain
water blue-orcein
Wayson stain
Weber-modified trichome stain
Weber stain

Weigert-Gram stain
Weigert-Pal stain
Weigert iron hematoxylin stain
Weigert stain
Weil myelin sheath stain
Wilder stain
Williams stain
Wright stain
Wright-Giemsa stain
xanthene dye
xylene cyanol FF
xylidine Ponceau 2 R
xylidine Ponceau stain
yellow corallin
Zenker formol
Ziehl stain
Ziehl-Neelsen stain
Zike flagella mordant

Appendix 4
Greek Alphabet

LOWER CASE	NAME	UPPER CASE
α	alpha	A
β	beta	B
γ	gamma	Γ
δ	delta	Δ
ε	epsilon	E
ζ	zeta	Z
η	eta	H
θ	theta	Θ
ι	iota	I
κ	kappa	K
λ	lamda	Λ
μ	mu	M
ν	nu	N
ξ	xi	Ξ
ο	omicron	O
π	pi	Π
ρ	rho	P
ς , σ	sigma	Σ
τ	tau	T
υ	upsilon	Y
	phi	Φ
χ	chi	X
ψ	psi	Ψ
ω	omega	Ω

Elements and Symbols

SYMBOL	ELEMENT	ELEMENT	SYMBOL
Ac	actinium	actinium	Ac
Ag	silver	aluminum	Al
Al	aluminum	americium	Am
Am	americium	antimony	Sb
Ar	argon	argon	Ar
As	arsenic	arsenic	As
At	astatine	astatine	At
Au	gold	barium	Ba
B	boron	berkelium	Bk
Ba	barium	beryllium	Be
Be	beryllium	bismuth	Bi
Bi	bismuth	boron	B
Bk	berkelium	bromine	Br
Br	bromine	cadmium	Cd
C	carbon	calcium	Ca
Ca	calcium	californium	Cf
Cd	cadmium	carbon	C
Ce	cerium	cerium	Ce
Cf	californium	cesium	Cs
Cl	chlorine	chlorine	Cl
Cm	curium	chromium	Cr
Co	cobalt	cobalt	Co
Cr	chromium	copper	Cu
Cs	cesium	curium	Cm
Cu	copper	dysprosium	Dy
Dy	dysprosium	einsteinium	Es
Er	erbium	erbium	Er
Es	einsteinium	europium	Eu
Eu	europium	fermium	Fe
F	fluorine	fluorine	F
Fe	fermium	francium	Fr
Fe	iron	gadolinium	Gd
Fr	francium	gallium	Ga
Ga	gallium	germanium	Ge
Gd	gadolinium	gold	Au
Ge	germanium	hafnium	Hf
H	hydrogen	helium	He

SYMBOL	ELEMENT	ELEMENT	SYMBOL
He	helium	holmium	Ho
Hf	hafnium	hydrogen	H
Hg	mercury	indium	In
Ho	holmium	iodine	I
I	iodine	iridium	Ir
In	indium	iron	Fe
Ir	iridium	krypton	Kr
K	potassium	lanthanum	La
Kr	krypton	lawrencium	Lr
La	lanthanum	lead	Pb
Li	lithium	lithium	Li
Lr	lawrencium	lutetium	Lu
Lu	lutetium	magnesium	Mg
Md	mendelevium	manganese	Mn
Mg	magnesium	mendelevium	Md
Mn	manganese	mercury	Hg
Mo	molybdenum	molybdenum	Mo
N	nitrogen	neodymium	Nd
Na	sodium	neon	Ne
Nb	niobium	nickel	Ni
Nd	neodymium	niobium	Nb
Ne	neon	nitrogen	N
Ni	nickel	nobellium	No
No	nobellium	osmium	Os
O	oxygen	oxygen	O
Os	osmium	palladium	Pd
P	phosphorus	phosphorus	P
Pa	protactinium	platinum	Pt
Pb	lead	plutonium	Pu
Pd	palladium	polonium	Po
Pm	promethium	potassium	K
Po	polonium	praseodymium	Pr
Pr	praseodymium	promethium	Pm
Pt	platinum	protactinium	Pa
Pu	plutonium	radium	Ra
Ra	radium	radon	Rn
Rb	rubidium	rhenium	Re
Re	rhenium	rhodium	Rh
Rh	rhodium	rubidium	Rb
Rn	radon	ruthenium	Ru
Ru	ruthenium	samarium	Sm

SYMBOL	ELEMENT	ELEMENT	SYMBOL
S	sulfur	scandium	Sc
Sb	antimony	selenium	Se
Sc	scandium	silicon	Si
Se	selenium	silver	Ag
Si	silicon	sodium	Na
Sm	samarium	strontium	Sr
Sn	tin	sulfur	S
Sr	strontium	tantalum	Ta
Ta	tantalum	technetium	Tc
Tb	terbium	tellurium	Te
Tc	technetium	terbium	Tb
Te	tellurium	thallium	Tl
Th	thorium	thorium	Th
Ti	titanium	thulium	Tm
Tl	thallium	tin	Sn
Tm	thulium	titanium	Ti
U	uranium	tungsten	W
Unh	unnilseptium	unnilpentium	Unp
Unp	unnilpentium	unnilquadium	Unq
Unq	unnilquadium	unnilseptium	Unh
V	vanadium	uranium	U
W	tungsten	vanadium	V
Xe	xenon	xenon	Xe
Y	yttrium	ytterbium	Yb
Yb	ytterbium	yttrium	Y
Z	zirconium	zinc	Zn
Zn	zinc	zirconium	Z

Appendix 6
Units of Measure for Pathology

Basic SI Units

Unit Name	SI Unit	Symbol
length	meter	m
mass	kilogram	kg
time	second	s
electric current	ampere	A
thermodynamic temperature	kelvin	K
amount of substance	mole	mol
luminous intensity	candela	cd

Derived SI Units

Unit Name	SI Unit	Symbol
frequency	hertz	Hz
force	newton	N
pressure	pascal	Pa
energy (all forms)	joule	J
power	watt	W
electric charge	coulomb	C
electric potential difference	volt	V
electrical capacitance	farad	F
electrical resistance	ohm	$\emptyset$
electrical conductance	siemens	S
magnetic flux	weber	Wb
magnetic induction	tesla	T
inductance	henry	H
luminous flux	lumen	lm
illumination	lux	lx
activity (of a radionuclide)	becquerel	Bq
absorbed dose	gray	Gy
dose equivalent	sievert	Sv
catalytic activity	katal	kat
Celsius temperature	degree Celsius	°C
plane angle	radian	rad
solid angle	steradian	sr

Sample Immunodiagnostic Panels

Arbovirus Competitive Enzyme Immunoassay (CEIA)
Eastern equine encephalitis IgM
St. Louis encephalitis IgM
LaCrosse encephalitis IgM
West Nile virus IgM Ab

Cat Scratch disease serology
Bartonella quintana
Bartonella henselae

Chlamydia-Gonorrhea Amplified Molecular Assay (AMA)
Neisseria gonorrhoeae
Chlamydia trachomatis

Cryptosporidium/Giardia Direct Fluorescence Antigen (DFA)
Cryptosporidium DFA
Giardia DFA

Hantavirus IgM and IgG
Hantavirus IgG
Hantavirus IgM

Hepatitis B Immune Status
Hepatitis B core antibody
Hepatitis B surface antibody

Hepatitis B Serodiagnosis
Hepatitis B surface antigen
Hepatitis B core antibody
Hepatitis B surface antibody

Lyme Disease
Lyme Disease Western blot IgM
Lyme Disease Western blot IgG

Measles Immunoglobulins
Measles IgM
Measles IgG

Mumps Immunoglobulins
Mumps IgM
Mumps IgG

Mycobacterium **Acid Fast Bacterium (AFB)**
Mycobacteriology smear
Mycobacteriology culture direct

Mycoplasma pneumoniae Enzyme Immunoassay (EIA)
Mycoplasma pneumoniae IgM
Mycoplasma pneumoniae IgG

Parvovirus B19
Parvovirus B19 IgG
Parvovirus B19 IgM

Prenatal Screen Panel
ABO group
Rh type
Blood factor antibody
VDRL
Hepatitis B surface antigen
Rubella IgG

Prenatal Screen Panel, Basic Plus HIV
Add: HIV prenatal

Prenatal Screen Panel, Basic Plus HIV/Toxoplasma
Add: HIV prenatal
Toxoplasma IgM serology
Toxoplasma IgG serology

Prenatal Screen Panel, Basic Plus Toxoplasma
Add: Toxoplasma IgM Serology Prenatal
Toxoplasma IgG Serology Prenatal

Q Fever Antibody
Q Fever phase 1
Q Fever phase 2

Rickettsia **Antibody**
Rickettsia antibody Rocky Mountain spotted fever
Rickettsia antibody typhus

Rubella Antibody
  Rubella IgM
  Rubella IgG

Toxoplasma Antibody
  Toxoplasma IgM
  Toxoplasma IgG

Varicella zoster Antibody
  Varicella zoster IgM
  Varicella zoster IgG

Common Lab Tests

Usage of various terms, both formal and what might appear to be slang, depend on the rules of the institution. Combinations of test components under a particular name might also depend on the institution or laboratory. For example, a chemistry panel at one hospital might routinely include glucose, while at another it would be considered an advanced or extra test. Units of measure may also vary by institution, method, and professionals' preference, and units of measure should be transcribed as above.

(See Tables following for selected range of values and units of measure.)

LAB TEST NAME	MAY BE HEARD AS	VALUES (SAMPLE)
BLOOD TESTS		
Complete Blood Count	*CBC, hemogram, blood count*	
Red blood cell count	*RBC, red cells*	4.2 to 6.2 (million)
White blood cell count	*WBC, white cells*	4.1 to 10.9 (thousand)
White blood cell differential	*diff, morphology*	% or #
granulocytes	*polymorphonuclear leukocytes*	
neutrophils	*segs, polys, PMNs*	% or #
immature neutrophils	*bands*	% increase = "left shift"
eosinophils	*eos*	% or #
basophils	*basos*	% or #
agranulocytes	*mononuclear leukocytes*	
lymphocytes	*lymphs*	% or #
monocytes	*monos*	% or #
Hemoglobin (first H of H&H)	*Hb, Hgb,*	12.0-18.0
Hematocrit (second H of H&H)	*crit, Hct, packed cell volume, PCV*	38–54
Platelets	*thrombocytes*	130 to 400 (thousand)
Reticulocytes	*retic*	%
Red blood cell indices		
mean corpuscular volume	*MCV*	80-99
mean corpuscular hemoglobin	*MCH*	27–31
mean corpuscular hemoglobin concentration MCHC		33–37
red cell distribution width	*RDW*	% or #

LAB TEST NAME	MAY BE HEARD AS	VALUES (SAMPLE)
Complete Blood Count (continued)		
Blood morphology	*peripheral smear*	descriptive
red blood cell smear	*blood smear*	**abnormalities:** *sickle cell, teardrop, elliptocyte, spherocyte, target cell, Mexican hat cell, ovalocyte*
white blood cell smear		
granulocyte		
neutrophil	*segmented neutrophils*	**abnormalities:** *segs, polys, PMN bands or immature neutrophils, toxic granulation, vacuolization, Döhle bodies, Auer bodies (Auer rod), hypersegmentation, Pelger-Huët nucleus, Alder-Reilly granules, Chédiak-Higashi malformation*
eosinophil, basophil	*eos, basos*	abnormalities: as above
agranulocytes		
lymphocytes	*lymphs*	abnormalities: reactive, hairy cell
monocytes	*monos*	descriptive
Other Blood Testing		
Electrolytes	*lytes, electrolyte panel*	
sodium	*Na*	136-145
potassium	*K*	3.5–5.1
chloride	*Cl*	98-107
bicarbonate	*CO2, bicarb, carbon dioxide, HCO3*	22-29
Anion gap (calculated value)	*base excess, base deficit*	#
(Na – (Cl + HCO3))		7–16
((Na + K) – (Cl + HCO3))		10–20

LAB TEST NAME	MAY BE HEARD AS	VALUES (SAMPLE)
Kidney Function Tests		
blood urea nitrogen	*BUN, urea nitrogen*	6–20
creatinine		0.6–1.3
Liver Function Tests		
alkaline phosphatase	*alk phos, ALP*	38–126
alanine amino transferase	*ALT, SGPT, transaminases*	10–40
aspartate amino transferase	*AST, SGOT, transaminases*	10–59
bilirubin	*bili*	
total bilirubin (blood component)	*t-bili, unconjugated*	0.2–1.2
direct bilirubin (liver component)	*direct bili, conjugated bili*	0.0–0.4
indirect bilirubin		calculated value, total minus direct
Lipid Panel	*lipids lipid profile, lipoprotein analysis, cholesterol test*	
total cholesterol	*cholesterol*	less than 200
HDL cholesterol	*HDL*	greater than 40
LDL cholesterol	*LDL*	less than 130
triglycerides		less than 150
Arterial Blood Gas		
pH		7.35 to 7.45
PO2		83 to 108
PCO2		32 to 48
bicarbonate	*CO2, HCO3, TCO2*	22 to 26
oxygen saturation	*sats, O2 sat, SAO2*	95 to 100%

LAB TEST NAME	MAY BE HEARD AS	VALUES (SAMPLE)

BLOOD CHEMISTRY PANELS (METABOLIC PROFILE)

Please refer to tables for values.

Chemistry panel	*chem panel, met profile, basic metabolic panel, BMP, chemistries, SMA, SMAC*	
Screening Chemistry Panel	*chem 6, chem 7, SMA 6, SMA 7, SMAC 6, SMAC 7*	#
components: **electrolytes** plus **kidney function tests**		
(sometimes) **glucose**	*blood glucose, blood sugar, sugars*	#
Comprehensive chemistry panel	*chem panel, metabolic panel, # SMA 12, SMA 20, SMAC 12, SMAC 20*	
components: **screening chemistry panel** plus **liver function tests**, **lipid panel** and may include:		
albumin		#
total protein		#
calcium	*Ca*	#
can also include:		
phosphorus	*P*	#
creatinine clearance	*CrCl*	#
total serum protein		#
lactic acid		#
uric acid		#
magnesium	*Mg, mag*	#
tests of pancreas function (amylase and lipase)		#
Cardiac Enzymes	AMI panel	
creatine kinase MB isoenzyme	*CK-MB*	0 to 7
troponin-I	*troponin "eye" or troponin "one"*	less than 0.04 (undetectable)
CPK	*creatinine phosphokinase, CK, CPK, TCK*	10-105

LAB TEST NAME	MAY BE HEARD AS	VALUES (SAMPLE)
Coagulation Studies	*coags, DIC panel*	
partial thromboplastin time, activated	*aPTT, PTT*	greater than 35 sec
prothrombin time	*PT, pro-time*	less than 20 sec
prothrombin time/international normalized ratio	*PT-INR*	birth–6 mo: 1.0–1.6 ±6 mo–adult: 0.9–1.2
Iron Studies		
iron	*Fe*	50–175
total iron binding capacity	*TIBC*	50–425
ferritin		10-322
Miscellaneous Blood Tests		
blood alcohol	*EtOH*	values per institution
serum pregnancy test	*beta-hCG*	positive or negative
triiodothronine	*T3*	0.8 to 2.7
thyroxine	*free T4*	5 to 12
thyroid stimulating hormone	*TSH*	0.4 to 4.2

LAB TEST NAME	MAY BE HEARD AS	VALUES (SAMPLE)

URINE TESTS

Urine Analysis (routine) *urine, urinalysis, dip*

Macroscopic

color		yellow, straw, red, brown, orange, green black
odor		fruity, fetid, maple syrup
appearance		clear, slightly hazy, hazy, slightly cloudy, cloudy, turbid
specific gravity	*specgrav*	one point ten, transcribed 1.010 ten-twenty, transcribed 1.020
pH		4.8-7.5 (normal range)
protein	*albumin*	negative, trace
glucose	*sugar*	normal, (or multiples of 50)
bilirubin	*bili*	negative, 1+, 2+, 3+
urobilinogen		0.1 to 0.8 (at 2 hours)
ketones		trace, 1+, 2+, 3+
leukocyte esterase	*leukesterase, leukoesterase*	small, moderate, large, negative
nitrite		positive, negative
blood	*gross blood*	negative, trace, small, large

Microscopic

RBCs per high-power field (HPF)		few, many, too numerous to count (TNTC)
WBCs per high-power field (HPF)		few, many, too numerous to count (TNTC)
epithelial cells per low-power field (LPF)	*squamous epithelial, epi*	rare, few, many
casts	*hyaline, granular, coarsely granular, finely granular, fatty, waxy, cellular cast (red cell, white cell, epithelial cell)*	negative, few, many
crystals		few, many, 1+, 2+, 3+

LAB TEST NAME	MAY BE HEARD AS	VALUES (SAMPLE)
yeast cells		rare, few, many, 1+, 2+, 3+
parasites		rare, few, many, 1+, 2+, 3+
bacteria		trace, few, many, 1+, 2+, 3+

Urine Toxicology Screen (values vary by test and place performed)

amphetamine

barbiturates

benzodiazepine

cocaine

heroin/opiates/morphine

marijuana

methadone

methamphetamine

phencyclidine   *PCP*

Blood Values

TEST	CONVENTIONAL UNITS	SI UNITS
acetone, serum		
Qualitative	Negative	Negative
Quantitative	0.3–2.0 mg/dL	0.05–0.34 mmol/L
acid hemolysis test (Ham test)	<5% lysis	<0.05 lysed fraction
adrenocorticotropin (ACTH), plasma		
8 am	<120 pg/mL	<26 pmol/L
Midnight (supine)	<10 pg/mL	<2.2 pmol/L
alanine aminotransferase (ALT, SGPT), serum		
Male	13–40 U/L (37°C)	0.22–0.68 µkat/L (37° C)
Female	10–28 U/L (37°C)	0.17–0.48 µkat/L (37° C)
albumin, serum		
Adult	3.5–5.2 g/dL	35–52 g/L
>60 y	3.2–4.6 g/dL Avg. of 0.3 g/dL higher in upright individuals	32–46 g/L Avg. of 0.3 g/dL higher in upright individuals
aldolase, serum	1.0–7.5 U/L (30° C)	0.02–0.13 µkat/L (30° C)
aldosterone, serum		
Supine	3–16 ng/dL	0.08–0.44 nmol/L
Standing	7–30 ng/dL	0.19–0.83 nmol/L
ammonia, plasma	9–33 µmol/L	9–33 µmol/L
amylase, serum	27–131 U/L	0.46–2.23 µkat/L
amylase:creatine clearance ratio	1–4%	0.01–0.04
androstenedione, serum		
Male	75–205 ng/dL	2.6–7.2 nmol/L
Female	85–275 ng/dL	3.0–9.6 nmol/L
anion gap		
$(Na - (Cl + HCO3))$	7–16 mEq/L	7–16 mmol/L
$((Na + K) - (Cl + HCO3))$	10–20 mEq/L	10–20 mmol/L

TEST	CONVENTIONAL UNITS	SI UNITS
alpha 1 antitrypsin, serum	78–200 mg/dL	0.78–2.00 g/L
apolipoprotein A1		
Male	94–178 mg/dL	0.94–1.78 g/L
Female	101–199 mg/dL	1.01–1.99 g/L
apolipoprotein B		
Male	63–133 mg/dL	0.63–1.33 g/L
Female	60–126 mg/dL	0.60–1.26 g/L
arsenic, whole blood	0.2–2.3 µg/dL	0.03–0.31 µmol/L
Chronic poisoning	10–50 µg/dL	1.33–6.65 µmol/L
Acute poisoning	60–930 µg/dL	7.98–124 µmol/L
ascorbic acid, plasma	0.4–1.5 mg/dL	23–85 µmol/L
aspartate aminotransferase (AST, SGOT), serum	10–59 U/L (37°C)	0.17–1.00 22 to 13 kat/L (37°C)
base excess, blood	–2 to +3 mmol/L	–2 to +3 mmol/L
bicarbonate, serum (venous) (bicarb, CO2, HCO3)	22–29 mmol/L	22–29 mmol/L
bilirubin, direct		
Birth–death	0.0–0.4 mg/dL	
bilirubin, total		
Birth–1 day	1.0–6.0 mg/dL	
1–2 days	6.0–7.5 mg/dL	
2–5 days	4.0–13.5 mg/dL	
5 days–death	0.2–1.2 mg/dL	
bilirubin, total, neonatal		
Birth–1 day	1.0–6.0 g/dL	
1–2 days	6.0–7.5 g/dL	
2–5 days	4.0– 13.5 g/dL	
5 days–1 month	0.0–1.8 g/dL	
1 month–death	0.0–1.8 g/dL	

Blood Values (continued)

TEST	CONVENTIONAL UNITS	SI UNITS
CA 125, serum	<35 U/mL	<35 kU/L
CA 15–3, serum	<30 U/mL	<30 kU/L
CA 19–9, serum	<37 U/mL	<37 kU/L
calcitonin, serum or plasma		
Male	≤100 pg/mL	≤100 ng/L
Female	≤30 pg/mL	≤30 ng/L
calcium, serum	8.6–10.0 mg/dL (Slightly higher in children)	2.15–2.50 mmol/L (Slightly higher in children)
calcium, ionized, serum	4.64–5.28 mg/dL	1.16–1.32 mmol/L
carbon dioxide (PCO2)	Male 35–48 mmHg	4.66–6.38 kPa
carbon dioxide, blood, arterial (ABG)	Female 32–45 mmHg	4.26–5.99 kPa
CO2, bicarb, HCO3- (electrolytes)	See bicarbonate, serum	See bicarbonate, serum
carboxyhemoglobin (HbCO, carbon monoxide, hemiglobin)		
Nonsmokers	0.5–1.5% total Hb	0.005–0.015 HbCO fraction
Smokers		
1–2 packs/d	4–5% total Hb	0.04–0.05 HbCO fraction
>2 packs/d	8–9% total Hb	0.08–0.09 HbCO fraction
Toxic	>20% total Hb	>0.20 HbCO fraction
Lethal	>50% total Hb	>0.50 HbCO fraction
carotene, serum	10–85 µg/dL	0.19–1.58 µmol/L
catecholamines, plasma		
Dopamine	<30 pg/mL	<196 pmol/L
Epinephrine	<140 pg/mL	<764 pmol/L
Norepinephrine	<1700 pg/mL	<10,047 pmol/L
carcinoembryonic antigen (CEA), serum		
Nonsmokers	<5.0 ng/mL	<5.0 µg/L

TEST	CONVENTIONAL UNITS	SI UNITS
CBC, blood cell counts, adult		
RBC Male	4.7–6.1 x 10^6/μL	4.7–6.1 x 10^{12}/L
Female	4.2–5.4 x 10^6/μL	4.2–5.4 x 10^{12}/L
WBC		
Total	4.8–10.8 x 10^3/μL	4.8–10.8 x 10^6/L
WBC Differential	Percentage	Absolute
Myelocytes	0	0/μL
Neutrophils		
Bands	3–5	150–400/μL 150–400 x 10^6/L
Segmented	54–62	3000–5800/μL 3000–5800 x 10^6/L
Lymphocytes	20.5–51.1	1.2–3.4 x 10^3/μL 1.2–3.4 x 10^9/L
Monocytes	1.7–9.3	0.11–0.59 x 10 0.11–0.59 x 10^9/L
Granulocytes	42.2–75.2	1.4–6.5 x 10^3/μL 1.4–6.5 x 10^9/L
Eosinophils	0.07 x 103/μL	0.07 x 10^9/L
Basophils	0–0.2 x 103/μL	0–0.2 x 10^9/L
Platelets	130–400 x 10^3/μL	130–400 x 10^9/L
Reticulocytes	0.5–1.5% red cells	0.005–0.015 of red cells
	24,000–84.000/μL	24–84 x 10^9/L
ceruloplasmin, serum	20–60 mg/dL	0.2–6.0 g/L
chloride (Cl)		
Serum or plasma	98–107 mmol/L	98–107 mmol/L
cholesterol, serum		
Adult desirable	<200 mg/dL	<5.2 mmol/L
borderline	200–239 mg/dL	5.2–6.2 mmol/L
high risk	≥240 mg/dL	≥6.2 mmol/L

Blood Values (continued)

TEST	CONVENTIONAL UNITS	SI UNITS
cholinesterase, serum	4.9–11.9 U/mL	4.9–11.9 kU/L
chorionic gonadotropin, intact (hCG)		
Serum or plasma		
Male and nonpregnant female	<5.0 mIU/mL	<5.0 IU/L
Pregnant female	Varies with gestational age	
coagulation tests (coags, clotting studies)		
Antithrombin III (synthetic substrate)	80–120% of normal	0.8–1.2 of normal
Bleeding time (Duke)	0–6 min	0–6 min
Bleeding time (Ivy)	1–6 min	1–6 min
Bleeding time (template)	2.3–9.5 min	2.3–9.5 min
Clot retraction, qualitative	50–100% in 2 h	0.5–1.0/2 h
coagulation time (Lee-White)	5–15 min (glass tubes)	5–15 min (glass tubes)
	19-60 min (siliconized tubes)	19-60 min (siliconized tubes)
cold hemolysin test (Donath-Landsteiner)	No hemolysis	No hemolysis
complement components		
Total hemolytic complement activity, plasma	75–160 U/mL	75–160 kU/L
Total complement decay rate	10–20%	Fraction decay rate: 0.10–0.20
(functional), plasma	Deficiency: >50%	>0.50
C1q, serum	14.9–22.1 mg/dL	149–221 mg/L
C1r, serum	2.5–10.0 mg/dL	25–100 mg/L
C1s(C1 esterase), serum	5.0–10.0 mg/dL	50–100 mg/L
C2, serum	1.6–3.6 mg/dL	16–36 mg/L
C3, serum	90–180 mg/dL	0.9–1.8 g/L

TEST	CONVENTIONAL UNITS	SI UNITS
C4, serum	10–40 mg/dL	0.1–0.4 g/L
C5, serum	5.5–11.3 mg/dL	55–113 mg/L
C6, serum	17.9–23.9 mg/dL	179–239 mg/L
C7, serum	2.7–7.4 mg/dL	27–74 mg/L
C8, serum	4.9–10.6 mg/dL	49–106 mg/L
C9, serum	3.3–9.5 mg/dL	33–95 mg/L
Coombs test		
Direct	Negative	Negative
Indirect	Negative	Negative
copper (Cu), serum		
Male	70–140 µg/dL	11–22 µmol/L
Female	80–155 µg/dL	13–24 µmol/L
RBC indices (corpuscular values) (values are for adults; in children values vary with age)		
Mean corpuscular hemoglobin (MCH)	27–31 pg	0.42–0.48 fmol
Mean corpuscular hemo- globin concentration (MCHC)	33–37 g/dL	330–370 g/L
Mean corpuscular volume (MCV)	Male 80–94 µ³	80–94 fL
cortisol, serum		
Plasma		
8 am	5–23 µg/dL	138–635 nmol/L
4 pm	3–16 µg/dL	83–441 nmol/L
10 pm	<50% of 8 AM value	<0.5 of 8 AM value
creatine kinase (CK), serum		
Male	15–105 U/L (30°C)	0.26–1.79 µkat/L (30°C)
Female	10–80 U/L (30°C)	0.17–1.36 µkat/L (30°C)

Note: Strenuous exercise or intramuscular injections may cause transient elevation of CK.

Blood Values (continued)

TEST	CONVENTIONAL UNITS	SI UNITS
creatine kinase MB isoenzyme (CK-MB), serum	0–7 ng/mL	0–7 µg/l
creatinine		
serum or plasma, adult		
Male	0.7–1.3 mg/dL	62–115 µmmol/L
Female	0.6–1.1 mg/dL	53–97 µmol/L
cryoglobulins, serum	0	0
cyanide		
Serum		
Nonsmokers	0.004 mg/L	0.15 µmol/L
Smokers	0.006 mg/L	0.23 µmol/L
Nitroprusside therapy	0.01–0.06 mg/L	0.38–2.30 µmol/L
Toxic	>0.1 mg/L	>3.84 µmol/L
Whole blood		
Nonsmokers	0.016 mg/L	0.61 µmol/L
Smokers	0.041 mg/L	1.57 µmol/L
Nitroprusside therapy	0.05–0.5 mg/L	1.92–19.20 µmol/L
Toxic	>1 mg/L	>38.40 µmol/L
cyclic AMP (cAMP)		
Plasma		
Male	4.6–8.6 ng/mL	14–26 nmol/L
Female	4.3–7.6 ng/mL	13–23 nmol/L
C-peptide, serum	0.78–1.89 ng/mL	0.26–0.62 nmol/L
C-reactive protein (CRP), serum	<0.5 mg/dL	<5 mg/L
dehydroepiandrosterone (DHEA), serum		
Male	180–1250 ng/dL	6.2–43.3 nmol/L
Female	130–980 ng/dL	4.5–34.0 nmol/L

TEST	CONVENTIONAL UNITS	SI UNITS
dehydroepiandrosterone sulfate, DHEAS, serum or plasma		
Male	59–452 µg/dL	1.6–12.2 µmol/L
Female		
Premenopausal	12–379 µg/dL	0.8–10.2 µmol/L
Postmenopausal	30–260 µg/dL	0.8–7.1 µmol/L
glucose (fasting)		
Blood	65–95 mg/dL	3.5–5.3 mmol/L
Plasma or serum	74–106 mg/dL	4.1–5.9 mmol/L
glucose, 2 h postprandial, serum	<120 mg/dL	<6.7 mmol/L
glucose-6-phosphate dehydrogenase, G6PD	12.1 ± 2.1 U/g Hb (SD)	0.78 ± 0.13 mU/mol Hb
in RBC, whole blood	351 ± 60.6 U/10^{12} RBC	0.35 ± 0.06 nU/RBC
gamma glutamyltransferase (GGT), serum		
Males	2–30 U/L (37°C)	0.03–0.51 µkat/L (37°C)
Females	1–24 U/L (37°C)	0.02–0.41 µkat/L (37°C)
glycated hemoglobin (hemoglobin A1C), whole blood	4.2%–5.9%	0.042–0.059
growth hormone, serum		
Male	<5 ng/mL	<5 µg/L
Female	<10 ng/mL	<10 µg/L
haptoglobin, serum	30–200 mg/dL	0.3–2.0 g/L
HDL-lipid panel		
cholesterol, HDL	>40 mg/dL	
cholesterol, LDL (calculated)		
optimal	<100 mg/dL	
near optimal	100–129 mg/dL	
borderline high	130–159 mg/dL	
high	>160 mg/dL	

Blood Values (continued)

TEST	CONVENTIONAL UNITS	SI UNITS
cholesterol, total		
0–1 y	50–120 mg/dL	
1–2 y	70–190 mg/dL	
2–16 y	120–220 mg/dL	
>16 y	0–199 mg/dL	
desirable	<200 mg/dL	
borderline	200–239 mg/dL	
high	>240 mg/dL	
triglycerides		
desirable	<150 mg/dL	
borderline high	150–199 mg/dL	
high	>200 mg/dL	
hematocrit (Hct)		
Males	42–52%	0.42–0.52
Females	37–47%	0.37–0.47
Newborns	53–65%	0.53–0.65
Children (varies with age)	30–43%	0.30–0.43
hemoglobin (Hb)		
Males	14.0–18.0 g/dL	2.17–2.79 mmol/L
Females	12.0–16.0 g/dL	1.86–2.48 mmol/L
Newborn	17.0–23.0 g/dL	2.64–3.57 mmol/L
Children (varies with age)	11.2–16.5 g/dL	1.74–2.56 mmol/L
hemoglobin, fetal	>1 y old: <2% of total Hb	>1 y old: <0.02% of total Hb
hemoglobin, plasma	<3 mg/dL	<0.47 mmol/L
hemoglobin electrophoresis, whole blood		
HbA	0.0095	>0.95 Hb fraction
HbA2	1.5–3.7%	0.015–0.37 Hb fraction
HbF	<2%	<0.02 Hb fraction
beta hydroxybutyric acids, serum, plasma	0.21–2.81 mg/dL	20–270 µmol/L

TEST	CONVENTIONAL UNITS	SI UNITS
immunoglobulins (Ig), serum		
IgG	700–1600 mg/dL	7–16 g/L
IgA	70–400 mg/dL	0.7–4.0 g/L
IgM	40–230 mg/dL	0.42.3 g/L
IgD	0–8 mg/dL	0–80 mg/L
IgE	3–423 mg/dL	3–423 kIU/L
insulin (Fe) plasma (fasting)	2–25 µU/mL	13–174 pmol/L
iron, serum		
Males	65–175 µg/dL	11.6–31.3 µmol/L
Females	50–170 µg/dL	9.0–30.4 µmol/L
iron binding capacity, total (TBIC), serum	250–425 µg/dL	44.8–71.6 µmol/L
iron saturation, serum		
Male	20–50%	0.2–0.5
Female	15–50%	0.15–0.5
L-lactate		
Plasma		
Venous	4.5–19.8 mg/dL	0.5–2.2 mmol/L
Arterial	4.5–14.4 mg/dL	0.5–1.6 mmol/L
Whole blood, at bed rest		
Venous	8.1–15.3 mg/dL	0.9–1.7 mmol/L
Arterial	<11.3 mg/dL	<1.3 mmol/L
lactate dehydrogenase (LDH)		
Total (L→P), 37°C, serum		
Newborn	290–775 U/L	4.9–13.2 µkat/L
Neonate	545–2000 U/L	9.3–34 µkat/L
Infant	180–430 U/L	3.1–7.3 µkat/L
Child	110–295 U/L	1.9–5 µkat/L
Adult	100–190 U/L	1.7–3.2 µkat/L
>60 y	110–210 U/L	1.9–3.6 µkat/L

Blood Values (continued)

TEST	CONVENTIONAL UNITS	SI UNITS
LDL-cholesterol (LDL-C), serum or plasma		
Adult desirable	<130 mg/dL	<3.37 mmol/L
borderline	130–159 mg/dL	3.37–4.12 mmol/L
high risk	≥ 160 mg/dL	≥ 4.13 mmol/L
lead (Pb)		
Whole blood	<25 μg/dL	<1.2 μmol/L
lipase, serum	23–300 U/L (37°C)	0.39–5.1 μkat/L (37°C)
luteinizing hormone (LH), serum or plasma		
Male	1.24–7.8 mIU/mL	1.24–7.8 IU/L
Female		
Follicular phase	1.68–15.0 mIU/mL	1.68–15.0 IU/L
Midcycle peak	21.9–56.6 mIU/mL	21.9–56.6 IU/L
Luteal phase	0.61–16.3 mIU/mL	0.61–16.3 IU/L
Postmenopausal	14.2–52.5 mIU/mL	14.2–52.3 IU/L
magnesium, serum	1.3–2.1 mEq/L	0.65–1.07 mmol/L
magnesium, serum	1.6–2.6 mg/dL	16–26 mg/L
mercury (Hg)		
Whole blood	0.6–59 μg/L	<0.29 μmol/L
Toxic	>150 μg/d	>0.75 μmol/d
methemoglobin, (MetHb), whole blood	0.06–0.24 g/dL or 0.78 ± 0.37% (SD)	9.3–37.2 μmol/L or mass fraction of total Hb: 0.0008 ± 0.0037 of total Hb (SD)
osmolality, serum	275–295 mOsm/kg serum water	275–295 mmol/kg serum water
osmotic fragility of RBC	Begins in 0.45–0.39% NaCl Complete in 0.33-0.30% NaCl	Begins in 77–67 mmol/L NaCl Complete in 56-61 mmol/L NaCl
oxygen (O2) blood, capacity	16–24 vol% (varies with hemoglobin)	7.14–10.7 mmol/L (varies with hemoglobin)

TEST	CONVENTIONAL UNITS	SI UNITS
O2 Content		
Arterial	15–23 vol%	6.69–10.3 mmol/L
Venous	10–16 vol%	4.46–7.14 mmol/L
O2 Saturation		
Arterial and capillary	95–98% of capacity	0.95–0.98 of capacity
Venous	60–85% of capacity	0.60–0.85 of capacity
O2 tension (partial pressure)		
PO2 arterial and capillary	83–108 mmHg	11.1–14.4 kPa
Venous	35–45 mmHg	4.6–6.0 kPa
P50 (blood O2 pressure at which (Hb) is half saturated with O2)	25–29 mmHg (adjusted to pH 7.4)	3.33–3.86 kPa
partial thromboplastin time activated (APTT)	<35 sec	<35 sec
pH		
Blood, arterial	7.35–7.45	7.35–7.45
phenylalanine, serum	0.8–1.8 mg/dL	48–109 μmol/L
phosphatase, alkaline (alkphos), total, serum	38–126 U/L (37°C)	0.65–2.14 μkat/L
phosphate, inorganic, serum		
Adults	2.7–4.5 mg/dL	0.87–1.45 mmol/L
Children	4.5–5.5 mg/dL	1.45–1.78 mmol/L
phospholipids, serum	125–275 mg/dL	1.25–2.75 g/L
potassium (K), plasma		
Males	3.5–4.5 mmol/L	3.5–4.5 mmol/L
Females	3.4–4.4 mmol/L	3.4–4.4 mmol/L
potassium (K), serum		
Premature		
Cord	5.0–10.2 mmol/L	5.0–10.2 mmol/L
48 h	3.0–6.0 mmol/L	3.0–6.0 mmol/L

Blood Values (continued)

TEST	CONVENTIONAL UNITS	SI UNITS
Newborn cord 5.6–12.0 mmol/L	5.6–12.0 mmol/L	
Newborn 3.7–5.9 mmol/L	3.7–5.9 mmol/L	
Infant 4.1–5.3 mmol/L	4.1–5.3 mmol/L	
Child 3.4–4.7 mmol/L	3.4–4.7 mmol/L	
Adult 3.5–5.1 mmol/L	3.5–5.1 mmol/L	
prealbumin (transthyretin), serum	10–40 mg/dL	100–400 mg/L
progesterone, serum		
Adult		
Male	13–97 ng/dL	0.4–3.1 nmol/L
Female		
Follicular phase	15–70 ng/dL	0.5–2.2 nmol/L
Luteal phase	200–2500 ng/dL	6.4–79.5 nmol/L
Pregnancy	Varies with gestational week	
prolactin, serum		
Males	2.5–15.0 ng/mL	2.5–15.0 µg/L
Females	2.5–19.0 ng/mL	2.5–19.0 µg/L
prostate-specific antigen (PSA), serum		
Male	<4.0 ng/mL	<4.0 µg/L
protein, serum		
Total	6.4–8.3 g/dL	64–83 g/L
Albumin	3.9–5.1 g/dL	39–51 g/L
Globulin		
alpha1	0.2–0.4 g/dL	2–4 g/L
alpha2	0.4–0.8 g/dL	4–8 g/L
beta	0.5–1.0 g/dL	5–10 g/L
gamma	0.6–1.3 g/dL	6–13 g/L
prothrombin, consumption	>20 sec	>20 sec

TEST	CONVENTIONAL UNITS	SI UNITS
prothrombin time-international normalized ratio (PT-INR)		
INR: birth–6 mo	1.0–1.6	
INR: ± mo–adult	0.9–1.2	
protoporphyrin, total, whole blood	<60 µg/dL	<600 µmg/L
pyruvate, blood	0.3–0.9 mg/dL	34–103 µmol/L
sedimentation rate, erythrocyte (ESR, sed rate)		
Westergren		
Male: 0–50 y	0–15 mm/h	
Male: ≥50 y	0–20 mm/h	
Female: 0–50 y	0–20 mm/h	
Female: ≥50 y	0–30 mm/h	
Wintrobe		
Males	<10 mm/h	
Females	<20 mm/h	
Critical value	>75 mm/h	
sodium (Na)		
Serum or plasma		
Premature		
Cord	116–140mmol/L	116–140 mmol/L
48 h	128–148 mmol/L	128–148 mmol/L
Newborn, cord	126–166 mmol/L	126–166 mmol/L
Newborn	133–146 mmol/L	133–146 mmol/L
Infant	139–146 mmol/L	139–146 mmol/L
Child	138–145 mmol/L	138–145 mmol/L
Adult	136–145 mmol/L	136–145 mmol/L
Normal	10–40 mmol/L	10–40 mmol/L
Cystic fibrosis	70–190 mmol/L	70–190 mmol/L

Blood Values (continued)

TEST	CONVENTIONAL UNITS	SI UNITS
testosterone, serum		
Male	280–1100 ng/dL	0.52–38.17 nmol/L
Female	15–70 ng/dL	0.52–2.43 nmol/L
Pregnancy	3–4 x normal	3–4 x normal
Postmenopausal	8–35 ng/dL	0.28–1.22 nmol/L
thyroid-stimulating hormone (TSH), serum	0.4–4.2 µU/mL	0.4–4.2 mU/L
thyroxine (T4), serum	5–12 µg/dL (varies with age, higher in children and pregnant women)	65–155 nmol/L (varies with age, higher in children and pregnant women)
thyroxine, free, (free T4), serum	0.8–2.7 ng/dL	10.3–35 pmol/L
thyroxine binding globulin (TBG), serum	1.2–3.0 mg/dL	12–30 mg/L
transferrin, serum		
Newborn	130–275 mg/dL	1.30–2.75 g/L
Adult	212–360 mg/dL	2.12–3.60 g/L
>60 yr	190–375 mg/dL	1.9–3.75 g/L
triglycerides, serum, fasting		
Desirable	<250 mg/dL	<2.83 mmol/L
Borderline high	250–500 mg/dL	2.83–5.67 mmol/L
Hypertriglyceridemia	>500 mg/dL	>5.65 mmol/L
triiodothyronine, total (T3) serum	100–200 ng/dL	1.54–3.8 nmol/L
troponin-I, cardiac, serum	undetectable	undetectable
troponin-T, cardiac, serum	undetectable	undetectable
urea nitrogen, (BUN), serum	6–20 mg/dL	2.1–7.1 mmol urea/L
urea nitrogen/creatinine ratio, (BUN:Cr), serum	12:1 to 20:1	48–80 urea/creatinine mole ratio

TEST	CONVENTIONAL UNITS	SI UNITS
uric acid		
Serum, enzymatic		
Male	4.5–8.0 mg/dL	0.27–0.47 mmol/L
Female	2.5–6.2 mg/dL	0.15–0.37 mmol/L
Child	2.0–5.5 mg/dL	0.12–0.32 mmol/L
viscosity, serum	1.00–1.24 cP	1.00–1.24 cP

Urine Values

TEST	CONVENTIONAL UNITS	SI UNITS
acetone, urine		
qualitative	Negative	Negative
albumin, urine		
qualitative	Negative	Negative
quantitative	50–80 mg/24 h	50–80 mg/24 h
aldosterone, urine		
alpha-aminolevulinic acid, urine	1.3–7.0 mg/24 h	10–53 µmol/24 h
amylase, urine		
cadmium, urine, 24 h	1–17 U/h	0.017–0.29 µkat/h
calcium, urine	<15 µg/d	<0.13 µmol/d
low calcium diet		
usual diet, trough	50–150 mg/24 h	1.25–3.75 mmol/24 h
catecholamines, urine	100–300 mg/24 h	2.50–7.50 mmol/24 h
dopamine		
epinephrine	65–400 µg/24 h	425–2610 nmol/24 h
norepinephrine	0–20 µg/24 h	0–109 nmol/24
chloride, urine, 24 h values vary greatly with Cl intake	15–80 µg/24 h	89–473 nmol/24
infant	2–10 mmol/24 h	2–10 mmol/24 h
child	15–40 nmol/24 h	15–40 mmol/24 h
adult	110–250 mmol/24 h	110–250 mmol/24 h
chorionic gonadotropin, intact, urine, qualitative		
male and nonpregnant female	Negative	Negative
pregnant female	Positive	Positive
copper, urine	3–35 µg/24 h	0.05–0.55 µmol/24 h
cortisol, free, urine	<50 µg/24 h	<138 mmol/24 h

TEST	CONVENTIONAL UNITS	SI UNITS
creatinine, urine		
male	14–26 mg/kg body	124–230 µmol/kg body
female	11–20 mg/kg body weight/24 h	97–177 µmol/kg body weight/24 h
creatinine clearance, serum or plasma and urine		
male	94–140 mL/min/1.73 m2	0.91–1.35 mL/s/m2
female	72–110 mL/min/1.73 m2	0.69–1.06 mL/s/m2
cyclic AMP, urine, 24 h	0.3–3.6 mg/d or 0.29–2.1 mg/g creatinine	100–723 mmol/d or 100–723 mmol/mol creatinine
cystine or cysteine, urine, qualitative	Negative	Negative
hemoglobin and myoglobin, urine, qualitative	Negative	Negative
homogentisic acid, urine, qualitative	Negative	Negative
17-hydroxycorticosteroids, urine		
males	3–10 mg/24 h	8.3–27.6 µmol/24 h (as cortisol)
females	2–8 mg/24 h	5.5–22 µmol/24 h (as cortisol)
5-hydroxylindoleacetic acid, urine		
qualitative	Negative	Negative
quantitative	2–7 mg/24 h	10.4–36.6 µmol/24 h
17-ketosteroids, urine		
males	10–25 mg/24 h	38–87 µmol/24 h
females	6–14 mg/24 h (decreases with age)	21–52 µmol/24 h (decreases with age)
L-lactate, urine, 24 h	496–1982 mg/d	5.5–22 mmol/d

Urine Values (continued)

TEST	CONVENTIONAL UNITS	SI UNITS
lead, urine, 24 h	<80 µg/d	<0.39µmol/d
magnesium, urine	6.0–10.0 mEq/24 h	3.0–5.0 mmol/24 h
mercury, urine, 24 h	<20 µg/d	<0.01 µmol/d
toxic	>150 µg/d	>0.75 µmol/d
metanephrines, total, urine	0.1–1.6 mg/24 h	0.5–8.1 µmol/24 h
osmolality, urine	50–1200 mOsm/kg water	50–1200 mmol/kg water
ratio, urine:serum	1.0–3.0, 3.0–4.7 after 12 h fluid restriction	1.0–3.0, 3.0–4.7 after 12 h fluid restriction
pH, urine	4.6–8.0 (depends on diet)	Same
penosulfonphthalein excretion (PSP), urine	28–51% in 15 min 13–24% in 30 min 9–17% in 60 min 3–10% in 2 h (After injection of 1 mL PSP IV)	0.28–0.51 in 15 min 0.13–0.24 in 30 min 0.09–0.17 in 60 min 0.03–0.10 in 2 h (After injection of 1 mL PSP IV)
phosphorus, urine	0.4–1.3 g/24 h	12.9–42 mmol/24 h
porphobilinogen, urine		
qualitative	Negative	Negative
quantitative	<2.0 mg/24 h	<9 µmol/24 h
porphyrins, urine		
coproporphyrin	34–230 µg/24 h	52–351 nmol/ 24 h
uroporphyrin	27–52 µg/24 h	32–63 nmol/ 24 h
potassium, urine		
24 h	25–125 mmol/d; varies with diet	25–125 mmol/d; varies with diet
protein, urine		
qualitative	Negative	Negative
quantitative	50–80 mg/24 h (at rest)	50–80 mg/24 h (at rest)
sodium, urine, 24 h	40–220 mEq/d (diet dependent)	40–220 mmol/d (diet dependent)

TEST	CONVENTIONAL UNITS	SI UNITS
specific gravity, urine	1.002–1.030	1.002–1.030
thiocyanate, urine		
nonsmoker	1–4 mg/d	17–69 µmol/d
smoker	7–17mg/d	120–292 µmol/d
uric acid, urine	250–750 mg/24 h (with normal diet)	1.48–4.43 mmol/24 h (with normal diet)
urobilinogen, urine	0.1–0.8 Ehrlich unit/2 h	0.1–0.8 EU/2 h
vanillylmandelic acid (VMA) (4-hydroxy-3-methoxy-mandelic acid), urine	1.4–6.5 mg/24h	7–33 µmol/d

Appendix 8

Other Values

TEST	CONVENTIONAL UNITS	SI UNITS
albumin, cerebrospinal fluid	10–30 mg/dL	100–300 mg/dL
bone marrow, differential cell count, adult		
undifferentiated cells	0–1%	0–0.01
myeloblast	0–2%	0–0.02
promyelocyte	0–4%	0–0.04
myelocytes		
neutrophilic	5–20%	0.05–0.20
eosinophilic	0–3%	0–0.03
basophilic	0–1%	0–0.01
metamyelocytes and bands		
neutrophilic	5–35%	0.05–0.35
eosinophilic	0–5%	0–0.05
basophilic	0–1%	0–0.01
segmented neutrophils	5–15%	0.05–0.15
pronormoblast	0–1.5%	0–0.015
basophilic normoblast	0–5%	0–0.05
polychromatophilic normoblast	5–30%	0.05–0.30
orthochromatic normoblast	5–10%	0.05–0.10
lymphocytes	10–20%	0.10–0.20
plasma cells	0–2%	0–0.02
monocytes	0–5%	0–0.05
chloride, sweat		
normal	5–35 mmol/L	5–35 mmol/L
cystic fibrosis	60–200 mmol/L	60–200 mmol/L
chloride, cerebrospinal fluid	118–332 mmol/L (20 mmol/L higher than serum)	118–332 mmol/L (20 mmol/L higher than serum)

TEST	CONVENTIONAL UNITS	SI UNITS
fat, fecal, 72 h		
infant, breast-fed	<1 g/d	
pediatrics (0–6 y)	<2 g/d	
adults	<7 g/d	
adult (fat-free diet)	<4 g/d	
lecithin:sphingomyelin ratio (L:S), amniotic fluid	2.0–5.0 indicates probable fetal lung maturity; >3.5 in diabetic patients	2.0–5.0 indicates probable fetal lung maturity; >3.5 in diabetic patients
occult blood, feces, random	Negative (<2 mL blood/150 g stool/d)	Negative (<13.3 mL blood/kg stool/d)
phosphatidylglycerol (PG), amniotic fluid		
fetal lung immaturity	Absent	Same
fetal lung maturity	Present	Same
potassium, premature, cord	5.0–10.2 mmol/L	5.0–10.2 mmol/L
potassium, newborn, cord	5.6–12.0 mmol/L	5.6–12.0 mmol/L
potassium, cerebrospinal fluid	70% of plasma level or 2.5–3.2 mmol/L; rises with plasma hyperosmolality	0.70 of plasma level; rises rises with plasma hyperosmolality
protein, cerebrospinal fluid, total	8–32 mg/dL	80–320 mg/dL
sodium, premature, cord	116–140mmol/L	116–140 mmol/L
sodium, premature, cord, 48 h	128–148 mmol/L	128–148 mmol/L
sodium, newborn, cord	126–166 mmol/L	126–166 mmol/L
sodium, sweat		
normal	10–40 mmol/L	10–40 mmol/L
cystic fibrosis	70–190 mmol/L	70–190 mmol/L

Dictation Samples

AMI PANEL
CPK was 1291, myoglobin was 171, troponin-I was 48, and CPK MB was 50.59.

ARTERIAL BLOOD GAS
ABG showed a pH of 7.19, a PCO2 of 65 and a PO2 of 45, bicarbonate of 24, and an oxygen saturation of 90%.

CBC WITH DIFFERENTIAL
Initial CBC showed a white blood cell count of 3800, hemoglobin of 13.2, hematocrit of 37.2, MCV of 86, and platelets of 224,000 with 63% segmented neutrophils, 28% lymphocytes, 4% monocytes, 4% eosinophils, and 2% basophils.

CHEM-7
On admission, sodium was 137, potassium was 4.4, chloride was 96, CO2 was 29, glucose was 110, BUN was 30, and creatinine was 1.2.

CHOLESTEROL PROFILE
Total cholesterol was 223 with an HDL of 51, triglycerides of 87, LDL of 155, and cholesterol/HDL ratio of 4.4.

ELECTROLYTE RESULTS
Sodium was 137, potassium was 4.4, chloride was 96, bicarbonate was 29.

KIDNEY FUNCTION TESTS
BUN was 30, and creatinine was 1.2.

LIVER FUNCTION TESTS
Liver function tests showed an SGOT of 61, alkaline phosphatase of 40, SGPT of 138, bilirubin of 9.

THYROID FUNCTION TESTS
The patient's T3 was 147, free T4 was 7, and TSH was 1.2.

URINALYSIS, ABNORMAL (dictated) (improper format; underlined terms need to be replaced with formal terms)
Urine dipped negative for ketones, spec grav of ten-twenty, 2+ protein, positive nitrates, positive leukesterase, large blood, white cells TNTC, red cells 500, many bacteria.

URINALYSIS, ABNORMAL (transcribed)
Dip urinalysis revealed negative ketones, specific gravity of 1.020, 2+ protein, positive nitrites, positive leukocyte esterase, large blood Microscopic showed white cells too numerous to count, 500 red cells, many bacteria.

URINALYSIS, NORMAL
Urinalysis revealed specific gravity of 1.010, negative protein, negative nitrites, negative leukocyte esterase. Microscopic showed 0-3 RBCs, 3-5 WBCs, few squamous epithelial cells.

Drugs of Abuse, Toxicology, and Therapeutic Drug Levels

DRUGS OF ABUSE
chloral hydrate
ethchlorvynol
phenolphthalein
salicylic acid
senna

CLASSES OF DRUGS
cannabinoids
cocaine metabolites
methadone
amphetamines
  amphetamine
  methamphetamine
  methylenedioxyamphetamine (MDA)
  methylenedioxymethamphetamine
  (MDMA)
barbiturates
  amobarbital
  butabarbital
  butalbital
  pentobarbital
  phenobarbital
  secobarbital

benzodiazepines
  alprazolambromazepam
  chlordiazepoxide
  clonazepam
  diazepam
  flunitrazepam
  flurazepam
  lorazepam
  midazolam
  nitrazepam
  oxazepam
  temazepam
  triazolam
opiates
  codeine
  hydrocodone
  morphine
  hydromorphone

INDIVIDUAL SUBSTANCES IDENTIFIED IN LABORATORY (list not intended to be exhaustive). These include medications, naturally occurring substances, poison, drugs of abuse. Generic names only.

acetaminophen
amantadine
amitriptyline
amobarbital
amoxapine
amphetamine
anileridine
benzocaine
benzoylecgonine
benztropine

benzydamine
biperiden
bromazepam
brompheniramine
bupivacaine
bupropion
buspirone
butacaine
butalbital
butorphanol

caffeine
canrenone
carbamazepine
carisoprodol
chlordiazepoxide
chlorophenylpiperazine
chloroquine
chlorpromazine
citalopram
clobazam

clomipramine
clonazepam
clonidine
clozapine
cocaethylene
cocaine
codeine
cotinine
cyclobenzaprine
desethylchloroquine
desipramine
dextromethorphan
diacetylmorphine
diazepam
diclofenac
diethylpropion
dilantin
diltiazem
diphenhydramine
disopyramide
doxepin
doxylamine
ecgonine methyl ester
EDDP
emetine
enalapril
ephedrine/pseu-
doephedrine
erythromycin
ethosuximide
fenfluramine
fenoprofen
fentanyl
fluconazole
flunitrazepam
fluoxetine
flurazepam
guaifenesin
heroin
hydrocodone
hydrocortisone
hydromorphone
hydroxyzine

ibuprofen
imipramine
indomethacin
ketamine
labetalol
lamotrigine
lidocaine
loratidine
lorazepam
loxapine
maprotiline
MDA
MDMA
meclizine
meclofenamic acid
mefenamic acid
meperidine
mephobarbital
mepivacaine
meprobamate
methadone
methamphetamine
methaqualone
methocarbamol
methotrimeprazine
methylphenidate
methylprednisolone
metronidazole
phencyclidine
pheniramine
phenmetrazine
phenobarbital
phentermine
phenylpropanolamine
phenyltolaxamine
phenytoin
prednisolone
primidone
procainamide
procaine
prochlorperazine
procyclidine
promethazine

propoxyphene
propranolol
pseudoephedrine
psilocin
pyrilamine
quetiapine
quinapril
quinidine
quinine
ranitidine
rofecoxib
ropivacaine
secobarbital
seroquel
sertraline
sildenafil
starnoc
strychnine
theophylline
thiopental
thioridazine
thymol
tolbutamide
topiramate
tramadol
tranylcypromine
trazodone
triamterene
triazolam
trihexyphenidyl
trimeprazine
trimethoprim
trimipramine
tripelennamine
tripolidine
valproate
venlafaxine
verapamil
xylometazoline
zaleplon
zimelidine
zolpidem
zopiclone

2-ethylidene-1,5-dimethyl3,3-diphenylpyrrolidine (EDDP)

Drug Values

TEST	CONVENTIONAL UNITS	SI UNITS
acetaminophen, serum or plasma		
therapeutic	10–30µg/mL	66–199 µmol/L
toxic	>200 µg/ml	>1324 µmol/L
amikacin, serum or plasma		
therapeutic		
peak	25–35 µg/mL	43–60 µmol/L
trough		
less severe infection	1–4 µg/mL	1.7–6.8µmol/L
life-threatening infection	4–8 µg/mL	6.8–13.7 µmol/L
toxic		
peak	>35–40 µg/mL	>60–68 µmol/L
trough	>10–15 µg/mL	>17–26 µmol/L
amitriptyline, serum or plasma		
trough ($\geq$12 h after dose)		
therapeutic	80–250 ng/mL	289–903 nmol/L
toxic	>500 ng/mL	>1805 nmol/L
arsenic		
whole blood	0.2–2.3 µg/dL	0.03–0.31 µmol/L
chronic poisoning	10–50 µg/dL	1.33–6.65 µmol/L
acute poisoning	60–930 µg/dL	7.98–124 µmol/L
urine, 24 h	5–50 µg/d	0.07–0.67 µmol/d
ascorbic acid, plasma	0.4–1.5 mg/dL	23–85 µmol/L
cadmium, whole blood	0.1–0.5 µg/dL	8.9–44.5 nmol/L
toxic	10–300 µg/dL	0.89–26.70 µmol/L
cadmium, urine, 24 h	<15 µg/d	<0.13 µmol/d
carbamazepine, serum or plasma, trough		
therapeutic	4–12 µg/mL	17–51 µmol/L
toxic	>15 µg/mL	>63 µmol/L
carotene, serum	10–85 µg/dL	0.19–1.58 µmol/L

Drug Values

TEST	CONVENTIONAL UNITS	SI UNITS
chloramphenicol, serum or plasma, trough		
therapeutic	10–25 µg/mL	31–77 µmol/L
toxic	>25 µg/mL	>77 µmol/L
clonazepam, serum or plasma, trough		
therapeutic	15–60 ng/mL	48–190 nmol/L
toxic	>80 ng/mL	>254 nmol/L
	weight/24 h	weight/24 h
female	11–20 mg/kg body weight/24 h	97–177 µmol/kg body weight/24 h
cyanide, serum		
nonsmokers	0.004 mg/L	0.15 µmol/L
smokers	0.006 mg/L	0.23 µmol/L
nitroprusside therapy	0.01–0.06 mg/L	0.38–2.30 µmol/L
toxic	>0.1 mg/L	>3.84 µmol/L
cyanide, whole blood		
nonsmokers	0.016 mg/L	0.61 µmol/L
smokers	0.041 mg/L	1.57 µmol/L
nitroprusside therapy	0.05–0.5 mg/L	1.92–19.20 µmol/L
toxic	>1 mg/L	>38.40 µmol/L
cyclosporine, whole blood, therapeutic, trough	100–200 ng/mL	83–166 nmol/L
desipramine, serum or plasma, trough		
12 h after last dose		
therapeutic	75–300 ng/mL	281–1125 nmol/L
toxic	>400 ng/mL	>1500 nmol/L
diazepam, serum or plasma, trough		
therapeutic	100–1000 ng/mL	0.35–3.51 µmol/L
toxic	>5000 ng/mL	>17.55 µmol/L
dibucaine inhibition	79–84%	0.79–0.84

TEST	CONVENTIONAL UNITS	SI UNITS
digitoxin, serum or plasma, 7.8 h after dose		
therapeutic	20–35 ng/mL	26–46 nmol/L
toxic	>45 ng/mL	>59 nmol/L
digoxin, serum or plasma, ≥12 h after dose		
therapeutic		
congestive heart failure	0.8–1.5 ng/mL	1.0–1.9 nmol/L
arrhythmias	1.5–2.0 ng/mL	1.9–2.6 nmol/L
toxic		
adult	>2.5 ng/mL	>3.2 nmol/L
child	>3.0 ng/mL	>3.8 nmol/L
disopyramide, serum or plasma, trough		
therapeutic arrhythmias		
atrial	2.8–3.2 µg/mL	8.3–9.4 µmol/L
aentricular	3.3–7.5 µg/mL	9.7–22 µmol/L
toxic	> 7 µg/mL	20.7 µmol/L
doxepin, serum or plasma, trough (≥12 h after dose)		
therapeutic	150–250 ng/mL	537–895 nmol/L
toxic	>500 ng/mL	>1790 nmol/L
ethanol, EtOH, (alcohol), whole blood or serum		
depression of CNS	>100 mg/dL	>21.7 mmol/L
fatalities reported	>400 mg/dL	>86.8 mmol/L
ethosuximide, serum or plasma, trough		
therapeutic	40–100 µg/mL	283–708 µmol/L
toxic	>150 µg/mL	1062 µmol/L
fluoride		
plasma	0.01–0.2 µg/mL	0.5–10.5 µmol/L
urine	0.2–3.2 µg/mL	10.5–168 µmol/L
urine, occupational exposure	<8 µg/mL	<421 µmol/L
fluoride inhibition	58–64%	0.58–0.64

Drug Values

TEST	CONVENTIONAL UNITS	SI UNITS
gentamicin, serum or plasma		
therapeutic		
peak		
less severe infection	5–8 µg/mL	10.4–16.7 µmol/L
severe infection	8–10 µg/mL	16.7–20.9 µmol/L
trough		
less severe infection	<1µg/mL	<2.1 µmol/L
moderate infection	<2 µg/mL	<4.2 µmol/L
severe infection	<2–4 µg/mL	<4.2–8.4 µmol/L
toxic		
peak	>10–12 µg/mL	>21–25 µmol/L
trough	>2–4 µg/mL	>4.2–8.4 µmol/L
imipramine, serum or plasma,		
trough ≥12 h after dose		
therapeutic	150–250 ng/mL	536–893 nmol/L
toxic	>500 ng/mL	>1785 nmol/L
lead		
whole blood	<25 µg/dL	<1.2 µmol/L
urine, 24 h	<80 µg/d	<0.39µmol/d
lidocaine, serum or plasma, **45 minutes after bolus**		
therapeutic	1.5–6.0 µg/mL	6.4–26 µmol/L
toxic		
CNS, cardiovascular depression	6–8 µg/mL	26–34.2 µmol/L
seizures, obtundation, decreased cardiac output	>8 µg/mL	>34.2µmol/L
lithium, serum or plasma, **12 h after last dose**		
therapeutic	0.6–1.2 mmol/L	0.6–1.2 mmol/L
toxic	>2 mmol/L	>2 mmol/L
lorazepam, serum or plasma therapeutic	50–240 ng/mL	156–746 nmol/L

TEST	CONVENTIONAL UNITS	SI UNITS
mercury		
whole blood	0.6–59 µg/L	<0.29 µmol/L
urine, 24 h	<20 µg/d	<0.01 µmol/d
toxic	>150 µg/d	>0.75 µmol/d
methotrexate, serum or plasma		
therapeutic	Variable	Variable
toxic		
1–2 wk after low-dose therapy	≥0.02 µmol/L	≥0.02 µmol/L
post-IV infusion 24 h	≥5 µmol/L	≥5 µmol/L
48 h	≥0.5 µmol/L	≥0.5 µmol/L
72 h	≥0.05 µmol/L	≥0.05 µmol/L
nortriptyline, serum or plasma, trough, ≥12 h after dose		
therapeutic	50–150 ng/mL	190–570 nmol/L
toxic	>500 ng/mL	>1900 nmol/L
N-acetylprocainamide, serum or plasma trough		
therapeutic	5–30 µg/mL	18–108 µmol/L
toxic	>40 µg/mL	>144 µmol/L
oxazepam, serum or plasma, therapeutic	0.2–1.4 µg/mL	0.70–4.9 µmol/L
pentobarbital, serum or plasma, trough		
therapeutic		
hypnotic	1.5 µg/mL	4–22 µmol/L
therapeutic coma	20–50 µg/mL	88–221 µmol/L
toxic	>10 µg/mL	>44 µmol/L
phenacetin, plasma		
therapeutic	1.30 µg/mL	6–167 µmol/L
toxic	50–250 µg/mL	279–1395 µmol/L

Drug Values

TEST	CONVENTIONAL UNITS	SI UNITS
phenobarbital, serum or plasma, trough		
therapeutic	15–40 µg/mL	65–172 µmol/L
toxic		
slowness, ataxia, nystagmus	35–80 µg/mL	151–345 µmol/L
coma with reflexes	65–117 µg/mL	280–504 µmol/L
coma without reflexes	>100 µg/mL	>430 µmol/L
phenytoin, serum or plasma, Itrough		
therapeutic	10–20 µg/mL	40–79 µmol/L
toxic	>20 µg/mL	>79 µmol/L
phosphatase, acid, prostatic, serum, RIA	<3.0 ng/mL	<3.0 µg/L
primidone, serum or plasma, trough		
therapeutic	5–12 µg/mL	23–55 µmol/L
toxic	>15 µg/mL	>69 µmol/L
procainamide, serum or plasma, trough		
therapeutic	4–10 µg/mL	17–42 µmol/L
toxic (also consider effect of metabolite NAPA)	>10–12 µg/mL	>42–51 µmol/L
propoxyphene, plasma		
therapeutic	0.1–0.4 µg/mL	0.3–1.2 µmol/L
toxic	>0.5 µg/mL	>1.5 µmol/
propranolol, serum or plasma, trough		
therapeutic	50–100 ng/mL	193–386 nmol/L
quinidine, serum or plasma, trough		
therapeutic	2–5 µg/mL	6–15 µmol/L
toxic	>6 µg/mL	>18 µmol/L

TEST	CONVENTIONAL UNITS	SI UNITS
salicylates, serum or plasma, trough		
therapeutic	150–300 µg/mL	1.09–2.17 mmol/L
toxic	>500 µg/mL	>3.62 mmol/L
theophylline, serum or plasma		
therapeutic		
bronchodilator	8–20 µg/mL	44–111 µmol/L
prem. apnea	6–13 µg/mL	33–72 µmol/L
toxic	>20 µg/mL	>110 µmol/L
thiocyanate, serum or plasma		
nonsmoker	1–4 µg/mL	17–69 µmol/L
smoker	3–12 µg/mL	52–206 µmol/L
therapeutic after nitroprusside infusion	6–29 µg/mL	103–499 µmol/L
urine		
nonsmoker	1–4 mg/d	7–69 µmol/d
smoker	7–17mg/d	120–292 µmol/d
thiopental, serum or plasma, trough		
hypnotic	1.0–5-0 µg/mL	4.1–20.7 µmol/L
coma	30–100 µg/mL	124–413 µmol/L
anesthesia	7–130 µg/mL	29–536 µmol/L
toxic concentration	>10 µg/mL	>41 µmol/L
tobramycin, serum or plasma		
therapeutic		
peak		
less severe infection	5–8 µg/mL	11–17 µmol/L
severe infection	8–10 µg/mL	17–21 µmol/L
trough		
less severe infection	<1 µg/mL	<2 µmol/L
moderate infection	<2 µg/mL	<4 µmol/L
severe infection	<2–4 µg/mL	<4–9 µmol/L

Drug Values

TEST	CONVENTIONAL UNITS	SI UNITS
toxic		
peak	>10–12 µg/mL	>21–26 µmol/L
trough	>2–4 µg/mL	>4–9 µmol/L
	0.5–4.0 EU/d	0.5–4.0 EU/d
valproic acid, serum or plasma, trough		
therapeutic	50–100 µg/mL	347–693 µmol/L
toxic	>100 µg/mL	>693 µmol/L
vancomycin, serum or plasma		
therapeutic		
peak	20–40 µg/mL	14–28 µmol/L
trough	5–10 µg/mL	3–7 µmol/L
toxic	>80–100 µg/mL	>55–69 µmol/L
vitamin A, serum	30–80 µg/dL	1.05–2.8 µmol/L
vitamin B12, serum	110–800 pg/mL	81–590 pmol/L
vitamin E, serum		
normal	5–18 µg/mL	12–42 µmol/L
therapeutic	30–50 µg/mL	69.6–116 µmol/L
zinc, serum	70–120 µg/dL	10.7–18.4 µmol/L

Sample Reports

AUTOPSY REPORT

MANNER OF DEATH: Homicide.

CAUSE OF DEATH: Exsanguination from multiple stab wounds and incised wounds of head, neck, trunk, and upper extremities.

FINDINGS
1. Generalized pallor and evidence of exsanguination.
2. Multiple stab and incised wounds of head, neck, trunk and upper extremities with 1 stab wound penetrating left skull into brain, 3 stab wounds penetrating right back into chest cavity and right lung, another stab wound at lateral right chest penetrating into right lung, and multiple wounds of upper extremities consistent with defensive injuries.
3. Left lower lateral chest wall abrasions and contusions with overlying rib fractures of left ribs 6, 7, and 8.
4. Subarachnoid hemorrhage of right cerebrum underlying one of the large, undermined right scalp incised wounds.
5. A few other minor blunt-force injuries of head and trunk.
6. Slight emphysematous changes of lungs.

LABORATORY RESULTS
1. Blood: Ethanol level of 0.14 g%. Cocaine present at less than 0.14 g/mL; quantity not sufficient for further examination.
2. Urine: Positive for cocaine and cocaine metabolite enzyme multiplied immunoassay test (EMIT) barbiturates screen.
3. Ocular fluid: Ethanol level of 0.14 g%.

GENERAL APPEARANCE: This is the body of a well-developed, well-nourished, adult black man who appears his stated age. Body height is 72 inches, and body weight is 175 pounds. At autopsy, rigor mortis is generalized. Livor mortis is posterior and blanching . The body is cool to touch. Artifacts of decomposition are absent. There is no evidence of medical or postmortem care. There is obvious evidence of sharp-force injury in multiple regions.

IDENTIFICATION: Identification of the decedent was established by circumstances of death and discovery of the body.

EXTERNAL EXAMINATION
Clothing and valuables: Body submitted to the morgue clothed, within a sheet and body bag. The hands are bagged.

The clothing is very bloody, with injuries matching those found on the trunk. Prior to removal of clothing, trace evidence was collected from the body and clothing by crime scene technician while I was in attendance. See section titled "Trace Evidence" found later in this report. Clothing consisting of white T-shirt, a pair of black slacks, black belt, black socks, and dress shoes. Valuables with the body include a Bic cigarette lighter, key ring containing 3 keys, cellular phone, and $22.38 in cash. Valuables are released to brother of decedent. The body is retained by law enforcement.

HEAD AND NECK: Head is of normal shape. Scalp hair is short, dark brown, and slightly curled. Head, face, neck, and shoulders show no suffusion. Irides are brown. The pupils are equal and round. The sclerae are white. Conjunctivae with no petechiae. No ecchymosis in the periorbital region. Facial hair is present. Nasal and oral cavities show presence of a small amount of bloody mucus. Multiple caries present; oral hygiene is poor. No petechiae in the oral cavity. Neck with normal range of motion, no crepitus or deformities.

TRUNK: Chest is not increased in the anteroposterior dimension. There is dried blood over the xiphoid and sternal regions. No gynecomastia present. No palpable masses or discharge from the nipples. Abdomen is soft and slightly protuberant. There is no discoloration of the external wall. There are no natural abnormalities of the back or buttocks. The anus is moderately dilated with reddish circumferential ecchymosis; there are no lacerations or scars visible. External genitalia normal for age, with no injuries.

EXTREMITIES: The extremities are symmetrical, without natural deformities. Lower extremities with no peripheral edema and no atrophy. Fingernails and short and even.

SCARS, TATTOOS, NEVI, AND INCIDENTAL FINDINGS: Midline scar, consistent with laparotomy. Scar found on the right hand in the web space between the 1st and 2nd digits. Left ankle with surgical scar on the lateral aspect.

INJURIES: Multiple incised and stab wounds are present on the head, neck, chest, back and upper extremities. The number of wounds is too numerous to count and detail. In general, however, there are 28 or more on the head, 13 or more on the chest and back, and about 45 defensive incised wounds at the right and left hands and forearms. Most of the sharp-force injuries present are incised wounds, and most of the stab wound are actually nonpenetrating of the body cavities, except as detailed below, and except for the deeper ones at the upper extremities. There are also some blunt-force injuries and some overlying rib fractures as noted below.

Many of the head wounds are irregular with slightly scalloped or curving borders, as discussed below. The forehead, the right face beside the nose, the lips on the right side, the left side of the head and ear, and the right side of the head have multiple incised wounds. At the forehead, the largest is 5 cm in length and is irregular and mostly vertical. Most of the incised wounds are diagonal, slanting from upper left to lower right, and are about 1.7 cm in length each. The longest, at the right face, is 5.3 cm long. Wounds on the lips are superficial. At the left side of the head are several marks, mostly diagonal downward and to the front and also passing along the left side of the forehead and the left side of the face. At the frontoparietal area is a V-shaped incision which appears to be 2 incisions crossing one another. There are also 5 short, jab-type incisions at the low left forehead. These just penetrate the outer table of the skull beneath this area, the largest being 0.3 x 0.2 cm. Just inferior and posterior to these jab wounds is a definite penetrating stab wound of the skull. At the skin this is diagonal, with the blunt end 0.1 cm to 0.2 cm in thickness, and being at the anteroinferior aspect of the diagonal stab wound, the acute angle at the superior-posterior aspect, and the wound is about 1.7 cm in length. At the skull, this makes a similar triangular-shaped wound, more horizontal over the left sphenoid bone, with a base thickness of 0.1 to 0.2 cm, with a length of 1.6 cm. The most anterior 1-cm aspect of this stab is the actual penetration of the skull. It passes approximately 3.6 cm through the skin and brain, passing into the brain at the inferolateral left frontal lobe, about 2 cm. This stab wound creates a permanent stab cavity 1-cm wide and 2-cm deep in that area. It just enters the tip of the left lateral ventricle and is accompanied by a slight intraventricular hemorrhage and also by a slight contusion of the white matter surrounding the injury.

The inferior border of the left ear has a prominent red band of abrasion and an upside-down, V-shape vertical incision, 6 cm in length, passing through the center of the abrasion and onto the upper lateral left neck. The longest incision of the left face is 5 cm in length.

At the right side of the head are multiple stab wounds varying from 1.1 to 5.7 cm in length and including a curving stab, 6.5 cm long, with undermining in the posterior direction. In front of the right ear is a 9.5-cm curving incision.

At the top of the head, located mostly on the right front side is another group of incised wounds, the most prominent having slightly scalloped edges, and being 2.2 cm long. At the upper lateral left side of the head are 3 wounds, 0.9 cm between each wound and parallel, each curving slightly and having slightly scalloped edges with the scalloping especially at the left, and with overlying, perpendicular, parallel, pale, reddish purple abrasion and contusion lines over a total area of 2 x 3 cm.

Beginning at the middle of the upper right sternocleidomastoid muscle, the right posterolateral and posterior neck have deep, muscular, incised wounds actually representing about 3 total cuts. The leftmost aspect has a 1-cm superficial cut while the major cut passing over to the right posterolateral region is 13.5 cm in length. A separate, 2-cm incision overlies the right posterolateral aspect of this incision and combines with the incision for an additional 9 cm to terminate at the right sternocleidomastoid muscle. More inferiorly, the right sternocleidomastoid muscle also has a smaller incision.

The head also has some blunt-force injuries although these may be ragged incised wounds from a dull object. The back of the head has 5 parallel, diagonal (upper left to lower right) lacerations with visible tissue bridging. The uppermost 2 wounds are the most superficial and may actually be incisions, these being 1.5 cm long and 4.2 cm long, respectively. The lowest 2 are mostly on the left side and are 2.7 and 1.7 cm long respectively, and they have prominent abrasion and contusion around the edges. The back of the right ear also has a reddish purple and reddish black abrasion and contusion. The nasal bridge and tip of the nose have some abrasions and contusions. The left scalp above the ear has a linear, vertical abrasion. The vertex of the head has a 2.3 x 0.6-cm irregular abrasion.

Inside the head, the right parietotemporal region of the cerebrum has a focal area of increased subarachnoid hemorrhage. Other than the stab wound at the left frontal lobe, the brain has no contusions, lacerations, subdural hematoma or other injuries. This does lie beneath the larger, curving, 6.5-cm incised wound discussed earlier. The spinal cord is not examined.

At the left midclavicular region of the upper left chest are some small, skip-like abrasions. The midregion of the right clavicle of the upper chest also has a small area of abrasion. At the right parasternal chest is a 5-cm stab wound. The inferior border is slightly curved and has some slight contusion with slightly undulating edges at the inferior one fourth of the stab wound. The upper edge of the stab wound at the skin is squared off, 0.3 cm wide. The stab passes through the sternum in a roughly diagonal fashion with blunt upper right edge and acute lower left edge, passing into the chest at the right 3rd intercostal space anteriorly. It passes posteriorly, slightly downward and to the right, and it just catches the outer edge of the right lung at the junction of the right upper and right middle lobes. The stab stops in the lung for a total of about 5 cm. Otherwise, the anterior chest has no stab wounds. Laterally, the right upper chest has a 1.7-cm stab wound, horizontal in orientation, with the posterior aspect acute and the anterior aspect blunt. This passes into the right posterolateral chest via the 3rd right intercostal space with no visible entry into the lung and with a depth of the stab greater than or equal to 6 cm.

The lateral left chest at the lower half has several irregular areas of mottled abrasions and contusions without pattern, the 2 largest being 3 x 0.3 cm and 1 x 1 cm. These overlie the fractures of the ribs with accompanying slight intercostal space contusion, mainly at the left lateral 6th rib, the left posterolateral 7th rib, and the left posterolateral 8th rib. The 7th rib has a parietal pleural perforation and the greatest amount of hemorrhage from contusion. These are injuries caused by blunt force. At the back, there are multiple shallow stabs and jab-type wounds along with some tiny superficial abrasions or incisions, all less than or equal to 0.3 cm. At the left upper shoulder posteriorly are 2 of the more prominent superficial stab wounds not passing into the chest, the upper right lateral wound being diagonally oriented and 2 cm long, and the more medial wound being 1.5 cm long and oriented horizontally. At the center of the back, slightly more on the right side of the spine than the left, are 7 parallel, diagonal stabs. These all have roughly the same appearance on the skin, although their upper and lower edges are less distinct than other stab wounds on the body.

Of these wounds, 3 are chosen for representative measurements. The uppermost right stab of this group is 1.8 cm long and appears to have the blunt edge downward with a V-shaped acute edge superiorly. Bringing the 2 edges of the wound together creates almost a double V, although the inferior aspect is more of a shallow V than is the upper V. The inferiormost right wound in this group is 1.5 cm long and has a prominent inferior V with an acute superior edge. Bringing the 2 sides together creates no V at the top at all, but instead makes the inferior V more prominent. The uppermost left wound of this group is 1.8 cm long and has a prominent upper blunt edge and an inferior acute edge. This wound, when the edges are brought together, is a simple slit. Three of the 4 stabs at the right side of this group penetrate the chest, with 1 stab wound going through the 6th posterior right intercostal space, one going through the 7th posterior right intercostal space, and 1 going through the 9th posterior right intercostal space. These go into the right chest cavity with 1 injury only penetrating the right lung for a total depth of greater than or equal to 5 cm. The 2 stab wounds to the left of the spine pass downward, medially and to the front, but they stop at the left lamina and left lateral side of the spinous processes of the back bone with a short overall distance for the stab of about 1.8 cm without penetration of the chest cavity.

As mentioned earlier, the upper extremities have multiple sharp-force injuries. At the anterior, distal right wrist are several abrasions and lacerations with slight reddish purple contusions, the longest 4.3 x 0.4 cm, and the most prominent being 1 x 1.5 cm. These are less clearly defined as incised wounds, although they may be from an irregular object. At the back of the right triceps area, almost exposing the bone, is a bloodless, 19.5-cm gaping and deeply incised wound. The lateral proximal right shoulder and proximal arm have 3 incisions, the longest more distal and 1.6 cm long, with an irregular distal border suggestive of an acute angle and with a proximal border squared off and 0.2 to 0.3 cm in width. The back of the right forearm has some small abrasions and some small incised wounds toward the wrist. The distal right biceps area, just above the antecubital fossa, has 1 small, incised wound.

The left distal forearm has a large, gaping incised wound of 3 x 5 cm in surface area, passing through the tendons. Just proximal to this is a 5 x 4-cm area of dried blood with abrasions and superficial incisions. Just proximal to that and more medial are 2 parallel, linear, thin abrasions.

The backs of the hands have multiple avulsed and oblique incisions and lacerations, mostly incisions, ranging from 1.5 to 3.2 cm in length. In addition, the back of the right hand has a larger, gaping wound that is 5.3 x 3 cm in length, and the right wounds and the left dorsal wrist wounds have superimposed purple contusions. On the medial edge of the right thumb is a 1.3-cm incised wound which continues onto the thumb pad itself. At the palmar surface of the left hand are approximately 78 oblique incised wounds, one being 3.5 cm long and having scalloped edges, and another being 2.5 cm long with the others varying. The hands do have clumps of straight, long, possibly blond hairs adherent, especially at the left palm. These are collected.

Overall, most of the incised wounds of the trunk suggest a single-edged, thin blade; however, a double-edged blade cannot be excluded. Many of the head wounds, as well as the hand and forearm injuries, suggest a scalloped edge or scalloped object, and the multiple injuries of the hands and forearms are consistent with defensive injuries.

Internally, there is almost no blood present in the heart and great vessels and tissues due to exsanguination from all of these multiple wounds. X-rays of the head and neck and also the chest and upper abdomen show no obvious fractures or foreign bodies. The internal structures of the neck, including the carotid arteries, show no injuries except for the large neck injury passing into the muscle, as mentioned above. The heart and liver have no injuries. See above for stabs of right lung, stab of brain, left rib fractures and right brain subarachnoid hemorrhage.

Internal Examination: In general, internal artifacts and injuries have been described above and will not be further detailed in this section.

The body cavities are opened in the standard autopsy fashion. The organs are present in their usual anatomic locations and relationships. Little blood is present in the pleural cavities, and there are some slight adhesions at the left upper lobe of the lung. There is no evidence of empyema, purulent exudate, or acute inflammation of the serous cavities. There is no tissue discoloration suggestive for carbon monoxide intoxication or jaundice. There is a slight smell suggestive of alcoholic beverages within the body.

The gallbladder contains the usual bile. The stomach contains 30 mL of grayish, mucoid fluid with curdled, small, soft, whitish lumps of mostly digested, unrecognizable food. There is no evidence of drug residue in the stomach. The vermiform appendix is present. The urinary bladder contains clear urine. In general, atherosclerosis is very mild. The heart has no evidence of infarction or scarring. The lungs have bullous emphysematous changes to a slight degree, mostly at the upper lobes. The right lung also has the stab wounds mentioned earlier. The liver appears pale but not fatty. The spleen, pancreas, kidneys, heart, adrenals, thyroid, pituitary, prostate and bladder are not, otherwise, remarkable. The testes show no contusions. The penis is circumcised.

Routine organ weights are as follows: heart, 365 g; right lung, 520 g; left lung, 570 g; liver, 1580 g; spleen 80 g; pancreas 165 g; right kidney 150 g; left kidney 170 g; brain 1450 g.

PROCEDURES AND SPECIMENS
TOXICOLOGY: Blood, bile, urine, ocular fluid, nasal swabs.

PHOTOGRAPHY: Slide identification pictures, 35-mm. Instant-print photos are also taken of the scene and of many of the injuries.

TRACE EVIDENCE: Trace materials on tape from right shoulder and chest. Possible small glass fragment from left upper chest. Trace materials on tape from left shoulder, neck, chest. Trace materials on tape from chest. Glass fragments from back. Possible glass fragments from chest. Hairs adherent to right and left sleeves of shirt. Hairs adherent to left hand. One hair from inside oral cavity. Clippings from right fingernails and left fingernails. Adherent hairs from right hand. Purple-topped and red-topped tubes of blood are also collected and sent to the lab.

CHEMISTRY AND CULTURES: None.

FIREARMS EXAMINATION: None performed.

X-RAYS: See section titled "Injuries."

MICROSCOPIC EXAMINATION: Representative sections of major organ systems have been obtained and routinely processed onto glass slides for histologic examination. These have been reviewed.

The liver, heart and kidney are not remarkable aside from some moderately advanced autolysis, especially at the kidney. The lungs show diffuse, moderate emphysematous changes including septal fibrosis and an increased number of macrophages, along with congestion. The cerebrum shows acute petechial hemorrhages at the directed section from the stab-wound area, but otherwise the cerebrum is not remarkable. The anoderm shows no contusion, but it does have dilated submucosal vessels without significant inflammation or scarring. There are no additional significant findings.

BONE MARROW ASPIRATE, BIOPSY, AND PERIPHERAL BLOOD SMEAR

INDICATIONS: Acute promyelocytic anemia. Biopsy taken recently revealed no morphologic evidence of residual disease.

PROCEDURE PERFORMED: Bone marrow biopsy.

GROSS EXAMINATION: The specimen labeled "left bone marrow biopsy" is received in Bouin's solution and consists of 1 elongated, cylindrical, tan-brown fragment of bony material that measures 1.5 x 0.3 x 0.4 cm. The specimen is submitted entirely between sponges in a single cassette following decalcification.

PERIPHERAL BLOOD SMEAR: Red blood cells are normochromic and range from microcytic to normocytic. There is occasional polychromasia. A few scattered teardrop forms are identified. Platelets are normal in number with occasional large and hypogranular forms. White blood cells are normal in number, with a normal absolute number of neutrophils. White blood cells are predominantly normal-appearing, segmented neutrophils, with fewer numbers of lymphocytes and monocytes.

BONE MARROW ASPIRATE: The bone marrow aspirate is adequate. Megakaryocytes are present in slightly higher than normal numbers but with normal morphology . The myeloid/erythroid (M:E) ratio is 2:1 to 3:1. Myeloid precursors are normal in number with a left shift, without a relative increase in the number of promyelocytes or blasts. Erythroid precursors are present in normal numbers, also with a slight shift to the left. Iron stores are present within histiocytes; no ringed sideroblasts are identified.

BONE MARROW BIOPSY: The bone marrow biopsy is mildly hypercellular for age, approximately 70%. Megakaryocytes are present in normal numbers and morphology. The M:E ratio is 3:1. Myeloid and erythroid precursors are normal in number and fully mature. The myeloid precursors have a slight left shift. There are no excess blasts. Notable, there is an area of fibrosis, which fibrosis appears to be associated with subcortical bone.

COMMENT: The bone marrow aspirate and biopsy reveal left-shifted myelogenesis and erythrogenesis. There is no relative increase in the number of promyelocytes or blasts. Since morphology is limited in distinguishing normal myelogenesis from residual disease, correlation with cytogenetic and/or molecular studies is recommended.

DIAGNOSIS: Bone marrow aspirate, biopsy, and peripheral blood smear. Mildly hypercellular marrow with left-shifted myeloid and erythroid maturation.

CARCINOMA OF THE STOMACH

INDICATIONS: Patient with history of gastric ulcer of long duration.

DIAGNOSIS: Carcinoma of stomach.

PROCEDURE PERFORMED: Vagotomy and subtotal gastrectomy.

GROSS DESCRIPTION: A total of 3 specimens were received.

Specimen #1 consisted of a portion of the stomach, measuring 13 x 7 x 2.5 cm. There was a portion of mesentery attached to the lesser curvature. There was a firm, indurated area in the wall of the lesser curvature. The serosal surface was smooth, glistening, and slightly hemorrhagic. On opening the specimen, a penetrating, well-circumscribed ulcer, 1 cm in diameter, was found in the wall of the lesser curvature. This ulcer penetrated to a depth of 1 cm. The ulcer was 3 cm from the proximal portion of the specimen and 4.5 cm from the distal portion. The edges of the ulcer were heaped up and firm, but the surround mucosa did not appear to be involved. The rugae or folds radiate toward the center of the ulcer from the superior side. The mucosa of the distal portion of the stomach was smooth.

Specimen #2 consisted of a portion of the left anterior vagus. The specimen consisted of a piece of pale, gray-white, soft tissue measuring 0.8 cm in length. The entire specimen was submitted for examination.

Specimen #3 was labeled "right posterior vagus" and consisted of a piece of soft, gray-white tissue measuring 2 cm in length and 0.4 cm in diameter. Entire specimen was submitted for examination.

MICROSCOPIC EXAMINATION: Microscopic examination reveals a ragged ulcer penetrating to within 5 mm of the serosal surface. The ulcer is surrounded by dense connective response and chronic inflammatory infiltrate. The edges are not heaped up; however, several sections of the ulcer reveal malignant changes. The tumor is superficial and composed of poorly formed glands and sheets of malignant cells. The cells are pleomorphic and contain small amounts of eosinophilic cytoplasm. The nuclei are either pyknotic or large with prominent nucleoli and clumped chromatin. Mitoses are rare. The tumor itself does not extend below the mucosa, but a single nest of malignant cells is seen in a submucosal lymphatic space. The surgical margins are free of tumor. There are 4 perigastric lymph nodes. These show no evidence of metastatic spread. There are 2 segments of the large peripheral nerve.

DIAGNOSES
1. Superficial, spreading carcinoma, rising in the margin of a gastric ulcer that is chronic in nature. The surgical margins appear free of tumor.
2. Four perigastric lymph nodes reveal no evidence of metastatic disease.

COLON POLYP BIOPSY

GROSS DESCRIPTION: Specimen sent to laboratory, labeled "polyp of sigmoid colon." This is an ovoid, smooth-surfaced, firm, pale-tan nodule that measures 0.7 x 0.5 x 0.3 cm. Specimen bisected and submitted in its entirety.

MICROSCOPIC DESCRIPTION: The sections show a polypoid structure consisting of a central fibrovascular core, surrounded by a mantle of mucosa showing an adenomatous architecture with a predominantly tubular pattern. The tubules are lined by tall, columnar epithelia showing nuclear pseudostratification, hyperchromasia, increased mitotic activity, and loss of cytoplasmic mucin. There is no evidence of stromal invasion.

DIAGNOSIS: Sigmoid colon, endoscopic biopsy, revealing tubular adenoma (adenomatous polyp).

INFILTRATING DUCTAL CARCINOMA OF BREAST

INDICATIONS: Patient with breast mass in left upper outer quadrant.

DIAGNOSIS: Breast carcinoma.

PROCEDURE PERFORMED: Left breast radical mastectomy.

SPECIMENS
1. Left breast tissue.
2. Apical axillary tissue.
3. Left radical mastectomy contents.

GROSS DESCRIPTION: Specimen #1 is labeled "left breast biopsy." This specimen is received fresh after a frozen section preparation. Specimen consists of a single, very firm nodularity measuring 3 cm in circular diameter and 1.5 cm in thickness. It is surrounded by adherent, fibrofatty tissue. On section examination, a pale gray, slightly mottled appearance is revealed. Numerous sections of this specimen are submitted for permanent pathology.

Specimen #2 is labeled "apical left axillary tissue" and is also received fresh. It consists of 2 amorphous, fibrofatty tissue masses with no grossly discernible lymph nodes. Both pieces are rendered into numerous sections and submitted for histology in their entirety.

Specimen #3 is labeled "contents of left radical mastectomy." This specimen is received fresh as well. Specimen consists of a large ellipse of skin overlying breast tissue, the ellipse measuring 20 cm in length and 14 cm in height. A freshly sutured incision extends 3 cm directly lateral from the areola, and this corresponds to the closure for removal of specimen #1, "left breast biopsy." Abundant amounts of fibrofatty connective tissue surround the entire breast. The deep aspect of the breast includes an 8-cm length of pectoralis minor muscle and a generous amount of overlying pectoralis major muscle. Incision from the deepest aspect of the specimen beneath the tumor mass reveals the tumor extending grossly to within 0.5 cm of the muscle.

Sections of this specimen are submitted according to the following code:
DE: Deep surgical resection margins.
SU, LA, INF, ME: Full-thickness radial, respectively.
NI: Nipple and subjacent tissue.

The lymph nodes are dissected free from axillary fibrofatty tissue levels 1, 2, and 3 and are labeled accordingly.

MICROSCOPIC EXAMINATION: Sections of specimen #1 confirm frozen section diagnosis of infiltrating ductal carcinoma. It is noted that the tumor cells show considerable pleomorphism, and mitotic figures are frequent (as many as 6 per high-power field). Many foci of calcification are present within this tumor.

Specimen #2 consists of fibrofatty tissue and a single, tiny lymph node that is free of disease.

Specimen #3 consists of 18 lymph nodes, 3 from level 3, 2 from level 2, and 13 from level 1. All these lymph nodes are free from disease except a single lymph node from level 1 that contains several masses of metastatic carcinoma.

All sections taken from the superficial center of the resection site, radially, fail to include tumor. This indicates the tumor originated deep within the breast parenchyma. Similarly, no malignancy is found in the nipple region or in the lactiferous sinuses.

Sections of the deep surgical margin demonstrate diffuse tumor infiltration of deep fatty tissues; however, there is no invasion of muscle. The primary tumor's total size is estimated to be 4 cm in greatest dimension.

DIAGNOSES
1. Left breast infiltrating ductal carcinoma.
2. Metastatic carcinoma of the left axillary lymph node, level 1.
3. No pathologic diagnosis of level 1 lymph nodes, 12 nodes total. No pathologic diagnosis of level 2 lymph nodes, 2 nodes total. No pathologic diagnosis of level 3 lymph nodes, 3 nodes total.

OVARIAN AND BREAST TISSUE ANALYSIS IN PATIENT WITH BREAST CANCER AND FAMILY HISTORY OF OVARIAN CANCER

SPECIMENS
1. Right tube and ovary.
2. Left tube and ovary.
3. Right breast and right axillary nodes.
4. Left breast.

GROSS EXAMINATION: Specimen #1, right tube and ovary, received in formalin. Specimen consists of a 3 x 1-cm fallopian tube segment with a well-healed surgical stump. There is a 4 x 2.3 x 2.2-cm ovary with a ruptured capsular surface, gray-pink in color. Cut section of the specimen shows a hemorrhagic corpus luteal cyst and an adjacent edematous ovarian stroma.

Specimen #2, left tube and ovary, also received in formalin. Specimen consists of a 2.8 x 1-cm fallopian tube stump, including the fimbriated end, with an adjacent 1.5 x 0.6-cm thin-walled cyst. The ovary is attached, size being 2.5 x 2 x 1.5 cm. Ovary has an intact, pale-yellow capsule that shows corpus luteal cyst on cut section.

The right side specimen, specimen #3, consists of right breast and right axillary nodes, taken from a modified radical mastectomy. The breast weighs 300 g with a 6-cm axillary tail. There is a tan skin ellipse overlying the specimen, 10 x 5 cm in size. The specimen has a centrally placed, everted nipple, and areola with multinodular appearance. Deep surgical margin is inked. Cut section shows lobules of yellow, soft adipose tissue with thin, rubbery white fibrous bands in the specimen. In the mid-portion of the breast tissue, 2 cm above the deep resection margin and 2 cm below the skin surface, is a palpable mass, 3 x 2 x 2 cm in size. On cut section this mass shows a granular cut surface, tan-gray color. Other masses are not identified in the specimen. The axillary tail is thin. Enlarged lymph nodes are not readily palpable or identified on gross examination.

Specimen #4 is tissue from the left side. This is from a modified radical mastectomy of the left breast. The breast weighs 280 g. The fatty breast tissue is lobulated and 15 x 14 x 6 cm in size. It has an axillary portion that is triangular in shape that measures

7 x 5 x 2 cm. On the superior surface is an ellipse of skin, 7 x 3.5 cm, with a normal-appearing, everted nipple. The deep surgical surface is covered by a white, fibrous membrane with some strands of skeletal muscle present. The breast tissue is sectioned in serial fashion and shows 85% lobulated homogenous fat with fibrous septa and a few areas of dense fibrous tissue beneath the areola. There are no large areas of cysts, tumor nodules, or fibrosis. Section of the axillary tail reveals no lymph nodes on gross examination.

MICROSCOPIC EXAMINATION: Section of the left and right fallopian tubes is unremarkable. Both ovaries show benign corpus luteal cysts.

Sections of the right nipple show no evidence of Paget disease or dermal lymphatic tumor spread. Sections of the tumor mid breast show poorly differentiated infiltrating ductal carcinoma with an area of necrosis in the center. The tumor extends into the adjacent adipose tissue. The tumor is not identified at the inked surgical margin. Extensive intraductal component is not identified. The tumor is composed of infiltrating trabecular sheets and nests of moderately pleomorphic oval epithelial cells which contain a large oval to angulated nucleus with coarsely clumped nuclear chromatin and a moderate amount of eosinophilic cytoplasm. There are 4 to 5 mitotic figures seen per high-power field. Sections of adjacent breast tissue show fibrocystic changes and duct ectasia with cyst formation. Axillary lymph nodes, 3 in total, show no evidence of metastasis.

Sections of the left nipple show no evidence of Paget disease or dermal lymphatic tumor spread. Sections of subareolar breast tissue show benign intraductal papilloma. There is mild, nonproliferative, fibrocystic changes of the breast tissue with stromal fibrosis and duct ectasia with small cyst formation. Atypical hyperplasia is not identified, nor is in situ and invasive malignancy.

DIAGNOSES
1. Right ovary and fallopian tube. Hemorrhagic corpus luteal cyst. Unremarkable fallopian tube.
2. Left ovary and fallopian tube. Benign physiologic cysts and ovary. Unremarkable fallopian tube.
3. Right breast and axillary lymph nodes from modified radical mastectomy.
   a. Infiltrating ductal carcinoma Bloom-Richardson grade 3.
      1. Tumor 3 x 2 x 2 cm in size.
      2. No evidence of tumor extension to deep surgical margins.
      3. Axillary lymph nodes (3 total) show no evidence of metastasis.
      4. No evidence of Paget disease or dermal lymphatic tumor spread.
      5. Pending hormone receptor and DNA analysis.
   b. Mild fibrocystic changes present.

4. Left breast, modified radical mastectomy.
  a. Benign intraductal papilloma.
  b. No evidence of Paget disease or dermal lymphatic tumor spread.
  c. Mild, nonproliferative changes, fibrocystic in nature, without atypia.

HORMONE RECEPTOR ANALYSIS: Immunoperoxidase stains for estrogen and progesterone receptors are applied to the paraffin-embedded tissue. No good positive and negative internal and external controls. Tumor cells from the right breast tumor show estrogen receptor negative (0% staining of tumor nuclei, histochemical score 0); progesterone receptor negative (0% staining of tumor cells).

PAP SMEAR

SOURCE OF SPECIMEN: Cervix.

LAST MENSTRUAL PERIOD: 01/01/2000.

MENSTRUAL STATUS: Regular menstrual periods.

RELEVANT MEDICAL HISTORY: Genital warts and pelvic inflammatory disease in the past.

NUMBER OF SLIDES SUBMITTED: One.

DESCRIPTION OF SPECIMEN ADEQUACY: Inadequate, due to excessive inflammation.

DIAGNOSIS: Unreliable Pap smear, due to inflammation.

RECOMMENDATION FOR FOLLOWUP: Recommend repeat smear.

PROSTATE CARCINOMA

DIAGNOSIS: Prostate carcinoma.

PROCEDURE PERFORMED: Prostatectomy.

GROSS DESCRIPTION: The specimen consists of 8 vials, each containing pink-tan prostate biopsies, each 1 mm in diameter. Specimens submitted in formalin in toto.

SPECIMENS
1. Prostate, right base, 1.8 cm in length.
2. Prostate, right mid, 2 cm in length.

3. Prostate, right mid lateral, 2.2 cm in length.
4. Prostate, right apex, 1.9 cm in length.
5. Prostate, left base, 1.8 cm in length.
6. Prostate, left mid, 1.7 cm in length.
7. Prostate, left mid lateral, 2 cm in length.
8. Prostate, left apex, 2 cm in length.

DIAGNOSES
1. Prostate, right base. Benign prostatic tissue.
2. Prostate, right mid. High-grade prostatic intraepithelial neoplasia.
3. Prostate, right mid lateral. Benign prostatic tissue, moderate atrophy, postatrophic hyperplasia.
4. Prostate, right apex. Adenocarcinoma, Gleason 4 + 4 = 8, involving 70% of the specimen.
5. Prostate, left base. Benign prostatic tissue, atypical adenomatous hyperplasia.
6. Prostate, left mid. Benign prostatic tissue, mild chronic inflammation.
7. Prostate, left mid lateral. Benign prostatic tissue.
8. Prostate, left apex. Benign prostatic tissue.

SPLEEN DISSECTION

GROSS DESCRIPTION: Specimen arrived, labeled "spleen." Specimen is an entire spleen, weighing 127 g, measuring 13 x 4.1 x 9.2 cm. The external surface is smooth, leathery, homogeneous, and dark purplish-brown in color. There are no defects in the capsule. The blood vessels of the hilum of the spleen are patent, with no thrombus or other abnormality. The hilar soft tissues contain a single, ovoid, 1.2-cm lymph node with a dark gray, cut surface. There are no focal lesions.

On section of the spleen at 2- to 3-mm intervals, there are 3 well-defined, pale-gray nodules on the cut surface, ranging from 0.5 to 1.1 cm in greatest dimension. The remainder of the cut surface is homogeneous, dark purple, and firm.

SPECIMENS
1. Hilar blood vessels.
2. Hilar lymph node, entirely submitted.
3. Spleen nodules, entirely submitted.
4. Spleen nodules, entirely submitted.
5. Spleen nodules, entirely submitted.
6. Spleen nodules, entirely submitted.
7. Spleen, away from nodules.
8. Spleen, away from nodules.

DIAGNOSIS: Normal-appearing spleen.

Squamous Cell Carcinoma of Left Floor of Mouth

Diagnosis: Left floor of mouth carcinoma.

Gross Description: A 3-part specimen was received fresh. Specimen #1 is labeled "? metastatic tumor in jugular vein lymph nodes." This specimen consists of an elliptical fragment of light, whitish-tan tissue that is approximately 0.3 x 0.2 x 0.2 cm in size. Specimen is examined by frozen section technique. Diagnosis is ganglion. Remainder of this specimen is submitted as frozen section control #1.

The 2nd part is labeled "resection of floor of mouth, continuous with tongue and mandible, plus left radical neck dissection." As received in the frozen section room, this specimen consists of an identifiable left radical neck dissection and also the entire left ascending ramus of the mandible, the posterior three fourths of the left mandible proper, the left lateral portion of the tongue, and the submental and submaxillary salivary glands. The main lesion is identified on the left side of the floor of the mouth. There is a lesion that is crater-like, measuring approximately 1.2 x 0.5 cm in greatest dimension. With the assistants, this specimen is properly oriented. There are 2 areas of interest defined. The initial area of interest is the anterior tongue margin. The 2nd area of interest is the medial tongue margin. Fragments from each of these areas are examined by the frozen section technique. The diagnosis on frozen section #2 (anterior tongue margin) noted as "no tumor seen." The diagnosis on frozen section #3 (medial tongue margin) is noted as "no tumor seen."

Two additional areas of special interest are also identified. The 1st of these is that portion of the left radical neck dissection which was nearest to the carotid artery. A fragment of tissue is excised from this area and submitted for sectioning labeled "CM." The 2nd area of interest is that portion of the left radical neck dissection bordering the anterior aspect of the vertebral column. A fragment of tissue is excised from this area and submitted for sectioning labeled "VM."

After having photographed the specimen in several positions, it is blocked further. A section is taken through the main tumor mass and submitted for sectioning labeled "T Post." Attention is directed to the left radical neck dissection proper. This part of the specimen is divided into the appropriate 5 levels. Each level is examined for lymph nodes, which are dissected free and submitted in their entirety for sectioning. The remainder of the specimen is saved.

The 3rd and final part of the specimen, labeled "anterior margin of inferior mandible," consists of an irregular fragment of fibrous connective and skeletal muscular tissues and measures approximately 1 x 0.5 x 0.2 cm. The specimen is submitted in its entirety for sectioning on 3 levels.

MICROSCOPIC DESCRIPTION: Examination of frozen section control #1 confirms the original frozen section diagnosis of ganglion. Microscopic examination of frozen section control #2 confirms the original frozen section diagnosis of no tumor seen. Microscopic examination of frozen section control #3 confirms the original frozen section diagnosis of no tumor seen.

Microscopic examination of 2nd part of the specimen reveals foci of moderately well-differentiated squamous cell carcinoma in the floor of the left side of the mouth. The residual tumor is surrounded by large amounts of dense, fibrous connective tissue. Microscopic examination of the section labeled CM, which represents the carotid margin, reveals squamous cell carcinoma that extends to within 0.1 cm of the surgical margin.

Microscopic examination of the section labeled VM, representing the vertebral margin, reveals no evidence of tumor in this location. Microscopic examination of the tissue in level 1 reveals a section of fibrotic and atrophic submaxillary salivary gland. There is also a single lymph node in level 1, being negative for metastatic tumor. Microscopic examination of the tissue in level 2 reveals sections of 11 lymph nodes. None of these lymph nodes contain squamous cell carcinoma. Microscopic examination of the tissue in level 4 reveals sections of 6 lymph nodes. These lymph nodes sections do not contain metastatic tumor. Microscopic examination of the tissue in level 5 reveals a single lymph node, negative for metastatic tumor.

DIAGNOSES
1. Left floor of mouth squamous cell carcinoma.
2. Squamous cell carcinoma in the extranodal connection tissue of neck, level 3.
3. No pathologic diagnosis in 19 cervical lymph nodes submitted.

TRANSITIONAL CELL CARCINOMA OF BLADDER

INDICATIONS: Multiple transurethral resection of bladder tumor resections for grade 2 transitional cell cancer.

PREOPERATIVE DIAGNOSIS: Bladder carcinoma; question of scalene lymph node metastasis.

POSTOPERATIVE DIAGNOSIS: Bladder carcinoma.

PROCEDURE PERFORMED: Bladder biopsy and left scalene lymph nodes.

SPECIMENS
1. Bladder tumor.
2. Left scalene lymph node.

GROSS DESCRIPTION: The specimen arrived to lab in 2 parts, labeled 1 as "biopsy bladder tumor," and 2 as "scalene node, left." Specimen #1 consists of several fragments of tissue, gray-brown in color. Tissue fragments appear slightly hemorrhagic. These are submitted in their entirety for processing. Specimen #2 consists of multiple fragments of tissue, fatty yellow in color. This tissue ranges in size from 0.2 cm to 1 cm in diameter. These tissue fragments are submitted in entirety for processing as well.

MICROSCOPIC EXAMINATION: This bladder specimen contains areas of transitional cell carcinoma; no areas of invasion can be identified. There is , acute and chronic, noted together with some necrosis. The section is examined in 6 levels. The scalene lymph node specimen contains normal nodal tissue with reactive germinal centers.

DIAGNOSES
1. Grade 2 papillary transitional cell carcinoma of bladder.
2. Inflammation, acute and chronic, of bladder, most consistent with recent biopsy procedure.
3. No pathologic diagnosis of left scalene lymph node.

Common Terms by Procedure

Autopsy Report

acute inflammation
adherent hair
anatomic location and relationship
anoderm
antecubital fossa
anteroposterior dimension
artifact of decomposition
atherosclerosis
barbiturate screen
bile
blanching
bloody mucus
blunt-force injury
body cavity
bullous emphysematous change
cerebrum
chest cavity
chest wall abrasion
cocaine metabolite
congestion
conjunctiva
contusion
crepitus
curving border
curving incision
decedent
defensive incised wound
defensive injury
dorsal wrist wound
drug residue
emphysematous change
enzyme multiplied immunoassay test
   (EMIT)
ethanol level
exsanguination
external genitalia
gallbladder
glass slide

head
histologic examination
homicide
incised wound
infarction
inferolateral left frontal lobe
intercostal space
internal structure of neck
intraventricular hemorrhage
jab-type wound
laceration
liver mortis
macrophage
middle lobe
mottled abrasion
mucoid fluid
nasal swab
natural deformity
neck
ocular fluid
oral cavity
organ weight
pallor
parietal pleural perforation
periorbital region
peripheral edema
petechia
petechial hemorrhage
pleural cavity
postmortem
purple-topped tube
red-topped tube
rib fracture
right middle lobe
right upper lobe
rigor mortis
scalloped border
scar
septal fibrosis

serous cavity
sharp-force injury
slide identification picture
slightly protuberant
sphenoid bone
spinal cord
spinous process
stab wound
sternal region
sternocleidomastoid muscle
subarachnoid hemorrhage
subdural hematoma
surgical scar
thumb pad
trace evidence
trace material
trunk
upper extremity
upper lobe
urinary bladder
vermiform appendix
xiphoid region

Bone Marrow Aspirate, Biopsy, and Peripheral Blood Smear
absolute number
acute promyelocytic anemia
blast
bone marrow aspirate
bone marrow biopsy
bony material
Bouin's solution
cytogenetic
decalcification
erythrogenesis
erythroid maturation
erythroid precursor
excess blast
fibrosis
histiocyte
hypercellular marrow
hypogranular form
iron store

left shift
left-shifted myelogenesis
lymphocyte
megakaryocyte
microcytic
molecular study
monocyte
morphologic evidence
morphology
myelogenesis
myeloid/erythroid (M:E) ratio
myeloid precursor
neutrophil
normocytic
platelet
polychromasia
promyelocyte
red blood cell
residual disease
ringed sideroblast
segmented neutrophil
subcortical bone
teardrop form
white blood cell

Carcinoma of the Stomach
carcinoma of stomach
chronic inflammatory infiltrate
clumped chromatin
eosinophilic cytoplasm
gastric ulcer
hemorrhagic
indurated area
lesser curvature
mesentery
metastatic spread
microscopic examination
mitosis
nest of malignant cells
penetrating ulcer
perigastric lymph node
peripheral nerve
pleomorphic

prominent nucleolus
proximal portion of specimen
pyknotic
ragged ulcer
ruga
serosal surface
sheet of malignant cells
spreading carcinoma
submucosal lymphatic space
subtotal gastrectomy
surgical margin
vagotomy
vagus
well-circumscribed ulcer

Colon Polyp Biopsy

adenomatous architecture
adenomatous polyp
bisected
central fibrovascular core
colon polyp
columnar epithelium
cytoplasmic mucin
endoscopic biopsy
fibrovascular core
hyperchromasia
mantle of mucosa
microscopic description
mitotic activity
nuclear pseudostratification
ovoid nodule
polypoid structure
sigmoid colon
stromal invasion
tubular adenoma
tubular pattern
tubule

Infiltrating Ductal Carcinoma of Breast

amorphous, fibrofatty tissue mass
areola
axillary tissue

breast carcinoma
breast mass
breast parenchyma
breast tissue
circular diameter
deep surgical margin
deep surgical resection margin
diffuse tumor infiltration
ellipse of skin
fibrofatty connective tissue
fibrofatty tissue
free of disease
freshly sutured incision
frozen section
frozen section diagnosis
focus of calcification
greatest dimension
grossly discernible lymph node
high-power field
infiltrating ductal carcinoma
lactiferous sinus
left radical mastectomy
left radical mastectomy
left upper outer quadrant
level 1 lymph node
level 2 lymph node
level 3 lymph node
lymph node
metastatic carcinoma
microscopic examination
mitotic figure
mottled appearance
nipple region
nodularity
pathologic diagnosis
pectoralis major muscle
pectoralis minor muscle
permanent pathology
pleomorphism
radical mastectomy
resection site
subjacent tissue
tumor cell
tumor infiltration

Ovarian and Breast Tissue Analysis in Patient with Breast Cancer and Family History of Ovarian Cancer

adipose tissue
adjacent adipose tissue
adjacent breast tissue
angulated nucleus
areola
atypical hyperplasia
axillary lymph node
axillary node
axillary tail
benign corpus luteal cyst
benign physiologic cyst
breast tissue
capsular surface
coarsely clumped nuclear chromatin
corpus luteal cyst
cut section
cyst formation
deep resection margin
deep surgical margin
dermal lymphatic tumor spread
DNA analysis
duct ectasia
edematous ovarian stroma
enlarged lymph node
eosinophilic cytoplasm
estrogen receptor
estrogen receptor negative
everted nipple
fallopian tube
fallopian tube stump
fibrocystic change
fibrosis
fibrous band
fibrous septum
fibrous tissue
fimbriated end
formalin
gross examination

hemorrhagic corpus luteal cyst
high-power field
histochemical score
homogenous fat
hormone receptor
immunoperoxidase stain
infiltrating ductal carcinoma
inked surgical margin
in situ
intraductal component
intraductal papilloma
invasive malignancy
left tube and ovary
lobulated homogenous fat
lobule
lymphatic tumor
metastasis
microscopic examination
mitotic figure
modified radical mastectomy
multinodular appearance
nest of pleomorphic oval epithelial cells
nuclear chromatin
ovarian stroma
Paget disease
palpable mass
paraffin-embedded tissue
poorly differentiated infiltrating ductal
   carcinoma
progesterone receptor
progesterone receptor negative
resection margin
right axillary node
right breast
right tube and ovary
ruptured capsular surface
serial fashion
skeletal muscle
skin ellipse
soft adipose tissue
stromal fibrosis
surgical margin

surgical stump
thin-walled cyst
trabecular sheet
tumor cell
tumor nodule
well-healed surgical stump

Pap Smear
cervix
excessive inflammation
genital wart
inadequate
last menstrual period
menstrual period
Pap smear
pelvic inflammatory disease
regular menstrual period
repeat smear
specimen adequacy

Prostate Carcinoma
adenocarcinoma
adenomatous hyperplasia
atrophy
atypical adenomatous hyperplasia
benign prostatic tissue
chronic inflammation
formalin
Gleason score
high-grade prostatic intraepithelial
    neoplasia
in toto
postatrophic hyperplasia
prostate biopsy
prostate carcinoma
prostatectomy

Spleen Dissection
blood vessel
external surface
focal lesion
greatest dimension

hilar soft tissue
hilum of spleen
homogeneous
leathery
lymph node
nodule
normal-appearing spleen
ovoid lymph node
soft tissue
spleen capsule
spleen dissection
spleen nodule
thrombus

Squamous Cell Carcinoma of Left Floor of Mouth
anterior margin
anterior tongue margin
ascending ramus of mandible
atrophic submaxillary salivary gland
carotid artery
carotid margin
dissected free
elliptical fragment
fibrous connective tissue
floor of mouth carcinoma
frozen section
frozen section diagnosis
frozen section technique
ganglion
greatest dimension
inferior mandible
irregular fragment
jugular vein lymph node
medial tongue margin
metastatic tumor
microscopic description
microscopic examination
moderately well-differentiated
    squamous cell carcinoma
no tumor seen
radical neck dissection

radical neck dissection proper
residual tumor
squamous cell carcinoma
sectioning
skeletal muscular tissue
submaxillary salivary gland
submental salivary gland
surgical margin
tongue margin
tumor mass
vertebral column
vertebral margin
well-differentiated squamous cell
   carcinoma
whitish-tan tissue

Transitional Cell Carcinoma of Bladder

bladder biopsy
bladder carcinoma
bladder specimen
bladder tumor
germinal center
inflammatory reaction
lymph node metastasis
marked inflammatory reaction
nodal tissue
papillary transitional cell carcinoma of
   bladder
scalene lymph node
tissue fragment
transitional cell cancer
transitional cell carcinoma
transurethral resection of bladder tumor